■   ■   ■

ACUTE
CORONARY
SYNDROMES

ACUTE CORONARY SYNDROMES

A Companion to Braunwald's Heart Disease

Pierre Théroux, MD
Professor of Medicine
Montreal Heart Institute and University of Montreal
Montreal, Quebec, Canada

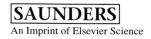

SAUNDERS
An Imprint of Elsevier Science

SAUNDERS
An Imprint of Elsevier Science (USA)

The Curtis Center
Independence Square West
Philadelphia, Pennsylvania 19106-3399

ACUTE CORONARY SYNDROMES   0-7216-9613-9

Notice

Medicine is an ever-changing field. Standard safety precautions must be followed, but as new research and clinical experience broaden our knowledge, changes in treatment and drug therapy may become necessary or appropriate. Readers are advised to check the most current product information provided by the manufacturer of each drug to be administered to verify the recommended dose, the method and duration of administration, and contraindications. It is the responsibility of the treating physician, relying on experience and knowledge of the patient, to determine dosages and the best treatment for each individual patient. Neither the Publisher nor the editor assume any liability for any injury and/or damage to persons or property arising from this publication.

The Publisher

Library of Congress Cataloging-in-Publication Data

Acute coronary syndromes: a companion to Braunwald's heart disease/editor, Pierre Théroux.—1st ed.
  p. cm.
  ISBN 0-7216-9613-9
    1. Coronary heart disease.   I. Théroux, Pierre   II. Title: Heart disease.

RC685.C6 A288 2003
616.1'23—dc21   2002030986

Publisher: Anne Lenehan
Senior Project Manager: Natalie Ware
Editorial Assistant: Vera Ginsburgs

KI/MVY

Printed in the United States of America.

Last digit is the print number: 9 8 7 6 5 4 3 2 1

To
Doris
Julie and Martin
Audrey, Marie Josée, and Michel

JEFFREY L. ANDERSON, MD
Professor of Medicine, Department of Medicine,
University of Utah; Associate Chief of Cardiology,
Division of Cardiology, and Co-Director,
Department of Cardiac Research, LDS Hospital,
Salt Lake City, Utah
The Role of Infection

ELLIOTT M. ANTMAN, MD
Associate Professor of Medicine, Harvard Medical
School; Director, Samuel A. Levine Cardiac Unit,
Cardiovascular Division, Brigham and Women's
Hospital, Boston, Massachusetts
*Risk Stratification in Non–ST-Segment Elevation Acute
Coronary Syndromes*

ANNEMARIE ARMANI, MD
Medical Director,
IntraMed Educational Group, New York,
New York
Antiplatelet Therapy

PAUL W. ARMSTRONG, MD
Professor of Medicine, Division of Cardiology, University
of Alberta; Attending Cardiologist, Division of
Cardiology, Department of Medicine, University of
Alberta Hospital; Director of Canadian VIGOUR Centre,
University of Alberta, Edmonton, Canada
*Electrocardiography, ECG Monitoring, and
Provocative Stress Testing in Acute Coronary
Syndromes*

HERBERT D. ARONOW, MD, MPH
Interventional Cardiology Fellow, Cleveland Clinic
Foundation, Cleveland, Ohio
*Identifying the Vulnerable Plaque and the Vulnerable
Patient*

RAMÓN ARROYO-ESPLIGUERO, MD
Research Fellow, Coronary Artery Disease Research
Unit, Department of Cardiological Sciences,
St. George's Hospital Medical School, London,
United Kingdom
Natural History and Prognosis

SHANNON M. BATES, MD, CM
Assistant Professor, Department of Medicine,
McMaster University; Active Staff, Hamilton Health
Sciences—McMaster Campus, Hamilton, Ontario,
Canada
Anticoagulant Therapy

RICHARD C. BECKER, MD
Professor of Medicine, University of Massachusetts
Medical School; Director, Cardiovascular Thrombosis
Research Center and Coronary Care Unit, University
of Massachusetts Medical Center, Worcester, Massachusetts
Antiplatelet Therapy

JACOB FOG BENTZON, MD
Research Associate, Institute of Experimental Clinical
Research, University of Aarhus; Department of
Cardiology, Aarhus University Hospital (Skejby),
Aarhus, Denmark
*Pathology of Stable and Acute Coronary
Syndromes*

MICHEL E. BERTRAND, MD, FRCP, FESC, FACC
Professor of Cardiology, Department of Medicine,
University of Lille; Cardiologic Hospital, Lille,
France
Guidelines of the European Society of Cardiology

LUIGI M. BIASUCCI, MD
Assistant Professor, Cardiovascular Medicine,
Catholic University of the Sacred Heart, Rome, Italy
Markers of Inflammation

MIMI SENGUPTA BISWAS, MD, MHSC
Clinical Fellow, Cardiovascular Disease, Duke University
Medical Center, Durham, North Carolina
*The Elderly, Women, and Patients with Diabetes
Mellitus*

XAVIER BOSCH, MD, FACC, FESC
Associate Professor of Medicine, Department of
Medicine, University of Barcelona; Consultant in
Cardiology, Coronary Care Unit, Cardiovascular
Institute, Hospital Clinic, Barcelona; Editor-in-Chief,
Revista Española de Cardiologia, Madrid, Spain
Continuous Risk Stratification

**EUGENE BRAUNWALD, MD, MD(HON), SCD(HON),
FRCP**
Distinguished Hersey Professor of Medicine and Faculty
Dean for Academic Programs, Brigham and Women's
and Massachusetts General Hospitals, Harvard Medical
School; Chief Academic Officer, Partners HealthCare
System, Boston, Massachusetts
*Foreword; Clinical Recognition of Acute Coronary
Syndromes; ACC/AHA 2002 Guidelines Update
for the Management of Patients with Unstable Angina
and Non-ST-Segment Elevation Myocardial
Infarction—Summary Article*

WANDA BRIDE, RN
Clinical Operations Director, III, Duke Heart Services,
Duke University Health System, Durham, North Carolina
The Modern Coronary Care Unit

KENNETH A. BROWN, MD, FACC
Professor, Department of Medicine, University of
Vermont College of Medicine; Director, Nuclear
Cardiology and Cardiac Stress Laboratories, Cardiology
Unit, Medical Center Hospital of Vermont—Fletcher
Allen HealthCare, Burlington, Vermont
*Nuclear Cardiology Techniques in Acute Coronary
Syndromes*

ADY BUTNARU, MD
Advanced Fellow in Echocardiography and Research,
Echo Department and Research Center, Montreal Heart
Institute, University of Montreal, Montreal, Quebec, Canada
Echocardiography in Acute Coronary Syndromes

ROBERT M. CALIFF, MD
Professor of Medicine, Department of Cardiology, Duke
University Medical Center; Director, Duke Clinical
Research Institute, Durham, North Carolina
The Modern Coronary Care Unit

CHRISTOPHER P. CANNON, MD
Associate Professor of Medicine, Harvard Medical
School; Cardiovascular Division, Brigham and Women's
Hospital, Boston, Massachusetts
Advantages and Hazards of Early Revascularization

RICHARD O. CANNON III, MD
Clinical Director, National Heart, Lung, and Blood
Institute, and Head, Clinical Cardiology, National
Institutes of Health, Bethesda, Maryland
*The Patient with Chest Pain Despite Normal Coronary
Angiography*

PATRICK J. COMMERFORD, MB, CHB
Professor of Cardiology, Department of Medicine,
University of Cape Town, and Division of Cardiology,
Groote Schuur Hospital, Cape Town, South Africa
*β-Blockers and Calcium Channel Blockers: Use in
Acute Coronary Syndromes*

C. RICHARD CONTI, MD, MACC
Professor of Medicine, Eminent Scholar (Cardiology),
Department of Medicine, Division of Cardiology,
University of Florida at Shands, Gainesville, Florida
*From Pre-infarction Angina to Acute Coronary
Syndromes: A Historical Perspective*

HOWARD A. COOPER, MD
Attending Physician, Coronary Care Unit, Washington
Hospital Center, Washington, DC
Clinical Recognition of Acute Coronary Syndromes

PIM J. DE FEYTER, MD
Professor, Cardiology and Radiology Departments,
Erasmus Medical Center, Rotterdam,
The Netherlands
*Computed Tomography in Coronary
Artery Disease*

ALI E. DENKTAS, MD
Interventional Cardiology Fellow, Division of
Cardiology, Mayo Clinic, Rochester, Minnesota
*New Surgical and Percutaneous Revascularization
Procedures*

ANIQUE DUCHARME, MD, MSc
Assistant Professor of Medicine, Department of
Medicine (Cardiology), University of Montreal;
Cardiologist, Director of the Heart Failure Clinic,
Montreal Heart Institute, Montreal, Quebec, Canada
Echocardiography in Acute Coronary Syndromes

VICTOR J. DZAU, MD
Hersey Professor of the Theory and Practice of Physic
(Medicine), Department of Medicine, Harvard Medical
School; Chairman, Physician in Chief, Director of
Research, Department of Medicine, Brigham and
Women's Hospital; Director of Academic Collaborations,
Partners HealthCare System, Inc., Boston, Massachusetts
Perspective for Gene and Cell-Based Therapy

ERLING FALK, MD, PhD
Professor of Cardiovascular Pathology, Institute of
Experimental Clinical Research, University of Aarhus;
Department of Cardiology, Aarhus University Hospital
(Skejby), Aarhus, Denmark
*Pathology of Stable and Acute Coronary
Syndromes*

NANCY FRASURE-SMITH, PhD
Associate Professor, Department of Psychiatry, McGill
University; Senior Research Associate, Montreal Heart
Institute, Montreal, Quebec, Canada
*What Cardiologists Need to Know on Depression in
Acute Coronary Syndromes*

YULING FU, MD
Assistant Professor, Department of Medicine, University
of Alberta; Canadian VIGOUR Centre, Edmonton,
Alberta, Canada.
*Electrocardiography, ECG Monitoring, and Provocative
Stress Testing in Acute Coronary Syndromes*

RICHARD GALLO, MD
Assistant Professor of Medicine, University of Montreal;
Interventional Cardiologist, Montreal Heart Institute,
Montreal, Quebec, Canada
*Emerging Diagnostic Procedures for the Vulnerable
Plaque*

DAVID GARCIA-DORADO, MD, PhD
Associate Professor, University Autonoma of Barcelona;
Section Chief, Laboratory of Cardiovascular
Investigation, General University Hospital,
Vall d'Hebron, Barcelona, Spain
*Myocardial Cell Protection in Acute Coronary
Syndromes*

JACQUES GENEST, MD, FRCP(C)
Professor, Faculty of Medicine, McGill University;
Novartis Chair in Medicine at McGill University;
Director, Division of Cardiology, McGill University
Health Center/Royal Victoria Hospital, Montreal,
Quebec, Canada
*Novel Risk Factors in Acute Coronary
Syndromes*

MARGARET A. GOODELL, PhD
Assistant Professor, Center for Cell and Gene Therapy,
Baylor College of Medicine, Houston, Texas
*Cardiovascular Regeneration and Stem Cell
Differentiation*

CHRISTOPHER B. GRANGER, MD
Associate Professor of Medicine, Department of
Medicine, Division of Cardiology, Duke University;
Director, Cardiac Care Unit, Department of Medicine,
Division of Cardiology, Duke Hospital, Durham,
North Carolina
The Modern Coronary Care Unit

CHRISTIAN W. HAMM, MD
Professor of Internal Medicine and Cardiology,
University of Hamburg, Hamburg; Professor of
Cardiology and Chief, Department of Cardiology,
Kerckhoff Heart Center, Bad Nauheim, Germany
Biochemical Markers of Myocardial Necrosis

CHRISTOPHER HEESCHEN, MD
Senior Scientist, Molecular Cardiology, University
of Frankfurt, Frankfurt, Germany
Biochemical Markers of Myocardial Necrosis

L. DAVID HILLIS, MD
Professor and Vice Chair, James M. Wooten Chair
in Cardiology, Department of Internal Medicine,
University of Texas Southwestern Medical Center,
Dallas, Texas
*Cocaine and Other Environmental Causes of Acute
Coronary Syndromes*

KAREN K. HIRSCHI, PhD
Assistant Professor, Departments of Pediatrics and
Cellular and Molecular Biology, Baylor College of
Medicine, Houston, Texas
*Cardiovascular Regeneration and Stem Cell
Differentiation*

JUDITH S. HOCHMAN, MD
Professor of Medicine, Columbia University,
College of Physicians and Surgeons; Director,
Cardiac Care Unit and Cardiac Research,
St. Luke's/Roosevelt Hospital Center, New York,
New York
*The Elderly, Women, and Patients with Diabetes
Mellitus*

JUDD E. HOLLANDER, MD, FACEP
Professor, Department of Emergency Medicine,
University of Pennsylvania; Clinical Research Director,
Department of Emergency Medicine, Hospital of
the University of Pennsylvania, Philadelphia,
Pennsylvania
*Acute Coronary Syndromes in the Emergency
Department: Diagnosis, Risk Stratification, and
Management*

DAVID R. HOLMES, JR., MD
Professor of Medicine, Mayo Medical School;
Director, Cardiac Catheterization Laboratory,
St. Mary's Hospital; Consultant in Cardiovascular
Diseases/Internal Medicine, Mayo Clinic, Rochester,
Minnesota
*New Surgical and Percutaneous Revascularization
Procedures*

PRISCILLA HSUE, MD
Assistant Professor, University of California,
San Francisco; Attending Physician,
San Francisco General Hospital, San Francisco,
California
Control of Risk Factors

KATHYJO A. JACKSON, PhD
Instructor, Center for Cell and Gene Therapy, Baylor
College of Medicine, Houston, Texas
*Cardiovascular Regeneration and Stem Cell
Differentiation*

JACOB JOSEPH, MD
Assistant Professor of Internal Medicine,
Department of Internal Medicine/Division of
Cardiovascular Medicine, University of Arkansas for
Medical Sciences; Staff Physician, Internal
Medicine/Division of Cardiovascular Medicine, Central
Arkansas Veterans Healthcare System, Little Rock,
Arkansas
Nitrates and Nitric Oxide Donors

JUAN CARLOS KASKI, MD, DSC, FRCP
Professor of Cardiovascular Science, St. George's
Hospital Medical School, University of London;
Consultant Cardiologist, St. George's Hospital, London,
United Kingdom
Natural History and Prognosis

GERHARD KONING, MSc
Division of Image Processing (LKEB), Department
of Radiology, Leiden University Medical Center, Leiden,
The Netherlands
*Coronary Angiography and the Culprit Lesion in
Acute Coronary Syndromes*

MICHAEL J. B. KUTRYK, MD, PhD, FRCPC
Assistant Professor, Department of Medicine, University
of Toronto; Staff Cardiologist/Clinical Scientist,
Department of Cardiology, Toronto, Ontario, Canada
Pharmacologic Revascularization

RICHARD A. LANGE, MD
Professor, Jonsson-Rogers Chair in Cardiology,
Department of Internal Medicine, University of Texas
Southwestern Medical Center, Dallas, Texas
*Cocaine and Other Environmental Causes of Acute
Coronary Syndromes*

FRANÇOIS LEDRU, MD
Senior Cardiologist, Cardiovascular Cardiology and
Radiology, European Hospital Georges Pompidou, Paris,
France
*Coronary Angiography and the Culprit Lesion in
Acute Coronary Syndromes*

JANE A. LEOPOLD, MD
Assistant Professor of Medicine, Boston University
School of Medicine, Whitaker Cardiovascular Institute;
Staff Interventional Cardiologist, Department of
Medicine, Boston Medical Center, Boston,
Massachusetts
Markers of a Thrombotic State

FRANÇOIS LESPÉRANCE, MD
Associate Professor of Research, Department of
Psychiatry, University of Montreal; Psychiatrist,
Department of Psychiatry, Centre Hospitalier de
l'Université de Montreal, Montreal, Quebec, Canada
*What Cardiologists Need to Know on Depression in
Acute Coronary Syndromes*

JACQUES LESPÉRANCE, MD
Associate Professor, Department of Radiology, University
of Montreal; Radiologist, Montreal Heart Institute,
Montreal, Quebec, Canada
*Coronary Angiography and the Culprit Lesion in
Acute Coronary Syndromes*

PETER LIBBY, MD
Mallinckrodt Professor of Medicine, Harvard Medical
School; Chief, Cardiovascular Medicine, Brigham and
Women's Hospital, Boston, Massachusetts
*Molecular Mechanisms of the Acute Coronary
Syndromes: The Roles of Inflammation and
Immunity*

GIOVANNA LIUZZO, MD, PhD
Assistant Professor, Department of Cardiology, Catholic
University of the Sacred Heart; Consultant, Cardiology,
Agostino Gemelli Polyclinic, Rome, Italy
Markers of Inflammation

GARY D. LOPASCHUK, PhD
Professor, Departments of Pediatrics and Pharmacology,
University of Alberta, Edmonton, Alberta, Canada
Metabolic Interventions

MICHEL DE LORGERIL, MD
Cardiologist and Nutritionist, UFR de Médecine,
Université Joseph Fourier, Grenoble; Researcher
(Principal Investigator), Département des Sciences de la
Vie, French National Center for Scientific Research
(CNRS), Paris, France
*Dietary Intervention in Coronary Care Units and in
Secondary Prevention*

JOSEPH LOSCALZO, MD, PhD
Wade Professor and Chairman, Department of
Medicine, and Director, Whitaker Cardiovascular
Institute, Boston University School of Medicine;
Physician-in-Chief, Boston Medical Center, Boston,
Massachusetts
Markers of a Thrombotic State

SUSAN M. MAJKA, PhD
Assistant Professor, Department of Pediatrics, University
of Colorado Health Sciences Center, Denver, Colorado
*Cardiovascular Regeneration and Stem Cell
Differentiation*

ABEEL A. MANGI, MD
Officer, Harvard Medical School; Resident, General
Surgery, Massachusetts General Hospital; Research
Fellow, Department of Medicine, Brigham and Women's
Hospital, Boston, Massachusetts
Perspective for Gene and Cell-Based Therapy

WINFRIED MÄRZ, PhD
Professor, Clinical Institute of Medical and Chemical
Laboratory Diagnostics, General and University
Hospital, Graz, Austria
*An Epidemiological Perspective: Society, Environment,
Risk Factors, and Genetics*

DARREN K. MCGUIRE, MD, MHSC
Assistant Professor of Medicine, Department of
Cardiology-Internal Medicine, University of Texas
Southwestern Medical Center at Dallas; Director,
Outpatient Cardiology Services, Parkland
Hospital and Health System; Cardiology-Internal
Medicine, St. Paul University Hospital, Dallas, Texas
*The Elderly, Women, and Patients with Diabetes
Mellitus*

JAWAHAR L. MEHTA, MD, PhD
Professor of Internal Medicine, Physiology, and
Biophysics, Stebbins Chair in Cardiology; Director,
Division of Cardiovascular Medicine, University of
Arkansas for Medical Sciences, Little Rock, Arkansas
Nitrates and Nitric Oxide Donors

LUÍS GABRIEL MELO, PhD
Associate Professor, Department of Physiology,
University of Saskatchewan, Saskatoon, Saskatchewan,
Canada
Perspective for Gene and Cell-Based Therapy

DAVID A. MORROW, MD, MPH
Instructor in Medicine, Harvard University; Associate
Physician, Cardiovascular Division, Brigham and
Women's Hospital, Boston, Massachusetts
*Risk Stratification in Non-ST-Segment Elevation Acute
Coronary Syndromes*

JOSEPH B. MUHLESTEIN, MD
Associate Professor, Department of Medicine, University
of Utah; Director of Cardiology Research, LDS Hospital,
Salt Lake City, Utah
The Role of Infection

JAMES E. MULLER, MD
Co-Director, CIMIT Vulnerable Plaque Program,
Massachusetts General Hospital, Harvard Medical
School, Boston, Massachusetts
Triggers to Acute Coronary Syndromes

L. KRISTIN NEWBY, MD, MHS
Associate Professor of Medicine, Department of
Medicine/Division of Cardiology, Duke University
Medical Center, Durham, North Carolina
*The Elderly, Women, and Patients with Diabetes
Mellitus; The Modern Coronary Care Unit*

KOEN NIEMAN, MD
Research Fellow, Thorax Center, Department of
Cardiology, Erasmus Medical Center, Rotterdam,
The Netherlands
Computed Tomography in Coronary Artery Disease

LIONEL H. OPIE, MD, DSC, FRCP, DPHIL
Professor of Medicine, Department of Medicine,
University of Cape Town Medical School; Director,
Cape Heart Centre, Hatter Institute, Cape Town,
South Africa
*β-Blockers and Calcium Channel Blockers: Use in
Acute Coronary Syndromes*

ALOK S. PACHORI, PhD
Research Fellow, Department of Medicine, Brigham and
Women's Hospital, Boston, Massachusetts
Perspective for Gene and Cell-Based Therapy

AUDREY H. RAPP, MD
Senior Fellow in Cardiology, Department of Internal
Medicine, University of Texas Southwestern Medical
Center, Dallas, Texas
*Cocaine and Other Environmental Causes of Acute
Coronary Syndromes*

JOHAN H. C. REIBER, PhD
Professor of Medical Imaging, Division of
Image Processing, Department of Radiology,
Leiden University Medical Center, Leiden,
The Netherlands
*Coronary Angiography and the Culprit Lesion in
Acute Coronary Syndromes*

MARC S. SABATINE, MD, MPH
Instructor in Medicine, Harvard Medical School;
Investigator, TIMI Study Group, Brigham and Women's
Hospital; Assistant in Cardiology, Massachusetts General
Hospital, Boston, Massachusetts
*Risk Stratification in Non-ST-Segment Elevation Acute
Coronary Syndromes*

PATRICIA SALEN, BSC
Dietitian and Clinical Assistant Researcher, UFR de
Médecine, Université Joseph Fourier, Grenoble,
France
*Dietary Intervention in Coronary Care Units and in
Secondary Prevention*

BALKRISHNA K. SINGH, MD
Assistant Professor of Medicine and Director, Section of
Echocardiography, University of Arkansas for Medical
Sciences; Staff Cardiologist, VA Medical Center,
Little Rock, Arkansas
Nitrates and Nitric Oxide Donors

JAGMEET P. SINGH, MD, DPHIL
Cardiac Arrhythmia Service, Massachusetts General
Hospital, Harvard Medical School, Boston, Massachusetts
Triggers to Acute Coronary Syndromes

SIDNEY C. SMITH, JR., MD
Professor of Medicine and Director, Center for
Cardiovascular Science and Medicine, University of
North Carolina at Chapel Hill, Chapel Hill,
North Carolina
*Acute Coronary Syndromes: National and
International Dimensions of the Problem*

CEZAR S. STANILOAE, MD
Interventional Cardiologist, Comprehensive
Cardiovascular Center, Saint Vincent Medical Center
of New York, New York Medical College, New York,
New York
*Emerging Diagnostic Procedures for the Vulnerable
Plaque*

DUNCAN J. STEWART, MD, FRCPC
Director, Division of Cardiology, Department of
Medicine, University of Toronto; Head, Division of
Cardiology, Department of Medicine, St. Michael's
Hospital, Toronto, Ontario, Canada
Pharmacologic Revascularization

JEAN-CLAUDE TARDIF, MD, FRCPC
Associate Professor of Medicine, Department of
Medicine, University of Montreal; Director of Clinical
Research and Cardiologist, Montreal Heart Institute,
Montreal, Quebec, Canada
Echocardiography in Acute Coronary Syndromes

UDHO THADANI, MD, MRCP, FRCP, FACC, FAHA
Professor Emeritus of Medicine, University of
Oklahoma Health Sciences Center; Consultant
Cardiologist, Oklahoma University Medical Center
and VA Medical Center, Oklahoma City,
Oklahoma
*The Patient with Disabling Angina Not Amenable to
Revascularization Procedures*

PIERRE THÉROUX, MD
Professor of Medicine, University of Montreal; Head,
Coronary Care Unit, Research Center, Montreal Heart
Institute, Montreal, Quebec, Canada
*Preface; Continuous Risk Stratification; Anti-
thrombotic Management*

PETER L. THOMPSON, MD, FRACP, FACP, FACC, MBA
Clinical Professor of Medicine and Public Health,
University of Western Australia; Cardiologist and
Director of Coronary Care, Sir Charles Gairdner
Hospital; Head of Cardiology, Joondalup Health
Campus; Deputy Director, Gairdner Campus, West
Australian Heart Research Institute, Perth, Western
Australia
Acute Plaque Passivation and Endothelial Therapy

FABRIZIO TOMAI, MD
Senior Staff Member, Cardiac Catheterization
Laboratory—Division of Cardiac Surgery, Tor Vergata
University of Rome, Rome, Italy
*ATP-Sensitive Potassium Channels, Adenosine, and
Preconditioning*

ERIC J. TOPOL, MD
Professor of Medicine, Cleveland Clinic Health Sciences
Center, Ohio State University School of Medicine,
Columbus; Provost and Chief Academic Officer
and Chairman, Department of Cardiovascular
Medicine, The Cleveland Clinic Foundation, Cleveland,
Ohio
*Identifying the Vulnerable Plaque and the Vulnerable
Patient*

JOAN C. TUINENBURG, MSc
Scientific Researcher, Division of Image Processing
(LKEB), Department of Radiology, Leiden University
Medical Center, Leiden, The Netherlands
*Coronary Angiography and the Culprit Lesion in
Acute Coronary Syndromes*

GALEN S. WAGNER, MD
Associate Professor of Medicine; Physician, Department
of Medicine, Duke University, Durham, North Carolina
The Modern Coronary Care Unit

LARS WALLENTIN, MD, PHD
Professor of Cardiology, Department of Medical Sciences,
Cardiology, Uppsala University; Consultant in Cardiology,
Cardiothoracic Centre, University Hospital; Director,
Uppsala Clinical Research Centre, Uppsala, Sweden
*Revascularization in Acute Coronary Syndromes:
Which Patients and When?*

DAVID D. WATERS, MD
Professor of Medicine, University of California, San
Francisco; Chief of Cardiology, San Francisco General
Hospital, San Francisco, California
Control of Risk Factors

JEFFREY I. WEITZ, MD, FRCP(C), FACP
Professor of Medicine, McMaster University; Director,
Experimental Thrombosis and Atherosclerosis Group,
Henderson Research Centre, Hamilton, Ontario, Canada
Anticoagulant Therapy

JAMES T. WILLERSON, MD
Professor of Medicine and President, University of Texas
Health Science Center at Houston; Medical Director,
Texas Heart Institute; Chief of Cardiology, St. Luke's
Episcopal Hospital; Editor, *Circulation*, Houston, Texas
Treatment of Cardiovascular Inflammation

BERNHARD R. WINKELMANN, MD
Assistant Professor, Department of Internal Medicine,
University Hospital, Frankfurt; Head of Cooperation Unit
Pharmacogenomics/Applied Genomics, University of
Heidelberg; Medical Faculty, University Hospital,
Heidelberg, Germany
*An Epidemiological Perspective: Society, Environment,
Risk Factors, and Genetics*

BRIAN Y. L. WONG, MD, FRCP(C)
Interventional Cardiology Fellow, Division of Cardiology,
Sunnybrook and Women's College Health Sciences
Center, University of Toronto, Toronto, Ontario, Canada
*Electrocardiography, ECG Monitoring, and Provocative
Stress Testing in Acute Coronary Syndromes*

HIROFUMI YASUE, MD
Director, Kumamoto Aging Research Institute,
Kumamoto City, Japan
Coronary Artery Spasm

At the beginning of the twentieth century, coronary artery disease was considered to be a serious condition, but the distinction between its two principal presentations, angina pectoris and acute myocardial infarction, was not clear. By the 1920s, the separate clinical and pathologic manifestations of chronic angina pectoris and acute myocardial infarction had been established and their differences recognized. In the 1930s, a condition characterized by prolonged chest pain that sometimes led to acute myocardial infarction was described, and by the 1940s a syndrome intermediate between angina pectoris and acute myocardial infarction, the so-called "intermediate syndrome" was deemed to be quite common. In the early 1970s, the term *unstable angina* was coined, and we now consider this designation to include patients with the new onset of severe angina, patients with accelerated angina, and those with angina at rest. As unstable angina became more clearly defined, increasing attention was directed to the separation of patients with acute myocardial infarction into those who presented with and those without electrocardiographic ST-segment elevation. It then became apparent that patients with unstable angina not infrequently developed the latter condition, i.e., non-ST-segment elevation myocardial infarction (NSTEMI).

By the 1990s, with the development of more sensitive biochemical markers of myocardial necrosis, the distinction between unstable angina and NSTEMI again became blurred. Indeed, an increasing percentage of patients with the former condition were shown actually to have the latter. By the end of the twentieth century, it became clear that from both pathophysiologic and clinical points of view these two conditions should be considered together, and they are now commonly referred to as "non-ST-segment elevation acute coronary syndromes," sometimes shortened simply to "acute coronary syndromes."

Research on acute coronary syndromes has exploded on many fronts, and this impressive book edited by Pierre Théroux masterfully captures the major developments. It carefully explores the many epidemiologic, clinical, pathophysiologic, and therapeutic advances in the field. The enormous frequency of this condition, and its seriousness, place it at the "heart" of cardiology. Indeed just about every cardiologist who treats adults—whether an invasive or a noninvasive cardiologist, whether primarily office- or hospital-based, whether specializing in hypertension, heart failure, prevention, or rehabilitation—encounters patients with acute coronary syndromes and must be comfortable with their diagnosis and management.

Cardiologists dealing with these patients will be indebted to Dr. Théroux and his talented authors for providing this important new book. My co-editors Douglas Zipes and Peter Libby and I are proud that it is a companion to *Heart Disease—A Textbook of Cardiovascular Medicine*.

Eugene Braunwald
Boston, Massachusetts

Acute Coronary Care: The Coronary Care Unit and Beyond

Pierre Théroux

A century of clinical observations and a wealth of knowledge gained in recent decades have propelled the acute coronary syndromes (ACSs) to the forefront of clinical practice and research in cardiology. Because of the increasingly high incidence of these acute syndromes and their serious prognosis, cardiologists must improve their knowledge and improve treatment strategies to prevent progression to irreversible myocardial damage and to counter the highly dynamic nature of ACSs.

Practice patterns in the coronary care unit (CCU) have undergone radical changes in recent years. For example, from 1990 to 2000, the total number of CCU admissions at the Montreal Heart Institute doubled from 800 patients to 1600. In 1990, 40% of patients were admitted for acute myocardial infarction and 45% for a non–ST-segment elevation ACS. In 2000, these proportions were 20% and 75%, respectively. Along with the aging of society, the mean age of patients has increased from 61 years to 64 years. Hospital stays have shortened from 8.5 days to 4.5 days. Encouragingly, mortality rates have decreased from 6% to 3%.

The traditional role of the CCU has also changed, encompassing new therapeutic goals, challenging concepts, and management strategies. Examples include the constant search for better and more rapid reperfusion techniques and cellular protection in ST-segment elevation myocardial infarction. Plaque passivation has become a focus in non–ST-segment elevation ACS; secondary prevention, with emphasis on control of risk factors, is now the rule in all patients. These targets are increasingly supported by novel therapeutic strategies.

Beyond atherosclerosis, and beyond the intravascular thrombus, there are active plaques in which inflammation and immunity are major players. Complex interactions exist between blood and vessel wall cells, cytokines, growth factors, and matrix metalloproteinases. As we further our knowledge, unknown interactions and triggers will certainly be uncovered. These interactions are fundamental to the biology of atherosclerosis and constitute targets for breakthrough therapies, each capable of acting at a specific site of the atherosclerotic cascade (Fig. 1). Accordingly, new diagnostic procedures and new therapies are needed and forthcoming.

The revolutionary changes and expanding costs in health care delivery necessitate the modern CCU to extend beyond its traditional confines. Today's CCU must change its goals and concepts to include pre-CCU care, prompt availability of cardiac catheterization and revas-

cularization procedures, and post-CCU care. At all levels, there is a need for a concerted multidisciplinary effort with a sharing of expertise and of diagnosis and treatment algorithms (Fig. 2).

The pre-CCU phase concerns all professionals involved in patient care, from physicians responding to patients with possible cardiac symptoms in their office to personnel in the 911/pre-hospital service and emergency departments. Risk stratification is inherent to diagnosis of an ACS and requires facilities for 12-lead ECG recording, troponin determination, and diagnostic provocative testing. Chest pain units and transition units have been developed in numerous hospitals to fill this role. Because time to treatment has become a survival issue, with a need for rapid to urgent or immediate intervention, the current effort is to bring the tools of diagnosis and treatment to the patient (Fig. 3).

The CCU, which copes with heavy workloads and preselected high-risk patients in a cost-controlled environment, is a place for action wherein diagnostic procedures and treatment, including revascularization procedures, are applied diligently, the aims being best therapy and cost-effectiveness. In this era, in which treatment often involves glamorous modern technology, one must not forget that patients are active participants in their own management. In addition, beyond acute-phase treatment strategies, treatment must also effectively control the disease process, preventing progression of atherosclerosis and improving survival and quality of life.

The average stay in the CCU is diminishing to barely longer than the time needed for outpatient cardiac catheterization; thus, a post-CCU phase is mandated. In this phase, the success or failure of treatment, as well as adequacy of and tolerance to prescribed medication, is reassessed. These measures can prevent excessive and unnecessary post-discharge consultations in the emergency department. Because patients retain limited information in an accelerated hospital stay, post-discharge re-education with emphasis on control of risk factors is required. Special needs and specific problems mandate appropriate patient orientation (Fig. 4).

Beyond usual care, modern cardiology care is fortunate in that physicians have the opportunity to remain at the forefront of knowledge and contribute to future medical discoveries and developments by participating actively in national and international clinical trials.

This book is structured according to these new concepts. There are sections on the dimension of the disease

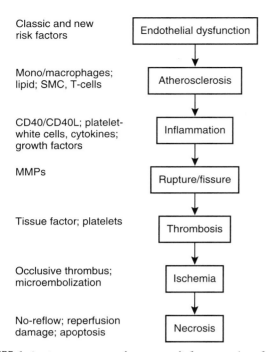

FIGURE 1. Acute coronary syndromes result from a series of pathophysiologic events that ultimately may result in cell death. Clinical manifestations occur relatively late in the cascade of events once the plaque is severely obstructed or a thrombus has formed with myocardial ischemia. There are numerous opportunities for modulating the disease process by acting at various levels. Current guidelines address the symptomatic phase. Emerging diagnostic procedures and therapies target earlier and later steps of the cascade. Mono, monocytes; MMPs, matrix metalloproteinases; SMC, smooth muscle cells.

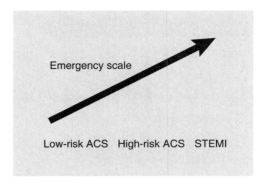

FIGURE 3. The importance of treatment as a function of time. The gradient is motivated by differences in treatment goals. For ST-segment elevation myocardial infarction (STEMI), time is of the essence to prevent rapid progression of the evolving ischemia to irreversible cell damage. In non–ST-segment elevation acute coronary syndromes (ACS), rapid passivation of the thrombotic process, attenuation of the triggers of thrombus formation, and revascularization of severe lesions are searched.

knowledge for the clinician is viewed from different perspectives, reflecting the pre-CCU, CCU, and post-CCU multidisciplinary approach. The book concludes with an outlook to the future and with a view to the new CCU before returning to daily practice with the latest guidelines for care from the European Society of Cardiology and from the American College of Cardiology and American Heart Association.

for both the individual and for society. Detailed attention is paid to pathophysiology, diagnosis, risk stratification, and pharmacologic and revascularization management strategies. Some themes are uniquely addressed. Practical

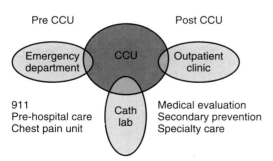

FIGURE 2. Management of acute coronary syndromes now extends to before and after the CCU phase. Concerted efforts among the various participants in the pre-CCU, CCU, and post-CCU phases and shared diagnostic and treatment algorithms yield the most effective patient care. Cath, catheterization.

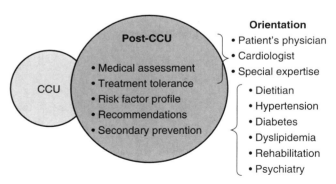

FIGURE 4. Post-CCU phase. Aggressive education and application of individualized preventive programs for the control of risk factors are imperative to ACS management. These patients have active atherosclerosis with a high risk of recurrence. Long-term risk is particularly high in patients with a non–ST-segment elevation acute coronary syndrome and in patients with uncontrolled risk factors. The cardiologist and the patient's physician can carry out the individualized programs and, as needed, in collaboration with various experts and specialized clinics.

CONTENTS

■ ■ ■ chapter 1

From Pre-infarction Angina to Acute Coronary Syndromes: A Historical Perspective

C. Richard Conti

The term *acute coronary syndrome* is a broad one encompassing several major groups of patients:

1. Patients with unstable angina at risk of myocardial infarction (pre-infarction angina)
2. Patients with non–ST-segment elevation myocardial infarction
3. Patients with ST-segment elevation myocardial infarction
4. Patients with angina pectoris in the immediate postinfarction state (postinfarction angina). Another group can be included:
5. Severe angina pectoris occurring during or after a percutaneous coronary intervention. This could be the result of dissection, coronary occlusion with thrombus, or distal coronary embolization.

The rationale for including the last group under the term *acute coronary syndrome* is based on the underlying pathophysiologic mechanisms that are responsible for the clinical presentation—a disruptive plaque resulting in platelet aggregation and thrombosis, which in turn produces a high-grade stenosis or occlusion of a coronary artery with or without associated emboli entering the microcirculation downstream.

This chapter focuses on patients who present with an acute ischemic syndrome prior to an ST-segment elevation myocardial infarction, that is, unstable angina and non–ST-segment elevation myocardial infarction.

UNSTABLE ANGINA: A COMPLEX CLINICAL CONDITION

There is a fine line between the labels of unstable angina and non–ST-segment elevation myocardial infarction. Generally, this line relates to the development of persistent electrocardiogram (ECG) changes plus the elevation of cardiac enzymes and other cardiac markers, such as troponin I or troponin T. The patient populations are not homogeneous. There are tremendous variations in coronary pathology, left-ventricular function, and markers of inflammation. However, the underlying pathology is similar for both conditions and the clinical presentations may be similar. Clinical trials frequently combine the two entities under the heading of acute coronary syndromes.

The underlying pathology can be a nonocclusive thrombus on a preexisting plaque, dynamic obstruction (coronary spasm or vasoconstriction), progressive mechanical obstruction, inflammation and/or infection (or both), and secondary causes resulting in increased myocardial oxygen consumption due to an underlying medical condition, for example, hyperthyroidism, anemia, hypoxia due to chronic obstructive pulmonary disease, tachycardias of any kind, and hypertension.

The plaque in the coronary arteries of patients with acute coronary syndromes is generally unstable. It is usually small, prone to rupture, and affected by multiple complex factors. The plaque generally has a thin cap and a lipid core that makes up greater than 50% of the overall plaque volume. There is high density of macrophages and high levels of expression of tissue factor and metalloproteinases as well as low densities of smooth muscle cells. The coronary lesion is generally not occlusive but may be if there are luxuriant collaterals to the distal circulation. It is highly probable that these plaques develop distal embolization of aggregates of platelets, undergo intermittent total occlusion, and often lead to spasm at the thrombus site (see Chapter 5).

Using coronary angiography (lumenography) itself, one cannot accurately and prospectively predict the site of future coronary occlusions or high-grade stenoses. Coronary angiography sometimes appears normal. In this circumstance, the mechanism for the development of the acute coronary syndrome is probably related to endothelial dysfunction and some vasospasm as well as some abnormal flow reserve.

In the unstable plaque that ruptures, there is deposition of platelet aggregates and thrombosis. As a result:

- There may be partial occlusions with lysis and repair and no symptoms. This also may result in rapid progression of atherosclerosis.

- There may be partial occlusion in which thrombolysis and thrombosis are at work; if thrombosis predominates, unstable angina or non–Q-wave myocardial infarction, or both, may result.
- Occlusion of the coronary artery generally results in Q-wave myocardial infarction. However, if collaterals are present, Q waves may not develop.

Thus, the term *unstable angina* describes a complex condition with varying clinical, electrocardiographic, and pathologic changes. In 1973, a simple clinical classification was proposed to characterize ischemic heart disease as unstable (Table 1-1).[1]

This classification served us well in the past but includes many patients who would be considered at low risk by today's criteria, for example, the patient whose mild-effort angina began 3 to 4 weeks before seeking medical attention. From the practical point of view, the patient with unstable angina admitted urgently to the hospital derives from two major patient pools. All of these patients have symptoms immediately preceding admission, that is, within the previous 24 hours, and include those whose angina has been increasing in frequency, severity, or duration from a previous stable state and those experiencing new onset of prolonged or recurrent (stuttering) rest angina. The major concern in these patients is whether or not a myocardial infarction is evolving or will evolve shortly.

In clinical practice, the patient who experiences new onset of mild nonprogressive angina 3 to 4 weeks before seeking medical care is rarely considered to be in unstable condition or admitted because of a suspected evolving myocardial infarction. If a physician is confronted with a patient whose new onset of angina is 1 or 2 days old, the patient could be considered to be in a precarious state and probably should be admitted for evaluation. The rationale is that it is not clear whether the angina will stabilize over the next several weeks and whether a myocardial infarction will evolve in the immediate future.

At the time of clinical presentation, several questions need to be addressed regarding the patient's symptoms (Table 1-2). These include:

- Are symptoms recurrent or are they an isolated single event?
- Are extracardiac factors (e.g., hypertension, tachycardia, anemia) present and do they contribute to the unstable state manifested as severe symptoms?
- Have symptoms occurred in a patient who was receiving anti-angina therapy before the condition became unstable?

■ ▫ ■

TABLE 1–1　ORIGINAL CLASSIFICATION OF UNSTABLE ANGINA

1. Recent onset of effort angina
2. Effort angina with a changing pattern, i.e., increased frequency, severity, or duration
3. Rest angina

■ ▫ ■

TABLE 1–2　QUESTIONS TO BE ADDRESSED ON CLINICAL PRESENTATIONS OF UNSTABLE ANGINA

1. Are symptoms recurrent or an isolated single event?
2. Are symptoms related to extracardiac factors?
3. Are symptoms occurring despite prior anti-angina therapy?
4. Are symptoms refractory to new anti-angina therapy?

After admission, it is important to know whether the patient's symptoms were responsive or refractory to new anti-angina therapy since prognosis and future therapy are determined by persistence of symptoms or myocardial ischemia, or both.

CLASSIFICATION OF THE UNSTABLE ANGINA PATIENT

The general classification of unstable angina has not changed much over the years. The following patterns of angina should be considered as unstable:

- Worsening angina: increasing severity and frequency compared with the patient's previous pattern; the chest pain, although similar to stable angina, may be more intense, may persist for longer periods of time, and may occur at minimal stress or at rest.
- New onset (hours or a few days) of prolonged rest angina: this can be a single episode or multiple recurrences.

A comprehensive definition of unstable angina encompassing the clinical manifestations, ECG changes, and cardiac serum markers was developed by Braunwald and recently updated by Braunwald and Hamm.[2,3] The original classification is summarized in Table 1-3. It was designed "to separate patients with unstable angina into a manageable number of meaningful and easily understood subgroups" based on severity of clinical manifestation, presence or absence of extracardiac conditions, presence or absence of ECG changes, and whether the patient was receiving intense medical therapy. The update subdivided patients into class IIIB (angina at rest within 48 hours of presentation) by troponin T or I elevation or not, with risks of death or infarction at 30 days of up to 20% and 2%, respectively.

FACTORS INFLUENCING RISK IN UNSTABLE ANGINA PATIENTS

The prognosis of unstable angina varies with factors related to clinical presentation (Table 1-4). Prognosis can be influenced by several factors, including age, previous treatment with aspirin, persistent pain, transient ST-segment shifts, left main coronary artery stenosis, silent myocardial ischemia, elevated troponin T and troponin I, elevated C-reactive protein and amyloid A, elevated fibrinogen levels, significant left-ventricular dysfunction associated with multivessel coronary disease,

■ ■ ■

TABLE 1–3   CLASSIFICATION OF UNSTABLE ANGINA

	CLINICAL CIRCUMSTANCES		
SEVERITY	A. Develops in Presence of Extracardiac Condition That Intensifies Myocardial Ischemia (Secondary UA)	B. Develops in Absence of Extracardiac Condition (Primary UA)	C. Develops Within 2 Weeks After AMI (Postinfarction UA)
I. New onset of severe angina or accelerated angina; no rest pain	IA	IB	IC
II. Angina at rest within past month but not within preceding 48 hr (angina at rest, subacute)	IIA	IIB	IIC
III. Angina at rest within 48 hr (angina at rest, acute)	IIIA	IIIB	IIIC

Patients with UA may also be divided into three groups depending on whether UA occurs (1) in the absence of treatment for chronic stable angina, (2) during treatment for chronic stable angina, or (3) despite maximal anti-ischemic drug therapy. These three groups may be designated by subscripts 1, 2, or 3, respectively.
Patients with UA may be further divided into those with and without transient ST-T wave changes during pain.
UA, unstable angina; AMI, acute myocardial infarction.
From reference 2.

extensive areas of ischemia as defined by radionuclide studies or dobutamine stress echo or exercise ECG testing, and multiple previous myocardial infarctions. These factors are discussed in detail in subsequent chapters.

In 2000, Antman and colleagues[4] devised a risk-scoring system (the Thrombolysis in Myocardial Ischemia [TIMI] risk score) that can be used by any physician since all of the variables are available at the time of clinical presentation. The authors analyzed data from the TIMI IIB and Efficacy and Safety of Subcutaneous Enoxaparin in Non-Q-wave Coronary Events (ESSENCE) trials regarding variables associated with prognosis in unstable coronary conditions. The composite end points of death, myocardial infarction, and recurrent ischemia at 14 days were assessed and related to relatively simple variables such as age greater than 65, three risk factors for coronary disease, prior 50% coronary stenosis, ST-segment change on admission, angina occurring twice in 24 hours, aspirin use within 7 days, and increased serum cardiac markers. If the patient had zero or one risk factor,

the 14-day composite end point was 4.7%. In contrast, if the patient had six or seven risk factors, the composite end point was 40.9% in 14 days. The gradient of risk depended on the number of risk factors (see Chapter 22).

One can add this TIMI risk score to severity of symptoms, extent of provoked ischemia, status of left-ventricular function, presence or absence of concurrent disease, and extent of coronary artery disease in order to determine appropriate treatment strategies for the patient with acute coronary syndrome. The patients in whom early angiography and revascularization may be of value include those with the following:

- High TIMI risk score
- Refractory angina
- Known multivessel coronary disease and left-ventricular dysfunction
- Suspicion of left main coronary artery stenosis
- Previous angioplasty followed by restenosis or previous coronary artery bypass graft followed by graft failure

■ ■ ■

TABLE 1–4   FACTORS INFLUENCING PROGNOSIS IN PATIENTS WITH UNSTABLE ANGINA

Age
Diabetes
Previous aspirin treatment
Persistent pain
Transient ST-segment shifts
Left main coronary artery stenosis
Silent myocardial ischemia
Elevated cardiac troponins
Elevated high-sensitivity C-reactive protein
Elevated serum amyloid A
Elevated fibrinogen levels
Left-ventricular dysfunction and multivessel disease
Extensive ischemia (radionuclide studies)
Low cardiac workload positive exercise test result
Multiple previous myocardial infarctions
TIMI risk score

SOME HISTORY OF UNSTABLE ANGINA

Table 1–5 summarizes some milestones in basic and clinical research that have paved the way to our actual understanding of unstable angina and the acute coronary syndromes. Heberden was probably the first physician to describe crescendo angina as he wrote in 1772 in reference to a patient with stable angina: "*There is a disorder of the breast marked with strong and peculiar symptoms and considerable for the kind of danger belonging to it.... The seat of it, and sense of strangling and anxiety with which it is attended, may make it not improperly be called Angina pectoris. Those who are afflicted with it, are seized, while they are walking, and more particularly when they walk soon after eating, with a painful an most disagreeable sensation in the breast, which seems as if it would take their life away, if it were to increase or to continue: the moment they*

■ ■ ■

TABLE 1–5   MILESTONES IN UNSTABLE ANGINA

CLINICAL PERSPECTIVES

1772	Clinical description of progression of angina symptoms to myocardial infarction and death[5]
1910	Description of "pre-infarction angina"[6]
1937	Observations on pre-infarction angina as a precursor of acute coronary occlusion and myocardial infarction[7,8]
1950-70	Prospective observations, description of natural history of pre-infarction angina[9-17]
1948	First intervention with an oral anticoagulant[12]
1971	Introduction of the terminology of "unstable angina"[17]
1973	The ECG for risk stratification[15]
1971-75	Revascularization with coronary artery bypass grafting[18-20]

MECHANISMS OF DISEASE

1966	Pathological description of plaque fissuring and underlying thrombus[21]
1970-75	Severity and extent of CAD[18-20]
1975-81	Dynamic occlusion and role of coronary vasospasm[22,23]
1980-85	Extensive pathological description of the unstable plaque and clinical correlates[24,25]
1981	Demonstration of an occluding thrombus in acute myocardial infarction in humans[26]
1988	Concept of acute coronary syndromes[30]
1989	Modern classification of unstable angina[2]
1990-95	Risk stratification
1992	Troponin (T or I)[33]
1994	C-reactive protein[34]
2000-...	The inflammation hypothesis[31,32]

stand still, all this uneasiness vanishes. After it has continued some months, it will not cease so instantaneously upon standing still; and it will come on, not only when the persons are walking, but when they are lying down."[5]

Subsequently, in his Lumleian lecture in 1910, Sir William Osler commented that myocardial infarction was often preceded by a progression of angina symptoms.[6]

Several other investigators have been associated with the acute coronary syndrome, including non–ST-segment elevation myocardial infarction. Multiple terms have been used to describe the acute coronary syndromes. These include crescendo angina, status anginosis, accelerated angina, coronary failure, acute coronary insufficiency, impending myocardial infarction, pre-infarction angina, and probably many more.

In 1937, Sampson and Eliaser[7] and Fiel[8] published on the diagnosis of impending acute coronary artery occlusion with angina attacks preceding the clinical picture of thrombosis by hours or days, usually 12 to 48 hours. Feil hypothesized that a gradually forming thrombosis could be the explanation for the preliminary pain and advised that "effort should be made to improve coronary artery flow."

In 1956, Levy discussed the natural history of the changing pattern of angina pectoris in 158 patients: 106 experienced sudden alteration in the pattern of angina pectoris as evidenced by pain precipitated more readily and with greater intensity or lesser degree of activity and occurring now at rest as well, and 52 patients experienced a sudden recurrence of angina pain after a period

of relative freedom of pain.[9] Anticoagulation for impending myocardial infarction was mentioned as a method of preventing subsequent infarctions.[9]

Beamish and Storrie published an article entitled "Impending Myocardial Infarction: Recognition and Management" in 1960.[10] They suggested that impending myocardial infarction can be recognized with a high degree of accuracy and that prompt administration of anticoagulants favorably influences the outcome. They proposed that impending myocardial infarction has three common presentations:

- Onset of ischemic cardiac pain in a patient previously free of symptoms; generally, this pain is prolonged
- Intensification of angina of effort in a patient with previous angina of several months' or years' duration
- Recurrence of pain in a patient with a recent previous myocardial infarction

In 1961, Vakil described the "intermediate coronary syndrome."[11] The various characteristics of this syndrome include:

- Pain, usually intermediate between that of angina and myocardial infarction
- Little or no alteration in blood pressure
- Absence of clinical laboratory and electrocardiographic signs of myocardial necrosis
- Absence of shock, embolization, and cardiac decompensation
- Characteristic ST-segment depression or T-wave inversion without reciprocal elevation
- Evidence of myocardial ischemia
- An uncomplicated recovery as a rule but with subsequent tendency to infarction

In 1961, Wood wrote that acute coronary insufficiency results when "physiologically the coronary circulation is insufficient to meet the full demands of the myocardium at rest, yet sufficient to prevent myocardial infarction."[13] He had also written in 1948 that "of a personal series of 25 patients with acute coronary insufficiency not treated with anticoagulants, no less than 12 developed acute cardiac infarction within 3 weeks and five of these died.[12] Of 33 similar cases treated with anticoagulants, only two developed cardiac infarction within the month neither of which died and a third steadily deteriorated and died suddenly a week after the onset of treatment." Obviously, Wood was a man ahead of his time.

In 1971, Fowler was the first to use the term *unstable angina* to describe this complex clinical condition. He pleaded for an objective definition and for a controlled clinical trial of the condition's management.[17]

In 1972, Krauss et al reported on the course and follow-up of patients with acute coronary insufficiency.[13] The clinical course of 100 patients with acute coronary insufficiency revealed only a single hospital death and six cases of myocardial infarction during hospitalization. Over a 20-month follow-up, 26 additional patients died, 8 from complications of myocardial infarction. The 1-year survival rate was 85%. Patients who presented with deterioration of chronic angina experienced significantly increased mortality over those with a recent onset of coronary pain.

In 1972, Fulton and colleagues reported on the natural history of 167 patients with unstable angina.[14] The authors defined unstable angina as "chest pain, suggestive of myocardial ischemia, occurring for the first time within the previous 4 weeks, or recurring within the previous 4 weeks after an interval of freedom, or abruptly and inexplicably increasing in frequency or severity in the last 4 weeks, in the absence of objective evidence of recent myocardial infarction." The authors concluded that approximately 14% of patients experienced acute myocardial infarction, and the symptoms of unstable angina lessened or disappeared in 50% when assessed at 3 months.

In 1973, Gazes et al were the first to report a prospective 10-year study discussing the prognostic significance of electrocardiographic changes and recurrent angina.[15] Of patients with persistent pain beyond 48 hours, 20% died within 1 month and 43% within 1 year. In contrast, there were no deaths within 1 month and only one death within 1 year among patients who had no persistent pain. Patients with T-wave inversion or normal-appearing ECGs had the best prognosis. The ECG abnormality associated with the worst prognosis was bundle branch block.

Clinical Trials

Reperfusion Therapy

The growing success of coronary artery bypass grafting in the early 1970s rapidly lead to the application of reperfusion procedures in unstable angina. Conti et al in 1971 reported on 57 consecutive patients presenting with unstable angina prospectively evaluated by clinical and angiographic studies and being considered for coronary artery bypass surgery.[18] The results suggested that symptomatic improvement can be obtained with either medical or surgical treatment in many patients with unstable angina. However, surgical survivors have a better chance of being pain-free than did medical survivors.

At the same time, Favalaro and colleagues reported a favorable experience with surgery in patients with an acute coronary syndrome and low mortality rates associated with surgery.[19]

In 1972, Ross and Conti and several members of the Myocardial Infarction Research Units proposed a randomized clinical trial of patients with unstable angina. This led to the unstable angina trial (sponsored by the National Heart, Lung and Blood Institute) comparing medical therapy of angina at the time with urgent coronary bypass graft surgery.[20] This trial showed that it was not necessary to perform immediate coronary angiography and coronary artery bypass graft surgery in the unstable angina patient and that crossover to surgery from medical therapy occurring later did not worsen mortality. Some patients received heparin, some received β-blockers, none received aspirin, and none received calcium antagonists since they were not available at the time of the study. This was the earliest randomized study comparing contemporary medical therapy with urgent coronary artery bypass graft surgery.

A larger randomized study—the Veterans Administration Cooperative Study—performed in the 1980s showed no benefit of coronary artery bypass surgery over medical management in the total population but significantly better survival in high-risk patients with depressed left-ventricular ejection fraction and multivessel disease.[35, 36]

Trials subsequently performed to evaluate invasive versus medical management shifted to compare routine coronary angiography with percutaneous intervention or coronary artery bypass surgery by coronary anatomy to angiography driven by uncontrolled symptoms or a positive provocative test result, mainly exercise testing.[37] Four such trials were performed. The two most recent, FRISC II[38] (performed in Scandinavian countries) and TACTICS-TIMI 18,[39] showed a statistically significant reduction in event rates with the invasive approach (see Chapter 35). In the FRISC II trial, Wallentin and colleagues showed a decrease in the composite end points of death or myocardial infarction after 6 months from 12.1% in the noninvasive group to 9.4% in the invasive group ($P = .031$). In TACTICS-TIMI 18, the primary end point (a composite of death, nonfatal myocardial infarction, and rehospitalization) occurred at 6 months in 19.4% of patients with the noninvasive strategy and in 5.9% of patients randomized to invasive strategy.

The lessons learned from the trial still apply. Clinical experience indicates that emergent myocardial revascularization (angioplasty or surgery) is not required in low-risk patients responding to various drug combinations such as antiplatelet agents, anticoagulants, nitrates, β-blockers, calcium antagonists, angiotensin-converting enzyme inhibitors, and statins. Today's patient with unstable angina is not exactly the same as patients entered into previous clinical trials. Many patients are now presenting with recurrent angina after a recent myocardial infarction, left main coronary stenosis, previous coronary bypass surgery or angioplasty, and often persistent angina on appropriate aggressive medical therapy, including intra-aortic balloon counterpulsation. All categories of patients were excluded from previous historically important clinical trials, including the Coronary Artery Surgery Study,[40] the Oregon study,[41] the National Heart, Lung and Blood Institute study,[20] and the Veterans Administration study.[35]

Drug Therapy

Drug therapy of acute coronary syndromes has evolved from the introduction of aspirin to combined antiplatelet and anticoagulant drugs, resulting in a striking reduction in event rates in cases managed medically as well as with interventions (Table 1–6).

Lewis et al conducted a multicenter double-blind, placebo-controlled, randomized trial of aspirin treatment for 12 weeks in 1266 men with unstable angina. The rate of nonfatal acute myocardial infarction was 50% lower in the aspirin group (21 patients vs. 44, $P = .005$.).[42]

Cairns and colleagues randomized 555 patients with unstable angina to aspirin 325 mg QID, sulfinpyrazone 200 mg QID, both, or neither. Follow-up was 2 years. Patients receiving aspirin showed a 51% risk reduction

■ ■ ■

TABLE 1–6   MILESTONES IN MANAGEMENT OF ACUTE CORONARY SYNDROMES

1987	Coronary artery bypass grafting[36]
1983–88	Aspirin therapy[42–45]
1988	Heparin and aspirin[44]
1997	Low molecular weight heparin (dalteparin) with aspirin[46]
1997	Enoxaparin better than unfractionated heparin[47,48]
1998	GPIIb/IIIa (eptifibatide and tirofiban) and heparin and aspirin[50,51]
1999–2001	Invasive management (PCI or CABG)[37–39]
2001	Clopidogrel with aspirin[52]

(P = .008). The rate of death from any cause was 3% in the groups given aspirin and 11.7% in the other groups—a risk reduction of 71% (P = .004).[43]

Theroux and colleagues tested the usefulness of aspirin (325 mg twice daily), heparin (1000 units per hour by intravenous infusion), and a combination of the two in the early management of acute unstable angina. Both aspirin and heparin reduced the rates of myocardial infarction, and heparin had the additional benefit of preventing recurrent ischemic events.[44]

The Risk of Myocardial Infarction and Death During Treatment with Low Dose Aspirin and Intravenous Heparin in Men with Unstable Coronary Artery Disease (RISC) study group confirms the efficacy of aspirin during the acute phase of unstable angina and for its secondary prevention.[45] The same group of Scandinavian investigators subsequently documented that the addition of dalteparin to aspirin reduced by 63% the risk of death or myocardial infarction occurring within 6 days compared with aspirin alone.[46]

Other investigators later directly compared a low-molecular-weight heparin formulation with unfractionated heparin. A benefit of enoxaparin was shown in the ESSENCE trial[47] that was subsequently confirmed by the TIMI IIB trial.[48] Direct thrombin inhibitors were also investigated in these syndromes, showing benefit during the acute phase but a higher incidence of bleeding complications.

In the mean time, antagonists of the GPIIb/IIIa receptors were introduced for clinical care, first for the prevention of complications associated with percutaneous intervention procedures[49] and subsequently for the medical management of acute coronary syndrome (see Chapter 31).[50,51] More recently, the CURE investigation showed that the addition of clopidogrel to aspirin effectively reduced the rate of death, myocardial infarction, or stroke in the acute phase with continuing benefit for 1 year.[52]

The concept of plaque passivation during the acute phase to prevent ischemic events was subsequently investigated. In the Atorvastatin Versus Revascularization Treatment Investigators (AVERT) trial, Pitt et al compared aggressive lipid lowering with atorvastatin versus revascularization treatments in selected stable patients referred for coronary angioplasty.[53] In these low-risk patients, lipid-lowering therapy was at least as effective as angioplasty and usual care in reducing the incidence of ischemic events. Subsequently, Schwartz et al randomized 3086 patients 24 and 96 hours after for admission for an acute coronary syndrome to atorvastatin 80 mg/day or matching placebo.[54] The primary end point of the trial was a combination of death, nonfatal myocardial infarction, cardiac arrest with resuscitation, or recurrence of symptomatic myocardial ischemia with objective evidence and requiring emergency hospitalization. Results indicated that for patients with acute coronary syndromes, lipid-lowering therapy with atorvastatin 80 mg/day reduced recurrent ischemic events in the first 16 weeks, mostly recurrent symptomatic ischemia requiring rehospitalization. The rates of death or myocardial infarction were unaffected, however. A number of trials using statins or other interventions are now ongoing in the line of plaque passivation.

Evolution of Pathophysiology of Unstable Angina

Our understanding of the pathophysiology of unstable angina has changed in recent decades (see Table 1-5).

In 1966, Constantinides described fissuring of atherosclerotic plaques leading to coronary artery thrombosis.[21] He studied 20 consecutive cases of fatal coronary thrombosis by histologic examination of serial sections of the coronary artery. In each instance, the thrombus was anchored in fissures in the surrounding atheromatous plaques. He pointed out that most of the plaque hemorrhage could be traced to an entry of blood from the lumen through the same or other cracks in the atherosclerotic artery wall, although some of them also resulted from rupture of plaque capillaries. Interestingly, no cracks in the wall could be found in 16 other atherosclerotic coronary arteries without thrombosis. The author concluded that the sudden break of the brittle lining of atherosclerotic coronary arteries is the major cause of human coronary thrombosis.

In the early 1980s, Davies et al and Falk used postmortem studies to demonstrate that patients dying because of unstable angina or myocardial infarction, or both, usually had atherosclerotic plaque fissuring or ulceration of plaques.[24,25] These so-called vulnerable plaques had thin fibrous caps over a lipid core containing inflammatory cells, principally monocyte-derived macrophages.

In 1981, Hirsh et al hypothesized that "an alteration in atherosclerotic plaque morphology led to platelet adhesion, thromboxane A_2 accumulation, growth of thrombus and dynamic vasoconstriction."[23] These changes were likely to result in conversion of a stable ischemic syndrome to an unstable ischemic syndrome.

Coronary angiography, first performed by Mason Sones in 1958, literally opened the door for the modern diagnosis and therapy of coronary artery disease and our understanding of coronary artery pathology and its relationship to clinical presentations.[26] Despite the fact that coronary angiography is lumenography, the analyses were expanded to morphologic assessment of plaques including contours of the lesions, presence or absence of ulcerations, thrombi, dissections, stenosis length, and stenosis symmetry.

In 1985, Ambrose and colleagues classified coronary stenoses according to angiographic morphology.[27] They found that patients presenting with acute coronary syndromes had an angina-producing lesion that appeared as an eccentric stenosis associated with sharp overhanging edges or irregular borders in more than 70% of patients. Histopathologic studies indicate that ruptured atherosclerotic plaques and partially occlusive thrombi cause these complicated stenoses.[28] DeWood et al introduced a new era in the management of acute coronary syndromes by performing angiography during the very acute phase.[26] An occluding thrombus was documented in most patients with ST-segment elevation myocardial infarction. From then on, coronary angiography became more and more routine procedure in acute myocardial infarction, first to assess success of thrombolytic therapy, then for interventional therapy and primary percutaneous intervention.

In the meantime, the role of intravascular thrombus formation on plaque rupture or fissure,[29] and of inflammation as a structural basis for rupture became more and more recognized, and the role of cellular elements, proinflammatory cytokines, and matrix metalloproteinases as well (see Chapter 6).[31,32] The concept of acute coronary syndromes was developed, encompassing the various clinical diagnoses related to the unstable active inflammatory plaques.[30] Markers of these different pathophysiological processes have been recognized, and their clinical validity for diagnosis, risk assessment, and treatment orientation has been documented. Troponin T and I are sensitive markers of an intravascular thrombotic process[33] and C-reactive protein of an inflammatory process.[34]

IMPORTANT CLINICAL POINTS

Previous experience has taught us some important clinical points regarding unstable angina.

1. Using arbitrary terms to define unstable angina, for example, onset less than 1 month in duration, is artificial and probably has little clinical significance if the angina is nonprogressive and has stabilized.

2. The patient with angina considered to be unstable may present with variable symptoms and different laboratory features. Thus, although most patients are limited by minimal-effort angina or by combination of minimal-effort and rest angina, a few patients (e.g., those with coronary artery spasm) have normal exercise tolerance and only recurrent rest angina.

3. Variable ECG changes compatible with myocardial ischemia, such as ST-segment depression or elevation or T-wave peaking or inversion, can occur during chest pain.

4. Results of coronary angiography may in rare cases be normal. Most commonly, significant coronary artery stenoses are visible in multiple vessels, although low-grade disruptive plaques are often visualized.

5. Extracardiac factors, such as hypertension, tachycardia, and anemia, also may accelerate ischemia in a patient with otherwise stable angina and proven coronary artery disease.

6. The variability of the clinical and laboratory expressions of the unstable state suggest that the complex entity known as unstable angina is not a homogeneous condition that can be defined simply.

7. If the patient's clinical condition stabilizes on aggressive medical therapy, as it does in 90% of treated hospitalized patients, the condition is by definition no longer clinically unstable. However, it is not known how long a ruptured, inflamed plaque that may have caused the problem remains unstable.

8. Valid blood markers of high-risk acute coronary syndromes patients have emerged: the troponin T or I levels, which have been associated with the presence of an intracoronary thrombus (see Chapter 14), and markers of an inflammatory state, mainly the C-reactive protein (see Chapter 16). Elevated levels of troponin and of C-reactive protein have been independently associated with mortality and cardiac events.

SUMMARY

The patient with unstable angina may have different clinical presentations, risk factors, electrocardiographic changes, and coronary artery disease. Troponin T or I combined with clinical features and ST-segment shifts are extremely useful in determining the degree of risk. High-sensitivity C-reactive protein testing results can be positive or negative. Left-ventricular function can be normal or abnormal, and coronary pathology can vary in the extent, location, severity, and morphology of the coronary lesions. Thus, there is no generic form of unstable angina.

The historical aspects of unstable angina began when Heberden described the clinical presentation of a patient with unstable angina, and the entity became progressively better defined as a clinical syndrome in the twentieth century (see Table 1-5). Over recent decades, numerous clinical trials have improved the management strategies of this condition and improved our understanding of the pathophysiologic mechanisms. Challenges that remain are identification of the plaques at risk of rupture and development of therapies effective in controlling the underlying disease processes that trigger plaque inflammation.

Controlled clinical trials provide us with guidelines for management strategies (see Table 1-6). Judgment is still necessary to make clinical decisions in the individual patient. Thus, more detailed information about the ECG, risk factors, extent of ischemia, serum troponin, high-sensitivity C-reactive protein, left-ventricular function, and angiographic coronary disease helps one to make clinical decisions on therapy.

REFERENCES

1. Conti CR, Brawley RK, Griffith LSC, et al: Unstable angina: morbidity and mortality in 57 consecutive patients evaluated angiographically. Am J Cardiol 1973;32:745–750.

2. Braunwald E: Unstable angina: A classification. Circulation 1989;80:410-414.

3. Hamm CW, Braunwald E. Classification of unstable angina revisited. Circulation 2000;102:118-122.

4. Antman EM, Cohen M, Bernink PJLM, et al: The TIMI risk score for unstable angina/non-ST elevation MI: A method for prognostication and therapeutic decision making. JAMA 2000;284:835.

5. Heberden W: Some account of a disorder of the breast. Med Trans Coll Physicians Lond 1772;2:59.

6. Osler W: The Lumleian lectures on angina pectoris. Lancet 1910;1:697-701.

7. Sampson JJ, Eliaser M Jr: The diagnosis of impending acute coronary artery occlusion. Am Heart J 1937;13:675-686.

8. Feil H: Preliminary pain in coronary thrombosis. Am J Med Sci 1937;193:42-48.

9. Levy H: The natural history of changing pattern of angina pectoris. Ann Intern Med. 1956;44:1123-1135.

10. Beamish RE, Storrie VM: Impending myocardial infarction: Recognition and management. Circulation 1960;21:1107-1115.

11. Vakil RJ: Intermediate coronary syndrome. Circulation 1961;24: 557-571.

12. Wood P: Therapeutic applications of anticoagulants. Trans Med Soc London 1948;13:80-85.

13. Krauss KR, Hutter AM, DeSanctis RW: Acute coronary insufficiency: Course and follow-up. Arch Intern Med 1972;129:808-813.

14. Fulton M, Lutz W, Donald KW, et al: Natural history of unstable angina. Lancet 1972;1:860.

15. Gazes PC, Mobley EM, Faris HM, et al: Preinfarction (unstable) angina—a prospective study—ten year follow-up: Prognostic significance of electrocardiographic changes. Circulation 1973;48: 331-337.

16. Wood P: Acute and sub-acute coronary insufficiency. Br Med J 1961;24:1779-1782.

17. Fowler NO: Preinfarction angina: A need for an objective definition and for a controlled clinical trial of its management. Circulation 1971;44:755-758.

18. Conti CR, Greene B, Pitt B, et al: Coronary surgery in unstable angina pectoris. Circulation 1971;44(Suppl 11):11-154.

19. Favaloro RG, Effler DB, Cheanvechai C, et al: Acute coronary insufficiency (impending myocardial infarction) and myocardial infarction: Surgical treatment by the saphenous vein graft technique. Am J Cardiol 1971;28:598.

20. Unstable Angina Pectoris—National Cooperative Study Group to Compare Surgical and Medical Therapy II: In hospital experience and initial follow-up results in patients with one, two and three vessel disease. Am J Cardiol 1978;42:839-848.

21. Constantinides P: Plaque fissuring in human coronary thrombosis. J Atheroscler Res 1966;6:1.

22. Maseri A, Mimmo R, Chierchia S, et al: Coronary spasm as a cause of acute myocardial ischemia in man. Chest 1975;68:625.

23. Hirsh PD, Hillis LD, Campbell WB, et al: Release of prostaglandins and thromboxane into the coronary circulation in patients with ischemic heart disease. N Engl J Med 1981;304:685-691.

24. Davies MJ, Thomas AEC: Plaque fissuring: The cause of acute myocardial infarction, sudden ischemic death, and crescendo angina. Br Heart J 1985;53:363.

25. Falk E: Plaque rupture with severe preexisting stenosis precipitating coronary thrombosis: characteristics of coronary atherosclerotic plaques underlying fatal occlusive thrombi. Br Heart J 1983;50:127.

26. DeWood MA, Spores J, Notske R, et al: Prevalence of total coronary occlusion during the early hours of transmural myocardial infarction. N Engl J Med 1980;303:897

26. Conti CR: Selective coronary angiography: 42 years later. Clin Cardiol 2001;24:269-270.

27. Ambrose JA, Winters SL, Stern A, et al: Angiographic morphology and the pathogenesis of unstable angina pectoris. J Am Coll Cardiol 1985;5:609-616.

28. Levin DC, Fallon JU: Significance of the angiographic morphology of localized coronary stenoses: Histopathologic correlations. Circulation 1982;66:3316-3320.

29. Theroux P, Fuster V: Acute coronary syndromes: unstable angina and non-Q-wave myocardial infarction. Circulation 1998;97: 1195-1206.

30. Fuster V, Badimon L, Cohen M, et al: Insights into the pathogenesis of acute ischemic syndromes. Circulation 1988;77:1213-1220.

31. Ross R: Atherosclerosis—an inflammatory disease. N Engl J Med 1999;340:115-120.

32. Libby P, Ridker PM, Maseri A: Inflammation and atherosclerosis. Circulation 2002;105:1135-1143.

33. Hamm CW, Ravkilde J, Gerhardt W, et al: The prognostic value of serum troponin T in unstable angina. N Engl J Med 1992;327: 146-150.

34. Liuzzo G, Biasucci LM, Gallimore JR, et al: The prognostic value of C-reactive protein in severe angina. N Engl J Med 1994;331:407.

35. Parisi AF, Khuri S, Deupress RH, et al: Medical compared with surgical management of unstable angina. Circulation 1989;80: 1176-1189.

36. Luchi RJ, Scott SM, Deupree RH, et al: Comparison of medical and surgical treatment for unstable angina pectoris. N Engl J Med 1987;316:977-984.

37. The TIMI IIIB Investigators. Effects of tissue plasminogen activator and a comparison of early invasive and conservative strategies in unstable angina and non-Q-wave myocardial infarction: results of TIMI IIIB trial. Circulation 1994;89:1545-1556.

38. FRagmin and fast revascularisation during InStability in Coronary artery disease investigators: Invasive compared with non-invasive treatment in unstable coronary-artery disease: FRISC II prospective randomised multicentre study. Lancet 1999;354:708-715.

39. Cannon CP, Weintraub WS, Demopoulos LA, et al: Comparison of early invasive and conservative strategies in patients with unstable coronary syndromes treated with glycoprotein IIB/IIIA inhibitor tirofiban. N Engl J Med 2001;344:1879-1887.

40. McCormick JR, Schick EC, McCabe CH, et al: Determinants of operative mortality and long term survival in patients with unstable angina. J Thorac Cardiovasc Surg 1985;89:683-688.

41. Rahimtoola SH, Nunley D, Grunkemeier G, et al: Ten year survival after coronary bypass surgery for unstable angina. N Engl J Med 1983;308:676-681.

42. Lewis HD Jr, Davis JW, Archibald DG, et al: Protective effects of aspirin against myocardial infarction and death in men with unstable angina: Result of a Veterans Administration Cooperative Study. N Engl J Med 1983;309:396-403.

43. Cairns JA, Gent M, Singer J, et al: Aspirin, sulfinpyrazone, or both in unstable angina: Results of a Canadian multicenter trial. N Engl J Med 1985;313:1369-1375.

44. Theroux P, Ouimet H, McCans J, et al: Aspirin, heparin, or both to treat acute unstable angina. N Engl J Med 1988;319:1105-1111.

45. The RISC Group: Risk of myocardial infarction and death during treatment with low-dose aspirin and intravenous heparin in men with unstable coronary artery disease. Lancet 1990;226: 827-830.

46. The FRISC Study Group: Low-molecular-weight heparin during instability in coronary artery disease. Lancet 1996;347: 561-568.

47. Cohen M, Demers C, Gurfinkel EP, et al: A comparison of low-molecular-weight heparin with unfractionated heparin for unstable coronary artery disease: Efficacy and Safety of Subcutaneous Enoxaparin in Non-Q-Wave Coronary Events Study Group. N Engl J Med 1997;337:447-452.

48. Antman EM, McCabe CH, Gurfinkel EP, et al: Enoxaparin prevents death and cardiac ischemic events in unstable angina/non-Q-wave myocardial infarction: Results of thrombolysis in myocardial infarction (TIMI) 11B trial. Circulation 1999;100:1593-1601.

49. EPIC Investigators: Use of a monoclonal antibody directed against the platelet glycoprotein IIb/IIIa receptor in high-risk coronary angioplasty. N Engl J Med 1997;336:1689-1696.

50. The PRISM-PLUS Study Investigators: Inhibition of the platelet glycoprotein IIb/IIIa receptor with tirofiban in unstable angina and non-Q-wave myocardial infarction: Platelet receptor inhibition in ischemic syndrome management in patients limited by unstable signs and symptoms. N Engl J Med 1998;338:1488-1497.

51. The PURSUIT Trial Investigators: Inhibition of platelet glycoprotein IIb/IIIa with eptifibatide in patients with acute coronary syndromes. N Engl J Med 1998;339:436-443.

52. Yusuf S, Zhao F, Mehta SR, et al: Effects of clopidogrel in addition to aspirin in patients with acute coronary syndromes without ST-segment elevation. N Engl J Med 2001;345:494-502.

53. Pitt B, Waters D, Brown WV, et al: Aggressive lipid-lowering therapy compared with angioplasty in stable coronary artery disease. Atorvastatin versus Revascularization Treatment Investigators. N Engl J Med 1999;341:70–76.

54. Schwartz GG, Olsson AG, Ezekowitz MD, et al: Effects of atorvastatin on early recurrent ischemic events in acute coronary syndromes—the MIRACL study: A randomized controlled trial. JAMA 2001;285:1711–1718.

Acute Coronary Syndromes: National and International Dimensions of the Problem

Sidney C. Smith, Jr.

The prevalence and treatment of coronary heart disease (CHD) worldwide has changed dramatically since the 1970s. In this setting, the acute coronary syndromes (ACSs), which include unstable angina (UA), non–ST-elevation myocardial infarction (NSTEMI), and ST-elevation myocardial infarction (STEMI), merit special consideration by physicians and their associated health care systems. ACSs present a major challenge because of their (1) urgent clinical presentation, (2) need for highly organized medical systems for treatment, and (3) significant morbidity and mortality.

PREVALENCE AND ECONOMIC IMPACT OF CORONARY HEART DISEASE AND THE IMPORTANCE OF ACUTE CORONARY SYNDROMES

Cardiovascular diseases (CVDs) are the leading cause of death in the United States, claiming 958,775 lives in 1999 and accounting for 40% of all deaths.[1] CHD is the major form of CVD in the United States, accounting for the largest number of deaths (529,659 in 1999). In the United States, the estimated cost of treating CHD (including both direct and indirect costs) during 2002 was $111.8 billion.[1] Much of the expense in treating CHD relates to therapies associated with the acute and chronic treatment of patients presenting with ACSs. In 1996 alone, the National Center for Health Statistics reported 1,433,000 hospital admissions in the United States for UA or NSTEMI.[2] In 1999, data from the United States National Discharge Survey revealed 449,000 Q-wave myocardial infarctions (STEMI), 530,000 non-Q-wave myocardial infarctions (NSTEMI), and 953,000 UA, yielding a total of 1,483,000 for NSTEMI/UA and a grand total of 1,932,000 for ACSs in terms of hospital discharges during 1999.[3] Clearly, the impact of ACSs on society in terms of patient mortality and morbidity and as seen from a financial perspective is immense.

CVDs are not only the leading cause of death, disability, and health care expense in the United States but also the leading cause of death worldwide.[4,5] According to World Health Organization estimates, CVD resulted in the death of 14.7 million persons in 1990 and 17 million in 1999.[4,6] In fact, CVDs are now the leading cause of mortality in every region of the world except sub-Saharan Africa, and it is anticipated that CVD mortality will exceed that of the current leader in that region, infectious disease, within the next few years.[4] Although accurate statistics on the economic burden of CHD and ACSs worldwide are not available, extrapolation based on their costs to the economy of the United States suggest that the direct and indirect costs of CHD and ACS will likely consume a major portion of global health care expenses in coming years.

TRENDS IN PRESENTATION AMONG PATIENTS WITH ACUTE CORONARY SYNDROMES

During the past few decades, CHD mortality rates began to decrease in many countries.[7-13] Although CHD has remained the leading cause of death in the United States, between 1985 and 1997, CHD mortality declined approximately 30% for both men and women.[14] Understanding the causes of the decline in CHD death rates involves knowledge of the rates of new and recurrent acute myocardial infarction (AMI); the relative frequency of STEMI, NSTEMI, and UA; changes in diagnostic practices; and changes in the use of acute and chronic medical therapies for ACSs. Prior to the use of reperfusion and revascularization strategies for NSTEMI, the 1-year mortality rate for patients with NSTEMI approached that for STEMI because of a high rate of reinfarction during the first year after hospital discharge.[15] Although expanded therapeutic options have significantly improved the discharge prognosis for patients with NSTEMI, it must be emphasized that these patients account for a major group at risk for future cardiovascular events.

Several investigators have noted an increased proportion of patients presenting with less severe forms of ACS or an increased number of patients with NSTEMI as compared with STEMI.[10,11,13,16-19] In the Finnish Monitoring Trends and Determinants in Cardiovascular Disease (FINMONICA) study, the proportion of electrocardiograms coded as definite and the proportion of patients with abnormal cardiac enzymes decreased for both women and men from 1983 to 1990.[13] In the Atherosclerosis Risk in Communities (ARIC) study, mean peak creatine kinase levels and the proportion of patients that met criteria for definite myocardial infarction decreased significantly from 1987 to 1994, suggesting a decreased severity of myocardial infarction in spite of the use of more sensitive cardiac enzyme detection over the study period.[16]

The National Registry of Myocardial Infarction (NRMI) 1, 2, and 3 data gathered from 1,514,292 patients during the period from 1990 through 1999 revealed an increase in the prevalence of non–Q-myocardial infarction (NSTEMI) from 45% in 1994 to 63% in 1999.[17] This registry also reported a decrease in patients presenting with ST elevation or left bundle branch block within 12 hours of the onset of symptoms (STEMI); the mean age increased from 65.3 to 68.0 years, and the percentage of women increased from 35.3% to 39.3%. In this registry, only NRMI-3 reported on the use of troponins, which increased significantly from 70.0% in 1998 to 84.3% in 1999.[17] These findings reflect the increased prevalence of NSTEMI among women and older patients. However, among patients of all ages, NSTEMI and UA occur more frequently than STEMI.

In a national cohort of 31,399 Medicare patients with confirmed AMI hospitalized during the period 1998 through 1999, the majority of patients presented with NSTEMI (19,278, 61.4%) as compared with STEMI (9304, 29.6%) and left bundle branch block or paced rhythms (2817, 9.0%).[18] Medicare patients with STEMI were younger than those with NSTEMI (mean age, 74.8 vs. 75.5 years, P <.0001) while patients with NSTEMI more frequently had a history of hypertension, diabetes, prior cardiac disease, stroke, or other comorbid conditions such as lung disease, anemia, or renal insufficiency. The expanded use of troponin testing, which is consistent with current guideline recommendations,[20] may account for part of the increase in the diagnosis of NSTEMI among this group of Medicare patients. In a sample of medical records drawn from Medicare, AMI hospitalizations during two distinct time periods, 1996 to 1997 (N = 2639) and 1998 to 1999 (N = 35,713), troponin testing increased significantly from 9% of patients to 59%; in 1998, elevated troponin levels were documented in 83% of patients with AMI.[21]

TRENDS IN TREATMENT FOR PATIENTS WITH ACUTE CORONARY SYNDROMES

In addition to the increased number of patients presenting with NSTEMI, improvements in the treatment of AMI and the implementation of secondary prevention therapies upon discharge likely contribute to the decline in mortality from CHD.[12] However, in spite of some improvement in the implementation of appropriate treatment strategies for patients with ACS, a significant number of patients remain untreated. They are more likely to suffer from recurrent events, thereby contributing to the expanding dimensions and clinical burden of ACSs. The relative increase in the number of patients presenting with NSTEMI has important implications for the clinician responsible for care of patients with ACSs. The patients with NSTEMI are often perceived to be at lower risk than those with STEMI and, as such, less likely to receive recommended secondary prevention medical

therapies,[22] although they could derive a large benefit (Table 2-1).[15]

Several national and international registries provide insight into the current application of recommended therapies for patients with ACSs. In NRMI-2 and -3, among the 805,341 AMI patients discharged from the hospital, there were clear trends for increasing prescription of aspirin, β-blockers, angiotensin-converting enzyme (ACE) inhibitors, anti-arrhythmic agents, and diuretic agents between 1994 and 1999.[17] The use of lipid-lowering therapy, recorded only in NRMI-3, increased from 29.2% in 1998 to 36.2% in 1999 (P = .0001). Despite these favorable trends the investigators recommend further improvement in the use of appropriate treatment strategies. Among the NRMI-2 and -3 patients with AMI receiving thrombolytic therapy, the rates of utilization of aspirin, β-blockers, and ACE inhibitors during the first 24 hours (93.5%, 66.9%, and 18.9%, respectively) were suboptimal.

The European Network for Acute Coronary Treatment (ENACT) study[23] reviewed data from European practices on the management of ACSs among 3092 patients from 29 countries. The patient population comprised 1431 (46%) with an initial diagnosis of UA/NSTEMI, 1205 (39%) with STEMI, and 445 (14%) with suspected ACS. The overall ratio of UA/NSTEMI to STEMI was 1.2:1 and similar across the various European countries. The rates of angiography and percutaneous coronary intervention, however, varied widely. Most patients with UA/NSTEMI received aspirin, nitrates, and heparin. There were large intercountry differences in the use of low-molecular-weight heparin and glycoprotein IIb/IIIa inhibitors. There were also national differences in the use of calcium antagonists, ACE inhibitors, and β-blockers.

To further evaluate the management of ACS, the European Society of Cardiology sponsored the Euro Heart Survey of Acute Coronary Syndromes,[24] a prospective survey of 10,484 patients from 25 countries. The survey confirmed a wide discordance between existing guideline recommendations for management of ACS and actual treatment applied.

The Global Registry of Acute Coronary Events (GRACE)[25] gathered information on the management of ACSs in 11,543 patients from 95 hospitals in 14 countries. The use of aspirin was similar across all hospital

■ ■ ■

TABLE 2–1 POSSIBLE CAUSES OF INCREASED INCIDENCE OF NON–ST-ELEVATION MYOCARDIAL INFARCTION

Aging population
Use of troponin assays to detect myocardial injury
Increased use of secondary prevention therapies (e.g., aspirin, statins, β-blockers, angiotensin-converting enzyme inhibitors)
Increased prevalence of diabetes
Earlier recognition of symptoms and arrival in emergency rooms
Change in spectrum of disease

types and geographic regions, with more than 91% of patients receiving therapy upon admission to the hospital. However, the use of medical therapies such as ACE inhibitors, β-blockers, and statins varied considerably. For example, statin use at hospital discharge was more frequent among teaching than nonteaching hospitals (51% vs. 37%). There was a 26% to 57% variation between countries. There was also wide variation between hospitals in the rate of percutaneous coronary intervention and glycoprotein IIb/IIIa inhibitor use; these were used more frequently in the United States and in teaching hospitals.

New data emerging from national and international registries clearly suggest a need for a major effort to coordinate treatment strategies for patients presenting with ACSs to ensure that effective therapies are uniformly available. The availability varies between countries and within countries for economic consideration and health care delivery systems. Nonetheless, one should try to derive optimal benefit from the facilities available.

FUTURE TRENDS AFFECTING PRESENTATION AND TREATMENT OF ACUTE CORONARY SYNDROMES

Several important trends are emerging that will further affect the incidence and prevalence of ACSs and the distribution of STEMI to NSTEMI and UA. These trends suggest that the number of patients presenting with NSTEMI or UA will be growing because of:

- Aging of the population (older patients are more likely to present with NSTEMI)
- Expanding use of troponins
- Increasing use of secondary prevention drugs such as aspirin, ACE inhibitors, and statin
- Increasing prevalence of diabetes (the presence of microvascular disease enhances the risk of NSTEMI)
- Earlier recognition of symptoms (enhanced by national efforts to patient education and an increasing number of patients who survive a first event

These trends will probably lead to an increasing need for chest pain centers and further refinement of targeted diagnostic, medical, and revascularization therapies. Physicians responsible for the care of patients with ACSs must remain informed about evolving diagnostic and treatment strategies for a complex and challenging disease.

REFERENCES

1. American Heart Association: 2002 Heart and Stroke Statistical Update. Dallas, American Heart Association, 2001.
2. National Center for Health Statistics: Detailed diagnoses and procedures: National Hospital Discharge Survey. Hyattsville, Md., National Center for Health Statistics, 1996.
3. Popovic JR: 1999 National Hospital Discharge Survey: Annual Summary with Detailed Diagnosis and Procedure Data. Vital Health Statistics, Vol. 13. Hyattsville, Md., National Center for Health Statisitics, 2001.
4. Murray CJ, Lopez AD: Mortality by cause for eight regions of the world. Global Burden of Disease Study. Lancet 1997;349: 1269-1276.
5. Howson CP, Reddy KS, Ryan TJ, et al (eds): Control of Cardiovascular Disease in Developing Countries: Research, Development, and Institutional Strengthening. Washington, D.C., National Academy Press, 1998.
6. World Health Report: Mental Health: New Understanding, New Hope. Geneva, World Health Organization, 2001, pp 144-149.
7. Marques-Vidal P, Ferrieres J, Metzger MH, et al: Trends in coronary heart disease morbidity and mortality and acute coronary care and case fatality from 1985-1989 in southern Germany and southwestern France. Eur Heart J 1997;18:816-821.
8. Brophy JM: The epidemiology of acute myocardial infarction and ischemic heart disease in Canada: Data from 1976 to 1991. Can J Cardiol 1997;13:474-478.
9. Beaglehole R, Stewart AW, Jackson R, et al: Declining rates of coronary heart disease in New Zealand and Australia, 1983-1993. Am J Epidemiol 1997;145:707-713.
10. McGovern PG, Pankow JS, Shahar E, et al: Recent trends in acute coronary heart disease—mortality, morbidity, medical care, and risk factors. The Minnesota Heart Survey Investigators. N Engl J Med 1996;334:884-890.
11. McGovern PG, Jacobs DR Jr, Shahar E, et al: Trends in acute coronary heart disease mortality, morbidity, and medical care from 1985 through 1997: The Minnesota Heart Survey. Circulation 2001;104:19-24.
12. Rosamond WD, Chambless LE, Folsom AR, et al: Trends in the incidence of myocardial infarction and in mortality due to coronary heart disease, 1987 to 1994. N Engl J Med 1998;339:861-867.
13. Salomaa V, Miettinen H, Kuulasmaa K, et al: Decline of coronary heart disease mortality in Finland during 1983 to 1992: Roles of incidence, recurrence, and case-fatality. The FINMONICA MI Register Study. Circulation 1996;94:3130-3137.
14. Mortality patterns: United States, 1997. MMWR Morbid Mortal Wkly Rep 1999;48:664-668.
15. Marmor A, Geltman, E, Schechtman K, et al: Recurrent myocardial infarction: Clinical predictors and prognostic implications. Circulation 1982;66:415-421.
16. Goff DC Jr, Howard G, Wang CH, et al: Trends in severity of hospitalized myocardial infarction: The atherosclerosis risk in communities (ARIC) study, 1987-1994. Am Heart J 2000;139:874-880.
17. Rogers WJ, Canto JG, Lambrew CT, et al: Temporal trends in the treatment of over 1.5 million patients with myocardial infarction in the US from 1990 through 1999: The National Registry of Myocardial Infarction 1, 2 and 3. J Am Coll Cardiol 2000;36: 2056-2063.
18. Foody J, Galusha D, Masoudi F, et al: Quality of care for older patients hospitalized with non–ST-elevation MI. Submitted for publication, 2002.
19. Roe M: Temporal trends in the management of patients with acute myocardial infarction. The National Myocardial Infarction-4 (NRMI-4) Registry. Submitted for publication, 2002.
20. Braunwald E, Antman AM, Beasley JW, et al: ACC/AHA Guideline Update for the Management of Patients with Stable and Unstable Angina and Non-ST Segment Elevation Myocardial Infarction—2002 Summary Article. A Report of the American College of Cardiology/American Heart Association Task Force on Practice Guidelines (Committee on the Management of Patients with Unstable Angina). Circulation 2002;106:1893-1900.
21. Foody J, Wang Y, Galusha D, et al: National trends and clinical implications of the use of troponin in the diagnosis of AMI. Submitted for publication, 2002.
22. Smith SC Jr, Blair SN, Bonow RO, et al: AHA/ACC Scientific Statement: AHA/ACC guidelines for preventing heart attack and death in patients with atherosclerotic cardiovascular disease: 2001 update: A statement for healthcare professionals from the American Heart Association and the American College of Cardiology. Circulation 2001;104:1577-1579.
23. Fox KA, Cokkinos DV, Deckers J, et al: The ENACT study: A pan-European survey of acute coronary syndromes. European Network for Acute Coronary Treatment. Eur Heart J 2000;21: 1440-1449.

24. Hasdai D, Behar S, Wallentin L, et al: A prospective survey of the characteristics, treatments and outcomes of patients with acute coronary syndromes in Europe and the Mediterranean basin; The Euro Heart Survey of Acute Coronary Syndromes (Euro Heart Survey ACS). Eur Heart J 2002;23:1190-1201.

25. Fox KA, Goodman SG, Klein W, et al: Management of acute coronary syndromes. Variations in practice and outcome; Findings from the Global Registry of Acute Coronary Events (GRACE). Eur Heart J 2002;23:1177-1189.

An Epidemiological Perspective: Society, Environment, Risk Factors, and Genetics

Bernhard R. Winkelmann
Winfried März

DEFINITION

The term *acute coronary syndrome (ACS)* has been introduced as a new clinical phenotype to adequately describe the full range of clinical manifestations resulting from atherosclerotic coronary plaque erosion, fissuring, or rupture leading to myocardial ischemia after incomplete or complete coronary artery thrombotic occlusion.[1-6] The initial working diagnosis is one of suspected ACS. The final diagnosis is readily applied in the setting of acute ST-elevation myocardial infarction (MI), for which therapeutic conduct is well established. In contrast, non–ST-elevation ACS remains a diagnostic and therapeutic challenge; further investigation for patient orientation, treatment, and final diagnosis is needed (Table 3-1).[7-8]

A diagnosis of definite ACS is established after a certain time course (i.e., hours to days) of serial ECGs, cardiac enzymes, and functional testing for myocardial ischemia or appropriate coronary imaging to demonstrate either evolution to MI or that symptoms of unstable angina (UA) coincide with objective signs of myocardial ischemia or of coronary atherosclerosis. Thus, the initial diagnosis of suspected ACS is either confirmed as definite ACS by its final outcome (as UA or MI) or is ruled out (Fig. 3-1). Noncardiac chest pain syndromes, secondary causes of angina, or variant angina occasionally coexists with "true"ACS.[9]

Rarely, vasospasm of Prinzmetal angina may be so severe that even in patients with normal coronary arteries, myocardial ischemia and angina, and even MI, may occur.[10-12] A diagnosis of UA requires that the patient's symptoms are actually caused by myocardial ischemia and that acute MI is ruled out during follow-up.[13] Troponin-positive MI has been redefined by the Joint European Society of Cardiology/American College of Cardiology Committee.[14-16] This change in definition will lead to an increase in the prevalence of MI but does not affect the definition of ACS, which includes all the acute ischemic phenotypes. However, troponin testing allows one to rapidly diagnose definite ACS, although certain limitations, as with any laboratory test, may apply.[17-19]

PREVALENCE AND INCIDENCE

Typically, the prevalence of coronary heart disease (CHD) increases with age. In North America or Northern Europe, the rate is 2% to 5% in men aged 45 to 54 years, increasing to 11% to 20% in men aged 65 to 74 years; in women, the rate is about 0.5% to 1% in premenopausal women aged 45 to 54 years, with the prevalence increasing after menopause to a level similar to that in men.[20] UA or MI is the first manifestation in about half of patients with CHD; the other half initially presents with stable angina.

Obviously, the prevalence of CHD in a population presenting with chest pain is the major determinant for definite ACS because underlying CHD is the prerequisite for that phenotype. Up to 30% to 50% of patients with chest pain presenting to an emergency department are hospitalized with an admission diagnosis of suspected ACS. Among those, again, about 30% to 50% are confirmed as having definite ACS. Vice versa, CHD and ACS are ruled out in about one third of patients with suspected ACS (Table 3-2).[21-28] The incidence of definite ACS is lower—and the incidence of no CHD higher—in low-risk subgroups of persons with suspected ACS, such as those with normal-appearing or nondiagnostic ECGs, whereas the opposite is true in high-risk populations, such as in participants of the Platelet Glycoprotein IIb/IIIa in Unstable Angina: Receptor Suppression Using Integrilin Therapy (PURSUIT) trial (see Table 3-2). Data from various sources demonstrate that the frequency of noncardiac, nonatherosclerotic causes of pain mimicking ACS varies considerably in relation with the characteristics of the population studied and the diagnostic methods and diagnostic criteria used.[29] In the International Global Registry of Acute Coronary Events (GRACE) trial, 27% of a total of 9251 patients admitted with a diagnosis of ACS had acute ST-segment elevation MI, 22% non–ST-elevation MI, 39% UA, and 7% no ACS in retrospect.[30]

Misdiagnosis of ACS as noncardiac chest pain or mislabeling of noncardiac disease as ACS in patients presenting to a hospital does not seem to be a major issue with adequate diagnostic testing. However, it can be estimated that a major proportion of MI or ACS will go undetected in the population as a whole. As many as one third of MIs went unrecognized in the population cohort of the Framingham study.[31] Sheifer and coauthors reported that at least one fourth of all MIs are clinically unrecognized and that their mortality is the same as that of recognized MI.[32] Similarly, in about one third of a cohort of patients in whom the mean age was

■ ■ ■

TABLE 3–1   CRITERIA FOR THE DEFINITION OF MYOCARDIAL INFARCTION (MI) AND ACUTE CORONARY SYNDROME (ACS) AND ASSOCIATED CLINICAL PHENOTYPES

KEY TERM	DEFINITION	CLINICAL PHENOTYPES
Suspected ACS	Working diagnosis on admission when symptoms and signs suggest underlying myocardial ischemia but definite objective evidence is still lacking	**Ischemic** Unstable angina (UA) MI Secondary causes of UA Variant angina **Nonischemic** Noncardiac chest pain syndromes
Definite ACS	Final diagnosis based on definite evidence	UA MI
MI	Defined by symptoms, ECG, and enzyme criteria	ST-segment elevation MI Non–ST-segment elevation MI Q-wave MI Non–Q-wave MI Anatomic location of MI (e.g., anterior, inferior, posterolateral)

53 years and CHD was unsuspected who were referred for catheter ablation therapy, angiography discovered diffuse coronary atherosclerosis of <50%; in addition, 7% of patients showed definite CHD with at least one major coronary vessel stenosed at least 50%.[33] In an earlier study, 105 of 2014 presumably healthy working men, aged 40 to 59 years, who underwent a comprehensive health screen were selected for coronary angiography because of a positive exercise test result. Among that subgroup, only one third had a normal-appearing coronary angiogram. Thus, the prevalence of CHD, based on invasive testing of those 105 patients alone, was 4% among all presumably healthy workers.[34]

It should be noted that the terms *non–ST-elevation* and *non–Q-wave* or *ST-elevation* and *Q-wave* as ECG descriptors of the initial or late phase of an MI are not entirely synonymous, although often viewed as such. The majority of patients with ST-segment elevation ultimately experience a Q-wave acute MI; a minority experience a non–Q-wave acute MI.[15,29] Of the patients who present without ST elevation, the majority are ultimately described as having UA (no development of cardiac markers diagnostic for MI) or acute non–Q-wave MI (cardiac markers diagnostic for MI). A minority of such patients experience a Q-wave MI (see Fig. 3–1). The concept of ACS also highlights the dynamic and life-threatening situation of patients with ischemic discomfort at rest regardless of whether or not they present with ST-segment elevation.[35,36]

Compared with patients with CHD and stable angina, patients presenting with ACS are at a much higher risk for coronary events within the first days after the onset of symptoms.[37] Five to 10% of patients with ACS reported in recent glycoprotein IIb/IIIa intervention studies will suffer from nonfatal MI within 1 month after onset of ACS, and about 2% to 5% die within that period.[38,39] Another 2% to 3% of such events will accumulate within the first year.[40-48] The risk of death remains highest in acute MI, where almost half of patients die before reaching the hospital.[49]

From an epidemiologic point of view (in terms of 1-year event rates), non–ST-elevation and ST-elevation MI carry the same long-term prognosis as non–Q-wave and Q-wave MI, respectively. Thus, a non–Q-wave MI is not as benign as often thought. Thus, the distinction into non–Q-wave and Q-wave MI is of no major value, if not to say meaningless, from an epidemiologic long-term perspective.[50]

EPIDEMIOLOGIC CONCEPTS

Incidence and prevalence rates are epidemiologic measures to quantify the occurrence of disease. *Prevalence* quantifies the proportion of patients having the disease in a population at a given point in time; *incidence* quantifies the number of new cases of disease that develop during a specified time interval.[51,52] Incidence is expressed as cumulative incidence or, more precisely, as incidence rate or incidence density (Table 3–3). Prevalence as an estimate of disease frequency depends on the rate at which new cases arise (incidence) and existing cases are removed (i.e., recover or die). CHD is a lifelong disease without recovery after its manifestation, but ACS is a condition ending in recovery or death. The duration of ACS is generally limited to days to weeks. Therefore, in cases of ACS, incidence is the appropriate measure; in cases of a chronic disease like CHD, incidence raises a number of problems. The incidence of (new) CHD may only be estimated by some specified manifestation or complication, whereas CHD prevalence

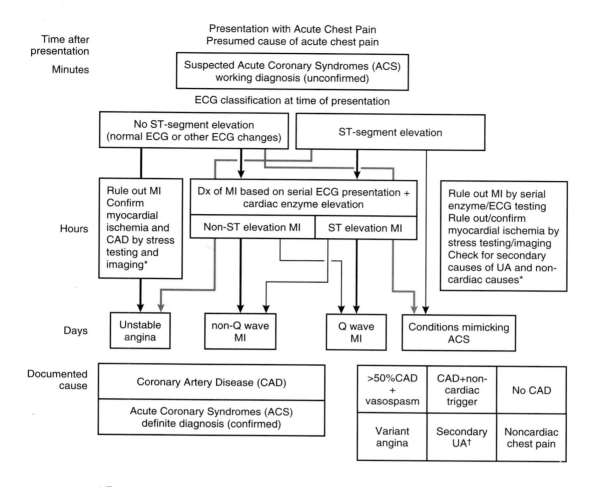

FIGURE 3–1. Nomenclature of acute coronary syndromes. Variant angina (Prinzmetal angina) with transient ST-segment elevations may occur in approximately 0.5% to 1% of patients admitted to the hospital with chest pain. Prinzmetal angina is a distinct entity associated with severe vasospasm but generally not with plaque rupture. CAD, coronary artery disease; MI, myocardial infarction; UA, unstable angina; *, Testing should be done as appropriate; several strategies apply (i.e., early invasive vs. conservative), depending on the patient's history and clinical risk assessment. †, Secondary UA is caused by conditions extrinsic to the coronary vasculature (e.g., tachycardia, fever, increase in left-ventricular afterload, severe hypertension, aortic stenosis, anemia, hypoxemia, or hyperviscosity).

may be estimated using any measure indicative of (chronic) CHD.

The incidence of ACS in a population is controlled by the prevalence of CHD as a necessary condition for evolution to ACS and the presence of generally unknown specific risk factors for ACS. Almost every CHD patient suffers at least one episode of ACS. Thus, CHD prevalence rates provide an estimate for a maximum incidence of ACS in a given population.

Published data on prevalence rates for CHD should always be scrutinized as to whether they meet certain epidemiologic standards (Table 3–4). True random samples provide the most accurate estimates for disease frequency in a given population, but such data are generally rare. Thus, in most instances, only biased data from various sources such as hospitals admissions, large phase III medication studies, or registries are available. Although such data may reflect true population rates, this should not be taken for granted. Especially important is that sample size estimates or confidence rates are based on the statistics of random error and cannot cope for systematic bias (Table 3–5). This holds particularly true for the flood of genetic epidemiologic case-control studies about associations of gene variants with disease, as discussed later in this chapter. Depending on the sample size, such a random variation can be decreased. However, rates in a sample will remain seriously flawed by the impact of a generally undetected systematic bias regardless of sample size.

Sole use of an accepted gold standard may not be a viable option in an epidemiologic setting (e.g., angiography for the diagnosis of CHD in populations). For

■ ▨ ■

TABLE 3–2   FREQUENCY OF NONCARDIAC CHEST PAIN AND SUSPECTED AND CONFIRMED ACUTE CORONARY SYNDROMES (ACSs)

POPULATION AND REFERENCE	PRESENTATION WITH ACUTE CHEST PAIN	STRATIFICATION OF ACUTE CHEST PAIN ON ADMISSION AS SUSPECTED ACS (%)	FINAL CLASSIFICATION OF SUSPECTED ACS AFTER DIAGNOSTIC TESTING	
			Confirmed (%)[*]	NO CHD (%)[†]
Emergency department (ED), Houston[21]	955	—	34 (including 12% MI)	—
ED, Olmsted County, MI[22]	6801	33	48[‡]	36[‡]
ED, Richmond, VA[23]	4162	52	27 (including 14% MI)	— (73% no ACS)
ED, Rotterdam[24]	417	100	74 (including 6% MI)	26
Chest pain clinic, Belfast, UK[25]	900	100	6[§]	55[§]
ED, New York, NY[26]	415	36 (with stress testing)	32	68
		64 (no stress testing)	13[‖]	28[‖]
ED[27]	292	100	78 (including 18% MI)	22
PURSUIT[28]	5767	100 (all with initial angiography)	94	6

MI, myocardial infarction.
Note: In cases of 100% suspected ACS, the total number of persons with any type of chest pain has not been reported.
[*]Category referred to as noncardiac chest pain or no coronary heart disease (CHD) based on a normal-appearing angiogram or functional test that rules out coronary ischemia (may occasionally include persons with stable CHD and with additional noncardiac chest pain mimicking ACS).
[†]Using all persons with an initial diagnosis of suspected ACS (or acute chest pain if the rate of suspected ACS was not reported) as the denominator.
[‡]Based on 795 patients undergoing angiography; another 16% had mild CHD defined as a maximum luminal narrowing of >0% to 49%.
[§]ACS 6%, stable CHD 19%, possible CHD 19%, no CHD 55%.
[‖]Using the subgroup with a normal or nondiagnostic ECG and normal enzymes on admission who were readmitted later (n = 60) as the denominator.

example, many tests and disease manifestations are indicative of CHD, but their presence or absence may be open to misinterpretation. Thus, in epidemiologic studies of populations in which angiography of apparently healthy subjects is not feasible, the prevalence of "silent" coronary artery stenosis will be significant whenever the prevalence of clinically manifest CHD is relatively high.[53]

TRADITIONAL CHD RISK FACTORS

Causative, predisposing, and nonmodifiable risk factors for CHD have been identified in the past 50 years based on epidemiologic long-term observations,[54] migrant studies,[55] autopsy studies,[56] intervention studies,[57,58]

and basic science evidence (Table 3–6). Causal risk factors fulfill the Bradford Hill criteria of causation (see Table 3–6) as opposed to risk markers that merely provide evidence of an association.[59]

Relative risk, risk ratio, and odds ratio are common epidemiologic measures for the strength of association of specific risk factors with disease. Although *relative risk* is a measure of the likelihood of disease in the group exposed to a risk factor relative to those not exposed and can only be assessed in prospective studies of disease incidence, *odds ratio* is an estimate of the relative risk in case-control studies, wherein the disease incidence is unknown (Table 3–7). For large numbers of controls compared with cases, the relative risk approaches the odds ratio as shown in Table 3–8.

■ ▨ ■

TABLE 3–3   KEY CONCEPTS IN EPIDEMIOLOGY—MEASURES OF DISEASE FREQUENCY

$$\text{Prevalence} = \frac{\text{Number of existing cases of a disease/condition}}{\text{Total study population [cases/population or \%]}} \text{ at a given point in time}$$

$$\text{(Cumulative) Incidence} = \frac{\text{Number of new cases of disease/condition}}{\text{Total study population at risk [cases/population or \% per time observed]}} \text{ during a given time period}$$

$$\text{Incidence Rate or Density} = \frac{\text{Number of new cases of disease/condition}}{\text{Total (=cumulated) person-time of observation [cases/person-years]}} \text{ during a given time period}$$

Modified from Hennekens CH, Buring JE: Epidemiology in Medicine. Boston, Little Brown, 1987.

TABLE 3–4 IMPORTANT EPIDEMIOLOGIC CONCEPTS IN THE STUDY OF DISEASE PREVALENCE IN POPULATIONS

CONCEPT	DEFINITION
Validity	Ability of a test to measure what it claims to measure
Sensitivity Proportion of true positives correctly identified (with only a few false negatives)	True positives identified by the test divided by all true positives defined by a reference method (true positives + false negatives)
Specificity Proportion of true negatives correctly identified (with only a few false positives)	True negatives identified by the test divided by all true negatives defined by a reference method (true negatives + false positives)
Predictive value The predictive value of even a relatively specific test (for example 95% specificity and 90% sensitivity) will be low and yield many false-positive results if the prevalence of the disease to be studied is low.	*Predictive value of a positive test* = probability that a person who tests positive actually has the disease; calculated as true positives divided by all tested as positive (true positive + false positives)

Prevalence (%)   *Predictive value (%)*
  0.1   2
  1   15
  5   49
  50   95
	Predictive value of a negative test = probability that a person with a negative test is disease free: true negatives divided by all tested as negative (true negatives plus false negatives)

Reliability/repeatability/precision	Repeated measures should remain consistent; influenced by true (biological) and technical (observer or measurement) variation
Standardization	Applies to every measure/method used
Measurement variation	Many factors contribute to variation, e.g., physiological fluctuation, environment, circadian, seasonal, temperature
Random error	For example, random misclassification is serious for the individual but less so for the group result; increases standard error of mean, can be reduced by increase in sample size, underestimates true effects
Bias (systematic error)	Conclusion about groups or comparisons will be distorted, not reduced, by increase in sample size; often remains unidentified

Modified from Rose GA, et al: Cardiovascular Survey Methods, 2nd ed. Geneva, World Health Organization, 1982.

TABLE 3–5 CALCULATION OF 95% CONFIDENCE LIMITS FOR SAMPLING VARIABILITY FOR VARIOUS RATES AND SIZES OF RANDOM SAMPLES OF PREVALENCE OR INCIDENCE STUDIES

ESTIMATED PERCENTAGE	95% CONFIDENCE INTERVAL FOR TWO SAMPLE SIZES	
	n = 500	n = 1000
2	1.0–3.7	1.2–3.1
4	2.5–6.1	2.9–5.4
6	4.1–8.5	4.6–7.7
8	5.8–10.7	6.4–9.9
10	7.5–13.0	8.2–12.0
12	9.3–15.2	10.1–14.2
14	11.1–17.4	11.9–16.3
20	16.6–23.8	17.6–22.6

Modified from Rose GA, et al: Cardiovascular Survey Methods, 2nd ed. Geneva, World Health Organization, 1982.

TABLE 3–6 RISK FACTORS FOR CORONARY HEART DISEASE AND BRADFORD HILL CRITERIA OF CAUSATION[59]

CAUSAL RISK FACTORS	PREDISPOSING RISK FACTORS*
Tobacco consumption	Physical inactivity
Dyslipidemia (elevated low-density lipoprotein and/or high-density lipoprotein cholesterol)	Obesity Diet **Nonmodifiable Risk Factors†**
High blood pressure	Male sex
Elevated glucose	Age

Bradford Hill Criteria of Causation

Strength of the association
Consistency of the association
Specificity of the association
Temporality of the association
Biological gradient (dose-response curve)
Biological plausibility
Coherence of evidence
Experimental evidence
Analogy to other causal settings

*Predisposing risk factors are presumed to work, at least in part, by affecting causal risk factors.
†Nonmodifiable risk factors may act as surrogate measures for the amount of exposure to causal risk factors. With increasing age, the male sex tends to lose its risk status compared with females once the females reach menopause.

■ ■ ■

TABLE 3–7 KEY CONCEPTS IN EPIDEMIOLOGY—MEASURES OF DISEASE ASSOCIATION WITH (RISK-FACTOR) EXPOSURE

TWO-BY-TWO TABLE		DISEASE	
		Yes (Case)	No (Control)
Risk-factor Exposure	Yes	a	b
	No	c	d

Relative Risk (Risk Ratio) = $RR = \dfrac{a/(a+b)}{c/(c+d)}$

Cumulative incidence in exposed/
Cumulative incidence in nonexposed

Relative Risk (Rate Ratio) =

Incidence rate in exposed/
Incidence rate in nonexposed

Likelihood of developing disease in the exposed group relative to those not exposed over a specified time interval; the relative risk changes with the length of observation

Attributable Risk (= Excess Risk) $a/(a+b) - c/(c+d)$

Risk difference of risk factor exposed and nonexposed (over a specified time period)

Odds Ratio $OR = \dfrac{a/c}{b/d} = \dfrac{a \times d}{b \times c}$

Ratio of the odds of risk factor exposure among cases to that among controls (at "one point in time"); OR is an estimate of the relative risk in case-control studies wherein the disease incidence is unknown

Modified from Hennekens CH, Buring JE: Epidemiology in Medicine. Boston, Little Brown, 1987.

Smoking

Consumption of tobacco, predominantly by smoking cigarettes, is the major avoidable cause of CHD and cardiovascular disease morbidity and mortality. The health care costs of smoking-related illnesses—estimated at $65 billion for the United States in 1985—are staggering.[60,61] Up to one half of all smokers will die because of their smoking habit.[62] In the "industrialized" countries, smoking is estimated to be the largest single cause of premature death, causing about 30% of deaths between ages 35 and 69 years, with an average loss of 23 years of life in those killed by tobacco.[63] Overall smoking is attributable for 20% of all deaths in established economies[63] as well as in developing economies like China.[64] Globally, there are more than 1 billion smokers; an estimated 6% of all deaths were attributable to tobacco in 1990. Figures are expected to double with the expected further rise in smoking rates in the developing economies (China, India, other Asian islands, the sub-Saharan Africa, Middle Eastern Crescent, Latin America, and the Caribbean) within the next 20 years.[65,66] Although the overall rate of smoking is declining in industrialized countries, from about 40% of adults smoking in 1965 in the United States to 23% in 1997,[67] the rates in young men and women are not.[68]

In the prospective Copenhagen City Heart Study of 20,000 men and women, the relative risk for first acute MI increased for smoking in a dose-dependent manner, 2% to 3% for each gram of tobacco (1 g equals one cigarette) smoked daily, and was higher in women than in men, with a relative risk ranging from 3.6 to 9.4, and 1.6 to 2.9, respectively, with an exposure of 1 to 14 g/day to 30 g/day of tobacco consumption.[69] Similar risk ratios have been found for women in the United States participating in the Nurses Health study, ranging from 2.4 to 10.8 for smoking 1 to 4 cigarettes per day to 45 per day, respectively.[70] As shown in survivors of MI in the International Studies of Infarct Survival (ISIS) studies,[71] the relative risk of MI associated with smoking is highest in the younger age groups and decreases with age (Fig. 3-2).

Smoking induces premature MI, with an onset of MI 8 to 13 years earlier than in nonsmokers as shown by the analyses of multinational trials of thrombolysis for MI (Table 3-9).[72-76] Because of their younger age and a more favorable profile of other risk factors generally, smokers surviving to the point of being admitted to the hospital fare better than their nonsmoking older counterparts with respect to the in-hospital event rate.[72,73] The higher mortality rates in nonsmokers compared with smokers have erroneously been labeled "smoker's paradox." These rates can be almost fully explained by

■ ■ ■

TABLE 3–8 SAMPLE CALCULATION TO DEMONSTRATE THE IMPACT OF A CHANGE IN THE SAMPLE SIZE OF THE CONTROL GROUP

The OR does not change with an increase in the number of controls if the proportions of exposure in cases and controls remain unchanged, while the relative risk will.

100 cases and 100 controls: a = 60, b = 40, c = 40, d = 60	OR = 60 × 60/40 × 40 = 2.25	RR = 60/(60+40)/40/(40+60) = 1.5
100 cases and 1000 controls: a = 60, b = 400, c = 40, d = 600	OR = 60 × 600/40 × 400 = 2.25	RR = 60/(60+400)/40/(40+600) = 2.1
For large number of controls (b, d) compared with cases (a, c), RR equals OR		$RR = \dfrac{a/(a+b)}{c/(c+d)} \sim \dfrac{a/b}{c/d} = \dfrac{a \times d}{b \times c}$

OR, odds ratio; RR, relative risk.

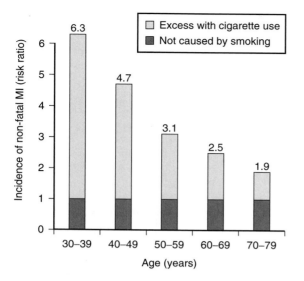

FIGURE 3–2. Occurrence of nonfatal myocardial infarction (MI) as a first event in the third International Study of Infarct Survival (ISIS-3) in persons without a previous history of major neoplastic or vascular disease. Relative risk for cigarette smokers compared with nonsmokers and ex-smokers for at least 10 years. (After Parish S, Collins R, Peto R, et al for the International Studies of Infarct Survival (ISIS): Cigarette smoking, tar yields, and non-fatal myocardial infarction: 14,000 cases and 32,000 controls in the United Kingdom. BMJ 1995;311:471–477.)

the differences in baseline risk. Smoking is associated with a premature need for coronary percutaneous procedures which are done on average 13 years earlier than in nonsmokers (see Table 3-9).[74-76] Despite the fact that many biomarkers of atherosclerosis are adversely affected by smoking,[77-84] the mechanisms by which smoking induces CHD and MI remain poorly understood.[85,86]

Smoking and Acute Coronary Syndromes

Tobacco smoking and a positive family history for MI are the two most common risk factors for premature CHD and MI in young adults.[87] A recent analysis of consecutive patients admitted to a large coronary care unit[88] found a surprising high proportion (25%) of young women (<46 years) with MI compared with previous data from the Gruppo Italiano por lo Studio della Streotochianasi nell'Infarto Miocardico (GISSI-2) studies, wherein the proportion of smokers was less than 10%.[89,90] Cigarette smoking in women is estimated to increase the risk of MI by two to six times compared with nonsmoking. Furthermore, the risk increases with the number of cigarettes smoked daily. Whether this increase in the proportion of young women experiencing MI is a play of chance or reflects recent trends to an increase in smoking rates among young girls remains to be established.[91]

Dyslipidemia

Elevated serum cholesterol levels increase the risk of CHD along a continuum. There does not seem to be a threshold level below which persons are free of risk and above which the risk of CHD suddenly begins.[92] The 6-year follow-up of 361,662 men screened for the Multiple Risk Factor Intervention Trial (MRFIT) study showed a steady increase in CHD mortality with increasing serum cholesterol.[93] Nevertheless, because CHD risk increases continuously with elevations in serum cholesterol, and because the number of people with slightly to moderately elevated levels is large, most CHD deaths still occur among those with almost "normal" cholesterol levels.[94] As a rule of thumb (derived from the results of the Lipid Research Clinics Program of lowering low-density lipoprotein (LDL) with cholestyramine[95,96] and the 30-year follow-up of the Framingham study[97]), a 1% reduction in total cholesterol translates into an approximate 2% reduction in CHD risk.[98] Although initially debated,[99] the large statin intervention trials confirmed those initial risk reduction estimates (Table 3-10).[101-108] It has been estimated from epidemiologic data of three large cohorts that cholesterol levels of less than 5.2 mmol/L (200 mg/dL) in younger men (39 years) are associated with a prolonged life expectancy of 4 to 9 years.[109]

■ ▪ ■

TABLE 3–9   SMOKING AND AVERAGE AGE OF ONSET OF MYOCARDIAL INFARCTION (MI) IN PARTICIPANTS OF MULTICENTER STUDIES OF THROMBOLYSIS FOR MI OR BALLON ANGIOPLASTY (PTCA) GROUPED BY SMOKING STATUS

STUDY ACRONYM (REFERENCE)	AGE AT ONSET OF MI OR PTCA (YEARS)		
	Smoker	Ex-Smoker	Nonsmoker
TpA/Streptokinase (Barbash, 1993)[72]	58 ± 11	64 ± 10	67 ± 10
GUSTO-I (Barbash, 1995)[73]	55 ± 11	64 ± 10	66 ± 12
TAMI 1-5 and 7 (Grines, 1995)[74]	54 (47 62)	—	62 (54 68)*
GUSTO IIb (Hasdai, 1999)[75]	55 (47 63)	66 (58 72)	68 (60 76)
PTCA† (Hasdai, 1997)[76]	55 ± 11	65 ± 10	67 ± 11

Data are mean ± standard deviation or median (25%, 75% percentile).
*Includes ex-smokers.
†All patients who underwent PTCA at the Mayo Clinic 1979 to 1995 without acute MI within 24 hours before the intervention.

■ ■ ■

TABLE 3–10   MAJOR RESULTS OF THE LANDMARK STATIN TRIALS

STUDY ACRONYM (REFERENCE)	BASELINE LDL-C, mmol/L (mg/dL)	ΔLDL-C (%)	EVENT RATE*		RRR = P – S/P (%)	ARR = P – S (%)	NNT = 1/ARR (1)
			Statin (S) (%)	Placebo (P) (%)			
4S[103]	4.9 (188)	35	19.4	28.0	31	8.6	12
LIPID[104]	3.9 (150)	25	12.3	15.9	23	3.6	28
HPS[105]	3.3 (128)	29	8.7	11.8	26	3.1	32
CARE[106]	3.6 (139)	32	10.2	13.2	23	3.0	33
WOSCOPS[107]	5.0 (192)	26	5.5	7.9	30	2.4	42
AFCAPS[58]	3.9 (150)	25	3.5	5.5	37	2.0	49

ARR, absolute risk reduction; LDL-C, low-density lipoprotein cholesterol; NNT, number needed to treat (= 100/ARR if ARR given in percentage); RRR, relative risk reduction.
*Primary end points: nonfatal myocardial infarction (MI), coronary death, or resuscitated cardiac arrest in 4S study; nonfatal MI or death from coronary heart disease in LIPID, APS, CARE, and WOSCOPS studies; nonfatal or fatal MI, unstable angina, or sudden cardiac death in AFCAPS study.
Adapted from Moriarty PM: Using both "risk reduction" and "number needed to treat" in evaluating primary and secondary clinical trials of lipid reduction. Am J Cardiol 2001;87:1206–1208.

Plaque fissuring inducing thrombus formation is presumably the cause of ACS. Elevated LDL cholesterol is associated with a higher risk of MI; thus hypercholesterolemia seems to be an important trigger of plaque rupture. Vice versa, cholesterol reduction is one important mechanism to stabilize a vulnerable plaque and prevent ACS in primary prevention and recurrent coronary events in stable CHD or ACS populations, regardless of whether the index event is UA or acute MI.[110] Aggressive cholesterol lowering applied during the acute phase of UA, and non–Q-wave MI was marginally effective in reducing recurrent ischemic events in the Myocardial Ischemia Reduction with Aggressive Cholesterol Lowering (MIRACL) study.[111]

Lipoprotein metabolism in humans is defined by three major pathways that are tightly interrelated:

- Transport of dietary (exogenous fat) with uptake in the intestine and transport in chylomicrons in the lymph to the liver
- Transport of hepatic (endogenous) fat via triglyceride-rich very-low-density lipoprotein, intermediate-density lipoprotein, and LDL particles to peripheral cells
- Reverse cholesterol transport pathway—the transfer and uptake of free cholesterol from the peripheral tissues, such as the arterial wall and its subsequent delivery to the liver by high-density lipoprotein (HDL) cholesterol[112]

HDL cholesterol is the most important lipid-related risk factor besides total cholesterol and LDL cholesterol and has been shown to be inversely and independently related to CHD risk. High levels are protective; low levels of HDL indicate increased risk.[113] Thus, the HDL/LDL cholesterol ratio is the most powerful lipoprotein predictor of future CHD.[114]

The role of triglycerides, which correlate inversely with HDL cholesterol values, as an independent CHD risk factor beyond the measurement of LDL and HDL cholesterol is controversial.[115-118] However, depending on the approach of statistical analysis, an independent gradient of risk for triglycerides stratified for HDL cholesterol may be obtained.[116,118] Because the day-to-day variability of triglycerides is higher than that of HDL cholesterol, the association between triglycerides and coronary risk tends to be underestimated.[119] Whether isolated hypertriglyceridemia is atherogenic is a matter of dispute; such phenotypes, however, are rare. From a population point of view, hypertriglyceridemia generally indicates risk-factor clustering associated with the metabolic syndrome; that is, hypertensive, overweight, and insulin-resistant individuals who are at high risk for CHD.[120-123] It has been estimated from population-based studies that hypertriglyceridemia independently increases the relative risk of cardiovascular disease by 14% for men and 37% for women after adjustment for HDL cholesterol.[124]

Apolipoproteins are major constituents of lipoprotein particles. Thus, apolipoproteins A to I may serve as a surrogate marker for HDL, and apolipoprotein B-100 may serve as a surrogate marker for LDL cholesterol. However, whether apolipoproteins are better markers of dyslipidemia risk than the conventional measures of cholesterol remains controversial,[125,126] and data on other apolipoproteins like A-II, C-III, or E are sketchy and incomplete.[127]

Hypertension

The physiologic variability in blood pressure makes detection of the risk factor phenotype of hypertension difficult. Furthermore, hypertension may be overdiagnosed by sole reliance on office readings ("white coat" hypertension), or it may go undetected in the many borderline cases. Ambulatory 24-hour blood pressure recording is a solution, but the method is time-consuming and other cutoffs for normal levels of blood pressure apply.[128,129] According to current guidelines,[130,131] systemic arterial hypertension is defined as a blood pressure of ≥140 mmHg systolic or ≥90 mmHg diastolic, or both, based on the average of two or more readings taken on at least two occasions after 5 minutes of quiet sitting. Different stages of severity apply (Table 3-11). Systolic blood pressure increases with age until about 80 years, whereas diastolic pressure declines sharply after the age of 55 years in men and 60 years in women (Fig. 3-3).[132] This widening in the pulse pressure (the increase in difference between systolic and diastolic pressure) is a consequence of arterial stiffening of the large conduit arteries with age.

In the National Health and Nutrition Examination Survey (NHANES) III, 43 million Americans (corresponding to 24% of the adjusted adult population of the United States) were identified as hypertensive.[133] Subtypes of hypertension are isolated systolic, isolated diastolic, and combined hypertension. Isolated systolic hypertension is a disease of the elderly and is, overall, the most common form of hypertension; isolated diastolic hypertension occurs predominantly in younger adults.[134] Combined systolic and diastolic hypertension was the most common form in adults 40 to 50 years old in NHANES III (Fig. 3-4).[133]

■ ■ ■

TABLE 3–11   DEFINITION AND CLASSIFICATION OF BLOOD PRESSURE LEVELS ACCORDING TO JOINT NATIONAL COMMITTEE[130] AND WORLD HEALTH ORGANIZATION[131] GUIDELINES

CLASSIFICATION	SYSTOLIC (mmHg)		DIASTOLIC (mmHg)
Optimal	<120	and	<80
Normal	<130	and	<85
High normal	130–139	or	85–89
Mild (hypertension stage 1)	140–159	or	90–99
Subgroup borderline hypertension	140–149	or	90–94
Moderate (hypertension stage 2)	160–179	or	100–109
Severe (hypertension stage 3)	≥180	or	≥110

If systolic and diastolic blood pressures fall into different categories, the highest category applies.

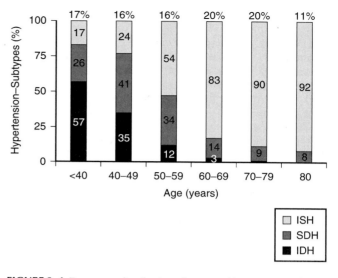

FIGURE 3–4. Frequency distribution of untreated hypertensives by age and hypertension subtype in the NHANES III survey. Numbers at the top of the bars represent the overall percentage of hypertension in that age group. IDH, isolated diastolic hypertension; ISH, isolated systolic hypertension; SDH, combined systolic/diastolic hypertension. (Adapted from Franklin SS, Jacobs MJ, Wong ND, et al: Predominance of isolated systolic hypertension among middle-aged and elderly US hypertensives. Analysis based on National Health and Nutrition Examination Survey [NHANES] III. Hypertension 2001;37:869–874.)

The phenotype *hypertension* is solely defined by blood pressure readings. However, according to etiology, primary hypertension is distinguished from secondary forms of elevated blood pressure. Essential or primary (systemic arterial) hypertension is a multifactorial disease and accounts for 95% of all hypertension cases in the population. However, essential hypertension can only be diagnosed by ruling out secondary forms of hypertension due to endocrine or renovascular disorders and rare monogenetic forms of hypertension. This distinction is important because other therapeutic options besides antihypertensive medication are available for most secondary forms. Up to 10% of patients with secondary hypertension were identified in a hypertension clinic, mostly referrals with unsatisfactory control of

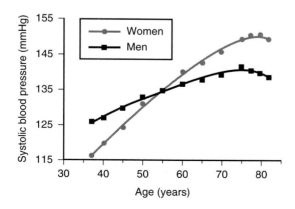

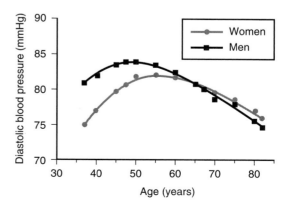

FIGURE 3–3. Cross-sectional age trends in systolic *(left panel)* and diastolic *(right panel)* blood pressure levels according to examinations 3 to 16 from the Framingham Study; actual values were fitted with a polynomial trendline. (Modified from Kannel WB: Historic perspectives on the relative contributions of diastolic and systolic blood pressure elevation to cardiovascular risk profile. Am Heart J 1999;138[Suppl]:205–210.)

their blood pressure: renovascular hypertension (3.1%), primary hypothyroidism (3%), renal insufficiency (1.8%), followed by primary aldosteronism (1.4%), Cushing syndrome (0.5%), and pheochromocytoma (0.3%), were diagnosed among 4429 patients.[135] Variations in at least 10 genes (among them aldosterone synthase, 11β- and 17α-hydroxylase, α-, β-, γ-subunits of the amiloride sensitive sodium channel and the sodium-chloride transporter) have been identified as causing rare mendelian single-gene forms of generally severe hypertension.[136]

The cause of essential (primary) hypertension is multifactorial and traceable to gene-environment interaction. About 30% to 40% of the variation in blood pressure among individuals is estimated to be due to complex (as opposed to monogenetic) genetic factors, most of which are presently unknown.[137] Lifestyle factors (salt intake, overweight, physical inactivity) act as modifiers on common genetic variants (polymorphisms) of candidate genes—with the role of many such genes still to be determined—together with gene–gene interactions in modulating blood pressure.[138,139]

Epidemiologic studies have established a strong and consistent link between elevated blood pressure and CHD risk.[140] In the MRFIT study, a similar relationship in magnitude of CHD risk was observed for diastolic blood pressure and hypercholesterolemia.[93] These findings are supported by the Framingham data, wherein CHD risk increased progressively over the entire range of systolic and diastolic blood pressure and cholesterol levels.[92] The increase in risk started at levels well below those typically regarded as hypertensive.[92,140] The latest reports of the Joint National Committee on Prevention, Detection, Evaluation, and Treatment of High Blood Pressure (JNC VI guidelines) and the World Health Organization and International Society of Hypertension (WHO-ISH guidelines) acknowledged those findings and lowered the threshold for an optimal blood pressure to less than 120 mmHg systolic and less than 85 mmHg diastolic for all age groups.[130,131] The strength and consistency of the association of hypertension as a dichotomous or blood pressure as a quantitative risk factor for new CHD suggests a direct causal relationship. Furthermore, hypertension is statistically independent from confounding factors like age, cholesterol, and smoking[140] and there is a direct relationship between the average reduction in blood pressure and a concomitant decrease in cardiovascular events, regardless of the approach to reducing blood pressure.[141,142]

Diastolic blood pressure offers no advantage over systolic pressure in predicting hypertension-associated cardiovascular risk (Fig. 3–5).[134] The risk of cardiovascular disease associated with hypertension is highest in combined hypertension, intermediate for the isolated systolic subtype, and lowest for isolated diastolic hypertension (Table 3–12). Based on 10-year data from the Framingham study, four categories of absolute risk have been defined (Table 3–13) and the impact of lowering blood pressure on CHD prevention has been estimated (Table 3–14).[131]

Because of the Gaussian distribution of blood pressure in the population (which is similar to that of cholesterol)—although there is a positive relationship between increasing values and increased risk (see Fig. 3–5, upper panels)—most of the risk, from a population perspective, occurs with mildly elevated values (see Fig. 3–5, lower panels).

However, in most patients with CHD, increased blood pressure is one factor among a cluster of other risk factors (i.e., smoking, diabetes, cholesterol) and lowering of high blood pressure will thus not remove entirely CHD risk in hypertensive patients. Thus, although it can be shown statistically that the risk generally increases with each of these risk factors, statistics cannot provide any causal proof. The link between hypertension and CHD is complex and not understood at the moment.[143,144] Data from the Boston Area Health Study showed that the apparent risk of hypertension was substantially attenuated by the addition of HDL cholesterol or triglycerides in the multivariate model.[145] It remains unknown whether hypertension and dyslipidemia affect MI and CHD risk independently, additively, or synergistically. The Framingham data demonstrated (1) that CHD risk in hypertensives concentrated in diabetic smokers with a high LDL/HDL cholesterol ratio and electrocardiographic signs of left-ventricular hypertrophy and (2) that risk factors clustered with increased body mass index (BMI).[134]

Diabetes Mellitus

Global statistics indicate that worldwide rates of diabetes mellitus will increase dramatically. In 1990, the prevalence for diabetes was calculated to be 118 million people worldwide.[146] According to WHO, rates are projected to increase to 300 million diabetics in 2025, with the largest increases occurring in China and India.[147] The most prevalent form of diabetes mellitus is type 2 diabetes—a polygenic disease, induced or aggravated by environmental factors—which constitutes more than 90% of all diabetics.[148,149] Although its precise cause is at present unknown, two underlying metabolic derangements are the hallmark of type 2 diabetes: impairment of insulin-mediated glucose disposal in peripheral tissues (insulin resistance) and defective insulin secretion of pancreatic beta cells.[150]

New Diagnostic Criteria for Diabetes

The previous WHO criteria published in 1985 defined diabetes based on a fasting plasma glucose of 140 mg/dL or greater or a 2-hour post-oGTT plasma glucose of 200 mg/dL or greater,[151,152] the provisional new WHO criteria[153,154] are identical to the American Diabetes Association criteria,[155] which lowered the threshold for diabetes to 126 mg/dL or greater for fasting (venous) plasma glucose. The threshold for the 2-hour value after oGTT for diabetes remained unchanged (≥200 mg/dL). Cutoffs are lower with venous whole blood or capillary blood.[153] The clinical diagnosis of diabetes mellitus may rest entirely on elevation of fasting plasma glucose to 126 mg/dL or greater (≥7.0 mmol/L) if the elevation is confirmed on a subsequent day. However, interchangeable diagnostic criteria for diabetes are a plasma glucose of 200 mg/dL or greater (≥11.1 mmol/L) 2 hours after

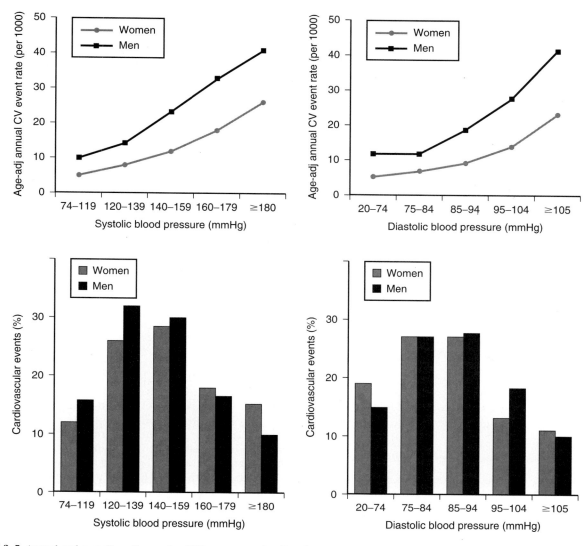

FIGURE 3–5. Annual and overall cardiovascular (CV) event rates by diastolic *(right panels)* and systolic *(left panels)* blood pressure in persons aged 35 to 64 years who were free of cardiovascular disease at baseline—38-year follow-up of the Framingham Heart Study. (From Kannel WB: Elevated systolic blood pressure as a cardiovascular risk factor. Am J Cardiol 2000;85:251–255.)

TABLE 3–12 RISK OF CARDIOVASCULAR EVENT BY HYPERTENSION SUBTYPE, SEX, AND AGE IN THE 36-YEAR FOLLOW-UP OF THE FRAMINGHAM STUDY

	AGE-ADJUSTED RISK RATIO*			
	35–64 yr		65–94 yr	
HYPERTENSION SUBTYPE	*Men*	*Women*	*Men*	*Women*
Isolated diastolic	1.8[†]	1.2	1.2[†]	1.6[§]
Isolated systolic	2.4[§]	1.9[‡]	1.9[‡]	1.4[‡]
Combined	2.7[§]	2.2[§]	2.2[§]	1.6[§]

*Reference group = normotensive individuals.
[†]*P* = .05.
[‡]*P* = .01.
[§]*P* = .001.
Adapted from Kannel WB: Elevated systolic blood pressure as a cardiovascular risk factor. Am J Cardiol 2000;85:251–255.

ingestion of 75 g glucose by oral glucose tolerance test or a casual plasma glucose of 200 mg/dL or greater (*casual* means a sample taken any time of the day) in the presence of symptoms of diabetes—polyuria, polydipsia, and unexplained weight loss—according to the revised American Diabetes Association and WHO criteria. The threshold for diabetes has been lowered from 140 mg/dL or greater in the previous WHO guidelines[151,152] to a fasting glucose of 126 mg/dL or greater in the new diabetes criteria in order to achieve a similar predictive value for diabetic complications from both fasting glucose (≥126 mg/dL) and the 2-hour post glucose load level (≥200 mg/dL).[153-155]

Simultaneous measurement of fasting and 2-hour post glucose challenge glucose will inevitably lead to diagnostic discrepancies. Therefore, the definition for diabetes allows one of the two parameters to be in the nondiabetic range. For epidemiologic purposes, estimates of diabetes prevalence and incidence may be

■ ▪ ■

TABLE 3–13   CARDIOVASCULAR RISK STRATIFICATION ACCORDING TO SEVERITY OF HYPERTENSION

	CARDIOVASCULAR RISK CATEGORY*		
	Mild Hypert. (Grade 1) 140–159/90–94†	Moderate Hypert. (Grade 2) 160–179/100–109†	Severe Hypert. (Grade 3) ≥180/≥110†
I Men < 55 yr, women < 65 yr and no other risk factor	Low	Medium	High
II 1-2 Risk factors	Medium	Medium	Very high
III ≥3 Risk factors or target-organ damage or diabetes‡	High	High	Very high
IV Cerebrovascular, cardiac, renal, or other vascular disease‡	Very high	Very high	Very high

*Ten-year cardiovascular risk estimates for cardiovascular death, nonfatal stroke, or myocardial infarction (major cardiovascular events) from Framingham data.
Low: Risk for major cardiovascular event < 15%
Medium: Risk for major cardiovascular event 15–20%
High: Risk for major cardiovascular event 20–30%
Very high: Risk for major cardiovascular event > 30%
†Systolic blood pressure/Diastolic blood pressure (mmHg).
‡See original publication for further details.
Adapted from Guidelines subcommittee: 1999 World Health Organization—International Society of Hypertension guidelines for the management of hypertension. J Hypertens 1999;17:151–183.

based on one single measurement and on the fasting glucose criteria alone. However, this approach leads to slightly lower estimates of prevalence than would be obtained from the combined use of both criteria.[167,169] The intermediate stage, not meeting the glucose criteria for normal or diabetic, is defined as impaired glucose tolerance or impaired fasting glucose if no oral glucose tolerance test has been performed (Table 3–15).[151-155]

Etiologic Classification of Diabetes Mellitus

Type 1 diabetes mellitus, previously known as *insulin-dependent diabetes*, is the second most prevalent subtype of diabetes (~5% to 10% of all diabetics) as opposed to the common type 2 diabetes, formerly called *non–insulin-dependent diabetes* or *adult-onset diabetes* (~90% prevalence of all diabetics). Type 1 diabetes typically begins early in life ("juvenile diabetes") following immunologic destruction of pancreatic beta cells. Type 1 diabetes is diagnosed if the initial manifestation of the disease included hyperglycemia and ketonuria and if insulin treatment was necessary less than 1 year after the diagnosis of hyperglycemia. Typically, islet cell-spe-

cific or glutamic acid decarboxylase autoantibodies, or both, are present, the latter in 85% to 90% of persons with type 1 diabetes.[153] However, a slowly progressive form of type 1 diabetes occurs in adults, called *latent autoimmune diabetes*, which is diagnosed with an onset of diabetes at 30 years, evolution to insulin deficiency after a period of insulin-independence, and the presence of autoantibodies to glutamic acid decarboxylase. It is important to note that the prevalence of latent autoimmune diabetes among type 2 diabetics not tested for glutamic acid decarboxylase antibodies may be up to 10% after such testing.[156] The prevalence of latent autoimmune diabetes misdiagnosed as type 2 diabetes decreases with age and weight, being more toward 15% to 20% in young (<45 years) or lean diabetics and approximately 5% in subjects who are 60 years and older or obese.[156]

Other subtypes of diabetes are rare (~1% to 5% of all persons with diabetes mellitus). However, similar to the secondary forms of hypertension, specific underlying defects or triggering conditions are known (i.e., gestational diabetes, diabetes secondary to diseases of the pancreas, endocrinopathies, infections). Rare genetic

■ ▪ ■

TABLE 3–14   CVD RISK AND TREATMENT EFFECT BY SEVERITY OF HYPERTENSION

PATIENT GROUP ACCORDING TO BASELINE RISK (SEE TABLE 3–13)	ABSOLUTE RISK (CVD EVENTS OVER 10 YEARS IN PERCENT)	ABSOLUTE TREATMENT EFFECT (NUMBER OF CVD EVENTS PREVENTED PER 1000 PATIENT-YEARS)	
		10/5 mmHg*	20/10 mmHg*
Low	<15%	<5	<9
Medium	15–20%	5–7	8–11
High	20–30%	7–10	11–17
Very high	>30%	>10	>17

*Average reduction of systolic/diastolic blood pressure.
Adapted from Guidelines subcommittee: 1999 World Health Organization—International Society of Hypertension guidelines for the management of hypertension. J Hypertens 1999;17:151–183.

■ ■ ■

TABLE 3–15 COMPARISON OF PREVIOUS WHO AND NEW WHO/ADA CRITERIA FOR THE CLASSIFICATION OF DIABETES MELLITUS AND IMPAIRED GLUCOSE TOLERANCE

GLUCOSE STATUS (REFERENCE)	PLASMA GLUCOSE mg/dL (mmol/L)		
	Fasting (0 hour)	1 Hour Post oGTT (only WHO 1980)	2 Hours Post oGTT
Normal (0 and 2 hr)			
ADA/WHO 1999[153-155]	<110 (<6.1)		<140 (<7.8)
WHO 1980/85[151,152]	<140 (<7.8)	<140 (<7.8)	<140 (<7.8)
Impaired fasting (0 hr) (new definition only)*	110-125 (6.1-6.9)	—	—
Impaired oGTT (0 and 2 hr)			
ADA/WHO 1999[153-155]	**<126 (<7.0)**		**140–199 (7.8–11.0)**
WHO 1980/85[151,152]	<140 (<7.8)	140-199 (7.8-11.0)	140-199 (7.8-11.0)
Diabetes (0 or 2 hr)			
ADA/WHO 1999[153-155]	**≥126 (>7.0)**		≥200 (≥11.1)
WHO 1980/85[151,152]	≥140 (7.8)	≥200 (≥11.1)	≥200 (≥11.1)

Conversion factor mg/dL in mmol/L: mg/dL * 0.05551 = mmol/L.
ADA, American Diabetes Association; oGTT, oral glucose tolerance test with a 75 g glucose load; WHO, World Health Organization.
*In cases of impaired fasting glucose, which by definition is based solely on fasting glucose, patients may eventually be diagnosed as having impaired glucose tolerance or diabetes if an oGTT were to be performed.

defects in insulin action and beta-cell function have been identified. The best known defect, *maturity-onset diabetes of the young*—characterized by families with autosomal dominant transmission of diabetes and at least one case of diabetes diagnosed before the age of 25—is caused by impaired insulin secretion due to genetic defects in the hepatic nuclear transcription factor genes (HNF1-4), in the glucokinase gene, or in the IPF-1 transcription factor.[153]

Thus, similar to the case of essential hypertension, the most common form of diabetes—type 2 diabetes—is a diagnosis made by ruling out type 1 diabetes and other rare subtypes of diabetes.

Undiagnosed Diabetes Mellitus

It has been estimated that the onset of diabetes occurs at least 5 to 7 years before its clinical diagnosis.[157] Thus, without rigorous blood glucose screening in the population, many cases of diabetes—estimates are up to 30% to 50% of all diabetics in a given population—remain undetected.[158-161] Thus, the United States has an estimated 15 million people with diabetes, one third of whom (5 million) remain undiagnosed.[162]

Diabetes and Cardiac Risk

Atherosclerosis or a history of clinical cardiovascular disease is common in persons suffering from diabetes mellitus. Cardiovascular disease accounts for about 75% to 80% of the total mortality in type 2 diabetes, and three fourths of these deaths are due to CHD.[162,163] Only 12% of all known diabetics of adults in the Cardiovascular Health study aged 65 years were free of clinical or subclinical cardiovascular disease as opposed to 25% of men and 33% of women with a normal glucose tolerance status.[164] Thus, it is not surprising that diabetics carry about a 1.5- to 4-fold higher risk of CHD death compared with nondiabetics and that their life expectancy is decreased

by 5 to 10 years.[165,166] The 30-day mortality rate after coronary artery bypass grafting in 1034 patients with diabetes was double the rate of 3350 nondiabetics, 5% and 2.5%, respectively.[167] The twofold increase in mortality for diabetes after coronary artery bypass grafting persisted over a 2-year observation period in a Swedish study.[168] Diabetes mellitus was the strongest predictor for future CHD events among the traditional risk factors in the West of Scotland Coronary Prevention Study of 6595 middle-aged men without prior MI.[169] Overall, the age-adjusted mortality in diabetic adults is approximately twice that of people without diabetes in population-based studies and in survivors of MI, and there is a 1.5- to 2-fold increase in the incidence of ACSs in the setting of ischemic heart disease.[170,171] The relative risk of cardiovascular and all-cause mortality during 12-year follow-up in the MRFIT trial for a self-reported history of diabetes in 347,000 men was 3.0 and 2.5, respectively.[172] In the Honolulu Heart study, the 12-year CHD risk progressively increased with increases in fasting glucose levels at baseline in men initially free from diabetes, treated hypertension, and CHD, indicating that even mild abnormalities in glucose tolerance are important.[173]

More important, though, diabetic subjects without previous MI have as high a risk of future MI as nondiabetic patients with prior MI have for recurrent MI (Fig. 3–6).[174] However, the incidence of atherosclerosis and CHD in diabetes seems to depend on the overall prevalence of CHD in the population and at least partly on the clustering of other cardiovascular risk factors in such populations.[175] Thus, mortality from diabetic nephropathy is increased in populations with a low CHD prevalence, such as the Pima Indians, Japanese, and Chinese.[176] Although the level of chronic hyperglycemia is the best established concomitant factor associated with diabetic complications, the mechanisms by which hyperglycemia causes complications remain unknown, and evidence for a uniform pathogenetic mechanism is far from established.[177]

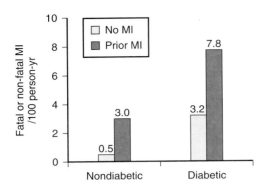

FIGURE 3–6. Risk of future fatal or nonfatal myocardial infarction (MI) in a Finnish population-based study during a 7-year observation period. (From Haffner SM, Lehto S, Rönnemaa T, et al: Mortality from coronary heart disease in subjects with type 2 diabetes and in nondiabetic subjects with and without prior myocardial infarction. N Engl J Med 1998;339:229–234.)

Genetic Predisposition

Type 2 diabetes is a multifactorial disease wherein the interplay of genetic predisposition with environmental stimuli leads to disease. The genetics of type 2 diabetes have been disappointing in the past. More than 250 candidate genes have been tested for association with or linkage to type 2 diabetes, but none has shown consistent results in different population studies.[178] Lately, the Calpain-10 gene has been implicated by the demonstration of an association with the risk for type 2 diabetes for certain haplotypes, that is, specific combinations of polymorphisms residing on the same allele, in Mexican Americans and Northern Europeans.[179] However, none of the candidate genes identified to date appears to act as a major susceptibility locus.[180,181] According to current thinking, type 2 diabetes is genetically and environmentally heterogeneous, that is, different individuals will have different combinations of subtle genetic defects of insulin secretion, insulin action, energy expenditure, or body fat metabolism that interact with different lifestyle factors (i.e., overeating, reduced physical activity, nutri-

tional toxins, glucose toxicity) that finally result in the disease.[182,183]

METABOLIC SYNDROME

Diagnostic Criteria for Metabolic Syndrome

Insulin resistance, which often develops from obesity, physical inactivity, and genetic predisposition, typically precedes the onset of type 2 diabetes. Insulin resistance is a condition describing impaired insulin action, that is, insulin produces a less-than-normal response or decreased insulin sensitivity. Pathophysiologically, insulin resistance must be distinguished from hepatic resistance (decreased hepatic extraction of insulin) and peripheral resistance (insufficient utilization of insulin). In other words, insulin resistance may be defined as a condition under which insulin causes a reduced blood glucose–lowering effect, the presence of which is estimated by measuring insulin sensitivity by various approaches including the gold-standard hyperinsulinemic euglycemic clamp, frequent intravenous sampling, or the oral glucose tolerance test. Circulating levels of insulin are widely used as a surrogate for insulin sensitivity, whereby hyperinsulinemia may be taken as an indicator of insulin resistance.[150,184-186]

Commonly, insulin resistance/hyperinsulinemia is accompanied by a cluster of risk factors, including obesity, hypertension, dyslipidemia characterized by low HDL cholesterol and high triglycerides, and a prothrombotic shift in the coagulation profile such as elevated PAI-1 and hyperfibrinogenemia.[187] Persons with such a cluster of risk factors have been described as having *metabolic syndrome*. This condition generally precedes type 2 diabetes by many years and is associated with increased risk of cardiovascular disease. Many definitions of metabolic syndrome have been used in the past,[120,188] but lately WHO has proposed diagnostic criteria (Table 3–16),[153,154] as has the National Cholesterol Education Program (Table 3–17).[189] Increased levels of uric acid (>480 μmol/L or >8.1 mg/dL) and fibrinogen (>3 g/L)

■ ■ ■

TABLE 3–16   WHO CRITERIA FOR THE DEFINITION OF METABOLIC SYNDROME

Impaired Fasting Glucose, Impaired Glucose Tolerance, or Diabetes and/or Insulin Resistance

and two or more further components among the items listed below

Impaired glucose regulation	Impaired fasting glucose or impaired glucose tolerance (as defined in Table 3–15)
Insulin resistance	Under hyperinsulinemic euglycemic conditions, defined as glucose uptake below the lowest quartile for the background population under investigation or estimated by the highest quartile of the $HOMA_{IR}$ index*
Hypertension	Antihypertensive treatment and/or elevated blood pressure (≥140 mmHg systolic and/or ≥90 mmHg diastolic)
Dyslipidemia	Triglycerides ≥ 150 mg/dL (≥1.7 mmol/L) and/or HDL < 35 mg/dL (<0.9 mmol/L) ♂ (♀: <39 mg/dL [<1.0 mmol/L])
Central obesity	Waist-to-hip ratio > 0.9 ♂, > 0.85 ♀ or BMI > 30 kg/m²
Microalbuminuria	≥20 μg/min urinary albumin excretion rate or albumin/creatinine ratio ≥ 20 mg/g

BMI, body mass index; HDL, high-density lipoprotein.
*Homeostasis model assessment (HOMA) may be applied to the fasting glucose and fasting insulin values as proxy measures of insulin resistance ($HOMA_{IR}$) and ß-cell function (HOMA ß-cell).[186] $HOMA_{IR}$ = fasting insulin (mU/l) × fasting glucose (mmol/L)/22.5; HOMA ß-cell = 20 × fasting insulin (mU/L)/(fasting glucose (mmol/L) – 3.5); although not suggested in the WHO report, plasma insulin > 15 mU/L may be used as a surrogate to indicate insulin resistance as well.
For more information, see references 153 and 154.

■ ■ ■

TABLE 3–17   NATIONAL CHOLESTEROL EDUCATION PROGRAM CRITERIA FOR METABOLIC SYNDROME[189]

ANY THREE OF THE FOLLOWING CHARACTERISTICS AFTER 3 MONTHS OF THERAPEUTIC LIFESTYLE CHANGES

Risk Factor	Defining Level
Fasting glucose	≥110 mg/dL
Abdominal obesity*	*Waist circumference*†
	Men: >102 cm
	Women: >88 cm
Triglycerides	≥150 mg/dL
HDL cholesterol	Men: <40 mg/dL
	Women: <50 mg/dL
Blood pressure	≥130/≥85 mmHg

HDL, high-density lipoprotein.

*Overweight and obesity are associated with insulin resistance and the metabolic syndrome. However, the presence of abdominal obesity is more highly correlated with the metabolic risk factors than is an elevated body mass index. Therefore, the simple measure of waist circumference is recommended to identify the body weight component of the metabolic syndrome.

†Some male patients can have multiple metabolic risk factors when the waist circumference is only marginally increased, e.g., 94–102 cm (37–39 in.). Such patients may have a strong genetic contribution to insulin resistance. They should benefit from changes in life habits, similarly to men with categorical increases in waist circumference.

and an increase of more than one standard deviation above normal values of plasma insulin, free testosterone, dihydroepiandrosterone, or von Willebrand factor have been proposed as additional components of the metabolic syndrome.[190] Clustering of these components is thought to be caused by environmental influences (i.e., being overweight, physical inactivity) modulated by genetic factors.[191,192] Whether there is a truly causal relationship or merely an association between insulin resistance and hypertension is a matter of debate.[193-195]

Clustering of Risk Factors and Cardiac Risk

Although 10 to 15 million Americans have diabetes mellitus, another over 45 million have asymptomatic hyperglycemia or a clustering of risk factors associated with insulin resistance and metabolic syndrome.[196] In 2906 Danish men, metabolic syndrome and the associated dyslipidemia (high triglycerides/low HDL cholesterol) were more predictive for CHD risk than blood pressure.[197] Metabolic syndrome is also the presumed cause of the excess risk for MI in South Asians (Indians, Pakistani, Bangladeshis) living abroad[198] and (in addition to high cholesterol) contributes to the progression of atherosclerosis after coronary artery bypass surgery.[199,200] Small dense LDL particles, which are a hallmark of metabolic syndrome and which are more atherogenic than larger LDLs, may be the most important determinant for the increased CHD risk associated with metabolic syndrome.[201] However, overall, the excess risk in metabolic syndrome can be explained by the individual effects of the defining risk factors in a multiple logistic model.[202,203] Factor analysis using the principal-components approach identified a central metabolic syndrome characterized by hyperinsulinemia, dyslipidemia,

and obesity and two other physiologic domains, impaired glucose tolerance and hypertension, which were linked together through mutual associations with hyperinsulinemia and obesity.[204]

The prevalence of overweight and obesity, which are major modifiable predisposing factors for metabolic syndrome and, subsequently, type 2 diabetes, has increased dramatically in westernized societies with the excess intake of nutritional calories. In the United States, rates have increased in recent decades from 43% to more than 55%.[205] In absolute terms, more than 97 million American adults are obese.[206] Overweight and obesity are on a continuum scale; overweight may be defined as excess fat of about 10% of total body weight and obesity as 25% fat mass of total body weight (men) and 30% (women).[207] Several techniques are available for determining body fat, ranging from simple anthropometric measures to underwater weighing, bioelectric impedance analysis, dual x-ray absorptiometry, or nuclear magnetic resonance imaging.[208] The most common surrogate measure for body fat used in clinical practice and epidemiologic studies is the BMI (or the Quetelet index). It is calculated by dividing a person's weight in kilograms by his or her height in meters squared. The *distribution* of body fat in terms of *central obesity*—accumulation of fat in the trunk and abdominal cavity (android obesity)—is specifically associated with the metabolic syndrome. The waist circumference and ratio of waist-to-hip circumference are indices of central obesity.[209] The BMI can be simply calculated from height and weight and is a well-established marker for the clustering of other risk factors and for increased CHD risk (Table 3–18).[209,210]

Whether weight alone is an independent risk factor is a matter of debate.[211] U-shaped mortality curves for cardiovascular disease (CVD), cancer, and all-causes, have been reported for men and women free of disease at baseline according to BMI.[212] Increased mortality associated with low weight or underweight has been explained by the presence of confounders, such as an acute or chronic disease, and smoking. A recent significant weight loss is associated with increased mortality. After controlling for such influences, the relationship between a low BMI and increased mortality tends to vanish.

According to Willett et al, obesity by itself, even after adjustment for obesity-related conditions, increases the risk for CHD.[211] Overweight and obesity, however, are rarely isolated, and the associated conditions are more of interest. Typically, the risk factors in the metabolic syndrome that are associated with overweight and obesity are impaired glucose tolerance/diabetes, hypertension, and low-HDL/high-triglyceride dyslipidemia. Among women who never smoked in the Nurses Health Study, there was an increase in risk of CHD and cancer mortality with increasing BMI that persisted after adjustment for hypertension, diabetes mellitus, and dyslipidemia.[213] The risk became J-shaped if smokers were included, with increased mortality at a low BMI. The 10-year CHD risk associated with the clustering of risk factors of metabolic syndrome can be estimated from Framingham risk scores (Fig. 3–7).[214]

■ ■ ■

TABLE 3–18   RISK OF CORONARY HEART DISEASE AND PREVALENCE OF RISK FACTORS IN 6987 MEN FROM THE NHANES III STUDY ACCORDING TO BODY MASS INDEX (BMI)

BMI (kg/m²)	CLASSIFICATION*	CHD RISK (%)	TYPE 2 DIABETES (%)	HIGH TOTAL CHOLESTEROL† (%)	HIGH BP‡ (%)
18.5–24.9	"Normal" weight	8.8	2.0	27	23
25.0–29.9	Overweight	9.6	4.9	36	34
30.0–34.9	Obese, grade 1	16.0	10.1	39	49
35.0–39.9	Obese, grade 2	10.2	12.3	34	65
≥40	Morbidly obese	14.0	10.7	37	65

A BMI < 18.5 kg/m² is classified as underweight or thin.
*Based on WHO guidelines on anthropometry.[209]
†Defined as total cholesterol > 240 mg/dL (treated with lipid-lowering medication).
‡BP, blood pressure; high BP is defined as BP > 140 mmHg systolic and/or > 90 mmHg diastolic or treated with antihypertensive medication.
Adapted from Must A, Spadano J, Coakley EH, et al: The disease burden associated with overweight and obesity. JAMA 1999;282:1523–1529.

Although hyperinsulinemia is a characteristic of the metabolic syndrome, the clinical impact of the relation between hyperinsulinemia and atherosclerosis remains to be defined. In a meta-analysis of epidemiologic studies, hyperinsulinemia remained a weak independent risk factor for cardiovascular disease.[215] Such a result is not surprising because most, if not all, risk associated with hyperinsulinemia in nondiabetics can be explained by the clustering with other cardiovascular risk factors, as shown in the 10-year follow-up of the Kupio Ischemic Heart Disease Risk Factor study.[216] Hyperinsulinemia was associated with a modest increase in cardiovascular mortality in middle-aged men, which was largely explained by obesity, hypertension, and dyslipidemia. The incidence of ACSs and stroke was not different among insulin quartiles.[216]

AGE AND SEX

Age and sex are so-called nonmodifiable risk factors for CHD (Fig. 3–8).[217] Life expectancy increased enormously in the last century; it is projected to increase even more so up to an average of 90 years in Japan by 2050.[218] However, the major impact of increasing age on CHD morbidity and mortality will persist, although it may shift toward older age in the future.

Although CHD morbidity and mortality is lower in premenopausal women than in men, rates are higher in elderly women than in men. Furthermore, contrasting with the decline in cardiovascular disease mortality observed in men during the recent decades in the United States, the rate in women continues to increase (Fig. 3–9).[219] A possible explanation is a change toward an

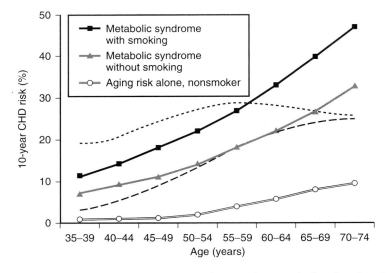

FIGURE 3–7. Ten year congestive heart disease (CHD) risk of metabolic syndrome and aging risk alone based on the Framingham risk scores published in 1998.[214] The *dashed lines* are fitted polynomial trendlines of the most recent version of the Framingham risk score, which adjusts CHD risk for the change in prevalence of hypercholesterolemia and smoking with age. The *upper dashed trendline* shows the risk estimate for a smoker with metabolic syndrome, the *lower dashed curve* for a nonsmoker. *Note:* Framingham point scores were calculated for metabolic syndrome with and without smoking using low-density lipoprotein cholesterol of 100 to 159 mg/dL; high-density lipoprotein < 35 mg/dL; blood pressure of 140 to 159 mmHg systolic and/or 90 to 99 mmHg diastolic; no diabetes[214] or total cholesterol 200 to 239 mg/dL; high-density lipoprotein cholesterol < 40 mg/dL; systolic blood pressure of 160 mmHg untreated, 130 to 159 mmHg treated; and aging risk alone for the Framingham risk scores published in the NCEP adult treatment panel III report. (From Expert Panel on Detection, Evaluation, and Treatment of High Blood Cholesterol in Adults: Executive summary of the third report of the national cholesterol education program [NCEP] Expert Panel on Detection, Evaluation, and Treatment of High Blood Cholesterol in Adults [adult treatment panel III]. JAMA 2001;285:2486–2497.)

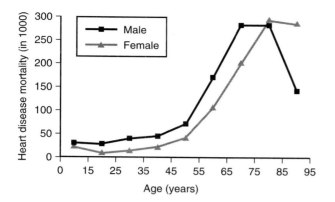

FIGURE 3–8. Mortality from diseases of the heart in United States residents according to the 1986 U.S. National Center of Health Statistics.[217] *Note:* Diseases of the heart is a cumulative grouping recommended by the World Health Organization for tabulating mortality data. It excludes categories such as cerebrovascular disease (stroke), atherosclerosis, or hypertension with or without renal disease, and thus this grouping only represents about three fourths of total cardiovascular mortality.

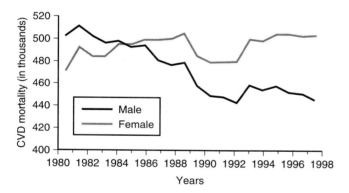

FIGURE 3–9. Cardiovascular disease (CVD) mortality trends for males and females in the United States, 1979 to 1998. (Data for the year 2000 from American Heart Association: 2001 Heart and Stroke Statistical Update. Dallas, American Heart Association, 2000.)

unhealthier lifestyle in women, with increasing rates of smoking whereas it fell in men, which will translate into an increase in CHD morbidity and mortality after a lag time of at least two to three decades.

Although the prevalence of the risk factors of hypertension and diabetes increases and that of smoking decreases with age, both in healthy populations and in CHD cohorts, this is not the case for cholesterol.[87,220,221] The average cholesterol is highest in young persons with CHD and decreases with age (Fig. 3–10),[221] whereas the opposite occurs in healthy persons, in whom cholesterol increases with age to levels matching those of persons with CHD at age 60.[220] This diverging pattern of cholesterol is a common finding in CHD cohorts.[221-223] This pattern is probably the consequence of a strong genetic risk of elevated cholesterol in young persons with the risk of premature death. This age pattern is similar for smoking, wherein the risk of MI decreases with age.[224]

The difference in CHD risk between men and women is largely caused by differences in major risk factors or age. Thus, differences in traditional cardiovascular risk factors explained a substantial part of the sex difference in CHD risk in a prospective study of 14,786 middle-aged Finnish men and women.[239] There was no difference between men and women in the rates of fatal and nonfatal MI in ACS after adjustment for differences in age.[240]

NEW RISK MARKERS

According to current concepts of the pathogenesis of the ACSs, new so-called "risk factors" are emerging. Whereas the term *risk factor* implies definite evidence for a causative involvement of this factor in disease, *risk marker* merely indicates an association with the disease. However, the evidence for all of the newer risk factors (or, more correctly, risk markers) is far from conclusive[227-229] and has yet to reach the level of evidence of the traditional risk factors that fulfill the Bradford Hill criteria[59] as shown in Table 3-6.

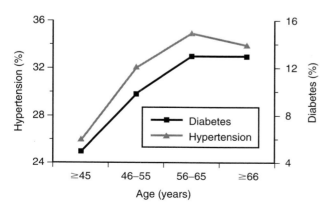

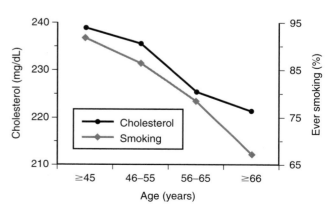

Coronary Artery Surgery Study (CASS) n = 12742 men

FIGURE 3–10. Distribution of traditional risk factors for congestive heart disease in 12,742 men participating in the Coronary Artery Surgery Study. (Data from Vlietstra RE, Kronmal RA, Frye RL, et al: Factors affecting the extent and severity of coronary artery disease in patients enrolled in the Coronary Artery Surgery Study. Arteriosclerosis 1982;2:208–215.)

TABLE 3–19 TRIGGERS OF PLAQUE RUPTURE AND NOVEL RISK FACTORS FOR ACUTE CORONARY SYNDROMES

Inflammation

Endothelium—Monocytes—Extracellular Matrix—Atherosclerotic Plaque

ACE activity in vascular tissue[234]
Asymmetrical dimethylarginine (ADMA)[235]
C-reactive protein (CRP)[236-241]
Serum amyloid A (SAA)[236]
Neopterin[242]
Secretory nonpancreatic type II phospholipase A$_2$[243]
Interleukin-1 receptor antagonist[244]
Interleukin-1β[245]
Interleukin-6[244,246-248]
Interleukin-8[249,250]
Decrease in interleukin-10[251]
Interleukin-18[252]
RANTES[250]
Macrophage inflammatory peptide 1α (MIP-1α)[250]
ENA-78[250]
GRO-α[250]
Intercellular adhesion molecule (ICAM)[241,253,254]
Vascular cell adhesion molecule (VCAM)[241]
Monocyte chemoattractant protein 1 (MCP-1)[250]
E-selectin[241]
L-selectin[253]
Leucocyte count[255]
Heat shock proteins[256]
Matrix proteins (collagen, proteoglycans, elastin)
Tenascin c
Plaque temperature[257]
Plaque instability due to multiple complex plaques[258,259]
Matrix metalloprotease 9 (MMP-9)[260]
Tissue inhibitor of metalloproteinase 1 (TIMP-1)[260]
Interferon-γ responsiveness of monocytes[261]
Tumor necrosis factors α[245]
Tumor growth factor β
Activated T lymphocytes (CD3 and HLA-DR–positive lymphocytes)[262]
Coronary calcification (electron beam computed tomography)[263]
Endothelial coronary artery dysfunction[264]
Shed membrane microparticles of endothelial origin[265]
CD146-positive microparticles[265]
CD31-positive microparticles[265]
Soluble CD14[266]
Monocyte migration[266]
Monocyte membrane fluidity[266]
Monoclonal CD28^{null} T-cell population in the vascular wall[267]
CD40[268]
CD40 ligand[268]
Soluble CD40 ligand[269]
CD64 upregulation on monocytes[267]

Coagulation and Thrombosis

Platelets

P-selectin[270]
Glycoprotein IIb/IIIa receptor
Monocyte-platelet aggregates (=CD 14+ CD61-positive particles)[271]

Coagulation Factor Concentration

von Willebrand factor antigen (vWF)[272-275]
Fibrinogen[237,275-277]
Factor II (prothrombin)[278]
Factor V[278]
Factor VII[275,276,278]
Factor VIII[274,275,279]
Factor X[278]
Factor XII[277]
Plasminogen[277]
Plasminogen activator inhibitor (PAI)[240,273]
Tissue-type plasminogen activator (tPA)[240,273]

Thrombomodulin[273]
Prekallikrein[277]
Kallikrein-like activity[277]
C$_1$-esterase inhibitor[277]

Coagulation Activation Markers

Factor VIIa[280,281]
Factor IX activation peptide[281]
Factor X activation peptide[281]
Factor XIIa[281]
Activated protein C resistance (APCR)
D-dimer[277,282]
Soluble fibrin[282]
Cross-linked fibrin
Fibrin degradation products
Prothrombin fragment 1+2[280,282]
Thrombin-antithrombin complex (TAT)[277,282]
Thrombin-thrombomodulin complex
Thrombin-activatable fibrinolysis inhibitor (TAFI)
Tissue factor[283]
Fibrinopeptide A[281]
Plasmin-α$_2$-antiplasmin complex
tPA/PAI-1 complex

Oxidative Stress

Superoxide anion (O$_2^-$)[250]
8-Isoprostane[250]
Decrease in β-carotene[250]
Decrease in vitamin C[250]
Decrease in vitamin E[250]
Angiotensin II[284]

Metabolism

Homocysteine[240,280,285]
Lipoprotein(a)[240,286]
Lipid pool within the plaque
Malondialdehyde (MDA)-modified LDL cholesterol[287]
Immunglobulin G class antibodies to oxidized low-density lipoprotein[239]
Immunoglobulin G[239]
Ceruloplasmin[239]
Insulin resistance[288]
Polycystic ovary syndrome[289]
Uric acid[290,291]

*Early Markers of Myocardial Necrosis**

Serum Markers

Troponin I and T[17,18,48,292,293]
Myoglobin[294]
Creatine kinase MB mass[294]

Infection

Viral and Bacterial Agents

Chlamydia pneumoniae[295]
Helicobacter[295,296]
Cytomegalovirus[295]
Herpesvirus
Ebstein-Barr virus
Upregulation of protease expression in the vessel wall

Lifestyle

Individual

Decreased physical activity[297]
Depression

Social

Emotional stress
Plasma catecholamines

LDL, low-density lipoprotein.
In some cases, negative study results were cited as well (e.g., *Helicobacter pylori*). In general, the markers listed are elevated in acute coronary syndromes; the associations of decreased levels of markers are indicated. All markers were measured in circulating blood unless indicated (reference values are listed in parentheses).
*Markers of myocardial infarction as the most severe stage of acute coronary syndrome.

A survey on CHD risk factors/markers revealed 246 potential candidates.[230] With respect to the recent growth in the molecular biology of the endothelium, its dysfunction, and the transition to atherosclerosis of the arterial vessel wall, a similar list of candidates exists for ACS.[231-233] Table 3-19 provides an overview of novel risk markers for ACS.[234-297] Some of these risk markers are discussed in further detail in Chapters 9, 30, and 43. However, it should be noted that plaque rupture by itself may be more common than previously thought, with only a certain percentage of lesions progressing to ACS and MI,[258,259,298] and that the nature and extent of the thrombotic response to plaque disruption and progression to ACS remain incompletely understood.[299]

SOCIETY AND ENVIRONMENT

Although cardiovascular disease rates declined in the 1990s, not only in the United States but in all established market economies (United States, Canada, Western Europe, Japan, Australia, and New Zealand), cardiovascular disease remains the leading cause of death in industrialized countries: An estimated 45% of all deaths are attributable to cardiovascular disease, and these rates are on the rise in virtually all other parts of the world.[300-303] Thus, despite the reductions achieved in industrialized countries—about half of the decline in CHD mortality was attributed to medical therapies and approximately half was attributed to reductions in major risk factors[300,302]—the global burden of cardiovascular disease will accelerate with the rate of urbanization and economic change in developing countries, which account for over 80% of the world's population. Atherosclerotic cardiovascular disease, CHD, and stroke are the dominating diseases of all cardiovascular disease. CHD alone accounts for more than half of all cardiovascular disease deaths, and ACS as an acute manifestation of CHD accounts for the major part of morbidity and mortality associated with CHD.

Susceptibility to CHD and its acute manifestation as ACS is influenced by "context-dependent effects," which are interactions among genes and environment (gene–environment interaction) or among genes alone (genetic epistasis). Typical exogenous factors may be protective (alcohol, exercise) or detrimental (cigarettes, high-fat diet, nutritional intake of excess calories). Apart from such rapidly avoidable "individual" environmental risk factors, persons are exposed to global risk factors such as the climate and the society they live in. MI and coronary death increase in cold weather. A 10°C decrease in temperature was associated with a 13% increase in coronary event rates in the Lille-WHO Monitoring Trends and determinants in Cardiovascular Disease (MONICA) survey.[304] Different populations show wide differences in cross-cultural CHD frequency.[305]

There is a North-South gradient in the incidence of CHD and ACS within the European countries[306] and a West-East gradient in Japanese men living in Japan,

Hawaii, and California.[307] Greenlandic Eskimos provide an example of a very low incidence of CHD in a cold climate.[308] It has been shown that with a change of culture and society, the low CHD risk in Japanese or Eskimos increases once they move into Western societies. Obviously, the change in diet and its adverse effect on plasma lipids seems to be the decisive factor for the increase in CHD risk,[307,309] but not the only one, as shown by the "French paradox"—low CHD rates despite a relatively high fat intake in the Mediterranean diet.[310] The societal impact on food consumption and subsequent decline in CHD risk was most obvious in countries afflicted with wartime restrictions in calories and foods containing fat during World War II.[311] Among the classic cardiovascular risk factors, cross-cultural differences in dietary fat and cholesterol intake—not withstanding gaps as shown earlier—explain most of the differences in frequency of CHD.[312] Most, but not all, of such differences in CHD and MI frequency can be explained by a change toward a healthier lifestyle and a reduction in the classic risk factors of dyslipidemia, cigarette smoking, hypertension, diabetes, and physical inactivity. This also holds true for the decline in CHD mortality observed in industrialized countries during the 1990s.[301,313]

Other factors that can affect clinical outcome are regional differences in the use of a variety of therapies for CHD and ACS around the world, both medical and invasive, that have been noted in recent large intervention trials like Global Utilization of Streptokinase and t-PA for Occluded Coronary Arteries (GUSTO) I[314-316] or PURSUIT[44,317] or registries like GRACE.[30]

Within societies, social risk factors that have been implicated with increased CHD risk are marital (single, widowed, or divorced) and socioeconomic class status (low-income housing, lack of education, unskilled worker).[318-320]

GENETICS

Although identical reproduction from generation to generation is an important feature of genes, human evolution would not have been possible without mutations in the gene pool. Allelic variation may occur in the gene regions that code for proteins (exons) or in the noncoding regions (introns). The simplest and most common variation is the exchange of one base pair (point mutation) or single nucleotide polymorphism (SNP). If the prevalence of a rare allele is ≥ 1% in a population, the mutation is called a *polymorphism*. Genetic variation may predispose to disease due to mutations in genes, with a functionally significant effect on the gene product itself (e.g., amino acid–altering mutation in the coding region of a gene) or on the response of a gene to the product of other genes (e.g., transcription factors) through mutations in the promoter or control sequence of a gene.

Table 3-20 provides a brief glossary of important genetic terms listed in alphabetical order. In a three-part series, Ellsworth and Manolio provide an excellent overview of genetic concepts and genetic epidemiology relevant for the study of complex genetic diseases like CHD and ACS.[321-323]

The common multifactorial diseases, including CHD, type 2 diabetes, and hypertension, are genetically complex non-mendelian diseases, that is, they are not heritable in mendelian recessive, dominant, or codominant transmission. Therefore, even in the case of an identical twin with an identical genotype, the disease may not develop in the other twin. According to current thinking, a combination of susceptibility or modifier alleles interact among themselves or with environmental stimuli to enhance or decrease the risk of disease and may modify the penetrance of putative disease-causing gene variants.

The remarkable human diversity at the genetic level is encoded by a variation of less than 0.1% in the human DNA between unrelated individuals. The human genome project has shown that about 1 of every 1000 base pairs shows a mutation in the DNA sequence between individuals. This translates to 3 million SNPs—SNPs being the most abundant mutation in the human genome—for the entire human genome of 3 billion nucleotides (3,000,000 ÷ 3,000,000,000 = 0.1%); in other words, unrelated humans still share 99.9% of identical genetic code.[324] SNPs can affect gene function, or they can be neutral. About 1% of all known SNPs are located in exons and encode a direct amino-acid change of the protein product that the specific gene is coding for. Such nonsynonymous SNPs (change in amino acid) are generally thought to be most relevant because a change in the amino acid sequence of a protein could affect its function. Indeed, many such instances are known. However, because current knowledge about the vast intergenic or introgenic regions of the human genome not directly coding for a protein is limited, it might be premature to conclude that a "non–protein-coding" SNP might be of lesser importance (Table 3-21).[325] Many processes affect gene expression and protein function that have yet to be fully explored, such as DNA methylation, alternative splicing, post-translational modification of proteins, gene duplication, and noncoding RNA.[326]

The estimation of a genetic component comes from family studies by comparing the risk in relatives of a patient with the general risk of disease in the population. Even then, familial aggregation may only indicate a common nongenetic environmental factor within the family. In such a case, genetically unrelated individuals such as spouses living in the same household may help to distinguish between genetic and nongenetic familial effects. Although the genetics of mendelian disease had to be focused on family studies, the genetic epidemiology of complex genetic diseases by using the family-based linkage disequilibrium approach to identify disease-related genes has not been very successful. However, linkage studies are the only way to map (identify) unknown disease susceptibility genes.

Genetic markers that cover the whole human genome are available; in theory, it is possible to localize any genomic region that contains a gene contributing to disease. However, depending on the number of markers used—typical microsatellite-based linkage studies use about 400 markers—the region identified by such a genome scan may still span over 10 million base pairs (10 cM), which need further fine-scale mapping or sequencing efforts. Because the collection of family data needs a lot of resources, the *affected sib-pair approach* (i.e., the study of siblings who both have the disease) has been advocated as a better family-based research strategy. Indeed, several large affected sib-pair studies (>1000 sib-pairs) are under way for the study of MI.[327] However, such studies are hampered by (1) the low relative risk of individual susceptibility gene variants contributing to the overall risk of the multifactorial disease, (2) the genetic heterogeneity of the disease, and (3) the many gene–gene and gene–environment interactions that modify disease penetrance.[328] A limiting factor is the sample size required for such studies in case of a low relative risk of about 1.5, as can be expected for most gene variants associated with CHD. The number of individuals to be studied generally needs to be in the thousands.[329-331] Newer approaches advocate the use of SNP-based genome-wide linkage studies, using thousands of biallelic SNPs as markers (up to 500,000 SNPs and more), which would allow a better resolution.[332] However, such studies have yet to be performed and await maturation of the technology and cost.

Currently, the majority of genetic studies use a case-control design and a candidate gene approach. Typically, DNA collections from cases and controls are compared with respect to the allelic frequencies of certain putative gene variants thought to be pathophysiologically implicated in the disease process itself or in disease susceptibility.[333,334] Although such studies are quite powerful if certain prerequisites are adhered to, especially sample size issues, precise phenotyping, and adequate definition of controls, the outcome after investigating many gene polymorphisms with respect to CHD or MI has been sobering and disappointing. After initial positive association studies, many findings could not be replicated in later, adequately powered studies.[335] Often, inconsistencies between studies are caused by inadequate study design, especially inadequate sample size, heterogeneity of the phenotype and population admixture, or errors in genotyping.[336] Guidelines have been proposed for performing genetic association studies in complex diseases.[335,337]

Nevertheless, the candidate gene approach has the potential to rapidly identify causative, susceptibility, or modifier gene variants in complex disease, especially if the entire pathophysiologic pathway is studied—for example, studying the expression (concentration) of the protein product of such a gene variant—the intermediate phenotype—and its association with disease, and studying the allelic frequency in disease—the distant phenotype—compared with controls.[338,339] Furthermore, environmental interaction needs to be accounted for in studies of genes of the coagulation pathway (in the case of smoking) or genes in the reverse cholesterol transport pathway ("HDL cholesterol") in the case of

■ ■ ■

TABLE 3–20   GLOSSARY OF IMPORTANT GENETIC TERMS*

Allele

Alleles are alternative forms of a *genetic locus* whereby each of the two alleles for one *locus* found in the diploid human individual is inherited separately from the parents. In other words, an allele is one form of a genetic locus that is distinguishable from other forms (alleles) by its particular *nucleotide* or *amino acid* sequence. Although one individual carries only two alleles—inherited from the father and mother—at a given locus, several different alleles may exist in the population if the locus is defined by more than one nucleotide (i.e., *microsatellites, haplotypes*). In contrast, *single nucleotide polymorphisms (SNPs)* are biallelic.

Base pair (bp)

The four *nucleotides* in *DNA* contain the purine bases: adenine (A), thymine (T), or—in the case of RNA—uracil (U), and the pyrimidine bases guanine (G) and cytosine (C). The two strands of the human DNA are held together in the shape of a double helix by weak bonds between adenine and thymine or guanine and cytosine that form base pairs.

Centimorgan (cM)

A unit of measure of recombination frequency. One centimorgan is equal to a 1% chance that a marker at one *genetic locus* will be separated from a marker at a second locus by crossing over (in a single generation). One cM is equivalent, on average, to 1 million *base pairs* in humans.

Chromosomes

Chromosomes are self-replicating genetic structures of cells containing DNA that bears in its linear nucleotide sequence the set of genes (i.e., the *genome*, the *genetic code*). Prokaryotes (i.e., bacteria) carry their genome in one circular chromosome. Eukaryotic genomes consist of a number of chromosomes (i.e., humans, N = 46).

Diploid

The full set of paired *chromosomes* (one chromosome set from each parent). The diploid human *genome* has 46 chromosomes (see also *haploid*).

DNA (deoxyribonucleic acid)

A double-stranded molecule held together by weak bonds between *base pairs* of *nucleotides* that encodes genetic information. The base sequence of each single strand can be deduced from that of its partner because base pairs form only between the bases A and T and between G and C.

DNA sequence

The relative linear order of *base pairs*, whether in a fragment of *DNA*, a *gene*, a *chromosome*, or an entire *genome*. The sequence is written by international definition from the 5'C atom of the sugar residue of a nucleotide to the 3'C atom of the next nucleotide.

Exon

DNA sequence portion of a *gene* that codes for the protein. Human genes consist of several exons that are separated by *introns*.

Gene

A gene is an ordered sequence of *nucleotides* located in a specific chromosomal *locus* (a segment of *DNA*) that contains all the information for the regulated biosynthesis of an RNA product, including *promoters, exons, introns*, and other untranslated regions that control expression and encodes particular products (i.e., RNA molecules, *proteins*). Fundamental physical and functional unit of heredity and evolution.

Gene expression

Entire process that translates the information coded in a *gene* into RNA and *proteins*. Expressed genes are transcribed into *mRNA* and subsequently translated into protein, or they are only transcribed into RNA (e.g., transfer and ribosomal RNAs).

Genetic code

Sequence of *nucleotides* along the *DNA* and coded in triplets (codons) along the *mRNA* that determines the sequence of amino acids in *protein* synthesis. The *DNA sequence* of a *gene* can be used to predict the mRNA sequence and subsequently to predict the amino acid sequence.

Genome

All the genetic material in the *chromosomes* of a particular organism. The size of a genome is generally given as its total number of *base pairs*.

Genotype

An unphased 5' to 3' sequence of *nucleotide* pair(s) found at one or more polymorphic sites in a *locus* on a pair of homologous *chromosomes* in an individual. Unphased means that the origin of the corresponding bases determining the *genotype* cannot be assigned to the father's or mother's chromosome.

Haploid

A single set of *chromosomes*. (In humans, the 23 chromosomes from either father or mother or the single set of chromosomes in their reproductive cells.) (See also *diploid*.)

Haplotype

A phased (belonging to one *chromosome*) 5' to 3' sequence of *nucleotides* found at one or more polymorphic sites on a single chromosome from a single individual. In general, genotyping methods determine the presence of individual *single nucleotide polymorphisms (SNPs)* in a diploid individual but cannot distinguish which chromosome of a *diploid* pair is associated with each SNP. The haplotype of an individual, however, describes specific *alleles* defined by the number of SNP loci associated with each chromosome. A haplotype can be defined on the level of a *gene*, a region of the chromosome, or any long *DNA* fragment. In case of n biallelic SNPs, the number of theoretically possible haplotypes is 2^n. However, because of linkage in humans, only a few of the theoretically possible haplotypes (in the range of 10 to 50) have empirically been identified in human genes (e.g., 18 biallelic SNPs could give rise to theoretically $2^{18} = 262,144$ haplotypes).

Continued

■ ▪ ■

TABLE 3–20   GLOSSARY OF IMPORTANT GENETIC TERMS*—CONT'D

Haplotype pair

The two *haplotypes* found for a locus in *diploid* organisms (e.g., humans). For example, the simplest haplotype is determined by two biallelic *SNPs* (Aa, Bb). Four different haplotypes are theoretically possible on each of the two *chromosomes*: AB, Ab, aB, ab (2^2). However, 10 different haplotype pairs may be found in diploid individuals: (1) AB/AB, (2) AB/Ab, (3) AB/aB, (4) AB/ab, (5) Ab/Ab, (6) Ab/aB, (7) Ab/ab, (8) aB/aB, (9) aB/ab, (10) ab/ab (discounting the origin of a haplotype, whether it originates from the father's or mother's chromosome, i.e., AB/Ab or Ab/AB count as one pair). Only two of the 10 haplotype pairs will represent *heterozygosity* at both loci (AB/ab and Ab/aB).

Heterozygosity

The presence of different *alleles* at one or more *loci* on homologous *chromosomes*.

Intron

DNA base sequence between *exons*, the protein-coding parts of a *DNA sequence* of a *gene*. Intronic sequence are transcribed into *mRNA*, but they are spliced out of the *RNA* molecule before the translation of RNA into *protein* (see also *exon*).

Kilobase (kb)

Kilo = thousand; unit of length for *DNA* fragments containing 1000 *nucleotides*.

Linkage

The closer two or more *markers* (e.g., *polymorphisms*) on a *chromosome* are together, the lower is the probability that they will be separated during *DNA* repair or replication. Therefore, the closer they are linked together, the greater the probability that they will be inherited together. The distance between markers is measured in *centimorgans (cM)*.

Locus

A location on a *chromosome* or *DNA* molecule corresponding to a *gene* or a physical or phenotypic feature.

Marker

An identifiable physical location on a *chromosome* (e.g., restriction enzyme cutting site, *gene*) whose inheritance can be monitored. Markers can be expressed regions of *DNA* (i.e., *genes*) or segments of DNA with no known coding function but whose pattern of inheritance can be determined (i.e., microsatellites).

Megabase (Mb)

Unit of length for *DNA* fragments containing 1 million *nucleotides*; roughly equal to 1 *cM*.

Messenger RNA (mRNA)

RNA that serves as a template for protein synthesis.

Mutation

Any change in *DNA sequence* that occurs by occasional error during *DNA* replication. Inherited mutations are transmitted through the generations via the parent's germ cells. Such common mutations are also called *polymorphisms*. The process of DNA replication is very accurate: Only once every 10^8–10^{12} bases does an error (mutation) occur during replication. Nevertheless, during human evolution, a large number of mutations have accumulated in the human *genome*, about 3 million, or one every 1000 *base pairs*. However, 3 million out of 3 billion bp of the entire human genome make up only a 0.1% difference between two unrelated individuals (i.e., they are still 99.9% identical in DNA sequence). Somatic mutations, in contrast, occurring in cancer are not heritable.

Nucleotide

A subunit of *DNA* or *RNA* consisting of a purine (adenine and guanine) or a pyrimidine base (thymine [*DNA* only], uracil [*RNA* only], and cytosine), a phosphate molecule, and a sugar molecule (deoxyribose in DNA and ribose in RNA).

Polymorphism

A common (i.e., ~ ≥1% prevalence of the minor *allele*) sequence variation observed at a *polymorphic site*. Polymorphisms include *nucleotide* substitutions, insertions, deletions, and microsatellites. They may be functional or silent, i.e., they do not result in detectable differences in *gene expression* or *protein* function.

Polymorphic site

A position within a *locus* at which at least two alternative sequences *(alleles)* are found in a population.

Promoter

A site on *DNA* to which *RNA* polymerase will bind and initiate transcription.

Protein

Molecules composed of one or more chains built from a set of 20 *amino acids* in humans. The order of amino acids is determined by the base sequence of *nucleotides* in the *gene* coding for the *protein*. *Proteins* are required for the structure, function, and regulation of the body's cells, tissues, and organs, and each *protein* has unique functions. Examples are hormones, enzymes, and antibodies. However, several factors may interact during the *transcription* process and result in different *proteins* being generated from the same genetic code (i.e., alternative splicing, epigenetic modification, distant control regions). Therefore, in humans, in general, one gene (with one single genetic code) does code for more than one protein (i.e., three to five proteins, many of which have yet to be linked to the corresponding gene), and the process can be modified by environmental stimuli.

Recombination

The process by which progeny derive a combination of *genes* different from that of either parent. In higher organisms, this is achieved by crossing over of *chromosomes*.

■ ■ ■

TABLE 3–20   GLOSSARY OF IMPORTANT GENETIC TERMS*—CONT'D

Ribonucleic acid (RNA)

Molecules including messenger RNA *(mRNA)*, transfer RNA *(tRNA)*, ribosomal RNA (rRNA), or small RNA. Messenger RNA serves as a template for *protein* synthesis and other biochemical processes of the cell. The structure of mRNA is similar to that of *DNA* except for the base thymidine being replaced by uracil.

Single Nucleotide Polymorphism (SNP)

DNA sequence variation due to a change in a single *nucleotide*. In *diploid* organisms, the specific pair of nucleotides observed at a single *polymorphic site*. In rare cases, three or four nucleotides may be found at the population level.

Transcription

The synthesis of an *RNA* copy from a sequence of *DNA* (i.e., a *gene*); the first step in *gene expression* (see also *translation*).

Transfer RNA (tRNA)

RNA with a triplet *nucleotide* sequence that is complementary to the triplet nucleotide coding sequences of *mRNA*. The role of tRNAs in *protein* synthesis is to bond with amino acids and transfer them to the ribosomes, where proteins are assembled according to the genetic code carried by mRNA.

Translation

Process of synthesizing *proteins* from amino acids based on the *genetic code* carried by *mRNA* with *tRNA* and *rRNA* in the ribosomes of the cell.

*Terms in italics indicate that a brief definition of that term is provided within the table.

alcohol, exercise, or smoking. For chronic diseases like CHD, different genes are almost certainly responsible for the development of disease and its progression to ACS. A particularly powerful approach in candidate gene studies could be the study of haplotypes, that is, not one single SNP in a gene but the inherited pattern of SNPs in a gene (see Table 3–20, haplotype pair).[340-345]

With the rapid development of high-throughput technology in genomics, future studies of complex disease will be able to look at not only the DNA (genome) but also, in parallel, at gene expression (transcriptome) by simultaneous monitoring of the expression of all genes with microarrays and at the proteome by monitoring the level and modification state of all proteins with mass spectrometry.[346]

Genetics of Acute Coronary Syndromes

From the point of view of genetic epidemiology, ACS, as a specific subset of CHD, is a complex multifactorial genetic disease as opposed to a monogenic disease. The definition of the phenotype ACS poses a major challenge in the study of this common multifactorial disease. Typically, ACS is characterized by (1) multiple phenotypic manifestations (multiplex ACS phenotype), (2) a high level of genetic complexity, with the interaction of multiple genes and environmental factors, and (3) penetrance of the underlying genotypes leading to disease, which depend on environmental factors such as diet, smoking, and drug therapy.

■ ■ ■

TABLE 3–21   TYPOLOGY OF SINGLE NUCLEOTIDE POLYMORPHISMS AND ESTIMATED PREVALENCE IN THE HUMAN GENOME

TYPE	DESCRIPTION	NUMBER
1	Coding, nonsynonymous,* nonconservative	60,000–100,000
2	Coding, nonsynonymous, conservative	100,000–180,000
3	Coding, synonymous†	200,000–400,000
4	Noncoding, 5′UTR	140,000
5	Noncoding, 3′UTR	300,000
6	Other noncoding	>1,000,000

UTR, untranslated region.
*Leads to a change in amino-acid sequence.
†Does not change the amino-acid sequence.
Adapted from Risch NJ: Searching for genetic determinants in the new millennium. Nature 2000; 405:847–856.

Multiplex Acute Coronary Syndrome Phenotype

By definition, ACS represents the three major clinical phenotypes UA, non–ST-segment elevation MI, and ST-segment elevation MI. Underlying coronary atherosclerosis is a prerequisite, and the "unstable coronary plaque" with imminent or manifest coronary artery occlusion by thrombus formation is generally viewed as the common denominator in ACS. Because of the dynamic evolution of these three phenotypes, their diagnosis remains challenging even with strict adherence to diagnostic guidelines. It is in the nature of a syndrome that it will not identify one single clinical condition, but a variety of similar disease entities. Although the underlying pathophysiology is tacitly assumed to be similar, the management strategy in ACS as one important environmental component is not. Various countries have major differences in medical systems and in health economics, and the management of ACS varies highly despite common official guidelines. Even within countries, management of ACS varies with the institution (tertiary care vs. community hospital) or the treating physician (specialist vs. nonspecialist). The wide range in medical treatment for ACS across Europe is exemplified in the European Network for Acute Coronary Treatment (ENACT) survey.[29] Therefore, whenever comparing ACS populations across different countries, the phenotypes may be quite different with regard to the impact of underlying genetic and environmental factors in the specific ACS population.

Even coronary atherosclerosis itself, as the necessary underlying causal condition for the development of ACS, is multifactorial. This holds true for known traditional (causal) risk factors such as cigarette smoking, hypertension, dyslipidemia, diabetes, and male gender or new risk markers such as inflammatory biomarkers and prothrombotic plasma proteins (e.g., C-reactive protein, fibrinogen). Therefore, any epidemiologic assessment of ACS needs to acknowledge not only that, by definition, the mix of phenotypes may vary widely in cohorts with a diagnosis of ACS—for example, predominantly consisting of either patients with UA or patients with MI—but also that, because of the multiplex phenotype of CHD itself, further variation is inherent in the ACS phenotype thanks to the variation in cardiovascular risk factors. Individual risk factors are further modulated by ethnicity and exposure to the respective cultural or societal environment. Finally, although the phenotype itself may not have changed, its definition may have, as has been exemplified by the recent consensus conference of redefining MI.[15] Some critics even question whether the reported recent decline in cardiovascular mortality in the United States and Europe is not largely an artifact due to changes in the coding of death certificates.[347]

Genetic Complexity of Acute Coronary Syndromes

Although certain aspects of the pathophysiology of ACS are understood, the relative importance and the interplay of various factors are poorly defined. Therefore, the number and relative importance of genes involved in the pathogenesis is speculative. According to current understanding, 15,000 to 30,000 genes (of a total of about 40,000 to 50,000 genes in the human genome) are expressed in any given cell.[324] Many genes are likely to be somehow involved in the disease process for CHD and subsequent ACS (Table 3–22).

The impact of genetics in CHD/ACS can be estimated from family studies. Among male twins, the relative hazard of death from CHD when one's twin died of CHD before the age of 55 years, as compared with the hazard when one's twin did *not* die before 55, was 8.1 for monozygotic and 3.8 for dizygotic twins in a Swedish study of 21,000 twins born between 1886 and 1925.[348] Furthermore, a family history of premature CHD or MI in first-degree relatives is an established risk factor for MI.[349-351]

As outlined earlier, several large affected sibling studies on premature MI are under way for a genome-wide search of chromosomal loci associated with MI.[327] The GeneQuest study of 398 families with premature CAD or MI by 45 years is the first among such studies to report its analysis of 72 SNPs drawn from 62 candidate genes.[352] Among the 62 candidate genes investigated, the thrombospondin family of five extracellular matrix glycoproteins emerged as the most significant finding. Particularly, one gene variant (THBS4 A387P) remained significant ($P < .10$) for the association with MI after correcting for 100 independent hypotheses. However, the research group failed to replicate the findings of two smaller series of patients with early-onset premature CHD.[352] The study did not find a significant association with gene variants of genes from the coagulation cascade, including the PL^{A2} allele (Leu33Pro) of the platelet glycoprotein IIb/IIIa receptor, multiple other variants from the lipid metabolism pathway, or genes involved in inflammation and adhesion.

Among the candidate genes studied most widely in ACS is the PL^{A2} allele of the platelet glycoprotein IIb/IIIa receptor HPA-1 gene. The glycoprotein IIb/IIIa receptor (integrin $\alpha_{IIb}\beta_3$) is the most abundant receptor on the platelet membrane surface with about 80,000 copies per platelet. The glycoprotein IIb/IIIa receptor is the

■ ▩ ■

TABLE 3–22   PARADIGMS IN THE GENETIC DISSECTION OF AN ACUTE CORONARY SYNDROME (ACS)

The genome type of an individual is the sum of all functionally relevant allelic variants.

The genome type is a necessary cause but not sufficient for the development of disease. Multiple environmental factors interact with multiple genes.

Confounding is due to genetic heterogeneity (different gene variants leads to the same clinical phenotype).

Confounding is due to a reduced penetrance of the disease (environment interacts with susceptible genes, and the risk associated with a gene variant may change depending on the surrounding genetic and environmental context).

Defining ACSs by discrete clinical end points (e.g., unstable angina, myocardial infarction) does not reflect the continuous nature of plaque erosion, fissuring, or rupture.

It is unlikely that many genes with a large, independent, average allelic effect exist.

It is likely that many genes with small, average allelic effects are involved in a disease.

Low values for odds ratios and relative risks (≤1.5) are to be expected in ACS for most gene variants.

Hundreds of genes are involved in the pathophysiology of coronary heart disease/ACS (e.g., receptors, enzymes, structural tissue components, regulation of blood pressure, lipid metabolism, coagulation, growth, and inflammation).

Genes with small, average effects can contribute to disease through gene-gene interaction.

Adapted from Winkelmann BR, Hager J, Kraus WE, et al: Genetics of coronary heart disease: Current knowledge and research principles. In: Granger CB, Kraus WE, Califf RM (eds): Proceedings of a Symposium Genetics of Coronary Heart Disease: Current Understanding and Future Prospects. Leesburg, Va., April 8–10, 1999. Am Heart J 2000;140(Suppl):S11–S26.

receptor for fibrinogen cross-linking of platelets and binding with von Willebrand factor to mediate platelet cohesion and thrombus formation. The PL[A2] gene variant is associated with increased binding to fibrinogen,[353] increased platelet aggregability,[354] enhanced thrombin formation,[355] and reduced inhibition by abciximab, a glycoprotein IIb/IIIa antagonist.[356] Despite demonstration of a functional impact of the gene polymorphism, the results of case-control association studies with MI and ACS conflict. After initial positive findings with ACS,[357] premature MI,[358] sudden death,[359] or stent thrombosis,[360] larger association studies reported negative findings with these phenotypes.[361-365] This gene variant also did not interact with the LDL receptor defect in familial hypercholesterolemia,[366] and a recent meta-analysis of 25 published studies did not find that the PL[A2] gene polymorphism increased the risk of MI.[367] Thus, after many studies, the situation seems to be confusing, despite the fact that some intermediate functional effect ("gain of receptor function") has been demonstrated for this gene variant. However, it should be noted that the phenotypes studied by different authors are quite heterogenous. Nevertheless, such a lack of consistency in results suggests that this gene variant cannot contribute in a major way to acute arterial disease.[368]

What has been found for the most widely studied polymorphism in ACS holds true for other gene variants involved in coagulation as well. Overall, the expectation that genetic risk factors appreciably explain arterial thrombosis has been largely unfulfilled, and expectations raised by early reports of positive associations have been tempered by inconsistent results with almost all genes studied, according to a recent overview of hemostatic gene polymorphisms.[369]

The glycoprotein Ia/IIa platelet membrane complex (integrin $\alpha_2\beta_1$) mediates platelet adhesion to collagen. A silent GP1a C807T (Phe[224]) polymorphism of the integrin α_2 gene (ITGA2) is known to be associated with an up to tenfold higher number of GP1a molecules on the platelet surface, correlates with platelet reactivity to collagen,[370] and has been implicated in an increased risk of MI[371,372] and ACS.[373] However, other studies have not confirmed this association.[374]

Other studies focused on the platelet receptor for von Willebrand receptor factor, GP1bα (HPA-2). A T (thymine) to C (cytosine) polymorphism at position (5 from the ATG start codon of the GP1bα gene, which influences the adjacent Kozak site and modulates expression of the protein, has been associated with ACS and predicted an increased risk of complications after percutaneous transluminal coronary angioplasty.[375] Other polymorphisms of the GP1bα (HPA-2) gene, Thr145Met and VNTR polymorphism, have also been associated with MI and sudden death.[376]

Finally, glycoprotein VI (GP VI) is a major glycoprotein (60 to 65 kDa) that has only recently been implicated in collagen binding. Gene variants of this putative glycoprotein collagen receptor have already been implicated as a new risk factor for MI.[377] However, the role of such isolated findings needs to be clarified in larger, well-standardized, prospective studies.[377] During endothelial damage or plaque rupture, collagens are exposed, von Willebrand factor adheres to exposed sites, and platelets undergo adhesion to the damaged vessel wall. This provides an ample pathophysiologic rationale for implicating such gene polymorphism in modifying outcome with ACS.[378] However, current clinical evidence has yet to meet epidemiologic standards set by the traditional cardiovascular risk factors with regard to consistency and strength of the findings.

The 4G allele of the plasminogen activator inhibitor (PAI-1) gene is associated with increased PAI-1 levels and has been associated with ACS[379] and risk of MI, although not consistently.[380] Other genes in the coagulation cascade have been investigated with varying results, including the tissue factor pathway inhibitor (TFPI),[381] fibrinogen, factor VII, and tissue plasminogen activator.[380] Generally, the relation between the gene polymorphism and the intermediate phenotype, the plasma level, or activity of the protein appeared consistent, but this did not translate into a consistent association with the clinical disease phenotype.

Other non–coagulation-related genes have been investigated in ACS,[382,383] and the number of studies of gene polymorphisms is expected to grow: Any gene coding for the proteins listed in Table 3–19 as a new risk marker for ACS is a putative candidate gene worthy of investigation. However, it is highly unlikely that single genetic polymorphisms will be major determinants of disease, and future studies should be designed to study entire pathways and adhere to strict standards for studies of genetic epidemiology.[335,337]

Gene–Environment Interaction

Many gene polymorphisms have been investigated in complex disease phenotypes like CHD, ACS, or MI. In contrast, with some strong but rare mutations (e.g., the LDL receptor defect as the basis for monogenic familial hypercholesterolemia) that have a strong genetic effect on disease, the real impact of common polymorphism is still poorly understood and, given our current knowledge, very small compared with other traditional risk factors. Thus, it is not surprising that studies in different clinical settings have yielded contrasting results in different populations and different study setups. Often, the risk associated with a polymorphism could only be found in a specific subgroup as an indication of the lack of an overall strong effect.

However, it is probably the wrong approach to expect a single gene polymorphism to make an appreciable independent contribution toward disease risk. Pathophysiologically, genes interact in pathways and they are up- or downregulated in response to environmental stimuli (i.e., nutrition, physical activity, smoking, medication). Therefore, the study of the impact of gene–environment interaction is of major relevance.

Lifestyle and socioeconomic status, that is, environmental factors, have a statistically significant impact on the level of certain coagulation factors, as has been shown for fibrinogen, factor VII antigen, and von Willebrand factor plasma levels in 300 healthy women.[384]

In the case of the PAI-1 4G/5G gene polymorphisms, gene–environment interactions are particularly strong in metabolic high-risk subgroups of subjects, that is, persons displaying features of the metabolic syndrome typically induced by lack of physical activity and intake of excess calories. Thus, triglyceride has been significantly associated with PAI-1 plasma levels only in type 2 diabetics or dyslipidemic subjects carrying the 4G/4G genotype.[485] The metabolic factors involved in insulin resistance (fasting insulin, body mass index, triglycerides, HDL cholesterol) explained a much larger part of the PAI-1 variability (30% to 50%) compared with gene polymorphism of PAI-1 (up to 3% only) in a study of 228 healthy families.[386]

A G-to-A sequence variation at position –455 of the promotor of the β-fibrinogen gene has been shown to be associated with higher plasma fibrinogen in the presence of the A^{-455} allele. In response to exercise as a moderate environmental stimulus, homozygous carriers of the A^{-455} allele experienced an acute rise in fibrinogen that was almost double the rise experienced by noncarriers of this allele, with heterozygous subjects displaying an intermediate response. Such an enhanced response could put persons at a greater-than-average risk for a thrombotic event.[387]

Finally, a significant interaction between smoking and the PL^{A2} allele of the platelet glycoprotein IIb/IIIa receptor HPA-1 gene has been reported. The risk of premature MI was not significant in nonsmoking carriers of at least one PL^{A2} allele but was doubled in smokers.[388] An interaction between smoking and the $PLA1^{A2}$ gene polymorphism has been confirmed in patients presenting with non–ST-elevation ACS, such that the MI risk in carriers of the PL^{A2} allele was significantly underrepresented in smokers.[389]

The polymorphisms studied until now seem to explain only a small portion of the global risk of CHD and ACS. Results should be improved by identifying the major gene–environment interactions for each of the respective candidate genes, by studying the genes of entire pathways (e.g., coagulation cascade, lipid metabolism, signaling, and adhesion), and by studying haplotypes instead of individual SNPs (i.e., several SNPs linked together as ancestral marker genotypes for the respective gene). Because environmental factors are a major determinant in gene expression and function, such factors always need to be identified and accounted for in the disentangling of complex genetic diseases.

REFERENCES

1. Théroux P, Fuster V: Acute coronary syndromes—unstable angina and non-Q-wave myocardial infarction. Circulation 1998;97:1195–1206.
2. Braunwald E, Antmann EM, Beasley JW, et al: ACC/AHA guidelines for the management of patients with unstable angina and non-ST-segment elevation myocardial infarction. J Am Coll Cardiol 2000;36:970–1062.
3. Hamm CW, Bertrand M, Braunwald E: Acute coronary syndromes without ST elevation: implementation of new guidelines. Lancet 2001;3258:1533–1538.
4. Davies MJ, Thomas AC: Plaque fissuring—the cause of acute myocardial infarction, sudden ischemic death, and crescendo angina. Br Heart J 1985;53:363–373.
5. Falk E: Unstable angina with fatal outcome: Dynamic coronary thrombosis leading to infarction and/or sudden death. Autopsy evidence of recurrent mural thrombosis with peripheral embolization culminating in total vascular occlusion. Circulation 1985;71:699–708.
6. Rauch U, Osende JI, Fuster V, et al: Thrombus formation on atherosclerotic plaques: pathogenesis and clinical consequences. Ann Intern Med 2001;134:224–238.
7. Braunwald E, Mark DB, Jones RH, et al: Unstable angina: Diagnosis and management—clinical practice guideline number 10 [AHCPR publication no. 94-0602]. Rockville, Md., U.S. Department of Health and Human Services, 1994.
8. Braunwald E, Antman EM, Beasley JW, et al: ACC/AHA guidelines for the management of patients with unstable angina and non-ST-segment elevation myocardial infarction: Executive summary and recommendations: A report of the American College of Cardiology/American Heart Association Task Force on Practice Guidelines (Committee on Management of Patients With Unstable Angina). Circulation 2000;102:1193–1209.
9. Braunwald E: Unstable angina—an etiologic approach to management. Circulation 1998;98:2219–2222.
10. Hillis LD, Braunwald E: Coronary-artery spasm. N Engl J Med 1978;299:695–702.
11. Maseri A, L'Abbate A, Baroldi G, et al: Coronary vasospasm as a possible cause of myocardial infarction. N Engl J Med 1978;299:1271–1277.
12. Conti CR: Coronary-artery spasm and myocardial infarction. N Engl J Med 1983;309:238–239.
13. Braunwald E: Unstable angina—a classification. Circulation 1989;80:410–414.
14. Hamm CW, Braunwald E: A classification of unstable angina revisited. Circulation 2000;102:118–122.
15. The Joint European Society of Cardiology/American College of Cardiology Committee: Myocardial infarction redefined—a consensus document of the Joint European Society of Cardiology/American College of Cardiology Committee for the redefinition of myocardial infarction. Eur Heart J 2000;21:1502–1513.
16. The Joint European Society of Cardiology/American College of Cardiology Committee: Myocardial infarction redefined—a consensus document of the Joint European Society of Cardiology/American College of Cardiology Committee for the redefinition of myocardial infarction. J Am Coll Cardiol 2000;36:959–969.
17. Hamm CW, Ravkilde J, Gerhardt W, et al: The prognostic value of serum troponin T in unstable angina. N Engl J Med 1992;327:146–150.
18. Lindahl B, Venge P, Wallentin L, for the FRISC study group: Relation between troponin T and the risk of subsequent cardiac events in unstable coronary artery disease. Circulation 1996;93:1651–1657.
19. Jaffe AS: Testing the wrong hypothesis: the failure to recognize the limitations of troponin assays. J Am Coll Cardiol 2001;38:999–1001.
20. Ford ES, Giles WH, Croft JB: Prevalence of nonfatal coronary heart disease among American adults. Am Heart J 2000;139:371–377.
21. Zimmerman J, Fromm R, Meyer D, et al: Diagnostic marker cooperative study for the diagnosis of myocardial infarction. Circulation 1999;99:1671–1677.
22. Mathew V, Farkouh M, Grill DE, et al: Clinical risk stratification correlates with the angiographic extent of coronary artery disease in unstable angina. J Am Coll Cardiol 2001;37:2053–2058.
23. Kontos MC, Ornato JP, Schmidt KL, et al: Incidence of high-risk acute coronary syndromes and eligibility for glycoprotein IIb/IIIa inhibitors among patients admitted for possible myocardial ischemia. Am Heart J 2002;143:70–75.
24. van Miltenburg-van Zijl AJM, Simoons ML, Veerhoek RJ, Bossuyt PMM: Incidence and follow-up of Braunwald subgroups in unstable angina pectoris. J Am Coll Cardiol 1995;25:1286–1292.
25. Dougan JP, Mathew T, Menown I, et al: Safety and efficacy of rapid access chest pain clinics for the triage of patients with acute chest [Scientific Sessions 2001, American Heart Association, November 11–14, 2001, Anaheim]. Circulation 2001;104(Suppl II):727.
26. Shoyeb A, Bokhari S, La Marca C, et al: Incidence of CAD in chest in patients from the hospital without provocative stress testing [Scientific Sessions 2001, American Heart Association, November 11–14, 2001, Anaheim]. Circulation 2001;104(Suppl II):727.
27. Meyer T, Binder L, Graeber T, et al: Superiority of combined CK-MB and troponin I measurements for the early risk stratification of

unselected patients presenting with acute chest pain. Cardiology 1998;90:286–290.

28. Roe MT, Harrington RA, Prosper DM, et al: Receptor Suppression Using Integrilin Therapy (PURSUIT) Trial Investigators. Clinical and therapeutic profile of patients presenting with acute coronary syndromes who do not have significant coronary artery disease. Circulation 2000;102:1101–1106.

29. Fox KAA, Cokkinos DV, Deckers J, et al on behalf of the ENACT (European Network for Acute Coronary Treatment) investigators. The ENACT study: A pan-European survey of acute coronary syndromes. Eur Heart J 2000;21:1440–1449.

30. Eagle KA, Goodman SG, Avezum A, et al for the GRACE investigators. Practice variation and missed opportunities for reperfusion in ST-segment-elevation myocardial infarction: Findings from the Global Registry of Acute Coronary Events (GRACE). Lancet 2002;359:373–377.

31. Kannel WB, Dannenberg AL, Abbott RD: Unrecognized myocardial infarction and hypertension: the Framingham study. Am Heart J 1985;109:581–585.

32. Sheifer SE, Manolio TA, Gersh BJ: Unrecognized myocardial infarction. Ann Intern Med 2001;135:801–811.

33. Enbergs A, Bürger R, Reinecke H, et al: Prevalence of coronary artery disease in a general population without suspicion of coronary artery disease: Angiographic analysis of subjects aged 40 to 70 years referred for catheter ablation therapy. Eur Heart J 2000;21:45–52.

34. Erikssen J, Enge I, Forfang K, Storstein O: False positive diagnostic tests and coronary angiography findings in 105 presumably healthy males. Circulation 1976;54:371–376.

35. Bertrand ME, Simoons ML, Fox KAA, et al: Management of acute coronary syndromes: acute coronary syndromes without persistent ST segment elevation [Task force report]. Eur Heart J 2000;21:1406–1432.

36. Braunwald E [chair]: Clinical practice guideline unstable angina: diagnosis and management [Quick reference guideline for clinicans. No. 10]. Rockville, Md., U.S. Department of Health and Human Services, Agency for Health Care Policy and Research. AHCPR publication no. 94-0603, 1994.

37. Cohen M, Antmann EM, Miurphy SA, Radley D: Mode and timing of treatment failures (recurrent ischemic events) after hospital admission for non-ST segment elevation acute coronary syndromes. Am Heart J 2002;143:63–69.

38. Winkelmann BR, Zahn R, Stilz HU: Overview of clinical trials with glycoprotein IIb-IIIa receptor antagonists in the prevention and management of coronary thrombosis. Exp Opin Invest Drugs 1997;6:1623–1642.

39. Boersma E, Harrington RA, Moliterno DJ, et al: Platelet glycoprotein IIb/IIIa inhibitors in acute coronary syndromes: A meta-analysis of all major randomised clinical trials. Lancet 2002;359:189–198.

40. Mulcahy R, Daly L, Graham I, et al: Unstable angina: natural history and determinants of prognosis. Am J Cardiol 1981;48:525–528.

41. Mulcahy R, Al Awadhi AH, de Buitleor M, et al: Natural history and prognosis of unstable angina. Am Heart J 1985;109:753–758.

42. Anderson HV, Cannon CP, Stone PH, et al for the TIMI IIIB investigators: One-year results of the thrombolysis in myocardial infarction (TIMI) IIIB clinical trial—a randomized comparison of tissue-type plasminogen activator versus placebo and early invasive versus early conservative strategies in unstable angina and non-Q wave myocardial infarction. J Am Coll Cardiol 1995;26:1643–1650.

43. Boden WE, O'Rourke RA, Crawford MH, et al for the Veterans Affairs Non-Q-Wave Infarction Strategies in Hospital (VANQWISH) trial investigators: Outcomes in patients with acute non-Q-wave myocardial infarction randomly assigned to an invasive as compared with a conservative management strategy. N Engl J Med 1998;338:1785–1792.

44. Boersma E, Pieper KS, Steyerberg EW, et al for the PURSUIT investigators: Predictors of outcome in patients with acute coronary syndromes without persistent ST-segment elevation. Circulation 2000;101:2557–2567.

45. Morrow DA, Cannon CP, Rifai N, et al for the TACTICS-TIMI 18 investigators: Ability of minor elevations of troponins I and T to predict benefit from an early invasive strategy in patients with unstable angina and non-ST elevation myocardial infarction—results from a randomized clinical trial. JAMA 2001;286:2405–2412.

46. Armstrong PW, Fu Y, Chang W-C, et al for the GUSTO-IIb investigators: Acute coronary syndromes in the GUSTO-IIb trial—prognostic insights and impact of recurrent ischemia. Circulation 1998;98:1860–1868.

47. Kaul P, Fu Y, Chang W-C, et al for the PARAGON-A and GUSTO-IIb investigators. Prognostic value of ST segment depression in acute coronary syndromes: Insights from PARAGON-A applied to GUSTO-IIb. J Am Coll Cardiol 2001;38:64–71.

48. Heidenreich PA, Alloggiamento T, Melsop K, et al: The prognostic value of troponin in patients with non-ST elevation acute coronary syndromes: A meta-analysis. J Am Coll Cardiol 2001;38:478–485.

49. Capewell S, MacIntyre K, Stewart S, et al: Age, sex, and social trends in out-of-hospital deaths in Scotland 1986–95: A retrospective cohort study. Lancet 2001;358:1213–1217.

50. Phibbs B, Marcus F, Marriott HJC, et al: Q-wave versus non-Q wave myocardial infarction: A meaningless distinction. J Am Coll Cardiol 1999;33:576–582.

51. Rose GA, Blackburn H, Gillum RF, Prineas RJ: Cardiovascular Survey Methods, 2nd ed. Geneva, World Health Organization, 1982.

52. Hennekens CH, Buring JE: Epidemiology in Medicine. Boston, Little Brown, 1987.

53. Kuller LE: Epidemiology of cardiovascular diseases: Current perspectives. Am J Epidemiol 1976;104:425–456.

54. Sytkowski PA, Kannel WB, D'Agostino RB: Changes in risk factors and decline in mortality from cardiovascular disease—the Framingham Heart Study. N Engl J Med 1990;322:1635–1641.

55. Kagan A, Harris BR, Winkelstein W Jr, et al: Epidemiologic studies of coronary heart disease and stroke in Japanese men living in Japan, Hawaii and California: Demographic, physical, dietary and biochemical characteristics. J Chron Dis 1974;27:345–364.

56. Solberg LA, Strong JP: Risk factors and atherosclerotic lesions—a review of autopsy studies. Arteriosclerosis 1983;3:187–198.

57. Multiple Risk Factor Intervention Trial Research Group: Multiple Risk Factor Intervention Trial—risk factor changes and mortality results. JAMA 1982;248:1465–1477.

58. Downs JR, Clearfield M, Weis S, et al for the AFCAPS/TexCAPS research group: Primary prevention of acute coronary events with lovastatin in men and women with average cholesterol levels—results of AFCAPS/TexCAPS. JAMA 1998;279:1615–1622.

59. Bradford Hill A: The environment and disease: Association or causation? Proc R Soc Med 1965;58:295–300.

60. Bartecchi CE, MacKenzie TD, Schrier RW: The human costs of tobacco use (first of two parts). N Engl J Med 1994;330:907–912.

61. MacKenzie TD, Bartecchi CE, Schrier RW: The human costs of tobacco use (second of two parts). N Engl J Med 1994;330:975–980.

62. Doll R, Peto R: Mortality in relation to smoking: 20 years' observations on male British doctors. Br Med J 1976;2:1525–1536.

63. Peto R, Lopez AD, Boreham J, et al: Mortality from tobacco in developed countries: Indirect estimation from national vital statistics. Lancet 1992;339:1268–1278.

64. Yuan J-M, Ross RK, Wang X-L, et al: Morbidity and mortality in relation to cigarette smoking in Shanghai, China—a prospective male cohort study. JAMA 1996;275:1646–1650.

65. World Health Report 1999: Making a Difference. Geneva, World Health Organization, 1999.

66. Tobacco or health: A global status report. Geneva, World Health Organization, 1997.

67. Cigarette smoking among adults—United States, 1997. MMWR Morbid Mortal Wkly Rep 1999;48:993–996.

68. Wechsler H, Rigotti NA, Gledhill-Hoyt J, Lee H: Increased levels of cigarette use among college students: A cause for national concern. JAMA 1998;280:1673–1678.

69. Nyboe J, Jensen G, Appleyard M, Schnohr P: Smoking and the risk of first acute myocardial infarction. Am Heart J 1991;122:438–447.

70. Willett WC, Green A, Stampfer MJ, et al: Relative and absolute excess risks of coronary heart disease among women who smoke cigarettes. N Engl J Med 1987;317:1303–1309.

71. Parish S, Collins R, Peto R, et al for the International Studies of Infarct Survival (ISIS): Cigarette smoking, tar yields, and non-fatal myocardial infarction: 14000 cases and 32000 controls in the United Kingdom. BMJ 1995;311:471–477.

72. Barbash GI, White HD, Diaz MR, et al for the investigators of the international tissue plasminogen activator/streptokinase mortality trial: Significance of smoking in patients receiving thrombolytic therapy for acute myocardial infarction. Experience gleaned from the International Tissue Plasminogen Activator/Streptokinase Mortality Trial. Circulation 1993;87:53–58.

73. Barbash GI, Reiner J, White HD, et al for the GUSTO-I investigators. Evaluation of paradoxical beneficial effects of smoking in patients receiving thrombolytics therapy for acute myocardial infarction: Mechanism of the "smoker's paradox" from the GUSTO-I trial, with angiographic insights. J Am Coll Cardiol 1995;26:1222-1229.

74. Grines CL, Topol EJ, O'Neill WW, et al: Effect of cigarette smoking on outcome after thrombolytic therapy for myocardial infarction. Circulation 1995;91:298-303.

75. Hasdai D, Lerman A, Rihal CS, et al: Smoking status and outcome after primary coronary angioplasty for acute myocardial infarction. Am Heart J 1999;137:612-620.

76. Hasdai D, Garratt KN, Grill DE, et al: Effect of smoking status on the long-term outcome after successful percutaneous coronary revascularization. N Engl J Med 1997;336:755-761.

77. Mead TW, Imeson J, Stirling Y: Effects of changes in smoking and other characteristics on clotting factors and the risk of ischaemic heart disease. Lancet 1987;2:986-988.

78. Nowak J, Murray JJ, Oates JA, FitzGerald GA: Biochemical evidence of a chronic abnormality in platelet and vascular function in healthy individuals who smoke cigarettes. Circulation 1987;76:6-14.

79. Newby DE, Wright RA, Labinjoh C, et al: Endothelial dysfunction, impaired endogenous fibrinolysis, and cigarette smoking—a mechanism for arterial thrombosis and myocardial infarction. Circulation 1999;99:1411-1415.

80. Adams MR, Jessup W, Celermajer DS: Cigarette smoking is associated with increased human monocyte adhesion to endothelial cells: Reversibility with oral L-arginine but not vitamin C. J Am Coll Cardiol 1997;29:491-497.

81. Craig WY, Palomaki GE, Haddow JE: Cigarette smoking and serum lipid and lipoprotein concentrations: An analysis of published data. Br Med J 1989;298:784-788.

82. Church DF, Pryor WA: Free-radical chemistry of cigarette smoke and its toxicological implications. Environ Health Perspect 1985;64:111-126.

83. Morrow JD, Frei B, Longmire AW, et al: Increase in circulating products of lipid peroxidation (F_2-isoprostanes) in smokers—smoking as a cause of oxidative damage. N Engl J Med 1995;332:1198-1203.

84. Nitenberg A, Antony I, Foult J-M: Acetylcholine-induced coronary vasoconstriction in young, heavy smokers with normal coronary arteriographic findings. Am J Med 1993;95:71-77.

85. Kannel WB: Update on the role of cigarette smoking in coronary artery disease. Am Heart J 1981;101:319-327.

86. Lakier JB: Smoking and cardiovascular disease. Am J Med 1992;93(Suppl 1A):8S-12S.

87. Mocecetti T, Malacrida R, Pasotti E, et al: Epidemiologic variables and outcomes of 1972 young patients with acute myocardial infarction: Data from the GISSI-2 database. Investigators of the Gruppo Italiano por lo Studio della Streotochianasi nell'Infarto Miocardico (GISSI-2). Arch Intern Med 1997;157:865-869.

88. Doughty M, Mehta R, Bruckman D, et al: Acute myocardial infarction in the young: The University of Michigan experience. Am Heart J 2002;143:56-62.

89. Gruppo Italiano por lo Studio della Streotochianasi nell'Infarto Miocardico (GISSI-2): A factorial design trial of alteplase vs streptokinase and heparin among 12,490 patients with acute myocardial infarction. Lancet 1990;336:65-71.

90. Gruppo Italiano por lo Studio della Streotochianasi nell'Infarto Miocardico (GISSI-3): Effect of lisinopril and transdermal glyceryl trinitrate singly and together on 6 week mortality and ventricular function after myocardial infarction. Lancet 1994;343:1115-1122.

91. Women and smoking: A report from the Surgeon General 2001. Http://www.cdc.gov/tobacco/sgr/sgr_women/ataglance.htm.

92. Levy D, Wilson PWF, Anderson KM, Castelli WP: Stratifying the patient at risk from coronary disease: New insights from the Framingham Heart Study. Am Heart J 1990;119:712-717.

93. Martin MJ, Hulley SB, Browner WS, et al: Serum cholesterol, blood pressure, and mortality: Implications from a cohort of 361 662 men. Lancet 1986;2:933-936.

94. Jousilahti P, Vartainen E, Pekkanen J, et al: Serum cholesterol distribution and coronary heart disease risk—observations and predictions among middle-aged population in Eastern Finland. Circulation 1998;97:1087-1094.

95. Lipid Research Clinics Program: The Lipid Research Clinics coronary primary prevention trial results: I. Reduction in incidence of coronary heart disease. JAMA 1984;251:351-364.

96. Lipid Research Clinics Program: The Lipid Research Clinics coronary primary prevention trial results: II. The relationship of reduction in incidence of coronary heart disease to cholesterol lowering. JAMA 1984;251:365-374.

97. Anderson KM, Castelli WP, Levy DL: Cholesterol and mortality: 30 years of follow-up from the Framingham study. JAMA 1987;257:2176-2180.

98. LaRosa JC, Hunnighake D, Bush D, et al: The cholesterol facts—a summary of the evidence relating dietary fats, serum cholesterol, and coronary heart disease. A joint statement by the American Heart Association and the National Heart, Lung, and Blood Institute. Circulation 1990;81:1721-1733.

99. Oliver MF: Reducing cholesterol does not reduce mortality. J Am Coll Cardiol 1988;12:814-817.

100. Gould AL, Roussow JE, Santanello NC, et al: Cholesterol reduction yields clinical benefit—impact of statin trials. Circulation 1998;97:946-952.

101. Bucher HC, Griffith LE, Guyatt GH: Systematic review on the risk and benefit of different cholesterol-lowering interventions. Arterioscler Thromb Vasc Biol 1999;19:187-195.

102. LaRosa JC, He J, Vupputuri S: Effects of statins on risk of coronary disease—a meta-analysis of randomized trials. JAMA 1999;282:2340-2346.

103. Scandinavian Simvastatin Survival Study Group: Randomized trial of cholesterol lowering in 4444 patients with coronary heart disease. Lancet 1994;344:1383-1389.

104. Long-term Intervention with Pravastatin in Ischemic Disease (LIPID) Study Group: Prevention of cardiovascular events and death with pravastatin in patients with coronary heart disease and a broad range of initial cholesterol levels. N Engl J Med 1998;339:1349-1357.

105. Heart Protection Study Collaborative Group: MRC/BHF Heart Protection Study of cholesterol lowering with simvastatin in 20536 high-risk individuals: A randomised placebo-controlled trial. Lancet 2002;360:7-22.

106. Sacks FM, Pfeffer MA, Moye LA, et al for the Cholesterol and Recurrent Events Trial Investigators: The effect of pravastatin on coronary events after myocardial infarction in patients with average cholesterol levels. 1996;335:1001-1009.

107. Shepherd J, Cobbe SM, Ford I, et al for the West of Scotland Coronary Prevention Study group: Prevention of coronary heart disease with pravastatin in men with hypercholesterolemia. N Engl J Med 1995;333:1301-1307.

108. Moriarty PM: Using both "relative risk reduction" and "number needed to treat" in evaluating primary and secondary clinical trials of lipid reduction. Am J Cardiol 2001;87:1206-1208.

109. Stamler J, Daviglus ML, Garside DB, et al: Relationship of baseline serum cholesterol levels in 3 large cohorts of younger men to long-term coronary, cardiovascular, and all-cause mortality and to longevity. JAMA 2000;284:311-318.

110. Tonkin AM, Colquhoun D, Emberson J, et al for the LIPID study group: Effects of pravastatin in 3260 patients with unstable angina: Results from the LIPID study. Lancet 2000;355: 1871-1875.

111. Schwartz GG, Olsson AG, Ezekowitz MD, et al for the Myocardial Ischemia Reduction with Aggressive Cholesterol Lowering (MIRACL) investigators: Effects of atorvastatin on early recurrent ischemic events in acute coronary syndromes: A randomized controlled trial. JAMA 2001;285:1711-1718.

112. Shah PK, Kaul S, Nilsson J, Cercek B: Exploiting the vascular protective effects of high-density lipoprotein and its apolipoproteins—an idea whose time for testing is coming, part I. Circulation 2001;104:2376-2383.

113. Kwiterovich PO: The aniatherogenic role of high-density lipoprotein cholesterol. Am J Cardiol 1998;82(Suppl Q):13-21.

114. Wang TD, Chen W-J, Chien KL, et al: Efficacy of cholesterol levels and ratios in predicting future coronary heart disease in a Chinese population. Am J Cardiol 2001;88:737-743.

115. Avins AL, Neuhaus JM: Do triglycerides provide meaningful information about heart disease risk? Arch Intern Med 2000;160:1937-1944.

116. Jeppesen J, Hein HO, Suadicani P, Gyntelberg F: Triglyceride concentration and coronary heart disease. An eight-year follow-up in the Copenhagen Male Study. Circulation 1998;97: 1029-1036.

117. Cullen P: Evidence that triglycerides are an independent coronary heart disease risk factor. Am J Cardiol 2000;86:943-949.

118. Assmann G, Cullen P, von Eckardstein A, et al: The importance of triglycerides as a significant risk factor. Eur Heart J Supplements. 1999;1(Suppl J):7-11.

119. Smith GD, Rhillips A: Declaring independence: Why we should be cautious. J Epidemiol Commun Health 1990;44:257-258.

120. Rantalla AO, Kauma H, Lilja M, et al: Prevalence of the metabolic syndrome in drug-treated hypertensive patients and control subjects. J Intern Med 1999;245:163-174.

121. Grundy SM: Hypertriglyceridemia, atherogenic dyslipidemia, and the metabolic syndrome. Am J Cardiol 1998;81(Suppl B): 19B-25B.

122. Kwiterovich PO: The metabolic pathways of high-density lipoprotein, low-density lipoprotein, and triglycerides: A current review. Am J Cardiol 2000;86(Suppl L):5-10.

123. Gotto AM. Triglyceride—the forgotten risk factor. Circulation 1998;97:1027-1028.

124. Hokanson JE, Austin ME: Plasma triglyceride is a risk factor for cardiovascular disease independent of high-density cholesterol level: A meta-analysis of population-based prospective studies. J Cardiovasc Risk 1996;3:216-219.

125. Rader DJ, Hoeg JM, Brewer HB: Quantification of plasma apolipoproteins in the primary and secondary prevention of coronary artery disease. Ann Intern Med 1994;120:1012-1025.

126. Sniderman AD, Genest J: The measurement of apolipoprotein B should replace the conventional lipid profile in screening for cardiovascular risk. Can J Cardiol 1992;8:133-140.

127. Alaupovic P: Use of apolipoprotein parameters and endpoints in drug development and approval process. Am J Cardiol 1998;81 (Suppl F):40-47.

128. Baumgart P, Walger P, Jürgens U, Rahn KH: Reference data for ambulatory blood pressure monitoring: What results are equivalent to the established limits of office blood pressure. Klin Wschr 1990;68:723-727.

129. Verdecchia P: Prognostic value of ambulatory blood pressure—current evidence and clinical implications. Hypertension 2000;35:844-851.

130. Joint National Committee on Prevention, Detection, Evaluation, and Treatment of High Blood Pressure: The sixth report of the Joint National Committee on Prevention, Detection, Evaluation, and Treatment of High Blood Pressure. Arch Intern Med 1997;157:2413-2446.

131. Guidelines subcommittee: 1999 World Health Organization—International Society of Hypertension guidelines for the management of hypertension. J Hypertens 1999;17:151-183.

132. Kannel WB: Historic perspectives on the relative contributions of diastolic and systolic blood pressure elevation to cardiovascular risk profile. Am Heart J 1999;138(Suppl):205-210.

133. Franklin SS, Jacobs MJ, Wong ND, et al: Predominance of isolated systolic hypertension among middle-aged and elderly US hypertensives. Analysis based on National Health and Nutrition Examination Survey (NHANES) III. Hypertension 2001;37: 869-874.

134. Kannel WB: Elevated systolic blood pressure as a cardiovascular risk factor. Am J Cardiol 2000;85:251-255.

135. Anderson GH, Blakeman N, Streeten DHP: The effect of age on prevalence of secondary forms of hypertension in 4429 consecutively referred patients. J Hypertens 1994;12:609-615.

136. Lifton RP: Molecular genetics of human blood pressure variation. Science 1996;272:676-680.

137. Gu C, Borecki I, Gagnon J, et al: Familial resemblance for testing blood pressure with particular reference to racial differences: Preliminary analyses from the HERITAGE Family Study. Hum Biol 1998;70:77-90.

138. Crews DE, Williams SR: Molecular aspects of blood pressure regulation. Hum Biol 1999;71:475-503.

139. Williams SM, Addy JH, Phillips JA III, et al: Combinations of variations in multiple genes are associated with hypertension. Hypertension 2000;36:2-6.

140. MacMahon S, Peto R, Cutler J, et al: Blood pressure, stroke and coronary heart disease, part I: Effects of prolonged differences in blood pressure. Evidence from nine prospective observational studies corrected for the regression dilution bias. Lancet 1990;335:765-774.

141. Staessen JA, Wang JG, Thijs L: Cardiovascular protection and blood pressure reduction: A meta-analysis. Lancet 2001;358:1305-1315.

142. Collins R, Peto R, MacMahon S, et al: Blood pressure, stroke, and coronary heart disease, part II: Effects of short-term reductions in blood pressure. An overview of the unconfounded randomised drug trials in an epidemiologic context. Lancet 1990;335:827-838.

143. Lembo G, Morisco C, Lanni F, et al: Systemic hypertension and coronary artery disease: The link. Am J Cardiol 1998;82(Suppl H):2-7.

144. Palù CD: Hypertension and atherosclerosis. J Hum Hypertens 1996;10(Suppl 3):89-92.

145. Gaziano JM, Sesso HD, Breslow JL, et al: Relation between systemic hypertension and blood lipids on the risk of myocardial infarction. Am J Cardiol 1999;84:768-773.

146. Murray CJL, Lopez AD: The Global Burden of Disease. Cambridge, Mass., Harvard School of Public Health, 1996.

147. King H, Aubert RE, Herman WH: Global burden of diabetes, 1995-2025: Prevalence, numerical estimates, and projections. Diabetes Care 1998;21:1414-1431.

148. Nathan DM, Meigs J, Singer DE: The epidemiology of cardiovascular disease in type 2 diabetes mellitus: How sweet it is...or is it? Lancet 1997;350(Suppl I):4-9.

149. National Diabetes Information Clearinghouse. National diabetes Statistics. Bethesda, Md, National Institute of Diabetes and Digestive and Kidney Diseases, NIH publication 02-3892, 2002.

150. DeFronzo RA, Ferraninni E: Insulin resistance—a multifaceted syndrome responsible for NIDDM, obesity hypertension, dyslipidemia, and atherosclerotic cardiovascular disease. Diabetes Care 1991;14:173-194.

151. World Health Organization: WHO expert committee on diabetes mellitus. 2nd report. Technical report series 646. Geneva, World Health Organization, 1980.

152. World Health Organization: Diabetes mellitus: Report of a WHO study group. Technical report series 727. Geneva, World Health Organization, 1985.

153. Alberti KGMM, Zimmet PZ for the WHO Consultation: Definition, diagnosis and classification of diabetes mellitus and its complications. Part 1: Diagnosis and classification of diabetes mellitus provisional report of a WHO consultation. Diabet Med 1998;15: 539-553.

154. World Health Organization: Definition, diagnosis and classification of diabetes mellitus and its complications. Report of a WHO consultation. Part 1: Diagnosis and classification of diabetes mellitus WHO/NCD/NCS/99. Geneva, World Health Organization, 1999.

155. The Expert Committee on the Diagnosis and Classification of Diabetes Mellitus: Report of the expert committee on the diagnosis and classification of diabetes mellitus. Diabetes Care 1997;20:1183-1197.

156. Tuomi T, Carlsson A, Li H, et al: Clinical and genetic characteristics of type 2 diabetes with and without GAD antibodies. Diabetes 1999;48:150-157.

157. Harris MI, Klein R, Welborn TA, Knuiman MW: Onset of NIDDM occurs at least 4-7 yr before clinical diagnosis. Diabetes Care 1992;15:815-819.

158. Harris MI, Hadden WC, Knowler WC, Bennett PH: Prevalence of diabetes and impaired glucose tolerance and plasma glucose levels in U.S. population aged 20-74 yr. Diabetes 1987;36: 523-534.

159. Harris MI: Undiagnosed NIDDM: Clinical and public health issues. Diabetes Care 1993;16:642-652.

160. Harris MI, Eastman RC: Early detection of undiagnosed non-insulin-dependent diabetes mellitus. JAMA 1996;276:1261-1262.

161. Eastman RC, Cowie CC, Harris MI: Undiagnosed diabetes or impaired glucose tolerance and cardiovascular risk. Diabetes Care 1997;20:127-128.

162. American Diabetes Association: Detection and management of lipid disorders in diabetes. Diabetes Care 1993;16:106-112.

163. Herlitz J, Malmberg K: How to improve the cardiac prognosis for diabetes. Diabetes Care 1999;22(Suppl):89-96.

164. Barzilay JI, Spiekerman CF, Kuller LH, et al: Prevalence of clinical and isolated subclinical cardiovascular disease in older adults with glucose disorders. Diabetes Care 2001;24:1233-1239.

165. Panzram G: Mortality and survival in type 2 (non-insulin-dependent) diabetes mellitus. Diabetologica 1987;30:123-131.

166. Laakso M, Lehto S: Epidemiology of macrovascular disease in diabetes. Diabetes Rev 1997;5:294-315.

167. Cohen Y, Raz I, Merin G, Mozes B for the Coronary Artery Bypass (ISCAB) study consortium: Comparison of factors associated with 30-d mortality after coronary artery bypass grafting in patients with versus without diabetes mellitus. Am J Cardiol 1998;81:7-11.

168. Herlitz J, Karlson BW, Wognsen GB, et al: Mortality and morbidity in diabetic and nondiabetic patients during a 2-year period after coronary artery bypass grafting. Diabetes Care 1996;19:698-703.

169. West of Scotland Coronary Prevention Study Group: Baseline risk factors and their association with outcome in the West of Scotland Coronary Prevention Study. Am J Cardiol 1997;79: 756-762.

170. Gu K, Cowie CC, Harris MI: Mortality in adults with and without diabetes in a national cohort of the U.S. population, 1971-1993. Diabetes Care 1998;21:1138-1145.

171. Aronson D, Rayfield EJ, Chesebro JH: Mechanisms determining course and outcome of diabetic patients who have had acute myocardial infarction. Ann Intern Med 1997;126:296-306.

172. Stamler J, Vaccaro O, Neaton JD, Wentworth D: Diabetes, other risk factors, and 12-yr cardiovascular mortality for men screened in the Multiple Risk Factor Intervention Trial. Diabetes Care 1993;16:434-444.

173. Donahue RP, Abbott RD, Reed DM, Yano K: Postchallenge glucose concentration and coronary heart disease in men of Japanese ancestry. Honolulu Heart Program. Diabetes 1987;36:689-692.

174. Haffner SM, Lehto S, Rönnemaa T, et al: Mortality from coronary heart disease in subjects with type 2 diabetes and in nondiabetic subjects with and without prior myocardial infarction. N Engl J Med 1998;339:229-234.

175. Kuller LH, Velentgas P, Barzilay J, et al: Diabetes mellitus—subclinical cardiovascular disease and risk of incident cardiovascular disease and all-cause mortality. Arterioscler Thromb Vasc Biol 2000;20:823-829.

176. Krolewski AS, Warram JH, Valsania P, et al: Evolving natural history of coronary artery disease in diabetes mellitus. Am J Med 1991;90(Suppl 2A):56-61.

177. Nathan DM: The pathophysiology of diabetic complications: how much does the glucose hypothesis explain? Ann Intern Med 1996;124(1 pt 2):86-89.

178. Ghosh S, Schork NJ: Genetic analysis of NIDDM. Diabetes 1996;45:1-14.

179. Horikawa Y, Oda N, Cox NJ, et al: Genetic variation in the gene encoding calpain-10 is associated with type 2 diabetes mellitus. Nat Genet 2000;26:163-175.

180. Elbein SC: The genetics of human noninsulin-dependent (type 2) diabetes mellitus. J Nutr 1997;127(Suppl):1891-1896.

181. Elbein SC: Genetics of diabetes—an overview for the millennium. Diabet Technol Ther 2000;2:391-400.

182. Groop LC, Tuomi T: Non-insulin-dependent diabetes mellitus—a collision between thrifty genes and an affluent society. Ann Med 1997;29:37-53.

183. Gerich JE: The genetic basis of type 2 diabetes mellitus: Impaired insulin secretion versus impaired insulin sensitivity. Endocrin Rev 1998;19:491-503.

184. Baba T, Neugebauer S: The link between insulin resistance and hypertension—effects of antihypertensive and antihyperlipidemic drugs on insulin sensitivity. Drugs 1994;47:383-404.

185. Ferrannini E, Mari A: How to measure insulin sensitivity. J Hypertens 1998;16:895-906.

186. Haffner SM, Miettinen H, Stern MP: The homeostasis model in the San Antonio Heart Study. Diabetes Care 1997;20:1087-1092.

187. Mykkanen L, Haffner SM, Rönnemaa T, et al: Low insulin sensitivity is associated with clustering of cardiovascular disease risk factors. Am J Epidemiol 1997;146:315-321.

188. Fagan TC, Deedwania PC: The cardiovascular dysmetabolic syndrome. Am J Med 1998;105(Suppl 1A):77S-82S.

189. Expert Panel on Detection, Evaluation, and Treatment of High Blood Cholesterol in Adults: Executive summary of the third report of the national cholesterol education program (NCEP) Expert Panel on Detection, Evaluation, and Treatment of High Blood Cholesterol in Adults (adult treatment panel III). JAMA 2001;285:2486-2497.

190. Hanefeld M, Scriba P: Das Metabolische Syndrom [Metabolic syndrome]. Internist (Berl) in 1996;377:679-680.

191. Grundy SM: Hypertriglyceridemia, insulin resistance, and the metabolic syndrome. Am J Cardiol 1999;83(Suppl F):25F-29F.

192. Grundy SM: Hypertriglyceridemia, atherogenic dyslipidemia, and the metabolic syndrome. Am J Cardiol 1998;81(Suppl B): 19B-25B.

193. Hall JE, Brands MW, Zappe DH, Galicia AG: Insulin resistance, hyperinsulinemia, and hypertension: Causes, consequences, or merely correlations? PSEBM 1995;208:317-329.

194. Mark AL, Anderson EA: Genetic factors determine the blood pressure response to insulin resistance and hyperinsulinemia: A call to refocus the insulin hypothesis of hypertension. Proc Soc Exp Biol Med 1995;208:330-336.

195. Reaven GM, Lithell H, Landsberg L: Hypertension and associated metabolic abnormalities—the role of insulin resistance and the sympathoadrenal system. N Engl J Med 1996;334:374-381.

196. Opara JU, Levine JH: The deadly quartet—the insulin resistance syndrome. South Med J 1997;90:1162-1168.

197. Jeppesen J, Hein HO, Suadicani P, Gyntelberg F: High triglycerides and low HDL cholesterol and blood pressure and risk of ischemic heart disease. Hypertension 2000;36:226-232.

198. McKeigue PM, Ferrie JE, Pierpoint T, Marmot MG: Association of early-onset coronary heart disease in South Asian men with glucose intolerance and hyperinsulinemia. Circulation 1993;87: 152-161.

199. Korpilahti K, Syvänne M, Engblom E, et al: Components of the insulin resistance syndrome are associated with progression of atherosclerosis in non-grafted arteries 5 years after coronary artery bypass surgery. Eur Heart J 1998;19:711-719.

200. Sprecher DL, Pearce GL: How deadly is the "deadly quartet"?—a post-CABG evaluation. J Am Coll Cardiol 2000;36:1159-1165.

201. Reaven GM, Chen I, Jeppesen J, et al: Insulin resistance and hyperinsulinemia in individuals with small, dense, low density lipoprotein particles. J Clin Invest 1993;92:141-146.

202. Yarnell JWG, Patterson CC, Bainton D, Sweetnam PM: Is metabolic syndrome a discrete entity in the general population? Evidence from the Caerphilly and Speedwell population studies. Heart 1998;79:248-252.

203. Zavaroni I, Bonini L, Gasparini P, et al: Hyperinsulinemia in a normal population as a predictor of non-insulin-dependent diabetes melitus, hypertension, and coronary heart disease: The Barilla Factory revisited. Metabolism 1999;48:989-994.

204. Meigs JB, D'Agostino RB, Wilson PWF, et al: Risk variable clustering in the insulin resistance syndrome—the Framingham offspring study. Diabetes 1997;46:1594-1600.

205. World Health Organization: Obesity: Preventing and managing the global epidemic. Report of a WHO consultation on obesity, Geneva, Switzerland, June 3-5, 1997. Geneva, WHO, 2000. WHO Technical Report Series No. 894 (available at http://whqlibdoc.int.hq/1998/WHO/NUT/NCD/98.1).

206. National Institutes of Health: Clinical guidelines on the identification, evaluation, and treatment of overweight and obesity in adults: The evidence report. Obes Res 1998;6(Suppl 2): 51-209.

207. Khaodhiar L, Blackburn GL: Obesity assessment. Am Heart J 2001;142:1095-1101.

208. Bray GA, Ryan GH: Clinical evaluation of the overweight patient. Endocrine 2000;13:167-186.

209. WHO expert committee: Physical status: The use and interpretation of anthropometry. WHO technical report series 854. Geneva, World Health Organization, 1995.

210. Must A, Spadano J, Coakley EH, et al: The disease burden associated with overweight and obesity. JAMA 1999;282:1523-1529.

211. Willett W, Dietz WH, Colditz GA: Primary care: Guidelines for healthy weight. N Engl J Med 1999;341:427-434.

212. Calle EE, Thun MJ, Petrelli JM, et al: Body-mass index and mortality in a propective cohort of US adults. N Engl J Med 1999;341: 1097-1110.

213. Manson JE, Willett WC, Stampfer MJ, et al: Body weight and mortality among women. N Engl J Med 1995;333:677-685.

214. Wilson PWF, D'Agostino RB, Levy D, et al: Prediction of coronary heart disease risk using risk factor categories. Circulation 1998;97:1837-1847.

215. Ruige JB, Assendelft WJJ, Dekker JM, et al: Insulin and risk of cardiovascular disease: A meta-analysis. Circulation 1998;97: 996-1001.

216. Lakka H-M, Lakka TA, Tuomilehto J, et al: Hyperinsulinemia and the risk of cardiovascular death and acute coronary and cerebrovascular events in men—the Kupio Ischemic Heart Disease Risk Factor study. Arch Intern Med 2000;160:1160-1168.

217. U.S. Bureau of Census: Table No. 118. In: Statistical abstract of the United States 1989. 109th edition. Washington, D.C., U.S. Bureau of Census, 1989, p 79.

218. Tuljapurkar S, Li N, Boe C: A universal pattern of mortality decline in the G7 countries. Nature 2001;405:789-792.

219. American Heart Association: 2001 Heart and Stroke Statistical Update. Dallas, American Heart Association, 2000.

220. Menotti A, Farchi G, Seccareccia F, and the RIFLE research group: The prediction of coronary heart disease mortality as a function of major risk factors in over 30 000 men in the Italian RIFLE pooling project. A comparison with the MRFIT primary screenees. J Cardiovasc Risk 1994;1:263-270.

221. Vlietstra RE, Kronmal RA, Frye RL, et al: Factors affecting the extent and severity of coronary artery disease in patients enrolled in the Coronary Artery Surgery Study. Arteriosclerosis 1982;2:208-215.

222. The Bezafibrate Infarction Prevention (BIP) Study Group, Israel: Lipids and lipoproteins in symptomatic coronary heart disease—distribution, intercorrelations, and significance for risk classification in 6700 men and 1500 women. Circulation 1992;86:839-848.

223. Köhler E, Fenzl R, Schönfeld R, Tataru MC: Untersuchungen über den Zusammenhang zwischen dem Risikoprofil und dem Schweregrad bzw. dem Manifestationsalter der koronaren Herzkrankheit (KHK)—Befunde von 3715 Patienten [Studies on the relationship between risk-profile and degree of severity resp. age at manifestation of coronary artery disease (CAD)—data of 3715 patients]. Z Kardiol 1992;81:310-319.

224. Prescott E, Hippe M, Schnohr P, et al: Smoking and the risk of myocardial infarction in women and men: Longitudinl population study. BMJ 1998;316:1043-1047.

225. Jousilahti P, Vartiainen E, Tuomilehto J, Puska P: Sex, age, cardiovascular risk factors, and coronary heart disease—a prospective follow-up study of 14 786 middle-aged men and women in Finland. Circulation 1999;99:1165-1172.

226. White AD, Rosamond WD, Chambless LE, et al for the Atherosclerosis Risk in Communities (ARIC) study investigators. Sex and race in short-term prognosis after acute coronary heart disease events: The Atherosclerosis Risk in Communities (ARIC) study. Am Heart J 1999;138:540-548.

227. Yusuf S, Reddy S, Ounpuu S, Anand S: Global burden of cardiovascular diseases. Part I: General considerations, the epidemiologic transition, risk factors, and impact of urbanization. Circulation 2001;104:2746-2753.

228. Hennekens CH: Increasing burden of cardiovascular disease: Current knowledge and future directions for research on risk factors. Circulation 1998;97:1095-1102.

229. Grundy SM, Balady GJ, Criqui MH, et al: Primary prevention of coronary heart disease: guidance from Framingham—a statement for healthcare professionals from the AHA task force on risk reduction. Circulation 1998;97:1876-1887.

230. Hopkins PN, Williams RR: A survey of 246 suggested coronary risk factors. Atherosclerosis 1981;40:1-52.

231. Libby P: Molecular basis of the acute coronary syndromes. Circulation 1995;91:2844-2850.

232. Libby P: Current concepts of the pathogenesis of the acute coronary syndromes. Circulation 2001;104:365-372.

233. Forrester JS: Role of plaque rupture in acute coronary syndromes. Am J Cardiol 2000;86(Suppl J):15J-23J.

234. Hoshida S, Kato J, Nishino M, et al: Increased angiotensin-converting enzyme activity in coronary artery specimens from patients with acute coronary syndrome. Circulation 2001;103:630-633.

235. Valkonen VP, Pälvä H, Salonen JT, et al: Risk of acute coronary events and serum concentrations of asymmetrical dimethylarginine. Lancet 2001;358:2127-2128.

236. Liuzzo G, Biasucci LM, Gallimore JR, et al: The prognostic value of C-reactive protein and serum amyloid A protein in severe unstable angina. N Engl J Med 1994;331:417-424.

237. Toss H, Lindahl B, Siegbahn A, Wallentin L, for the FRISC study group: Prognostic influence of increased fibrinogen and C-reactive protein levels in unstable coronary artery disease. Circulation 1997;96:4204-4210.

238. Yokoya K, Takatsu H, Suzuki T, et al: Process of progression of coronary artery lesions from mild to moderate stenosis to moderate or severe stenosis—a study based on four serial coronary angiograms per year. Circulation 1999;100:903-909.

239. Kervinen H, Palosuo T, Manninen V, et al: Joint effects of C-reactive protein and other risk factors on acute coronary events. Am Heart J 2001;141:580-585.

240. Bogaty P, Poirier P, Simard S, et al: Biological profile in subjects with recurrent acute coronary events compared with subjects with long-standing stable angina. Circulation 2001;103:3062-3068.

241. Blankenberg S, Rupprecht HJ, Bickel C, et al for the AtheroGene investigators: Circulating cell adhesion molecules and death in patients with coronary artery disease. Circulation 2001;104:1336-1342.

242. Schumacher M, Halwachs G, Tatzber F, et al: Increased neopterin in patients with chronic and acute coronary syndromes. J Am Coll Cardiol 1997;30:703-707.

243. Kugiyama K, Ota Y, Sugiyama S, et al: Prognostic value of plasma levels of secretory type II phopholipase A_2 in patients with unstable angina pectoris. Am J Cardiol 2000;86:718-722.

244. Biasucci LM, Liuzzo G, Fantuzzi G, et al: Increasing levels of interleukin (IL)-1RA and IL-6 during the first 2 days of hospitalization in unstable angina are associated with increased risk of in-hospital events. Circulation 1999;99:2079-2084.

245. Appels A: Inflammation and the mental state before an acute coronary event. Ann Med 1999;31(Suppl 1):41-44.

246. Woods A, Brull DJ, Humphries SE, Montgomery HE: Genetics of inflammation and risk of coronary artery disease: The central role of interleukin-6. Eur Heart J 2000;21:1574-1583.

247. Lindmark E, Diderholm E, Wallentin L, Siegbahn A: Relationship between interleukin 6 and mortality in patients with unstable coronary artery disease—effects of an early invasive or noninvasive strategy. JAMA 2001;286:2107-2113.

248. Ikeda U, Ito T, Shimada K: Interleukin-6 and acute coronary syndromes. Clin Cardiol 2001;24:701-704.

249. Kanda T, Hirao Y, Oshima S, et al: Interleukin 8 as a sensitive marker of unstable coronary artery disease. Am J Cardiol 1996;77:304-307.

250. Aukrust P, Berge RK, Ueland T, et al: Interaction between chemokines and oxidative stress: Possible pathogenic role in acute coronary syndromes. J Am Coll Cardiol 2001;37:485-491.

251. Smith DA, Irving SD, Sheldon J, et al: Serum levels of the anti-inflammatory cytokine interleukin-10 are decreased in patients with unstable angina. Circulation 2001;104:746-749.

252. Mallat Z, Henry P, Fressonnet R, et al: Plasma levels of interleukin (IL)-18 are increased in patients with acute coronary syndromes and are associated with increased mortality at follow-up. Scientific sessions 2001, Anaheim [Abstract]. Circulation 2001 (Suppl II);104:390.

253. Haught WH, Mansour M, Rothlein R, et al: Alterations in circulating intercellular adhesion molecule-1 and L-selectin: Further evidence for chronic inflammation in ischemic heart disease. Am Heart J 1996;132:1-8.

254. Ogawa H, Yasue H, Miyao Y, et al: Plasma soluble intercellular adhesion molecule-1 levels in coronary circulation in patients with unstable angina. Am J Cardiol 1999;83:38-42.

255. Furman MI, Davidson MC, Anderson FA, et al: Relationship between elevated leukocyte count and hospital clinical events in patients with acute coronary syndromes: Findings from the Global Registry of Acute Coronary Events. Scientific sessions 2001, Anaheim [Abstract]. Circulation 2001(Suppl II);104:650.

256. Roma P, Catapano AL: Stress proteins and atherosclerosis. Atherosclerosis 1996;127:147-154.

257. Stefanadis C, Toutouzas K, Tsiamis E, et al: Increased local temperature in human coronary atherosclerotic plaques: An independent predictor of clinical outcome in patients undergoing a percutaneous coronary intervention. J Am Coll Cardiol 2001;37:1277-1283.

258. Goldstein JA, Demetriou D, Grines CL, et al: Multiple complex coronary plaques in patients with acute myocardial infarction. N Engl J Med 2000;343:915-922.

259. Gilles R, Finet G, Rossi R, et al: Does more than one plaque rupture in acute coronary syndromes? A three-vessel IVUS study. Scientific sessions 2001, Anaheim [Abstract]. Circulation 2001(Suppl II);104:650.

260. Inokubo Y, Hanada H, Ishizaka H, et al: Plasma levels of matrix metalloproteinase-9 and tissue inhibitor of metalloproteinase-1 are increased in the coronary circulation in patients with acute coronary syndrome. Am Heart J 2001;141:211-217.

261. Liuzzo G, Vallejo AN, Kopecky SL, et al: Molecular fingerprint of inferon-γ signaling in unstable angina. Circulation 2001;103:1509-1514.

262. Caligiuri G, Liuzzo G, Biasucci LM, Maseri A: Immune system activation follows inflammation in unstable angina: Pathogenetic implications. J Am Coll Cardiol 1998;32:1295-1304.

263. Taylor AJ, Burke AP, O'Malley PG, et al: A comparison of the Framingham risk index, coronary artery calcification, and culprit plaque morphology in sudden cardiac death. Circulation 2000;101:1243-1248.

264. Al Suwaidi J, Hamasaki S, Higano ST, et al: Long-term follow-up of patients with mild coronary artery disease and endothelial dysfunction. Circulation 2000;101:948-954.

265. Mallat Z, Benamer H, Hugel B, et al: Elevated levels of shed membrane microparticles with procoagulant potential in the peripheral circulating blood of patients with acute coronary syndromes. Circulation 2000;101:841-843.

266. Zalai CV, Koloziejczyk D, Pilarski L, et al: Increased circulating monocyte activation in patients with unstable coronary syndromes. J Am Coll Cardiol 2001;38:1340-1347.

267. Liuzzo G, Goronzy JJ, Yang H, et al: Monoclonal T-cell proliferation and plaque instability in acute coronary syndromes. Circulation 2000;102:2883-2888.

268. Mach F, Schönbeck U, Bonnefoy J-Y, et al: Activation of monocyte/macrophage functions related to acute atheroma complication by ligation of CD40. Circulation 1997;96:396-399.

269. Schönbeck U, Varo N, Libby P, et al: Soluble CD40L and cardiovascular risk in women. Circulation 2001;104:2266-2268.

270. Ikeda H, Takajo Y, Ichiki K, et al: Increased soluble form of P-selectin in patients with unstable angina. Circulation 1995;92: 1693-1696.

271. Furman MI, Barnard MR, Krueger LA, et al: Circulating monocyte-platelet aggregates are an early marker of acute myocardial infarction. J Am Coll Cardiol 2001;38:1002-1006.

272. Montalescot G, Philippe F, Ankri A, et al for the French investigators of the ESSENCE trial: Early increase of von Willebrand factor predicts adverse outcome in unstable coronary artery disease. Circulation 1998;98:294-299.

273. Thögersen AM, Jansson J-H, Boman K, et al: High plasminogen activator inhibitor and tissue plasminogen activator levels in plasma precede a first acute myocardial infarction in both men and women—evidence for the fibrinolytic system as an independent primary risk factor. Circulation 1998;98: 2241-2247.

274. Rumley A, Lowe GDO, Sweetnam PM, et al: Factor VIII, von Willebrand factor and the risk of major ischaemic heart disease in the Caerphilly Heart study. Br J Haematol 1999;105:110-116.

275. Saito I, Folsom AR, Brancati FL, et al: Nontraditional risk factors for coronary heart disease incidence among patients with diabetes: The Atherosclerosis Risk in Communities (ARIC) study. Ann Intern Med 2000;133:81-91.

276. Meade TW, Brozovic M, Chakrabarti RR, et al: Hemostatic function and ischaemic heart disease: Principal results of the Northwick Park Heart study. Lancet 1986;2:533-537.

277. Hoffmeister HM, Jur M, Wendel HP, et al: Alterations of coagulation and fibrinolytic and kallikrein-kinin systems in the acute and postacute phases in patients with unstable angina pectoris. Circulation 1995;91:2520-2527.

278. Redondo M, Watzke HH, Stucki B, et al: Coagulation factors II, V, VII, and X, prothrombin gene 20120G→A transition, and factor V Leiden in coronary artery disease—high factor V clotting activity is an independent risk factor for myocardial infarction. Arterioscler Thromb Vasc Biol 1999;19:1020-1025.

279. Kamphuisen PW, Eikenboom JCJ, Bertina RM: Elevated factor VIII levels and the risk of thrombosis. Arterioscler Thromb Vasc Biol 2001;21:731-738.

280. Al-Obaidi MK, Philippou H, Stubbs PJ, et al: Relationship between homocysteine, factor VIIa, and thrombin generation in acute coronary syndromes. Circulation 2000;101:372-377.

281. Cooper JA, Miller GJ, Bauer KA, et al: Comparison of novel hemostatic factors and conventional risk factors for prediction of coronary heart disease. Circulation 2000;102:2816-2822.

282. Oldgren J, Linder R, Grip L, et al: Coagulation activity and clinical outcome in unstable coronary artery disease. Arterioscler Thromb Vasc Biol 2001;21:1059-1064.

283. Misumi K, Ogawa H, Yasue H, et al: Comparison of plasma tissue factor levels in unstable and stable angina pectoris. Am J Cardiol 1998;81:22-26.

284. Serneri GGN, Boddi M, Poggesi L, et al: Activation of cardiac renin-angiotensin system in unstable angina. J Am Coll Cardiol 2001;38:49-55.

285. Stubbs PJ, Al-Obaidi MK, Conroy RM, et al: Effect of plasma homocysteine concentration on early and late events in patients with acute coronary syndromes. Circulation 2000;102:605-610.

286. Stubbs P, Seed M, Lane D, et al: Lipoprotein(a) as a risk predictor for cardiac mortality in patients with acute coronary syndromes. Eur Heart J 1998;19:1355-1364.

287. Holvoet P, Vanhaecke J, Janssens S, et al: Oxidized LDL and malondialdehyde-modified LDL in patients with acute coronary syndromes and stable coronary artery disease. Circulation 1998;98: 1487-1494.

288. Andreotti F, Sciahbasi A, de Gaetano A, et al: Comparison of insulin response to intravenous glucose in healed myocardial infarction, in "cooled-off" unstable and stable angina pectoris, and in healthy subjects. Am J Cardiol 1999;84:870-875.

289. Lobo RA, Carmina E: The importance of diagnosing the polycystic ovary syndrome. Ann Intern Med 2000;132:989-993.

290. Culleton BF, Larson MG, Kannel WB, Levy D: Serum uric acid and risk for cardiovascular disease and death: The Framingham Heart Study. Ann Intern Med 1999;131:7-13.

291. Johnson RJ, Tuttle KR: Much ado about nothing, or much to do about something? The continuing controversy over the role of uric acid in cardiovascular disease. Hypertension 2000;35: e10-e12.

292. Heeschen C, Van den Brand MJ, Hamm CW, Simoons ML, for the Capture investigators: Angiographic findings in patients with refractory unstable angina according to troponin T status. Circulation 1999;104:1509-1514.

293. Newby LK, Christenson RH, Ohman M, et al for the GUSTO-IIa investigators: Value of serial troponin T measures for early and late risk stratification in patients with acute coronary syndromes. Circulation 1998;98:1853-1859.

294. Holmvang L, Lüscher MS, Clemmensen P, et al and the TRIM study group: Very early risk stratification using combined ECG and biochemical assessment in patients with unstable coronary artery disease (Thrombin Inhibition in Myocardial Ischemia [TRIM]) substudy. Circulation 1998;98:2004-2009.

295. Camm AJ, Fox KM: Chlamydia pneumonia (and other infective agents) in atherosclerosis and acute coronary syndromes—how good is the evidence? Eur Heart J 2000;21:1046-1051.

296. Zhu J, Quyyumi AA, Muhlestein JB, et al: Lack of association of Helicobacter pylori infection with coronary artery disease and frequency of acute myocardial infarction or death. Am J Cardiol 2002;89:155-158.

297. Wannamethee SG, Shaper AG, Walker M: Changes in physical activity, mortality, and incidence of coronary heart disease in older men. Lancet 1998;351:1603-1608.

298. Ojio S, Takatsu H, Tanaka T, et al: Considerable time from the onset of plaque rupture and/or thrombi until the onset of acute myocardial infarction in humans—coronary angiographic findings within 1 week before the onset of infarction. Circulation 2000;102: 2063-2069.

299. Rentrop KP: Thrombi in acute coronary syndromes—revisited and revised. Circulation 2000;101:1619-1626.

300. Hunink MGM, Goldman L, Tosteson ANA, et al: The recent decline in mortality from coronary heart disease, 1980-1990. JAMA 1997;277:535-542.

301. Rosamond WD, Chambless LE, Folsom AR, et al: Trends in the incidence of myocardial infarction and in mortality due to coronary heart disease, 1987 to 1994. N Engl J Med 1998;339:861-867.

302. Capewell S, Beaglehole R, Sedon M, McMurray J: Explanation for the decline in coronary heart disease mortality rates in Auckland, New Zealand, between 1982 and 1993. Circulation 2000;102: 1511-1516.

303. Gaziano M: Global burden of cardiovascular disease. In: Braunwald E, Zipes DP, Libby P (eds): Heart Disease—A Textbook of Cardiovascular Medicine, 6th ed. Philadelphia, W.B. Saunders, 2000, pp 1-18.

304. Danet S, Richard F, Montaye M, et al: Unhealthy effects of atmospheric temperature and pressure on the occurrence of myocardial infarction and coronary deaths—a 10-year survey: The Lille-World Health Organization MONICA project (Monitoring Trends and Determinants in Cardiovascular Disease). Circulation 1999;100:e1-e7.

305. Yusuf S, Reddy S, Ounpuu S, Anand S: Global burden of cardio-vascular diseases. Part II: Variations in cardiovascular disease by specific ethnic groups and geographic regions and prevention strategies. Circulation 2001;104:2855-2864.

306. Chambless L, Keil U, Dobson A, et al for the WHO MONICA project: Population versus clinical view of case fatality from acute coronary heart disease. Circulation 1997;96:3849-3859.

307. Marmot MG, Syme SL, Kagan A, et al: Epidemiologic studies of coronary heart disease and stroke in Japanese men living in Japan, Hawaii and California: Prevalence of coronary artery disease and associated risk factors. Am J Epidemiol 1975;102:514-525.

308. Bang HO, Dyerberg J, Nielsen AB: Plasma lipid and lipoprotein pattern in Greenlandic west-coast Eskimos. N Engl J Med 1971;1:1143-1146.

309. Bang HO, Dyerberg J: Plasma lipids and lipoproteins in Greenlandic west-coast Eskimos. Acta Med Scand 1972;192:85-94.

310. Artaud-Wild SM, Connor SL, Sexton G, Connor WE: Differences in coronary mortality can be explained by differences in cholesterol and saturated fat intakes in 40 countries but not in France and Finland: A paradox. Circulation 1993;88:2771-2779.

311. Strom A, Jensen RA: Mortality from circulatory diseases in Norway 1940-1945. Lancet 1951;1:126-129.

312. Epstein FH: Cardiovascular disease epidemiology—a journey from the past into the future. Circulation 1996;93:1755-1764.

313. Goldman L, Cook EF: The decline in ischemic heart disease mortality rates—an analysis of the comparative effects of medical interventions and changes in lifestyle. Ann Intern Med 1984;101:825-836.

314. Mark DB, Naylor CD, Hlatky MA, et al: Use of medical resources and quality of life after acute myocardial infarction in Canada and the United States. N Engl J Med 1994;331:1130-1135.

315. Pilote L, Califf RM, Sapp S, et al for the GUSTO-1 investigators: Regional variation across the United States in the management of acute myocardial infarction. N Engl J Med 1995;333:565-572.

316. Holmes DR, Califf RM, van de Werf F, et al for the GUSTO-I investigators: Difference in countries' use of resources and clinical outcome after myocardial infarction: Results from the GUSTO trial. Lancet 1997;349:75-78.

317. Harrington RA: Clinical trials in acute coronary syndromes: Lessons from PURSUIT. Eur Heart J Suppl 1999;1(Suppl R):R28-R34.

318. Koskenvuo M, Kaprio J, Kesäniemi A, Sarna S: Differences in mortality from ischemic heart disease by marital status and social class. J Chron Dis 1980;33:95-106.

319. Salomaa V, Niemelä M, Miettinen H, et al: Relationship of socioeconomic status to the incidence and prehospital, 28-day, and 1-year mortality rates of acute coronary events in the FINMONICA myocardial infarction register study. Circulation 2000;101:1913-1918.

320. Cooper R, Cutler J, Desvigne-Nickens P, et al: Trends and disparities in coronary heart disease, stroke, and other cardiovascular diseases in the United States—findings of the national Conference on Cardiovascular Disease Prevention. Circulation 2000;102:3137-3147.

321. Ellsworth DL, Manolio TA: The emerging importance of genetics in epidemiologic research. I: Basic concepts in human genetics and laboratory technology. Ann Epidemiol 1999;9:1-16.

322. Ellsworth DL, Manolio TA: The emerging importance of genetics in epidemiologic research. II: Issues in study design and gene mapping. Ann Epidemiol 1999;9:75-90.

323. Ellsworth DL, Manolio TA: The emerging importance of genetics in epidemiologic research. III: Bioinformatics and statistical genetic methods. Ann Epidemiol 1999;9:207-224.

324. Wang DG, Fan J-B, Siao C-J, Berno A, et al: Large-scale identification, mapping, and genotyping of single-nucleotide polymorphisms in the human genome. Science 1998;280:1077-1082.

325. Risch NJ: Searching for genetic determinants in the new millennium. Nature 2000;405:847-856.

326. Subramanian G, Adams MD, Venter JG, Broder S: Implications of the human genome for understanding human biology and medicine. JAMA 2001;286:2296-2307.

327. Kraus WE: Genetic approaches for the investigation of genes associated with coronary heart disease. In: Granger CB, Kraus WE, Califf RM (eds): Proceedings of a Symposium Genetics of Coronary Heart Disease: Current Understanding and Future Prospects. Leesburg, Va., April 8-10, 1999. Am Heart J 2000;140(Suppl):S27-S35.

328. Cambien F, Poirier O, Mallet C, Tiret L: Coronary heart disease and genetics: An epidemiologist's view. Mol Med Today 1997;May:197-203.

329. Lander ES, Schork NJ: Genetic dissection of complex traits. Science 1994;265:2037-2048.

330. Lander E, Kruglyak L: Genetic dissection of complex traits: Guidelines for interpreting and reporting linkage results. Nat Genet 1995;11:241-247.

331. Risch N, Merikangas K: The future of genetic studies of complex human diseases. Science 1996;273:1516-1517.

332. Kruglyak L: Prospects for whole-genome linkage disequilibrium mapping of common diseases. Nat Genet 1999;22:139-144.

333. Clayton D, McKeigue PM: Epidemiological methods for studying genes and environmental factors in complex disease. Lancet 2001;358:1356-1360.

334. Grimes DA, Schulz KF: An overview of clinical research: The lay of land. Lancet 2002;359:57-61.

335. Winkelmann BR, Hager J, Kraus WE, et al: Genetics of coronary heart disease: Current knowledge and research principles. In: Granger CB, Kraus WE, Califf RM (eds): Proceedings of a Symposium Genetics of Coronary Heart Disease: Current Understanding and Future Prospects. Leesburg, Va., April 8-10, 1999. Am Heart J 2000;140(Suppl):S11-S26.

336. Anonymous: Freely associating. Nat Genet 1999;22:1-2.

337. Cardon LR, Bell JI: Association study designs for complex diseases. Nat Rev Genet 2001;2:91-99.

338. Sing CF, Haviland MB, Templeton AR, et al: Biological complexity and strategies for finding DNA variations responsible for inter-individual variation in risk of a common chronic disease, coronary artery disease. Ann Med 1992;24:539-547.

339. Sing CF, Haviland MB, Reilly SL: Genetic architecture of common multifactorial disease. In: Ciba Foundation Symposium 197. Variation in the Human Genome. Chichester, Wiley, 1996, pp 211-232.

340. Keavney B, McKenzie CA, Connell JMC, et al: Measured haplotype analysis of the angiotensin-I converting enzyme gene. Hum Mol Genet 1998;7:1745-1751.

341. Brookes AJ: The essence of SNPs. Gene 1999;234:177-186.

342. Fallin D, Cohen A, Essioux L, et al: Genetic analysis of case/control data using estimated haplotype frequencies: Application to APOE locus variation and Alzheimer's disease. Genome Res 2001;11:143-151.

343. Johnson GCL, Esposito L, Barratt BJ, et al: Haplotype tagging for the identification of common disease genes. Nat Genet 2001;29:233-237.

344. Bader JS: The relative power of SNPs and haplotypes as genetic markers for association tests. Pharmacogenomics 2001;2:11-24.

345. Schork NJ, Fallin D, Thiel B, et al: The future of genetic case-control studies. Adv Genet 2001;42:191-211.

346. Lander ES: The new genomics: Global view of biology. Science 1996;274:536-539.

347. Stehbens WE: An appraisal of the epidemic rise of coronary heart disease and its decline. Lancet 1987;1:606-611.

348. Marenberg ME, Risch N, Berkman LF, et al: Genetic susceptibility to death from coronary heart disease in a study of twins. N Engl J Med 1994;330:1041-1046.

349. Jousilahti P, Puska P, Vartainen E, et al: Parental history of premature coronary heart disease: An independent risk factor of myocardial infarction. J Clin Epidemiol 1996;49:497-503.

350. Ciruzzi M, Schargrodsky H, Rozlosnik J, et al for the Argentine FRICAS (Factores de Riesgo Coronario en America del Sur) investigators: Frequency of family history of acute myocardial infarction. Am J Cardiol 1997;80:122-127.

351. Sesso HD, Lee IM, Gaziano JM, et al: Maternal and paternal history of myocardial infarction and risk of cardiovascular disease in men and women. Circulation 2001;104:393-398.

352. Topol EJ, McCarthy J, Gabriel S, et al for the GeneQuest investigators and collaborators: Single nucleotide polymorphisms in multiple novel thrombospondin genes may be associated with familial premature myocardial infarction. Circulation 2001;104:2641-2644.

353. Goodall AH, Curzen N, Panesar M, et al: Increased binding of fibrinogen to glycoprotein IIIa-proline 33 (HPA-1b, Pl^{A2}, Zw^b) positive platelets in patients with cardiovascular disease. Eur Heart J 1999;20:742-747.

354. Feng DL, Lindpaintner K, Larson MG, et al: Increased platelet aggregability associated with platelet GPIIIaPl^{A2} polymorphism—

the Framingham Offspring study. Arterioscler Thromb Vasc Biol 1999;19:1142–1147.

355. Undas A, Brummel K, Musial J, et al: Pl^{A2} polymorphism of β_3 integrins is associated with enhanced thrombin generation and impaired antithrombotic action of aspirin at the site of microvascular injury. Circulation 2001;104:2666–2672.

356. Wheeler GL, Braden GA, Bray PF, et al: Reduced inhibition by abciximab in platelets with the Pl^{A2} polymorphism. Am Heart J 2002;143:76–82.

357. Weiss EJ, Bray PF, Tayback M, et al: A polymorphism of a platelet glycoprotein receptor as an inherited risk factor for coronary thrombosis. N Engl J Med 1996;334:1090–1094.

358. Zotz RB, Winkelmann BR, Nauck M, et al: Polymorphism of platelet membrane glycoprotein IIIa: Human platelet antigen (HPA-1b/PLa2) is an inherited risk factor for premature myocardial infarction in coronary artery disease. Thromb Haemost 1998;79:731–735.

359. Mikkelsson J, Perola M, Laippala P, et al: Glycoprotein IIIa Pl$^{a1/a2}$ polymorphism and sudden cardiac death. J Am Coll Cardiol 2000;36:1317–1323.

360. Walter DH, Schächinger V, Elsner M, et al: Platelet glycoprotein IIIa polymorphisms and risk of coronary stent thrombosis. Lancet 1997;350:1217–1219.

361. Herrmann SM, Poirier O, Marques-Vidal P, et al: The Leu^{33}/Pro polymorphism (Pl^{A1}/ Pl^{A2}) of the glycoprotein IIIa (GPIIIa) receptor is not related to myocardial infarction in the ECTIM study. Thromb Haemostas 1997;77:1179–1181.

362. Ridker PM, Hennekens CH, Schmitz C, et al: Pl$^{a1/a2}$ polymorphism of platelet glycoprotein IIIa and risks of myocardial infarction, stroke, and venous thrombosis. Lancet 1997;349:385–388.

363. Aleksic N, Juneja H, Folsom AR, et al: Platelet Pl^{A2} allele and incidence of coronary heart disease—results from the Atherosclerosis Risk in Communities (ARIC) study. Circulation 2000;102: 1901–1905.

364. Kastrati A, Koch W, Gawaz M, et al: Pl^a polymorphism of glycoprotein IIIa and risk of adverse events after coronary stent placement. J Am Coll Cardiol 2000;36:84–89.

365. Laule M, Cascorbi I, Stangl V, et al: A1/A2 polymorphism of the glycoprotein IIIa and associations with excess procedural risk for coronary catheter interventions: A case-controlled study. Lancet 1999;353:708–712.

366. Cenarro A, Casao E, Civeira F, et al: PLA1/^{A2} polymorphism of platelet glycoprotein IIIa and risk of acute coronary syndromes in heterozygous familial hypercholesterolemia. Atherosclerosis 1999;143:99–104.

367. Zhu MM, Weedon J, Clark LT: Meta-analysis of the association of platelet glycoprotein IIIa PlA1/A2 polymorphism with myocardial infarction. Am J Cardiol 2000;86:1000–1005.

368. Williams MS, Bray PF: Genetics of arterial prothrombotic risk states. Exp Biol Med 2001;226:409–419.

369. Lane DA, Grant PJ: Role of hemostatic gene polymorphism in venous and arterial thrombotic disease. Blood 2000;95: 1517–1532.

370. Beer JH, Pederiva S, Pontiggia L: Genetics of platelet receptor single-nucleotide polymorphisms: Clinical implications in thrombosis. Ann Med 2000;32(Suppl 1):10–14.

371. Mosfegh K, Wuillemin WA, Redondo M, et al: Association of two silent polymorphisms of platelet glycoprotein Ia/IIa receptor with risk of myocardial infarction: A case-control study. Lancet 1998;353:351–354.

372. Santoso S, Kunicki TJ, Kroll H, et al: Association of the platelet glycoprotein Ia C$_{807}$T gene polymorphism with nonfatal myocardial infarction in younger patients. Blood 1999;93:2449–2453.

373. Casorelli I, de Stefano V, Leone AM, et al: The C807T/G873A polymorphism in the platelet glycoprotein Ia gene and the risk of acute coronary syndrome in the Italian population. Br J Haematol 2001;114:150–154.

374. Bray PF: Platelet glycoprotein polymorphisms as risk factors for thrombosis. Curr Opin Hematol 2000;7:284–289.

375. Meisel C, Afshar-Kharghan V, Cascorbi I, et al: Role of Kozak sequence polymorphism of platelet glycoprotein Ibα as a risk factor for coronary artery disease and catheter interventions. J Am Coll Cardiol 2001;38:1023–1027.

376. Mikkelsson J, Perola M, Penttilä A, Karhunen PJ: Platelet glycoprotein Ibα HPAA-2 Met/VNTR B haplotype as a genetic predictor of myocardial infarction and sudden death. Circulation 2001;104: 876–880.

377. Croft SA, Samani NJ, Teare MD, et al: Novel platelet membrane glycoprotein VI Dimorphism is a risk factor for myocardial infarction. Circulation 2001;104:1459–1463.

378. Kunicki TJ: The influence of platelet collagen receptor polymorphisms in hemostasis and thrombotic disease. Arterioscler Thromb Vasc Biol 2002;22:14–20.

379. Iwai N, Shimoike H, Nakamura Y, et al: The 4G/5G polymorphism of the plasminogen activator inhibitor gene is associated with the time course to acute coronary syndromes. Atherosclerosis 1998;136:109–114.

380. Iacoviello L, Zito F, di Castelnuovo A, et al: Contribution of factor VII, fibrinogen and fibrinolytic components to the risk of ischaemic cardiovascular disease: Their genetic determinants. Fibrinol Proteolys 1998;12:259–276.

381. Moatti D, Seknadji P, Galand C, et al: Polymorphisms of the tissue factor pathway inhibitor (TFPI) gene in patients with acute coronary syndromes and in healthy subjects—impact of the V264M substitution on plasma levels of TFPI. Arterioscler Thromb Vasc Biol 1999;19:862–869.

382. Park HY, Kwon HM, Kim D, et al: The angiotensin converting enzyme genetic polymorphism in acute coronary syndrome—ACE polymorphism as a risk factor of acute coronary syndrome. J Korean Med Sci 1997;12:391–397.

383. Snapir A, Heinonen P, Tuomainen TP, et al: An insertion/deletion polymorphism in the α_{2B}-adrenergic receptor gene is a novel genetic risk factor for acute coronary events. J Am Coll Cardiol 2001;37:1516–1522.

384. Wamala SP, Murray MA, Horsten M, et al: Socioeconomic status and determinants of hemostatic function in healthy women. Arterioscler Thromb Vasc Biol 1999;19:485–492.

385. Burzotta F, di Castelnuovo A, Amore C, et al: 4G/5G promoter PAI-1 gene polymorphism is associated with plasmatic PAI-1 activity in Italians: A model of gene-environment interaction. Thromb Haemostas 1998;79:354–358.

386. Henry M, Tregouet DA, Alessi MC, et al: Metabolic determinants are much more important than genetic polymorphism in determining the PAI-1 activity and antigen plasma concentrations—a family study with part of the Stanislas cohort. Arterioscler Thromb Vasc Biol 1998;18:84–91.

387. Humphries SE, Panahloo A, Montgomery HE, et al: Gene-environment interaction in the determination of levels of haemostatic variables involved in thrombosis and fibrinolysis. Thromb Haemostas 1997;78:457–461.

388. Ardissino D, Mannucci PM, Merlini PA, et al: Prothrombotic genetic risk factors in young survivors of myocardial infarction. Blood 1999;94:46–51.

389. Barakat K, Kennon S, Hitman GA, et al: Interaction between smoking and the glycoprotein IIIA PL^{A2} polymorphism in non-St-elevation acute coronary syndromes. J Am Coll Cardiol 2001;38: 1639–1643.

chapter 4

Natural History and Prognosis

Juan Carlos Kaski
Ramón Arroyo Espliguero

In the United States alone, unstable angina (UA) accounted for more than 1 million hospital admissions in 1996.[1] Patients with UA constitute a heterogeneous group because of the diversity of pathogenic mechanisms responsible for the condition and the different clinical manifestations of the syndrome. Although most patients with UA have obstructive coronary artery disease (CAD), the severity of the coronary lesions varies markedly and coronary arteriograms appear normal in a sizable proportion of patients. The most common pathogenic mechanism in UA is atheromatous plaque disruption with subsequent acute coronary thrombosis,[2,3] a mechanism shared with other acute coronary syndromes.

The term *acute coronary syndrome* is currently used to describe the spectrum of conditions that includes UA, non–ST-segment elevation myocardial infarction (NSTEMI) and ST-segment elevation myocardial infarction (STEMI).[4] Pathogenesis and clinical manifestations are similar in patients with UA and in those with NSTEMI. The two diagnoses are distinguished mainly by the results of cardiac enzyme levels or other specific tests of myocardial damage such as cardiac troponins T and I.

Prognosis may vary markedly among patients with UA; this may be explained by the heterogeneous nature of the condition. As a clinical syndrome, unstable angina pectoris encompasses a variety of clinical presentations associated with transient episodes of acute myocardial ischemia. These episodes are caused by obstructions to coronary blood flow and involve different pathophysiologic mechanisms, including intracoronary atheromatous plaque rupture, platelet aggregation, thrombus formation, and increased vasomotor tone.[5,6] Few data are available on the prognosis of "real life" patients with UA because reports have often focused on selected patient subgroups,[7-12] which makes comparison among studies difficult. On average, however, patients with UA are at high risk for major cardiovascular events as shown by the fact that approximately 6% to 8% of patients suffer a nonfatal myocardial infarction (MI) or die within the first year after diagnosis.[13,14] In other series, progression to MI has been reported to occur in 7% to 16% of patients.[15-17] The risk in a given patient depends on the underlying pathophysiology and clinical presentation.[7,8,17-22] It has been reported that the incidence of MI and cardiac death is higher in the first 6 to 8 weeks after the onset of UA.[23] The successful management of UA requires appropriate risk stratification and fast effective treatment.

From a historical perspective, although regarding risk stratification and management of typical Q-wave MI has seen steady progress, it has taken cardiologists much longer to systematically characterize a syndrome that is intermediate in severity between chronic stable angina and NSTEMI. The heterogeneity of UA and the lack of a clear agreed-on definition gave way to a large number of denominations to describe this syndrome associated with severe transient myocardial ischemia.[24-27] What could be considered to represent the first formal report on the condition that we now know as UA goes back to 1923, when Wearn[28] described the presence of prolonged attacks of angina pectoris preceding the development of acute MI. Later, in 1937, Sampson and Eliaser[29] and Feil[30] separately described a syndrome consisting of severe prolonged angina that often led to acute MI and named it *impending acute MI*. Other terms that have been used to label this condition and describe its prognostic importance include *preinfarction angina, crescendo or accelerated angina,* and *intermediate coronary syndrome.* Indeed, in most series,[32] 30% to 60% of patients who experience acute MI also experience a prodrome of UA. The prognostic importance of UA is now well established as it has become apparent that only a minority of patients recover from the condition without experiencing either serious cardiovascular complications or chronic forms of angina pectoris.[27,32,33]

This chapter focuses on the prognostic implications of UA and discusses some of the mechanisms responsible for impaired patient outcome. Other more specific aspects, such as patient risk stratification, the prognostic role of markers of myocardial damage and inflammation, and clinical classifications of UA, are not addressed here because they are discussed in other specific chapters.

NATURAL HISTORY AND PROGNOSIS

As a diagnostic category, UA includes patients at different levels of risk for an unfavorable outcome. Of approximately 7 million people attending emergency departments with chest pain suggestive of acute coronary syndrome in the United States, 20% to 25% have a confirmed diagnosis of acute coronary syndrome (UA or MI).[34,35] The diagnosis is based on the patient's description of chest pain suggestive of acute myocardial ischemia. A diagnosis of NSTEMI is based on the presence of both a clinical presentation compatible with UA and abnormal concentrations of circulating markers of myocardial damage (such as cardiac troponin T or I or cardiac enzymes).[36] As expected, given the heterogeneous nature of UA, prognosis differs markedly among patients and ranges from an excellent to a high risk of MI and death. This depends on a number of factors that include clinical presentation, gender, pathogenic mechanisms, previous history of CAD, presence of risk factors, electrocardiogram (ECG) changes, the extent of CAD, the state of the left ventricular function, and biochemical markers of myocardial damage.

The natural history of UA/NSTEMI follows, on average, a more benign course than that of STEMI.[37-40] However, certain subgroups of patients with UA appear to have a much worse prognosis than others. Prospective studies have reported a 2.4% mortality rate at 42 days of follow-up and 2.9% incidence of new or recurrent MI. The actual patient mortality rate is higher, ranging from 3.5% to 4.5% at 30 days. The new or recurrent MI rate has been reported to be 6% to 12% in different studies.[41-44]

A unique study carried out by Mulcahy et al[22] in Ireland in the late 1970s is perhaps the most representative investigation of the natural history of UA. This study described the clinical outcome of patients with UA who were treated conservatively without the routine use of β-adrenergic blocking agents, calcium antagonists, anticoagulant agents, or nitrates. This prospective study included 101 consecutive patients with UA (70 men, mean age 57 years and 31 women, mean age 61 years) admitted to the coronary care unit at St. Vincent's Hospital in Dublin from July 1975 to June 1977. The diagnosis of UA was based on the presence of typical chest pain, transient ST-segment and T-wave changes, and normal cardiac enzyme levels. Patients entered the study if no clinical, ECG, or biochemical evidence of MI was found within 24 hours of admission. Drugs were administered for symptomatic reasons only and included β-adrenergic blockers (5 patients), anticoagulants (2 patients), and bed rest; such treatment was continued until the patient was free of pain for 24 hours. Patients were subdivided in three groups according to clinical presentation: (1) chronic exertional angina with recent deterioration of symptoms and pain at rest, (2) recent onset of angina on effort with pain at rest, and (3) recent onset of pain at rest. The study showed a 28-day mortality rate of 4% and a total 1-year cardiac mortality rate of 10%. Nonfatal MI developed in 9% of patients during the first 28 days and in 12% at 1 year of follow-up (Table 4-1).

Lessons From Recent Trials and Registries

Large-scale trials assessing pharmacologic agents, mainly low-molecular-weight heparins and platelet glycoprotein

TABLE 4–1 CARDIAC MORBIDITY AND MORTALITY AT 28 DAYS AND 1 YEAR IN UNTREATED PATIENTS WITH UNSTABLE ANGINA

	NONFATAL MI (n)	DEATH (n)	TOTAL (n)
28 days	9	4	13
1 year*	3	6†	11
Total	12	10	24

MI, myocardial infarction.
*One patient lost to follow-up. Only two patients underwent coronary angiography and coronary artery bypass surgery during the first year.
†One patient who died late had a nonfatal myocardial infarction during the first 28 days.
From Mulcahy D, Daly L, Graham I, et al: Unstable angina: Natural history and determinants of prognosis. Am J Cardiol 1981;48:525–528, with permission.

IIb/IIIa blockers, have provided useful information regarding prognosis in patients with UA.[42-50] The rate of death or MI at 30 days ranged from 5.5% to 15.7% in selected patients recruited in these studies (data are summarized in Tables 4-2 and 4-3). Important information has been reported by the Global Registry of Acute Coronary Events (GRACE) Investigators[51] regarding outcome of patients with UA/NSTEMI (Fig. 4-1). The GRACE registry is the largest multinational registry (14 countries) to date, encompassing the whole spectrum of acute coronary syndromes. Patients entered into GRACE are representative of the general population with acute coronary syndromes and cover the full spectrum of hospital facilities (94 hospitals) and therapeutic approaches. Each center in the Registry recruited the first 10 to 20 consecutive patients with CAD presenting with qualifying symptoms.

The aim of the study was to provide clear and accurate information on demographics, practice strategies, and patient outcome in subjects presenting with UA, NSTEMI, and STEMI. Up to 2001, over 12,000 patients had been recruited, of whom 40% had UA, 28% had NSTEMI, and 32% had STEMI. Regarding in-hospital outcome, death occurred in 7% of patients with STEMI, 6% of patients with NSTEMI, and 3% of patients with UA. Reinfarction developed in 3%, 2%, and 0.2% of patients, respectively, and recurrent angina with ST-segment changes occurred in 12%, 15%, and 14% of patients, respectively (see Fig. 4-1A). In-hospital to 6-month rates of death were 12% in STEMI, 13% in NSTEMI, and 8% in patients with UA (see Fig. 4-1B). An important finding in this study is that patients with UA considered to be at low risk for serious cardiovascular events—i.e., those without ECG changes, troponin elevations, or hemodynamic abnormalities—experienced an impaired outcome at 6 months. Readmission with angina occurred in 17%, revascularization was required in 9%, and angiography was required in 51%. Death occurred in 2.2% of cases, and MI developed in 0.2% of patients (see Fig. 4-1C).

TABLE 4–2 INCIDENCE OF DEATH AND MYOCARDIAL INFARCTION IN CLINICAL TRIALS OF LARGE LOW-MOLECULAR-WEIGHT HEPARIN

TRIAL	STUDY DRUG	N	Death 6 days (%)	Death or MI 6 days (%)	Death 40 days (%)	Death or MI 40 days (%)	Death 150 days (%)	Death or MI 150 days (%)
FRISC[45]	Dalteparin	741	0.9	1.8	2.6	8.0	5.4	14.0
	Placebo	757	1.1	4.8	3.0	10.7	5.5	15.5

TRIAL	STUDY DRUG	N	Death 48 hours (%)	Death, MI, or UA 48 hours (%)	Death 14 days (%)	Death, MI, or UA 14 days (%)	Death 30 days (%)	Death, MI, or UA 30 days (%)
ESSENCE[46]	Enoxaparin	1607	0.5	6.2	2.2	16.6	2.9	19.8
	UFH	1564	0.4	7.4	2.3	19.8	3.6	23.3

TRIAL	STUDY DRUG	N	Death 48 hours (%)	Death or MI 48 hours (%)	Death 14 days (%)	Death or MI 14 days (%)	Death 43 days (%)	Death or MI 43 days (%)
TIMI 11B[47]	Enoxaparin	1953	0.6	1.7	2.2	5.7	3.8	7.9
	UFH	1957	0.3	2.1	2.8	6.9	4.0	8.9

MI, myocardial infarction; N, number of patients; UA, unstable angina; UFH, unfractionated heparin.

■ ■ ■

TABLE 4–3 INCIDENCE OF DEATH AND MYOCARDIAL INFARCTION IN CLINICAL TRIALS OF LARGE GLYCOPROTEIN IIB/IIA INHIBITORS

TRIAL	STUDY DRUG	N	DEATH 30 DAYS (%)	DEATH OR MI 30 DAYS (%)	DEATH OR MI 6 MONTHS (%)
PRISM[43]	Tirofiban	1616	3.6	5.8	
	Placebo	1616	2.3	7.1	
PRISM-PLUS[44]	Tirofiban	773	3.6	8.7	12.3
	Placebo	797	4.5	11.9	15.3
PARAGON-A[48]	Lamifiban (low dose)	755	3.0	10.6	13.7
	Lamifiban (high dose)	769	3.6	12.0	16.4
	Placebo	758	2.9	11.7	15.3
PURSUIT[42]	Eptifibatide	4722	3.5	14.2	
	Placebo	4739	3.7	15.7	
PARAGON-B[49]	Lamifiban	2600	2.9	10.6	
	Placebo	2569	3.3	11.5	
GUSTO IV[50]	Abciximab (24 h)	2590	3.4	8.2	
	Abciximab (48 h)	2612	4.3	9.1	
	Placebo	2598	3.9	8.0	

MI, myocardial infarction.

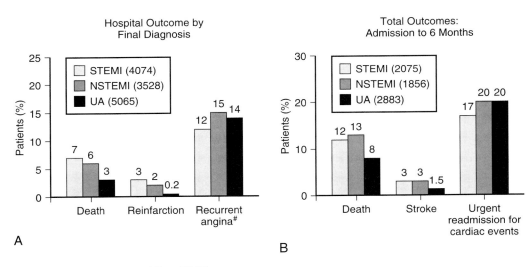

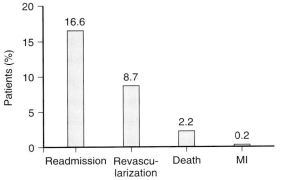

FIGURE 4–1. Preliminary results from the Global Registry of Acute Coronary Events (GRACE). *A,* Hospital outcome by final diagnosis. *B,* Total outcomes: admission to 6 months. *C,* Outcome of "low-risk" patients with ACS at 6 months. #, Recurrent angina: symptoms plus ST-segment deviation; *, Low-risk: absence of dynamic ECG changes, no troponin elevation, no arrhythmia, and no hypotension. ACS, acute coronary syndromes; ECG, electrocardiogram; MI, myocardial infarction; NSTEMI, non–ST-segment elevation myocardial infarction; STEMI, ST-segment elevation myocardial infarction; UA, unstable angina. (From Fox KAA, et al: Preliminary data from the Global Registry of Acute Coronary Events [GRACE]. Presented at XXII European Society of Cardiology Annual Congress, Amsterdam, The Netherlands, August, 2000.)

Outcome According to Clinical Presentation

It has been suggested that a comprehensive clinical classification of UA may help to identify patients at higher risk for MI and sudden death and may provide clues as to possible disease mechanisms.[33,52-54] For a clinical classification to be useful, it should provide prognostic information, help to identify patients who are at high risk, and guide management.

In 1989, Braunwald proposed a clinical classification of UA,[33] which has been widely used in the clinical setting to categorize patients according to the severity of clinical manifestations. Briefly, the Braunwald classification includes several categories based on the presence of acute angina while at rest (within the 48 hours before presentation), "subacute" angina while at rest (within the previous month but not within the 48 hours before presentation), or new onset of accelerated (progressively more severe) angina; and the clinical circumstances in which UA develops, defined as angina in the *presence* or *absence* of other conditions (e.g., anemia, fever, hypoxia, tachycardia, or thyrotoxicosis) or angina occurring within 2 weeks after an acute MI.

Several studies have validated the clinical usefulness of the classification,[55-57] which allows identification of patients at high risk for cardiovascular events. In the Thrombolysis in Myocardial Ischemia (TIMI) III registry, which recruited over 3000 consecutive patients with UA/NSTEMI, the Braunwald classification provided an accurate prediction of risk.[57] Patients at higher risk for death and MI at 1 year were identified by the severity of their angina and the clinical circumstances related to the development of UA. Very-high-risk patients with UA were those with acute angina at rest and post-MI UA.[57]

Bertolet et al[58] conducted a clinical study of UA (recent-onset UA, crescendo angina, and postinfarction UA) in a relatively small number (N = 129) of patients who were followed for over 12 months after discharge from the hospital. Coronary angiographic features were similar in these patient subgroups. This study confirmed that mortality was significantly higher in post-MI

patients with UA (7.7%) compared with those in the other categories (1.1%). However, contrary to findings in other more recent, well-designed studies, subclassification of patients based on clinical characteristics at presentation in the Bertolet et al[58] study was not useful in predicting MI or recurrent angina requiring revascularization. Moreover, cardiac risk factors were present in a majority of these patients but neither their presence nor their number correlated with future events. Another intriguing finding of the study was that patients without ST-segment changes at admission, frequently considered to represent a relatively low-risk group, were just as likely to experience cardiac events as other subgroups. The GRACE Investigators[51] have reported similar findings.

Another prospective study[56] assessed the prognostic value of clinical classification in 417 consecutive patients admitted to hospital for acute chest pain suggestive of myocardial ischemia but without MI. Two hospitals in Rotterdam, The Netherlands, created a prospective registry over a 7-month period between 1988 and 1989. A final diagnosis was established using all information obtained during admission. Patients with confirmed UA were classified according to Braunwald,[33] and it was found that 74% of patients belonged to class III. Follow-up data (6 months) were available in 97% of patients. Recurrent pain developed in 137 patients within 48 hours after admission; this finding was more frequent in class III patients compared with those in class I or II (P = .0001) (Fig. 4-2). The strongest predictor of recurrent ischemia was the time elapsed from the previous episode. The probability of new recurrent pain rapidly decreased to less than 10% after 3 days. Progression to MI or death during the in-hospital period was more common in class III patients and in those with post-MI angina (class C) (Table 4-4). Figure 4-3 shows survival, survival without infarction, and MI-free survival without intervention at the 6-month follow-up in the different patient subgroups.

This study[56] also showed that old age, male gender, post-MI UA (class C), and maximal anti-anginal therapy were independent predictors of mortality. One of the

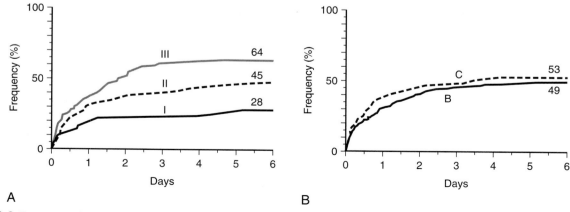

FIGURE 4-2. Frequency of recurrent ischemia in unstable angina subgroups, according to Braunwald's classification. *A,* Recurrent ischemia after admission was more frequent in patients with acute angina at rest (class III) compared with those in class I or II (P < .0001). *B,* There was no significant difference between patients with primary (class B) and postinfarction (class C) angina. (From van Miltenburg-van Zijl AJM, Simoons ML, Veerhoek RJ, et al: Incidence and follow-up of Braunwald subgroups in unstable angina pectoris. J Am Coll Cardiol 1995;25:1286-1292.)

■ ▪ ■

TABLE 4–4   CLINICAL EVENTS AND INTERVENTION DURING HOSPITAL ADMISSION IN DIFFERENT BRAUNWALD SUBGROUPS

CLASS	TOTAL	AMI/DEATH	ANGIOGRAPHY*	PTCA/CABG*
Severity				
I	55	2 (4)	22 (40)	19 (35)
II	100	4 (4)	15 (15)	10 (10)
III	127	14 (11)[†]	100 (79)[*‡]	71 (56)[‡]
Clinical Circumstances				
B	236	13 (6)	104 (44)	77 (33)
C	46	7 (46)[†]	33 (72)[*‡]	23 (50)[†]
Total	282	20	137	100

AMF, acute myocardial infarction; CABG, coronary artery bypass graft; PTCA, percutaneous transluminal coronary angioplasty.
*Including both emergency and elective procedures.
[†]P <.05.
[‡]P <.01.
Data presented are number (%) of patients.
From van Miltenburg-van Zijl AJM, Simoons ML, Veerhoek RJ, et al: Incidence and follow-up of Braunwald subgroups in unstable angina pectoris. J Am Coll Cardiol 1995;25:1286–1292.

strengths of this study is that the whole spectrum of UA was represented in the registry. This contrasts with previous studies on UA, which only included selected patients or restricted analysis to specific subgroups.[8,18,19,59-62] In this Dutch population with mainly class III UA, the rate of death or MI was 4.3% during the in-hospital period and 9.6% at 6-month follow-up. Survival without MI varied between 80% and 91%, depending on clinical severity. This outcome compares favorably with other reports[8,22,61,63,64] and may be due to the intensive medical therapy and high intervention rate (35%) in these institutions. Prognosis was found to

correlate with class severity; the worst prognosis was found in classes III and C.

Outcome According to ECG Changes at Presentation

The importance of the ECG as a marker of risk in UA is well established. Transient ischemic ST-segment changes have been shown to be useful markers of impaired patient outcome in several studies (Table 4–5).[65-67] T-wave changes, however, appear to be of lesser value than ST shifts in terms of risk stratification according to

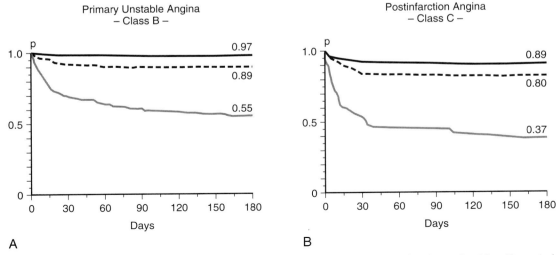

FIGURE 4–3. Six-month follow-up outcomes for *(A)* primary unstable angina (class B) and *(B)* postinfarction angina (class C): survival *(solid lines)*, infarct-free survival *(dashed lines)*, and infarct-free survival without intervention *(lighter solid lines)*. P, probability. (From van Miltenburg-van Zijl AJM, Simoons ML, Veerhoek RJ, et al: Incidence and follow-up of Braunwald subgroups in unstable angina pectoris. J Am Coll Cardiol 1995;25:1286–1292.)

■■■

TABLE 4–5 ROLE OF ECG CHANGES: RISK OF DEATH OR MYOCARDIAL INFARCTION DURING THE 30-DAY, 6-MONTH, AND 1-YEAR FOLLOW-UP

	DEATH OR MYOCARDIAL INFARCTION		
	30-Day[*] (n)	6-Month[*] (n)	1-Year[†] (n)
ST-segment **elevation**	9.4% (P <.01)[‡]	12.3% (P <.01)	16.1% (P <.05)[§]
ST-segment **depression**	10.5% (P <.01)	15.4% (P <.01)	18.1% (P <.01)
ST-segment **elevation** and **depression**	12.4% (P <.01)	15.7% (P <.01)	25.6% (P <.001)
Isolated T-wave **inversion**	5.5% (P <.01)	8.1% (P <.01)	13.6% (P <.05)

[*]Risk of death or myocardial infarction during the 30-day and 6-month follow-up by electrocardiographic category (N = 12.124).

[†]The P values are a test for differences across the four electrocardiographic categories, based on likelihood ratio chi-square test.

(Data from Savonitto S, Ardissino D, Grangr CB, et al: Prognostic value of the admission electrocardiogram in actue coronary syndromes: The GUSTO IIb Investigators. JAMA 1999;281:707–713.)

[‡]Risk of death or myocardial infarction during 1-year follow-up with regard to different ST-T segment changes in ECG at rest obtained during the initial 3 days of hospitalization (N = 911).

[§]Significant differences compared to patients with normal ECG during the initial 3 days of hospitalization, who had a 7.6% 1-year risk of MI or death.

(Data from Nyman I, Areskog M, Areskog NH, et al: Very early risk stratification by electrocardiogram at rest in men with suspected unstable coronary artery disease: The RISC Study Group. J Intern Med 1993;234:293–301.)

recent data.[68,69] New or transient ST-segment shifts of 0.5 mm or the presence of left bundle branch block at admission with UA were shown to be associated with increased 1-year risk of MI or death (15.8% compared with 8.2% in patients without ECG abnormalities).[67,68]

According to the TIMI III report[68] and the findings of Hyde et al,[69] ST-segment depression of 0.5 mm on the admission ECG is associated with increased risk of death not only at 1-year (risk ratio 2.8, P < .001) but also at 4- year follow-up. It has been shown that the greater the ST-segment shift, the higher the risk (see Figure 13-3).[69,70] Similar findings were reported by the GUSTO (Global Use of STrategies to Open occluded coronary arteries) IIb trial.[67] In GUSTO IIb,[67] the presence of ST-segment depression of 0.5 mm was found to be associated with poor outcome at 30 and 180 days (see Fig. 13-2).

Results of these large investigation registries have confirmed previous reports by other authors. Patel et al[23] assessed the occurrence of death, MI, and need for revascularization over a median follow-up of 2.6 years in 212 patients with UA (presenting within 24 hours of angina) who received standardized medical therapy. The risk of death or MI in these patients was greatest in the first 6 to 8 weeks after admission. ST-segment depression in the admission ECG and the presence of transient ischemia predicted increased risk of subsequent death or MI, whereas a normal ECG predicted a good prognosis. Severi et al[71] also studied the prognostic significance of basal ECG and exercise tests in 374 patients with UA.

They reported that 54 patients with a normal basal ECG and an exercise test result negative for ischemia had experienced no deaths at 1 year and that 86 patients who had a normal basal ECG but a positive exercise test result experienced a 97% probability of survival at 1 year. Langer et al[72] found ST-segment shifts on the admission ECG in 60 of 135 patients who had rest or prolonged angina. In these patients, the incidence of death, MI, or need for urgent revascularization during hospital stay was 55% compared with 25% in patients without ST changes (P < .005). Similarly, 89 patients who had symptomatic or silent ST-segment shifts on 24-hour Holter monitoring had a poorer prognosis than patients without ST shifts (48% rate of unfavorable events vs. 20%; P < .005). Larger studies such as the RISC (Risk of Myocardial Infarction and Death during Treatment with Low-Dose Aspirin and Intravenous Heparin in Men with Unstable Coronary Artery Disease) trial[65] and the PEPA (Unstable Angina in the Elderly) registry[66] have confirmed the prognostic importance of ECG changes in patients with UA (Table 4–6).

Prognostic Role of Recurrent Angina and Silent Ischemia

A recurrence of chest pain after admission appears to identify patients at higher risk for future events. Betriu et al[73] reviewed 10 representative series of patients with UA involving a total of almost 2000 patients.[7,11,12,22,62,63,74–77] Of these, 53% had ECG changes as inclusion criteria. The in-hospital mortality rate ranged between 2% and 8%; at 1 year, the mean survival rate was 90%. The event-free probability (probability of survival without MI) rate was 89% at 1 month and 79% at 1 year (Fig. 4-4). In a prospective study of 140 patients, Gazes et al[7] found that the probability of survival at 1 year was significantly decreased (from 96% to 57%) in 54 patients who had persistent angina within 48 hours after hospital admission. Similarly, Mulcahy et

■■■

TABLE 4–6 INDEPENDENT PREDICTORS OF MORTALITY AT 90-DAY FOLLOW-UP IN PATIENTS WITH UNSTABLE ANGINA

	CHI-SQUARE	RELATIVE RISK (CI 95%)	P
ST-segment **depression**	15.18	1.48 (1.21–1.80)	.0001
Age ≥ 80 y	13.50	1.48 (1.21–1.80)	.0002
CHF at admission	13.24	1.51 (1.22–1.85)	.0003
Diabetes	7.91	1.33 (1.09–1.62)	.005
PVD	1.07	1.13 (0.89–1.42)	NS
Females	0.19	0.96 (0.78–1.17)	NS
Prior infarct	0.07	1.03 (0.85–1.27)	NS

CHF, congestive heart failure; NS, nonsignificant difference; PVD, peripheral vascular disease.

Multivariate analysis with Cox-model showing mortality independent predictors at 90-day follow-up in patients with unstable angina.

(From Bermejo-García J, López de Sá E, López Sendón JL, et al: Unstable angina in the elderly: Clinical, profile, management and mortality at three months. The PEPA Registry Data. Rev Esp Cardiol 2000;53:1564–1572.)

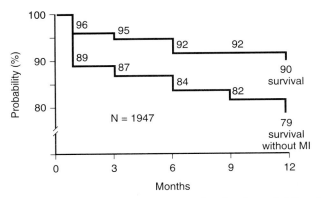

FIGURE 4–4. Kaplan-Meier actuarial curve showing the probability of survival and survival without myocardial infarction (MI) for the first 12 months after progressive or prolonged angina. N, number of patients. (From Betriu A, Heras M, Cohen M, et al: Unstable angina: Outcome according to clinical presentation. J Am Coll Cardiol 1992;19: 1659-1663.)

al[22] observed that compared with 79 unstable patients without recurrent angina during admission, the event-free probability rate was reduced from 87% to 65% in 22 patients with repeated episodes of chest pain after admission to the coronary care unit. Bosch et al[78] studied 449 patients with UA treated in the coronary care unit. During a mean follow-up of 14 months, patients with early angina had a significantly lower survival rate (92% vs. 83%; $P = .01$) compared with patients without angina.

Overall, patients with UA have a high incidence of acute coronary events and myocardial revascularization. Unrecognized (silent) persistent myocardial ischemia may be responsible for the high incidence of events observed within a few months after discharge from coronary care units in patients with UA. Studies have suggested that transient myocardial ischemia detected by Holter monitoring, but not necessarily chest pain, is the best predictor of unfavorable short-term clinical outcome.[79]

Gottlieb et al[80] studied the prognostic significance of silent myocardial ischemia in 70 patients with UA who were receiving standard medical treatment. Compared with 33 patients without silent ischemia, the 37 patients with silent ischemia showed a fivefold increase in the relative risk of acute MI or bypass surgery for recurrent angina at 30 days. Nademanee et al[81] reported a similar prognostic value of silent ischemia in 49 patients with UA who were followed for 6 months. The incidence of cardiac death, MI, or urgent revascularization was higher in patients with silent ischemia. Patients with greater than 60 minutes of silent ischemia in 24 hours had a higher event rate (94%) than patients with less than 60 minutes of ischemia (27%) or without silent ischemia (5%). It is important to mention that most of these studies were carried out at a time when patients received less aggressive antiplatelet, anti-anginal, and antithrombotic therapy than present standards dictate. Currently, with more effective patient management, transient ST-segment depression occurs in a minority of patients (<15%)[82] and Holter monitoring may offer relatively little help in risk stratification. The message derived from

these findings, however, is that the persistence of myocardial ischemia, whether silent or symptomatic, is a powerful marker of risk.

Cardiac Troponins

The role of markers of myocardial damage such as cardiac troponin I and troponin T is well established and this subject is specifically discussed in Chapter 14. Briefly, however, a number of studies have shown that patients with UA who have high serum levels of cardiac troponins or creatinine kinase MB (CK-MB) (NSTEMI) carry a worse long-term prognosis than those with UA with normal troponin or CK-MB concentrations.[11,65,83-88] Patients with "microinfarction"[89] or "minor myocardial damage"[90,91] (i.e., those with abnormal troponin T[92-100] or troponin I levels[99,101-104] meeting the new criteria for MI) constitute a high-risk group. This is as shown by the fact that these patients have a higher risk of subsequent cardiac mortality (Fig. 4-5).[92-103,105,106] There is a direct correlation between serum troponin T or I and cardiovascular risk. Thus, troponins T and I are clinically useful markers of risk in patients with acute UA/NSTEMI.

Inflammatory Markers—C-Reactive Protein

In recent years, evidence has accumulated that inflammatory markers (i.e., interleukin-6,[107] CD40 ligand,[108] CD4/CD28[null,109] and acute phase reactants such as amyloid A[110] and C-reactive protein [CRP]) are useful markers of risk in patients with UA/NSTEMI. High CRP levels appear to predict death, MI, the need for urgent

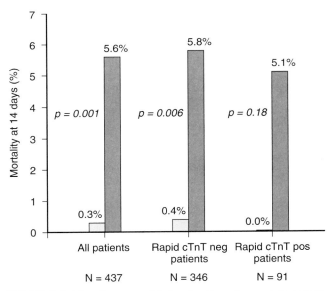

FIGURE 4–5. Mortality rate at 14 days by C-reactive protein concentration (*light bars*, <1.55 mg/dL; *dark bars*, >1.55 mg/dL) in all patients and in those with negative and positive rapid cTnT assays. CTnT, cardiac-specific troponin T; Neg, negative; N, number of patients; Pos, positive. (From Morrow DA, Rifai N, Antman EM, et al: C-reactive protein is a potent predictor of mortality independently of and in combination with troponin T in acute coronary syndromes: A TIMI IIA substudy. J Am Coll Cardiol 1998;31:1460-1465.)

revascularization, or a combination of these.[111-118] In TIMI IIA, the 14-day mortality rate in patients with CRP level of 1.55 mg/dL was significantly higher than that of patients with normal CRP levels (5.6% *vs.* 0.3%) (Fig. 4–6).[119] CRP appears to provide independent risk assessment: Even in patients with negative troponin T, a high CRP concentration identified a high-risk group in TIMI IIA.[119] CRP measured at the time of hospital discharge has been found to be a strong predictor of outcome to 3 to 12 months in other studies.[120,121] The combined use of CRP and troponin T for risk assessment has been shown to be useful in the clinical setting.[116,118,119] Indeed, in TIMI IIA, patients in whom both markers were negative had a very low risk (mortality rate, 0.4%), whereas patients with both high CRP levels and abnormal troponin concentrations had a higher mortality rate (9.1%).[119] In another recent study, however, CRP was not predictive of in-hospital events but was strongly associated with 30-day and 6-month cardiac events.[117]

Combined Risk Assessment Scores

An integrated approach using comprehensive risk scores has been developed using clinical, ECG, and biochemical variables. The TIMI risk score[122] was recently developed using multivariate analysis, which identified seven independent risk factors: age 65 years or older, more than three CAD risk factors, documented CAD, ST-segment shifts greater than 0.5 mm, more than two episodes of angina in the last 24 hours, use of aspirin within the prior week, and elevated cardiac markers. This scoring system was able to risk-stratify patients across a tenfold gradient of risk, from 4.7% to 40.9% ($P < .001$). These findings are discussed in Chapter 22.

PROGNOSIS IN DIFFERENT SUBSETS OF PATIENTS WITH UNSTABLE ANGINA

Understanding the natural history and prognosis of acute coronary syndromes, particularly UA, may be helpful in guiding management. Past studies suffered from several limitations such as the lack of an agreed definition of angina, differences in the condition of patients entered in each study, small patient numbers, lack of angiographic information in many series, and differences in both the length of follow-up and the treatment received.

Recently, registries and trials involving large numbers of well-characterized patients have provided useful information in this regard. Patients in most of these UA/NSTEMI studies were systematically investigated and treated, and outcome variables were identified prospectively.[42-44,48-50,123] Among the large registries, the TIMI III registry[39] was an observational study carried out between October 1990 and April 1993 to assess the natural history and effects of treatment in patients with

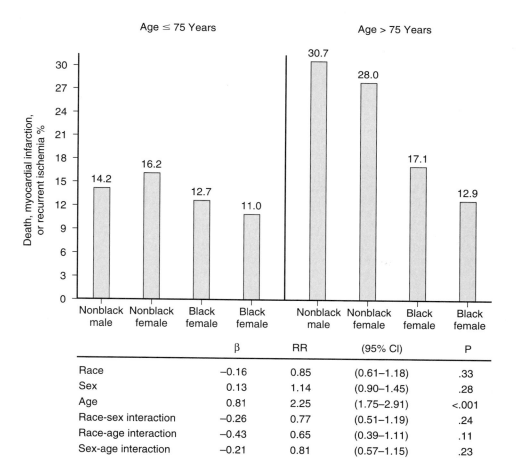

FIGURE 4–6. Specific 42-day event (death, myocardial infarction, or recurrent angina) rates by demographic group. The accompanying tables describe the risk ratios for each end point based on race, sex, and age as well as the interactions among demographic groups. CI, confidence interval. (From Stone PH, Thompson B, Anderson V, et al: Influence of race, sex, and age on management of unstable angina and non-Q-wave myocardial infarction. The TIMI III Registry. JAMA 1996;275: 1104–1112.)

	β	RR	(95% CI)	P
Race	−0.16	0.85	(0.61–1.18)	.33
Sex	0.13	1.14	(0.90–1.45)	.28
Age	0.81	2.25	(1.75–2.91)	<.001
Race-sex interaction	−0.26	0.77	(0.51–1.19)	.24
Race-age interaction	−0.43	0.65	(0.39–1.11)	.11
Sex-age interaction	−0.21	0.81	(0.57–1.15)	.23

UA or non–Q-wave MI. One of the missions of this registry was to provide information regarding specific patient subgroups—namely, blacks, women, and elderly patients (older than 75 years). Thus, a sampling strategy was used to recruit at least 500 blacks, 500 women, and 500 patients older than 75 years. Patients were included if they had an episode of angina on effort, defined as new-onset angina (<2 months) or an accelerating pattern of angina, or chest pain at rest (5 minutes in duration) suggestive of myocardial ischemia and occurring within 96 hours before study entry. Patients with persistent ST-segment elevation Q-wave MI occurring within 48 hours of the qualifying episode of pain, pericarditis, pain suggestive of aortic dissection, or noncardiac pain were not included. The TIMI III registry[39] prospectively studied the history, management, and outcome of representative patients.

The incidence of death or MI at 6 weeks after entry was assessed in black versus nonblack patients, women versus men, and elderly versus younger patients. Other "softer" end points were also assessed, such as recurrent ischemia and the composite outcome of death, MI, and recurrent ischemia at 6 weeks. Patient groups were compared with respect to baseline characteristics, medical history, clinical characteristics, and treatment received during the initial 6-week observation period. The primary end point for this study was the time to death or MI; all other clinical end points were considered secondary. Of the initial 8676 admissions in the enumeration roster, 7731 represented the first hospitalization of a TIMI III registry patient. Of these, 3318 accepted to participate in the prospective study and were enrolled.

Main findings of the study were as follows:

- Black patients were more likely than nonblacks to have arterial hypertension and diabetes mellitus but less likely to have a family history of CAD, hypercholesterolemia, or prior MI. They had less exertional or accelerating angina but were more likely to have a non–Q-wave MI with their qualifying episode. In the hospital, black patients were less likely to be treated with intensive anti-ischemic medication or undergo coronary angiography (OR, 0.49; 95% CI, 0.42 to 0.578; $P < .001$ compared with nonblacks). At 6 weeks, outcome for death and MI was similar in blacks and nonblacks.
- Women were less likely than men to have a history of smoking but more likely to have a history of arterial hypertension and diabetes mellitus and a family history of CAD. Women were less likely to receive intensive anti-ischemic therapy for their qualifying episode of angina and much less likely to undergo coronary angiography compared with men (OR, 0.59; 95% CI, 0.51 to 0.68; $P < .001$). As observed in blacks, women were found to have less severe and extensive coronary disease. Outcome by 42 days, in terms of death, MI, or recurrent ischemia, was similar in men and women (see Fig. 4-6).
- Elderly patients were more likely to have a history of MI, but they were less likely to have other major risk factors. At 6 weeks, they were much less likely to undergo coronary angiography, but those who did

undergo the test had more severe and extensive CAD than younger patients. They were also found to be at a higher risk for death, MI, and recurrent myocardial ischemia. Findings at the 42-day follow-up period are summarized in Figure 4-6. Age greater than 75 years was an independent marker of clinical outcome with relative risk of death being 3.76 (95% CI, 2.456 to 5.749; $P < .001$); of MI, 2.05 (95% CI, 1.372 to 3.074; $P = .001$); and of death, MI, or recurrent ischemia, 1.91 (95% CI, 1.607 to 2.272; $P < .001$).

Although previous studies reported important differences in the natural history and in the medical and surgical management of blacks and nonblacks presenting with acute coronary syndrome,[124-129] these studies did not specifically focus on the course and outcome of patients with UA but mainly concentrated on patients with MI.

As the investigators pointed out, the observation that several risk factors such as smoking, family history of CAD, and hypercholesterolemia occurred less frequently in the elderly perhaps indicates that the persons with these risk factors had died of CAD at a younger age. Elderly patients underwent fewer revascularization procedures and had a worse in-hospital course with increased mortality and recurrent ischemia. Previous studies in patients with chronic stable CAD and acute MI[66,127-134] have shown that old age is the most important independent risk marker for mortality. The TIMI III registry[39] reported a similar effect of advanced age for patients with UA and non–Q-wave MI. Another interesting finding in TIMI III is that outcome was similar in women and men, despite the fact that women had less severe angiographic CAD. The reasons for this finding remain to be investigated.

Pathogenesis and Prognosis

Coronary arteriography has shown that rapid progression of coronary stenosis often precedes UA[135] and that stenoses that progress rapidly are frequently those caused by eccentric, irregular lesions[136] often associated with filling defects indicative of coronary thrombi.[137-140] Also, evidence shows that abnormal coronary vasoconstriction[141] and activation of platelets[142] and the clotting system[24] have a pathogenic role in UA.[143] Unstable angina occurring soon after acute MI is particularly dangerous as it often heralds MI extension and is associated with a high incidence of serious cardiovascular events.[144-147] Coronary atheromatous plaque activity with local inflammatory activity, increased vasomotor tone, and platelet activation appear to be the mechanisms underlying clinical instability in patients presenting with UA. Systemic inflammation also contributes to alterations in the homeostatic and coagulation pathways that have been reported in patients with acute coronary syndromes and may play a part in the initiation of the intermittent thrombotic mechanism that is characteristic of UA.[148-150] Inflammatory acute-phase reactants, cytokines, chronic infections, and increased catecholamine production may provide a systemic stimulus for enhancing production of tissue factor, procoagulant activity, and platelet hyperaggregability.

Disruption of a formed plaque is a complex pathologic process that is central to the initiation of the acute coronary syndromes. Local thrombosis occurring after plaque disruption results from complex interactions among the lipid core, smooth muscle cells, macrophages, and collagen matrix.[151-153] The arterial lesions of patients with UA frequently have complex morphologic features on coronary angiography, which have been found to represent ruptured plaque with superimposed thrombus.[136,154-157] As part of the response to any type of disruption of the endothelial wall, platelets aggregate and release granular contents that result in vasoconstriction, further platelet aggregation, thrombus formation, and platelet embolization to microvessels. An association has been reported between complex stenosis morphology and markers of myocardial damage (cardiac troponin),[158-159] suggesting that platelet microemboli can cause minor myocardial damage. Markers of ischemic myocardial damage are thus also a marker of plaque instability and may predict further cardiac events (see Fig. 4-5).

Angiographic Morphology and Acute Coronary Events

Progression of CAD as occurs in patients with UA/NSTEMI is rapid and unpredictable.[135,160] It has been shown that stenosis progression, whether clinically silent or associated with acute coronary events, is a strong predictor of cardiovascular risk.[2,3] In patients with acute coronary syndromes, atheromatous plaques characteristically show fibrous cap disruption, which appears to be responsible for acute intracoronary thrombosis.[160] Other mechanisms such as endothelial erosion have been also shown to be associated with rapid CAD progression in patients with UA.[161] "Culprit" plaques in patients with UA/NSTEMI, usually called *vulnerable* or *unstable,* have well-defined anatomopathologic characteristics.[160] These plaques have a large lipid core and a thin fibrous cap, which may alter plaque biophysical properties and reduce plaque stability. More importantly, these plaques have high concentrations of inflammatory cells that contribute to plaque instability,[162-164] as discussed in detail in Chapter 5. It is important from a prognostic point of view that patients may have, on average, 20 or more plaques in a single coronary artery, none of which will be identical to others in terms of inflammatory activity and pathologic characteristics.[163]

There is no strict correlation between stenosis severity and plaque vulnerability, and the majority of vulnerable plaques may not be apparent at coronary arteriography.[163] Indeed, plaque disruption and endothelial erosion do not necessarily occur in the most severe stenoses but in those that show only mild or moderate severity but harbor intense inflammatory activity.[161,162,165,166] Angiographic studies by Ambrose et al[136,157] showed that "complex" (irregular, hazy edges and filling defects) coronary artery stenoses are more common in patients who experience acute MI or UA compared with patients who have stable angina. Complex plaques are likely to represent ulcerated or disrupted plaques and may have increased thrombogenic activity.[167] Davies et al[168] found a strong correlation between postmortem stenosis morphology and hospital outcome in patients with MI. Moreover, several angiographic studies have shown that complex lesion morphology is associated with increased cardiovascular risk and represents an independent determinant of stenosis progression and acute coronary events.[157,167-174]

Briefly, in 1995 we studied the role of complex stenosis morphology in rapid disease progression in 94 consecutive patients awaiting routine coronary angioplasty (PCI).[166] Coronary arteriography was repeated at 8 ± 3 months' follow-up, immediately preceding routine PCI (68 patients), or after an acute coronary event (26 patients). Disease progression was assessed by computerized angiography in 217 stenoses, of which 79 (36%) were complex and 138 (64%) were "smooth." At presentation, 63 patients had stable angina pectoris and 31 had UA that settled rapidly with medical therapy. At follow-up, 23 patients (24%) had progression of preexisting stenoses and 71 (76%) had no progression. Patients with stenosis progression did not differ from those without progression with regard to risk factors, previous MI, or severity and extent of CAD. Twenty-three lesions (11%) progressed, 15 to total occlusion (11 complex and 4 smooth—65%). Progression occurred in 17 of the 79 complex stenoses (22%) and in 6 of the 138 smooth lesions (4%) ($P = .002$). The mean reduction in stenosis diameter was also significantly greater in complex than in smooth lesions (11.6% vs. 3.9% change; $P < .001$). Acute coronary events occurred in 57% of patients with progression compared with 18% of those without progression ($P < .001$) and were more frequent in patients who presented with UA ($P = .002$). Our study thus showed that rapid progression of preexisting stenoses was relatively common in patients with moderate or severe CAD who were on a waiting list for PCI. Indeed, approximately 25% of our patients showed significant stenosis progression while on the waiting list. This was a prospective study that included consecutive patients with CAD who can be considered to represent the patient population that undergoes coronary angioplasty in a general hospital.

The observation that complex lesions are more likely to progress than smooth stenoses of similar severity both in patients with stable angina and in those presenting with UA indicates that the morphologic appearance of a stenosis is an independent factor in determining stenosis progression.[171] Studies have shown that in patients with UA, angiographic stenosis complexity predicts subsequent in-hospital instability.[175,176] However, because it is customary in UA to rapidly intervene with PCI or coronary artery bypass surgery when significant disease is demonstrated, the natural history of unstable coronary lesions is largely undetermined in this setting.

The question as to whether complex stenosis morphology is a predictor of poor outcome in patients with UA whose condition stabilizes rapidly on conventional medical therapy was addressed by Chen et al[171] in a prospective angiographic study. In this study, which took advantage of the existence of waiting lists in the United Kingdom, 85 consecutive patients with UA who experienced stabilization on medical therapy were found to require PCI for treatment of CAD. Angiography was carried out at admission, and patients were put on a waiting list and restudied 8 ± 4 months (mean ± SD) later, prior to scheduled PCI. Culprit stenoses were classified as complex (irregular borders, overhanging edges, or thrombus) or smooth (absence of complex features). Stenosis progression, defined as 20% diameter reduction or new total occlusion, was assessed by automated edge detection. At initial angiography, there were 198 stenoses (50%, 102 cases), of which 85 (54 complex and 31 smooth) were culprit lesions. At restudy, 21 culprit stenoses and 8 non–ischemia-related stenoses progressed (25% vs. 7%; $P = .001$). Seventeen of the 21 culprit stenoses progressed to total occlusion compared with 3 of the 8 non–ischemia-related stenoses ($P = .02$). Increase in stenosis severity was significantly larger in culprit stenoses versus non–ischemia-related stenoses ($P < .03$). Regarding morphology, 34% of complex stenoses progressed, compared with 10% smooth lesions ($P = .02$). During follow-up, 1 patient died and 25 patients had nonfatal coronary events that were associated with progression of culprit stenoses in 14 (56%).

This study showed that in patients with UA that stabilizes with medical treatment, subsequent rapid stenosis progression and coronary events are common. Thus, the unstable coronary lesion (particularly complex stenoses) is often not stabilized and continues to progress over the ensuing months. The relatively short time in which significant stenosis progression took place in these studies suggests that acute changes, rather than slow linear events, occurred at the stenosis site. This is in agreement with current knowledge that vascular injury and thrombus formation are key events in the pathogenesis of acute coronary syndromes. In fact, available data[3,135,136,157,160,166,171] indicate that in patients with angina (particularly, but not exclusively, patients with UA), active plaques exist that progress rapidly, leading to total vessel occlusion and acute coronary events. These clinical findings have a pathologic substrate as shown by Mann et al,[177] who observed that plaque disruption and subsequent healing is a mechanism responsible for recurrent angina and CAD progression in patients with UA. Burke et al[178] have endorsed these findings and provided evidence that subclinical plaque rupture and subsequent healing has a role in plaque progression.

Why are complex stenoses more likely to continue to progress over time, even after the acute symptoms have subsided? Complex lesions are associated with increased platelet activation and vasoconstriction.[179,180] Episodic vasospasm may contribute to vascular instability via an alternative mechanism of lumen narrowing leading to further thrombosis, increased oxidative stress, and endothelial injury.[181]

During the acute phase of UA and MI, patients exhibit increased procoagulant activity. Over the following 6 months, even patients with an uneventful clinical course show a persistent hypercoagulable state that may contribute to future adverse events.[182]

Markers of macrophage activation such as serum neopterin showed a significant correlation with the number of complex coronary artery stenoses in patients with UA.[183] Neopterin has also been shown to be associated with rapid CAD progression and coronary events in patients with stable angina and acute coronary syndromes.[184-186]

New Markers of Risk

New markers of risk have been identified in patients with acute coronary syndromes—i.e., pregnancy-associated plasma protein A (PAPP-A)[187] and brain (B-type) natriuretic peptide (BNP).[188] The latter, in particular, opens new and interesting pathophysiologic links between cardiac neurohumoral activation and disease activity.

Brain Natriuretic Peptide as a Marker of Risk in Unstable Angina

In a recent study, de Lemos et al[188] observed that BNP levels predict outcome in patients with acute coronary syndrome. The authors assessed BNP levels in 2525 patients with acute coronary syndromes (ST-elevation MI, 825; non–ST-segment elevation, 565; and UA, 1133). BNP plasma levels correlated with the risk of death, heart failure, and MI at both 1- and 10-month follow-up. A significant association was found between BNP and risk of events in the different patient subgroups. In other words, BNP levels predicted risk in patients with ST-elevation MI and in those with no ST-elevation MI as well as in the patients with UA. The positive association between BNP levels and outcome remained significant after correcting for confounding factors. The odds ratio for death at 10 months' follow-up in the second, third, and fourth BNP quartiles were 3.8, 4.0, and 5.8, respectively. BNP levels were also predictive of new MI ($P < .01$) and new or worsening heart failure ($P < .001$) at 10 months of follow-up.

It is interesting that a single measurement of BNP, performed during hospital admission, gives independent prognostic information across the whole spectrum of acute coronary syndromes. BNP, a marker of neurohumoral activity, has been previously shown to predict clinical outcome in patients with heart failure.[189,190] de Lemos et al[188] speculate that cardiac neurohumoral activation may be the unifying feature regarding the prognostic ability of BNP in patients with acute coronary syndromes. Recently, an association has been postulated between activation of the renin-angiotensin system and inflammation,[191,192] which may be relevant to the findings of de Lemos et al.

Pregnancy-Associated Plasma Protein A (PAPP-A)

Bayés-Genís et al[187] reported that PAPP-A, a pro-atherogenic metalloproteinase, was found to be elevated in the blood of patients with acute coronary syndromes compared with patients with stable angina pectoris and control subjects. In this study, PAPP-A levels correlated with plasma CRP levels, which is a marker of systemic inflammation and a predictor of risk in UA.[193] Interestingly, PAPP-A levels did not correlate with cardiac troponin levels. This finding suggests that PAPP-A is a marker of inflammatory activity rather than a marker of myocardial damage. Bayés-Genís et al[187] also found that PAPP-A is abundantly expressed in plaques showing signs of instability, such as endothelial erosion and fibrous cap fissuring, but not in stable, inactive plaques. This finding suggests that PAPP-A is expressed in response to local vascular inflammation. It is therefore conceivable that in view of its enzymatic properties, PAPP-A could play a pathogenic role in the acute coronary syndrome, perhaps through plaque disruption. This, however, is currently speculative and requires confirmation. The Bayés-Genís study[187] supports the importance of inflammation in the genesis of the acute coronary syndrome and has identified the presence of a new protein that may be a useful marker of risk. However, this pilot study was carried out in a small number of subjects, and thus its findings must be confirmed. Both the study of Bayés-Genís et al and that of de Lemos et al[187,188] have opened interesting avenues in the search for new clinically relevant markers of cardiovascular risk.

REFERENCES

1. Graves E: National Hospital Discharge Survey: Annual Survey 1996. Washington, D.C.: National Center for Health Statistics, Series 13, No. 4, 1998.
2. Rosch J, Antonovic R, Trenouth RS, et al: The natural history of coronary artery stenosis: A longitudinal angiographic assessment. Radiology 1976;119:513-520.
3. Bruschke AV, Wijers TS, Kolsters W, et al: The anatomic evolution of coronary artery disease demonstrated by coronary arteriography in 256 nonoperated patients. Circulation 1981;63:527-536.
4. Yeghiazarians Y, Braunstein JB, Askari A, et al: Unstable angina pectoris. N Engl J Med 2000;342:101-104.
5. Forrester JS, Litvack F, Grundfest W, et al: A perspective of coronary disease seen through the arteries of living man. Circulation 1987;75:505-513.
6. Theroux P: A pathophysiologic basis for the clinical classification and management of unstable angina pectoris. Circulation 1987;75(Suppl V):v-103.
7. Gazes PC, Mobley EM, Faris HM, et al: Preinfarctional (unstable) angina—a prospective study—ten year follow-up: Prognostic significance of electrocardiographic changes. Circulation 1973;48:331-337.
8. Wilcox I, Freedman B, McCredie RJ, et al: Risk of adverse outcome in patients admitted to the coronary care unit with suspected unstable angina pectoris. Am J Cardiol 1989;64:845-848.
9. Timmis AD, Griffin B, Crick JC, et al: Early percutaneous transluminal coronary angioplasty in the management of unstable angina. Int J Cardiol 1987;14:25-31.
10. de Feyter PJ, Suryapranata H, Serruys PW, et al: Coronary angioplasty for unstable angina: Immediate and late results in 200 consecutive patients with identification of risk factors for unfavorable early and late outcome. J Am Coll Cardiol 1988;12:324-333.
11. Luchi RJ, Scott SM, Deupree RH: Comparison of medical and surgical treatment for unstable angina pectoris: Results of a Veteran Administration Cooperative Study. N Engl J Med 1987;316:977-984.
12. Unstable Angina Pectoris Study Group: Unstable angina pectoris: National Cooperative Study Group to compare surgical and medical therapy. II: In-hospital experience and initial follow-up results in patients with one, two or three vessel disease. Am J Cardiol 1978;42:839-848.
13. Lincoff AM, Tcheng JE, Califf RM, et al: Sustained suppression of ischemic complications of coronary intervention by platelet GP IIb/IIIa blockade with abciximab: One-year outcome in the EPILOG trial. Circulation 1999;99:1951-1958.
14. Gibson CM, Goel M, Cohen DJ, et al: Six-month angiographic and clinical follow-up of patients prospectively randomized to receive either tirofiban or placebo during angioplasty in the RESTORE trial. J Am Coll Cardiol 1998;32:28-34.
15. Nattel S, Warnica W, Ogilvie RI: Indications for admission to a coronary care unit in patients with unstable angina. Can Med Assoc J 1980;122:180-184.
16. Fahri J-I, Cohen M, Fuster V: The broad spectrum of unstable angina pectoris and its implications for future controlled trials. Am J Cardiol 1986;58:547-550.
17. Conti RC, Brawley RK, Griffith LSC, et al: Unstable angina pectoris: Morbidity and mortality in 57 consecutive patients evaluated angiographically. Am J Cardiol 1973;32:745-750.
18. Ouyang P, Brinker JA, Mellits ED, et al: Variables predictive of successful medical therapy in patients with unstable angina: Selection by multivariate analysis from clinical, electrocardiographic, and angiographic evaluations. Circulation 1984;70:367-376.
19. Olson HG, Lyons KP, Aronow WS, et al: The high-risk angina patient: Identification by clinical features, hospital course, electrocardiography and technetium-99m stannous pyrophosphate scintigraphy. Circulation 1981;64:674-685.
20. Krauss KR, Hutter AM, DeSanctis RW: Acute coronary insufficiency: Course and follow-up. Arch Intern Med 1972;129:808-813.
21. Severi S, Michelassi C, Orsini E, et al: Long-term prognosis of transient acute ischemia at rest. Am J Cardiol 1989;64:889-895.
22. Mulcahy R, Daly L, Graham I, et al: Unstable angina: Natural history and determinants of prognosis. Am J Cardiol 1981;48:525-528.
23. Patel DJ, Knight CJ, Holdright DR, et al: Long-term prognosis in unstable angina: The importance of early risk stratification using continuous ST segment monitoring. Eur Heart J 1998;19:240-249.
24. Patterson DLH: Unstable angina. Postgrad Med J 1988;64:196-200.
25. Patterson DLH: Management in unstable angina. Postgrad Med J 1988;64:271-277.
26. Bertolasi CA, Tronge JE, Mon GA, et al: Clinical spectrum of "unstable angina." Clin Cardiol 1979;2:113-120.
27. Julian DG: The natural history of unstable angina. In Hugenholtz PG, Goldman BS (eds): Unstable Angina: Current Concepts and Management. Stuttgart, Schattauer, 1985, pp 65-70.
28. Wearn JT: Thrombosis of the coronary arteries, with infarction of the heart. Am J Med Sci 1923;165:250-276.
29. Sampson JJ, Eliaser M Jr: The diagnosis of impending acute coronary artery occlusion. Am Heart J 1937;13:675-686.
30. Feil H: Preliminary pain in coronary thrombosis. Am J Med Sci 1937;193:42-48.
31. Harper RW, Kennedy G, DeSanctis RW, et al: The incidence and pattern of angina prior to acute myocardial infarction: A study of 577 cases. Am Heart J 1979;97:178-183.
32. National Center for Health Statistics: Vital and Health Statistics: Detailed Diagnosis and Procedures for Patients Discharged from Short Stay Hospitals. Hyattsville, Md.: US Department of Health and Human Services, Public Health Service, Series 13, No. 90, 1987.
33. Braunwald E: Unstable angina: A classificaction. Circulation 1989;80:410-414.
34. Pope JH, Ruthazer R, Beshanky JR, et al: Clinical features of emergency department patients presenting with symptoms suggestive of acute myocardial ischemia: A multicenter study. J Throm Thrombolysis 1998;6:63-74.
35. Kontos MC, Ornato JP, Tatum JL, et al: How many patients are eligible for treatment with GP IIb/IIIa inhibitors? Results from a clinical data-base [abstract]. Circulation 1999;100(Suppl I):I-775.
36. Braunwald E, Antman EM, Beasley JW, et al: ACC/AHA guidelines for the management of patients with unstable angina/non-ST segment elevation myocardial infarction: A report for the American College of Cardiology/American Heart Association Task Force on Practice Guidelines (Committee on the Management of Unstable Angina and Non-ST Segment Elevation Myocardial Infarction). J Am Coll Cardiol 2000;36:970-1062.
37. Hochman JS, McCabe CH, Stone PH, et al: Outcome and profile of women and men presenting with acute coronary syndromes: A report from TIMI IIIB. J Am Coll Cardiol 1997;30:141-148.
38. Hochman JS, Tamis JE, Thompson TD, et al: Sex, clinical presentation, and outcome in patients with acute coronary syndromes: Global Use of Strategies to Open Occluded Coronary Arteries in Acute Coronary Syndromes IIb Investigators. N Engl J Med 1999;341:226-232.
39. Stone PH, Thompson B, Anderson HV, et al: Influence of race, sex, and age on management of unstable angina and non-Q-wave myocardial infarction: The TIMI III Registry. JAMA 1996;275:1104-1112.

40. The Global Use of Strategies to Open Occluded Coronary Arteries (GUSTO) IIb Investigators: A comparison of recombinant hirudin with heparin for the treatment of acute coronary syndromes. N Engl J Med 1996;335:775–782.

41. Antman EM, Cohen M, Radley D, et al: Assesment of the treatment effect of enoxaparin for unstable angina/non-Q-wave myocardial infarction: TIMI IIB-ESSENCE Meta-Analyisis. Circulation 1999;100:1602–1608.

42. The PURSUIT Trial Investigators: Inhibition of platelet glycoprotein IIb/IIIa with eptifibatide in patients with acute coronary syndromes. N Engl J Med 1998;339:436–443.

43. The Platelet Receptor Inhibition for Ischemic Syndrome Management (PRISM) Study Investigators: A comparison of aspirin plus tirofiban with aspirin plus heparin for unstable angina. N Engl J Med 1998;338:1498–1505.

44. The Platelet Receptor Inhibition for Ischemic Syndrome Management in Patients Lmited by Unstable Sigs and Symptoms (PRISM-PLUS) Trial Investigators: Inhibition of the platelet glycoprotein IIb/IIIa receptor with tirofiban in unstable angina and non-Q-wave myocardial infarction. N Engl J Med 1998;338:1488–1497.

45. FRagmin during InStability in Coronary artery disease (FRISC) study group: Low-molecular-weight heparin during instability in coronary artery disease. Lancet 1996;347:561–568.

46. Cohen M, Demers C, Gurfinkel EP, et al: A comparison of low-molecular-weight heparin with unfractionated heparin for unstable coronary artery disease: Efficacy and Safety of Subcutaneous Enoxaparin in Non-Q-Wave Coronary Events (ESSENCE) Study Group. N Engl J Med 1997;337:447–452.

47. Antman EM, McCabe CH, Gurfinkel EP, et al: Enoxaparin prevents death and cardiac ischemic events in unstable angina/non-Q-wave myocardial infarction: Results of the Thrombolysis in Myocardial Infarction (TIMI) IIB Trial. Circulation 1999;100:1593–1601.

48. The PARAGON Investigators: International, randomized, controlled trial of lamifiban (a platelet glycoprotein IIb/IIIa inhibitor), heparin, or both in unstable angina: The Platelet IIb/IIIa Antagonism for the Reduction of Acute Coronary Syndrome Events in a Global Organization Network. Circulation 1998;97:2386–2395.

49. The PARAGON-B Investigators: Randomized, placebo-controlled trial of titrated intravenous lamifiban for acute coronary syndromes: The Platelet IIb/IIIa Antagonism for the Reduction of Acute coronary syndrome events in a Global Organization Network. Circulation 2002;105:316–321.

50. The GUSTO-IV ACS Investigators: Effect of glycoprotein IIb/IIIa receptor blocker abciximab on outcome in patients with acute coronary syndromes without early coronary revascularization: The GUSTO IV-ACS randomised trial. Lancet 2001;357:1915–1924.

51. Fox KAA, et al: Preliminary data from the Global Registry of Acute Coronary Events (GRACE): XXII European Society of Cardiology Annual Congress, Amsterdam, The Netherlands, August, 2000.

52. Chierchia S, Brunelli C, Simonetti I, et al: Sequence of events in angina at rest: Primary reduction in coronary flow. Circulation 1980;61:659–667.

53. Davies MJ, Thomas A: Thrombosis and acute coronary lesions in sudden cardiac ischemic death. N Engl J Med 1984;310:1137–1140.

54. Chesebro JH, Fuster V: Thrombosis in unstable angina. N Engl J Med 1992;327:192–194.

55. Calvin JC, Klein LW, VanderBerg BJ, et al: Risk stratification in unstable angina: Prospective validation of the Braunwald classification. JAMA 1995;273:136–144.

56. van Miltenburg-van Zilj AJM, Simmons ML, Veerhoek RJ, et al: Incidence and follow-up of Braunwald subgroups in unstable angina pectoris. J Am Coll Cardiol 1995;25:1286–1292.

57. Cannon CP, McCabe CH, Stone PH, et al: Prospective validation of the Braunwald classification of unstable angina: Results from the Thrombolysis In Myocardial Infarction (TIMI) III Registry [abstract]. Circulation 1995;92(Suppl I):I–19.

58. Bertolet BD, Dinerman J, Hartke R, et al: Unstable angina: Relationship of clinical presentation, coronary artery pathology, and clinical outcome. Clin Cardiol 1993;16:116–122.

59. de Feyter PJ, Serruys W: Coronary angioplasty for patients with unstable angina pectoris. In Topol EJ (ed): Acute Coronary Interventions. New York, Alan R. Liss, 1988, pp 215–229.

60. Heng MK, Norris RM, Singh BN, et al: Prognosis in unstable angina. Br Heart J 1976;38:921–925.

61. The Holland Interuniversity Nifedipine/Metoprolol Trial (HINT) Research Group: Early treatment of unstable angina in the coronary care unit: A randomised, double bind placebo controlled comparison of recurrent ischemia in patients treated with nifedipine or metoprolol or both. The HINT Research Group. Br Heart J 1986;56:400–413.

62. Lewis HD, Davis JW, Archibald DG, et al: Protective effects of aspirin against acute myocardial infarction and death in men with unstable angina: Results of a Veteran Administration Cooperative Study. N Engl J Med 1983;309:396–403.

63. Theroux P, Ouimet H, McCans J, et al: Aspirin, heparin, or both to treat acute unstable angina. N Engl J Med 1988;319:1105–1111.

64. Balsano F, Rizzon P, Violi F, et al: Antiplatelet treatment with ticlopidine in unstable angina: A controlled multicenter trial. Circulation 1990;82:17–26.

65. Nyman I, Areskog M, Areskog NH, et al: Very early risk stratification by electrocardiogram at rest in men with suspected unstable coronary artery disease: The RISC Study Group. J Intern Med 1993;234:293–301.

66. Bermejo-García J, López de Sá E, López-Sendón JL, et al: Unstable angina in the elderly: Clinical profile, management and mortality at three months. The PEPA Registry Trial. Rev Esp Cardiol 2000;53:1564–1572.

67. Savonitto S, Ardissino D, Granger CB, et al: Prognostic value of the admission electrocardiogram in acute coronary syndromes: The GUSTO IIb Investigators. JAMA 1999;281:707–713.

68. Cannon CP, McCabe CH, Stone PH, et al: The electrocardiogram predicts one-year outcome of patients with unstable angina and non-Q wave myocardial infarction: Results of the TIMI III Registry ECG Ancillary Study. J Am Coll Cardiol 1997;30:133–140.

69. Hyde TA, French JK, Wong CK, et al: Four-year survival of patients with acute coronary syndromes without ST-segment elevation and prognostic significance of 0.5-mm ST-segment depression. Am J Cardiol 1999;84:379–385.

70. Kaul P, Fu Y, Chang WC, et al: Prognostic value of ST segment depression in acute coronary syndromes: Insights from PARAGON-A applied to GUSTO-IIb. J Am Coll Cardiol 2001;38:64–71.

71. Severi S, Orsini E, Marracini P, et al: The basal electrocardiogram and the exercise stress test in assessing prognosis in patients with unstable angina. Eur Heart J 1988;9:441–446.

72. Langer A, Freeman MR, Armstrong PW: ST segment shift in unstable angina: pathophysiology and association with coronary anatomy and hospital outcome. J Am Coll Cardiol 1989;13:1495–1502.

73. Betriu A, Heras M, Cohen M, et al: Unstable angina: Outcome according to clinical presentation. J Am Coll Cardiol 1992;19:1659–1663.

74. Cairns JA, Gent M, Singer J, et al: Aspirin, sulfinpyrazone, or both in unstable angina. N Engl J Med 1985;313:1369–1375.

75. Fulton M, Lutz W, Donald KW, et al: Natural history of unstable angina. Lancet 1972;1:860–865.

76. Roberts KD, Califf RM, Harrel FE, et al: The prognosis for patients with new-onset angina who have undergone cardiac catheterization. Circulation 1983;68:970–978.

77. Alison HW, Russell RO, Mantle JA, et al: Coronary anatomy and arteriography in patients with unstable angina pectoris. Am J Cardiol 1978;451:204–209.

78. Bosch X, Theroux P, Waters DD, et al: Early postinfarction ischemia; clinical, angiographic, and prognostic significance. Circulation 1987;75:988–995.

79. Bugiardini R, Borghi A, Pozzati A, et al: Relation of severity of symptoms to transient myocardial ischemia and prognosis in unstable angina. J Am Coll Cardiol 1995;25:597–604.

80. Gottlieb SO, Weisfeldt ML, Ouyang P, et al: Silent ischemia as a marker for early unfavorable outcomes in patients with unstable angina. N Engl J Med 1986;314:1214–1219.

81. Nademanee K, Intarachot V, Josephson MA, et al: Prognostic significance of silent myocardial ischemia in patients with unstable angina. J Am Coll Cardiol 1987;10:1–9.

82. Stone PH: The role of ST-segment monitoring in the management of patients with unstable angina. In Rutherford JD (ed): Unstable Angina Pectoris. New York, Marcel Dekker, 1991, pp 105–120.

83. The TIMI IIIB Investigators: Effects of tissue plasminogen activator and a comparison of early invasive and conservative strategies in unstable angina and non-Q-wave myocardial infarction: Results of the TIMI IIIB Trial. Circulation 1994;89:1545–1556.

84. Anderson HV, Cannon CP, Stone PH, et al: One-year results of the Thrombolysis In Myocardial Infarction (TIMI) IIIB clinical trial: A randomized comparison of tissue-type plasminogen activator versus placebo and early invasive versus conservative strategies in unstable angina and non-Q-wave myocardial infarction. J Am Coll Cardiol 1995;26:1643–1650.

85. Cohen M, Xiong J, Parry G, et al: Prospective comparison of unstable angina versus non-Q-wave myocardial infarction during antithrombotic therapy. J Am Coll Cardiol 1993;22:1338–1343.

86. Gibson RS, Boden WE, Theroux P, et al: Diltiazem and reinfarction in patients with non-Q-wave myocardial infarction: Results of a double-bind, randomized, multicenter trial. N Engl J Med 1986; 315:423–429.

87. Gheorghiade M, Schultz L, Tilley B, et al: Natural history of the first non-Q-wave myocardial infarction in the placebo arm of the Beta-Blocker Heart Attack Trial. Am Heart J 1991;122:1548–1553.

88. Gibson RS: Non-Q-wave myocardial infarction: Prognosis, changing incidence, and management. In Gersh BJ, Rahimtoola SH (eds): Acute Myocardial Infarction. New York, Elsevier Science, 1991, pp 284–307.

89. Antman EM, Grudzien C, Mitchell RN, et al: Detection of unsuspected myocardial necrosis by rapid bedside assay for cardiac troponin T. Am Heart J 1997;133:596–598.

90. Rottbauer W, Greten T, Muller-Bardorff M, et al: Troponin T: A diagnostic marker for myocardial infarction and minor cardiac cell damage. Eur Heart J 1996;17(Suppl F):3–8.

91. Simmons ML, van der Brand M, Lincoff M, et al: Minimal myocardial damage during coronary intervention is associated with impaired outcome. Eur Heart J 1999;20:1112–1119.

92. Ohman EM, Armstrong P, Christenson RH, et al: Cardiac troponin T levels for risk stratification in unstable myocardial ischemia. N Engl J Med 1996;335:1333–1341.

93. Hamm CW, Goldmann BU, Heeschen C, et al: Emergency room triage of patients with acute chest pain by means of rapid testing for cardiac troponin T or troponin I. N Engl J Med 1997;337: 1648–1653.

94. Hamm CW, Ravkilde J, Gerhardt W, et al: The prognostic value of troponin T in unstable angina. N Engl J Med 1992;327:146–150.

95. Ravkilde J, Nissen H, Horder M, et al: Independent prognostic value of serum creatine kinase isoenzyme MB mass, cardiac troponin T and myosin light chain levels in suspected acute myocardial infarction: Analysis of 28 months of follow-up in 196 patients. J Am Coll Cardiol 1995;25:574–581.

96. Lindahl B, Venge P, Wallentin L, for the FRISC Study Group: Relation between troponin T and the risk of subsequent cardiac events in unstable coronary artery disease. Circulation 1996;93:1651–1657.

97. Newby LK, Christenson RH, Ohman EM, et al: Value of serial troponin T measurements for early and late risk stratification in patients with acute coronary syndromes: The GUSTO-IIa Investigators. Circulation 1998;98:1853–1859.

98. Hamm CW, Heeschen C, Goldman B, et al: Benefit of abciximab in patients with refractory unstable angina in relation to serum troponin T levels: C7E3 Fab Antiplatelet Therapy in Unstable Refractory Angina (CAPTURE) Study Investigators. N Engl J Med 1998;340:1623–1629.

99. Heeschen C, Hamm CW, Goldman B, et al: Troponin concentrations for stratification of patients with acute coronary syndromes in relation to therapeutic efficacy of tirofiban: PRISM Study Investigators. Platelet Receptor Inhibition in Ischemic Syndrome Management. Lancet 1999;354:1757–1762.

100. Stubbs P, Collinson P, Moseley D, et al: Prospective study of the role of cardiac troponin T in patients admitted with unstable angina. BMJ 1996;313:262–264.

101. Antman EM, Tanasijevic MJ, Thompson B, et al: Cardiac-specific troponin I levels to predict the risk of mortality in patients with acute coronary syndromes. N Engl J Med 1996;335:1342–1349.

102. Galvani M, Ottani F, Ferrini D, et al: Prognostic influence of elevated values of cardiac troponin I in patients with unstable angina. Circulation 1997;95:2053–2059.

103. Olatidoye AG, Wu AH, Feng YJ, et al: Prognostic role of troponin T versus troponin I in unstable angina pectoris for cardiac events with meta-analysis comparing published studies. Am J Cardiol 1998;81:1405–1410.

104. Adams JE, Bodor GS, Davila-Roman VG, et al: Cardiac troponin I: A marker with high specificity for cardiac injury. Circulation 1993;88:101–106.

105. Morrow DA, de Lemos JA, Rifai N, et al: Troponin I predicts early need for revascularization in acute coronary syndromes: A TIMI IIB substudy [abstract]. Circulation 1999;100(Suppl I): I-775.

106. Antman EM, Sacks DB, Rifai N, et al: Time to positivity of a rapid bedside assay for cardiac-specific troponin T predicts prognosis in acute coronary syndromes: A Thrombolysis in Myocardial Infarction (TIMI) IIA Substudy. J Am Coll Cardiol 1998;31: 326–330.

107. Biasucci LM, Liuzzo G, Fantuzzi G, et al: Increasing levels of interleukin (IL)-1Ra and IL-6 during the first 2 days of hospitalization in unstable angina are associated with increased risk of in-hospital coronary events. Circulation 1999;99:2079–2084.

108. Aukrust P, Muller F, Ueland T, et al: Enhanced levels of slouble membrane-bounded CD40 ligand in patients with unstable angina: Possible reflection of T lymphocyte and platelet involvement in the pathogenesis of acute coronary syndromes. Circulation 1999;100:614–620.

109. Liuzzo G, Kopecky SL, Frye RL, et al: Perturbation of the T-cell repertoire in patients with unstable angina. Circulation 1999;100:2135–2139.

110. Morrow DA, Antman EM, Rifai N, et al: Serum amyloid A and rapid troponin independently predict mortality in acute coronary syndromes. J Am Coll Cardiol 2000;35:358–362.

111. Berk BC, Weintraub WS, Alexander RW: Elevation of C-reactive protein in "active" coronary artery disease. Am J Cardiol 1990;65: 168–172.

112. Liuzzo G, Biasucci LM, Gallimore JR, et al: The prognostic value of C-reactive protein and serum amyloid A protein in severe unstable angina. N Engl J Med 1994;331:417–424.

113. Haverkate F, Thompson SG, Pyke SDM, et al: Production of C-reactive protein and risk of coronary events in stable and unstable angina. Lancet 1997;349:462–466.

114. Bickel C, Rupprecht HJ, Blankenberg S, et al: Relation of markers of inflammation (C-reactive protein, fibrinogen, von Willebrand factor, and leukocyte count) and statin therapy to long-term mortality in patients with angiographically proven coronary artery disease. Am J Cardiol 2002;89:901–908.

115. Toss H, Lindahl B, Siegbahn A, et al: Prognostic influence of increased fibrinogen and C-reactive protein levels in unstable coronary artery disease. Circulation 1997;96:4204–4210.

116. Rebuzzi AG, Quaranta G, Liuzzo G, et al: Incremental prognostic value of serum of troponin T and C-reactive protein on admission in patients with unstable angina pectoris. Am J Cardiol 1998;82: 715–719.

117. Heeschen C, Hamm CW, Jens B. Predictive value of C-reactive protein and troponin T in patients with unstable angina: A comparative analysis [abstract]. Circulation 1999;1000(Suppl I):I-371.

118. de Winter RJ, Bholasingh R, Lijmer JG, et al: Independent prognostic value of C-reactive protein and troponin I in patients with unstable angina or non-Q-wave myocardial infarction. Cardiovasc Res 1999;42:240–245.

119. Morrow DA, Rifai N, Antman EM, et al: C-reactive protein is a potent predictor of mortality independently and in combination with troponin T in acute coronary syndromes: A TIMI IIA substudy. J Am Coll Cardiol 1998;31:1460–1465.

120. Ferreiros ER, Boissonnet CP, Pizarro R, et al: Independent prognostic value of elevated C-reactive protein in unstable angina. Circulation 1999;100:1958–1963.

121. Biasucci LM, Liuzzo G, Grillo RL, et al: Elevated levels of C-reactive protein at discharge in patients with unstable angina predict recurrent instability. Circulation 1999;99:855–860.

122. Antman EM, Cohen M, Bernink PJLM, et al: The TIMI risk score for unstable angina/non-ST elevation MI: A method for prognostication and therapeutic decision making. JAMA 2000; 284: 835–842.

123. Boersma E, Harrington RA, Moliterno DJ, et al: Platelet glycoprotein IIb/IIIa in acute coronary syndromes: A meta-analysis of all major randomised clinical trials. Lancet 2002;359:189–198.

124. Roig E, Castaner A, Simmons B, et al: In-hospital mortality rates from acute myocardial infarction by race in US hospitals: Findings from the National Hospital Discharge Survey. Circulation 1987;76:280–288.

125. Maynard C, Litwin PE, Martin JS, et al: Characteristics of black patients admitted to coronary care units in metropolitan Seattle: Results from the Myocardial Infarction Triage and Intervention Registry (MITI). Am J Cardiol 1991;67:18–23.

126. Goldberg KC, Hartz AJ, Jacobsen SJ, et al: Racial and community factors influencing coronary artery bypass graft surgery rates for all 1986 Medicare patients. JAMA 1992;267:1473-1477.

127. Johnson PA, Lee TH, Cook EF, et al: Effect of race on the presentation and management of patients with acute chest pain. Ann Intern Med 1993;118:593-601.

128. Taylor HA, Chaitman BR, Rogers WJ, et al: Race and prognosis after myocardial infarction: results of the Thrombolysis in Myocardial Infarction (TIMI) Phase II Trial. Circulation 1993;88:1484-1494.

129. Peterson ED, Wright SM, Daley J, et al: Racial variation in cardiac procedure use and survival following acute myocardial infarction in the Department of Veterans Affairs. JAMA 1994;271:1175-1180.

130. Smith SC, Gilpin E, Ahnve S, et al: Outlook for acute myocardial infarction in the very elderly compared with that in patients 65-75 years. J Am Coll Cardiol 1990;16:784-792.

131. Montague TJ, Ikuta RM, Wong RY, et al: Comparison of risk and patterns of practice in patients older and younger than 70 years with acute myocardial infarction in a two-year period (1987-1989). Am J Cardiol 1991;68:843-847.

132. Udvarhelyi IS, Gatsonis C, Epstein AM, et al: Acute myocardial infarction in the Medicare population: Process of care and clinical outcomes. JAMA 1992;268:2530-2536.

133. Goldberg RJ, Gore JM, Gurwitz JH, et al: The impact of age on the incidence and prognosis of initial acute myocardial infarction: The Worcester Heart Attack Study. Am Heart J 1989;117:543-549.

134. Karlson BW, Herlitz J, Pettersson P, et al: One-year prognosis in patients hospitalized with a history of unstable angina. Clin Cardiol 1993;16:397-402.

135. Moise A, Theroux P, Taeymans Y, et al: Unstable angina and progression of coronary atherosclerosis. N Engl J Med 1983;309:685-689.

136. Ambrose JA, Winters SL, Arora RR, et al: Angiographic evolution of coronary artery morphology in unstable angina. J Am Coll Cardiol 1986;7:472-478.

137. Holmes DR Jr, Hartzler GO, Smith HC, et al: Coronary artery thrombosis in patients with unstable angina. Br Heart J 1981;45:411-416.

138. Vetrovec GW, Cowley MJ, Overton H, et al: Intracoronary thrombus in syndromes of unstable myocardial ischemia. Am Heart J 1981;102:1202-1208.

139. Capone G, Wolf NM, Meyer B, et al: Frequency of intracoronary filling defects by angiography in angina pectoris at rest. Am J Cardiol 1985;56:403-406.

140. Gotoh K, Katoh K, Fukui S, et al: Angiographic visualization of coronary thrombus during anginal attack in unstable angina [abstract]. Circulation 1985;72(Suppl III):III-112.

141. Maseri A: Pathogenetic classifications of unstable angina as a guideline to individual patient management and prognosis. Am J Med 1986;80(Suppl 4C):48-55.

142. Fitzgerald DJ, Roy L, Catella F, et al: Platelet activation in unstable coronary disease. N Engl J Med 1986;315:983-989.

143. Haerem JW: Mural platelet microthrombi and major acute lesions of main epicardial arteries in sudden coronary death. Atherosclerosis 1974;19:529-541.

144. Ross J Jr, Gilpin EA, Madsen EB, et al: A decision scheme for coronary angiography after acute myocardial infarction. Circulation 1989;79:292-303.

145. Ross J Jr, Bradenburg RO, Dinsmore RE, et al: Guidelines for coronary angiography: Report of the Joint American College of Cardiology/American Heart Association Task Force on Assessment of Cardiovascular Procedures. J Am Coll Cardiol 1987;10:935-950 and Circulation 1987;76:963A-977A.

146. Breyer RH, Engelman RM, Rousou JA, et al: Postinfarction angina: An expanding subset of patients undergoing coronary artery bypass. J Thorac Cardiovasc Surg 1985;90:532-540.

147. DeBusk RF, Blonqvist CG, Kochoukos NT, et al: Identification and treatment of low-risk patients after acute myocardial infarction and coronary artery bypass graft surgery. N Engl J Med 1986;314:161-166.

148. Cermak J, Key NS, Bach RR, et al: C-reactive protein induces human peripheral blood monocytes to synthesise tissue factor. Blood 1993;82:513-520.

149. Ridker PM, Glynn RJ, Hennekens CH: C-reactive protein adds to the predictive value of total and HDL cholesterol in determining risk of first myocardial infarction. Circulation 1998;97:2007-2011.

150. Ridker PM, Cushman M, Stampfer MJ, et al: Plasma concentration of C-reactive protein and risk of developing peripheral vascular disease. Circulation 1998;97:425-428.

151. Fernández-Ortiz A, Badimón JJ, Falk E, et al: Characterisation of the relative thrombogenicity of atherosclerotic plaque components: Implications for consequences of plaque rupture. J Am Coll Cardiol 1994;23:1562-1569.

152. Moreno PR, Bernardi VH, López-Cuéllar J, et al: Macrophages, smooth muscle cells, and tissue factor in unstable angina: Implications for cell-mediated thrombogenicity in acute coronary syndromes. Circulation 1996;94:3090-3097.

153. Wilcox JN, Smith KM, Schqartz SM, et al: Localisation of tissue factor in the normal vessel wall and in the atherosclerotic plaque. Proc Natl Sci U S A 1989;86:2839-2843.

154. Ambrose JA, Tannenbaum MA, Alexopoulos D, et al: Angiographic progression of coronary artery disease and the development of myocardial infarction. J Am Coll Cardiol 1988;12:56-62.

155. Alison HW, Russell RO Jr, Mantle JA, et al: Coronary anatomy and arteriography in patients with unstable angina pectoris. Am J Cardiol 1978;41:204-209.

156. Fuster V, Frye RL, Connolly DC, et al: Arteriographic patterns early in the onset of coronary syndromes. Br Heart J 1975;37:1250-1255.

157. Ambrose JA, Winters SL, Stern A, et al: Angiographic morphology and the pathogenesis of unstable angina pectoris. J Am Coll Cardiol 1985;5:609-616.

158. Benamer H, Steg PG, Benessiano J, et al: Elevated cardiac troponin I predicts a high-risk angiographic anatomy of the culprit lesion in unstable angina. Am Heart J 1999;137:815-820.

159. Heeschen C, van Den Brand MJ, Hamm CW, et al: Angiographic findings in patients with refractory unstable angina according to troponin T status. Circulation 1999;100:1509-1514.

160. Davies MJ: Stability and instability: Two faces of coronary atherosclerosis. Circulation 1996;94:2013-2020.

161. van der Wal AC, Becker AE, van der Loos CM, et al: Site of intimal rupture or erosion of thrombosed coronary atherosclerotic plaques is characterized by an inflammatory process irrespective of the dominant plaque morphology. Circulation 1994;89:36-44.

162. Ross R. Atherosclerosis—an inflammatory disease. N Engl J Med 1999;340:115-126.

163. Davies MJ: The evolving cholesterol knowledge base. Stability and instability: Two faces of coronary atherosclerosis. ACCEL 1995;27:36-37.

164. Davies MJ: Reactive oxygen species, metalloproteinases and plaque stability. Circulation 1998;97:2382-2383.

165. Little W, Constantinescu M, Applegate RJ, et al: Can coronary angiography predict the site of a subsequent myocardial infarction in patients with mild-to-moderate coronary artery disease? Circulation 1988;78:1157-1166.

166. Kaski JC, Chester MR, Chen L, et al: Rapid angiographic progression of coronary artery disease in patients with angina pectoris: The role of complex stenosis morphology. Circulation 1995;92:2058-2065.

167. Levin DC, Fallon JT: Significance of the angiographic morphology of localized coronary stenoses: Histopathologic correlations. Circulation 1982;66:316-320.

168. Davies SW, Marchant B, Lyons JP, et al: Irregular coronary lesion morphology after thrombolysis predicts early clinical instability. J Am Coll Cardiol 1991;18:669-674.

169. Ellis S, Alderman EL, Cain K, et al: Morphology of left anterior descending coronary territory lesions as a predictor of anterior myocardial infarction: A CASS registry study. J Am Coll Cardiol 1989;13:1481-1491.

170. Wilson R, Holida M, White C: Quantitative angiographic morphology of coronary stenoses leading to myocardial infarction or unstable angina. Circulation 1985;73:286-293.

171. Chen L, Chester MR, Redwood S, et al: Angiographic stenosis progression and coronary events in patients with "stabilized" unstable angina. Circulation 1995;91:2319-2324.

172. Kaski JC, Chen L, Chester M: Rapid angiographic progression of "target" and "nontarget" stenoses in patients awaiting coronary angioplasty. J Am Coll Cardiol 1995;26:416-421.

173. Chester MR, Chen L, Tousoulis D, et al: Differential progression of complex and smooth stenoses within the same coronary tree in men with stable coronary artery disease. J Am Coll Cardiol 1995;25:837-842.

174. Chester MR, Chen L, Kaski JC: The natural history of unheralded complex coronary plaques. J Am Coll Cardiol 1996;28: 604–608.

175. Williams AE, Freeman MR, Chisholm RJ, et al: Angiographic morphology in unstable angina pectoris. Am J Cardiol 1988;62: 1024–1027.

176. Bugiardini R, Pozzati A, Borghi A, et al: Angiographic morphology in unstable angina and its relation to trasient myocardial ischemia and hospital outcome. Am J Cardiol 1991;67:460–464.

177. Mann J, Kaski JC, Pereira WI, et al: Histological patterns of atherosclerotic plaques in unstable angina patients vary according to clinical presentation. Heart 1998;80:19–22.

178. Burke AP, Kolodgie FD, Farb A, et al: Healed plaque ruptures and sudden coronary death: Evidence that subclinical rupture has a role in plaque progression. Circulation 2001;103:934–940.

179. Tomai F, Crea F, Gaspardone A, et al: Unstable angina and elevated C-reactive protein levels predict enhanced vasoreactivity of the culprit lesion. Circulation 2001;104:1471–1476.

180. Bogaty P, Poisier P, Simard S, et al: Biological profiles in subjects with recurrent acute coronary events compared with subject with long-standing stable angina. Circulation 2001;103: 3062–3068.

181. Farb A, Burke AP, Tang AL, et al: Coronary plaque erosion without rupture into a lipid core: A frequent cause of coronary thrombosis in sudden coronary death. Circulation 1996;93:1354–1363.

182. Merlini PA, Bauer KA, Oltrona L, et al: Persistent activation of coagulation mechanism in unstable angina and myocardial infarction. Circulation 1994;90:61–68.

183. Garcia-Moll X, Coccolo F, Cole D, Kaski JC: Serum neopterin and complex stenosis morphology in patients with unstable angina. J Am Coll Cardiol 2000;35:956–962.

184. Gupta S, Fredericks S, Schwartzman RA, et al: Serum neopterin in acute coronary syndromes [research letter]. Lancet 1997;349: 1252.

185. Schumacher M, Halwachs G, Tatzber F, et al: Increased neopterin in patients with chronic and acute coronary syndromes. J Am Coll Cardiol 1997;30:703–707.

186. Kaski JC: Increased neopterin in patients with chronic and acute coronary syndromes. J Am Coll Cardiol 1998;31:1215–1216.

187. Bayés-Genís A, Conover CA, Overgaard MT, et al: Pregnancy-associated plasma protein A as a marker of acute coronary syndromes. N Engl J Med 2001;345:1022–1029.

188. de Lemos JA, Morrow DA, Bentley JH, et al: The prognostic value of B-type natriuretic peptide in patients with acute coronary syndromes. N Engl J Med 2001;345:1014–1021.

189. Yasue H, Yoshimura M, Sumida H, et al: Localisation and mechanism of secretion of B-type natriuretic peptide in comparison with those of A-type natriuretic peptide in normal subjects and patients with heart failure. Circulation 1994;90:194–203.

190. Cheng V, Kazanagra R, Garcia A, et al: A rapid bedside test for B-type peptide predicts treatment outcomes in patients admitted for decompensated heart failure: A pilot study. J Am Coll Cardiol 2001;37:386–391.

191. Tummala PE, Chen XL, Sundell CL, et al: Angiotensin II induces vascular cell adhesion molecule-1 expression in rat vasculature: a potential link between the renin-angiotensin system and atherosclerosis. Circulation 1999;100:1223–1229.

192. Harrison DG: Endothelial function and oxidant stress. Clin Cardiol 1997;20(Suppl II):II-11–II-17.

193. Ridker PM, Rifai N, Pfeffer MA, et al: Inflammation, pravastatin, and the risk of coronary events after myocardial infarction in patients with average cholesterol levels. Circulation 1998;98:839–844.

■ ■ ■ chapter 5

Pathology of Stable and Acute Coronary Syndromes

Jacob Fog Bentzon
Erling Falk

Atherosclerosis is a chronic inflammatory disease of the intima of large- and medium-sized arteries. This condition has existed at least from ancient times, with the oldest pathologic findings in Egyptian mummies from the third millennium BC,[1] and thus has probably been encountered by every pathologist throughout history. However, the common nature of atherosclerosis, its wide heterogeneity, and the inconsistent relationship between symptoms and atherosclerotic lesions found after death long hampered the recognition of atherosclerosis as a cause of death and disability.

Edward Jenner, who also introduced vaccination, proposed coronary artery disease to be the cause of stable angina pectoris in 1786, and his friend, Caleb Hillier Parry, soon thereafter hypothesized that reduced blood flow was the underlying pathophysiologic culprit.[2] For the acute manifestations, progress was much slower. Though James Herrick had documented occlusive thrombosis of severely atherosclerotic coronary arteries as the cause of acute myocardial infarction (AMI) in 1912,[3] it would take 50 years until the careful autopsy studies by Constantinides, Chapman, and Friedman in the mid-1960s described the steps leading from atherosclerosis to coronary thrombosis.[4-6] These investigators demonstrated that the great majority of coronary thrombi are precipitated by atherosclerotic *plaque rupture* whereby highly thrombogenic plaque components are exposed to the flowing blood. Later it was established that such thrombi can also form on de-endothelialized but otherwise intact plaques, and the term *plaque erosion* was introduced to describe this phenomenon.[7]

Today we know that not only AMI but also unstable angina and most cases of sudden death are caused by thrombosis superimposed on ruptured or eroded plaques. The understanding of this shared pathogenic entity is reflected in the use of the collective clinical term *acute coronary syndromes (ACS)*.

Data from the Duke Cardiovascular Databank illustrate the differences in severity and progression between the modes of presentation of coronary atherosclerosis (Fig. 5-1).[8]

An ACS starts abruptly with a many-fold increment in mortality followed by a gradual decline of risk, reaching that of stable angina in a few months. This chapter reviews the evidence that it is acute thrombosis, usually precipitated by plaque rupture, that initiates the syndrome and gradual healing of the complicated plaque that ends it. By comparison, stable angina is a relatively benign disease. Thus, if the devastating thrombotic complications of plaques could be avoided, atherosclerosis would be a rather harmless disease. Why do some plaques present clinically as stable angina, whereas others cause acute and life-threatening luminal thrombosis? The issue is addressed at the end of the chapter through an account of the concept of plaque vulnerability. The first sections describe the formation and classification of atherosclerotic plaques and the pathogenesis of stenoses in stable angina.

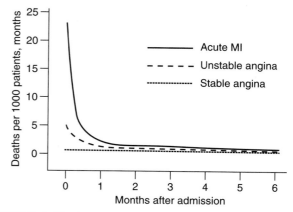

FIGURE 5–1. The beginning and end of acute coronary syndromes. The rate of cardiac death in 21,761 patients grouped by admission diagnosis and treated for coronary artery disease without interventional procedures at Duke University Medical Center between 1985 and 1992. (Redrawn from Braunwald E, Mark DB, Jones RH, et al: Unstable Angina: Diagnosis and Management. Rockville, Md, Agency for Health Care Policy and Research and the National Heart, Lung, and Blood Institute, US Public Health Service, US Department of Health and Human Services, 1994, p 1. AHCPR Publication No 94-0602 [amended]).

CLASSIFICATION AND PROGRESSION OF ATHEROSCLEROSIS

Atherosclerosis is a chronic inflammatory disorder of the intima of large- and medium-sized arteries characterized by recruitment of monocytes and T lymphocytes and the induction of fibrosis with smooth muscle cell (SMC) proliferation and matrix synthesis.[9]

In their series of reviews of autopsy data from persons of different ages, the Committee on Vascular Lesions of the Council on Atherosclerosis, American Heart Association (AHA), has proposed that atherosclerosis develops through morphologically differentiable lesion types and has adopted a recommendation on nomenclature of these lesions.[10] The lesion types depicted in Figure 5-2 derive from this important publication, although their inter-relationships do not completely follow the AHA classification. The patient with clinically significant coronary atherosclerosis has a mixture of all of these plaque types (Fig. 5–3).

Fatty Streaks

The central proinflammatory instigator in atherosclerosis appears to be retention of lipoproteins, primarily low-density lipoprotein (LDL), in the arterial intima.[11] At sites of branching of the arterial tree where low shear stress, high wall tension, or both prevail, normal arteries have intimal thickenings most likely as a physiologic adaptive response. These sites are affected early during atherogenesis, that is, they are *atherosclerosis-prone*. With further progression of atherosclerosis, adjacent intima is also involved so that the majority of the coronary arterial tree is affected in persons dying from an ACS in old age.[12]

At atherosclerosis-prone sites, extracellular lipid droplets of fused LDL particles in the proteoglycan-rich subendothelial layer form as the first morphologic sign of atherosclerosis. The fusion of LDL particles and their retention to proteoglycans of the intimal matrix may be facilitated by the modifying action of hydrolytic enzymes, such as type IIa secretory nonpancreatic phospholipase A_2 and secretory sphingomyelinase.[13,14] Native LDL particles do not have these properties.[14]

Subendothelial oxidative modification of native and fused LDL particles by radical species yields a range of bioactive lipids.[15] Macrophages are proficient producers of oxidizing radical species and may be the quantitatively more important in this process, although endothelial cells and SMCs may be essential in early steps before intimal macrophages appear.[15] The oxidized LDL moieties, in turn, are proinflammatory mediators that (1) are chemoattractant for blood monocytes[9]; (2) stimulate recruitment and replication of monocyte-derived macrophages through induction of adhesion molecules (e.g., vascular cell adhesion molecule [VCAM]-1), chemoattractants (e.g., monocyte chemoattractant protein [MCP]-1, transforming growth factor [TGF]-β), and growth factors (e.g., granulocyte-macrophage colony-stimulating factor)[9]; and/or (3) activate macrophages (after ingestion), increasing their ability to oxidize more lipoproteins.[16] In the face of hypercholesterolemia, the inflammatory response may not be able to effectively neutralize oxidized LDL, and instead continuing cycles of inflammation, modification of lipoproteins, and further inflammation are maintained in the arterial intima. T lymphocytes are present in atherosclerotic lesions early on, and immune responses probably augment the vicious cycle of ongoing inflammation,[17] as does hypertension and diabetes through poorly understood mechanisms.

Macrophages and SMCs avidly ingest oxidized, but not native, LDL particles through scavenger receptors. As a result, their cytoplasm become packed with droplets of cholesteryl esters,[18] giving them the appearance of *foam cells*. This accumulation of cholesterol is counteracted by the reverse cholesterol transport mechanism.[19] Nascent high-density lipoproteins (HDL) that pass through the endothelium accept excess cholesterol by an interaction between apolipoprotein A-I and the adenosine triphosphate–binding cassette transporter 1 in foam cell membranes. Cholesterol is incorporated into HDL particles by lecithin:cholesterol acyl transferase and ultimately cleared from the circulation by means of hepatic scavenger receptor BI or after cholesteryl ester transfer protein–mediated transfer to very-low-density lipoprotein (VLDL) and LDL particles through hepatic VLDL and LDL receptors.[19] The balance between these processes may ultimately be the key determinant for the rate of foam cell generation. Small accumulations of foam cells are present in half of infants in the first 6 months of life, but the number declines in subsequent years and probably reflects risk factors of the mother.[20,21] At puberty, fatty streaks develop in two thirds of persons and is soon followed by the appearance of lipid pools

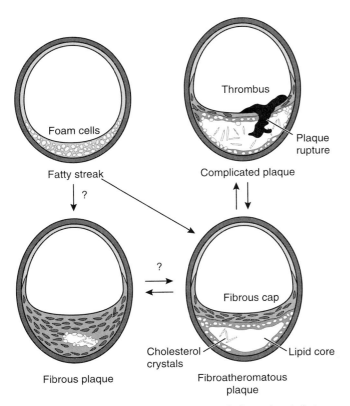

FIGURE 5–2. Classification and progression of atherosclerotic lesions.

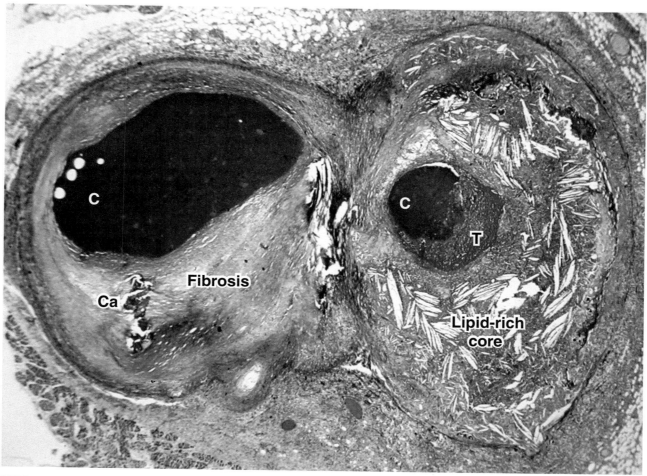

FIGURE 5–3. Severe atherosclerosis: a variable mixture of lesion types. Cross-sectioned coronary artery bifurcation illustrating a fibrous plaque *(left)* and a complicated plaque with a nonocclusive thrombosis in the greatly enlarged side branch *(right)*. Elastin-trichrome stain. C, contrast in the lumen; Ca, calcification; T, thrombosis.

and incipient calcification in high-susceptibility locations.[21]

Fibroatheromatous Plaques

As atherosclerosis progresses, confluent areas of extracellular lipid pools form in the deep parts of lesions. This has often been called the *necrotic core.* However, continuing LDL particle fusion and retention in the proteoglycan matrix is probably more important than cell degeneration and is further facilitated by the absence of lymph drainage in the arterial intima.[13] Biochemical studies show that the fatty acid composition and the ratio of free to esterified cholesterol comply with the composition of LDL particles.[22] Cell death, both oncosis and apoptosis, has been documented by electron microscopy at the margin of the lipid pool,[23] and studies using immunohistochemical and TUNEL staining techniques have identified macrophage-specific antigens and apoptotic nuclear fragments within the core, indicating that cell death contributes to its formation or growth, or both.[24,25] Apoptosis of foam cells may be particularly important in determining the thrombogenicity of the lipid core. Perfusion chamber studies have identified the lipid core as the most thrombogenic part of the ath-

erosclerotic plaque and have linked its thrombogenic potential closely to the expression of tissue factor.[26] Tissue factor is expressed in a subpopulation of foam cells, but tissue factor activity is highly dependent on the presence of anionic phospholipids, chiefly phosphatidylserine, which is confined to the internal layer of the cell membrane in the living cell. During apoptosis, phosphatidylserine is redistributed to the external membrane layer, conferring potent procoagulant activity to membrane microparticles arising from apoptotic cell fragmentation. It has been shown that these apoptotic microparticles account for almost all tissue factor activity of the lipid-rich pool.[27]

SMCs respond to the intimal injury by migrating, proliferating, and synthesizing collagen-rich matrix, thereby producing the fibrous component of the developing fibroatheromatous plaque. Literally, both softening and hardening are present in this advanced atherosclerotic plaque in the form of a soft, hypocellular, lipid-rich core (*athére*—Greek for "gruel" or "porridge") walled off by a hard, fibrous capsule (*skleros*—Greek for "hard"). The part of the fibrous tissue that separates the lipid core from the lumen is called the *fibrous cap.* It has a high content of type I collagen arranged in a densely woven pattern interspersed with groups of SMCs.

Sometimes, several layers of fibrous tissue are present intertwined by lipid cores (multilayered fibroatheromatous plaque).[10]

The SMCs produce the connective tissue matrix proteins, including the collagens, under the control of growth factors such as TGF-β and platelet-derived growth factor (PDGF). Both factors are upregulated in the atherosclerotic plaque but generally not expressed in normal intima.[28] The importance of TGF-β in inducing the fibrous reparative response was underlined in a study in the apoE-deficient mouse model of atherosclerosis, wherein inhibition of TGF-β signaling using neutralizing antibodies favored development of plaques with increased inflammatory component and decreased collagen content.[29] Inhibition of PDGF signaling in the same model led to decreased smooth muscle content in plaques but also decreased plaque development overall, complicating the interpretation.[30]

Granules of calcium deposits are found scattered throughout the lesion, both extracellularly among lipid droplets and cell remnants and intracellularly in SMC organelles.[31] These initially microscopic foci of calcification expand and fuse to form larger lumps and plates of calcium deposits; osseus metaplasia may occur as a late step.[31] Neovascularization, often expressing leukocyte adhesion molecules and associated with inflammatory cell infiltration, is frequently present at the stage of fibroatheroma, and it has been suggested that these new vessels could play an active role in the recruitment of leukocytes into plaques and thus contribute to disease progression.[32]

Beyond doubt, fatty streaks form the substrate on which fibroatheromatous plaques develop. This is solidly documented in animal models of atherosclerosis, e.g., the apoE-deficient mouse, in which smooth transition types are observed. However, there may be dissociation between the stimuli that cause fatty streaks to generate and those that cause them to progress to advanced stages. Females have more aortic fatty streaks than males early in life despite the fact that males develop more advanced lesions later in life.[33] Similarly, the thoracic aorta has more fatty streaks than the abdominal aorta early in life but the opposite applies for advanced lesions later in life.[34] This seems confusing, but may on the other hand not be surprising given the shift in plaque biology that occurs with progression beyond the fatty streak stage with increasing involvement of SMCs and fibrous matrix.

Fibrous Plaques

The majority of plaques examined at autopsy are not fibroatheromatous but fibrous plaques with an absent or minimal atheromatous component.[12] Their genesis is not fully understood. It is possible that the balance between the fibroproliferative response and the processes that lead to lipid core formation vary widely in location and time. Fibrous plaques may thus represent an analogue to fibroatheromatous plaques in which fibroproliferation has severely dominated over core growth, and time-dependent alterations in the balance may cause fibroatheromatous plaques to turn into fibrous plaques

and vice versa. The view of an intimate relationship between fibrous and fibroatheromatous plaques is substantiated by the fact that sequential sectioning of atherosclerotic lesions often yields both sections in which a large atheromatous component is present and sections in which the lesion appears completely fibrotic. On the other hand, some pathologists think that fibrous plaques may have a separate genesis, developing in the absence of a preceding fatty streak.

Complicated Plaques

When thrombus is present, with or without luminal obstruction, the lesion is denoted a *complicated plaque* and is further subdivided by the presence or absence of *plaque rupture*. With rupture (also known as *plaque fissuring*), the thrombus is in direct connection with the highly thrombogenic lipid core of a fibroatheromatous plaque through a disruption of the fibrous cap. When no such rupture can be identified despite a thorough search, the term *plaque erosion* is used.[7] Both fibrous and fibroatheromatous plaques may be complicated by plaque erosion. Note that plaque erosion, being an diagnosis of exclusion, does not reflect a uniform pathophysiologic entity, and although erosion (endothelial denudation) is generally present this is not documented as the precipitating thrombogenic mechanism. *Plaque disruption* is sometimes used synonymously with *plaque rupture* and sometimes as a collective term for rupture and erosion.

STABLE ANGINA

Myocardial ischemia results from flow obstruction by plaque, thrombosis on plaque, vasoconstriction (spasm), or a combination thereof; flow obstruction by plaque is characteristic for stable angina, thrombosis on plaque being typical for ACS and vasoconstriction important in both.

The severity of chronic flow obstruction in atherosclerotic arteries depends on plaque size and *remodeling* of the vessel wall. Rather than being a static structure, the media and adventitia of diseased segments may both dilate to preserve lumen (*positive remodeling*, also known as *outward remodeling* or *compensatory enlargement*) or shrink to diminish it (*negative remodeling*, also known as *paradoxical shrinkage*) (Fig. 5–4). This has been known for decades from autopsy studies, but knowledge and interest in this area were sparse before the introduction of intravascular ultrasonography (IVUS) and its ability to assess dynamic aspects of remodeling in vivo. In prospective studies, remodeling of a lesion site is defined dynamically as the ratio between the areas within the external elastic lamina (EEM area) at two successive measurements. More often, a cross-sectional design is used and remodeling is indirectly assessed as the ratio between the EEM area at the lesion site to the EEM area at a proximal reference site minimally affected by atherosclerosis. Positive remodeling is defined as a remodeling ratio greater than 1.0 (or 1.05) and negative remodeling as remodeling ratio less than

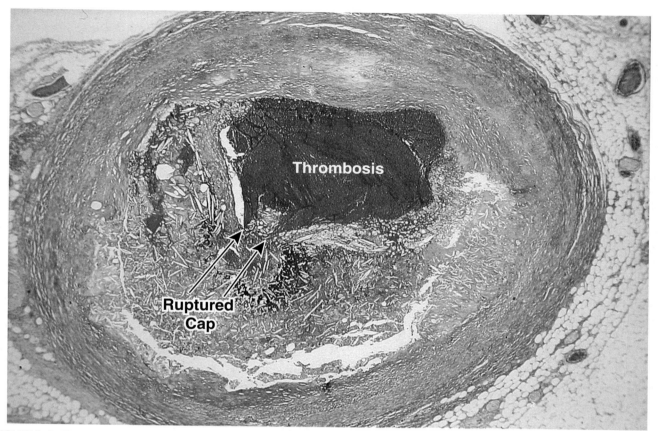

FIGURE 5–4. Plaque rupture. Cross-section of a ruptured plaque with superimposed occlusive thrombosis. Elastin-trichrome stain.

1.0 (or 0.95). In a recently published autopsy study, Varnava et al examined 389 coronary segments with plaque formation but no (acute) thrombotic complications in men dying from sudden cardiac death.[35] They found positive remodeling of the vessel wall in 317 of 389 of the segments examined and negative remodeling in 72 of 389 segments. In this material, remodeling ratio was a stronger determinant of lumen stenosis than plaque size, a finding also reported by others.[36]

Stenosis Formation

Rather than being caused by linear plaque growth, stenosis formation often takes on an episodic course in which positive remodeling long preserves the lumen and rapid plaque growth or negative remodeling, or both, hastily attenuate it. Although some stenotic sites visible at angiography performed at regular intervals in patients with stable angina show gradual narrowing, more arise rapidly, with newly developed high-grade stenoses at sites that had preserved lumen the year before.[37]

Resting blood flow through a stenosed artery is not significantly affected until the lumen area is reduced by approximately 80% (or the diameter by 50%), although the flow reserve is decreased with less reduction.[38] At autopsy, a plaque causing chronic stenoses of this magnitude is often a multilayered fibroatheromatous plaque with high collagen content and relatively small lipid cores.[39] A proportion of these plaques have residual

thrombus as evaluated by atherectomy,[40] and post mortem there may be evidence of previous occlusive thrombosis with the development of a multichannel lumen suggesting recanalization or myocardial scarring in the region supplied by the artery.[39] Furthermore, a special nonuniform pattern of dense (older) and loosely arranged (younger) collagen, judged to indicate healed plaque rupture, has been identified in many coronary plaques, particularly in those that cause chronic high-grade stenoses.[41] Often, several healed rupture sites are present in plaques and the number of healed ruptures correlates with the severity of stenosis.[42] Indeed, plaque rupture is a common event that often does not lead to symptomatic thrombosis. Davies et al found ruptured plaques without luminal thrombosis in 9% of persons who died from noncardiac causes, and this figure increased to 22% (including 5% with nonocclusive luminal thrombosis) if an atherosclerosis-related disease such as diabetes or hypertension was present.[43]

The emerging message is that subclinical plaque rupture and superimposed thrombosis are common in the development of stenoses, contradicting the traditional dogma of stable ischemic symptoms reflecting a stable atherosclerotic process. Hypothetically, plaque rupture and subsequent repair with fibrous tissue deposition and contraction may be the central pathophysiologic mechanism of severe stenosis formation. First of all, this would explain the episodic rather than gradual development of stenoses observed in angiographic studies. Rapid growth of the fibrous plaque component may result from incorporation and organization of overlying thrombus and a fibroproliferative response induced by growth factors, such as PDGF and TGF-β, that are released from degranulating platelets during superimposed thrombosis.[44] As in general wound healing, this is likely followed by scar-like contraction resulting in negative remodeling (see Fig. 5-4).

Whether or not caused by plaque rupture and repair processes, some kind of contraction (indicated by negative remodeling) does occur in stenosis formation, and this is associated with the presence of a large fibrous plaque component. Varnava et al found no or negative remodeling in 72 of the 389 lesions examined, and Mintz et al identified that 15% of lesions responsible for stable angina at preinterventional IVUS were inadequately or negatively remodeled after correcting for normal vessel tapering.[35,45] Recently, a combined angioscopy and IVUS study showed that negative remodeling was much more prevalent in plaques that appeared white by angioscopy (indicating fibrous plaque) than in yellow plaques (indicating lipid-rich plaque), in which positive remodeling was the rule.[46]

Coronary angioplasty or atherectomy may be viewed as an experimental means of gaining insight into the dynamics and mechanisms of plaque repair. Restenosis after balloon angioplasty or atherectomy occurs in 30% to 50% of patients as the result of negative remodeling (beyond that of elastic recoil) and neointima formation with proliferation of SMCs and organization of thrombus.[47] Of these, negative remodeling accounts for more than half of the postinterventional lumen loss.[48]

Although these procedures do not mimic frank plaque rupture,[47] the ensuing reparative processes may be similar. An SMC-rich plaque component, histologically indistinguishable from postangioplasty neointima, is found in nearly half of primary plaques debulked by coronary atherectomy from patients with unstable angina and is found in specimens from patients in clinically stable condition.[40,49] Furthermore, TGF-β signaling, which has been suggested to be important in controlling fibrous cap formation, is equally important in postangioplastic negative remodeling and neointima formation, at least in the rat.[50]

Investigation into the putative role of plaque rupture and repair in the pathogenesis of stable angina would be greatly facilitated if a reliable animal model of spontaneous plaque rupture could be developed.

ACUTE CORONARY SYNDROMES

ACSs, with or without ST-segment elevation, are almost always caused by a luminal thrombus imposed on a ruptured or eroded atherosclerotic plaque, with or without concomitant vasoconstriction.[51] Rare causes include emboli, artery dissection, vasculitis, cocaine abuse, and trauma.[52] Sudden coronary death is associated with the finding of acute or organized thrombus in more than 70% of cases; the rest die with severe coronary disease in the absence of thrombosis.[51] In ST-segment elevation myocardial infarction, the thrombus is occlusive and sustained, whereas in ACS without ST-segment elevation and sudden cardiac death, the thrombus is usually incomplete and dynamic.[53,54]

■ ▩ ■

TABLE 5-1 PLAQUES UNDERLYING FATAL THROMBI IN ACUTE CORONARY SYNDROMES

STUDY	SYNDROME	SEX	N	RUPTURE n	RUPTURE %	REFERENCE
Chapman, 1965			19	19	100%	5
Constantinides, 1966			17	17	100%	4
Friedman, 1966			40	30	75%	6
Tracy, 1985[55]			21	18	86%	55
Falk, 1983[56]	AMI	M	37	32	86%	56
		F	12	8	67%	
van der Wal, 1994[57]	AMI		20	12	60%	57
Arbustini, 1999[58]	AMI	M	184	150	82%	58
		F	107	67	63%	
Kojima, 2000[59]	AMI	M	74	63	85%	59
		F	26	18	69%	
Farb, 1996	SCD	M	34	23	68%	7
		F	16	5	31%	
Davies, 1997[60]	SCD	M	134	113	84%	60
		F	27	16	59%	
Burke, 1997[61]	SCD	M	59	41	69%	61
Burke, 1998[62]	SCD	F, ≤ 50 yr	16	1	6%	62
		F, ≥ 50 yr	10	7	70%	
All, N > 900	Sex unknown		213	184	86%	
	Males		522	422	81%	
	Females*		182	116	63%	
	Females, < 50 y		16	1	6%	

Where information is lacking, it was not given in the original publication.
AMI, acute myocardial infarction; SCD, sudden coronary death.
*Excluding young females in Farb et al (7) and Burke et al (62).

Table 5-1 offers an overview that, although far from complete, sketches the relative importance of rupture and erosion in provoking fatal coronary thrombosis in different studies and patient groups. Regardless of the type of ACS, thrombus is formed on a ruptured plaque in about 80% and 60% of cases in men and postmenopausal women, respectively. Absence of plaque rupture (i.e., plaque erosion) seems to be more prevalent in females, especially the young,[62] and in patients with preceding stable angina.[59]

The magnitude of the thrombotic response and hence the form of clinical presentation has not been linked to characteristics of the underlying ruptured or eroded plaques in autopsy studies. This is especially intriguing in the case of plaque rupture because we know it is a common event but has an extremely varied outcome. The determinants are probably those of the classic triad of Virchow: (1) thrombogenicity of the exposed plaque material, (2) local flow disturbances, and (3) systemic thrombotic propensity. With plaque rupture, cap collagen and the highly thrombogenic lipid core, enriched in tissue factor-expressing apoptotic microparticles, are exposed to the thrombogenic factors of the blood.[51] The mechanism of thrombus formation on eroded plaques is more controversial. Van der Wal et al identified superficial infiltration of activated macrophages at the site of erosion in all eight coronary thrombi examined,[57] whereas Farb et al found that the sites of erosion were enriched in SMCs and proteoglycans rather than macrophages.[7] Whatever the cause of endothelial denudation, it is a relatively week thrombogenic stimulus and thus flow disturbances and systemic thrombotic propensity may be particularly important in this setting.

The time relationship between plaque rupture and syndrome onset is not easily assessed because rupture in itself is asymptomatic and the following thrombotic process highly unpredictable. Plaque material is sometimes found interspersed in the thrombus,[57] indicating that severe thrombosis followed immediately after plaque rupture. In other cases, superimposed thrombosis seems to be a highly dynamic process of alternating thrombus growth and lysis, causing intermittent flow obstruction and the formation of a layered thrombus developing over days (Figs. 5-5 and 5-6).[63,64] Prodromal chest pain within 7 days before AMI onset occurs in about one fourth of patients regardless of whether the precipitating event is plaque rupture or erosion.[59] While blood flow continues over the culprit lesion, microemboli of plaque material and thrombus may be washed away, with the potential to produce downstream microembolic vascular obstruction with compromised tissue perfusion (see Figs. 5-5 and 5-6).[63,65] Such microembolization has been associated with an aggravated prognosis for patients with AMI and unstable angina.[65-67]

PLAQUE VULNERABILITY

Plaque rupture is fundamental in eliciting ACSs and probably a key element in the cause of stable angina. If rupture could be prevented, the gradual growth of

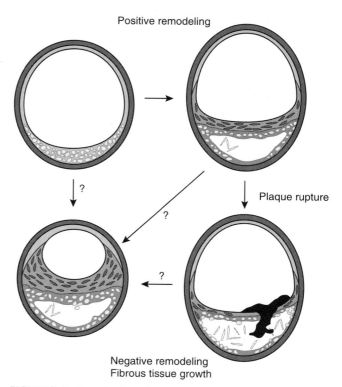

Positive remodeling

Plaque rupture

Negative remodeling
Fibrous tissue growth

FIGURE 5–5. Hypothesis: pathways to coronary stenosis. *Left,* Plaque growth with inadequate or negative vascular remodeling compromising the lumen. *Right,* Positive remodeling originally occurred but is negated by plaque rupture and subsequent plaque repair with scarlike contraction.

atherosclerosis would rarely cause symptoms and these would be more easily manageable because they would lack the most feared complication: the acuteness of thrombosis.

Rupture of the plaque surface tends to occur at the cap margin or "shoulder region" where the cap is thinnest and therefore weakest.[68-70] Thus, plaque rupture is probably the result of a dynamic interaction between intrinsic plaque vulnerability and mechanical forces imposed on the plaque (triggers).

Comparing ruptured plaques with intact plaques, pathologists have begun to characterize this as the *vulnerable plaque* type. Plaque vulnerability is a morphologic term covering plaque features frequently encountered in culprit plaques of ACS at autopsy. The term is applied to plaques assumed to be predisposed to rupture and should be distinguished from terms that refer to a plaque with actual superimposed thrombosis *(complicated plaque).*

The risk of plaque rupture seems to depend primarily on plaque morphology, less on plaque size, and not on severity of stenosis. Fibrosis with SMC proliferation and collagen synthesis hardens the plaque, stabilizing it against rupture, whereas inflammation leading to degradation of the fibrous cap and growth of the soft core predisposes the plaque to rupture (Figs. 5-7 and 5-8).

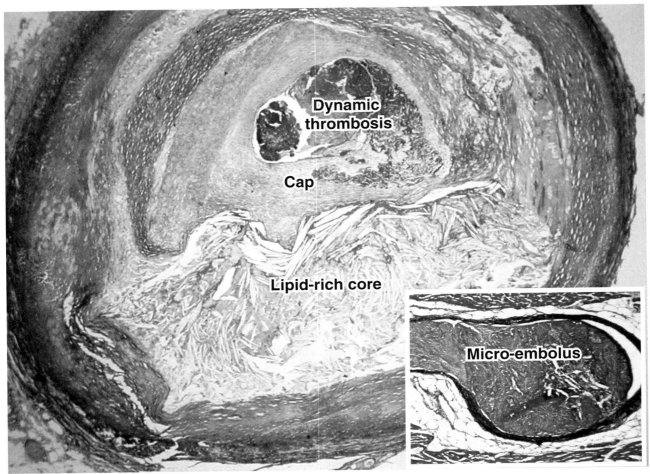

FIGURE 5–6. Dynamic thrombosis. In acute coronary syndromes, the thrombotic process is dynamic (indicated by a layered structure morphologically) and often accompanied by local vasoconstriction and distal thromboembolism (inset: microemboli downstream in the myocardium) that may prevent optimal myocardial perfusion despite a patent culprit artery.

Plaque Inflammation and Fibrosis

Nonspecific but sensitive markers of the inflammatory cascade (C-reactive protein, interleukin-6, P-selectin, TNF-β)

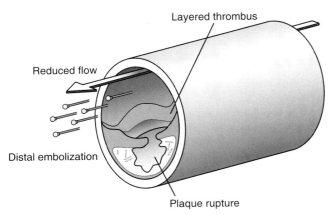

FIGURE 5–7. The culprit lesion of unstable angina. Plaque rupture with superimposed dynamic thrombosis. Layering of thrombus reveals the stepwise progression. Microscopic distal emboli are seeded to the myocardium supplied by the artery.

are risk factors for ACS in prospective studies.[71] The level of these systemic markers reflects the sum of inflammatory activity in all parts of the body, and it has been speculated whether the limited amount of atherosclerotic tissue could affect such global levels or if the atherosclerotic process rather fed on inflammatory cytokines produced elsewhere in the body. That plaque inflammation does matter is suggested by the fact that attenuation of plaque inflammation with statin treatment reduces levels of C-reactive protein.[71] Furthermore, the systemic markers have been associated directly to local activity in vivo in coronary plaques. By using a thermography catheter to measure surface temperature of plaques, a Greek group demonstrated that heat production, indicating macrophage activity,[72] was increased in plaques responsible for unstable angina (vs. stable angina) and that the increase was closely related to systemic markers of inflammation.[73] This finding is consistent with a study of atherectomy specimens from culprit lesions responsible for stable angina, unstable resting angina, or non–Q-wave infarction.[74] Lesions responsible for the ACSs contained significantly more macrophages than did lesions responsible for stable angina (14% vs. 3% of

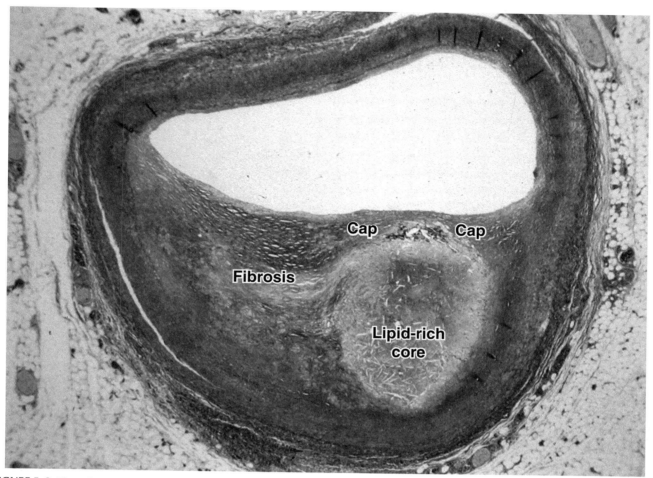

FIGURE 5–8. The vulnerable plaque. Large lipid-rich core covered by a thin fibrous cap.

plaque tissue occupied by macrophages). The inverse relationship between the extent of inflammatory activity in culprit plaque tissues and the clinical stability of the ischemic syndrome was later confirmed by others.[75]

One way that inflammation could precipitate ACS is by stimulating plaque rupture. The thickness and collagen content of the cap is important for its strength and stability: The thinner the cap is, the more rupture-prone the plaque seems to be.[68,70,76] Infiltration of macrophages and T lymphocytes into the fibrous cap might lead to degradation of the collagen-rich cap matrix[76] and apoptosis of the matrix-producing SMCs.[77] Ruptured caps examined at autopsy are usually heavily infiltrated by macrophage foam cells[68] and contain fewer SMCs and less collagen than intact caps,[78,79] and SMCs are usually absent at the actual site of rupture.[57] The link between these characteristics and mechanical fibrous cap weakening was confirmed in a rabbit model of ex vivo plaque rupture.[80]

Macrophages may weaken the extracellular cap matrix by secreting proteolytic enzymes such as plasminogen activators and a family of matrix metalloproteinases (MMPs: collagenases, gelatinases, and stromelysins).[81] The MMPs are secreted in the form of latent zymogens

that require extracellular activation, after which they are capable of degrading virtually all components of the extracellular matrix. Indeed, cultured human macrophages can degrade the mature collagen present in advanced aortic plaques while expressing MMP-1 (interstitial collagenase) and inducing MMP-2 (gelatinolytic) activity in the culture medium.[76] The MMPs are highly regulated, partly through the required transformation from the zymogenic form and partly by co-secretion of tissue inhibitors of matrix proteinases (TIMP-1 and TIMP-2). Despite their low numbers in atherosclerosis, activated mast cells may play a role by secreting powerful proteolytic enzymes that can activate pro-MMP factors secreted by other cells (e.g., macrophages). Most cells are present in shoulder regions of mature plaques and at sites of rupture,[82] and their density is related to the stability of the clinical syndrome.[83]

The increased cap inflammation associated with plaque rupture may be controlled by an immune response. T lymphocytes in stable plaques are polyclonal, probably reflecting variable antigenic backgrounds in the atherosclerotic plaque, but during phases of instability, T lymphocytes are clonally expanded, a phenomenon that suggests the direct involvement of a limited number of antigens in plaque rupture.[84] Oxidized LDL is one plausible antigen,[84] but it is also possible that infective pathogens (e.g., *Chlamydia pneumoniae*) could exacerbate the inflammatory process and provoke plaque rupture.[85]

The lipid-rich core of a plaque is a soft, hypocellular gruel totally devoid of supporting collagen.[68] Thus, the core has low tensile strength and the stress of the overlying fibrous cap is proportionally higher.[70] Not surprisingly, the size of this soft core seems to be critical for plaque stability. At autopsy, Gertz et al found much larger soft cores in coronary plaques with ruptured (vs. intact) surfaces,[86] and Felton et al found a strong relation between core size and plaque rupture in the aorta.[87] Besides death of lipid-filled macrophages, growth of the lipid core is probably largely the result of LDL hydrolysis by the action of hydrolytic enzymes such as secretory phospholipase A_2 and secretory sphingomyelinases,[13,14] which are highly expressed in inflamed tissues and can be measured systemically as acute-phase reactants.[14] Thus, large lipid cores may be yet another marker of severe plaque inflammation.

All the known characteristics of the vulnerable plaque seem to link together as reflecting one single entity: plaque inflammation. An elevated level of LDL particles with subsequent generation of raised concentrations of oxidized LDL subendothelially is probably the primary inflammatory instigator with secondary (1) growth of the lipid core (after subendothelial enzymatic hydrolysis), (2) weakening of the fibrous cap, and (3) elevation of systemic markers of inflammation. Consistent with this idea, statin treatment aimed at lowering LDL cholesterol attenuates all of these harmful elements.[71,88] Also consistent is the observation that oxidative stress in the vessel wall (the balance between reactive radical production capable of oxidizing LDL and endogenous antioxidant defenses) seems to predict future acute coronary events.[89]

Plaque Size

Surprisingly, the basic question of whether plaque size is a determinant of plaque vulnerability has not been well addressed until recently. It has generally been judged that plaque size was not an important issue, but this notion more or less evolved out of the observation that stenosis has little predictive value for the occurrence of ACS, before the concept of remodeling was fully appreciated. Recently, an autopsy study[90] found that larger plaques were more frequently associated with rupture than small ones, confirming an observation made by Yamagishi et al in their prospective IVUS study.[91] However, plaque size is not an independent variable of plaque vulnerability because size of ruptured plaques correlates positively to macrophage count and the relative size of the lipid core and negatively to the area of fibrosis.[90]

Severity of Stenosis

In autopsy studies, fatal thrombi have generally been judged to form in modest to severely stenotic segments, but this is probably due to the failure of past autopsy studies to account for the effect of remodeling because individual cross-sections were studied. When looked at in retrospective angiographic studies, nearly two thirds of coronary thrombi are precipitated by plaques that were not seen to be causing hemodynamically significant stenosis in a prior angiogram obtained weeks or months before.[68] The greater overall risk enforced by nonobstructive plaques can be accounted for in three ways. First, nonobstructive plaques greatly outnumber obstructive ones.[37,68] Second, preservation of the lumen by positive remodeling may be tightly linked to plaque vulnerability,[90-92] both being fundamentally a result of severe inflammation. Third, thrombotic occlusion of an already severely compromised lumen may be subclinical because of well-developed collateral blood flow.[93]

Positive remodeling has been hypothesized to be either a homeostatic response to maintain normal shear stress and wall tension or a pathophysiologic process in which matrix MMPs expressed by macrophages cause the media to thin or yield, or both.[94] The latter hypothesis is supported by the fact that medial thinning and elastolysis is present beneath plaques in both humans and animal models, and overdilation of the vessel in response to atherosclerotic plaque formation is not rare in either setting.[35,94] As stated by Crawford and Levene in 1953 in what must have been an inspired moment, "*In this way the triad of atheroma, thrombosis and aneurysm become linked in one continuous pathological process.*"[95]

Limitations of Current Knowledge

What we know about plaque rupture has been inferred mainly from autopsy studies that describe the morphologic features of ruptured plaques. Not surprisingly, however, these features (fibrous cap inflammation, large lipid core, lack of SMCs) are commonly observed in intact plaques as well.[68,96] Pathologists would call these plaques vulnerable, but are they in fact rupture-prone? Without the ability to conduct prospective studies, which are limited by the difficulties in imaging plaques in vivo, we cannot answer that. Increased resolution of IVUS and magnetic resonance imaging techniques, and perhaps most of all the development of an animal model of plaque rupture, would boost our insight into mechanisms of plaque rupture and subsequent thrombosis.

Plaque Vulnerability: Focal or Systemic?

It is generally assumed that the same atherosclerotic plaque is responsible for unstable angina and subsequent AMI and similarly for AMI and early reinfarction. However, the fact that multiple complicated plaques are present in many patients who present with an ACS challenges this "single-culprit" concept. Goldstein et al found multiple angiographically complex plaques (indicating rupture) in 40% of 253 patients with AMI and reported that the risk of a recurrent ACS was 10 times higher in these patients as in patients a single complex plaque. Patients with multiple and single complex plaques did not differ in mean age, sex ratio, or the frequency of coronary risk factors.[97]

In autopsy studies, the prevalence of multiple ruptured plaques is even higher, probably because of a combination of selection bias (patients harboring multiple ruptured plaques are more likely to die) and the higher sensitivity of autopsy in detecting ruptured plaques compared with angiography. In 47 patients who died from coronary atherosclerosis, 103 ruptured coronary plaques were identified (an average of 2.2 per patient); only 40 of these patients had superimposed obstructive, and probably fatal, luminal thrombosis. The remaining 63 ruptures were covered by a small nonobstructive thrombus.[56] None of these ruptures had healed, an observation that suggested that they had developed within a relatively short period before death, although not necessarily simultaneously. Consistently, Frink found more than one rupture with or without luminal thrombosis in 71% (and more than three in 20%) of 83 patients who suffered acute coronary death,[98] and Arbustini et al reported multiple coronary thrombi in 29 (10%) of the cases in a large autopsy series of 298 consecutive patients with AMI.[58] Thus, multiple ruptured plaques are the rule rather than the exception in patients who die from atherosclerosis, and multiple luminal thrombi are not rare.

Do these observations indicate acute pancoronary destabilization of plaques preceding clinical symptoms? Although thought-provoking, these numbers of plaque rupture with or without luminal thrombi should really be compared with a control group with similar presumptive ACS risk dying from noncardiac causes, and this is complicated foremost by the difficulties in assessing ACS risk. To our knowledge, the highest number of observed plaque ruptures in noncardiac deaths applying the most sensitive method (autopsy) was 0.22 ruptures per patient as observed by Davies et al in patients with diabetes or hypertension.[43] This suggests that, although ruptures are frequent, the number of plaque ruptures in patients dying with severe coronary atherosclerosis does not at all reach the number observed in some patients dying from an ACS. Candidates for the potential systemic plaque destabilization include systemic inflammation or simultaneous triggering of rupture-prone plaques, and in the setting of multiple thrombi, simultaneous thrombosis on thrombosis-prone (eroded or unhealed ruptured) plaques precipitated by a systemic thrombophilic state. If plaque vulnerability changes for the entire arterial tree as a whole, rather than focally, systemic treatment modalities are indicated.

PERSPECTIVE

Plaque rupture occurs frequently in patients with atherosclerosis. The event is often subclinical but may serve as a substrate for accelerated stenosis formation and the development of stable angina. In other patients, rupture is a catastrophic incident precipitating the emergency situation of an ACS. Systemic inflammatory markers, in vivo heat production in coronary plaques, and histologic features of ruptured plaques brought to light in postmortem studies suggest that increased plaque inflammation predisposes coronary plaques to rupture. The mechanisms for these inflammatory exacerbations are unknown, but they may include a systemic element. This element is suggested by the frequent finding of multiple unhealed plaque ruptures in patients who die from atherosclerosis. Regardless of the reason, the multiplicity of complicated plaques indicates the need for a systemic approach to diagnosis and treatment. Invasive techniques may be needed to achieve rapid, complete, and sustained reperfusion of infarct-related arteries or to stabilize plaques that pose a particularly high short-term risk in unstable angina. However, a target lesion-based approach will not eliminate the threat posed by all the other existing plaques, and their overall risk determines the prognosis in the long term.

REFERENCES

1. Sandison AT: Degenerative vascular disease. In Brothwell D, Sandison AT (eds): Diseases in Antiquity: A Survey of the Diseases, Injuries and Surgery of Early Populations. Springfield, Ill, Charles C Thomas, 1967, p 474.
2. Fye WB: A historical perspective on atherosclerosis and coronary artery disease. In Fuster V, Ross R, Topol EJ (eds): Atherosclerosis and Coronary Artery Disease. Philadelphia, Lippincott-Raven 1996, p 1.
3. Herrick J: Landmark article (JAMA 1912): Clinical features of sudden obstruction of the coronary arteries. JAMA 1983;250:1757.
4. Constantinides P: Plaque fissures in human coronary thrombosis. J Atheroscler Res 1966;6:1.
5. Chapman I: Morphogenesis of occluding coronary artery thrombosis. Arch Pathol 1965;80:256.
6. Friedman M, Van den Bovenkamp: The pathogenesis of a coronary thrombus. Am J Pathol 1966;48:19.
7. Farb A, Burke AP, Tang AL, et al: Coronary plaque erosion without rupture into a lipid core: A frequent cause of coronary thrombosis in sudden coronary death. Circulation 1996;93:1354.
8. Braunwald E, Mark DB, Jones RH, et al: Unstable angina: Diagnosis and management. Rockville, Md, Agency for Health Care Policy and Research and the National Heart, Lung, and Blood Institute, US Public Health Service, US Department of Health and Human Services; 1994, p 1. AHCPR Publication No 94-0602 (amended).
9. Ross R: Atherosclerosis—an inflammatory disease. N Engl J Med 1999;340:115.
10. Stary HC, Chandler AB, Dinsmore RE, et al: A definition of advanced types of atherosclerotic lesions and a histological classification of atherosclerosis: A report from the Committee on Vascular Lesions of the Council on Arteriosclerosis, American Heart Association. Arterioscler Thromb Vasc Biol 1995;15:1512.
11. Williams KJ, Tabas I: The response-to-retention theory of early atherogenesis. Arterioscler Thromb Vasc Biol 1995;15:551.
12. Roberts WC: Coronary atherosclerosis: Is the process focal or diffuse among patients with symptomatic or fatal myocardial ischemia? Am J Cardiol 1998;82:41T.
13. Hakala JK, Öörni K, Markku OP, et al: Lipolysis of human secretory phospholipase A$_2$ induces particle fusion and enhances the retention of LDL to human aortic proteoglycans. Arterioscler Thromb Vasc Biol 2001;21:1053.
14. Guyton JR: Phospholipid hydrolytic enzymes in a "cesspool" of arterial intima lipoproteins. Arterioscler Thromb Vasc Biol 2001;21:884.
15. Chisolm GM, Steinberg D: The oxidative modification hypothesis of atherogenesis: An overview. Free Radic Biol Med 2000;28:1815.
16. Nguyen-Khoa T, Massy ZA, Witko-Sarsat V, et al: Oxidized low-density lipoprotein induces macrophage respiratory burst via its protein moiety: A novel pathway in atherogenesis? Biochem Biophys Res Commun 1999;263:804.
17. Ludewig B, Freigang S, Jaggi M, et al: Linking immune-mediated arterial inflammation and cholesterol-induced atherosclerosis in a transgenic mouse model. Proc Natl Acad Sci U S A 2000;97:12752.
18. Hajjar DP, Haberland ME: Lipoprotein trafficking in vascular cells. Molecular Trojan horses and cellular saboteurs. J Biol Chem 1997;272:22975–22978.

19. von Eckardstein A, Nofer JR, Assmann G: High density lipoproteins and arteriosclerosis: Role of cholesterol efflux and reverse cholesterol transport. Arterioscler Thromb Vasc Biol 2001;21:13.

20. Napoli C, D'Armiento FP, Mancini FP, et al: Fatty streak formation occurs in human fetal aortas and is greatly enhanced by maternal hypercholesterolemia: Intimal accumulation of low density lipoprotein and its oxidation precede monocyte recruitment into early atherosclerotic lesions. J Clin Invest 1997;100:2680.

21. Stary HC: Lipid and macrophage accumulations in arteries of children and the development of atherosclerosis. Am J Clin Nutr 2000;72(Suppl):1297S.

22. Guyton JR, Klemp KF: Development of the atherosclerotic core region: chemical and ultrastructural analysis of microdissected atherosclerotic lesions from human aorta. Arterioscler Thromb 1994;14:1305.

23. Crisby M, Kallin B, Thyberg J, et al: Cell death in human atherosclerotic plaques involves both oncosis and apoptosis. Atherosclerosis 1997;130:17.

24. Ball RY, Stowers EC, Burton JH, et al: Evidence that the death of macrophage foam cells contributes to the lipid core of atheroma. Atherosclerosis 1995;114:45.

25. Björkerud S, Björkerud B: Apoptosis is abundant in human atherosclerotic lesions, especially in inflammatory cells (macrophages and T cells), and may contribute to the accumulation of gruel and plaque instability. Am J Pathol 1996;149:367.

26. Badimon JJ, Lettino M, Toschi V, et al: Local inhibition of tissue factor reduces the thrombogenicity of disrupted human atherosclerotic plaques: Effects of tissue factor pathway inhibitor on plaque thrombogenicity under flow conditions. Circulation 1999;99:1780.

27. Mallat Z, Hugel B, Ohan J: Shed membrane particles with procoagulant potential in human atherosclerotic plaques. Circulation 1999;99:348.

28. Ross R: The pathogenesis of atherosclerosis: A perspective for the 1990s. Nature 1993;362:801.

29. Mallat Z, Gojova A, Marchiol-Fournigault C, et al: Inhibition of transforming growth factor-beta signaling accelerates atherosclerosis and induces an unstable plaque phenotype in mice. Circ Res 2001;89:930.

30. Sano H, Sudo T, Yokode M, et al: Functional blockade of platelet-derived growth factor receptor-beta but not of receptor-alpha prevents vascular smooth muscle cell accumulation in fibrous cap lesions in apolipoprotein E-deficient mice. Circulation 2001;103:2955.

31. Stary HC: Natural history of calcium deposits in atherosclerosis progression and regression. Z Kardiol 2000;89(Suppl 2):II28.

32. O'Brien KD, McDonald TO, Chait A, et al: Neovascular expression of E-selectin, intercellular adhesion molecule-1, and vascular cell adhesion molecule-1 in human atherosclerosis and their relation to intimal leukocyte content. Circulation 1996;93:672.

33. McGill HC Jr, McMahan CA, Malcolm GT, et al: Effects of serum lipoproteins and smoking on atherosclerosis in young men and women—the PDAY Research Group: Pathobiological Determinants of Atherosclerosis in Youth. Arterioscler Thromb Vasc Biol 1997;17:95.

34. McGill HC Jr: George Lyman Duff memorial lecture. Persistent problems in the pathogenesis of atherosclerosis. Arteriosclerosis 1984;4:443.

35. Varnava AM, Davies MJ: Relation between coronary artery remodelling (compensatory dilation) and stenosis in human native coronary arteries. Heart 2001;86:207.

36. Pasterkamp G, Schoneveld AH, van Wolferen W, et al: The impact of atherosclerotic arterial remodeling on percentage of luminal stenosis varies widely within the arterial system: A postmortem study. Arterioscler Thromb Vasc Biol 1997;17:3057.

37. Alderman E, Corley S, Fisher L, et al: Five-year angiographic follow-up of factors associated with progression of coronary artery disease in the coronary artery surgery study (CASS). J Am Coll Cardiol 1993;22:1141.

38. Ganz P, Ganz W: Coronary blood flow and myocardial ischemia. In Braunwald E, Zipes DP, Libby P (eds): Heart Disease: A Textbook of Cardiovascular Medicine, 6th ed, vol II. Philadelphia, WB Saunders, 2001, p 1087.

39. Davies MJ: The pathology of coronary atherosclerosis. In Schlant RC, Alexander RW (eds): Hurst's The Heart, 8th ed. New York, McGraw-Hill, 1994, p 1009.

40. Escaned J, van Suylen R, MacLeod D, et al: Histological characteristics of tissue excised during directional coronary atherectomy in stable and unstable angina pectoris. Am J Cardiol 1993;71:1442.

41. Mann J, Davies MJ: Mechanisms of progression in native coronary artery disease: Role of healed plaque disruption. Heart 1999;82:265.

42. Burke AP, Kolodgie FD, Farb A, et al: Healed plaque ruptures and sudden coronary death: Evidence that subclinical rupture has a role in plaque progression. Circulation 2001;103:934.

43. Davies MJ, Bland JM, Hangartner JRW, et al: Factors influencing the presence or absence of acute coronary artery thrombi in sudden ischaemic death. Eur Heart J 1989;10:203.

44. Border WA, Noble NA: Transforming growth factor β in tissue fibrosis. N Engl J Med 1994;331:1286.

45. Mintz GS, Kent KM, Pichard AD, et al: Contribution of inadequate arterial remodeling to the development of focal coronary stenoses. Circulation 1997;95:1791.

46. Takano M, Mizuno K, Okamatsu K, et al: Mechanical and structural characteristics of vulnerable plaques: Analysis by coronary angioscopy and intravascular ultrasound. J Am Coll Cardiol 2001;38:99.

47. de Feyter PJ: Catheter-based techniques to treat ischemic heart disease. In Crawford MH, DiMarco JP (eds): Cardiology. London, Mosby, 2001.

48. Kimura T, Kaburagi S, Tamura T, et al: Remodeling of human coronary arteries undergoing coronary angioplasty or atherectomy. Circulation 1997;96:475.

49. Miller MJ, Kuntz RE, Friedrich SP, et al: Frequency and consequences of intimal hyperplasia in specimens retrieved by directional atherectomy of native primary coronary artery stenoses and subsequent restenoses. Am J Cardiol 1993;71:652.

50. Lindner V: Vascular repair processes mediated by transforming growth factor-beta. Z Kardiol 2001;90(Suppl 3):17.

51. Davies MJ: The pathophysiology of acute coronary syndromes. Heart 2000;83:361.

52. Antman EM, Braunwald E: Acute myocardial infarction. In Braundwald E, Zipes DP, Libby P (eds): Heart Disease: A Textbook of Cardiovascular Medicine, 6th ed, vol II. Philadelphia, WB Saunders, 2001, p 1115.

53. Wallentin L, Lindahl B, Siegbahn A: Unstable coronary artery disease. In Crawford MH, DiMarco JP (eds): Cardiology. London, Mosby, 2001.

54. DeWood MA, Stifter WF, Simpson CS, et al: Coronary arteriographic findings soon after non-Q-wave myocardial infarction. N Engl J Med 1986;315:417.

55. Tracy RE, Devaney K, Kissling G: Characteristics of the plaque under a coronary thrombus. Virchows Arch A Pathol Anat Histopathol 1985;405:411.

56. Falk E: Plaque rupture with severe pre-existing stenosis precipitating coronary thrombosis: Characteristics of coronary atherosclerotic plaque underlying fatal occlusive thrombi. Br Heart J 1983;50:127.

57. van der Wal AC, Becker AE, van der Loos CM, et al: Site of intimal rupture or erosion of thrombosed coronary atherosclerotic plaques is characterized by an inflammatory process irrespective of the dominant plaque morphology. Circulation 1994;89:36.

58. Arbustini E, Bello BD, Morbini P, et al: Plaque erosion is a major substrate for coronary thrombosis in acute myocardial infarction. Heart 1999;82:269.

59. Kojima S, Nonoogi H, Miyao Y, et al: Is preinfarction angina related to the presence or absence of coronary plaque rupture? Heart 2000;83:64.

60. Davies MJ: The composition of coronary-artery plaques. N Engl J Med 1997;336:1312.

61. Burke AP, Farb A, Malcolm GT, et al: Coronary risk factors and plaque morphology in men with coronary disease who died suddenly. N Engl J Med 1997;336:1276.

62. Burke AP, Farb A, Malcolm GT, et al: Effect of risk factors on the mechanism of acute thrombosis and sudden coronary death in women. Circulation 1998;97:2110.

63. Falk E: Unstable angina with fatal outcome: Dynamic coronary thrombosis leading to infarction and/or sudden death. Autopsy evidence of recurrent mural thrombosis with peripheral embolization culminating in total vascular occlusion. Circulation 1985;71:699.

64. Ojio S, Takatsu H, Tanaka T, et al: Considerable time from the onset of plaque rupture and/or thrombi until the onset of acute myocardial infarction in humans. Circulation 2000;102:2063.

65. Topol EJ, Yadav JS: Recognition of the importance of embolization in atherosclerotic vascular disease. Circulation 2000;101:570.

66. Wu K, Zerhouni EA, Judd RM, et al: Prognostic significance of microvascular obstruction by magnetic resonance imaging in patients with acute myocardial infarction. Circulation 1998;97:765.

67. Hamm CW, Heeschen C, Goldman B, et al: Benefit of abciximab in patients with refractory unstable angina in relation to serum troponin T levels. N Engl J Med 1999;340:1623.

68. Falk E, Shah PK, Fuster V: Coronary plaque disruption. Circulation 1995;92:657.

69. Richardson PD, Davies MJ, Born GVR: Influence of coronary configuration and stress distribution on fissuring of coronary atherosclerotic plaques. Lancet 1989;2:941.

70. Loree HM, Kamm RD, Stringfellow RG, et al: Effects of fibrous cap thickness on peak circumferential stress in model atherosclerotic vessels. Circ Res 1992;71:850.

71. Blake GJ, Ridker PM: Novel clinical markers of vascular wall inflammation. Circ Res 2001;89:763.

72. Casscells W, Hathorn B, David M, et al: Thermal detection of cellular infiltrates in living atherosclerotic plaques: Possible implications for plaque rupture and thrombosis. Lancet 1996;347:1447.

73. Stefanadis C, Diamantopoulos L, Dernellis J, et al: Heat production of atherosclerotic plaques and inflammation assessed by the acute phase proteins in acute coronary syndromes. J Mol Cell Cardiol 2000;32:43.

74. Moreno PR, Falk E, Palacios IF, et al: Macrophage infiltration in acute coronary syndromes: Implications for plaque rupture. Circulation 1994;90:775.

75. van der Wal AC, Becker AE, Koch KT, et al: Clinically stable angina pectoris is not necessarily associated with histologically stable atherosclerotic plaques. Heart 1996;76:312.

76. Shah PK, Falk E, Badimon JJ, et al: Human monocyte–derived macrophages induce collagen breakdown in fibrous caps of atherosclerotic plaques: Potential role of matrix-degrading metalloproteinases and implications for plaque rupture. Circulation 1995;92:1565.

77. Geng YJ, Henderson LE, Levesque EB, et al: Fas is expressed in human atherosclerotic intima and promotes apoptosis of cytokine-primed human vascular smooth muscle cells. Arterioscler Thromb Vasc Biol 1997;17:2200.

78. Davies MJ, Richardson PD, Woolf N, et al: Risk of thrombosis in human atherosclerotic plaques: Role of extracellular lipid, macrophage, and smooth muscle cell content. Br Heart J 1993;69:377.

79. Burleigh MC, Briggs AD, Lendon CL, et al: Collagen types I and III, collagen content, GAGs and mechanical strength of human atherosclerotic plaque caps: Span-wise variations. Atherosclerosis 1992;96:71.

80. Rekhter MD, Hicks GW, Brammer DW, et al: Hypercholesterolemia causes mechanical weakening of rabbit atheroma: Local collagen loss as a prerequisite of plaque rupture. Circ Res 2000;86:101.

81. Galis ZS, Sukhova GK, Lark MW, et al: Increased expression of matrix metalloproteinases and matrix degrading activity in vulnerable regions of human atherosclerotic plaques. J Clin Invest 1994;94:2493.

82. Kovanen PT, Kaartinen M, Paavonen T: Infiltrates of activated mast cells at the site of coronary atheromatous erosion or rupture in myocardial infarction. Circulation 1995;92:1084.

83. Kaartinen M, van der Wal AC, van der Loos CM, et al: Mast cell infiltration in acute coronary syndromes: Implications for plaque rupture. J Am Coll Cardiol 1998;32:606.

84. Caligiuri G, Paulsson G, Nicoletti A, et al: Evidence for antigen-driven T-cell response in unstable angina. Circulation 2000; 102:1114.

85. Zhu J, Nieto J, Horne BD, et al: Prospective study of pathogen burden and risk of myocardial infarction and death. Circulation 2001;103:45.

86. Gertz SD, Roberts WC: Hemodynamic shear force in rupture of coronary arterial atherosclerotic plaques. Am J Cardiol 1990;66:1368.

87. Felton CV, Crook D, Davies MJ, et al: Relation of plaque lipid composition and morphology to the stability of human aortic plaques. Arterioscler Thromb Vasc Biol 1997;17:1337.

88. Crisby M, Nordin-Fredriksson G, Shah PK, et al: Pravastatin treatment increases collagen content and decreases lipid content, inflammation, metalloproteinases, and cell death in human carotid plaques: Implications for plaque stabilization. Circulation 2001;103:926.

89. Heitzer T, Schlinzig T, Krohn K, et al: Endothelial dysfunction, oxidative stress, and risk of cardiovascular events in patients with coronary artery disease. Circulation 2001;104:2673.

90. Bezerra HG, Higuchi ML, Gutierrez PS, et al: Atheromas that cause fatal thrombosis are usually large and frequently accompanied by vessel enlargement. Cardiovasc Pathol 2001;10:189.

91. Yamagishi M, Terashima M, Awano K, et al: Morphology of vulnerable coronary plaque: Insights from follow-up of patients examined by intravascular ultrasound before an acute coronary syndrome. J Am Coll Cardiol 2000;35:106.

92. Pasterkamp G, Schoneveld AH, van der Wal AC, et al: Relation of arterial geometry to luminal narrowing and histologic markers for plaque vulnerability: The remodeling paradox. J Am Coll Cardiol 1998;32:655.

93. Mason MJ, Walker SK, Patel DJ, et al: Influence of clinical and angiographic factors on development of collateral channels. Coron Artery Dis 2000;11:573.

94. Ward MR, Pasterkamp G, Yeung AC, et al: Arterial remodeling: Mechanisms and clinical implications. Circulation 2000;102:1186.

95. Crawford T, Levene CI: Medial thinning in atheroma. J Pathol Bacteriol 1953;66:19.

96. Pasterkamp G, Schoneveld AH, van der Wal AC, et al: Inflammation of the atherosclerotic cap and shoulder of the plaque is a common and locally observed feature in unruptured plaques of femoral and coronary arteries. Arterioscler Thromb Vasc Biol 1999;19:54.

97. Goldstein JA, Demetriou D, Grines CL, et al: Multiple complex coronary plaques in patients with acute myocardial infarction. N Engl J Med 2000;343:915.

98. Frink RJ: Chronic ulcerated plaques: New insights into the pathogenesis of acute coronary disease. J Invas Cardiol 1994;6:173.

Molecular Mechanisms of the Acute Coronary Syndromes: The Roles of Inflammation and Immunity

Peter Libby

Histologic observations have taught us much regarding the pathophysiology of the acute coronary syndromes. Pathoanatomic examination of atheromas that provoke fatal thrombosis reveals much about the mechanisms of this extreme form of an acute coronary syndrome.[1-6] Although the role of thrombosis in producing the acute coronary syndromes has intermittently been controversial,[7] such a role is now rarely disputed.

Four distinct microanatomic mechanisms can precipitate the acute coronary syndromes (Fig. 6-1). Plaque rupture, the most common and perhaps the best understood, causes two thirds to three quarters of fatal acute myocardial infarctions (Fig. 6-1A). Superficial erosion without a frank rupture in the plaque's fibrous cap underlies some 20% of fatal acute coronary thrombi (Fig. 6-1B),[6,8] and erosions around calcium nodules account for a few acute coronary thromboses. Another mechanism of rapid plaque expansion, intraplaque hemorrhage, may also play a role in precipitating some cases of acute coronary syndromes.

Beyond these structural microanatomic substrates, which usually involve a disruption of the plaque, functional changes can also influence the thrombotic potential and stability of clots. A balance between procoagulant and anticoagulant factors prevails at any particular moment in the vascular compartment (Fig. 6-2). Likewise, pro- and anti-fibrinolytic factors may regulate the stability of clots. In addition to fluctuations in the blood compartment in the determinants of thrombosis, local regulation at the level of the arterial wall in these regulatory pathways may determine the consequences of any given plaque disruption.

We recognize increasingly that inflammation is a fundamental and common theme in the structural and functional pathways to thrombosis.[9] Furthermore, molecules and cells involved in both the innate and adaptive arms of the immune response may participate in many of the processes that precipitate the acute coronary syndromes.[10,11] These new insights aid our understanding of the pathophysiology of the acute coronary syndromes; they have prognostic and therapeutic implications as well. This chapter describes recent advances in the pathophysiology of the acute coronary syndromes, emphasizing the practical clinical import of these new concepts.

PLAQUE RUPTURE

Many human coronary atheromas contain a lipid-rich central core. In addition to extracellular lipid debris, the lipid core contains foamy macrophages, many of which have surfaces studded with the potent procoagulant, tissue factor.[12-15] A collagenous fibrous cap overlies the typical lipid core and serves as a barrier between the blood compartment, which contains proteins of the coagulation cascade, and thrombogenic material in the lipid core.[2,16]

In plaque rupture, a thinned and friable fibrous cap fractures. The contact between blood and tissue factor in the lipid core unleashes the clotting cascade. Collagen uncovered during plaque disruption can promote platelet adherence and activation. Resistance of the fibrous cap to rupture depends largely on the integrity of the interstitial collagen in the extracellular matrix.[4,17] Collagen fibrils lend biomechanical strength to the fibrous cap. In general, interstitial collagen has considerable stability and turns over slowly, if at all. Moreover, until recently, most regarded the atheroma as a metabolically inactive "graveyard" for excess cholesterol stuck in the artery wall. We now understand that the atheroma teems with living cells whose functions and exchanged messages may dictate the clinical consequences of the atheromatous lesion. Inflammation has also emerged as a unifying concept in the pathogenesis of atherosclerosis and its complications.[18]

Therefore, in the early 1990s, we hypothesized that the collagenous skeleton of the plaque depended on a dynamic balance between ongoing collagen synthesis and degradation. The arterial smooth muscle cell synthesizes the great majority of the collagen in this structure, and expression of interstitial collagen genes by smooth muscle cells depends on the inflammatory milieu. Gamma interferon (IFN-γ), a cytokine produced in plaques, virtually halts procollagen gene expression by cultured smooth muscle cells.[19] Atherosclerotic plaques contain IFN-γ. When activated, the T lymphocyte produces high levels of IFN-γ.

Other cells found in the atheroma can also elaborate IFN-γ under certain circumstances. For example, smooth muscle cells and macrophages exposed to a combination of cytokines found in the plaque (interleukin [IL]-12 and IL-18) can secrete IFN-γ.[20] These observations

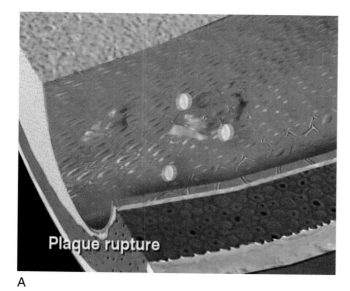

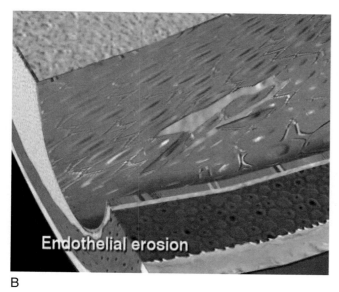

FIGURE 6–1. Depiction of a cross-section of a coronary artery shows *(A)* an intimal flap corresponding to a ruptured fibrous cap or *(B)* a patch of desquamating endothelial cells corresponding to superficial erosion.

Anticoagulant, Antithrombotic Profibrinolytic Local Hemostatic Balance

- ↓ Tissue Factor
- ↓ Plasminogen activator inhibitor (PAI-1)
- ↓ Fibrinogen
- ↓ Platelet-activating factor

- ↑ Plasminogen activators (tPA, uPA)
- ↑ Thrombomodulin
- ↑ Prostacyclin

A

Procoagulant, Prothrombotic, Antifibrinolytic Local Hemostatic Balance

- ↓ Plasminogen activators (tPA, uPA)
- ↓ Thrombomodulin
- ↓ Prostacyclin

- ↑ Tissue Factor
- ↑ Plasminogen activator inhibitor (PAI-1)
- ↑ Fibrinogen
- ↑ Platelet-activating factor

B

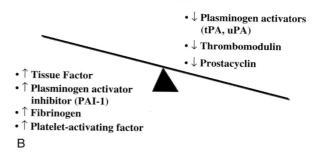

FIGURE 6–2. *A,* In the normal endothelium, anticoagulant, profibrinolytic, and antithrombotic molecules *(right)* outweigh the procoagulant, antifibrinolytic factors *(left)*. *B,* In the activated, or dysfunctional, endothelium, the procoagulant, prothrombotic, and antifibrinolytic factors prevail, tipping the balance toward an environment that favors clot formation and stability.

led to the hypothesis that T cells may locally inhibit collagen synthesis in regions of the atherosclerotic plaque. In the mid-1980s, Jonasson and colleagues localized T cells in atherosclerotic plaques, particularly in the shoulder region, where tears in the plaque often cause rupture.[21] Indeed, computational analysis of the biomechanical forces impinging on a plaque reveal maxima in circumferential stresses at the shoulders of plaques.[22] Rekhter and colleagues painstakingly enumerated cell types in various regions of the plaque and simultaneously assessed rates of interstitial collagen gene expression by in situ hybridization.[23] They found a highly significant coincidence of T cells within regions of lower levels of interstitial collagen gene expression. In

Amsterdam, Van der Wal and colleagues carefully enumerated cell types at sites of actual disruptions of human coronary plaques that caused fatal thrombosis and found abundant T cells in the vicinity of the site of plaque disruption.[8]

Taken together, these results indicate that IFN-γ derived from T cells in the shoulder region of inflamed plaques can impede the synthesis of new collagen by smooth muscle cells. Inhibition of interstitial collagen synthesis would interfere with the ability of the smooth muscle cell to repair and maintain the all-important fibrous cap. Results of recent experiments in mice rendered scorbutic by genetic engineering show that vitamin C (ascorbic acid) deficiency impairs the collagenous structure of the plaque. Because vitamin C promotes the cross-linking of collagen chains, this finding supports a role for collagen protein production in determining the structure of the plaque's fibrous cap.[24,25]

Intact collagen fibrils resist degradation by all but a few enzymes, known as *interstitial collagenases.* These entities were first discovered in the context of resorption of the tadpole tail; our knowledge of the biochemistry of collagenolysis is now considerable. Humans produce three interstitial collagenases. These three enzymes belong to a broader family of proteinases that are dependent on zinc atoms and are thus known as *matrix metalloproteinases (MMPs)*.[26]

In 1991, Henney and colleagues detected messenger RNA encoding one MMP—stromelysin, or MMP-3—in human atherosclerotic plaques.[27] In 1994, we first described overexpression of an interstitial collagenase in human atheroma.[28] We found the prototypical interstitial collagenase, MMP-1, in macrophage foam cells and smooth muscle–derived foam cells in regions of human atherosclerotic plaques shown to be particularly vulnerable by biomechanical and pathologic studies. In observations made on experimental atheroma in rabbits, we subsequently showed the importance of the macrophage as a source of interstitial collagenase.[29] Further studies yielded similar results for another interstitial collagenase, MMP-13.[30]

Most recently, we made the surprising observation that many cells in human atheroma overexpress the third form of human interstitial collagenase, MMP-8.[31] Human atheromata harbor few if any polymorphonuclear leukocytes, the classic source of neutrophil collagenase (MMP-8). In the course of transcriptional profiling experiments that screened for genes overexpressed in human macrophages stimulated with the pro-inflammatory cytokine, CD40 ligand, we found that macrophages can express this so-called neutrophil collagenase. We then sought overexpression of MMP-8 in atheromas and determined that macrophages, smooth muscle cells, and endothelial cells within human atherosclerotic plaques can overexpress this unexpected form of interstitial collagenase. This latter observation has particular importance because MMP-8 degrades type I collagen more efficiently than MMP-1 or MMP-13. Type I collagen accounts for the bulk of collagen in the atheroma. Therefore, MMP-8 has a substrate specificity that may render it one of the most important proteinases in degrading collagen in the atheroma. In other studies, we established overexpression of a non-metalloenzyme, cathepsin-S, in the atherosclerotic plaque.[32] Although chiefly implicated in elastolysis, cathepsin-S may exhibit interstitial collagenase activity as well.

The overexpression of messenger RNA and protein corresponding to interstitial collagenases does not necessarily translate into increased enzyme activity. Proteinase cascades important in biologic control undergo regulation at several levels. MMPs, first synthesized as inactive precursors, require activation to attain their enzymatic function (Fig. 6–3). Moreover, widely distributed endogenous inhibitors can limit the action of any activated form of the MMPs. Four members of the *tissue inhibitor of MMP (TIMP)* family exist, and vascular lesions can contain all four.[28,33,34] Also, we described the expression in human arteries of tissue factor pathway inhibitor 2 (TIMP-2), which also inhibits collagenases.[35] This homologue of TIMP-2 actually inhibits tissue factor poorly but blocks the action of collagenases as potently as TIMPs. Even if active molecules of the interstitial collagenase were to exist in the plaque, they could not digest collagen unless they outnumbered these endogenous inhibitors. Unfortunately, none of the available immunologic reagents can distinguish the inactive zymogen form of the interstitial collagenases from their active counterparts.

REGULATION OF MATRIX METALLOPROTEINASE ACTIVITY

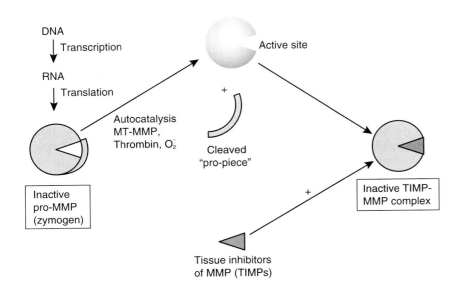

FIGURE 6–3. Multiple levels of control of activity of extracellular matrix metalloproteinases (MMPs). MMPs, first synthesized as inactive zymogen precursors, require processing to gain enzymatic activity. Cleavage of the "pro" portion of nascent protease can occur autocatalytically or heterocatalytically, involving other MMPs, including MT-MMP, thrombin, or reactive oxygen species in the case of MMP-2. Cleavage or unfolding of the pro portion of the molecule allows the active site of enzyme to access substrates and degrade them. Ubiquitously distributed tissue inhibitors of MMPs (known as TIMPs 1 through 4) can bind to active protease, blocking the active site and rendering enzyme inactive. Thus, control of MMP activity depends on gene transcription, translation, post-translational control of zymogen activation, and the balance between proteases and their endogenous inhibitors, TIMPs. (Adapted from Libby P, Lee RT: Matrix matters. Circulation 2000;102:1874–1876.)

Thus, the mere presence of immunoreactive interstitial collagenases in plaques does not imply that they actively participate in collagenolysis in situ. To prove this point, our laboratory assessed collagen degradation directly in situ using an antibody that selectively recognizes collagen that has undergone cleavage by interstitial collagenase. This study established that active collagen breakdown occurred in advanced human atheromas and, further, co-localized MMP-1 and MMP-13 within regions of collagenolysis in situ.[30] These observations all suggest that enhanced breakdown of interstitial collagen due to the action of MMPs may contribute to thinning and weakening of the fibrous cap and hence to the pathogenesis of plaque rupture. Therapies that limit the acute coronary syndromes may act in part by stabilizing plaques by interfering with collagen breakdown and increasing collagen synthesis. In rabbits with dietary or endogenous hyperlipidemia, lowering of cholesterol by dietary or pharmacologic means can reduce expression of interstitial collagenase and promote collagen accumulation within plaques.

Given the principal role of the smooth muscle cell in collagen synthesis in the artery wall, the level of collagen in a plaque may depend on the number of smooth muscle cells. Indeed, the regulation of collagen gene expression in smooth muscle cells varies with the prevailing mediator milieu. For example, platelet-derived growth factor and transforming growth factor β, protein mediators released from platelets at sites of thrombosis but also produced by many other cells, augment interstitial collagen gene expression in human smooth muscle cells.[19] Thus, smooth muscle cells, when present, promote plaque stability. Histopathologic observations have shown an inverse correlation between smooth muscle cells and plaque ruptures: Plaques that have ruptured have few smooth muscle cells.[8,36] Hence, we proposed that the smooth muscle cell was the "guardian of the integrity of the plaque's fibrous cap."[4] We now recognize that smooth muscle cells in the plaque can die. Cell death may cause "dropout" of smooth muscle cells in atherosclerotic plaques, eventually making a plaque more vulnerable.[37]

Smooth muscle cells within the plaque can die by several mechanisms, including apoptosis, or programmed cell death.[38] Smooth muscle cells exposed to pro-inflammatory mediators found in the atheroma can die by apoptosis. Notably, cocktails of pro-inflammatory cytokines can promote smooth muscle cell apoptosis.[39] The members of the surface-based cell death signaling dyad, Fas/Fas ligand, also operate in plaques.[40] These observations strengthen the link between inflammation and impaired stability of the fibrous cap in human atheroma.

These observations all support the concept that dynamic regulation of collagen levels contributes to plaque stability. Recent experiments in genetically altered mice provide direct evidence that collagenolysis influences the levels of collagen accumulating in atherosclerotic plaques. Genetic manipulation has permitted the construction of mice that express type I collagen, which resists cleavage by collagenases due to a mutation introduced into its cleavage site. Further genetic manipulation introduced this collagen mutation onto a background susceptible to atherosclerosis. The atherosclerotic mice expressing collagenase-resistant collagen showed increased collagen levels in the atheroma.[41] These "loss of function" experiments rigorously establish that plaque collagenolysis plays a role in determining the structure of plaques in vivo.

Superficial Erosion

Another form of physical disruption of the atherosclerotic plaque contributes to many coronary thromboses. A superficial erosion, rather than a frank fissure, in the fibrous cap accounts for approximately one quarter to one third of fatal coronary thrombi.[6] Superficial erosion appears more commonly than fibrous cap fracture in younger persons, women, and those with hypertriglyceridemia or diabetes. The molecular pathways underlying superficial erosion have received less attention than those regulating the friability of the fibrous cap. Not all experts agree on the degree to which inflammation participates in superficial erosion. Virmani and colleagues emphasized the bland, noninflammatory nature of sites of superficial erosion in human coronary arteries.[6,8] The Amsterdam group consistently finds evidence for the coexistence of T cells and macrophages at sites of plaque disruption due to both superficial erosion and rupture of the cap.[8]

Although the underlying mechanisms remain speculative, some mechanistic commonality may exist between these two most common forms of plaque disruption. In superficial erosion, endothelial cells may detach because the connections that tether them to the underlying basement membrane loosen. Type IV collagen, the major type of collagen in the subendothelial basement membrane, may also undergo proteolytic degradation. In contrast with the fibrillar collagens that make up the plaque's fibrous cap, type IV collagen in the basement membrane does not form fibrils. Type IV collagen also can undergo catabolism by MMPs. However, instead of the interstitial collagenases, this nonfibrillar type of collagen undergoes degradation by MMP-2, a form of gelatinase. Like the other MMPs, MMP-2 requires activation from a zymogen precursor to cleave its substrate, type IV collagen. Another MMP bound to the surface of cells and known as membrane-type MMP, or MT-MMP (MMP-14), participates in the activation of MMP-2.[26,42] Pro-inflammatory cytokines and oxidized low-density lipoprotein can augment the expression by endothelial cells of the MT-1-MMP/MMP-14 that can activate MMP-2.[43] Moreover, reactive oxygen species released from vascular cells and infiltrating inflammatory cells in inflamed plaques can activate MMPs directly.[44] Thus, active degradation of the subendothelial basement membrane due to the proteinases regulated by inflammation may promote endothelial desquamation. Such a scenario could provide one mechanism for superficial erosion as a source of coronary thrombi.

In addition, endothelial cells may detach because they die. As in the case of smooth muscle cells, endothelial cells can undergo death by apoptosis.[45] Some inflammatory mediators encountered by endothelial cells may promote resistance to apoptosis, partially by inducing the anti-apoptotic pathway involving nuclear factor κB (NF-κB). However, other pro-inflammatory stimuli may sensitize endothelial cells to programmed cell death. Thus, increased endothelial cell death, regulated in part by inflammatory mediators, may contribute to the pathogenesis of superficial erosion.

Erosion Due to Calcium Nodules

Erosion due to mineral collections, niduses of calcification, provides another route to coronary thrombosis. This mechanism accounts for only 4% to 7% of fatal coronary thromboses. Calcification in atherosclerotic plaques depends on tightly regulated biochemical processes. Proteins such as osteopontin and bone morphogenetic proteins may regulate the accretion of calcium mineral in atheroma.[46-48] Just as the level of collagen in the plaque depends on the balance of synthesis and degradation, the level of calcium mineral depends on a similar balance. Bone morphogenetic protein likely enhances the formation of bony metaplasia in atherosclerotic plaques. On the other hand, macrophages may break down deposits of calcium. Indeed, macrophages in human atherosclerotic plaques can express some of the enzymes implicated in bone resorption by osteoclasts, including cathepsins S and K. Observations in mice with mutations that affect the number and function of macrophages illustrate in vivo the importance of the catabolism of calcified tissue in atheroma. Specifically, mice lacking macrophage colony-stimulating factor and that are thus unable to produce mature macrophages show increased levels of calcium in experimentally produced atheroma.[49] These observations show how the degree of calcification in atheroma depends in part on inflammatory signaling within the lesion.

Plaque Hemorrhage

Intraplaque hemorrhage with rapid lesion expansion may also precipitate the acute coronary syndromes. Many earlier pathologic studies viewed intraplaque hemorrhage as a major pathway to coronary thrombosis. However, later pathologic studies involving painstaking serial sectioning has identified ruptures of the plaque's fibrous cap as the primary lesion, with blood collection within the atheroma often secondary.

The amount of microvessels within the plaque may influence its biology in several ways. In the same way that growth of tumors depends on formation of new blood vessels, the progression of atheroma may depend in part on neovascularization. Experiments with inhibitors of angiogenesis have shown attenuated lesion formation in mice.[50] Atherosclerotic lesions express a number of angiogenic factors. For example, acidic fibroblast growth factor correlates with microvessel formation in plaques and co-localizes with inflammatory cells.[51] Vascular endothelial growth factor, basic fibroblast growth factor, and other angiogenic proteins may promote plaque neovascularization.

Although intraplaque hemorrhage probably causes very few acute coronary syndromes by itself, the phenomenon may yet have important consequences for plaque evolution. Thrombosis in situ due to rupture friable neovessels in the plaque would lead to local thrombin generation. Thrombin potently stimulates smooth muscle cell migration, replication, and collagen synthesis. In this manner, intraplaque hemorrhage might promote the evolution of fibrous atherosclerotic plaques. In addition, iron derived from hemosiderin in extravasated blood within the plaque may promote oxidative processes. Notably, the production of reactive oxygen substances by the Fenton reaction requires transition metal cations such as iron. The presence of microvessels within plaques and the potential role of intraplaque hemorrhage in lesion expansion and growth sound a cautionary note in the context of angiogenic therapy for myocardial ischemia. Administration of angiogenic growth factors in the regions of atherosclerotic plaques might actually enhance plaque neovascularization and favor intraplaque hemorrhage with its attendant adverse consequences for plaque formation. If angiogenic therapy has a similar effect on the atheroma, plaque growth and instability could result from increased nourishment of ischemic myocardium.

REGULATION OF THROMBOSIS

Thus far, our discussion has centered on the mechanisms of plaque disruption. Such episodes permit the blood compartment contact with thrombogenic materials. The consequences of a given plaque disruption, however, may depend on prevailing levels of proteins governing thrombosis in blood (see Fig. 6-2). Atherosclerotic events may correlate with levels of fibrinogen, the substrate of thrombin and the principal constituent of many intravascular thrombi. Fibrinogen, produced by the liver in response to systemic inflammation (the acute phase response), may thus help determine whether a given plaque disruption leads to a sustained and propagated thrombus (Fig. 6-4). In addition, the levels of inhibitors of fibrinolysis, such as plasminogen activator inhibitor 1 (PAI-1), can determine the operation of endogenous fibrinolytic pathways that combat the stability of thrombi. Elevated levels of PAI-1 in diabetic patients may explain in part their predilection to thrombosis.[52]

Coagulation depends not only on factors circulating in blood but also on local levels within the atherosclerotic lesion. For example, the amount of tissue factor in the core of a disrupted plaque may determine the degree of resultant thrombosis. Inflammatory mediators such as CD40 ligand increase the expression of tissue factor in plaques.[53] Inflammatory mediators regulate the antifibrinolytic balance in plaques as well.[54] Thus, inflammation regulates both the fluid phase and "solid state" factors that control thrombus formation. Therapies that reduce

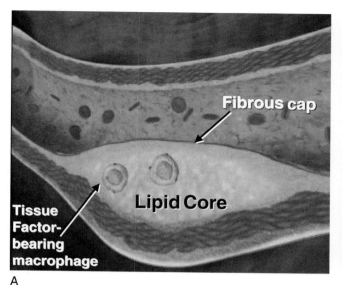

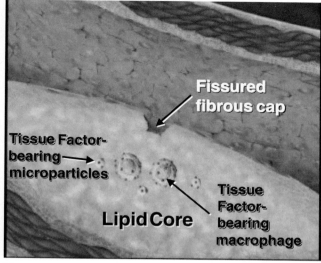

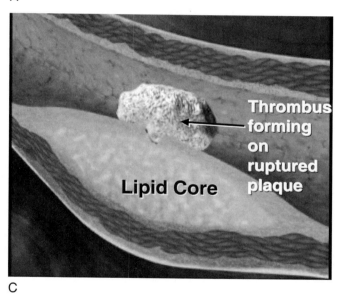

FIGURE 6–4. Depiction of the sequence of events in plaque rupture and thrombosis. *A,* The vulnerable, or high-risk, atheroma has a thin fibrous cap overlying a large lipid core that contains tissue factor–bearing macrophages. *B,* When the fibrous cap fissures, tissue factor–bearing macrophages and microparticles become accessible to the coagulation proteins in blood. *C,* This triggers thrombus formation on the ruptured plaque, which can lead to partial or transient coronary artery occlusion (clinically manifested as unstable angina) or a persistent and occlusive thrombus (leading to acute myocardial infarction).

thrombotic complications of atherosclerosis—particularly lipid lowering and statins—may reduce events by decreasing thrombogenicity and increasing endogenous fibrinolysis. For example, dietary lipid lowering decreases tissue factor expression in rabbits.[55] Statins can decrease PAI-1 production by vascular cells and, under some circumstances, increase the production of plasminogen activators.[56] The decrease in tissue factor noted with lipid lowering goes hand in hand with a decrease in the tissue factor inducer CD40 ligand and its receptor CD40.[55] In experimental atheroma, lipid lowering by statins can also decrease PAI-1 expression in situ.[41]

CONCLUSIONS

Contemporary research has enabled a molecular approach to understanding the molecular bases of the acute coronary syndromes. Many pathways of evidence have converged on inflammatory processes as a unifying theme in the pathophysiology of the acute coronary syndromes. Pro-inflammatory mediators important in regulating these functions include pro-inflammatory cytokines, a major effector limb of innate immunity. However, much recent evidence indicates that the T lymphocyte may orchestrate the cytokine symphony in atherogenesis. Activated T cells localize to regions of plaque disruption and decreased collagen synthesis in situ. T cells produce high levels of CD40 ligand and IFN-γ, pro-inflammatory mediators of particular interest in regulation of plaque stability and thrombosis. These observations indicate an important role for the pathways of adaptive, antigen-specific immunity in the pathogenesis of the acute coronary syndromes. Candidate antigens for stimulating an immune response during atherogenesis include oxidatively modified lipoprotein and heat shock proteins 60/65 expressed in stressed tissues, including atheroma, and by infectious organisms occasionally found in atheroma, such as *Chlamydia pneumoniae*.[10] β_2-Glycoprotein I, a target of antiphospholipid antibodies, may also figure in autoimmunity during atherogenesis.[57]

These novel concepts of the molecular signaling involved in the acute coronary syndromes have enhanced our understanding of basic pathophysiology. More practically, the insight that inflammation links to coronary events has opened new avenues for risk stratification and prognostication. A consistent and rapidly accumulating body of evidence suggests that persons with signs of low-level inflammation are at heightened risk for future acute coronary events. Studies with the acute-phase reactant C-reactive protein and other markers of vascular cell activation, including IL-6 and soluble intercellular adhesion molecule 1, show that inflammation is linked at several levels with future risk of atherosclerotic complications (Fig. 6–5).[58,59]

In addition to providing new tools for prognostication, the emerging molecular biology of plaque thrombosis has therapeutic implications. The link between inflammation and plaque stability has prompted experimental studies that shed new light onto the mechanisms by which existing therapeutic strategies may effectively reduce thrombotic complications of atherosclerosis.

Identification of novel targets by probing the molecular mechanisms of plaque disruption and thrombosis may also identify novel targets for therapy in the future. The emerging molecular biology of the acute coronary syndromes may thus pave the way for novel therapies that will permit us to more effectively reduce the residual burden of atherosclerotic events.

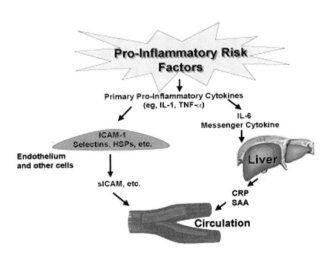

FIGURE 6–5. The pathway that generates inflammatory markers in the blood. Pro-inflammatory risk factors elicit the production of primary pro-inflammatory cytokines such as the soluble proteins interleukin-1 (IL-1) or tumor necrosis factor α (TNF-α). These primary cytokines can stimulate production of interleukin-6 (IL-6), a "messenger" cytokine, from a variety of cell types including vascular smooth muscle cells. IL-6 can change the program of hepatic protein synthesis from one that produces primarily "housekeeping" proteins (e.g., albumin) to one that favors production of acute-phase reactants such C-reactive protein (CRP), serum amyloid-A (SAA), and fibrinogen (not shown). These soluble acute-phase reactants enter the bloodstream, where they can be sampled in venipuncture. The left side of this diagram depicts augmented expression of adhesion mo'ecules such as the selectins or intercellular adhesion molecule 1 by endothelial and other cells in response to the primary pro-inflammatory cytokines. The adhesion molecules can be shed from the surface of the endothelial cell and enter the bloodstream, where they also can be sampled by venipuncture. In this way, the peripheral blood serves as a mirror of pro-inflammatory risk factors. (After Libby P, Ridker PM: Novel inflammatory markers of coronary risk: Theory versus practice. Circulation 1999;100:1148–1150.)

REFERENCES

1. Davies MJ, Thomas AC: Plaque fissuring—the cause of acute myocardial infarction, sudden ischemic death, and crescendo angina. Br Heart J 1985;53:363.
2. Davies MJ: Stability and instability: The two faces of coronary atherosclerosis. The Paul Dudley White Lecture, 1995. Circulation 1996;94:2013.
3. Falk E, Shah P, Fuster V: Coronary plaque disruption. Circulation 1995; 92:657.
4. Libby P: The molecular bases of the acute coronary syndromes. Circulation 1995; 91 (11): 2844.
5. Libby P: Current concepts of the pathogenesis of the acute coronary syndromes. Circulation 2001;104:365.
6. Farb A, Burke A, Tang A, et al: Coronary plaque erosion without rupture into a lipid core: A frequent cause of coronary thrombosis in sudden coronary death. Circulation 1996;93:1354.
7. Roberts WC: Relationship between coronary thrombosis and myocardial infarction. Mod Concepts Cardiovasc Dis 1972;41:7.
8. van der Wal AC, Becker AE, van der Loos CM, et al: Site of intimal rupture or erosion of thrombosed coronary atherosclerotic plaques is characterized by an inflammatory process irrespective of the dominant plaque morphology. Circulation 1994; 89:36.
9. Libby P, Simon DI: Inflammation and thrombosis: The clot thickens. Circulation 2001;103:1718.
10. Hansson GK: Immune mechanisms in atherosclerosis. Arterioscler Thromb Vasc Biol 2001;21:1876.
11. Hansson GK, Libby P, Schonbeck U, et al: Innate and adaptive immunity in the pathogenesis of atherosclerosis. Circ Res 2002;91(4):281–291.
12. Wilcox JN, Smith KM, Schwartz SM, et al: Localization of tissue factor in the normal vessel wall and in the atherosclerotic plaque. Proc Natl Acad Sci U S A 1989;86:2839.
13. Drake TA, Morrissey JH, Edgington TS: Selective cellular expression of tissue factor in human tissues: Implications for disorders of hemostasis and thrombosis. Am J Pathol 1989;134:1087.
14. Taubman MB, Fallon JT, Schecter AD, et al: Tissue factor in the pathogenesis of atherosclerosis. Thromb Haemost 1997;78:200.
15. Thiruvikraman SV, Guha A, Roboz J, et al: In situ localization of tissue factor in human atherosclerotic plaques by binding of digoxigenin-labeled factors VIIa and X. Lab Invest 1996;75:297.
16. Kolodgie FD, Burke AP, Farb A, et al: The thin-cap fibroatheroma: A type of vulnerable plaque: The major precursor lesion to acute coronary syndromes. Curr Opin Cardiol 2001;16:285.
17. Lee R, Libby P: The unstable atheroma. Arterioscler Thromb Vasc Biol 1997;17:1859.
18. Libby P, Ridker PM, Maseri A: Inflammation and atherosclerosis. Circulation 2002;105:1135.
19. Amento EP, Ehsani N, Palmer H, et al: Cytokines and growth factors positively and negatively regulate interstitial collagen gene expression in human vascular smooth muscle cells. Arterioscler Thromb 1991;11:1223.
20. Gerdes N, Sukhova GK, Libby P, et al: Expression of interleukin (IL)-18 and functional IL-18 receptor on human vascular endothelial cells, smooth muscle cells, and macrophages: Implications for atherogenesis. J Exp Med 2002;195:245.
21. Jonasson L, Holm J, Skalli O, et al: Regional accumulations of T cells, macrophages, and smooth muscle cells in the human atherosclerotic plaque. Arteriosclerosis 1986;6:131 .
22. Cheng GC, Loree HM, Kamm RD, et al: Distribution of circumferential stress in ruptured and stable atherosclerotic lesions: A structural analysis with histopathologic correlation. Circulation 1993;87:1179.

23. Rekhter M, Zhang K, Narayanan A, et al: Type I collagen gene expression in human atherosclerosis: Localization to specific plaque regions. Am J Pathol 1993;143:1634.

24. Nakata Y, Maeda N: Vulnerable atherosclerotic plaque morphology in apolipoprotein E-deficient mice unable to make ascorbic acid. Circulation 2002;105:1485.

25. Libby P, Aikawa M: Vitamin C, collagen, and cracks in the plaque. Circulation 2002;105:1396.

26. Brinckerhoff CE, Matrisian LM: TIMELINE: Matrix metalloproteinases: A tail of a frog that became a prince. Nat Rev Mol Cell Biol 2002;3:207.

27. Henney AM, Wakeley PR, Davies MJ, et al: Localization of stromelysin gene expression in atherosclerotic plaques by in situ hybridization. Proc Natl Acad Sci U S A 1991;88:8154.

28. Galis Z, Sukhova G, Lark M, et al: Increased expression of matrix metalloproteinases and matrix degrading activity in vulnerable regions of human atherosclerotic plaques. J Clin Invest 1994;94:2493.

29. Galis Z, Sukhova G, Kranzhöfer R, et al: Macrophage foam cells from experimental atheroma constitutively produce matrix-degrading proteinases. Proc Natl Acad Sci U S A 1995;92:402.

30. Sukhova GK, Schonbeck U, Rabkin E, et al: Evidence for increased collagenolysis by interstitial collagenases-1 and -3 in vulnerable human atheromatous plaques. Circulation 1999;99:2503.

31. Herman MP, Sukhova GK, Libby P, et al: Expression of neutrophil collagenase (matrix metalloproteinase-8) in human atheroma: A novel collagenolytic pathway suggested by transcriptional profiling. Circulation 2001;104:1899.

32. Sukhova GK, Shi GP, Simon DI, et al: Expression of the elastolytic cathepsins S and K in human atheroma and regulation of their production in smooth muscle cells. J Clin Invest 1998;102:576.

33. Fabunmi RP, Sukhova GK, Sugiyama S, et al: Expression of tissue inhibitor of metalloproteinases-3 in human atheroma and regulation in lesion-associated cells: A potential protective mechanism in plaque stability. Circ Res 1998;83:270.

34. Dollery CM, McEwan JR, Wang M, et al: TIMP-4 is regulated by vascular injury in rats. Ann N Y Acad Sci 1999;878:740.

35. Herman MP, Sukhova GK, Kisiel W, et al: Tissue factor pathway inhibitor-2 is a novel inhibitor of matrix metalloproteinases with implications for atherosclerosis. J Clin Invest 2001;107:1117.

36. Davies MJ, Richardson PD, Woolf N, et al: Risk of thrombosis in human atherosclerotic plaques: Role of extracellular lipid, macrophage, and smooth muscle cell content. Br Heart J 1993;69:377.

37. Geng Y-J, Libby P: Evidence for apoptosis in advanced human atheroma: Co-localization with interleukin-1 b-converting enzyme. Am J Pathol 1995;147:251.

38. Bennett MR, Evan GI, Newby AC: Deregulated expression of the c-myc oncogene abolishes inhibition of proliferation of rat vascular smooth muscle cells by serum reduction, interferon-gamma, heparin, and cyclic nucleotide analogues and induces apoptosis. Circ Res 1994;74:525.

39. Geng Y-J, Wu Q, Muszynski M, et al: Apoptosis of vascular smooth muscle cells induced by in vitro stimulation with interferon-gamma, tumor necrosis factor-alpha, and interleukin-1-beta. Arterioscler Thromb Vasc Biol 1996;16:19.

40. Geng Y-J, Henderson L, Levesque E, et al: Fas is expressed in human atherosclerotic intima and promotes apoptosis of cytokine-primed human vascular smooth muscle cells. Arterioscler Thromb Vasc Biol 1997;17:2200.

41. Fukumoto Y, Libby P, Rabkin E, et al: Genetically determined resistance to collagenase action alters content of collagen and smooth muscle cells in atheroma [abstract 410-1]. J Am Coll Cardiol 2002;39(Suppl A).

42. Kridel SJ, Sawai H, Ratnikov BI, et al: A unique substrate binding mode discriminates membrane type-1 matrix metalloproteinase (MT1-MMP) from other matrix metalloproteinases. J Biol Chem 2002;16:16.

43. Rajavashisth TB, Liao JK, Galis ZS, et al: Inflammatory cytokines and oxidized low density lipoproteins increase endothelial cell expression of membrane type 1-matrix metalloproteinase. J Biol Chem 1999;274:11924.

44. Rajagopalan S, Meng XP, Ramasamy S, et al: Reactive oxygen species produced by macrophage-derived foam cells regulate the activity of vascular matrix metalloproteinases in vitro: Implications for atherosclerotic plaque stability. J Clin Invest 1996;98:2572.

45. Slowik MR, Min W, Ardito T, et al: Evidence that tumor necrosis factor triggers apoptosis in human endothelial cells by interleukin-1-converting enzyme-like protease-dependent and -independent pathways. Lab Invest 1997;77:257.

46. Bostrom K, Watson KE, Horn S, et al: Bone morphogenetic protein expression in human atherosclerotic lesions. J Clin Invest 1993;91:1800.

47. Giachelli CM, Liaw L, Murry CE, et al: Osteopontin expression in cardiovascular diseases. Ann N Y Acad Sci 1995;760:109.

48. Bostrom K, Demer LL: Regulatory mechanisms in vascular calcification. Crit Rev Eukaryot Gene Expr 2000;10:151.

49. Qiao JH, Tripathi J, Mishra NK, et al: Role of macrophage colony-stimulating factor in atherosclerosis: Studies of osteopetrotic mice. Am J Pathol 1997;150:1687.

50. Moulton KS, Heller E, Konerding MA, et al: Angiogenesis inhibitors endostatin or TNP-470 reduce intimal neovascularization and plaque growth in apolipoprotein E-deficient mice. Circulation 1999;99:1726.

51. Brogi E, Winkles J, Underwood R, et al: Distinct patterns of expression of fibroblast growth factors and their receptors in human atheroma and non-atherosclerotic arteries: Association of acidic FGF with plaque microvessels and macrophages. J Clin Invest 1993;92:2408.

52. Sobel BE: The potential influence of insulin and plasminogen activator inhibitor type 1 on the formation of vulnerable atherosclerotic plaques associated with type 2 diabetes. Proc Assoc Am Physicians 1999;111:313.

53. Mach F, Schoenbeck U, Bonnefoy J-Y, et al: Activation of monocyte/macrophage functions related to acute atheroma complication by ligation of CD40: Induction of collagenase, stromelysin, and tissue factor. Circulation 1997;96:396.

54. Bevilacqua MP, Schleef R, Gimbrone MAJ, et al: Regulation of the fibrinolytic system of cultured human vascular endothelium by IL-1. J Clin Invest 1986;78:587.

55. Aikawa M, Libby P: Lipid lowering reduces proteolytic and pro-thrombotic potential in rabbit atheroma. Ann N Y Acad Sci 2000;902:140.

56. Bourcier T, Libby P: HMG CoA reductase inhibitors reduce plasminogen activator inhibitor-1 expression by human vascular smooth muscle and endothelial cells. Arterioscler Thromb Vasc Biol 2000;20:556.

57. Harats D, George J: Beta2-glycoprotein I and atherosclerosis. Curr Opin Lipidol 2001;12:543.

58. Ridker PM, Hennekens CH, Buring JE, et al: C-reactive protein and other markers of inflammation in the prediction of cardiovascular disease in women. N Engl J Med 2000;342:836.

59. Ridker PM: Novel risk factors and markers for coronary disease. Adv Intern Med 2000;45:391.

The Role of Infection

Jeffrey L. Anderson
Joseph B. Muhlestein

INFLAMMATION IN THE PATHOPHYSIOLOGY OF CORONARY ARTERY DISEASE AND THE ACUTE CORONARY SYNDROMES

Epidemiology

At the beginning of the 21st century, cardiovascular disease remains the leading cause of death.[1] Cardiovascular disease claimed 950,000 lives in the United States in 1998, accounting for over 40% of all deaths. Coronary artery disease (CAD) is the leading cause of cardiovascular death, with 460,000 fatalities annually; 220,000 of these deaths occur suddenly, out of the hospital. Over 12,400,000 Americans are living with clinical CAD.

Attributable Risk

Despite ambitious research efforts, our understanding of the pathophysiology of CAD is incomplete. Several CAD risk factors have long been known (dyslipidemia, hypertension, smoking, diabetes, family history), but traditional risk factors explain only about one half of attributable risk.[2] Additional environmental and genetic risk factors remain to be discovered and placed into a comprehensive pathophysiologic framework.

Inflammation

Our understanding of CAD pathophysiology has undergone a paradigm shift in recent years. Atherosclerosis has come to be recognized as an active, inflammatory process rather than simply the passive infiltration of lipids.[3,4] Acute coronary syndromes (ACSs) are precipitated by erosion or rupture of atheromatous plaques.[5-8] Disruption often occurs at the plaque's intersection with normal arterial wall, a shoulder region rich in T lymphocytes and macrophages that actively secrete inflammatory cytokines, chemokines, and matrix-degrading metalloproteinases.[9,10] The consequence is expansive hemorrhage into plaque and occlusive luminal thrombosis triggered by contact of blood elements with collagen, tissue factor, and other thrombogenic substances. Recognizing the inflammatory nature of atherosclerosis raises the question of the primary stimuli for inflammation.

GENESIS OF THE "INFECTION THEORY" OF ATHEROSCLEROSIS

Older Theories and Models

Speculation on an association between infectious agents and atherosclerosis dates back to the late 19th century.[11] Huchard (1891), followed by Weisel and Klotz (1906), proposed a relation between early atherosclerosis in animals and humans and various common infections, including typhoid fever, scarlet fever, measles, and sepsis. In his classic textbook of medicine (1908), Osler wrote of a potential link between infection and atherosclerosis.[12] Discovery of the association of infection with the Marek disease virus and atherosclerosis in chickens provided an experimental proof of principle by the mid-20th century.[13] (Marek disease virus is a herpes family DNA virus that causes avian T-cell lymphomatosis.) Subsequent work with this model by Fabricant, Minick, Hajjar, and coworkers established that Marek disease virus infection caused vascular wall injury and altered cellular lipid metabolism.[14-18] Infection stimulated low-density lipoprotein (LDL) cholesterol uptake and reduced cholesterol ester hydrolytic activity. Aortic cholesterol, cholesterol ester, triglyceride, and phospholipid accumulated, resulting in marked atherosclerosis. Relative to human disease, Melnick et al reported in 1983 on the presence of antigen from the herpes family cytomegalovirus (CMV) in smooth muscle cells (SMCs) from carotid and aortic plaques of patients undergoing vascular surgery.[19]

Recent Insights: *Helicobacter pylori* and *Chlamydia pneumoniae*

Interest in infection as an atherogenic factor was reawakened in the early 1990s after the surprising discovery of a pivotal role for *Helicobacter pylori* in gastritis and peptic ulcer disease.[20] Acid peptic diseases had been considered to be noninfectious inflammatory and degenerative processes. *H. pylori* organisms, whose presence had been occasionally described in the stomach's mucosal lining, had previously been ignored or considered to be a harmless commensal.

About the same time, reports of a common organism of respiratory infection, *Chlamydia pneumoniae*, were published.[21,22] Initial serologic studies claimed to show an association between *C. pneumoniae* exposure and myocardial infarction (MI).[23,24] Subsequently, *Chlamydia* organisms were found within human atherosclerotic plaque.[25,26] The current era of the infection theory of atherosclerosis was underway.

PROPOSED TRIGGERS OF VASCULAR INFLAMMATION: NONINFECTIOUS AND INFECTIOUS FACTORS

Studies of both local (within plaque) and circulating (systemic) factors support an inflammatory process for atherosclerosis.[27] Histologic studies show accumulation of activated inflammatory cells (macrophages, T lymphocytes, mast cells) in atherosclerotic plaque (especially unstable and disrupted plaques, the substrate for ACSs). At the same time, elevations in circulating markers of inflammation (e.g., C-reactive protein [CRP], interleukins) are present. The specific triggers for the vascular inflammatory responses observed in atherosclerosis are uncertain. Noninfectious as well as infectious stimuli have been implicated.

Noninfectious Factors

A number of noninfectious factors, many related to standard risk factors, lead to oxidative stress and stimulation of vascular inflammation.[4,27,28] These include oxidized LDLs and other modified non–high-density lipoproteins, hypertension, diabetes, cigarette smoking, physical or emotional distress associated with sympathoadrenal activation, increased angiotensin-II levels, and hyperhomocystinemia (Table 7–1).

Infectious Factors

Infection is a classic stimulus for inflammation, which is directed at eradication or containment of the offending organism. A role for infection as an inflammatory stimulus of chronic diseases, such as rheumatoid arthritis or atherosclerosis, is more speculative but gaining support.[4,29-31] Clearly, infection can lead to induction of the

■ ■ □

TABLE 7–1 PROPOSED INFLAMMATORY TRIGGERS OF ATHEROSCLEROSIS AND ACUTE CORONARY SYNDROMES

Noninfectious

Modified lipoproteins (e.g., oxidized low-density lipoproteins)
Diabetes
Hypertension (mechanical stress)
Products of cigarette smoke
Sympathoadrenal activation (physical, emotional stress)
Neuroendocrine factors (increased angiotensin-II)
Hyperhomocysteinemia
Renal insufficiency, uremic factors
Other inflammatory mediators, cytokines, oxidants

Infectious (see Table 7–2)

■ ■ □

TABLE 7–2 CANDIDATE PRO-ATHEROGENIC INFECTIOUS ORGANISMS

Bacteria

Chlamydia pneumoniae
Helicobacter pylori
Periodontal disease (e.g., *Porphyromonas gingivalis*, *Streptococcus sanguis*, *Streptococcus viridans*)
Mycoplasma pneumoniae
Haemophilus influenzae
Chronic bacterial respiratory, urinary, dental, other infections

Viruses

Cytomegalovirus
Herpes simplex viruses (HSV-1, HSV-2)
Epstein-Barr virus
Hepatitis A
Human immunodeficiency virus (HIV)
Influenza

molecular and cellular events involved in vascular inflammation and atherosclerosis.[4,29-31] Whether, when, and to what extent infection plays a role in human disease remains to be established.[32] The list of infectious agents that might play a role in atherogenesis, directly or indirectly, continues to grow (Table 7–2).

POTENTIALLY ATHEROGENIC PATHOGENS

Chlamydia pneumoniae

Chlamydia are specialized, intracellular gram-negative bacteria that lack the ability to synthesize high-energy phosphates.[33] They have been described as "energy parasites," depending on host eukaryotic cells to provide the adenosine triphosphate and guanosine triphosphate essential to metabolism.

Four species belong to the *Chlamydia* genus.[33] *C. trachomatis* causes human infections of the epithelial surfaces of the ocular or genital tracts and is a suspected immunologic trigger of reactive oligoarthritis. *C. psittaci* and *C. pecorum* are agents of veterinary disease, affecting a wide range of birds as well as mammals, arthropods, and mollusks. *C. pneumoniae*, the most recently recognized species, is a major cause of acute respiratory tract infections and is being investigated for its potential role in several chronic diseases, including asthma, sarcoidosis, Alzheimer-type dementia,[34] and atherosclerosis and myocardial infarction.

C. pneumoniae isolates from respiratory infections were first reported in 1986.[21] Subsequent epidemiologic studies found *C. pneumoniae* to be the cause of 5% to 10% of respiratory infections in adults and children, making it the third most common etiologic agent.[22] Antibody prevalence studies suggest that over 50% of adults have been exposed worldwide.[35]

The life cycle of *Chlamydia* is unique (Fig. 7–1).[33,36] Chlamydia exist outside of cells in a sporelike form called an *elementary body (EB)*. Chlamydial replication begins with the attachment of an infectious EB to the host cell surface. The chlamydial major outer membrane protein (MOMP), a dominant surface protein of the EB, is a candidate adhesin in this process, although the details of cell adhesion and endocytosis have not been clearly defined. Once inside its host, the EB uses the cell's metabolic machinery for its development into a metabolically active but noninfectious form called the *reticulate body*. In this form, the bacterium can divide and proliferate. Differentiation back to EB forms eventually may occur with cell lysis, EB expulsion, and invasion of neighboring cells. Alternatively, under metabolically limiting conditions, reticulate bodies may remain within the cell and convert into a metabolically inactive form called a *persistent body*. In this state, chlamydia can remain within the cell for extended periods. In the persistent state, chlamydia may be difficult for the immune system to recognize and unresponsive to antibiotics that interfere with bacterial metabolism. Under more favorable metabolic conditions and with various stressors, infectious reactivation may occur in association with a transition back to the active reticulate body form.

Other Bacterial Pathogen Candidates

Helicobacter pylori

H. pylori, the etiologic agent of peptic ulcer disease, has received attention as a potential risk factor for atherosclerosis and MI.[37] *H. pylori* is a gram-negative, spiral, flagellated bacillus that naturally infects humans and monkeys.[38] It is noninvasive, living in the gastric mucosa.[38,39] Animal models have not yet demonstrated a pathologic role.[11] One[40] but not other studies[11,41] found *H. pylori* or its antigen in atherosclerotic plaque. However, the organism can induce platelet aggregation and may increase CRP levels, raising the possibility that it might increase risk at a distance through induction of circulating procoagulant and pro-inflammatory factors.[11]

The serologic prevalence of *H. pylori* infection is about 30% in the United States and other developed countries and about 80% in most developing countries.[39] About 50% of Americans have evidence of prior *H. pylori* infection by age 60. Most studies show that spontaneous acquisition or loss of infection in adulthood is uncommon, so most infections are likely acquired in childhood.

Periodontal Infection

Bacterial periodontal disease has attracted attention as a possible risk factor for CAD and MI. Patients with poor dentition have frequent episodes of bacteremia.[42,43] The infectious agents involved in gingivitis include gram-negative bacteria, such as *Porphyromonas gingivalis* and *Streptococcus viridans*.[43] Periodontal disease and other dental infections also increase the risk of endocarditis.[42] Initial reports of associations between periodontal disease and CAD and MI sparked interest in this chronic infection and CAD risk.[44]

Other Common Bacterial Infections

Many other common bacterial infections, acting at a distance and in some cases locally within arteries, may be involved in atherogenesis.[45] Seropositivity (immunoglob-

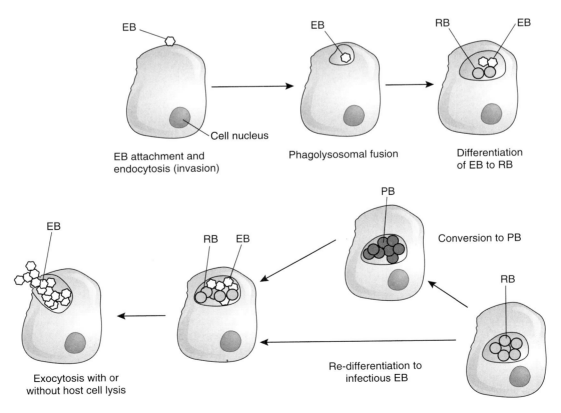

FIGURE 7–1. Schematic of life cycle of *Chlamydia*. EB, elementary body; PB, persistent body; RB, reticulate body.

ulin A [IgA]) to *Mycoplasma pneumoniae*, another common cause of respiratory infection, predicted coronary artery disease (CAD) prevalence in our preliminary report.[46]

Cytomegalovirus and Other Herpesviridae

Cytomegalovirus

CMV, a member of the herpes family of DNA viruses, is a common human pathogen.[11] Exposure (based on antibody prevalence) approximates age: 15% of adolescents, 50% of adults, and 70% of the elderly are seropositive.[47] CMV causes a wide range of human disorders spanning infancy to old age. As with other herpesviruses, CMV persists indefinitely in the host. However, unlike herpes simplex and varicella zoster, which develop latent infections at specific sites, the sites of latency of CMV are uncertain and the virus may reside in a variety of tissues and cell types, including bone marrow, mononuclear cells, and vascular cells.[11] CMV has been proposed to enhance cardiac allograft atherosclerosis, coronary restenosis, and native atherosclerosis. Evidence for these conjectures includes serologic associations, the presence of viral products at sites of vascular disease, and animal models.

Other Herpesviridae

Other herpesviruses that establish chronic latent infections include herpes simplex virus 1 (HSV-1), HSV-2, varicella zoster, Epstein-Barr virus (EBV), and human herpesvirus 6. Several of these also appear to have the potential to promote atherosclerosis alone and in aggregate.[48,49]

Hepatitis Viruses

Hepatitis viruses, even if not harbored in vascular lesions, can establish chronic infection and induce autoimmune disease (perhaps through molecular mimicry) and may provoke atherogenesis indirectly.[49]

Human Immunodeficiency Virus

The worldwide impact of HIV is increasing, and HIV should be considered a candidate pathogen of atherosclerosis.

ASSOCIATIONS OF ATHEROSCLEROSIS WITH SEROLOGY AND ACTIVE INFECTION

C. pneumoniae

Ironically, although early reports of associations of *C. pneumoniae* seropositivity with MI launched current interest in the infectious theory of atherosclerosis,[23,24] more recent studies have been less supportive of a strong link between seropositivity and CAD risk.[50-52] As noted, *C. pneumoniae* infection is highly prevalent worldwide, with antibody prevalence studies suggesting exposure in over 50% of adults.[35]

A problem in serologic studies is differentiating persistent infection from resolved infection with persistent antibody.[53] Primary infection is characterized by an IgM response followed by an IgG response and a weak or absent IgA response. Re-infection, more common in adults, is associated with IgG and IgA responses, and diagnosis requires paired sampling. Serologic criteria for chronic persistent infection are poorly established. High-titer, persistently elevated specific IgA and IgG antibodies may indicate chronic infection because IgA is thought to have a much shorter half-life than IgG.[53] Serologic diagnosis of chronic infection is further limited by individual variability in antibody response, differing assay methods, varying criteria for seropositivity, differing populations, and differing statistical approaches to adjustment for confounding factors.[54] These considerations may help to explain discrepancies in serologic associations.

C. pneumoniae *and Acute Coronary Syndromes*

The first seroepidemiologic study investigated paired sera from 40 men with MI, 30 with chronic CAD and 41 controls.[23] Elevated anti–*C. pneumoniae* IgG titers (1:128) or IgA titers (1:32), or both, were more common in MI and chronic CAD patients (68% and 50%, respectively) than in controls (17%). Seroconversion was common after acute MI but not with chronic CAD or in controls. Multiple serologic studies from several centers and sites around the world have since been performed. The presence and strength of associations with CAD and MI have varied but are generally less than in this initial report.[52,55-58]

The possibility that only very high antichlamydial titers are predictive of ACSs has been raised.[59] Among a consecutive series of patients, a strong association was observed only between very high serotiters ($\geq$1:1024) and ACS. Thus, recent re-infection, reactivation, or an exaggerated immune response to *C. pneumoniae* may be an etiologic factor for ACS, and therapeutic interventions might be specifically targeted to these patients.

Persistent *C. pneumoniae* infection also may characterize patients with unstable angina. *C. pneumoniae* antibodies (and elevated fibrinogen) were more common among 256 patients with unstable angina than in controls (36% vs. 19%).[60]

Not all studies have found antibody positivity to be predictive of CAD or ACS. We studied 363 patients undergoing coronary angiography and found seropositivity in 68% with CAD but also in 65% without; also, seropositivity was found in 75% with a history of MI compared with 60% without.[50] The Physicians' Health Study prospectively measured IgG antibodies against *C. pneumoniae* in 343 participants who had a first MI and 343 age- and smoking-matched controls without vascular events during a 12-year follow-up; the prevalence of seropositivity for *C. pneumoniae* was the same in both groups.[61] In a large women's study, seropositivity also was not predictive.[51] Another nested case control study of 496 men who experienced a coronary event and 989 men without found an odds ratio for CAD events of just 1.22 associated with top tertile of IgG antibody titers after adjustment for smoking and socioeconomic status.[52] A meta-analysis of 15 prospective trials including 3169 subjects yielded a combined odds ratio of only 1.15 (95% CI, 0.97 to 1.36).[52]

Future *C. pneumoniae* serologic studies might focus on specific patient subgroups such as young patients with ACS. A recent Italian study supported the hypothesis that *C. pneumoniae* seropositivity is a risk predictor primarily for premature MI in a pro-inflammatory setting (age ≤ 50 years, smoker, elevated anti-CMV titer).[62]

C. pneumoniae *and Asymptomatic Atherosclerosis*

Positive *C. pneumoniae* titers have been associated with asymptomatic atherosclerosis assessed by carotid ultrasonography (adjusted odds ratio, 2.0).[63] An autopsy study in Alaskan natives with stored sera linked *C. pneumoniae* in coronary tissue to IgG antibody titers of 1:256 (adjusted odds ratio, 9.4).[64] *C. pneumoniae* seropositivity was associated with an atherogenic lipid profile in Finnish and British studies.[65,66]

C. pneumoniae *and Restenosis*

Restenosis after coronary angioplasty is characterized by excessive proliferation of vascular SMCs. Some serologic evidence suggests that *C. pneumoniae* may increase restenosis after coronary angioplasty.[67] Antibiotics may reduce restenosis in patient subgroups with very high *C. pneumoniae* titers (discussed later).[68]

C. pneumoniae *and Ischemic Stroke*

C. pneumoniae IgA seropositivity was associated with risk of a first ischemic stroke (adjusted odds ratio, 4.5) in a study of 89 patients and 89 controls.[69] The association with IgG was weaker (odd ratio, 2.6).

H. pylori *and Coronary Artery Disease*

Evidence for an association between *H. pylori*, the etiologic organism of peptic ulcer disease, and atherosclerosis has been primarily serologic. An initial British study reported that 59% of 111 patients with documented CAD were seropositive for *H. pylori*, compared with 39% of age-matched and sex-matched controls.[37] At least 25 epidemiologic studies have followed. Some studies have reported positive associations,[70,71] but the majority have been negative,[51,71-76] suggesting that an association, if present, is small. Some of these epidemiologic studies made little adjustment for possible confounding variables such as socioeconomic status. Studies that did adjust generally reported weaker or absent associations.

Danesh et al reported a meta-analysis of primarily European *H. pylori* serologic studies.[71,77] *H. pylori* seropositivity did not significantly predict CAD (odds ratio, 1.1; 95% CI, 0.9 to 1.4). Another meta-analysis by Ridker et al of 10 prospective studies found an odds ratio of only 1.15 (99% CI, 0.96 to 1.37).[78] Studies in the United States also have generally been negative.[50,51,75,78] Exposure to the virulent strain of *H. pylori* producing CagA, an antigen that enhances gastric inflammatory response, has been associated with CAD in some but not

all studies.[79-81] Thus, a role for *H. pylori* in CAD has not been firmly established by serologic associations, and any true association is likely to be of small magnitude. The most promising group for further study might be patients with early-onset (before age 50) MI.[71,80]

Periodontal Infection and Coronary Artery Disease

Some but not all studies have found an association between periodontal disease and CHD and MI. In this case, "exposure" is based on dental examination rather than serologic testing. In 1989, Mattila et al reported a strong association between dental disease and MI.[44] A subsequent study of 9760 healthy males reported that periodontitis at initial screening increased the risk of a cardiac ischemic event during follow-up by 25%.[82] Data from the Normative Aging and the Dental Longitudinal studies also suggested that men with significant periodontal disease were at increased risk for fatal CAD or stroke.[83] Still another study reported an association between periodontal disease and peripheral vascular disease.[84]

In contrast, the prospective U.S. Physician's Health Study in over 22,000 men found no link between self-reported gum disease and MI.[85,86] Likewise, the National Health and Nutrition Examination Survey I (NHANES I) study of over 8000 subjects followed for up to 20 years found no convincing association between periodontal disease and CAD risk.[87] Insufficient control for smoking history, socioeconomic status, and health awareness was proposed as an explanation for the results of previous positive studies. Finally, a meta-analysis of five epidemiologic studies comparing prevalence of dental disease in those with and without CAD showed only a weak association with CAD, with an odds ratio of 1.2 (1.1 to 1.4).[77] Nevertheless, mouth organisms, such as *P. gingivalis* and *S. sanguis*, have been identified in carotid atherosclerotic plaques.[42] Therefore, the question of a true relationship between periodontal disease and CAD remains to be more clearly defined.

Serologic Associations of Cytomegalovirus with Coronary Artery Disease

The association of CMV seropositivity with angiographic CAD also has been inconsistent or negative. Among 11 case-control studies, 4 showed a strong association of CMV antibody positivity with CAD, whereas the other 7 showed little or no association.[88] CMV correlates with age and socioeconomic class, which may confound apparent associations.

CMV seropositivity did not predict primary CAD risk in our database.[50] CMV seropositivity also was not predictive of primary risk in several larger studies.[51,88-90] Similarly, a meta-analysis of three *prospective* prevention studies found an odds ratio of 0.91 (95% CI, 0.69 to 1.19).[77] In the Atherosclerosis Risk in Communities (ARIC) study, a primary CAD event was predicted by CMV seropositivity but only at the highest antibody levels (top quintile).[91]

In contrast with the study of primary risk, CMV seropositivity did predict outcomes (death or MI) in those with angiographic CAD in our database.[92] Mortality risk was particularly evident in those with both elevated CRP and positive serology to CMV ($P < .0001$).[92] Consistent with this finding, CMV seropositivity was a univariate but not a multivariate risk predictor in the European AtheroGene study.[93] However, in those with elevated interleukin-6, an inflammatory cytokine, CMV seropositivity marked a 3.2-fold ($P < .01$) increased risk of death, suggesting that the atherosclerotic effects of CMV are mediated through an underlying inflammatory response.[93]

Given the variability of CMV and CAD associations, Zhu et al postulated that patterns of inflammation and sex might influence CMV induction of atherosclerosis.[94] Among 238 subjects evaluated for CAD, elevation of CRP was a strong predictor in men and CMV seropositivity was associated with elevated CRP. In contrast, in women, CMV seropositivity was independently predictive of CAD and CRP was less predictive. In addition, CAD prevalence was higher in women with serologic or mixed but not a cellular (T cell)-only response to CMV. Thus, gender and other host-specific immune responses may determine the role of CMV in individual patients. Young age (≤50) in a pro-inflammatory setting is a subgroup worthy of further investigation of CMV serology as a risk marker for MI.[71]

A role for CMV in restenosis after coronary angioplasty has been proposed. CMV antibody is associated with elevated CRP,[95] which in turn is predictive of restenosis.[96] In one clinical report, patients undergoing atherectomy or angioplasty who were CMV-seropositive experienced a higher rate of angiographic restenosis (43% vs. 8%).[97] On the other hand, we were unable to associate clinical restenosis with CMV seropositivity.[98]

Serologic Associations for Herpes Simplex and Other Viruses

Antibodies to herpes simplex virus have been measured in several studies. Among patients in the Helsinki Heart Study, antibody to HSV-1 showed the strongest association with primary CAD risk (2.1 in the highest HSV quartile) of six serologic tests (the others being adenovirus, enterovirus, CMV, *C. pneumoniae*, and *H. pylori*).[90] Risk increased further in those with both HSV-1 antibody and elevated CRP. In contrast, HSV-1 antibodies were not predictive of primary risk in the U.S. Physician's Health, Women's Health, and ARIC studies.[51,88,91] In two secondary prevention studies, however, herpesviruses contributed to risk both individually and as part of an aggregate score ("pathogen burden"; see later).[48,49] Potential risk associations with HSV-2, EBV, and hepatitis A virus serologic responses also were raised by these studies.

PATHOGEN BURDEN, ATHEROGENESIS, AND ACUTE CORONARY SYNDROMES

Epstein et al introduced the concept of "total pathogen burden" as a CAD risk factor.[30] Exposure to a single atherogenic infectious agent might increase risk modestly, but multiple infectious exposures could combine to substantially raise the aggregate risk of CAD. An initial study evaluated the relationship of pathogen burden, assessed by the aggregate number of a panel of five pathogens to which patients showed serologic exposure, to primary CAD risk assessed angiographically.[99] The study cohort consisted of 233 patients, of whom 68% were found to have angiographic CAD. Pathogens tested were *C. pneumoniae*, CMV, hepatitis A virus, HSV-1, and HSV-2. After multivariate analysis, the prevalence of CAD was 48%, 69%, and 85% in persons with antibodies to two pathogens, three to four pathogens, or all five pathogens, respectively. The adjusted odds ratio for CAD was 6.1 for those with five antibodies versus those with two antibodies.

To prospectively test the pathogen burden hypothesis and extend it to secondary cardiovascular risk, an independent patient cohort (N = 890) with angiographically documented CAD was tested for antibodies to *C. pneumoniae*, CMV, HSV-1, HSV-2, hepatitis A virus, and *H. pylori* and followed for up to 5 years for the outcomes of death or MI.[49] Compared with patients positive for zero to one antibody, those positive for two, three, four, five, or six had fully adjusted relative hazard rates for incident MI or death of 2.4, 3.0, 4.9, 6.5, and 6.3, respectively ($P = .0005$) (Fig. 7–2). Individually, CMV, HSV-1, HSV-2, and hepatitis A virus were significantly associated with risk (hazard ratio, 1.5 to 2.0) after adjustment for traditional risk factors, whereas *C. pneumoniae* and *H. pylori* alone were not.

European investigators also have found an association between the number of infectious pathogen exposures and long-term prognosis in patients with documented CAD.[48] The AtheroGene study tested IgG and IgA antibodies to HSV-1, HSV-2, CMV, EBV, *Haemophilus influenzae*, *C. pneumoniae*, *Mycoplasma pneumoniae*, and *H. pylori* in 1018 patients with angiographically demonstrated CAD. Patients were followed for cardiovascular events over a mean of 3.1 years. Increasing pathogen

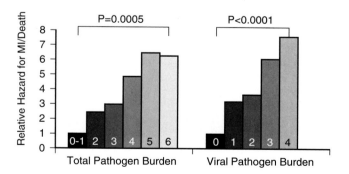

FIGURE 7–2. Pathogen burden and secondary risk of myocardial infarction and death according to Zhu et al.[46] Relative hazard rates of MI or death by number of positive IgG antibodies to all 6 infectious agents (*C. pneumoniae*, *H. pylori* [Hpyl], and 4 viruses) (left) or to the 4 viruses alone (HSV-1, HSV-2, CMV, Hepatitis A) (right). Hazard ratios are adjusted for age, sex, number of affected vessels, presentation (stable angina, unstable angina, MI), diabetes, smoking, hyperlipidemia, hypertension, family history, renal failure. (Data are from Zhu J, Nieto FJ, Horne BD, et al: Prospective study of pathogen burden and risk of myocardial infarction or death. Circulation 2001;103:48.)

burden was highly predictive of long-term prognosis ($P < .0001$) (Fig. 7–3): Cardiovascular mortality ranged from 3.7% to 12.6% for seropositivity to zero to three versus seropositivity to six to eight. The result was primarily driven by seropositivity to the Herpesviridae (CMV, HSV-1, HSV-2, EBV) (adjusted hazard ratio, 5.6; $P < .0001$). Risk predictions were independent of CRP, which also predicted mortality.

Thus, a greater prevalence of serologic exposures to selected pathogens, particularly to viral pathogens, leads to an increased probability of CAD as well as an increased probability of a clinical event (death or MI).

COMMON BACTERIAL INFECTION, INFLAMMATORY MARKERS, AND RISK OF CORONARY ARTERY DISEASE

The possibility that common chronic bacterial infections, acting at a distance, can accelerate atherosclerosis has gained recent support from the Bruneck study.[45] The Bruneck study assessed 5-year changes in carotid atherosclerosis by high-resolution duplex ultrasonography in 826 men and women initially 40 to 79 years old. The presence of chronic respiratory, urinary tract, dental, and other infections was ascertained. Chronic infections amplified the risk of atherosclerosis development and progression. For those free of carotid disease at baseline, chronic infection independently increased the hazard of developing new lesions by over four times ($P < .0001$). Infection increased risk even in the absence of other vascular risk factors. Relative CRP elevation (>1 mg/L) also increased the risk of early atherogenesis and added to the risk of chronic infection (Fig. 7–4). The combination of chronic infection with an inflammatory response (elevated CRP) was associated with a fivefold relative risk of incident carotid atherosclerosis.

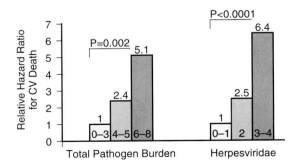

FIGURE 7–3. Pathogen burden and secondary risk of myocardial infarction and death according to Rupprecht et al.[44] Relative hazard rates for cardiovascular (CV) death of total pathogen burden (number of antibodies positive to 8 bacterial—*Cpn, Hpyl, H influenzae, M pneumoniae*—or viral infectious agents), left, or herpesviridae pathogen burden alone (HSV-1, HSV-2, CMV, Epstein-Barr virus), right. Hazard rate ratios are adjusted for age, sex, diabetes, smoking, HDL cholesterol, ejection fraction (<30%), and CRP. Data are from Rupprecht HJ, Blankenberg S, Bickel C, et al: Impact of viral and bacterial infectious burden on long-term prognosis in patients with coronary artery disease. Circulation 2001;104:29.)

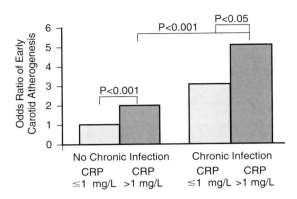

FIGURE 7–4. Chronic bacterial infection, inflammation (C-reactive protein), and coronary risk.[41] Odds ratios for new carotid plaque detection by chronic infection status and C-reactive protein (CRP) level. 1 mg/L represents the 60th percentile. Number of subjects with incident atherosclerosis per number at risk in the 4 categories (left to right) are: 109/403, 76/155, 93/132, 112/136. (Adapted from Kiechl S, Egger G, Mayr M, et al: Chronic infections and the risk of carotid atherosclerosis: Prospective results from a large population study. Circulation 2001;103:1068.)

PATHOGENS IN VASCULAR TISSUES

C. pneumoniae

C. pneumoniae has been localized to coronary and carotid atherosclerotic plaque as well as to occluded saphenous vein grafts.

Evidence for the organism was initially found in coronary and aortic atheromas taken from a limited number of South African autopsy cases tested by immunocytochemistry (ICC), electron microscopy, and the polymerase chain reaction (PCR).[25,26,100] In a study of 90 consecutive patients with symptomatic CAD undergoing coronary atherectomy, we detected chlamydial antigen by direct immunofluorescence in 66 (73%); another 5 (6%) were borderline-positive.[101] In contrast, only 1 of 24 control specimens (4%) was positive.

Several authors have assessed the distribution of *C. pneumoniae* within the body as a whole and within vascular tissues. Jackson et al tested 38 autopsy cases by ICC and PCR.[102] *C. pneumoniae* was detected more frequently in coronary artery specimens (34%) than lung (13%), liver (10%), spleen (5%), and granulomatous tissue (9%). Noncardiovascular presence usually was associated with cardiovascular presence. In an autopsy study of 60 patients, Ericson et al found *C. pneumoniae* more frequently in areas of severe atherosclerotic disease than mild disease (80% to 86% vs. 6% to 38%).[103] Similarly, Vink et al found *C. pneumoniae* to be more prevalent in arteries typically involved with atherosclerosis (67% in the aorta, 41% in the iliac arteries, 33% in the coronary arteries) than in arteries with a low prevalence of atherosclerosis (0% in the radial and 2% in the cerebral arteries).[104] In contrast, another postmortem study failed to find a correlation between the distribution of *C. pneumoniae* and the severity and extent of coronary disease.[105]

Maass et al studied 70 patients undergoing coronary artery endarterectomy and recovered viable chlamydia organisms from 16% of patients and detected chlamydial DNA in 30%.[106,107] In contrast, *C. pneumoniae* was not detected in any of the nonatherosclerotic control patients who were undergoing revascularization because of restenosis.

Ramirez cultured *C. pneumoniae* from a native atherosclerotic coronary vessel explanted at the time of cardiac transplantation.[108] In contrast, Weiss et al were unable to find culture or DNA evidence for *C. pneumoniae* in atherectomy specimens.[109]

C. pneumoniae produces a large amount of heat shock protein (HSP) during chronic persistent infections, which co-localizes with human HSP in macrophages found within human atherosclerotic plaques.[110] These HSPs have a variety of actions that could promote the development of atherosclerosis, including activation of vascular SMCs and induction of the expression of tumor necrosis factor α and matrix-degrading metalloproteinases by macrophages.[110,111]

C. pneumoniae also has been linked to carotid artery atherosclerosis. In one study, tissue obtained at carotid endarterectomy was examined by ICC and PCR for the presence of *C. pneumoniae*.[112] All five of the fresh endarterectomy specimens were positive for *C. pneumoniae* by ICC (three of the five were positive by PCR). A total of 56 archival formalin-fixed, paraffin-embedded carotid endarterectomy tissues were then examined by ICC; 32 were positive. In comparison, all 13 normal carotid arterial sections from six patients were negative for *C. pneumoniae*.

C. pneumoniae vasculitis may play a role in saphenous vein graft occlusion after coronary artery bypass surgery. One study of 38 occluded saphenous vein grafts found chlamydial DNA in 25%; viable *C. pneumoniae* organisms were recovered from 16%.[113] In contrast, only 1 of 20 native saphenous veins had evidence of chlamydial infection. No evidence was found for CMV infection of occluded grafts.

Studies assessing the presence of *C. pneumoniae* within vascular tissues and atherosclerotic plaque are summarized in Table 7-3.

Cytomegalovirus and Herpes Simplex Virus and Atherosclerosis

Native Vessel Atherosclerosis

CMV and other herpesviruses or viral antigens also have been found in atherosclerotic arteries, although the database is less robust and less consistent than for *C. pneumoniae*.[19,114,115] CMV DNA also has been demonstrated in restenotic coronary lesions.[116] Yamashiroya et al found HSV or CMV but not EBV (by DNA hybridization or immunoperoxidase methods) in the aorta or coronary arteries at autopsy in 7 and 8 of 20 young trauma patients, respectively.[115] HSV or CMV was observed at sites overlying endothelial cells, SMCs, and early atheroma laden with macrophages. No infectious virus

■ ■ ■

TABLE 7-3 PATHOLOGIC EVIDENCE OF *CHLAMYDIA PNEUMONIAE* WITHIN VASCULAR AND ATHEROSCLEROTIC TISSUE

AUTHOR AND DATE	NO. SAMPLES—TISSUE(S)	METHODS	NO. POSITIVE
Shor,* 1992	7—Autopsy coronary artery	ICC, PCR	71%
Kuo, 1993	21—Aorta	ICC	33%
Kuo, 1993	36—Autopsy coronary artery	ICC, PCR, EM	56%
Kuo, 1995	18—Autopsy coronary artery	ICC, PCR	39%
Grayston, 1995	56—Carotid artery	ICC, PCR	57%
Campbell, 1995	38—Coronary atherectomy	ICC, PCR	53%
Muhlestein, 1996	90—Coronary atherectomy	DIF	79%
Blasi, 1996	51—Abdominal aortic aneurysm	PCR	51%
Weiss, 1996	58—Coronary atherectomy	PCR, EM	2%
Kuo, 1997	23—Femoral artery	ICC, PCR	48%
Jackson, 1997	16—Carotid artery	ICC, PCR, EM	69%
Jackson, 1997	38—Coronary artery	ICC, PCR	34%
Juvonen, 1997	12—Abdominal aortic aneurysm	ICC, PCR	100%
Davidson, 1998	60—Autopsy coronary artery	ICC, PCR	37%
Shor, 1998	24—Autopsy various arteries	ICC, PCR, EM	71%
Maass, 1998	238—Various arterial plaques	PCR	21%
Maass, 1998	158—Coronary artery	PCR	22%
Ouchi, 1998	39—Coronary, iliac arteries	ICC, PCR	64%
Paterson, 1998	49—Coronary, carotid arteries	PCR	0%
Lindholt, 1998	20—Abdominal aortic aneurysm	PCR	0%
Yamashita, 1998	20—Carotid artery	ICC	55%
Wong, 1999	49—SVG, IMAG	PCR	38%
Virok, 2001	15—MCA	PCR	33%

See text and references for details.[38]

DIF, direct immunofluorescence; EM, electron microscopy; ICC, immunocytochemistry; IMAG, internal mammary arterial graft; MCA, middle cerebral artery; PCR, polymerase chain reaction; SVG, saphenous vein graft.

was detected, suggesting abortive infection and colonization.

Hendrix et al examined arterial or aortic autopsy samples from patients undergoing vascular surgery and found CMV nucleic acid by dot hybridization in one half of samples from patients with atherosclerosis compared with 22% from CMV-seropositive patients without atherosclerotic disease (P = NS).[117] In a follow-up study using more sensitive PCR techniques, CMV nucleic acid sequences were detected in 90% of patients with atherosclerosis compared with 53% without significant atherosclerosis (P = .001). CMV was distributed throughout all major arteries in seropositive patients. These findings suggested widespread arterial presence of virus with the potential for reactivation of latent infection.

Cytomegalovirus and Allograft Atherosclerosis

Both CMV infection and accelerated CAD of the cardiac allograft are common after heart transplantation.[118] In the Stanford University experience (N = 387), one third of patients showed evidence of CMV infection, and graft atherosclerosis developed earlier and more frequently than in uninfected patients and was associated with higher CAD-related death rates (30% vs. 10% at 10 years).[119] Observations from the University of Minnesota program support the same conclusion.[120] CMV within spindle cells and lymphocytes has been found more commonly (67% vs. 30%) in allografts with atherosclerosis.[121] Finally, favorable effects of antiviral therapy have been reported in an animal model,[122] suggesting the potential for prevention (e.g., with ganciclovir) in human transplant recipients.

Cytomegalovirus and Coronary Restenosis

Coronary angioplasty causes vessel wall injury; vascular "response to injury" leads to SMC proliferation and restenosis. Reactivation of latent CMV may play a role in this process. Speir et al[116] noted increased frequency of CMV, of tumor suppression protein p53, and of early viral gene expression (which inhibits p53) in restenotic tissue. In a subsequent clinical study, restenosis was more common in CMV-seropositive patients (43% vs. 8%).[97] The hypothesis that activation of CMV at the time of angioplasty is a mechanism of restenosis is mechanistically attractive, but this explanation has been inconsistent and requires confirmation.[98]

Pathogen Delivery to Vascular Wall

It has been postulated but not clearly proved that CMV and *C. pneumoniae* are delivered to the arterial wall by circulating monocytes, CMV from myelomonocytic precursor cell reservoir, and *C. pneumoniae* from a pulmonary alveolar macrophage reservoir.[30] Arterial transport of *C. pneumoniae* directly as EBs from lung to arterial sites or within other cell types (e.g., T lymphocytes) also is theoretically possible.

CELLULAR AND MOLECULAR MECHANISMS IN VASCULAR TISSUES AND ATHEROMAS

C. pneumoniae and CMV infect vascular wall cells and may provoke or accelerate atherosclerosis by a variety of cellular and molecular mechanisms.[30,123] *C. pneumoniae* readily infects and replicates in endothelial cells, monocyte/macrophages, and vascular SMCs,[124-128] and *C. pneumoniae* shows tropism toward vascular tissue.[129] Its residence in these cells presents the opportunity to accelerate progression of atherosclerosis by a variety of mechanisms. CMV and other Herpesviridae also infect vascular cells.[30,130] CMV is thought to infect monocyte precursors in bone marrow, with the viral genome persisting in these cells.[30,131,132] After differentiation of monocytes to macrophages in the subintimal space,[133] CMV reactivation may occur with induction of pathogen-related atherogenic effects. Vascular SMCs support abortive CMV infection, leading to proliferation and accumulation.[134,135]

Epstein et al summarized a number of cellular and molecular mechanisms by which infectious agents may directly affect vascular atherosclerosis and thrombosis.[30] Selected proposed mechanisms are described in the following paragraphs (Table 7-4).

Inflammation: Provocation of General and Specific Immune Responses

Inflammation, provoked by infection, is a major mechanism by which atherosclerosis may be promoted by

■ ▦ ■

TABLE 7–4 MOLECULAR AND CELLULAR MECHANISMS BY WHICH INFECTIOUS AGENTS MAY PROMOTE ATHEROSCLEROSIS

Stimulate Inflammation

↑Local and circulating inflammatory mediators
  ↑Chemokines, cytokines, adhesion molecules
    ↑Matrix-degrading proteases
Pathogen (or pathogen-product) directed immune responses
Host-directed (auto-immune) responses (molecular mimickry)

Lipid Accumulation

↑Scavenger receptor activity
↓Cholesterol esterase activity

Endothelial Dysfunction

Impaired vasodilator function
↓Anticoagulant activity, ↑procoagulant effects

Smooth Muscle Cell (SMC) Accumulation

↑SMC proliferation
  p53 inhibition
  Growth factor/receptor expression
↑SMC migration
↓SMC apoptosis
  p53 inhibition

Modified after Epstein et al., Circulation 1999;100:e20-9.[30]

infection. Inflammation is triggered by vascular oxidative stress and "injury."[3] These stressors include hyperlipidemia, elevated homocysteine, cytokines, free radicals, circulating products of smoking, and biomechanical stresses such as hypertension.

The endothelium reacts to these noninfectious stressors by producing reactive oxygen species, cytokines, chemokines, and cellular adhesion molecules. Reactive oxygen species lead to oxidation of LDL. Chemokines attract monocytes, and adhesion molecules secure their attachment to the vessel wall. After migration to the subintimal space, these monocytes transform into macrophages and begin to secrete pro-inflammatory, prothrombotic, and matrix-degrading molecules, promoting atherogenesis.

Infection facilitates expression of reactive oxygen species and other oxidation and inflammation-related molecules.[136-139] Specifically, Dechend et al showed that *C. pneumoniae* infection of vascular SMCs and endothelial cells activates nuclear factor κB (NF-κB) and induces expression of tissue factor, interleukin-6, and plasminogen activator inhibitor 1.[128] These pro-inflammatory and pro-coagulant mechanisms may lead to plaque destabilization, disruption, thrombosis, and precipitation of ACSs.

Atherosclerosis has features of a delayed-time hypersensitivity immune response (Th-1) and has been compared with rheumatoid arthritis.[9,29,30,128] The role of specific T-cell subgroups in directing this response (including natural killer–type cells) also has been proposed.[29]

Induction of specific immune responses by pathogens may be directed initially at infectious antigens and subsequently at target host peptides through molecular mimicry.[140,141]

HSPs may be not only a target antigen for an (auto)immune response promoting atherosclerosis but also an inflammatory stimulus.[142] HSPs act as chaperones for newly synthesized proteins and are induced in response to cellular stresses (heat, biomechanical stress, oxidants) and act to prevent protein denaturation. Common risk factors for atherosclerosis, such as oxidized LDL and hypertension, as well as infections, cause overexpression of HSPs by endothelial cells, SMCs, and macrophages. Soluble HSPs bind to the Toll-like receptor 4/CD14 complex, initiating an innate immune response. HSPs are highly conserved across species, including bacteria (e.g., chlamydia), and show substantial homology.

Growing evidence suggests that HSPs play a central role in the pathogenesis of atherosclerosis.[142-149] Indeed, HSPs may serve as a link between infections and the atherosclerotic process.[142] Through induction of host and pathogen-related HSPs, infection could induce autoantibodies and autoreactive cells against HSPs. Moreover, HSPs may act through induction of adhesion molecule expression by endothelial cells, proliferation of SMCs, and secretion of pro-inflammatory cytokines by macrophages.[142]

Differences in host inflammatory response to infection make up another potentially important but poorly studied factor modifying the inflammatory response to infection, a factor that is ripe for further research.[30,45,48,49,59,90,92,93,95,150]

Several studies highlight the concept that markers of inflammation (e.g., CRP, interleukin-6) are additive and complementary to but are not a surrogate for markers of infection (e.g., serologic studies, evidence of active infection).[45,48-50,93,95] Although increasing infectious exposure often is associated with higher CRP levels, the degree of correlation is low. Only a variable part of associated risk of infectious markers has been explained by adjusting for inflammatory markers. Pathogen burden up to eight organisms (viral and bacterial) and CRP were independent and additive risk factors in the AtheroGene study (see Fig. 7-3).[48] The Bruneck Study,[45] discussed earlier, found independent and additive risk of elevated CRP and evidence for chronic bacterial infection (see Fig. 7-4). Among 985 patients with angiographic CAD, we found that both elevated CRP and seropositivity to CMV were independent risk factors. However, risk was concentrated and greatest in those with both elevated CRP and CMV (Fig. 7-5).[92,93] These observations suggest the hypothesis that infection may promote atherosclerosis through activation of a chronic inflammatory response.[49] Neither CRP (and interleukin-6 or other inflammatory markers) nor infectious markers fully capture this risk, whereas a combination of both appears to provide the best risk assessment.

Lipid Accumulation

Lipid accumulation is a second general mechanism promoting atherosclerosis. Marek disease of chicken, the classic animal model of infection-related atherosclerosis, is caused by an avian herpesvirus and is characterized by marked vascular accumulation of lipids.[14,15,17,18,151] The likely mechanism for this effect, demonstrated in human SMCs infected with herpes simplex virus, is decreased cellular cholesterol ester hydrolytic activity.[18]

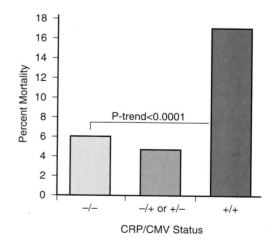

FIGURE 7–5. Risk interactions between seropositivity to CMV and inflammation (C-reactive protein).[71] Mortality among 985 patients with angiographic CAD after a mean of 2.7 years based on relative elevation of C-reactive protein (CRP) (2nd and 3rd tertiles) and/or seropositivity to CMV. Modified after Muhlestein JB, Horne BD, Carlquist JF, et al: Cytomegalovirus seropositivity and C-reactive protein have independent and combined predictive value for mortality in patients with angiographically demonstrated coronary artery disease. Circulation 2000; 102:1912.)

Enhanced scavenger receptor activity of SMCs and macrophages is another mechanism by which pathogens may increase lipid accumulation. This has been demonstrated for human SMCs infected with CMV.[97] An early IE gene product appears to be responsible. We have found that CMV also upregulates scavenger receptor activity in macrophages.[152] C. pneumoniae infection of macrophages incubated with LDL leads to increased cholesteryl ester accumulation and foam cell formation, although the mechanism may not be mediated by scavenger receptors.[127]

Endothelial Dysfunction

Endothelial dysfunction is a third general mechanism by which infection may facilitate atherosclerosis. The endothelium produces a number of antithrombotic substances, including nitric oxide, prostacyclin, plasminogen activator, thrombomodulin, and heparin sulfate. A number of laboratories have shown the ability of infectious agents (e.g., HSV, CMV, and C. pneumoniae) to change this phenotype from anticoagulant to procoagulant.[18, 153-157] In cell culture studies at our institution, Fryer et al[126] demonstrated that infection of human vascular endothelial cells induced procoagulant activity through a marked increase in production of tissue factor and enhancement of platelet adhesion.

Modulation of vascular tone by endothelial cells, critical to normal vascular function, is impaired by prior CMV or C. pneumoniae infection and may occur by both nitric oxide–dependent and –independent pathways.[158]

Smooth Muscle Cell Accumulation

SMC accumulation through proliferation, migration, and inhibition of apoptosis may be promoted, increasing atherosclerotic plaque size. Abortive CMV infection leads to SMC proliferation.[134,135] An intriguing molecular mechanism is through inhibition (binding) of the tumor suppressor gene p53 by an early CMV gene product (IE2-84).[116,159-161] Another mechanism associated with CMV infection is increased expression of growth factors (bFGF, aFGF, PDGF-BB) and growth factor receptors (i.e., for PDGF).[134,135,162,163] CMV and chlamydia inhibit apoptosis of infected cells.[130,164] Early viral gene products (i.e., IE2-84) are involved in CMV inhibition of apoptosis in human endothelial and HeLa cells.[116,130,159,161,165,166] SMC accumulation is promoted by migration from media and adventitia to neointima. Migration is enhanced by CMV infection of SMCs.[134]

NONVASCULAR INFECTIONS ASSOCIATED WITH RISK

H. pylori gastric disease and gingivitis are two examples of candidate infections discussed earlier that are potentially associated with atherosclerosis and CHD and are postulated to act systemically. The Bruneck study suggested that other common and chronic infections of the respiratory and urinary tract and other sites foster new carotid atherosclerosis.[45] Low-grade infection may induce circulating procoagulant and pro-inflammatory factors that act at a distance to enhance atherosclerosis progression and the initiation of acute ischemic syndromes.[30,45,167]

CIRCULATING FACTORS INDICATING INFECTION OR MEDIATING VASCULAR EFFECTS

Circulating C. pneumoniae DNA

The predictive value for CAD of circulating antibodies to the candidate infectious agents has been discussed. Circulating C. pneumoniae DNA also has been proposed as a circulating infectious marker. C. pneumoniae DNA has been detected within peripheral blood mononuclear cells (PBMCs) of patients with CAD and proposed to mark active vascular infection. In a study of 1025 subjects undergoing coronary angiography, circulating C. pneumoniae DNA was found within mononuclear cells in 9% of men with CAD compared with 3% of men with normal coronary arteries (odds ratio, 3.2; 95% CI, 1.1 to 8.9).[168] In another study, C. pneumoniae DNA was detected in both atherosclerotic tissue and circulating PBMCs in 39% of 41 patients undergoing resection of an abdominal aortic aneurysm but rarely (<8%) in either site separately, suggesting circulating DNA as a marker of vascular infection.[169] Still another study found the presence of C. pneumoniae DNA in PBMCs by PCR in 46% (13 of 28) of patients with CAD compared with 26% (5 of 19) of healthy blood bank donors (P = .08). Interestingly, the PCR signal in nonadherent cells was found within the CD3+ T-lymphocyte cell fraction (CD8+ subfraction).[170] A Swedish study also found C. pneumoniae DNA to be commonly present (59%) by nested PCR in PBMCs of patients with CAD and in middle-aged blood donors (46%).[171] Assay difficulties and variability in results have prevented current widespread use of C. pneumoniae DNA as a marker, but additional research may increase its utility.

Circulating Factors Promoting Infection at a Distance

Infection might cause vascular injury and facilitate atherosclerosis in the absence of resident pathogens in the vessel wall. Indeed, Zhou et al found that rats infected with CMV manifested increased neointimal proliferation in response to vascular injury despite the absence of virus from the injured segment.[167] CMV was isolated instead from salivary gland and spleen. The circulating factors responsible for these vascular effects were not determined, but they could include cytokines, acute-phase reactants, procoagulants, white blood cells, and cross-reactive antibodies. Similar mechanisms may be operative in humans who show increased vascular risk associated with chronic nonvascular bacterial infections[45] or with bacterial or viral organisms contributing to pathogen burden but not causing vascular infection.[48,49] A number of procoagulant and pro-inflammatory factors that act at a distance to enhance atherosclerosis progression and the initiation of acute ischemic syndromes have been proposed,[30] but an in-depth review of these is beyond the scope of this chapter.

ANIMAL MODELS

Animal models may be useful for determining the potential for atherosclerosis causality of infectious agents and in assessing the role of antibiotic therapy. The association of Marek disease virus infection and atherosclerosis in chickens, first discovered over 50 years ago, provided the first experimental proof of principle for a viral cause of atherosclerosis.[151,172] A variety of animal models also have evaluated a potential role of bacterial infection with *C. pneumoniae* in atherosclerosis.

Rabbit Models

C. pneumoniae causes pneumonitis in the rabbit,[173] and the cholesterol-fed rabbit is an established model for accelerated atherosclerosis.[174] Fong et al demonstrated the potential for nasally infected rabbits to experience early and intermediate histologic lesions of atherosclerosis.[174,175] We hypothesized that repeated infections and the addition of a small supplement of dietary cholesterol would consistently accelerate atherosclerosis and that antibiotic therapy would suppress this process.[176] Thirty New Zealand White rabbits were fed a 0.25% cholesterol diet and infected with three separate intranasal inoculations of either *C. pneumoniae* or saline. Weekly injections of azithromycin or no therapy were given for 7 weeks, and the animals were sacrificed 3 months after infection. Aortic maximal intimal thickness (Fig. 7–6), the percentage of involved luminal circumference, and plaque area index all increased in infected rabbits compared with uninfected controls. Antibiotic therapy of infected rabbits significantly suppressed atherosclerosis.

Murine Models

Wild-type C57BL/6J mice and both apo-E and LDL receptor–deficient mice have been successfully infected with *C. pneumoniae* through the intranasal route with subsequent detection of the organism within arterial walls in association with accelerated atherosclerosis.[177-179] In murine infection, *C. pneumoniae* was shown to be systemically disseminated via macrophages.[178] Moazed et al subsequently reported that *C. pneumoniae* infection causes progression of atherosclerosis in apolipoprotein E-deficient mice.[179] Hu et al studied the atherogenic effects of chlamydia in mice deficient in LDL receptors.[180] Atherogenesis was found to be specific to *C. pneumoniae* and to depend on dietary cholesterol.[180] Both low-cholesterol and high-cholesterol dietary conditions were studied. *C. pneumoniae* but not *C. trachomatis* exacerbated atherogenesis (increased lesion area and severity), but it did so only in the presence of hypercholesterolemia. The permissive role of hypercholesterolemia was postulated to relate to the necessity for initial lesion formation before *C. pneumoniae* could successfully infect aortic tissues.

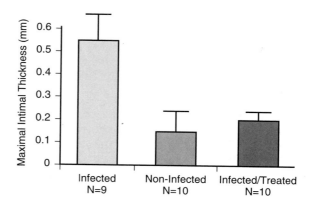

FIGURE 7–6. Acceleration of atherosclerosis by *C. pneumoniae* and suppression of atherosclerosis with azithromycin in a rabbit model.[155] Maximal aortic intimal thickness (mean of 9 or 10 animals), given in mm (mean ± SE). (Data from Muhlestein JB, Anderson JL, Hammond EH, et al: Infection with Cpn accelerates the development of atherosclerosis and treatment with azithromycin prevents it in a rabbit model. Circulation 1998;97:634.)

In contrast, Caligiuri et al did not detect induction of atherosclerosis by *C. pneumoniae* infection in wild-type C57BL/6J mice or in chow-fed apoE-KO mice,[181] perhaps the result of differences in diet and study design. Liuba et al observed the appearance of endothelial dysfunction after repeated *C. pneumoniae* infection in apolipoprotein E-knockout mice, suggesting that *C. pneumoniae* may hamper endothelial NO production.[182]

In summary, several but not all animal models have shown acceleration of atherosclerosis with *C. pneumoniae* infection, and it appears that some degree of hyperlipidemia must be induced before the atherosclerotic process is accelerated. Additionally, no animal model of atherosclerosis exactly mimics human disease. Therefore, these studies, although generally supportive of the infectious hypothesis of atherosclerosis, do not by themselves prove that intravascular infection with *C. pneumoniae* plays a causative role in human cardiovascular disease.

THERAPEUTIC INITIATIVES TARGETING INFECTIOUS AND INFLAMMATORY FACTORS

Antibiotics Directed at *C. pneumoniae*

Chlamydia are sensitive to macrolides, tetracyclines, and fluoroquinolones,[183] and these antibiotics have been considered for antibiotic trials directed against chronic vascular inflammation and atherosclerosis associated with *C. pneumoniae*.

Azithromycin is taken up into atherosclerotic plaque,[184] has been effective in animal models,[176] and has been used in several antibiotic trials for CAD. Azithromycin is approved for sexually transmitted *C. trachomatis* infection and is effective for acute upper respiratory and skin infections caused by *C. pneumoniae*. Azithromycin is rapidly absorbed and widely distributed into tissues. Its tissue half-life is prolonged (about 72 hours), and a single dose may require 10 days for elimination. This property has allowed azithromycin to be given once weekly (after initial loading) in clinical trials. Azithromycin has been generally well tolerated during long-term prophylaxis[185]; its most common adverse effects are gastrointestinal upset and superinfection (e.g., candidiasis).[185,186]

Another macrolide, roxithromycin, has been used in other trials. Finally, the quinolones have the advantage of greater cytotoxic (as opposed to cytostatic) potential, and gatifloxacin[187] currently is being tested in a large multicenter trial.

Indirect evidence of the benefit of some of these drugs comes from a population-based case-control study of 3315 patients with a first acute MI and over 12,000 controls.[188] Patients with MI were less likely than controls to have used a tetracycline antibiotic (adjusted odds ratio, 0.7) or a quinolone (odds ratio, 0.45). In contrast, MI risk was not affected by previous use of macrolides, sulfonamides, penicillins, or cephalosporins.

Another population-based study found *no* reduction in risk for a first MI with the use of erythromycin, tetracycline, or doxycycline during the previous 5 years, arguing against the use of these agents for primary prevention.[189]

Given the potential for confounding in observational study results, prospective randomized trials are required.

Antibiotic Trials in Acute Coronary Syndromes

The Roxithromycin Ischemic Trial (ROXIS), the first randomized antibiotic trial in ACS, randomized 202 Argentine patients with unstable angina or non–Q-wave MI to roxithromycin (150 mg BID) or placebo for 30 days.[190] At the end of the treatment period, the rates of recurrent ischemia (1.1% vs. 5.4%), MI (0% vs. 2.2%), and ischemic death (0% vs. 2.2%) were reduced in the patients treated with roxithromycin (adjusted $P = .064$ for the composite event rate). No major drug-related adverse effects occurred. At 6 months, individual and composite event rates remained lower in the roxithromycin group (8.7% vs. 14.6%), but the differences were no longer significant.[191]

The South Thames trial of Antibiotics in Myocardial Infarction and unstable Angina (STAMINA) was a second randomized antibiotic trial in ACS.[192] STAMINA randomized 325 patients to one of three regimens, each lasting 1 week: (1) azithromycin 500 mg/day, omeprazole 20 mg BID, and metronidazole 400 mg BID (designed to be antichlamydial), (2) amoxicillin 500 mg BID, omeprazole 20 mg BID, and metronidazole 400 mg BID (designed to be anti-*Helicobacter*), or (3) placebo. Follow-up extended for 1 year. All patients received standard treatment for CHD. There was no statistically significant difference in frequency or timing of major adverse cardiac events between either the azithromycin or the amoxicillin groups and placebo. However, when combined, subjects receiving either one or the other antibiotic-containing regimens experienced a 36% reduction in major events at 12 weeks compared with placebo ($P = .02$). The benefit persisted through 1 year. Seropositivity to *C. pneu-*

moniae or *H. pylori* did not impact the treatment effect. Given STAMINA's limited size and power, benefits related to the antimicrobial or anti-inflammatory properties of the specific regimens could not be distinguished. Larger clinical trials were recommended.

The Azithromycin in Acute Coronary Syndromes (AZACS) trial, the largest trial to date in ACS (N ≈1450 patients), was recently completed at Cedars of Sinai Medical Center, Los Angeles.[32] Patients were entered regardless of whether serologic tests for *C. pneumoniae* were positive or negative. Treatment was given for 5 days; duration of follow-up was 6 months. The preliminary results of AZACS, presented early in 2002, indicated no benefit of therapy.[193]

Antibiotic Trials in Chronic Coronary Artery Disease

In an initial pilot clinical trial, 60 survivors of an acute MI with persistently elevated anti–*C. pneumoniae* antibody titers (1:64) were randomized to receive placebo, a single 3-day course of azithromycin (500 mg/day), or two courses 3 months apart.[194] Anti–*C. pneumoniae* titers fell at 6 months to less than 1:16 in more patients receiving azithromycin than placebo (43 vs. 10%; $P = .02$). Azithromycin treatment apparently reduced cardiovascular events (from 28% to 8%; odds ratio, 0.2; $P = .03$) compared with those receiving placebo and a nonrandomized group of patients with high anti–*C. pneumoniae* titers. Outcomes were similar with one and two courses of azithromycin.

The Azithromycin in Coronary Artery Disease: Elimination of Myocardial Infection with Chlamydia (ACADEMIC) trial, performed by our group, examined markers of inflammation and subsequent cardiovascular events in 302 seropositive patients randomized to azithromycin (500 mg daily for 3 days, then weekly) or placebo for 3 months.[186,195] After 6 months, azithromycin reduced a global index of four systemic markers of inflammation (CRP, tumor necrosis factor α, interleukins-1 and -6) compared with placebo, reaching significance for CRP and interleukin-6; antibody titers were unchanged. Cardiovascular events were infrequent and similar in the two groups. Clinical events in ACADEMIC were assessed after 2 years. Cardiovascular event rates were not significantly different in treated patients and controls (22% vs. 25%; hazard ratio, 0.9; 95% CI, 0.5 to 1.6; $P = .7$), although a trend toward a reduction in events in the azithromycin arm was noted during the second year of the study (hazard ratio, 0.6; 95% CI, 0.23 to 1.5; $P = .26$).

These results, if combined with the two previous randomized trials, leave open the potential for a modest to moderate antibiotic benefit (of the order of 20% to 30% event reduction) of antibiotics in CAD and ACS (Table 7-5),[196] but this possibility requires prospective testing in very large studies.

Antibiotics to Prevent Restenosis

Restenosis is a common problem following coronary intervention. Although distinct from native CAD,

TABLE 7–5   CORONARY ARTERY DISEASE (CAD) EVENT REDUCTIONS IN EARLY RANDOMIZED ANTIBIOTIC TRIALS

TRIAL (MONTHS FOLLOW-UP)	STUDY POPULATION	ANTIBIOTIC GROUP (EVENTS/PATIENTS)	CONTROL GROUP (EVENTS/PATIENTS)
Gupta et al (British)[194]	Chronic CAD	3/40	5/20[*]
ROXIS (Argentine)[191]	Acute coronary syndrome	9/100	15/102
ACADEMIC (United States)[195]	Chronic CAD	22/150	25/152
Total	OR = 0.72 (CI 0.45–1.16)	34/290 (11.7%)	45/274 (16.4%)

OR, odds ratio; CI, 95% confidence interval.
[*]Randomized patients only.

restenosis after angioplasty also involves excessive proliferative, inflammatory, and prothrombotic responses. Cellular infection with *C. pneumoniae* activates these responses,[128] and *C. pneumoniae* might be a cofactor in promoting restenosis.[197]

The Intracoronary Stenting and Antibiotic Regimen 3 (ISAR-3) trial investigated roxithromycin, an effective antichlamydial macrolide, for the prevention of restenosis after coronary stent deployment.[67,68] A total of 1010 patients with successful coronary stenting were randomized to receive roxithromycin, 300 mg daily for 4 weeks, or placebo. The primary end point was the frequency of restenosis (≥50%) at 6-month follow-up angiography. A secondary end point was target vessel revascularization during the year after stenting.

Overall in ISAR-3, there was no significant difference in the roxithromycin and placebo groups in terms of 6-month angiographic restenosis rate (31% vs. 29%), target vessel revascularization (19% vs. 17%), or 1-year rate of death or MI (7% vs. 6%). However, a significant interaction was found between *C. pneumoniae* titers and treatment, both for restenosis and for revascularization. Roxithromycin was favored for patients with high titers (adjusted odds ratio, 0.44 for titers ≥1:512) but was ineffective at lower titers. These (and other) results raise the intriguing possibility that antibiotics may be selectively beneficial in a subgroup of patients with an active infection and a vigorous immune response.

Ongoing or Planned Antibiotic Studies

Based on the results of these preliminary studies, several large trials of sufficient size and duration to answer the question of a small to moderate but worthwhile clinical benefit are underway in patients with chronic CAD and ACS (Table 7–6).[198,199]

The Weekly Intervention with Zithromax for Atherosclerosis and its Related Disorders (WIZARD) trial, expected to be completed in 2002, has enrolled over 7000 stable patients with a history of MI and seropositivity to *C. pneumoniae* and randomized them to receive either placebo or 3 months of treatment with azithromycin (600 mg per week).[198,199] The primary clinical end point is the composite of death, MI, hospitalization for unstable angina, or need for repeat revascularization at 3 years. In a preliminary report early in 2002, the primary clinical end point was not significant at study end, although a reduction in death or nonfatal MI was observed through 6 months, during and shortly after antibiotics were administered.[200]

The Azithromycin and Coronary Events Study (ACES), sponsored by the National Institutes of Health, is a randomized, double-blind, placebo-controlled trial of azithromycin among adults with stable CAD.[198] ACES does not require seropositivity to *C. pneumoniae*, although serology is assessed. Participants are randomized to azithromycin, 600 mg orally once a week for 1

TABLE 7–6   LARGE ANTIBIOTIC SECONDARY PREVENTION TRIALS: ONGOING AND RECENTLY COMPLETED

TRIAL	N	POPULATION	ANTIBIOTIC	DURATION RX//FOLLOW-UP	STATUS
AZACS[32]	1450	Acute coronary syndrome	Azithomycin	5 da/6 mo	Completed
WIZARD[199]	7000+	Post-myocardial infarction	Azithomycin	3 mo/3 yr	Completed
ACES[198]	4000+	Coronary artery disease	Azithomycin	12 mo/4 yr	Into follow-up
MARBLE[199]	1200	CABG-list	Azithomycin	3 mo	Enrolling
ISAR-3[68]	1000+	PCI	Roxithromycin	1 mo/6–12 mo	Completed
ANTIBIOS[199]	4000	Post-myocardial infarction	Roxithromycin	6 wk	Enrolling
PROVE-IT[32]	4200	Coronary artery disease	Gatifloxacin	18 mo	Enrolling

CABG, coronary artery bypass graft; PCI, percutaneous coronary interventions.

year, or placebo. Follow-up will extend for a mean of 4 years. The primary end point is a composite of CHD death, nonfatal MI, hospitalization for unstable angina, or coronary revascularization. Secondary objectives will assess relationships among antibody titers, inflammatory markers, treatment status, and outcome. More than 4000 patients have been enrolled in ACES and are into the follow-up period.

The PRavastatin or AtorVastatin Evaluation and Infection Therapy (PROVE-IT) trial is a study enrolling over 3000 patients presenting with ACS. Randomization follows a 2×2 factorial design.[199] Treatments include one of two statin regimens (pravastatin or atorvastatin) and an intermittent course of gatifloxacin or placebo. The primary end point is major cardiovascular clinical events after at least 18 months of follow-up. The two statin therapies have different lipid-lowering potencies but potentially similar anti-inflammatory effects. Quinolone therapy offers potentially bactericidal antimicrobial (i.e., antichlamydial) activity. PROVE-IT addresses a number of questions regarding the role and therapy of inflammation and infection in the pathogenesis of ACS.

Other trials in ACS or MI with roxithromycin and with planned bypass surgery also are ongoing, and results will be of interest.

Antiviral Therapeutic Trials

No antiviral drug trials for the prevention of CHD have been conducted. However, favorable effects of antiviral therapy have been reported in one animal model,[122] suggesting the potential for treatment (e.g., with ganciclovir) in human disease.

Of recent interest, vaccination against influenza has been reported to reduce the risk of recurrent MI.[201] A case-control study was performed on 218 patients with CAD in a single center during the influenza season. The relative risk of MI, adjusted for multiple baseline variables, was found to be 0.33 (95% CI, 0.13 to 0.82; $P = .02$). The mechanism of benefit was not determined, but nine potential anti-inflammatory and anti-infectious effects, both specific and nonspecific, were proposed.

Another study compared the vaccination histories of 342 subjects who experienced sudden cardiac death in King County, Washington, with 549 randomly selected controls.[202] Those who had received vaccination against influenza within the previous year were 51% less likely to experience primary cardiac arrest. Because sudden cardiac death is commonly precipitated by an acute ischemic event, this study also supports a protective effect of vaccination against ACS.

Others also have proposed vaccination as a therapeutic strategy to prevent atherosclerosis progression and ACS,[203] and future vaccine trials against purported viral and bacterial pathogens can be expected.

EXPECTATIONS OF ANTIBIOTIC TRIALS

Enthusiastic expectations of these antibiotic trials for proving the infection hypothesis of atherosclerosis and ACS and establishing therapy must be tempered by a number of limitations and uncertainties (Table 7-7). Negative outcomes might be explained by not only an incorrect hypothesis (infection does not cause CAD) and an inadequate study size or design but also an ineffective antibiotic regimen. Indeed, Gieffers et al found *C. pneumoniae* infection in circulating monocytes to be refractory to antibiotics.[204] Blood monocytes from healthy volunteers were obtained before and after oral therapy with azithromycin or rifampin, inoculated with *C. pneumoniae*, and cultured in the presence of the antibiotic. Circulating monocytes from patients with CAD who were undergoing experimental therapy with azithromycin also were cultured. Antibiotics did not inhibit chlamydial growth within monocytes. After withdrawal of antibiotics, *C. pneumoniae* could be cultured from the monocyte cell lines. In contrast, antibiotics eliminated *C. pneumoniae* from epithelial cells.

Thus, prevention or elimination of vascular infection with antibiotics may be problematic if *C. pneumoniae* residing in circulating monocytes, which can carry and disseminate the organism, are antibiotic-resistant. Negative results in antibiotic studies might be explained if reactivation of *C. pneumoniae* from a persistent state, stimulation of pro-inflammatory mediator production, and promotion of atherosclerosis can occur despite an "effective" course of antibiotics.

On the other hand, if the results of studies are positive, the hypothesis is not entirely proved: A nonspecific anti-inflammatory effect or an anti-infective action against another organism might be operative. This uncertainty already has arisen in attempting to explain the benefits of minocycline therapy for rheumatoid arthritis.[205] The infectious theory of atherosclerosis does not lend itself well to proof using Koch's classic postulates. Thus, new and innovative experimental approaches are required to gain adequate insight into the role of infection in atherosclerosis and its therapy.

■ ■ ■

TABLE 7-7   POTENTIAL IMPLICATIONS AND LIMITATIONS OF ANTIBIOTIC TRIALS

Negative Trial

Infection hypothesis false?
False negative; study underpowered
Treatment incorrect: too short, dose inadequate, drug ineffective
Treatment-resistant organism (e.g., *Cpn* in persistent state) or resistant reservoir (e.g., monocytes/macrophages)
Wrong organism targeted; multiple organisms involved
Wrong stage of disease targeted (late versus early, acute versus chronic)
Wrong population tested (what markers predict active/latent atherogenic infection?)

Positive Trial

Infection hypothesis true?
False positive (small study, chance result)
Nonspecific anti-inflammatory effect
Nonspecific anti-infective effect

CONCLUSIONS

The recent recognition that atherosclerosis is inflammatory has raised the intriguing question of the inflammatory triggers. In particular, inflammation underlies the plaque instability and disruption that occurs in ACSs. Although noninfectious factors (e.g., oxidized LDL) clearly play a pro-inflammatory role, interest is increasing in the possibility that these triggers may include infections.

Cellular and molecular studies have demonstrated that infectious agents can trigger several key pathways involved in vascular infection, atherosclerosis, and ACSs. Animal models, beginning with Marek disease, also show the potential for infection to accelerate and anti-infective treatment to suppress atherosclerosis.

The possibility that infection might explain chronic inflammatory degenerative diseases previously regarded as noninfectious is well exemplified by the recent discovery that *H. pylori* is an etiologic factor in human peptic ulcer disease. The finding of *C. pneumoniae*, CMV, and other infectious agents within human atherosclerotic tissue has best raised this issue for atherosclerosis and has forced us to address the question of "innocent bystander versus dangerous pathogen." Serologic studies have shown high antibody prevalence for these agents among persons with CHD and ACSs. Nevertheless, associations have varied and confounding has been suspected. Aggregate exposure to many candidate infectious agents (pathogen burden) appears to be a stronger, more consistent risk marker. Better markers than serologic testing of active or latent as opposed to past resolved infection are needed. HSPs and anti-HSP antibodies appear to be one promising possibility.[206]

Although *C. pneumoniae* and CMV have received the most attention as infectious risk factors, others are likely involved, including common nonvascular infections acting at a distance through pro-inflammatory and pro-thrombotic factors.

In coming years, several well-powered antibiotic and (potentially) vaccine trials will be completed. These will provide additional insight into the role of infection in atherosclerosis and its therapy. Even so, these trials will also have limitations. Currently, antibiotic therapy directed at prevention of CHD and ACSs is unproven and inappropriate. In contrast, innovative research efforts are to be encouraged.

REFERENCES

1. American Heart Association: 2001 Heart and Stroke Statistical Update. Dallas, Tex, American Heart Association, 2000.
2. Wilson PW, D'Agostino RB, Levy D, et al: Prediction of coronary heart disease using risk factor categories. Circulation 1998;97:1837–1847.
3. Ross R: Atherosclerosis—an inflammatory disease. N Engl J Med 1999;340:115–126.
4. Morrow DA, Ridker PM: Inflammation in cardiovascular disease. In Topol EJ (ed): Textbook of Cardiovascular Medicine. Cedar Knolls, NJ, Lippincott Williams & Wilkins, 1999, pp 1–12.
5. Davies MJ, Thomas AC: Plaque fissuring—the cause of acute myocardial infarction, sudden ischaemic death, and crescendo angina. Br Heart J 1985;53:363–373.
6. van der Wal AC, Becker AE, van der Loos CM, Das PK: Site of intimal rupture or erosion of thrombosed coronary atherosclerotic plaques is characterized by an inflammatory process irrespective of the dominant plaque morphology. Circulation 1994;89:36–44.
7. Fuster V, Lewis A: Conner Memorial Lecture. Mechanisms leading to myocardial infarction: Insights from studies of vascular biology. Circulation 1994;90:2126–2146.
8. Shah PK: Plaque disruption and coronary thrombosis: New insight into pathogenesis and prevention. Clin Cardiol 1997;20:II-38-II-44.
9. Libby P: Molecular bases of the acute coronary syndromes. Circulation 1995;91:2844–2850.
10. Shah PK, Galis ZS: Matrix metalloproteinase hypothesis of plaque rupture: Players keep piling up but questions remain. Circulation 2001;104:1878–1880.
11. Kuvin JT, Kimmelstiel CD: Infectious causes of atherosclerosis. Am Heart J 1999;137:216–226.
12. Osler W: Diseases of the arteries. In Osler W (ed): Modern Medicine: Its Practice and Theory. Philadelphia, Lea & Febiger, 1908, pp 429–447.
13. Paterson JC, Cottral GE: Experimental coronary sclerosis: Lymphomatosis as a cause of coronary sclerosis in chickens. Arch Pathol 1950;49:699–709.
14. Fabricant CG, Fabricant J, Litrenta MM, Minick CR: Virus-induced atherosclerosis. J Exp Med 1978;148:335–340.
15. Minick CR, Fabricant CG, Fabricant J, Litrenta MM: Athero-arteriosclerosis induced by infection with a herpesvirus. Am J Pathol 1979;96:673–706.
16. Fabricant CG, Hajjar DP, Minick CR, Fabricant J: Herpesvirus infection enhances cholesterol and cholesteryl ester accumulation in cultured arterial smooth muscle cells. Am J Pathol 1981;105:176–184.
17. Hajjar DP, Fabricant CG, Minick CR, Fabricant J: Virus-induced atherosclerosis. Herpesvirus infection alters aortic cholesterol metabolism and accumulation. Am J Pathol 1986;122:62–70.
18. Hajjar DP, Pomerantz KB, Falcone DJ, et al: Herpes simplex virus infection in human arterial cells. Implications in arteriosclerosis. J Clin Invest 1987;80:1317–1321.
19. Melnick JL, Petrie BL, Dreesman GR, et al: Cytomegalovirus antigen within human arterial smooth muscle cells. Lancet 1983;2:644–647.
20. Bernersen B, Johnsen R, Bostad L, et al: Is *Helicobacter pylori* the cause of dyspepsia? BMJ 1992;304:1276–1279.
21. Grayston JT, Kuo CC, Wang SP, Altman J: A new *Chlamydia psittaci* strain, TWAR, isolated in acute respiratory tract infections. N Engl J Med 1986;315:161–168.
22. Grayston JT: Infections caused by *Chlamydia pneumoniae* strain TWAR. Clin Infect Dis 1992;15:757–761.
23. Saikku P, Leinonen M, Mattila K, et al: Serological evidence of an association of a novel *Chlamydia*, TWAR, with chronic coronary heart disease and acute myocardial infarction. Lancet 1988;2:983–986.
24. Saikku P, Leinonen M, Tenkanen L, et al: Chronic *Chlamydia pneumoniae* infection as a risk factor for coronary heart disease in the Helsinki Heart Study. Ann Intern Med 1992;116:273–278.
25. Shor A, Kuo CC, Patton DL: Detection of *Chlamydia pneumoniae* in coronary arterial fatty streaks and atheromatous plaques. S Afr Med J 1992;82:158–161.
26. Kuo CC, Shor A, Campbell LA, et al: Demonstration of *Chlamydia pneumoniae* in atherosclerotic lesions of coronary arteries. J Infect Dis 1993;167:841–849.
27. Chyu K-Y, Shah PK: The role of inflammation in plaque disruption and thrombosis. Rev Cardiovasc Med 2001;2:82–91.
28. Libby P, Ridker PM, Maseri A: Inflammation and atherosclerosis. Circulation 2002;105:1135–1143.
29. Libby P, Egan D, Skarlatos S: Roles of infectious agents in atherosclerosis and restenosis: An assessment of the evidence and need for future research. Circulation 1997;96:4095–4103.
30. Epstein SE, Zhou YF, Zhu J: Infection and atherosclerosis: Emerging mechanistic paradigms. Circulation 1999;100:e20–e28.
31. Shah PK: Plaque disruption and thrombosis: Potential role of inflammation and infection. Cardiol Clin 2000;17:271–281.
32. Shah PK: Link between infection and atherosclerosis: Who are the culprits: Viruses, bacteria, both, or neither? Circulation 2001;103:5–6.
33. Ward ME: The immunobiology and immunopathology of chlamydial infections. APMIS 1995;103:769–796.

34. Balin BJ, Gerard HC, Arking EJ, et al: Identification and localization of *Chlamydia pneumoniae* in the Alzheimer's brain. Med Microbiol Immunol (Berl) 1998;187:23–42.

35. Aldous MB, Grayston JT, Wang SP, Foy HM: Seroepidemiology of *Chlamydia pneumoniae* TWAR infection in Seattle families, 1966–1979. J Infect Dis 1992;166:646–649.

36. Grayston JT: Background and current knowledge of *Chlamydia pneumoniae* and atherosclerosis. J Infect Dis 2000;181(Suppl 3):S402–S410.

37. Mendall MA, Goggin PM, Molineaux N, et al: Relation of *Helicobacter pylori* infection and coronary heart disease. Br Heart J 1994;71:437–439.

38. Goodwin CS, Worsley BW: Microbiology of *Helicobacter pylori*. Gastroenterol Clin North Am 1993;22:5–19.

39. Goodwin CS, Mendall MM, Northfield TC: *Helicobacter pylori* infection. Lancet 1997;349:265–269.

40. Ameriso SF, Fridman EA, Leiguarda RC, Sevlever GE: Detection of *Helicobacter pylori* in human carotid atherosclerotic plaques. Stroke 2001;32:385–391.

41. Blasi F, Denti F, Erba M, et al: Detection of *Chlamydia pneumoniae* but not helicobacter pylori in atherosclerotic plaques of aortic aneurysms. J Clin Microbiol 1996;34:2766–2769.

42. Loesche WJ: Association of the oral flora with important medical diseases. Curr Opin Periodontol 1997;4:21–28.

43. Lamont RJ, Jenkinson HF: Life below the gum line: Pathogenic mechanisms of *Porphyromonas gingivalis*. Microbiol Mol Biol Rev 1998;62:1244–1263.

44. Mattila KJ, Valtonen VV, Rasi RP, et al: Association between dental health and acute myocardial infarction. BMJ 1989;298:779–781.

45. Kiechl S, Egger G, Mayr M, et al: Chronic infections and the risk of carotid atherosclerosis: Prospective results from a large population study. Circulation 2001;103:1064–1070.

46. Horne BD, Muhlestein JB, Carlquist JF, et al: IgA seropositivity to *Mycoplasma pneumoniae* predicts the diagnosis of coronary artery disease [Abstract]. J Am Coll Cardiol 2000;35:312A.

47. Melnick JL, Adam E, DeBakey ME: Possible role of cytomegalovirus in atherogenesis. JAMA 1990;263:2204–2207.

48. Rupprecht HJ, Blankenberg S, Bickel C, et al: Impact of viral and bacterial infectious burden on long-term prognosis in patients with coronary artery disease. Circulation 2001;104:25–31.

49. Zhu J, Nieto FJ, Horne BD, et al: Prospective study of pathogen burden and risk of myocardial infarction or death. Circulation 2001;103:45–51.

50. Anderson JL, Carlquist JF, Muhlestein JB, et al: Evaluation of C-reactive protein, an inflammatory marker, and infectious serology as risk factors for coronary artery disease and myocardial infarction. J Am Coll Cardiol 1998;32:35–41.

51. Ridker PM, Hennekens CH, Buring JE, et al: Baseline IgG antibody titers to *Chlamydia pneumoniae*, *Helicobacter pylori*, herpes simplex virus, and cytomegalovirus and the risk for cardiovascular disease in women. Ann Intern Med 1999;131:573–577.

52. Danesh J, Whincup P, Walker M, et al: *Chlamydia pneumoniae* IgG titres and coronary heart disease: Prospective study and meta-analysis. BMJ 2000;321:208–213.

53. Wong YK, Gallagher PJ, Ward ME: *Chlamydia pneumoniae* and atherosclerosis. Heart 1999;81:232–238.

54. Epstein SE, Zhu J: Lack of association of infectious agents with risk of future myocardial infarction and stroke: Definitive evidence disproving the infection/coronary artery disease hypothesis? Circulation 1999;100:1366–1368.

55. Gupta S, Leatham EW, Carrington D, et al: Elevated *Chlamydia pneumoniae* antibodies, cardiovascular events, and azithromycin in male survivors of myocardial infarction. Circulation 1997;96:404–407.

56. Strachan DP, Carrington D, Mendall MA, et al: Relation of *Chlamydia pneumoniae* serology to mortality and incidence of ischaemic heart disease over 13 years in the caerphilly prospective heart disease study. BMJ 1999;318:1035–1039.

57. Nieto FJ, Folsom AR, Sorlie PD, et al: *Chlamydia pneumoniae* infection and incident coronary heart disease: The Atherosclerosis Risk in Communities Study. Am J Epidemiol 1999;150:149–156.

58. Siscovick DS, Schwartz SM, Corey L, et al: *Chlamydia pneumoniae*, herpes simplex virus type 1, and cytomegalovirus and incident myocardial infarction and coronary heart disease death in older adults: The Cardiovascular Health Study. Circulation 2000;102:2335–2340.

59. Chandra HR, Choudhary N, O'Neill C, et al: *Chlamydia pneumoniae* exposure and inflammatory markers in acute coronary syndrome (CIMACS). Am J Cardiol 2001;88:214–218.

60. Toss H, Gnarpe J, Gnarpe H, et al: Increased fibrinogen levels are associated with persistent *Chlamydia pneumoniae* infection in unstable coronary artery disease. Eur Heart J 1998;19:570–577.

61. Ridker PM, Kundsin RB, Stampfer MJ, et al: Prospective study of *Chlamydia pneumoniae* IgG seropositivity and risks of future myocardial infarction. Circulation 1999;99:1161–1164.

62. Gattone M, Iacoviello L, Colombo M, et al: *Chlamydia pneumoniae* and cytomegalovirus seropositivity, inflammatory markers, and the risk of myocardial infarction at a young age. Am Heart J 2001;142:633–640.

63. Melnick SL, Shahar E, Folsom AR, et al: Past infection by *Chlamydia pneumoniae* strain TWAR and asymptomatic carotid atherosclerosis. Atherosclerosis Risk in Communities (ARIC) Study Investigators. Am J Med 1993;95:499–504.

64. Davidson M, Kuo CC, Middaugh JP, et al: Confirmed previous infection with *Chlamydia pneumoniae* (TWAR) and its presence in early coronary atherosclerosis. Circulation 1998;98:628–633.

65. Laurila A, Bloigu A, Nayha S, et al: Chronic *Chlamydia pneumoniae* infection is associated with a serum lipid profile known to be a risk factor for atherosclerosis. Arterioscler Thromb Vasc Biol 1997;17:2910–2913.

66. Murray LJ, O'Reilly DP, Ong GM, et al: *Chlamydia pneumoniae* antibodies are associated with an atherogenic lipid profile. Heart 1999;81:239–244.

67. Neumann FJ, Kastrati A, Miethke T, et al: Previous cytomegalovirus infection and restenosis after coronary stent placement. Circulation 2001;104:1135–1139.

68. Neumann F, Kastrati A, Miethke T, et al: Treatment of *Chlamydia pneumoniae* infection with roxithromycin and effect on neointima proliferation after coronary stent placement (ISAR-3): A randomised, double-blind, placebo-controlled trial. Lancet 2001;357:2085–2089.

69. Elkind MS, Lin IF, Grayston JT, Sacco RL: *Chlamydia pneumoniae* and the risk of first ischemic stroke: The Northern Manhattan Stroke Study. Stroke 2000;31:1521–1525.

70. Zimmer C: Do chronic diseases have an infectious root? Science 2001;293:1974–1977.

71. Danesh J, Wong Y, Ward M, Muir J: Chronic infection with *Helicobacter pylori*, *Chlamydia pneumoniae*, or cytomegalovirus: Population based study of coronary heart disease. Heart 1999;81:245–247.

72. Whincup PH, Mendall MA, Perry IJ, et al: Prospective relations between *Helicobacter pylori* infection, coronary heart disease, and stroke in middle aged men. Heart 1996;75:568–572.

73. Strandberg TE, Tilvis RS, Vuoristo M, et al: Prospective study of *Helicobacter pylori* seropositivity and cardiovascular diseases in a general elderly population. BMJ 1997;314:1317–1318.

74. Wald NJ, Law MR, Morris JK, Bagnall AM: *Helicobacter pylori* infection and mortality from ischaemic heart disease: Negative result from a large, prospective study. BMJ 1997;315:1199–1201.

75. Folsom AR, Nieto FJ, Sorlie P, et al: *Helicobacter pylori* seropositivity and coronary heart disease incidence. Atherosclerosis Risk In Communities (ARIC) Study Investigators. Circulation 1998;98:845–850.

76. Pieniazek P, Karczewska E, Duda A, et al: Association of *Helicobacter pylori* infection with coronary heart disease. J Physiol Pharmacol 1999;50:743–751.

77. Danesh J: Coronary heart disease, *Helicobacter pylori*, dental disease, *Chlamydia pneumoniae*, and cytomegalovirus: Meta-analyses of prospective studies. Am Heart J 1999;138:S434–S437.

78. Ridker PM, Danesh J, Youngman L, et al: A prospective study of *Helicobacter pylori* seropositivity and the risk for future myocardial infarction among socioeconomically similar U.S. men. Ann Intern Med 2001;135:184–188.

79. Danesh J, Whincup P, Walker M, et al: High prevalence of potentially virulent strains of *Helicobacter pylori* in the general male British population. Gut 2000;47:23–25.

80. Gunn M, Stephens JC, Thompson JR, et al: Significant association of cagA positive *Helicobacter pylori* strains with risk of premature myocardial infarction. Heart 2000;84:267–271.

81. Murray LJ, Bamford KB, Kee F, et al: Infection with virulent strains of *Helicobacter pylori* is not associated with ischaemic heart

disease: Evidence from a population-based case-control study of myocardial infarction. Atherosclerosis 2000;149:379–385.

82. DeStefano F, Anda RF, Kahn HS, et al: Dental disease and risk of coronary heart disease and mortality. BMJ 1993;306:688–691.

83. Beck J, Garcia R, Heiss G, et al: Periodontal disease and cardiovascular disease. J Periodontol 1996;67:1123–1137.

84. Mendez MV, Scott T, LaMorte W, et al: An association between periodontal disease and peripheral vascular disease. Am J Surg 1998;176:153–157.

85. Christen WG, Hennekens CH, Ajani U, Ridker PM: Periodontal disease and coronary heart disease risk. Circulation 1998;97.

86. Howell TH, Ridker PM, Ajani UA, et al: Periodontal disease and risk of subsequent cardiovascular disease in U.S. male physicians. J Am Coll Cardiol 2001;37:445–450.

87. Hujoel PP, Drangsholt M, Spiekerman C, DeRouen TA: Periodontal disease and coronary heart disease risk. JAMA 2000;284:1406–1410.

88. Ridker PM, Hennekens CH, Stampfer MJ, Wang F: Prospective study of herpes simplex virus, cytomegalovirus, and the risk of future myocardial infarction and stroke. Circulation 1998;98:2796–2799.

89. Strachan DP, Carrington D, Mendall MA, et al: Cytomegalovirus seropositivity and incident ischaemic heart disease in the Caerphilly prospective heart disease study. Heart 1999;81:248–251.

90. Roivainen M, Viik-Kajander M, Palosuo T, et al: Infections, inflammation, and the risk of coronary heart disease. Circulation 2000;101:252–257.

91. Sorlie PD, Adam E, Melnick SL, et al: Cytomegalovirus/herpesvirus and carotid atherosclerosis: The ARIC Study. J Med Virol 1994;42:33–37.

92. Muhlestein JB, Horne BD, Carlquist JF, et al: Cytomegalovirus seropositivity and C-reactive protein have independent and combined predictive value for mortality in patients with angiographically demonstrated coronary artery disease. Circulation 2000;102:1917–1923.

93. Blankenberg S, Rupprecht HJ, Bickel C, et al: Cytomegalovirus infection with interleukin-6 response predicts cardiac mortality in patients with coronary artery disease. Circulation 2001;103:2915–2921.

94. Zhu J, Shearer GM, Norman JE, et al: Host response to cytomegalovirus infection as a determinant of susceptibility to coronary artery disease: Sex-based differences in inflammation and type of immune response. Circulation 2000;102:2491–2496.

95. Zhu J, Quyyumi AA, Norman JE, et al: Cytomegalovirus in the pathogenesis of atherosclerosis: The role of inflammation as reflected by elevated C-reactive protein levels. J Am Coll Cardiol 1999;34:1738–1743.

96. Buffon A, Liuzzo G, Biasucci LM, et al: Preprocedural serum levels of C-reactive protein predict early complications and late restenosis after coronary angioplasty. J Am Coll Cardiol 1999;34:1512–1521.

97. Zhou YF, Guetta E, Yu ZX, et al: Human cytomegalovirus increases modified low density lipoprotein uptake and scavenger receptor mRNA expression in vascular smooth muscle cells. J Clin Invest 1996;98:2129–2138.

98. Muhlestein JB, Carlquist JF, Horne BD, et al: No association between prior cytomegalovirus infection and the risk of clinical restenosis after percutaneous coronary interventions. Circulation 1997;96:I–650.

99. Zhu J, Quyyumi AA, Norman JE, et al: Effects of total pathogen burden on coronary artery disease risk and C-reactive protein levels. Am J Cardiol 2000;85:140–146.

100. Kuo CC, Gown AM, Benditt EP, Grayston JT: Detection of Chlamydia pneumoniae in aortic lesions of atherosclerosis by immunocytochemical stain. Arterioscler Thromb 1993;13:1501–1504.

101. Muhlestein JB, Hammond EH, Carlquist JF, et al: Increased incidence of Chlamydia species within the coronary arteries of patients with symptomatic atherosclerotic versus other forms of cardiovascular disease. J Am Coll Cardiol 1996;27:1555–1561.

102. Jackson LA, Campbell LA, Schmidt RA, et al: Specificity of detection of Chlamydia pneumoniae in cardiovascular atheroma: Evaluation of the innocent bystander hypothesis. Am J Pathol 1997;150:1785–1790.

103. Ericson K, Saldeen TG, Lindquist O, et al: Relationship of Chlamydia pneumoniae infection to severity of human coronary atherosclerosis. Circulation 2000;101:2568–2571.

104. Vink A, Poppen M, Schoneveld AH, et al: Distribution of Chlamydia pneumoniae in the human arterial system and its relation to the local amount of atherosclerosis within the individual. Circulation 2001;103:1613–1617.

105. Thomas M, Wong Y, Thomas D, et al: Relation between direct detection of Chlamydia pneumoniae DNA in human coronary arteries at postmortem examination and histological severity (Stary grading) of associated atherosclerotic plaque. Circulation 1999;99:2733–2736.

106. Maass M, Bartels C, Engel PM, et al: Endovascular presence of viable Chlamydia pneumoniae is a common phenomenon in coronary artery disease. J Am Coll Cardiol 1998;31:827–832.

107. Maass M, Bartels C, Kruger S, et al: Endovascular presence of Chlamydia pneumoniae DNA is a generalized phenomenon in atherosclerotic vascular disease. Atherosclerosis 1998;140(Suppl 1):S25–S30.

108. Ramirez JA: Isolation of Chlamydia pneumoniae from the coronary artery of a patient with coronary atherosclerosis. The Chlamydia pneumoniae/Atherosclerosis Study Group. Ann Intern Med 1996;125:979–982.

109. Weiss SM, Roblin PM, Gaydos CA, et al: Failure to detect Chlamydia pneumoniae in coronary atheromas of patients undergoing atherectomy. J Infect Dis 1996;173:957–962.

110. Kol A, Sukhova GK, Lichtman AH, Libby P: Chlamydial heat shock protein 60 localizes in human atheroma and regulates macrophage tumor necrosis factor-alpha and matrix metalloproteinase expression. Circulation 1998;98:300–307.

111. Kol A, Bourcier T, Lichtman AH, Libby P: Chlamydial and human heat shock protein 60s activate human vascular endothelium, smooth muscle cells, and macrophages. J Clin Invest 1999;103:571–577.

112. Grayston JT, Kuo CC, Coulson AS, et al: Chlamydia pneumoniae (TWAR) in atherosclerosis of the carotid artery. Circulation 1995;92:3397–3400.

113. Bartels C, Maass M, Bein G, et al: Detection of Chlamydia pneumoniae but not cytomegalovirus in occluded saphenous vein coronary artery bypass grafts. Circulation 1999;99:879–882.

114. Chiu B, Viira E, Tucker W, Fong IW: Chlamydia pneumoniae, cytomegalovirus, and herpes simplex virus in atherosclerosis of the carotid artery. Circulation 1997;96:2144–2148.

115. Yamashiroya HM, Ghosh L, Yang R, Robertson AL Jr: Herpesviridae in the coronary arteries and aorta of young trauma victims. Am J Pathol 1988;130:71–79.

116. Speir E, Modali R, Huang ES, et al: Potential role of human cytomegalovirus and p53 interaction in coronary restenosis. Science 1994;265:391–394.

117. Hendrix MG, Dormans PH, Kitslaar P, et al: The presence of cytomegalovirus nucleic acids in arterial walls of atherosclerotic and nonatherosclerotic patients. Am J Pathol 1989;134:1151–1157.

118. Gao SZ, Alderman EL, Schroeder JS, et al: Accelerated coronary vascular disease in the heart transplant patient: Coronary arteriographic findings. J Am Coll Cardiol 1988;12:334–340.

119. Grattan M: Accelerated graft atherosclerosis following cardiac transplanatation: Clinical perspectives. Clin Cardiol 1991; 14:16–20.

120. McDonald K, Rector TS, Braulin EA, et al: Association of coronary artery disease in cardiac transplant recipients with cytomegalovirus infection. Am J Cardiol 1989;64:359–362.

121. Hruban RH, Wu TC, Beschorner WE, et al: Cytomegalovirus nucleic acids in allografted hearts. Hum Pathol 1990;21:981–982.

122. Lemstrom K, Sihvola R, Bruggeman C, et al: Cytomegalovirus infection-enhanced cardiac allograft vasculopathy is abolished by DHPG prophylaxis in the rat. Circulation 1997;95:2614–2616.

123. Muhlestein JB: Chronic infection and coronary artery disease. Med Clin North Am 2000;84:123–148.

124. Godzik KL, O'Brien ER, Wang SK, Kuo CC: In vitro susceptibility of human vascular wall cells to infection with Chlamydia pneumoniae. J Clin Microbiol 1995;33:2411–2414.

125. Gaydos CA, Summersgill JT, Sahney NN, et al: Replication of Chlamydia pneumoniae in vitro in human macrophages, endothelial cells, and aortic artery smooth muscle cells. Infect Immun 1996;64:1614–1620.

126. Fryer RH, Schwobe EP, Woods ML, Rodgers GM: *Chlamydia* species infect human vascular endothelial cells and induce procoagulant activity. J Invest Med 1997;45:168-174.

127. Kalayoglu MV, Byrne GI: Induction of macrophage foam cell formation by *Chlamydia pneumoniae*. J Infect Dis 1998;177:725-729.

128. Dechend R, Maass M, Gieffers J, et al: *Chlamydia pneumoniae* infection of vascular smooth muscle and endothelial cells activates NF-kappaB and induces tissue factor and PAI-1 expression: A potential link to accelerated arteriosclerosis. Circulation 1999;100:1369-1373.

129. Jackson LA, Campbell LA, Kuo CC, et al: Isolation of *Chlamydia pneumoniae* from a carotid endarterectomy specimen. J Infect Dis 1997;176:292-295.

130. Kovacs A, Weber ML, Burns LJ, et al: Cytoplasmic sequestration of p53 in cytomegalovirus-infected human endothelial cells. Am J Pathol 1996;149:1531-1539.

131. Minton EJ, Tysoe C, Sinclair JH, Sissons JG: Human cytomegalovirus infection of the monocyte/macrophage lineage in bone marrow. J Virol 1994;68:4017-4021.

132. Kondo K, Kaneshima H, Mocarski ES: Human cytomegalovirus latent infection of granulocyte-macrophage progenitors. Proc Natl Acad Sci U S A 1994;91:11879-11883.

133. Ibanez CE, Schrier R, Ghazal P, et al: Human cytomegalovirus productively infects primary differentiated macrophages. J Virol 1991;65:6581-6588.

134. Zhou YF, Yu ZX, Wanishsawad C, et al: The immediate early gene products of human cytomegalovirus increase vascular smooth muscle cell migration, proliferation, and expression of PDGF beta-receptor. Biochem Biophys Res Commun 1999;256:608-613.

135. Lemstrom KB, Aho PT, Bruggeman CA, Hayry PJ: Cytomegalovirus infection enhances mRNA expression of platelet-derived growth factor–BB and transforming growth factor–beta 1 in rat aortic allografts. Possible mechanism for cytomegalovirus-enhanced graft arteriosclerosis. Arterioscler Thromb 1994;14:2043-2052.

136. Grundy JE, Downes KL: Up-regulation of LFA-3 and ICAM-1 on the surface of fibroblasts infected with cytomegalovirus. Immunology 1993;78:405-412.

137. Span AH, Mullers W, Miltenburg AM, Bruggeman CA: Cytomegalovirus induced PMN adherence in relation to an ELAM-1 antigen present on infected endothelial cell monolayers. Immunology 1991;72:355-360.

138. Burns LJ, Pooley JC, Walsh DJ, et al: Intercellular adhesion molecule-1 expression in endothelial cells is activated by cytomegalovirus immediate early proteins. Transplantation 1999;67:137-144.

139. Speir E, Yu ZX, Ferrans VJ, et al: Aspirin attenuates cytomegalovirus infectivity and gene expression mediated by cyclooxygenase-2 in coronary artery smooth muscle cells. Circ Res 1998;83:210-216.

140. Oldstone MB: Molecular mimicry and autoimmune disease. Cell 1987;50:819-820.

141. Bachmaier K, Neu N, de la Maza LM, et al: *Chlamydia* infections and heart disease linked through antigenic mimicry. Science 1999;283:1335-1339.

142. Xu Q: Role of heat shock proteins in atherosclerosis. Arterioscler Thromb Vasc Biol 2002;22:1547-1559.

143. Burian K, Kis Z, Virok D, et al: Independent and joint effects of antibodies to human heat-shock protein 60 and *Chlamydia pneumoniae* infection in the development of coronary atherosclerosis. Circulation 2001;103:1503-1508.

144. Mayr M, Metzler B, Kiechl S, et al: Endothelial cytotoxicity mediated by serum antibodies to heat shock proteins of *Escherichia coli* and *Chlamydia pneumoniae*: Immune reactions to heat shock proteins as a possible link between infection and atherosclerosis. Circulation 1999;99:1560-1566.

145. Schett G, Xu Q, Amberger A, et al: Autoantibodies against heat shock protein 60 mediate endothelial cytotoxicity. J Clin Invest 1995;96:2569-2577.

146. Xu Q, Willeit J, Marosi M, et al: Association of serum antibodies to heat-shock protein 65 with carotid atherosclerosis. Lancet 1993;341:255-259.

147. Xu Q, Kleindienst R, Schett G, et al: Regression of arteriosclerotic lesions induced by immunization with heat shock protein 65-containing material in normocholesterolemic, but not hypercholesterolemic, rabbits. Atherosclerosis 1996;123:145-155.

148. Birnie DH, Holme ER, McKay IC, et al: Association between antibodies to heat shock protein 65 and coronary atherosclerosis. Possible mechanism of action of *Helicobacter pylori* and other bacterial infections in increasing cardiovascular risk. Eur Heart J 1998;19:387-394.

149. George J, Shoenfeld Y, Afek A, et al: Enhanced fatty streak formation in C57BL/6J mice by immunization with heat shock protein-65. Arterioscler Thromb Vasc Biol 1999;19:505-510.

150. Kiechl S, Lorenz E, Reindl M, et al: Toll-like receptor 4 polymorphisms and atherogenesis. N Engl J Med 2002;347:185-192.

151. Fabricant CG, Fabricant J: Atherosclerosis induced by infection with Marek's disease herpesvirus in chickens. Am Heart J 1999;138:S465-S468.

152. Horne BD, Carlquist JF, Habashi J, et al: Cytomegalovirus infection of human macrophages induces increased expression of scavenger receptor CD36 gene and cell surface glycoprotein [Abstract]. J Am Coll Cardiol 2000;35:268A.

153. Vercellotti GM: Effects of viral activation of the vessel wall on inflammation and thrombosis. Blood Coagul Fibrinolysis 1998;9:S3-S6.

154. Visser MR, Tracy PB, Vercellotti GM, et al: Enhanced thrombin generation and platelet binding on herpes simplex virus–infected endothelium. Proc Natl Acad Sci U S A 1988;85:8227-8230.

155. Key NS, Vercellotti GM, Winkelmann JC, et al: Infection of vascular endothelial cells with herpes simplex virus enhances tissue factor activity and reduces thrombomodulin expression. Proc Natl Acad Sci U S A 1990;87:7095-7099.

156. Etingin OR, Silverstein RL, Friedman HM, Hajjar DP: Viral activation of the coagulation cascade: Molecular interactions at the surface of infected endothelial cells. Cell 1990;61:657-662.

157. van Dam-Mieras MC, Muller AD, van Hinsbergh VW, et al: The procoagulant response of cytomegalovirus infected endothelial cells. Thromb Haemost 1992;68:364-370.

158. Prasad A, Zhu J, Mincemoyer R, et al: Cytomegalovirus infection is a determinant of endothelial dysfunction and coronary flow reserve [Abstract]. Circulation 1998;98:I-244.

159. Levine AJ: p53, the cellular gatekeeper for growth and division. Cell 1997;88:323-331.

160. Yonemitsu Y, Kaneda Y, Tanaka S, et al: Transfer of wild-type p53 gene effectively inhibits vascular smooth muscle cell proliferation in vitro and in vivo. Circ Res 1998;82:147-156.

161. Tsai HL, Kou GH, Chen SC, et al: Human cytomegalovirus immediate-early protein IE2 tethers a transcriptional repression domain to p53. J Biol Chem 1996;271:3534-3540.

162. Gonczol E, Plotkin SA: Cells infected with human cytomegalovirus release a factor(s) that stimulates cell DNA synthesis. J Gen Virol 1984;65:1833-1837.

163. Alcami J, Barzu T, Michelson S: Induction of an endothelial cell growth factor by human cytomegalovirus infection of fibroblasts. J Gen Virol 1991;72:2765-2770.

164. Fan T, Lu H, Hu H, et al: Inhibition of apoptosis in chlamydia-infected cells: blockade of mitochondrial cytochrome c release and caspase activation. J Exp Med 1998;187:487-496.

165. Tanaka K, Zou JP, Takeda K, et al: Effects of human cytomegalovirus immediate-early proteins on p53-mediated apoptosis in coronary artery smooth muscle cells. Circulation 1999;99:1656-1659.

166. Zhu H, Shen Y, Shenk T: Human cytomegalovirus IE1 and IE2 proteins block apoptosis. J Virol 1995;69:7960-7970.

167. Zhou YF, Shou M, Guetta E, et al: Cytomegalovirus infection of rats increases the neointimal response to vascular injury without consistent evidence of direct infection of the vascular wall. Circulation 1999;100:1569-1575.

168. Wong YK, Dawkins KD, Ward ME: Circulating *Chlamydia pneumoniae* DNA as a predictor of coronary artery disease. J Am Coll Cardiol 1999;34:1435-1439.

169. Blasi F, Boman J, Esposito G, et al: *Chlamydia pneumoniae* DNA detection in peripheral blood mononuclear cells is predictive of vascular infection. J Infect Dis 1999;180:2074-2076.

170. Kaul R, Uphoff J, Wiedeman J, et al: Detection of *Chlamydia pneumoniae* DNA in CD3+ lymphocytes from healthy blood donors and patients with coronary artery disease. Circulation 2000;102:2341-2346.

171. Boman J, Soderberg S, Forsberg J, et al: High prevalence of *Chlamydia pneumoniae* DNA in peripheral blood mononuclear cells in patients with cardiovascular disease and in middle-aged blood donors. J Infect Dis 1998;178:274-277.

172. Paterson DL, Hall J, Rasmussen SJ, Timms P: Failure to detect *Chlamydia pneumoniae* in atherosclerotic plaques of Australian patients. Pathology 1998;30:169–172.

173. Moazed TC, Kuo C, Patton DL, et al: Experimental rabbit models of *Chlamydia pneumoniae* infection. Am J Pathol 1996;148:667–676.

174. Fong IW, Chiu B, Viira E, et al: Rabbit model for *Chlamydia pneumoniae* infection. J Clin Microbiol 1997;35:48–52.

175. Fong IW, Chiu B, Viira E, et al: De novo induction of atherosclerosis by *Chlamydia pneumoniae* in a rabbit model. Infect Immun 1999;67:6048–6055.

176. Muhlestein JB, Anderson JL, Hammond EH, et al: Infection with *Chlamydia pneumoniae* accelerates the development of atherosclerosis and treatment with azithromycin prevents it in a rabbit model. Circulation 1998;97:633–636.

177. Moazed TC, Kuo C, Grayston JT, Campbell LA: Murine models of *Chlamydia pneumoniae* infection and atherosclerosis. J Infect Dis 1997;175:883–890.

178. Moazed TC, Kuo CC, Grayston JT, Campbell LA: Evidence of systemic dissemination of *Chlamydia pneumoniae* via macrophages in the mouse. J Infect Dis 1998;177:1322–1325.

179. Moazed TC, Campbell LA, Rosenfeld ME, et al: *Chlamydia pneumoniae* infection accelerates the progression of atherosclerosis in apolipoprotein E-deficient mice. J Infect Dis 1999;180:238–241.

180. Hu H, Pierce GN, Zhong G: The atherogenic effects of chlamydia are dependent on serum cholesterol and specific to *Chlamydia pneumoniae*. J Clin Invest 1999;103:747–753.

181. Caligiuri G, Rottenberg M, Nicoletti A, et al: *Chlamydia pneumoniae* infection does not induce or modify atherosclerosis in mice. Circulation 2001;103:2834–2838.

182. Liuba P, Karnani P, Pesonen E, et al: Endothelial dysfunction after repeated *Chlamydia pneumoniae* infection in apolipoprotein E-knockout mice. Circulation 2000;102:1039–1044.

183. Chirgwin K, Roblin PM, Hammerschlag MR: In vitro susceptibilities of *Chlamydia pneumoniae* (*Chlamydia* sp. strain TWAR). Antimicrob Agents Chemother 1989;33:1634–1635.

184. Schneider CA, Diedrichs H, Riedel KD, et al: In vivo uptake of azithromycin in human coronary plaques. Am J Cardiol 2000;86:789–791.

185. Havlir DV, Dube MP, Sattler FR, et al: Prophylaxis against disseminated *Mycobacterium avium* complex with weekly azithromycin, daily rifabutin, or both. California Collaborative Treatment Group. N Engl J Med 1996;335:392–398.

186. Anderson JL, Muhlestein JB, Carlquist J, et al: Randomized secondary prevention trial of azithromycin in patients with coronary artery disease and serological evidence for *Chlamydia pneumoniae* infection: The Azithromycin in Coronary Artery Disease: Elimination of Myocardial Infection with Chlamydia (ACADEMIC) study. Circulation 1999;99:1540–1547.

187. Fish KN, North DS: Gatifloxacin, an advanced 8-methoxy fluoroquinolone. Pharmacotherapy 2001;21:35–59.

188. Meier CR, Derby LE, Jick SS, et al: Antibiotics and risk of subsequent first-time acute myocardial infarction. JAMA 1999;281:427–431.

189. Jackson LA, Smith NL, Heckbert SR, et al: Past use of erythromycin, tetracycline, or doxycycline is not associated with risk of first myocardial infarction. J Infect Dis 2000;181(Suppl 3):S563–S565.

190. Gurfinkel E, Bozovich G, Daroca A, et al: Randomised trial of roxithromycin in non-Q-wave coronary syndromes: ROXIS Pilot Study. ROXIS Study Group. Lancet 1997;350:404–407.

191. Gurfinkel E, Bozovich G, Beck E, et al: Treatment with the antibiotic roxithromycin in patients with acute non-Q-wave coronary syndromes. The final report of the ROXIS Study. Eur Heart J 1999;20:121–127.

192. Stone ASM, Mendall M, Kaski JC, et al: Effect of treatment for *Chlamydia pneumoniae* and *Helicobacter pylori* on markers of inflammation and cardiac events in patients with acute coronary syndromes. Circulation 2002;106.

193. Anderson JL: Commentary: The effect of short-term treatment with azithromycin on recurrent ischemic events in patients with acute coronary syndrome: The AZACS Trial. J Am Coll Cardiol 2002;40:7.

194. Gupta S, Camm AJ: Chronic infection in the etiology of atherosclerosis—the case for *Chlamydia pneumoniae*. Clin Cardiol 1997;20:829–836.

195. Muhlestein JB, Anderson JL, Carlquist JF, et al: Randomized secondary prevention trial of azithromycin in patients with coronary artery disease: Primary clinical results of the ACADEMIC study. Circulation 2000;102:1755–1760.

196. Muhlestein JB: Secondary prevention of coronary artery disease with antimicrobials: Current status and future directions. Am J Cardiovascular Drugs 2002;2:107–118.

197. Zhou YF, Leon MB, Waclawiw MA, et al: Association between prior cytomegalovirus infection and the risk of restenosis after coronary atherectomy. N Engl J Med 1996;335:624–630.

198. Grayston JT: Secondary prevention antibiotic treatment trials for coronary artery disease. Circulation 2000;102:1742–1743.

199. Dunne M: WIZARD and the design of trials for secondary prevention of atherosclerosis with antibiotics. Am Heart J 1999;138:S542–S544.

200. Anderson JL: Commentary: Weekly intervention with zithromax for atherosclerosis and its related disorders: Preliminary results of the WIZARD Study. J Am Coll Cardiol 2002;40:8.

201. Naghavi M, Barlas Z, Siadaty S, et al: Association of influenza vaccination and reduced risk of recurrent myocardial infarction. Circulation 2000;102:3039–3045.

202. Siscovick DS, Raghunathan TE, Lin D, et al: Influenza vaccination and the risk of primary cardiac arrest. Am J Epidemiol 2000;152:674–677.

203. Capron L: How to design vaccination trials to prevent atherosclerosis. Am Heart J 1999;138:S558–S559.

204. Gieffers J, Fullgraf H, Jahn J, et al: *Chlamydia pneumoniae* infection in circulating human monocytes is refractory to antibiotic treatment. Circulation 2001;103:351–356.

205. Tilley BC, Alarcon GS, Heyse SP, et al: Minocycline in rheumatoid arthritis. A 48-week, double-blind, placebo-controlled trial. MIRA Trial Group. Ann Intern Med 1995;122:81–89.

206. Mahdi OS, Horne BD, Mullen K, et al: Serum immunoglobulin G antibodies to chlamydial heat shock protein 60 but not to human and bacterial homologs are associated with coronary artery disease. Circulation 2002;106:1659–1663.

Triggers to Acute Coronary Syndromes

Jagmeet P. Singh
James E. Muller

Atherosclerotic cardiovascular disease remains the leading cause of death and disability in the industrialized world and is assuming increased importance in the developing world. Despite considerable insight into long-term risk factors for coronary disease and the dramatic improvement in acute in-hospital therapy during recent decades, the number of coronary deaths remains high and continues to increase in many countries. Identification of triggering factors associated with acute coronary syndromes helps us understand the pathologic processes that lead to clinically manifest coronary atherosclerosis. Epidemiologic observations of newly identified acute and chronic risk factors for coronary artery disease, as well as pathophysiologic studies of converting chronic coronary disease to an acute event, have in turn greatly expanded our knowledge of triggering mechanisms. Identification and modification of the triggers of cardiovascular events is a relatively new approach to the prevention of death and disability.

PATHOPHYSIOLOGY OF ACUTE CORONARY SYNDROMES

It is now well recognized that coronary arterial plaques become vulnerable and then disrupt, leading to coronary thrombosis,[1-3] which in turn may lead to unstable angina pectoris, acute myocardial infarction (MI), or sudden cardiac death. Since the first angiographic observation that most coronary events result from disruption of vulnerable plaques that are not severely stenotic,[4] much has been learned about the process that leads to plaque disruption. Retrospective autopsy studies suggest that most vulnerable plaques have a characteristic composition that renders them at risk for disruption when exposed to triggering activity.[1]

Despite the great clinical importance of plaque disruption, very little is known about the mechanism through which it occurs. A series of recent studies of the activities of persons who experience nonfatal MI provide some insight into the mechanisms of disruption. It is well-documented that initiation of activity in the morning, heavy physical exertion, anger, sexual activity, and cocaine can lead to a nonfatal MI.[5-9] Because all of these triggers are associated with an increase in systemic arterial pressure, it is possible that the pressure increase causes increased stress on the plaque, leading to disruption.

The idea of triggering as a cause of disruption has recently been supported by a study of autopsy findings among men dying suddenly. Subjects dying during exertion were much more likely to demonstrate a plaque with a ruptured cap than were those dying at rest.[1] The association between external triggers and MI onset (relative risk of 2 to over 20 times) is well beyond what is to be expected by chance alone and comparable with that of the known long-term risk factors for cardiac disease. An understanding of triggering by patient activity and exposures may clarify mechanisms of plaque disruption and suggest measures to sever the linkage between a potential trigger and its pathologic consequence.

The onset of an acute coronary syndrome might result from an interaction between a vulnerable plaque, a trigger, and acute risk factors (Fig. 8-1). As noted, the coronary plaque suspected to be most vulnerable to rupture is lipid-rich and has a thin fibrous cap that is weakest at its junction with the intima,[10] probably because of increased inflammatory cellular activity with elaboration of metalloproteinases.[11] Triggers, either physical or mental, produce acute risk factors defined as vasoconstrictive, hemodynamic, and hemostatic forces that, in turn, provoke disruption of the vulnerable plaque and lead to occlusive coronary thrombosis.

Plaque Disruption

Speculation about the causes of disruption has centered on three mechanisms: hemodynamic stress, vasomotor tone increases, and biochemical processes within the plaque.

Hemodynamic Forces

There has been debate as to whether arterial pressure disrupts the plaque from the luminal surface or whether the forces are transmitted to the interior of the plaque via the vasa vasorum and cause it to rupture.[12] The luminal forces trigger plaque disruption by causing circumferential stress that exceeds the tensile strength of the cap.[13] In addition to disruption brought on by a relatively infrequent extreme hemodynamic stress, the routine stresses produced by each cardiac contraction may eventually lead to disruption through a fatigue mechanism.[13]

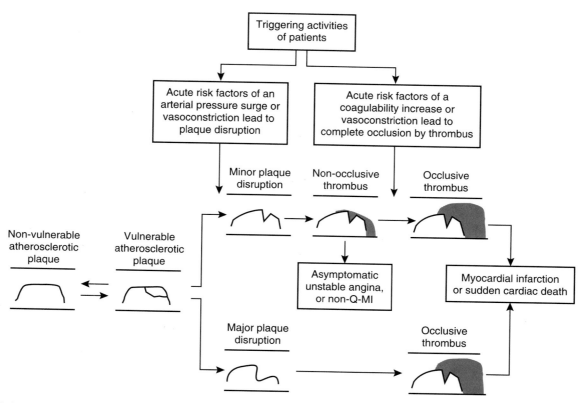

FIGURE 8–1. Hypothetical method by which daily activities and exposures may trigger coronary thrombosis. Three triggering mechanisms are presented: physical or mental stress producing hemodynamic changes leading to plaque rupture, activities or exposures causing a coagulability increase, and stimuli leading to vasoconstriction. The scheme depicting the role of coronary thrombosis in unstable angina, myocardial infarction (MI), and sudden cardiac death has been well described by numerous authors. The novel portion of this figure is the addition of triggers. (Adapted from Muller JE, Tofler GH, Stone PH: Circadian variation and triggers of onset of acute cardiovascular disease. Circulation 1989;79:733–743.)

Increased Vascular Tone

Supportive data are not available, but it is possible that increased vascular tone at the site of the vulnerable plaque may cause disruption. Vessels with atherosclerotic plaques demonstrate severe impairment of vasomotor regulation, presumably due to the loss of normal nitric oxide function or excessive release of vasoconstrictor substances such as endothelin-1.[14] Inappropriate vasoconstriction at the site of atherosclerotic lesions could exert both direct and shear stress on the cap of the plaque, thereby precipitating disruption.

Intraplaque Factors

It is likely that plaque disruption often results primarily from cellular and biochemical processes contained within the plaque. Accumulation of macrophages, mast cells, and other inflammatory cells within the fibrous cap has been demonstrated to lead to increased activity of several proteolytic enzymes, in turn leading to accelerated destruction of the cap of the vulnerable plaque.[11] Work is ongoing to define the roles of acute and chronic infections with agents such as *Chlamydia pneumoniae*, cytomegalovirus, and herpes simplex virus in plaque inflammation.[15]

Triggering of Coronary Thrombosis

Triggers may induce the onset of infarction by multiple concomitant pathways. Significant physical activity or emotional stress may lead to:

- Hemodynamic stress of hypertension and tachycardia from sympathetic stimulation
- Endothelial dysfunction-induced coronary vasoconstriction with increased shear forces
- A prothrombotic state characterized by platelet activation, a reduced fibrinolytic response, and reduced prostacyclin release

An acute coronary syndrome might be triggered by a stressor that produces a hemodynamic response sufficient to cause a major plaque disruption, exposing collagen and atheromatous core contents to coronary blood that results in thrombus formation at the site of the plaque. If the thrombus is large yet does not totally obstruct coronary blood flow, unstable angina or non–Q-wave MI may result clinically. If the thrombus is large and totally occludes the coronary vessel, acute MI is likely except in the rare case of extensive collateral circulation.

A synergistic combination of triggering activities may account for thrombosis in a setting in which each activity alone may not exceed the threshold for causation of infarction. For example, heavy physical exertion producing a minor plaque disruption in a sedentary cigarette smoker (associated with an increase in coronary artery vasoconstriction and a hypercoagulable state)[16] may be needed to cause occlusive thrombosis and disease onset. However, in a patient with an extremely vulnerable plaque, even the nonstrenuous activities of daily living may be sufficient to trigger the cascade leading to the cardiovascular event.

There is considerable support for the hypothesis that acute coronary syndromes and sudden cardiac death are "triggered events" occurring nonrandomly with circadian (daily), circaseptan (weekly), and circannual (seasonal) variations.[17-21] Several studies permit an estimate of the relative importance of external activities versus processes internal to the plaque in causing disruption.[5,7,22] At present, triggers can be found for approximately 20% of nonfatal MIs. With additional studies, it is likely that approximately one third of all events will have an identifiable trigger. An additional third are likely to have a trigger (such as psychological stress) too subtle to identify with the limited historical means available. In a final third, it is likely that the clinical events (and in most cases the disruption that caused it) resulted from processes internal to the plaque alone.

CYCLICAL PATTERN OF MYOCARDIAL INFARCTION ONSET

MI and sudden cardiac death demonstrate a marked circadian variation, with an increased risk during the morning after awakening and arising. The recognition of the morning increase of acute cardiovascular events has convinced many that such events may be triggered by morning activities. However, cardiovascular events occur throughout the day, even if at lower frequency compared with the morning. There is a strong association between external triggers and the onset of MI and sudden cardiac death beyond what is to be expected by chance alone. The magnitude of this association (relative risk, two to three times) is comparable with the known long-term risk factors of cardiac disease. The pathophysiologic links between external triggers and the onset of cardiovascular events are important in addressing the question of a causal relationship between triggers and disease onset and perhaps in improving preventive strategies.

Circadian Variation of Acute Coronary Syndromes

Myocardial Infarction

Although the peak incidence of infarct onset occurs in the morning, it is likely that similar physiologic processes trigger disease onset at other times of the day. The peak morning incidence of infarct onset probably results from the synchronization of potential triggers in the morning; a secondary evening peak in the infarct onset (observed in the Multicenter Investigation of

Limitation of Infarct Size Study[17]) may result from synchronization of the population for an additional potential trigger.

Serum creatine phosphokinase measurements, obtained from 703 subjects in the Multicenter Investigation of Limitation of Infarct Size Study,[17] were used to demonstrate a marked circadian variation in the incidence of MI, with a threefold increase at 9 AM compared to 11 PM. In the Intravenous Streptokinase in Acute Myocardial Infarction Study (ISAM),[20] Willich et al used clinical criteria and serial creatine phosphokinase measurements to identify the time of onset of MI in all 1741 patients enrolled. A morning peak in the onset of MI was reported with a 3.8-fold increase in frequency noted between 8 AM and 9 AM as compared with the period between midnight and 1 AM. The morning was a risk period for patients with mild as well as severe coronary artery disease (Fig. 8-2).

Goldberg et al[18] examined the times of onset of acute MI in relation to awakening in 137 patients with confirmed acute MI. Approximately 23% of patients reported onset of initial symptoms of MI within 1 hour after awakening. Willich et al,[23] using the community-based Triggers and Mechanisms of Myocardial Infarction pilot data, supported this finding with the observation that the increased incidence of MI occurred within the first 3 hours after awakening. Of the 3339 patients entered into the Thrombolysis in Myocardial Infarction II (TIMI II) trial,[24] 34.4% of the heart attacks occurred between 6 AM and noon versus 15.4% between midnight and 6 AM. Genes et al[25] reviewed the data on 2563 patients and noted that 30.6% of the acute cardiac events occurred between 6 AM and noon, whereas only 20.1% occurred between midnight and 6 AM.

Cannon and associates[26] examined the time of onset of myocardial ischemic pain in 7731 patients who were

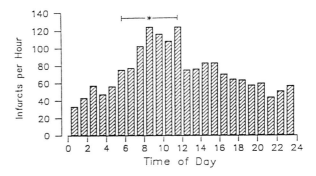

FIGURE 8–2. Bar graph of incidence of myocardial infarction of 1741 patients of the Intravenous Streptokinase in Acute Myocardial Infarction Study. There is a marked circadian variation, with a peak during the morning hours. Myocardial infarction occurred 1.8 times more frequently between 6:00 AM and 12:00 noon compared with the average of other quarters of the day. The risk of myocardial infarction in the afternoon and evening was approximately equally distributed, whereas a trough period occurred during the night. (Adapted from Willich SN, Linderer T, Wegscheider K, et al: Increased morning incidence of myocardial infarction in the ISAM Study: Absence with prior beta-adrenergic blockade. ISAM Study Group. Circulation 1989; 80:853–858.)

prospectively identified in the TIMI III Registry. The authors documented a statistically significant circadian variation in the incidence of onset of unstable angina and evolving non–Q-wave MI, with a peak occurrence rate between 6 AM and noon. Thompson et al[27] and others[27-31] have suggested that in the evening hours (between 6 PM and 12 midnight), a secondary peak of onset of MI occurs. This may relate to the evening meal or other triggers concentrated in those hours.

Transient Myocardial Ischemia

Transient myocardial ischemia occurring during daily life has a circadian variation with a peak in the morning waking hours, and a trough at night, which corresponds with the circadian variations in onset of acute coronary syndromes. All the known parameters that influence the ischemic picture surge after waking and commencing activities, and therefore it is not surprising that ischemic activity peaks at his time (Fig. 8–3).[32] Delayed rising and commencement of activities delay the surge in heart rate and in ischemic activity, suggesting an important cause-and-effect relationship between activation of the sympathetic adrenergic system and transient ischemic activity but also implying that the circadian rhythm of myocardial ischemia is primarily activity-related rather than an intrinsic rhythm.

Much evidence supports the activation of the sympathetic adrenergic system as an important pathophysiologic mechanism in a majority of such ischemic episodes, especially those occurring in the morning waking hours. This finding is supported by several pharmacologic studies, which have demonstrated the effectiveness of β-adrenergic blocking agents in reducing the frequency of ischemic episodes and blunting the morning surge.[33,34] The increase in catecholamines, in addition to exerting its effect on heart rate, blood pressure, and contractility, may also cause increased coronary vasoconstriction with a resultant reduction in myocardial oxygen supply, thus producing ischemia or reducing the threshold for ischemia.[35-37] Autonomic changes consistent with vagal withdrawal can act as a precipitating factor for ischemia in daily life, particularly in activities triggered by mental activities.[38]

Pathophysiology of Morning Increase in Acute Coronary Syndromes

A variety of factors both related to and independent of activity level may create the milieu at the level of the coronary plaque that leads to an increased incidence of onset of MI in the morning hours (Fig. 8–4). A morning systemic surge in blood pressure related to increased cortisol and catecholamine secretion,[39] in combination with increased coronary artery tone,[40] could promote disruption of a vulnerable plaque. Increased coronary artery tone alone could worsen the flow reduction produced by fixed stenoses. Prothrombotic processes, including increased platelet adhesion and aggregability,[41] increased factor VII and plasminogen activator inhibitor activity,[42] and increased blood viscosity[43] have been implicated in the onset of acute cardiac events and have been associated with decreased effectiveness of heparin and thrombolytics in the morning hours.[4,44] Predisposition to plaque disruption and subsequent thrombosis added to reduced fibrinolytic activity in the morning could increase the likelihood that an otherwise harmless mural thrombus overlying a small plaque fissure would propagate and occlude the coronary lumen.

Epidemiologic and physiologic evidence suggests that the diurnal periodicity of MI onset is likely based primarily on the daily rest/activity cycle. Endogenous circadian rhythms may play a small role in events, but supporting data are limited. Cortisol secretion, a determinant of systemic blood pressure, is an established endogenous circadian process independent of daily activity, whereas enhanced platelet aggregability[41] and in vitro platelet responsiveness to adenosine diphosphate and epinephrine[45] increase only after the patient awakens and assumes the upright posture. It is likely that the peak morning incidence of MI results from the synchronization of adverse pathophysiologic processes, primarily driven by activity of the patient.

Weekly Variations of Acute Myocardial Infarction

Numerous authors have reported a circaseptan (weekly) variation of MI, with a peak incidence on Monday.[46-51] Willich et al[49] noted this increase to be primarily in the working population, with a 33% increase in relative risk of MI on this day of the week. In contrast, Spielberg et al[46] observed a Monday increase in both the working and retired subgroups of patients who were studied. Some researchers noted an increased incidence of MI on the weekend[52,53] whereas others reported a weekend nadir.[46-50]

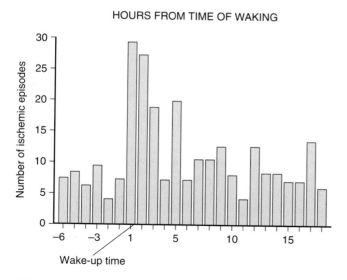

HOURS FROM TIME OF WAKING

Wake-up time

FIGURE 8–3. Circadian variation in frequency of transient ischemic episodes in patients with stable angina, when frequency of episodes is corrected for the time of awakening. (Adapted from Rocco MB, Barry J, Campbell S, et al: Circadian variation of transient myocardial ischemia in patients with coronary artery disease. Circulation 1987;75:395–400.)

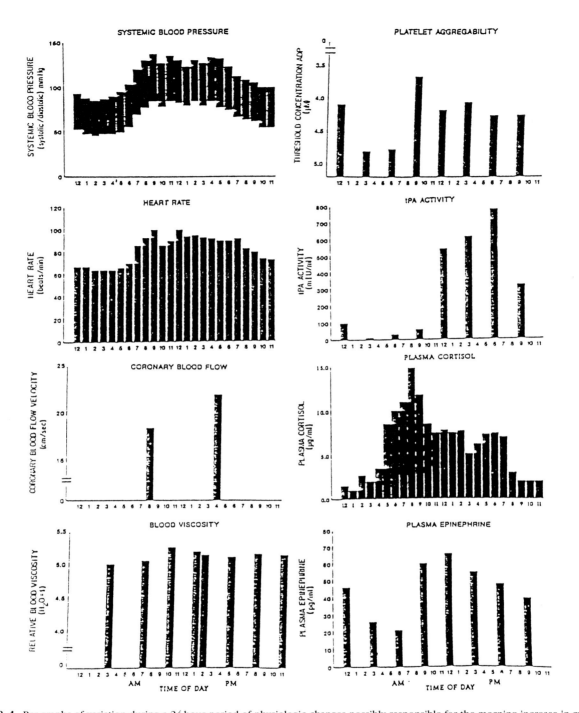

FIGURE 8–4. Bar graphs of variation during a 24-hour period of physiologic changes possibly responsible for the morning increase in myocardial infarction. tPA, tissue plasminogen activator. (Adapted from Muller JE, Tofler GH, Stone PH: Circadian variation and triggers of onset of acute cardiovascular disease. Circulation 1989;79:733–743.)

Seasonal Variations in Coronary Deaths

Several investigators have reported a circannual (seasonal) variation, with a peak in the incidence of onset of acute MI and cardiac mortality in winter.[19,54-57] Of the 83,541 subjects entered into the National Registry of Myocardial Infarction (NRMI) database between 1990 and 1993, 10% more acute cardiac events occurred in winter or spring than in summer.[58] Spencer et al[59]

reviewed the data on 259,891 patients reported to the second NRMI during the 25-month period beginning July 1, 1994. The authors noted that over 50% more cases of MI were reported in the peak winter month of January than during the summer month of July.

Sayer et al[57] prospectively obtained data on 1225 consecutive patients with acute MI admitted to a general hospital. Overall, a winter peak in the incidence of onset of MI was noted. However, the subgroups of patients who were diabetic, South Asian, or taking β-blockers or aspirin on admission did not demonstrate a seasonal variation. Marchant et al[54] noted a winter peak in the 633 consecutive patients with acute MI admitted to the cardiac care unit during a 4-year period. Interestingly, the authors noted an excess of infarctions on colder days in both winter and summer, suggesting the additional environmental influence of temperature on the onset of this disease. Colder weather has been shown to alter hemodynamic (arterial pressure, sympathetic tone) and hematologic (platelet count, fibrinogen) factors favoring plaque disruption and arterial thrombosis.[60,61]

However, the increase in cardiac events does not appear to be simply temperature-dependent. Even in the milder climate of Los Angeles County, a study of 220,000 subjects revealed a peak cardiac death rate in December and January.[21] Possible roles for dietary and psychological changes around the holidays, as well as the seasonal decrease in number of daylight hours, are under investigation.

Nocturnal Triggers and Acute Myocardial Infarction

Normal sleep is a dynamic process involving complex regulation of autonomic nervous system activity punctuated by episodes of rapid eye movement (REM) sleep and catecholamine secretion that rivals the awakened state.[62] In the United States, annually, more than 250,00 acute MIs and more than 38,000 sudden cardiac deaths occur at night during sleep. This rate is less than observed during the daytime hours, but several factors make events during sleep of interest. First, this pattern demonstrates that events can occur at a time of reduced environmental stresses; second, the distribution of onset of cardiac events at night during sleep is not uniform, suggesting the existence of triggers.

Lavery et al[63] performed an extensive literature review on the incidence of acute cardiac episodes between the hours of midnight and 5:59 AM and identified 19 studies of acute MI, 7 on automatic implantable cardioverter-defibrillator (AICD) discharges and 12 on sudden cardiac death. The peak incidence of MI and AICD discharge occurred between midnight and 0:59 AM, and the peak incidence of sudden cardiac deaths took place between 1:00 AM and 1:59 AM. The lowest incidence of MI and AICD discharge occurred between 3:00 AM and 3:59 AM, and the trough for sudden cardiac deaths was between 4:00 AM and 4:59 AM. Interpretation of these temporal data would be enhanced if sleep status of the individuals at any given hour was more accurately known. Further research on sleep state–dependent fluctuations in autonomic nervous system activity may make it possible to identify the mechanisms responsible and subsequently reduce acute cardiac events during sleep.

TRIGGERS OF CARDIOVASCULAR EVENTS

The Myocardial Infarction Onset Study (MIOS) investigators and others have characterized several activities and exposures that serve as triggers of MI onset, including heavy physical exertion, anger, mental stress, sexual activity, cocaine use, marijuana use, and exposure to air pollution.[5-9,22,64]

Anger

The lethal effects of anger are attributed to its activation of high-gain central neurocircuitry and the sympathetic nervous system, leading to acute sinus tachycardia, hypertension, impaired myocardial perfusion, and a high degree of cardiac electrical instability. Reich et al[65] noted that anger was the probable trigger for 15% of the life-threatening arrhythmias identified in 117 patients. Fear, anxiety, and bereavement have also been implicated in increased vulnerability to cardiac events.[66,67]

The Determinants of Myocardial Infarction Onset Study investigators interviewed 1623 subjects approximately 4 days after an acute MI to assess the intensity and timing of anger (and other triggers) during the 26 hours before the acute event.[7] Anger was objectively assessed by the onset anger scale (Table 8–1, a single-item, seven-level, self-reported scale) and the state anger subscale of the State-Trait Personality Inventory. The onset anger scale identified 39 patients (2.4%) who experienced anger within the 2 hours prior to onset of MI.

Heavy Exertion

In the MILIS,[68] TIMI II,[24] and MIOS[5] trials, heavy physical exertion was identified as a trigger of acute MI. In the MILIS trial,[68] 14% of patients engaged in moderate physical activity and 9% engaged in heavy physical activity prior to sustaining a MI. In the TIMI II trial,[24] moderate or marked physical activity was reported to occur at onset of MI in 18.7% of patients. Compared with patients whose infarction occurred at rest or during mild activity, those with exertion-related infarction had fewer coronary vessels with greater than 60% stenosis and were more likely to have an occluded infarct-related vessel after thrombolytic therapy.

Fifty-four (4.4%) of 1228 patients enrolled in the MIOS trial[5] reported heavy exertion (six or more metabolic

■ ■ ■

TABLE 8–1   ONSET STUDY ANGER SCALE USED TO ASSESS EPISODES OF ANGER IN THE MYOCARDIAL INFARCTION ONSET STUDY

ANGER LEVEL	DESCRIPTION
1	Calm
2	Busy, but not hassled
3	Mildly angry, irritated and hassled, but it does not show
4	Moderately angry, so hassled it shows in the voice
5	Very angry, body tense, clenching fists or teeth
6	Furious, almost out of control, very angry, pounds table, slams door
7	Enraged! Loses control, throwing objects, hurting oneself or others

Data from Mittleman MA, Maclure M, Tofler GH, et al: Triggering of acute myocardial infarction by heavy physical exertion. Protection against triggering by regular exertion. Determinants of Myocardial Infarction Onset Study Investigators. N Engl J Med 1993;329:1677–1683.

equivalents, or METS) within 1 hour of the onset of MI. The cardiac symptoms often began during the activity. The estimated relative risk of MI in the hour after heavy physical activity was almost six times higher as compared with less strenuous or no physical exertion (Fig. 8–5). Habitually sedentary persons were at greatest risk for MI after heavy exertion, and increasing levels of regular physical exercise were associated with progressively lower coronary risk. This same exercise-related protection also appears to hold true for sudden cardiac death associated with heavy physical exertion.[69,70]

Proposed mechanisms for triggering of MI onset by heavy exertion include increased sympathetic nervous system activation leading to increased myocardial demand[71] and increased platelet activation in sedentary patients and those with prior MI.[72] Interestingly, heavy exertion does not cause platelet activation in healthy active volunteers, which may contribute to the protective effect of regular exercise. Additional benefits of regular exercise include blunted upregulation of the sympathetic nervous system during exertion and activation of the fibrinolytic system.[73] Thus, a patient's propensity for triggering MI in the setting of heavy exertion appears to depend, in part, on the degree of sympathetic activity and a balance between prothrombotic and fibrinolytic effects. Despite the proposed importance of sympathetic activation and a potential net prothrombotic effect, it remains unclear whether β-blockers or aspirin decreases the relative risk of MI triggered by exertion.

Sexual Activity

Decreased frequency of sexual intercourse after MI, largely due to patient and partner anxiety, remains a significant problem, affecting an estimated 70% of married men 3 years post MI and a large proportion of patients who have undergone coronary artery bypass grafting.[74] Given the impact of anecdotal reports linking MI and sexual activity, investigators of the MIOS study sought to assess the magnitude of the risk of MI after sexual activity.[9] Of the more than 1700 patients participating in the study, 858 (48%) agreed to answer questions about sexual activity. Of these, 3% reported sexual activity within the 2 hours before MI onset. Case-crossover analysis yielded a relative risk of 2.5 for onset of MI during this period. The relative risk of MI immediately following sexual activity is no different for patients with known cardiac disease than for people without heart disease—a finding that may reassure patients during cardiac rehabilitation.

Although sexual activity doubles the acute risk of MI, patients should be reassured that the absolute risk increase is small because the baseline risk is low, the risk is transient, and the activity is relatively infrequent.[74] Regular exercise has been shown to decrease the cardiac work associated with sexual activity and the risk of triggering of MI onset.[9] Patients who remain sedentary after an MI and those with persistent unstable angina or advanced congestive heart failure require full medical evaluation before sexual activity can be safely recommended. Because only two cases of MI associated with sexual activity were reported in the MIOS study among patients who were able to achieve 6 METS on exercise testing,[9] patient performance on an exercise tolerance test can be of help to clinicians in assessing cardiac safety of sexual activity when indicated.

Mental Stress

Acute mental stress may be a trigger of transient myocardial ischemia,[75,76] MI,[77] and sudden cardiac death.[78,79] People who possess a high potential for hostility in response to a mental stress and an inability to express that anger outwardly appear to be at significant risk for coronary artery disease.[80]

Bairey et al[75] noted that 75% of 29 patients with CAD and exercise-induced myocardial ischemia also demonstrated mental stress–induced wall-motion abnormalities by radionuclide ventriculography.

Behar et al[77] studied 1818 consecutive patients with acute MI. Exceptional heavy physical work, a violent quarrel at work or at home, and unusual mental stress were the three most frequent possible triggers of MI that occurred within 24 hours of symptom onset. Within the first week of missile attacks on Israel during the 1991 Iraqi war, 20 people experienced an acute MI at one hospital compared with 8 MIs during a control period.[81] Leor and Kloner[82] identified a 35% increase in the number of hospital admissions for acute MI in Southern California in the week following the 1994 Northridge earthquake. Most of these events were associated with mental rather than physical stress. Numerous authors have noted an increase in sudden cardiac death triggered by mental stress, including psychological stress, occupational stress, and natural disasters,[44,83-85] probably due to neural/neurohormonal activation and sympathetic

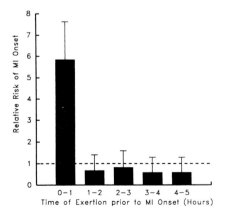

FIGURE 8–5. Time to onset of myocardial infarction after an episode of heavy physical exertion (induction time). Each of the five hours before the onset of myocardial infarction (MI) was assessed as an independent hazard period, and exertion during each hour was compared with that during the control period. Only exertion during the hour immediately before the onset of MI was associated with an increase in the relative risk, suggesting that the induction time for MI is less than 1 hour. The error bars indicate 95% confidence limits. The *dotted line* indicates the baseline risk. (Adapted from Mittleman MA, Maclure M, Tofler GH, et al: Triggering of acute myocardial infarction by heavy physical exertion. Protection against triggering by regular exertion. Determinants of Myocardial Infarction Onset Study Investigators. N Engl J Med 1993;329:1677–1683.)

stimulation precipitating malignant arrhythmias or plaque rupture and thrombosis in susceptible persons.[80,83,86]

An increase in coagulation factors VII, VIII, fibrinogen, von Willebrand factor, and platelet activity has also been observed in patients subjected to mental stress and may play a role in precipitating acute cardiac events.[83]

Other Triggers

Cocaine and Marijuana

Cocaine and marijuana use remain relatively common in the United States: More than 30 million Americans have used cocaine at least once and more than 72 million have tried marijuana.[6,64] Nine of the 3946 patients interviewed in the Onset Study reported cocaine use in the hour prior to MI.[6] One hundred twenty-four (3.2%) of the 3882 patients interviewed in the MIOS study reported marijuana use in the prior year, 37 within 24 hours, and 9 within 1 hour of MI onset.[64] The case crossover method[87] was used to assess the risk of MI onset, which was elevated 23.7 and 4.8 times over baseline in the 60 minutes after cocaine or marijuana use, respectively, with a rapid decrease in risk thereafter. Cocaine users were more likely to be male, tobacco smokers, and minority group members. Marijuana users were more likely to be male, tobacco smokers, and obese.

These agents may trigger the onset of MI via several pathways. Cocaine, a blocker of the presynaptic reuptake of norepinephrine and dopamine, leads to coronary vasoconstriction and increased myocardial oxygen demand via increased heart rate, contractility, and systemic blood pressure. In addition, cocaine causes accelerated atherosclerosis and enhanced platelet aggregability, thus increasing the propensity for vulnerable plaque formation and occlusive thrombus formation following disruption.[6] The effects of marijuana—increased heart rate, postural hypotension, and hypertension when supine—are primarily mediated by the activation of cannabinoid receptors located in the central nervous system and heart. Decreased oxygen-carrying capacity caused by increased serum carboxyhemoglobin and exposure to airborne particulates and gaseous compounds, along with marijuana action at cannabinoid receptors located in the spleen and immune cells, may also play a role in triggering of MI onset by marijuana.[64] Both marijuana and cocaine use are *rare* triggers of MI and result in only a small number of cases of MI onset.

Air Pollution

Ambient particulate air pollution has been epidemiologically linked to acute cardiac events. In a recent report from the MIOS group, fluctuations in hourly concentrations of particle mass were measured in Boston and the risk of MI onset was assessed in relation to increases in air pollution.[64] In a study of 772 patients, the risk of MI onset increased (odds ratio, 1.69) in association with elevated concentrations of fine particles in the previous 2 hours. Potential pathways by which inhaled particles could lead to acute exacerbation of cardiovascular disease include triggering of pulmonary and systemic inflammation with resulting hypercoagulability.[64]

TRIGGERING AND PREVENTION

Epidemiologic studies now indicate that an identifiable trigger is present in approximately 20% of cases. An even larger number of infarcts are likely to have a trigger that could not be identified by the relatively insensitive methods available. Hence, triggering plays a role in a very large number of cardiac events. Intervention aimed at reducing triggers may become part of a program to reduce the impact of cardiovascular disease, along with proven prevention programs aimed at reducing established cardiovascular disease risk factors and risk of adverse events. It is hoped that further understanding of the role of triggering factors will lead to the identification of tailored pharmacologic and lifestyle intervention strategies in persons who are at increased risk for acute coronary syndromes.

Although most external triggers for plaque disruption and thrombosis are unavoidable, it may be possible to sever the link between a potential trigger and disruption of a vulnerable plaque leading to an event. A relatively vulnerable lesion might be prevented from causing a clinical event, either because the disruption was prevented or because the hypercoagulability or vasoconstrictive forces of the potential trigger were blocked. In such a manner, "activities that trigger infarction" could be converted into "activities that would have triggered infarction."

Modulating Triggers of Acute Coronary Syndromes

Results of triggering research should not be routinely used to recommend avoidance of a potential triggering situation, but information is available that is useful for individual patient management. There are patients in whom an avoidable potential trigger occurs with such regularity that the accumulated risk becomes substantial and intervention may be helpful. For instance, a patient who experiences anger, a known trigger, many times per day may benefit from stress management instruction.

Physical Activity

Physical activity has a favorable effect on the lipid profile by lowering total serum cholesterol and triglycerides and raising HDL cholesterol. In addition, physical activity is associated with reduced blood pressure, improved glucose tolerance, increased insulin sensitivity, and reduced blood coagulability.[88] The higher rate of infarction in the morning hours has raised concerns about the desirability of physical activity during this period. Murray and colleagues[89] found no difference in risk of cardiac events between persons who attended cardiac rehabilitation programs in the morning and those who attended in the afternoon. In fact, regular physical activity appears to be protective against triggering of MI onset by heavy exertion and sexual activity.[9]

Pharmacologic Therapy

Given the compelling data on the circadian variation of myocardial event onset, it is prudent to provide pharmacologic protection during the morning hours for patients already receiving anti-ischemic and antihypertensive therapy. The current absence of a reliable method to measure plaque vulnerability in living patients has precluded direct studies of agents that might "stabilize" plaques. However, it is suspected that at least some of the agents documented to prevent acute coronary events do so by rendering a plaque less likely to disrupt. There are varying levels of evidence that the four classes of agents most commonly administered to prevent acute coronary events (lipid-lowering agents, angiotensin-converting enzyme inhibitors, β-adrenergic blocking agents, and aspirin) act via trigger modulation. Aspirin use was associated with a reduced risk of anger-triggered MI onset, but further study is necessary to define the role of additional agents in trigger modulation.[7]

Knowledge of potential triggering mechanisms has modified the clinician's approach to certain patients at risk for an acute coronary syndrome. Triggering activity data are also useful to provide reassurance to patients that an activity is highly unlikely to cause an infarct. A method to identify and stabilize the vulnerable plaque would also be of great benefit in the prevention of triggering.

CONCLUSIONS

Despite recent progress in the prevention of coronary heart disease, approximately 50% of deaths continue to occur out of the hospital. Many major cardiac events occur in persons not previously known to be at risk. This has led to great interest in attempting to identify the triggers that may cause acute coronary syndromes and sudden cardiac death. Since the initial observations that the incidence of MI depended on time and activity with circadian variation, it has been demonstrated that events can be caused by heavy exertion, sexual activity, anger, mental stress, cocaine and marijuana use, and exposure to air pollution. Study of the pathophysiologic changes produced by these triggers may provide novel therapeutic and preventive targets via a more thorough understanding of vulnerable plaque disruption and coronary thrombosis.

REFERENCES

1. Burke AP, Farb A, Malcom GT, et al: Plaque rupture and sudden death related to exertion in men with coronary artery disease. JAMA 1999;281:921-926.
2. Falk E, Shah PK, Fuster V: Coronary plaque disruption. Circulation 1995;92:657-671.
3. Fuster, V, Badimon J, Chesebro JH, Fallon JT: Plaque rupture, thrombosis, and therapeutic implications. Haemostasis 1996;26 (Suppl 4):269-284.
4. Hackett D, Davies G, Maseri A: Pre-existing coronary stenoses in patients with first myocardial infarction are not necessarily severe. Eur Heart J 1988;9:1317-1323.
5. Mittleman MA, Maclure M, Tofler GH, et al: Triggering of acute myocardial infarction by heavy physical exertion. Protection against triggering by regular exertion. Determinants of Myocardial Infarction Onset Study Investigators. N Engl J Med 1993;329:1677-1683.
6. Mittleman MA, Mintzer D, Maclure M, et al: Triggering of myocardial infarction by cocaine. Circulation (Online) 1999;99:2737-2741.
7. Mittleman MA, Maclure M, Sherwood JB, et al: Triggering of acute myocardial infarction onset by episodes of anger. Determinants of Myocardial Infarction Onset Study Investigators. Circulation 1995;92:1720-1725.
8. Muller JE, Abela GS, Nesto RW, Tofler GH: Triggers, acute risk factors and vulnerable plaques: The lexicon of a new frontier. J Am Coll Cardiol 1994;23:809-813.
9. Muller JE, Mittleman MA, Maclure M, et al: Triggering myocardial infarction by sexual activity. Low absolute risk and prevention by regular physical exertion. Determinants of Myocardial Infarction Onset Study Investigators. JAMA 1996;275:1405-1409.
10. Richardson PD, Davies MJ, Born GV: Influence of plaque configuration and stress distribution on fissuring of coronary atherosclerotic plaques. Lancet 1989;2:941-944.
11. Libby P: Molecular basis of the acute coronary syndromes. Circulation 1995;91:2844-2850.
12. Barger AC, Beeuwkes R: Rupture of coronary vasa vasorum as a trigger of acute myocardial infarction. Am J Cardiol 1990;66: 41G-43G.
13. Loree HM, Kamm RD, Stringfellow RG, Lee RT: Effects of fibrous cap thickness on peak circumferential stress in model atherosclerotic vessels. Circ Res 1992;71:850-858.
14. Lerman A, Holmes DR, Bell MR, et al: Endothelin in coronary endothelial dysfunction and early atherosclerosis in humans. Circulation 1995;92:2426-2431.
15. Epstein SE, Zhou YF, Zhu J: Infection and atherosclerosis: emerging mechanistic paradigms [review] [130 refs]. Circulation 2001;27; 100:e20-e28, 1999; e20-e28.
16. Belch JJ, McArdle BM, Burns P, et al: The effects of acute smoking on platelet behaviour, fibrinolysis and haemorheology in habitual smokers. Thrombosis Haemostasis 1984;51:6-8.
17. Muller JE, Stone PH, Turi ZG, et al: Circadian variation in the frequency of onset of acute myocardial infarction. N Engl J Med 1985;313:1315-1322.
18. Goldberg RJ, Brady P, Muller JE, et al: Time of onset of symptoms of acute myocardial infarction. Am J Cardiol 1990;66:140-144.
19. Beard CM, Fuster V, Elveback LR: Daily and seasonal variation in sudden cardiac death, Rochester, Minnesota, 1950-1975. Mayo Clin Proc 1982;57:704-706.
20. Willich SN, Linderer T, Wegscheider K, et al: Increased morning incidence of myocardial infarction in the ISAM Study: Absence with prior beta-adrenergic blockade. ISAM Study Group. Circulation 1989;80:853-858.
21. Kloner RA, Poole WK, Perritt RL: When throughout the year is coronary death most likely to occur? A 12-year population-based analysis of more than 220,000 cases. Circulation (Online) 1999;100: 1630-1634.
22. Peters A, Dockery DW, Muller JE, Mittleman MA: Increased particulate air pollution and the triggering of myocardial infarction. Circulation (Online) 2001;103:2810-2815.
23. Willich SN, Lowel H, Lewis M, et al: Association of wake time and the onset of myocardial infarction. Triggers and mechanisms of myocardial infarction (TRIMM) pilot study. TRIMM Study Group. Circulation 1991;84:VI62-VI67.
24. Tofler GH, Muller JE, Stone PH, et al: Modifiers of timing and possible triggers of acute myocardial infarction in the Thrombolysis in Myocardial Infarction Phase II (TIMI II) Study Group. J Am Coll Cardiol 1992;20:1049-1055.
25. Genes N, Vaur L, Renault M, et al: Circadian rhythm in myocardial infarct in France. Results of the USIK study. Presse Med 1997;26:603-608.
26. Cannon CP, McCabe CH, Stone PH, et al: Circadian variation in the onset of unstable angina and non-Q-wave acute myocardial infarction (the TIMI III Registry and TIMI IIIB). Am J Cardiol 1997;79:253-258.

27. Thompson DR, Blandford RL, Sutton TW, Marchant PR: Time of onset of chest pain in acute myocardial infarction. Int J Cardiol 1985;7:139–148.

28. Hjalmarson A, Gilpin EA, Nicod P, et al: Differing circadian patterns of symptom onset in subgroups of patients with acute myocardial infarction. Circulation 1989;80:267–275.

29. Peters RW, Zoble RG, Liebson PR, et al: Identification of a secondary peak in myocardial infarction onset 11 to 12 hours after awakening: The Cardiac Arrhythmia Suppression Trial (CAST) experience. J Am Coll Cardiol 1993;22:998–1003.

30. Hansen O, Johansson BW, Gullberg B: Circadian distribution of onset of acute myocardial infarction in subgroups from analysis of 10,791 patients treated in a single center. Am J Cardiol 1992;69:1003–1008.

31. Kono T, Morita H, Nishina T, et al: Circadian variations of onset of acute myocardial infarction and efficacy of thrombolytic therapy. J Am Coll Cardiol 1996;27:774–778.

32. Rocco MB, Barry J, Campbell S, et al: Circadian variation of transient myocardial ischemia in patients with coronary artery disease. Circulation 1987;75:395–400.

33. Imperi GA, Lambert CR, Coy K, et al: Effects of titrated beta blockade (metoprolol) on silent myocardial ischemia in ambulatory patients with coronary artery disease. Am J Cardiol 1987;60:519–524.

34. Stone PH, Gibson RS, Glasser SP, et al: Comparison of propranolol, diltiazem, and nifedipine in the treatment of ambulatory ischemia in patients with stable angina. Differential effects on ambulatory ischemia, exercise performance, and anginal symptoms. The ASIS Study Group. Circulation 1990;82:1962–1972.

35. Panza JA, Diodati JG, Callahan TS, et al: Role of increases in heart rate in determining the occurrence and frequency of myocardial ischemia during daily life in patients with stable coronary artery disease. J Am Coll Cardiol 1992;20:1092–1098.

36. Quyyumi AA, Panza JA, Diodati JG, et al: Circadian variation in ischemic threshold. A mechanism underlying the circadian variation in ischemic events. Circulation 1992;86:22–28.

37. Muller JE, Tofler GH, Stone PH: Circadian variation and triggers of onset of acute cardiovascular disease. Circulation 1989;79:733–743.

38. Kop WJ, Verdino RJ, Gottdiener JS, et al: Changes in heart rate and heart rate variability before ambulatory ischemic events. J Am Coll Cardiol 2001;38:742–749.

39. Millar-Craig MW, Bishop CN, Raftery EB: Circadian variation of blood-pressure. Lancet 1978;1:795–797.

40. Panza JA, Epstein SE, Quyyumi AA: Circadian variation in vascular tone and its relation to alpha-sympathetic vasoconstrictor activity. N Engl J Med 1991;325:986–990.

41. Tofler GH, Brezinski D, Schafer AI, et al: Concurrent morning increase in platelet aggregability and the risk of myocardial infarction and sudden cardiac death. N Engl J Med 1987;316:1514–1518.

42. Kapiotis S, Jilma B, Quehenberger P, et al: Morning hypercoagulability and hypofibrinolysis: Diurnal variations in circulating activated factor VII, prothrombin fragment F1 + 2, and plasmin-plasmin inhibitor-complex. Atherosclerosis 1997;134:192.

43. Ehrly AM, Jung G: Circadian rhythm of human blood viscosity. Biorheology 1973;10:577–583.

44. Kurnik PB: Circadian variation in the efficacy of tissue-type plasminogen activator. Circulation 1995;91:1341–1346.

45. Brezinski DA, Tofler GH, Muller JE, et al: Morning increase in platelet aggregability. Association with assumption of the upright posture. Circulation 1988;78:35–40.

46. Spielberg C, Falkenhahn D, Willich SN, et al: Circadian, day-of-week, and seasonal variability in myocardial infarction: Comparison between working and retired patients. Am Heart J 1996;132:579–585.

47. Gnecchi-Ruscone T, Piccaluga E, Guzzetti S, et al: Morning and Monday: Critical periods for the onset of acute myocardial infarction. The GISSI 2 Study experience. Eur Heart J 1994;15:882–887.

48. Thompson DR, Pohl JE, Sutton TW: Acute myocardial infarction and day of the week. Am J Cardiol 1992;69:266–267.

49. Willich SN, Lowel H, Lewis M, et al: Weekly variation of acute myocardial infarction. Increased Monday risk in the working population. Circulation 1994;90:87–93.

50. Ohlson CG, Bodin L, Bryngelsson IL, et al: Winter weather conditions and myocardial infarctions. Scand J Social Med 1991;19:20–25.

51. Peters RW, Brooks MM, Zoble RG, et al: Chronobiology of acute myocardial infarction: Cardiac arrhythmia suppression trial (CAST) experience. Am J Cardiol 1996;78:1198–1201.

52. Zhou RH, Xi B, Gao HQ, et al: Circadian and septadian variation in the occurrence of acute myocardial infarction in a Chinese population. Jpn Circ J 1998;62:190–192.

53. van der Palen J, Doggen CJ, Beaglehole R: Variation in the time and day of onset of myocardial infarction and sudden death. N Z Med J 1995;108:332–334.

54. Marchant B, Ranjadayalan K, Stevenson R, et al: Circadian and seasonal factors in the pathogenesis of acute myocardial infarction: The influence of environmental temperature. Br Heart J 1993;69:385–387.

55. Baker-Blocker A: Winter weather and cardiovascular mortality in Minneapolis-St. Paul. Am J Public Health 1982;72:261–265.

56. Rogers WJ, Bowlby LJ, Chandra NC, et al: Treatment of myocardial infarction in the United States (1990 to 1993). Observations from the National Registry of Myocardial Infarction. Circulation 1994;90:2103–2114.

57. Sayer JW, Wilkinson P, Ranjadayalan K, et al: Attenuation or absence of circadian and seasonal rhythms of acute myocardial infarction. Heart (British Cardiac Society) 1997;77:325–329.

58. Ornato JP, Peberdy MA, Chandra NC, Bush DE: Seasonal pattern of acute myocardial infarction in the National Registry of Myocardial Infarction. J Am Coll Cardiol 1996;28:1684–1688.

59. Spencer FA, Goldberg RJ, Becker RC, Gore JM: Seasonal distribution of acute myocardial infarction in the second National Registry of Myocardial Infarction. J Am Coll Cardiol 1998;31:1226–1233.

60. Keatinge WR, Coleshaw SR, Cotter F, et al: Increases in platelet and red cell counts, blood viscosity, and arterial pressure during mild surface cooling: Factors in mortality from coronary and cerebral thrombosis in winter. Br Med J (Clin Res Ed) 1984;289:1405–1408.

61. Woodhouse PR, Khaw KT, Plummer M, et al: Seasonal variations of plasma fibrinogen and factor VII activity in the elderly: Winter infections and death from cardiovascular disease. Lancet 1994;343:435–439.

62. Verrier RL, Muller JE, Hobson JA: Sleep, dreams, and sudden death: The case for sleep as an autonomic stress test for the heart. Cardiovasc Res 1996;31:181–211.

63. Lavery CE, Mittleman MA, Cohen MC, et al: Nonuniform nighttime distribution of acute cardiac events: A possible effect of sleep states. Circulation 1997;96:3321–3327.

64. Mittleman MA, Lewis RA, Maclure M, et al: Triggering myocardial infarction by marijuana. Circulation 2001;103:2805–2809.

65. Reich P, DeSilva RA, Lown B, Murawski BJ: Acute psychological disturbances preceding life-threatening ventricular arrhythmias. JAMA 1981;246:233–235.

66. Verrier RL, Mittleman MA: Cardiovascular consequences of anger and other stress states. Bailliere Clin Neurol 1997;6:245–259.

67. Verrier RL, Mittleman MA: Life-threatening cardiovascular consequences of anger in patients with coronary heart disease. Cardiol Clin 1996;14:289–307.

68. Tofler GH, Stone PH, Maclure M, et al: Analysis of possible triggers of acute myocardial infarction (the MILIS study). Am J Cardiol 1990;66:22–27.

69. Ledru F, Theroux P, Lesperance J, et al: Geometric features of coronary artery lesions favoring acute occlusion and myocardial infarction: A quantitative angiographic study. J Am Coll Cardiol 1999;33:1353–1361.

70. Vuori, I: The cardiovascular risks of physical activity. Acta Med Scand Suppl 1986;711:205–214.

71. Kohl HW, Powell KE, Gordon NF, et al: Physical activity, physical fitness, and sudden cardiac death. Epidemiol Rev 1992;14:37–58.

72. Douste-Blazy P, Sie P, Boneu B, et al: Exercise-induced platelet activation in myocardial infarction survivors with normal coronary arteriogram. Thromb Haemost 1984;52:297–300.

73. Winther K, Hillegass W, Tofler GH, et al: Effects on platelet aggregation and fibrinolytic activity during upright posture and exercise in healthy men. Am J Cardiol 1992;70:1051–1055.

74. Muller JE: Triggering of cardiac events by sexual activity: Findings from a case-crossover analysis. Am J Cardiol 2000;86:14F–18F.

75. Bairey CN, Krantz DS, Rozanski A: Mental stress as an acute trigger of ischemic left ventricular dysfunction and blood pressure elevation in coronary artery disease. Am J Cardiol 1990;66:28G–31G.

76. Barry J, Selwyn AP, Nabel EG, et al: Frequency of ST-segment depression produced by mental stress in stable angina pectoris from coronary artery disease. Am J Cardiol 1988;61:989–993.

77. Behar S, Halabi M, Reicher-Reiss H, et al: Circadian variation and possible external triggers of onset of myocardial infarction. SPRINT Study Group. Am J Med 1993;94:395–400.

78. Davis AM, Natelson BH: Brain-heart interactions. The neurocardiology of arrhythmia and sudden cardiac death. Texas Heart Institute Journal (from the Texas Heart Institute of St Luke's Episcopal Hospital, Texas Children's Hospital) 1993;20:158–169.

79. Lown B, Verrier RL, Rabinowitz SH: Neural and psychologic mechanisms and the problem of sudden cardiac death. Am J Cardiol 1977;39:890–902.

80. Manuck SB, Kaplan JR, Matthews KA: Behavioral antecedents of coronary heart disease and atherosclerosis. Arteriosclerosis (Dallas, Tex) 6:2–14, 2001.

81. Meisel SR, Kutz, I, Dayan KI, et al: Effect of Iraqi missile war on incidence of acute myocardial infarction and sudden death in Israeli civilians. Lancet 1991;338:660–661.

82. Leor J, Kloner RA: The Northridge earthquake as a trigger for acute myocardial infarction. Am J Cardiol 1996;77:1230–1232.

83. Frimerman A, Miller HI, Laniado S, Keren G: Changes in hemostatic function at times of cyclic variation in occupational stress. Am J Cardiol 1997;79:72–75.

84. Frasure-Smith N, Lesperance F, Talajic M: Depression following myocardial infarction. Impact on 6-month survival. JAMA 1993;270:1819–1825.

85. Leor J, Poole WK, Kloner RA: Sudden cardiac death triggered by an earthquake. N Engl J Med 1996;334:413–419.

86. Schwartz PJ, Zaza A, Locati E, Moss AJ: Stress and sudden death. The case of the long QT syndrome. Circulation 1991;83:II71–II80.

87. Maclure M: The case-crossover design: A method for studying transient effects on the risk of acute events. Am J Epidemiol 1991;133:144–153.

88. Rauramaa R, Salonen JT, Kukkonen-Harjula K, et al: Effects of mild physical exercise on serum lipoproteins and metabolites of arachidonic acid: A controlled randomised trial in middle aged men. Br Med J 1984;288:603–606.

89. Murray PM, Herrington DM, Pettus CW, et al: Should patients with heart disease exercise in the morning or afternoon? Arch Intern Med 1993;153:833–836.

Novel Risk Factors in Acute Coronary Syndromes

Jacques Genest, Jr.

As earlier chapters have emphasized, heart disease is the major cause of mortality and morbidity worldwide and is expected to remain so for at least the next 20 years, assuming current social trends continue.[1-3] Aging of the population and the partial eradication of major infectious diseases of childhood have been important forces contributing to the epidemiologic increase in cardiovascular diseases. Other factors, especially urbanization, increased dietary fat intake, cigarette smoking, pollution, stress and, in wealthy societies, a dramatic increase in obesity, diabetes, and concomitant metabolic abnormalities contribute to erode gains made in the reduction of the prevalence of cardiovascular diseases in the Western world.[2-9]

Coronary artery disease (CAD) accounts for two thirds of cardiovascular deaths. Atherosclerosis, the cause of CAD, is a systemic, chronic disease that does not result in clinical symptoms until hypoxemic symptoms develop. Unfortunately, the initial presentation of CAD is often sudden cardiac death or an acute coronary syndrome (ACS).[10] Current public health strategies for the prevention of cardiovascular diseases in North America and Europe are designed to identify high-risk persons and to treat risk factors in order to prevent a first myocardial infarction or a recurrent event.[4,11,12]

Despite decades of epidemiologic studies, risk stratification in individual subjects is only approximate. Preventive therapies must be initiated in a large group of persons within the same risk category in order to prevent a limited number of events. This is often referred to as the *number to treat* in intervention studies. The search for novel risk factors (Table 9–1) has the potential to direct therapy more specifically in moderate- to high-risk patients and to identify subjects at high risk who would otherwise be missed by the current guidelines. This approach has led to the identification of C-reactive protein (CRP) as a novel risk factor and as a predictor of response to therapy (see Chapter 16).[13,14]

A cardiovascular risk factor is currently defined as a variable (a biochemical measurement, a genotype, and an anthropometric or psychological trait) that can be measured in a standardized fashion and that has been associated in prospective studies to be an independent predictor of the development of CAD. This definition will likely undergo refinement in the future, but it emphasizes the need for scientific rigor when applying screening and treatment algorithms in clinical practice. The characterization of a trait as a risk factor is a slow and methodical process. Initial observations in case-control studies must be confirmed in large-scale prospective studies wherein problems inherent to selection bias can be accounted for. The number of subjects observed and the duration of observation, the statistical power of the study, and the questions asked (as well as the interpretation of the answers) are essential design criteria. A single study is rarely sufficient to change medical practice and determine public health issues. Confirmation from other cohorts is sought; only when the data are solid and reproducible can a trait be considered as a risk factor.

For CAD, male gender, increasing age, elevated plasma cholesterol, decreased plasma levels of high-density lipoprotein (HDL) cholesterol, elevated blood pressure, and diabetes constitute the categorical risk factors (see Chapter 3) and form the basis of the current approach toward controlling the CAD pandemic.[11,12]

Many other risk factors, however, have not fulfilled these criteria or are still under intense scientific scrutiny. As such, they have not yet been included in the current guidelines for the prevention of CAD and are considered as emergent or conditional risk factors.[4] A set of postulates must be met before a novel risk factor is included within public health guidelines for screening and treatment: The trait must be shown in several prospective studies to be causally related to the disease; it must be safely treatable; and modification of the trait must lead to increased survival.

Epidemiologic studies of CAD were initiated in the 1950s and have shown the importance of risk factors for CAD. Long-term observational studies such as the Framingham and Procam studies have provided sufficient prospective data to develop mathematical models that allow the prediction of CAD in groups of asymptomatic subjects. Individual risk is far more difficult to determine, but physicians can apply preventive measures in specific patients in order to decrease overall cardiovascular risk. This approach now forms the basis of the National Cholesterol Education Program Adult Treatment Panel III (NCEP III), the European Guidelines for the prevention of CAD, and the Canadian Guidelines for the treatment of dyslipidemias.[4,11,12] Recent epidemiologic studies have shown the importance of and interrelationships among visceral obesity, insulin resistance, plasma lipoprotein disorders, high blood pressure, and multiple systemic effects affecting almost all markers of cardiovascular disease and contributing to much of the increase in cardiovascular risk in our society.[8,15,16]

■ ▦ ■

TABLE 9–1 NOVEL RISK FACTORS FOR CORONARY ARTERY DISEASE

Metabolic syndrome
Lipoprotein factors (discussed in Chapter 3)
   High-density lipoprotein C
   Low-density lipoprotein particle size
   Apolipoproteins AI, B, and E
   Triglyceride-rich lipoprotein
   Lipoprotein (a)
Homocysteine
Infectious (discussed in Chapter 7)
   Chlamydia pneumoniae
   Helicobacter pylori
Inflammatory (discussed in Chapters 6 and 16)
   C-reactive protein
   Interleukins, tumor necrosis factor α, interferon-γ
   Markers of plaque fragility
Coagulation factors
   Fibrinogen
   von Willebrand factor
   Factors VII, VIII, IX, X, XII
   Fibrinopeptide A
Fibrinolysis factors
   Tissue plasminogen activator
   Plasminogen activator inhibitor
   D-dimer
Cell adhesion molecule
   Intracellular cell adhesion molecule
   Vascular cell adhesion molecule
   E-selectin
   P-selectin
Genetic predisposition (discussed in Chapter 3)
Psychological factors (discussed in Chapter 10)

NOVEL RISK FACTORS AS POTENTIAL PREDICTORS OF RECURRENT EVENTS IN ACUTE CORONARY SYNDROMES

Compared with chronic stable CAD, patients with ACSs have a markedly elevated short-term increase in cardiovascular events. To date, none of the traditional cardiovascular risk factors has helped determine which patients will sustain another event in the weeks following presentation with an ACS. Because the pathophysiological processes leading to the formation of an unstable atherosclerotic plaque involve many factors related to inflammation, cytokines, adhesion molecules, matrix metallo-proteinases, and several proteins transiently expressed during an inflammatory reaction, measurements of one or more of these factors might help predict recurrent events and perhaps guide therapy. The list of such potential predictors is constantly lengthening as new evidence is published in the literature. Identifying such markers will require the design of epidemiologic studies that account for the clinical condition of the patient during which blood was drawn for measurement, the accuracy and the biologic variability of the biochemical measurement, the possibility of circadian variation, gender and hormonal differences, and the overall systemic state

of the individual (with respect to other inflammatory processes such as transient viral illness, nutritional status, presence of arthritis or systemic inflammatory reactions, and other parameters that can influence acute phase reactants). Also under consideration will be the severity of the ACS at the time of presentation and the statistical power of the study under consideration as well as the multivariate analysis to eliminate confounding bias. To date, few studies fulfill these criteria. Therefore, many of the molecules, proteins, and markers examined in this chapter have yet to be prospectively associated with a worse prognosis in ACS; furthermore, it remains unclear what specific action their detection should trigger in terms of patient management.

CATEGORICAL RISK FACTORS

The NCEP guidelines recognize categorical risk factors for risk prediction.[11] These include increasing age, male gender, diabetes, cigarette smoking, elevated blood pressure, elevated total cholesterol (or low-density lipoprotein [LDL] cholesterol), and decreased HDL cholesterol (Table 9–2). These parameters are used in a cardiovascular disease prevention program to determine the overall risk of a cardiovascular event in the next 10 years in subjects not known to have atherosclerosis. From a global score, derived from the presence and severity of these risk factors, a patient's risk is determined to be very high, high, or moderate. In turn, this determines the goals of therapy. Major changes in the 2001 guidelines of the NCEP ATP III, compared with previous versions, include raising the threshold for HDL-C as a risk factor to less than 40 mg/dL and the inclusion of diabetic patients in the very-high-risk category, regardless of other risk factors or the absence of atherosclerotic vascular disease. The realization that clustering of risk factors characteristic of the insulin resistance syndrome and including multiple biochemical abnormalities predisposes to atherosclerotic heart disease has led the NCEP to better define this syndrome and provide guidelines for treatment.

■ ▦ ■

TABLE 9–2 CATEGORICAL RISK FACTORS (NCEP III)

Age
Male gender
Diabetes
Cigarette smoking
Elevated blood pressure
Elevated total (or low-density lipoprotein) cholesterol
Decreased high-density lipoprotein C (40 mg/dL or ~1.0 mmol/L)
Physical inactivity
Obesity
Metabolic syndrome
Family history

METABOLIC SYNDROME

Affluent societies bear the burden of the wages of their sins, medically speaking. In developed countries, urbanization, physical inactivity, overabundance of food, and loss of the balance between caloric intake and energy expenditure have led to an explosion in the prevalence of obesity, insulin resistance, and diabetes mellitus and contribute to reverse the tremendous gains made in the decreased incidence of CAD in the past 50 years. The pattern of distribution of adipose tissue appears to be a key determinant of the metabolic consequences associated with obesity. A gynecoid distribution of fat is predominantly subcutaneous and does not confer a major increase in cardiovascular risk. An android fat distribution, which is predominantly visceral (i.e., around the mesentery), increases the waist/hip ratio. This latter type of obesity is associated with many of the categorical risk factors and several metabolic abnormalities that confer additional cardiovascular risk. Subjects with abdominal obesity have higher blood pressure, a lower HDL cholesterol level, higher total cholesterol, insulin resistance, and abnormal glucose metabolism. In addition, elevated plasma triglycerides, the presence of small dense LDL particles, increased fibrinogen, altered fibrinolysis, and increased CRP are part of the metabolic syndrome.[4,5,8,17,18]

The complex interrelationships between abdominal obesity and cardiovascular risk factors makes it difficult to assess individual risk factors in the overall determination of risk. This is due to the statistical analysis process in multivariate regression models that eliminate the variable "obesity" as a risk factor. Clinicians now recognize that visceral obesity is a major health problem and that its incidence grows in tandem with that of diabetes. The revised guidelines now propose a novel approach designed to stem the epidemic of obesity and its associated consequences. Under the acronym *TLC,* which stands for *t*herapeutic *l*ifestyle *c*hanges, the aim is to use a targeted approach at weight control, exercise, and diet.[11]

The metabolic syndrome has been difficult to define accurately in terms of strict cut-points but it is by far the most prevalent phenotype identifiable in subjects at high risk for CAD.

LIPOPROTEIN FACTORS

The conventional lipid profile used in the diagnosis and treatment of most disorders of lipoproteins include total plasma cholesterol, triglyceride levels, and HDL cholesterol, from which the LDL-C level is calculated using the Friedewald formula.[19] This approach is accurate when plasma triglyceride levels are below 400 mg/dL (4.5 mmol/L). The rare exception to the use of the Friedewald formula, other than moderate and severe hypertriglyceridemia, occurs in patients with the rare type III hyperlipoproteinemia. In such cases, LDL-C must be measured with the use of ultracentrifugation or direct LDL-C measurement. There has been intense debate in recent decades as to the predictive value of other measurements of lipoprotein composition, apolipoprotein (apo) content, or specific lipoproteins. To date, lipoprotein (a) has shown some promise as an independent variable. The use of total cholesterol or LDL cholesterol for the determination of cardiovascular risk has recently assumed a lesser importance. Many studies have shown that the LDL-C level is a better predictor of disease than total cholesterol but the total cholesterol is easier to use in screening programs and in algorithms. The total cholesterol/HDL-C ratio is a better predictor than either variables and is currently considered a secondary target in the Canadian guidelines for the treatment of dyslipidemias. The NCEP ATP III has rather focused on the secondary target of non-HDL cholesterol. This measurement includes cholesterol contained within very-low-density lipoproteins (VLDLs), intermediate-density lipoproteins (and remnant particles), and LDLs. This measurement is a more global index of atherogenic lipoprotein cholesterol. Some authorities have argued that because each of these lipoproteins contain one molecule of apo B, the measurement of apo B is a better reflection of atherogenic lipoproteins.

HDL-C

As mentioned in Chapter 3, a reduced plasma level of HDL cholesterol is considered a major risk factor for the development of CAD and is part of the current recommendations for cardiovascular risk stratification. The revised NCEP guidelines now state that a HDL-C level of less than 40 mg/dL (~1 mmol/L) is a categorical risk factor.[11] HDL particles have multiple beneficial effects on vascular tissue, especially on vascular endothelial cells.[20] Prospective epidemiologic studies have attempted to identify subfractions or components of HDL particles as variables that would increase the predictive value of HDLs. In this light, subfractions HDL3 and HDL2, HDL particle size, HDL phospholipid content, and apo content (more specifically apo AI and apo AII) have not been shown to be better predictors that total HDL cholesterol.[21]

The therapeutic action that should be implemented in the presence of a low HDL-C level is debated. Current lipid-modifying drugs do not raise HDL-C levels significantly (Table 9–3). Drugs aimed at raising HDL-C levels by modulating key steps in HDL metabolism are being investigated. Inhibition of cholesteryl ester transfer protein raises HDL-C levels significantly, but the effect on CAD is currently not known. Drugs aimed at raising the adenosine triphosphate–binding cassette transported A1 (ABCA1)-mediated cellular cholesterol efflux are under active scrutiny. Because a low HDL-C level is a component of the metabolic syndrome, another approach has been to target lifestyle changes, including a reduction in visceral obesity, a reduction in the relative and absolute quantities of saturated fat consumed toward monounsaturated fats, and an increase in physical exercise. Moderate alcohol intake has a beneficial effect on HDL-C levels.[22] Epidemiologic studies have supported the concept that moderate alcohol consumption is

■ ■■ ■

TABLE 9–3   CHANGE IN HIGH-DENSITY LIPOPROTEIN C (HDL-C) CLINICAL STUDIES AND RELATION WITH CARDIOVASCULAR EVENTS

	HDL-C CHOLESTEROL	
STUDY	**HDL-C % Change**	**Relation to CVE**
Primary Prevention		
Helsinki Heart Study (gemfibrozil)	+11%	*P* <.001
AF/TexCAPS	+6%	NS
WOSCOPS	+5%	NS
Secondary Prevention		
CARE (pravastatin)	+5%	NS
4S (simvastatin)	+8%	*P* = .001
VA-HIT (gemfibrozil)	+6%	*P* < .05
BIP (bezafibrate)	+18%	NS*
DAIS (fenofibrate)	+6%	?
HAT (simvastatin + niacin)	+26%	ND

CVE, cardiovascular events; ND, no data; NS, not significant.

associated with reduced cardiovascular and total mortality. Excessive alcohol intake, however, exerts a terrible toll in violent deaths, liver disease, and social ills in general.

Lipoprotein Subfractions

The search for better markers of cardiovascular disease has triggered a search for lipoprotein fractions that are "atherogenic," the measurement of which would allow better discrimination between subjects at risk for vascular disease and those not at risk. To date, however, the data with subfractions of HDLs, VLDLs, remnant particles, or LDL particles have not been convincing. The measurement of LDL particle size showed initial promise and is a component of the metabolic syndrome.[18] Most studies, however, have not shown that LDL particle size is an independent cardiovascular risk factor. In large-scale population studies, such as the Framingham study, LDL particle size is determined by plasma triglyceride and HDL-C levels.

The identification of cholesteryl ester–rich remnant lipoproteins in the intermediate lipoprotein density range as being atherogenic has led to novel techniques for their measurement. Remnant lipoprotein cholesterol can be directly measured in plasma.[23,24] Case-control studies have shown that remnant lipoprotein cholesterol is a risk factor for CAD but correlates strongly with other lipoprotein measurements.[26-30] It is too early to recommend such measurement in cardiovascular risk stratification.

Plasma sphingomyelin levels have also been identified as a cardiovascular risk factor. Interestingly, sphingomyelin levels correlate with remnant cholesterol levels and might thus indicate an increase in remnant lipoproteins in plasma.[31] Lipoprotein-associated phospholipase A_2 has been shown to be associated with increased cardiovascular risk. Mechanistically, these observations can be reconciled by a hypothesis put forth by Williams and Tabas whereby atherogenic lipoproteins aggregate and contribute to the atherogenesis "response to retention" hypothesis.[32]

Apolipoproteins AI, B, and E

Apo AI is the major protein constituent of HDL particles and accounts for approximately 70% of HDL protein mass. Some earlier studies suggested that apo AI was a better discriminator that HDL-C levels, but this has not withstood statistical scrutiny.[33] Apo B has been considered as a potential candidate either to replace total and LDL cholesterol levels or to be used in screening and treatment algorithms. Apo B is a large protein present as a single copy on VLDL, intermediate-density lipoprotein, and LDL particles. Apo B is therefore a very good index of the number of atherogenic lipoproteins in plasma. In conditions wherein the LDL-C level may be relatively normal (especially in the presence of elevated plasma triglycerides and reduced HDL-C levels, which produce a small LDL particle with reduced cholesterol content), apo B may be an index of an atherogenic state. Opinions on the usefulness of apo B vary, but current recommendations have not included its measurement in clinical practice. Apo E is a major apolipoprotein on triglyceride-rich lipoprotein and remnant particles. Three isoforms—apo E2, E3, and E4—exist in humans, giving rise to six possible phenotypes (E2/2, 2/3, 2/4, 3/3, 3/4, 4/4). Apo E2/2 is required for the development of type III hyperlipoproteinemia. This rare lipoprotein disorder is associated with a marked increase in remnant particles and an increase in atherosclerosis.[27] The apo E4/4 phenotype is associated with early manifestations of Alzheimer disease and predisposes in the long term to atherosclerosis. The effects on cardiac risk, however, are in part explained by lipoprotein changes in apo E4/4 subjects. Apo E phenotype of genotype is not currently recommended for cardiovascular risk stratification.

Experienced clinicians have long considered plasma triglyceride levels to be a risk factor. The relationship between plasma triglycerides and CAD, however, is not linear and is complex. Because of the close relationship between plasma triglyceride and HDL-C levels, the former has often been dropped from multivariate models of cardiovascular risk.[33,34] The search for a class of triglyceride-rich lipoproteins that adds further information to that provided by the conventional lipid profile has led to various measurements that have yet to show their clinical usefulness. These include the measurement of "remnant lipoprotein cholesterol",[24] VLDL subfractions, and apolipoprotein-specific lipoprotein measurement (such as lipoprotein B:E or lipoprotein B:CIII particles).[33] Despite their conceptual appeal, none of these particles is part of conventional cardiovascular risk profiling tools. In the Cholesterol And Recurrent Events (CARE) trial, VLDL, VLDL apo B, VLDL apo CIII, and VLDL apo E were shown to predict recurrent cardiovascular risk.[33a,35] It should be emphasized that participants in the CARE trial had relatively low plasma LDL-C levels. In such circumstances, lipoproteins other that LDL appear to confer relatively more risk. This was shown in the Veteran's Administration HDL intervention Trial (VA-HIT), wherein reducing of plasma triglycerides and raising HDL-C levels with gemfibrozil (a fibric acid derivative) decreased recurrent cardiovascular events and strokes.[36] Thus, patients with elevated plasma triglycerides and reduced HDL-C levels in the presence of a normal LDL-C level benefit from a reduction in plasma triglyceride–rich lipoproteins and raised HDL-C levels.

Lipoprotein a

Lipoprotein (a) is a lipoprotein that shares many of the characteristics as LDL particles.[37] The structure of lipoprotein (a) consists of one LDL particle to which is covalently linked one molecule of apo (a) through a cystine bond.[38,39] The apo (a) gene is located on chromosome 6, close to that of plasminogen and an apo (a) pseudogene. The structure of the apo (a) gene resembles that of plasminogen in that repetitive motifs called *kringles* are visible in both proteins, with a high degree of homology. Apo (a), the protein encoded by the apo (a) gene is a highly glycosylated protein that shares homology with plasminogen.[38] Unlike plasminogen, apo (a) does not have an active serine esterase proteolytic cleavage site. Plasminogen is formed of five kringle motifs, and apo (a) has multiple copies of kringle 4. The gene is highly polymorphic, and plasma lipoprotein (a) levels are highly negatively correlated with the number of repetitive kringle IV domain present in the mature apo (a). The molecular weight of apo (a) varies between 300 and 800 kDa, reflecting the number of kringle 4 repeats, which can vary between 3 and 48. Plasma levels of lipoprotein (a) are highly heritable, with almost all of the genetic variability being accounted for by DNA sequence variations within the apo (a) gene.[38,40-45] This genetic variability is explained in great part by the number of kringle repeats but also by apo (a) haplotypes that are not associated with kringle repeat number. As a trait, lipoprotein (a) is one of the most genetically determined risk factors for CAD. Population studies show that the distribution of lipoprotein (a) is markedly skewed to the right.

Interspecies differences in lipoprotein (a) levels remain unexplained on the basis of the known genetic variability of the apo (a) gene.[43-46] In African Americans, for instance, the median plasma lipoprotein (a) levels are nearly three times higher than in Caucasians.

Apo (a) is synthesized in the liver, and production rates determine some of the differences in lipoprotein (a) levels in plasma. The mechanisms by which lipoprotein (a) is formed has been the matter of some debate. The current concept is that the assembly of lipoprotein (a) takes place after secretion of apo (a) from the liver (and therefore, after protein glycosylation) in a two-step process. First, apo (a) associates noncovalently with the apo B moiety of LDL particles; second, apo (a) is covalently linked by a cystine bridge from a kringle 4 domain of apo (a) to residue 4326 of apo B on LDL.[38,47-49] Catabolism of lipoprotein (a) and apo (a) remains somewhat of a puzzle. A relatively small portion of plasma lipoprotein (a) is taken up by receptor-mediated endocytosis via the LDL receptor and possibly by the VLDL receptor. The kidney appears to be a major site of lipoprotein (a) degradation. Some factors modulate plasma lipoprotein (a) levels. Plasma lipoprotein (a) levels are lower in patients using estrogens or testosterone, in hyperthyroidism, or with the use of drugs such as nicotinic acid (niacin) or metformin. Conversely, renal insufficiency, inflammation (acute-phase reactant), menopause, orchiectomy, hypothyroidism, and drugs such as isotretinoin and troglitazone are associated with increased lipoprotein (a) levels.

Clinical studies, first in the form of case-control studies, initially associated plasma lipoprotein (a) levels with atherosclerosis.[50,51] Conflicting results were then reported in prospective studies, mostly in the form of nested case-control studies.[52-55] Major epidemiologic flaws have hampered the interpretation of these studies. A major concern is the lack of an appropriate standard for the measurement of lipoprotein (a). Other considerations include the lack of control for confounders listed earlier, difference in population studied, condition of plasma storage, and selection bias inherent in some studies. A recent meta-analysis of prospective studies reveal that lipoprotein (a) is a risk factor for CAD even after adjustment for confounding variables.[56]

Lipoprotein (a) may be causal in the pathogenesis of atherosclerosis by a variety of mechanisms[58-65]: the lipoprotein is an LDL-sized lipoprotein and can thus be oxidized and cause an inflammatory reaction and be taken up by macrophages; lipoprotein (a) interacts with endothelial cells, increases the expression of cell adhesion molecules, and promotes the recruitment of inflammatory cells. The apo (a) moiety competes with plasminogen for its cell surface receptor, thereby preventing the formation of activated plasmin. Oxidized lipoprotein (a) is taken up by scavenger receptors on macrophages and increases foam cells. An interesting finding has been that the reduced generation of plasmin leads to a reduction in the generation of transforming growth factor β, leading to an increase in smooth muscle cell proliferation, and lipoprotein (a) may interfere with endothelial cell proliferation. Lipoprotein (a) may also promote angiogenesis.[66]

The initial enthusiasm for measuring lipoprotein (a) in a preventive setting has been dampened by the lack of coherence between studies and the lack of effective treatment. Currently, no drug specifically lowers lipoprotein (a) levels, although niacin and estrogens are used for that purpose. In the absence of controlled clinical trials that specifically address the issue of lowering lipoprotein (a) to prevent the development of atherosclerosis, current guidelines do not include lipoprotein (a) as a parameter to be included in screening strategies. When available, the measurement of apo A may shed some light in cases of unexplained atherosclerosis. What to do with an elevated lipoprotein (a) remains controversial. Although niacin reduces lipoprotein (a) levels, its use is hampered by lack of tolerance and side effects. Estrogen replacement is not recommended in secondary prevention in women because of the results of the Heart and Estrogen/Progestin Replacement (HERS) study. Another strategy in patients with elevated lipoprotein (a) is to markedly lower LDL-C levels and to give aspirin. This strategy has little effect on lipoprotein (a) levels but might reduce the risk attributable to lipoprotein (a) when LDL-C is low.

HOMOCYSTEINE

Homocysteine is a nonessential amino acid formed during the demethylation of methionine. Homocysteine is found in plasma in the free form (~1%), as homocystine (5% to 10%) or the homocysteine-cysteine mixed disulfide (5% to 10%), or as protein-bound homocysteine (~80% to 90%). Collectively, these forms are called *total plasma homocysteine* or *tHcy*. Methionine is obtained from the diet or during protein turnover and donates its methyl group to form s-adenosyl methionine. In turn, this methyl group is used in over 100 different biochemical reactions, including DNA methylation, synthesis of norepinephrine and phospholipids (phosphatidyl choline), and creatine metabolism. The resultant molecule, s-adenosyl homocysteine, is then recycled into adenosine and homocysteine. At plasma concentrations that exceed the norm (usually approximately 10 μM), homocysteine is associated with endothelial dysfunction and, at high concentrations, appears to mediate several prothrombotic mechanisms. Inborn errors of metabolism of the methionine-homocysteine pathway, especially homocystinuria and hyperhomocysteinemia, cause widespread venous and arterial thrombosis and are a major cause of morbidity and mortality in affected persons. The association between homocysteine and CAD was initially examined over 30 years ago by Wilken and subsequently by Malinow and colleagues.[67,68]

The major determinant of plasma homocysteine level is the status of vitamins B_{12}, B_6, and folate. These vitamins are essential in the metabolism of homocysteine. Homocysteine can be metabolized by two distinct but coordinately regulated pathways. Homocysteine can be used to form cysteine or can be methylated to form methionine. Vitamin B_6 is a cofactor in the sulfoconjugation of homocysteine and serine to form γ-cystathionine, a step catabolized by cystathionine β-synthase. Folic acid and cyanocobalamin (vitamin B_{12}) are used in the remethylation reaction of homocysteine to form methionine. The rate-limiting step in this reaction is 5, 10-methylene tetrahydrofolate reductase (MTHFR). Nutritional deficiencies of any of these three vitamins can cause elevated homocysteine levels.

From a population standpoint, plasma levels of tHcy are determined by levels of vitamins B_{12}, B_6, and folate. Conversely, in mild to moderate hyperhomocystinemia, dietary supplementation with these vitamins can often lower homocysteine levels. Mutations of the genes coding for enzymes involved in homocysteine metabolism have been associated with severe homocystinemia and homocystinuria. Polymorphisms within these genes have also been associated with altered plasma homocysteine levels. The best-characterized polymorphism is the MTHFR C677T that causes thermolability of the enzyme and increased plasma homocysteine levels, especially in conditions wherein folate is low. Interestingly, subjects with the MTHFR C677T polymorphism have normal homocysteine levels when supplemented with dietary folate. This is an example of gene/environment interaction wherein a genetic predisposition (MTHFR C677T) can be corrected by environmental intervention (folate supplementation).

To date, at least 80 case-control studies have shown an association between tHcy and vascular disease (carotid, coronary, and peripheral). A meta-analysis of some of the case-control studies concluded that in both men and women, cardiovascular risk was increased significantly for each 5 μM increase in plasma tHcy.[69,70] Data from prospective studies, mostly in the form of nested case-control investigations, have not been as consistent.[71-74] Indeed, the prospective data have lead to a more conservative evaluation of tHcy as a cardiovascular risk factor.[75-78,79] In subjects with diabetes, homocysteine appeared to confer additional risk.[80,81] Plasma homocysteine levels have been found to correlate with D-dimer, fibrinogen, and von Willebrand factor, among others.[73] Epidemiologically, it has not been possible to determine whether homocysteine is an independent cardiovascular risk factor. In patients with established CAD, especially postmyocardial infarction, tHcy is a strong and independent predictor of mortality.[74-82] It is conceivable that homocysteine may be a marker of disease rather than a predictive cardiovascular risk factor.

The mechanisms by which tHcy mediates cardiovascular disease are not clear. Homocysteine has been shown to increase protein C activation, thrombomodulin surface expression, and tissue plasminogen activator binding; to alter heparan sulfate expression; to increase factor V activation and tissue factor expression; and to promote lipoprotein (a) binding to fibrin. In vitro experiments using cultured endothelial cells have shown that homocysteine has a procoagulant effect and promotes smooth muscle cell proliferation and decreases endothelial cell proliferation. The experimental conditions under which many of these experiments have been carried out have, in retrospect, been the subject of criticism.

The treatment of mild to moderate hyperhomocystinemia has not yet been shown to reduce cardiovascular risk. There are currently a dozen trials of CAD and stroke prevention by vitamins B_{12}, folate, and B_6 that include an aggregate of 65,000 subjects. Results of these trials are expected between 2003 and 2005. The mainstay of treatment is vitamin supplementation. Although intervention thresholds and goals of therapy have not been determined and the benefit of vitamin supplementation has not been shown, no recommendation can be made for the screening of and treatment for elevated homocysteine levels. In patients with vascular disease with an elevated tHcy level, a therapeutic goal of less than 10 μM tHcy has been proposed by some authorities. Dietary supplementation with folate (0.8 to 5 mg/day), alone or in combination with vitamin B_{12} (0.5 to 1 mg/day) and vitamin B_6 (25 mg/day), has been proposed. This regimen significantly lowers tHcy levels in the majority of subjects by 20% to 50%. Patients with renal failure and those on hemodialysis have markedly elevated tHcy levels and do not respond to dietary vitamin supplementation. High-dose folic acid has been shown to reduce tHcy in end-stage renal disease, although not to proposed therapeutic goals.

Agencies such as the American Heart Association, the International Task Force for the Prevention of Cardiovascular Diseases (based in Europe), and the Canadian Cardiovascular Society state that data are insufficient to recommend the measurement of plasma tHcy levels for cardiovascular disease prevention. In the secondary prevention of cardiovascular disease, some authorities recommend vitamin supplementation (folate alone or in combination with vitamins B_{12} and B_6). The argument that treatment is innocuous and might be helpful should not be used in a context of public health. Clinical trials will soon provide conclusive data on this issue. In the interim, clinical judgment is warranted.

INFECTIOUS FACTORS

The potential direct or indirect role of bacterial or viral infections in precipitating coronary artery disease is discussed in Chapter 7.

INFLAMMATORY FACTORS

The importance of inflammatory markers has been highlighted by the work of Ridker et al.[84] CRP is one of the most promising new cardiovascular risk factors. In multiple nested case-control prospective studies, CRP has been shown to confer additional cardiovascular risk and to add to the conventional risk factors. In addition, the response to the statin class of lipid-lowering medications can be predicted, in part, by the measurement of CRP levels.[84] This topic is dealt with in detail in Chapter 16.

COAGULATION FACTORS

Fibrinogen

Coagulation factors, especially fibrinogen,[85] have been shown to be associated with CAD in prospective studies.

Meta-analyses have shown that such factors are an independent cardiovascular risk factor. In the Prospective Cardiovascular Study, Münster (PROCAM) study, the relative risk of patients in the top tertile of plasma fibrinogen was 2.4 times higher than those in the bottom tertile; even after correction for confounding variables, this relation was statistically significant.[86] Similarly, combined results from the Caerphilly and Speedwell studies in the United Kingdom have shown that subjects with fibrinogen levels in the top quintile experienced a 4.1-fold increase in cardiovascular risk.[87-92] In the Framingham offspring study, Stec et al[91] showed that plasma fibrinogen levels are closely correlated with age, body mass index, smoking, the presence of diabetes, total cholesterol, HDL cholesterol, and triglycerides. Measurement techniques seem to influence results. The more recent immunoprecipitation method (American Biogenic Sciences) appears more specific than the functional Clauss method. The weight of the data suggests that fibrinogen is an independent risk factor, even after correction for confounding variables. It is not clear, however, whether the measurement of fibrinogen should influence clinical decision-making. Nor has it been established whether interventions aimed at lowering plasma fibrinogen levels can decrease overall cardiovascular risk. Current guidelines do not recommend the routine measurement of fibrinogen to determine cardiovascular risk.[93]

Plasma levels of activated VIII, factor VII, and fibrinopeptide A have been shown to be associated with atherosclerotic vascular disease in many studies. Similarly, prothrombin fragments 1 and 2, fibrinopeptide A, factor IX, and factor X, and activated factor XII have been associated with myocardial infarction in prospective studies.[94-102] However, after adjustment for other cardiovascular risk factors, such as apo AI and activated factor VII, these factors were no longer statistically significantly associated with acute MI.[97] Interestingly, there is a strong relationship between altered plasma levels of hemostatic factors and obesity.[103]

FIBRINOLYSIS FACTORS

The endothelium has multiple functions but can be conceptually grouped in two major functions: to *vasodilate* in response to physiologic demands and to *keep blood liquid*. The latter mechanism is provided by a complex interplay between the need to form blood clots when the endothelium has been broken and dissolving these clots to restore normal blood flow. Fibrinolysis is controlled by tissue plasminogen activator (t-PA) and urokinase-type plasminogen activator (u-PA) and their endogenous inhibitors—mainly, plasminogen activator inhibitor 1 (PAI-1). PAI-1 levels are increased in patients with CAD and may reflect an increased propensity for altered fibrinolysis.

Tissue Plasminogen Activator

Tissue Plasminogen Activator (t-PA) is secreted by the endothelium in response to a noxious stimulus. The role of t-PA is to enhance clot lysis. Several studies have shown an association between CAD and reduced levels of t-PA.[104-106] Conversely, plasma levels of PAI-1 are associated with increased cardiovascular risk. PAI-1 levels correlate positively with plasma triglyceride levels.[107-111] PAI-1 is produced not solely be vascular endothelial cells and platelets but by adipocytes as well. In patients affected with the metabolic syndrome and abdominal obesity, PAI-1 levels are elevated.[112-114] The data thus indicate that an imbalance between decreased fibrinolysis and increased fibrinolysis inhibition constitutes a risk for atherosclerosis. Plasma measurement of PAI-1 depends on proper technique in order to avoid release of PAI-1 from platelets during phlebotomy. In addition, PAI-1 levels in plasma follow circadian variations, with peak levels encountered in the morning.[115] Clot lysis time is a reflection of plasminogen activators and inhibitors and reflects the physiologic counterpart to the direct measurement of these parameters. Clot lysis time is also a predictor of coronary risk.

D-Dimer

The measurement of serum levels of D-dimer is a marker of fibrinogen breakdown and turnover. D-dimer may therefore reflect enhanced propensity for clot formation (and subsequent lysis). Prospective studies and a recent meta-analysis suggest that serum D-dimer levels are positively correlated with CAD. A significant correlation was observed between D-dimers with CRP and serum amyloid A but not with smoking, lipoprotein lipids, and blood pressure.[95,116] Despite the sound biologic and pathophysiologic basis for their measurement, fibrinolysis factors appear to add little to the overall prediction of cardiovascular risk.

CELL ADHESION MOLECULES

Cell adhesion molecules are proteins expressed on the surface of cells, including the vascular endothelial cells, platelets, and leukocytes. They mediate the slowing, rolling, and adhesion of blood-borne cells to the endothelium. Intracellular cell adhesion molecule (ICAM-1) and vascular cell adhesion molecule (VCAM-1) are membrane proteins that are expressed by a dysfunctional endothelium. They can be cleaved from the membrane and measured in serum by highly sensitive assays. Similarly, E-selectin and P-selectin, respectively expressed on endothelial cells and platelets, are two other CAMs that can be identified in plasma in their soluble forms. They are implicated in the initial stages of atherosclerosis when endothelial dysfunction first appears. CAMs mediate the adhesion and migration of monocytes to the subendothelial layer, where they come into contact with oxidized lipoproteins and initiate the formation of the atherosclerotic plaque. CAMs are expressed in more complicated lesions and contribute to the cellular inflammatory component of the plaque, which may contribute to plaque instability.

Several studies have prospectively examined the soluble forms of ICAM-1, VCAM-1, E-selectin, and P-selection

as potential risk factors.[117-119] Results from several studies have suggested that ICAM-1 and E-selectin are both predictors of CAD; the data are less strong for VCAM-1.[117-119] The pattern of expression of VCAM-1 and ICAM-1 differ in atherosclerosis plaques, suggesting that they may have different roles during the atherosclerosis process. Conflicting results have been published on the value of CAMs in their ability to predict ACSs. In one study by O'Malley et al, soluble ICAM was considered to represent a potential marker for ACSs.[119] These conclusions have been challenged by the results of a moderately large prospective study of ICAM-1, VCAM-1, E-selectin, and P-selectin in 643 patients with CAD and 1278 controls in a nested-control prospective study design. In addition, the authors performed a meta-analysis of these CAMs based on published reports. Only ICAM-1 was considered a significant predictor of CAD (odds ratio, 1.68; 95% CI, 1.32 to 2.14). However, this odds ratio decreased to 1.11 (95% CI, 0.75 to 1.64) after adjustment for conventional risk factors and socioeconomic status. A trend was also observed for E-selectin, but after correction for possible confounders, VCAM, E-selectin, and P-selectin were not shown to be significant predictors of CAD. On the basis of their findings and the results of their meta-analysis, the authors concluded that the measurement of CAMs in plasma is unlikely to add much predictive information over that provided by more established risk factors.[118]

At present, therefore, the measurement of the soluble form of the CAMs ICAM-1, VCAM-1, E-selectin, and P-selectin should be considered more in a research context and do not appear to add further information in terms of cardiovascular risk stratification. It remains to be established whether direct inhibition of these CAMs will prevent atherosclerosis or its sequelae.

GENETIC PREDISPOSITION

A family history of CAD has long been considered a cardiovascular risk factor. Family studies of MI survivors and patients with premature CAD have identified familial forms of lipoprotein disorders. Monogenic disorders such as familial hypercholesterolemia are strongly associated with premature CAD. A family history of CAD is no longer considered a cardiovascular risk factor in the NCEP III guidelines.[11] The major reason for this change from earlier versions of the NCEP is the difficulty in defining family history of CAD and to discern a genetic contribution that is independent from conventional risk factors. For example, in familial hypercholesterolemia, the strong family history can be accounted for by the elevated levels of LDL-C in affected family members. Conversely, a strong family history can be due to the "shared household" effect, such as poor diet or cigarette smoking. Studying the genetics of CAD has been a major challenge in recent decades, when the genes coding for known proteins associated with various risk factors were cloned and sequenced and genetic polymorphisms were identified for population studies.

The genetics of CAD can be examined at three levels:

- *Monogenic disorders.* Many rare genetic disorders are associated with premature CAD, but the most important is familial hypercholesterolemia due to defects in the LDL receptor gene. This occurs in 3% to 5% of premature CAD cases. Rare lipoprotein disorders, including type III hyperlipoproteinemia due to a mutant apo E, familial HDL deficiency (Tangier disease) due to mutations in the ABCA1 gene, and mutations in the structural apolipoprotein genes (apo AI, apo E), account for less than 0.01% of premature CAD cases.
- *Disease susceptibility genes.* Functional mutations within genes coding for proteins involved in lipoprotein metabolism, diabetes, hypertension, and vascular biology have been identified in recent decades. Association studies have yielded important information on the link between these genes and CAD: Often the increase in risk is wholly (or in great part) attributable to the biologic effect of a measurable substance. For example, mutations at the lipoprotein lipase gene LPLGly188Glu are associated with a 78% increase in plasma triglyceride levels and a 0.25 mmol/L decrease in HDL-C. In a meta-analysis of LPL mutations and CAD, the presence of the LPLGly188Glu mutations is associated with a 4.9 (95% CI, 1.2 to 19.6) increase in CAD risk. Much of this risk is thought to be associated with changes in lipoprotein lipid levels, although an independent effect of LPL function on endothelial function cannot be excluded. Another example is the presence of the apolipoprotein E4 allele. Long-term follow-up of the Framingham Heart Study showed that subjects carrying the apo E4 allele experienced decreased survival at 30 years compared with subjects carrying the apo E2 or E3 alleles.
- *Association studies of genetic polymorphisms.* Despite over 20 years of research since the first genetic polymorphisms were identified, enthusiasm for such association studies has been somewhat dampened by the lack of consistency among studies, the effects of populations studied, the lack of a physiologic effect of the polymorphism observed, confounding variables and, very often, the lack of statistical power to answer the question.

PSYCHOLOGICAL FACTORS

Psychological factors are discussed in Chapter 10.

CONCLUSIONS

Recent years have seen an explosion in the knowledge of the biologic processes that lead to atherosclerotic plaque.[120] Refined analytical techniques have permitted the measurement of many molecules involved in endothelial dysfunction, adhesion of leukocytes, inflammatory mediators, coagulation, and fibrinolysis parameters in addition to refinement in the biochemical markers of conventional risk factors.[121] Large-scale epidemiologic studies (usually in the form of nested case-control studies) have been used to assess individual parameters found to be of interest in case-control studies without the bias typical of such studies. The analysis of candidate gene polymorphisms has uncovered very large

amounts of mutations and polymorphisms that are associated with CAD. Despite this wealth of information, current guidelines do not recommend screening for these factors for the prediction of a first coronary event (primary prevention).

CRP shows a strong, reproducible link with the development of CAD and may soon be part of screening algorithms. The usefulness of biochemical markers for recurrent events is obvious in clinical practice. Despite the vast gain in knowledge, clinical application of the parameters mentioned in this chapter to predict future coronary events remains uncertain. Epidemiologic data may be very strong for several of these markers of atherosclerosis, but it remains unclear how these markers will alter clinical practice. Furthermore, clinical studies are needed to assess the potential gains in terms of reductions in morbidity and mortality that these actions will have triggered.

New syndromes of cardiovascular risk factor clustering are being uncovered in patients with HIV infections treated with protease inhibition. This syndrome resembles the metabolic syndrome.[122-125] The epidemiology of CAD is complex, and the pathophysiology of the disease is still not fully identified. Great advances have been made in predicting which persons are at risk for atherosclerosis. Novel factors—such as the pregnancy-associated protein A,[126] cysteine,[127] novel inflammatory factors,[128,129] and infection[130,131]—must undergo rigorous scientific evaluation before they influence clinical decision-making. There is overwhelming evidence that atherosclerosis starts in childhood.[132] Preventive measures initiated early can only have beneficial long-term consequences on cardiovascular health.

REFERENCES

1. Morrow RH, Hyder AA, Murray CJ, Lopez AD: Measuring the burden of disease. Lancet 1998;352:1859–1861.
2. Lopez AD, Murray CC: The global burden of disease. 1998;11:1241–1243.
3. Murray CJ, Lopez AD: Global mortality, disability, and the contribution of risk factors: Global burden of disease study. 1997;349:1436–1442.
4. Coronary Heart Disease: Reducing the Risk; The scientific background for primary and secondary prevention of coronary heart disease. International Task Force for the Prevention of CAD. Nutr Metab Cardiovasc Dis 1999;2:1–89.
5. Despres JP, Lamarche B, Mauriege P, et al: Hyperinsulinemia as an independent risk factor for ischemic heart disease. N Engl J Med 1996;334:952–957.
6. Kannel W, McGee D: Diabetes and glucose tolerance as risk factors for cardiovascular disease. The Framingham Study: Diabetes Care 1979;2:120–126.
7. Peters A, Dockery DW, Muller JE, Mittleman MA: Increased particulate air pollution and the triggering of myocardial infarction. Circ 2001;103:2810.
8. Reaven GM. Banting Lecture 1988. Role of insulin resistance in human disease. Nutrition 1997;13:64–66.
9. Stamler J, Stamler R, Neaton JD, et al: Low risk factor profile and long-term cardiovascular and noncardiovascular mortality and life expectancy: findings for 5 large cohorts of young adult and middle-aged men and women. JAMA 1999;282:2012–2018.
10. Chambless L, Keil U, Dobson A, et al: Population versus clinical view of case fatality from acute coronary heart disease: results from the WHO MONICA Project 1985-1990. Multinational MONItoring of Trends and Determinants in CArdiovascular Disease. Circulation 1997;96:3849–3859.

11. Executive summary of the Third Report of the National Cholesterol Education Program (NCEP) Expert Panel on Detection, Evaluation, and Treatment of high blood cholesterol in Adults (Adult Treatment Panel III). JAMA 2001;285:2486-2497.

12. Fodor G, Frohlich J, Genest J Jr, McPherson R: Recommendations for the management and treatment of dyslipidemias. Report of the working group on hypercholesterolemia and other dyslipidemias. Can Med Ass J 2000;162:1441-1447.

13. Ridker PM: High-sensitivity C-reactive protein. Potential adjunct for global risk assessment in the primary prevention of cardiovascular disease. Circ 2001;103:1813.

14. Ridker PM, Rifai N, Clearfield M, et al: Measurement of c-reactive protein for the targeting of statin therapy in the primary prevention of acute coronary events. N Engl J Med 2001;344(26): 1959-1965.

15. Kannel WB, D'Agostino RB, Wilson PW, et al: Diabetes, fibrinogen, and risk of cardiovascular disease. The Framingham experience. Am Heart J 1990;120:672-676.

16. Grundy SM: Small LDL, atherogenic, dyslipidemia, and the metabolic syndrome. Circ 1997;95:1-4.

17. Juhan-Vague I, Thompson SG, Jespersen J: Involvement of the hemostatic system in the insulin resistance syndrome: A study of 1500 patients with angina pectoris. The ECAT Angina Pectoris Study Group. Arterioscler Thromb 1993;13:1865-1873.

18. Lamarche B, Tchernof A, Moorjani S, et al: Small, dense low-density lipoprotein particles as a predictor of the risk of ischemic heart disease in men. Prospective results from the Quebec Cardiovascular Study. Circ 1997;95:69-75.

19. Friedewald WT, Levy RI, Fredrickson DS: Estimation of the concentration of low-density lipoprotein cholesterol in plasma, without use of the preparative ultracentrifuge. Clin Chem 1972;18: 499-502.

20. O'Connell B, Genest J: High density lipoproteins and endothelial function. Circ 2001;104;1978-1983.

21. Genest JJ, Marcil M, Denis M, et al: High-density lipoproteins in health and in disease. J Invest Med 1999;47:31-42.

22. Goldberg IJ, Mosca L, Piano MR, Fisher EA: Wine and your heart. A science Advisory for Healthcare Professionals from the Nutrition Committee, Council on Epidemiology and Prevention, and Council on Cardiovascular Nursing of the American Heart Association. Circulaiton 2001;103:472.

23. Nakajima K, Saito T, Tamura A, et al: Cholesterol in remnant-like lipoproteins in human serum using monoclonal anti apo B-100 and anti apo A-1 immunoaffinity mixed gels. Clin Chem Acta 1993;223:53-71.

24. Nakajima K, Okazaki M, Tanaka A, et al: Separation and determination of remnant-like particles in human serum using monoclonal antibodies to apo B-100 and apo A-I. J Clin Ligand Assay 1996;19: 177-183.

26. Havel RJ: Remnant lipoproteins as therapeutic targets. Curr Opin Lipidol 2000;11:615-620.

27. Mahley RW, Ji ZS: Remnant lipoprotein metabolism: Key pathways involving cell-surface heparin sulfate proteoglycans and apolipoprotein E. J Lipid Res 1999;40:1-16.

28. Marcoux C, Tremblay M, Nakajima K, et al: Characterization of remnant-like particles isolated by immunoaffinity gel from the plasma of type III and type IV hyperlipoproteinemic patients. J Lipid Res 1999;40:636-647.

29. Masuoka H, Ishikura K, Kamei S, et al: Predictive value of remnant-like particles cholesterol/high-density lipoprotein cholesterol ratio as a new indicator of coronary artery disease. Am Heart J 1998;136:226-230.

30. Masuoka H, Kamei S, Wagayama H, et al: Association of remnant-like particles: cholesterol in patients with normal total cholesterol levels. Am Heart J 2000;139:305-310.

31. Jiang XC, Paultre F, Pearson TA, et al: Plasma sphingomyelin level as a risk factor for coronary artery disease. Arterioscler Thromb Vasc Biol 2000;20:2614-2618.

32. Williams KJ, Tabas I: The response-to-retention hypothesis of early atherosclerosis. Arterioscler Thromb Vasc Biol 1995;15:551-561.

33. Genest J Jr, McNamara JR, Ordovas JM, et al: Lipoprotein cholesterol, apolipoprotein a-i and b and lipoprotein (a) abnormalities in men with premature coronary artery disease. J Am Coll Cardiol 1992;19:792-802.

33a. Genest J Jr, Bard JM, Fruchart J-C, et al: Plasma apolipoproteins A-I, A-II, B, E and CIII containing particles in men with premature coronary artery disease. Atherosclerosis 1991;90:149-157.

34. Austin MA, McKnight B, Edwards KL, et al: Cardiovascular disease mortality in familial forms of hypertriglyceridemia: A 20-year prospective study. Circulation 2000;101:2777.

35. Sacks FM, Alaupovic P, Moye LA, et al: VLDL, apoproteins B, CIII, and E, and risk of recurrent coronary events in the cholesterol and recurrent (CARE) trial. Circulation 2000;102:1886.

36. Rubins HB, Robins SJ, Collins D, Fye CL, Anderson JW, et al: Gemfibrozil for the secondary prevention of coronary heart disease in men with low levels of high-density lipoprotein cholesterol. N Engl J Med 1999;341:410-418.

37. Berg K: A new serum type system in man—Lp system. Acta Pathol Microbiol Scand 1963;59:369-382.

38. Hobbs HH, White AL: Lipoprotein (a): Intrigues and insights. Curr Opin Lipidol 1999;10:225-236.

39. Koschinsky ML, Cote GP, Gabel B, Van der Hoek YY: Identification of the cysteine residue in Apolipoprotein (a) that mediates extracellular coupling with Apolipoprotein B-100. J Biol Chem 1993;268:19819-19825.

40. Boerwinkle E, Leffert CC, Lin J, et al: Apolipoprotein(a) gene accounts for greater than 90% of the variation in plasma lipoprotein(a) concentrations. J Clin Invest 1992;90:52-60.

41. Cohen JC, Chiesa G, Hobbs HH: Sequence polymorphisms in the Apolipoprotein(a) gene. Evidence for dissociation between Apolipoprotein(a) size and plasma lipoprotein(a) levels. J Clin Invest 1993;91:1630-1636.

42. Miles LA, Fless GM, Levin EG, et al: A potential basis for the thrombotic risks associated with lipoprotein(a). Nature 1989;339:301-303.

43. Wade DP, Lindahl GE, Lawn RM. apolipoprotein(a) gene transcription is regulated by liver-enriched trans-acting factor hepatocyte nuclear factor 1 alpha. J Biol Chem 1994;269:19757-19765.

44. Mooser V, Mancini FP, Boop S, et al: Sequence polymorphisms in the apo(a) gene associated with specific levels of Lp(a) in plasma. Hum Mol Genet 1995;4:173-181.

45. Puckey LH, Lawn RM, Knight BL: Polymorphisms in the apolipoprotein(a) gene and their relationship to allele size and plasma lipoprotein(a) concentration. Hum Mol Genet 1997;6: 1099-1107.

46. Rader DJ, Cain W, Zech LA, et al: Variation in lipoprotein(a) concentrations among individuals with the same Apolipoprotein(a) isoform is determined by the rate of lipoprotein(a) production. J Clin Invest 1993;91:443-447.

47. Sandholzer C, Hallman DM, Saha N, et al: Effects of the Apolipoprotein(a) size polymorphism on the lipoprotein(a) concentration 7 ethnic groups. Hum Genet 1991;86:607-614.

48. Wade DP, Puckey LH, Knight BL, et al: Characterization of multiple enhancer regions upstream of the apolipoprotein(a) gene. J Biol Chem 1997;272:30387-30399.

49. White AL, Lanford RE: Cell surface assembly of lipoprotein(a) in primary cultures of baboon hepatocytes. J Biol Chem 1994;269: 28716-28723.

50. Armstrong WW, Cremer P, Eberle E, et al: The association between serum Lp(a) concentrations and angiographically assessed coronary atherosclerosis; dependence on serum DL levels. Atherosclerosis 1986;62:249-257.

51. Genest J Jr, Jenner JL, McNamara JR, et al: Prevalence of lipoprotein (a) (Lp[a]) excess in coronary artery disease. Am J Cardiol 1991;67: 1039-1045.

52. Cremer P, Nagel D, Labrot B, et al: Lipoprotein Lp(a) as predictor of myocardial infarction in comparison to fibrinogen, LDL cholesterol and other risk factors: Results from the prospective Gottingen Risk Incidence and Prevalence Study (GRIPS). Eur J Clin Invest 1994;24:444-453.

53. Jauhianen M, Koskinen P, Ehnholm C, et al: Lipoprotein(a) and coronary heart disease risk: A nested case-control study of the Helsinki heart Study participants. Atherosclerosis 1991;89: 59-67.

54. Ridker PM, Hennekens CH, Stampfer MJ: A prospective study of lipoprotein(a) and the risk of myocardial infarction. JAMA 1993;270:2195-2199.

55. Schaefer EJ, Lamon-Fava S, Jenner JL, et al: Lipoprotein(a) levels and risk of coronary heart disease in men: The Lipid Research Clinics Coronary Primary Prevention Trial. JAMA 1994;271: 999-1003.

56. Danesh J, Collins R, Peto R: Lipoprotein (a) and coronary heart disease. Meta-analysis of prospective studies. Circulation 2000;102: 1082-1085.

57. Etingin OR, Hajjar KA, et al: Lipoprotein(a) regulates plasminogen activator inhibitor-1 expression in endothelial cells: A potential

mechanism in thrombogenesis. J Biol Chem 1991;266: 2459-2465.

59. Wild SH, Fortmann SP, Marcovina SM: A prospective case-control study of lipoprotein(a) levels and apo(a) size and risk of coronary heart disease in Stanford Five-City Project participants. Arterioscler Thromb Vasc Biol 1997;17:239-245.

60. Grainger DJ, Kemp PR, Liu AC, et al: Activation of transforming growth-factor-B is inhibited in transgenic Apolipoprotein(a) mice. Nature 1994;370:460-462.

61. Haberland ME, Fless GM, Scanu AM, Fogelman AM: Malondialdehyde modification of lipoprotein(a) produces avid uptake by human monocyte-macrophages. J Biol Chem 1992;267:4143-4151.

62. Hajjar KA, Gavish D, Breslow JL, et al: Lipoprotein(a) modulation of endothelial cell surface fibrinolysis and its potential role in atherosclerosis. Nature 1989;339:303-305.

63. Hajjar KA, Nachman RL: The role of lipoprotein(a) in atherogenesis and thrombosis. Ann Rev Med 1996;47:423-442.

64. Kojima S, Harpel PC, Rifkin DB: Lipoprotein(a) inhibits the generation of transforming growth factor beta: An endogenous inhibitor of smooth muscle cell migration. J Cell Biol 1991;113:1439-1445.

65. Meade TW, Ruddock V, Stirling Y, et al: Fibrinolytic activity, clotting factors and long-term incidence of ischaemic heart disease in the Northwick Park Heart Study. Lancet 1993;342:1076-1079.

66. Poon M, Zhang X, Dunsky KG, et al: Apolipoprotein(a) induces monocyte chemotactic activity in human vascular endothelial cells. Circulation 1997;96:2514-2519.

67. Ribatti D, Vacca A, Giacchetta F, et al: Lipoprotein(a) induces angiogenesis on the chick embryo chorioallantoic membrane. Eur J Clin Invest 1998;28:533-537.

68. Welch GN, Loscalzo J: Homocysteine and atherothrombosis. N Engl J Med 1998;338:1042-1050.

69. Hankey GJ, Eikelboom JW: Homocysteine and vascular disease. Lancet 1999;354:407-413.

70. Boushey CJ, Beresford SA, Omenn GS, et al: A quantitative assessment of plasma homocysteine as a risk factor for vascular disease. Probable benefits of increasing folic acid intakes. JAMA 1995;274:1049-1057.

71. Eikelboom JW, Lonn E, Genest J Jr, et al: Homocyst(e)ine and cardiovascular disease: A critical review of the epidemiologic evidence. Ann Intern Med 1999;131:363-375.

72. Genest J Jr, McNamara JR, Salem DN, et al: Plasma homocyst(e)ine levels in men with premature coronary artery disease. J Am Coll Cardiol 1990;16:1114-1119.

73. Graham IM, Daly LE, Refsum HM, et al: Plasma homocysteine as a risk factor for vascular disease: The European Concerted Action Project. JAMA 1997;277:1775-1781.

74. Anderson JL, Muhlestein JB, Benjamin D, et al: Plasma homocysteine predicts mortality independently of traditional risk factors and c-reactive protein in patients with angiographically defined coronary artery disease. Circulation 2000;102:1227.

75. Stubbs PJ, Al-Obaidi MK, Conroy RM, et al: Effect of plasma homocysteine concentration on early and late events in patients with acute coronary syndromes. Circulation 2000;102:605.

76. Wald NJ, Watt HC, Law MR, et al: Homocysteine and ischemic heart disease: Results of a prospective study with implications regarding prevention. Arch Intern Med 1998;281:1817-1821.

77. Stampfer MJ, Malinow MR, Willett WC, et al: A prospective study of plasma homocyst(e)ine and risk of myocardial infarction in US physicians. JAMA 1992;268:877-881.

78. Evans RW, Shaten BJ, Hempel JD, et al: Homocyst(e)ine and risk of cardiovascular disease in the Multiple Risk Factor Intervention Trial. Arterioscler Thromb Vasc Biol 1997;17:1947-1953.

79. Folsom AR, Nieto FJ, McGovern PG, et al: Prospective study of coronary heart disease incidence in relation to fasting total homocysteine, related genetic polymorphisms, and B vitamins: The Atherosclerosis Risk in Communities (ARIC) study. Circulation 1998;98:204-210.

80. Lentz SR: Does homocysteine promote atherosclerosis? Arterioscler Thromb Vasc Biol 2001;21:1385-1386.

81. Hoogeveen EK, Kostense PJ, Jakobs C, et al: Hyperhomocysteinemia increases risk of death, especially in type 2 diabetes. Circulation 2000;101:1506.

82. Audelin M-C, Genest J Jr: Homocysteine and cardiovascular disease in diabetes mellitus. Atherosclerosis 2001;159:497-511.

83. Nygard O, Nordrehaug JE, Refsum H, et al: Plasma homocysteine levels and mortality in patients with coronary artery disease. N Engl J Med 1997;337:230-236.

84. Ridker PM, Hennekens CH, Miletich JP: G20210A mutation in prothrombin gene and risk of myocardial infarction, stroke, and venous thrombosis in a large cohort of US men. Circulation 1999;99:999-1004.

85. Ridker PM, Rifai N, Pfeffer MA, et al: Long-term effects of pravastatin on plasma concentration of c-reactive protein. Circulation 1999;100:230-235.

86. Ernst E, Resch KL: Fibrinogen as a cardiovascular risk factor: A meta-analysis and review of the literature. Ann Intern Med 1993;118:956-963.

87. Heinrich J, Balleisen L, Schulte H, et al: Fibrinogen and factor VII in the prediction of coronary risk: Results from the PROCAM study in healthy men. Arterioscler Thromb 1994;14:54-59.

88. Maresca G, Di Blasio A, Marchioli R, et al: Measuring plasma fibrinogen to predict stroke and myocardial infarction: An update. Arterioscler Thromb Vasc Biol 1999;19:1368-1377.

89. Ma J, Hennekens CH, Ridker PM, et al: A prospective study of fibrinogen and risk of myocardial infarction in the Physicians' Health Study. J Am Coll Cardiol 1999;33:1347-1352.

90. Kannel WB, Wolf PA, Castelli WP, et al: Fibrinogen and risk of cardiovascular disease: The Framingham Study. JAMA 1987;258:1183-1186.

91. Stec JJ, Silbershatz H, Tofler GH, et al: Association of fibrinogen with cardiovascular risk factors and cardiovascular disease in the Framingham Offspring population. Circulation 2000;102: 1634.

92. Wu KK, Folsom AR, Heiss G, et al: Association of coagulation factors and inhibitors with carotid artery atherosclerosis: Early results of the Atherosclerosis Risk in Communities (ARIC) Study. Ann Epidemiol 1992;2:471-480.

93. Woodward M, Lowe GD, Rumley A, et al: Fibrinogen as a risk factor for the Scottish Heart Health Study. Eur Hear J 1998;18:53-62.

94. Danesh J, Collins R, Appleby P, et al: Association of fibrinogen, C-reactive protein, albumin, or leukocyte count with coronary heart disease: Meta-analyses of prospective studies. JAMA 1998;279: 1477-1482.

95. Cooper JA, Miller GJ, Bauer KA, et al: Comparison of novel hemostatic factors and conventional risk factors for prediction of coronary heart disease. Circulation 2000;102:2816.

96. Danesh J, Whincup P, Walker M, et al: Fibrin D-Dimer and coronary heart disease. Prospective study and meta-analysis. Circulation 2001;103:2323.

97. Feng D, Tofler GH, Larson MG, et al: Factor VII gene polymorphism, factor VII levels, and prevalent cardiovascular disease. Arterio Thromb Vasc Biol 2000;50:593.

98. Folsom AR, Wu KK, Rosamond WD, et al: Prospective study of hemostatic factors and incidence of coronary heart disease: The Atherosclerosis Risk in Communities (ARIC) Study. Circulation 1997;96:1102-1108.

99. Porreca E, Di Febbo C, Amore C, et al: Effect of lipid-lowering treatment on factor VII profile in hyperlipidemic patients. Thromb Haemost 2000;84:789-793.

100. Meade TW, Mellows S, Brozovic M, et al: Hemostatic function and ischaemic heart disease: Principal results of the Northwich Park Heart Study. Lancet 1986;2:533-537.

101. Redondo M, Watzke HH, Stucki B, et al: Coagulation factors II, V, VII, and X, prothrombin gene 20210G-A transition, and factor V leiden in coronary artery disease. Arterioscler Thromb Vasc Biol 1999;19:1020-1025.

102. Thompson SG, Kienast J, Pyde SD, et al: Hemostatic factors and the risk of myocardial infarction or sudden death in patients with angina pectoris. European Concerted Action on Thrombosis and Disabilities Angina Pectoris Study Group. N Engl J Med 1995;332:635-641.

103. Zito F, Drummond F, Bujac SR, et al: Epidemiological and genetic associations of activated factor XII concentration with factor VII activity, fibrinopeptide a concentration, and risk of coronary heart disease in men. Circulation 2000;102:2058.

104. Juan-Vague I, Thompson SG, Jesperson J, et al: Involvment of the hemostatic system in the insulin resistance syndrome. Arterioscler Thromb 1993;13:1933-1941.

105. Jansson JH, Olofsson BO, Nilsson TK: Predictive value of tissue plasminogen activator mass concentration on long-term mortality in patients with coronary artery disease: A 7-year follow-up. Circulation 1993;88:2030-2034.

106. Ridker PM, Hennekens CH, Stampfer MJ, et al: Prospective study of endogenous tissue plasminogen activator and risk of stroke. Lancet 1994;343:940-943.

107. Thogersen AM, Jansson JH, Boman K, et al: High plasminogen activator inhibitor and tissue plasminogen activator levels in plasma precede a first acute myocardial infarction in both men and women: Evidence for the fibrinolytic system as an independent primary risk factor. Circulation 1998;98:2241-2247.

108. Hamsten A, Wiman B, de Faire U, Blombeck M: Increased plasma levels of a rapid inhibitor of tissue plasminogen activator in young survivors of acute myocardial infarction. N Engl J Med 1983;313:1557-1561.

109. Hamsten A, de Faire U, Walldius G, et al: Plasminogen activator inhibitor in plasma: Risk factor for recurrent myocardial infarction. Lancet 1987;2:3-9.

110. Landgren CH, Brown SL, Nordt TK, et al: Elaboration of type-1 plasminogen activator inhibitor from adipocytes: A potential pathogenetic link between obesity and cardiovascular disease. Circulaiton 1996;93:106-110.

111. Scarabin PY, Aillaud MF, Amouyel P, et al: Associations of fibrinogen, factor VII and PAI-1 with baseline findings among 10,500 male participants in a prospective study of myocardial infarction—the PRIME Study. Prospective Epidemiological Study of Myocardial Infarction. Thromb Haemost 1998;80:749-756.

112. Alessi MC, Peiretti F, Morange P, et al: Production of plasminogen activator inhibitor 1 by human adipose tissue. Possible link between visceral fat accumulation and vascular disease. Diabetes 1997;46:860-867.

113. Potter van Loon BJ, Kluft C, Raddr JK, et al: The cardiovascular risk factor plasminogen activator inhibitor type 1 is related to insulin resistance. Metabolism 1993;42:945-949.

114. Shimomura I, Funahashi T, Takahashi M, et al: Enhanced expression of PAI-1 in visceral fat: Possible contributor to vascular disease in obesity. Nat Med 1996;2:800-803.

115. Angleton P, Chandler WL, Schmer G: Diurnal variation of tissue-type plasminogen activator and its rapid inhibitor (PAI-1). Circulation 1989;79:101-106.

116. Ridker PM, Hennekens CH, Cerskus A, et al: Plasma concentration of cross-linked fibrin degradation product (D-dimer) and the risk of future myocardial infarction among apparently healthy men. Circulation 1994;90:2236-2240.

117. Blankenberg S, Rupprecht HJ, Bickel C, et al: Circulating cell adhesion molecules and death in patients with coronary artery disease. Circulation 2001;104:1336-1342.

118. Malik I, Danesh J, Whincup P, et al: Soluble adhesion molecules and prediction of coronary heart disease: A prospective study and meta-analysis. Lancet 2001;358:971-976.

119. O'Malley T, Ludlam CA, Riemermsa RA, Fox KA: Early increase in levels of soluble inter-cellular adhesion mole 1 (sICAM-1): Potential risk factor for the acute coronary syndromes. Eur Heart J 2001;22:1155-1159.

120. Libby P: Current concepts of the pathogenesis of the acute coronary syndromes. Circulation 2001;104:365-372.

121. Ridker PM, Hennekens CH, Buring JE, Rifai N: C-reactive protein and other markers of inflammation in the prediction of cardiovascular disease in women. N Engl J Med 2000;342:836-843.

122. Carr A, Samaras K, Thorisdottir A, et al: Diagnosis, prediction, and natural course of HIV-1 protease-inhibitor associated lipodystrophy, hyperlipidemia, and diabetes mellitus. A cohort study. Lancet 1999;353:2093-2099.

123. Echevarria KL, Hardin TC, Smith JA: Hyperlipidemia associated with protease inhibitor therapy. Ann Pharmacother 1999;33:859-863.

124. Periard D, Telenti A, Sudre P, et al: Atherogenic dyslipidemia in HIV-infected individuals treated with protease inhibitors. The Swiss HIV Cohort Study. Circulation 1999;100:700-705.

125. Purnell JQ, Zambon A, Knopp RH, et al: Hyperlipidemia and insulin resistance are induced by protease inhibitors independent of changes in body composition in patients with HIV infection. J AIDS 2000;23:35-43.

126. Bayes-Genis A, Conover CA, Overgaard MT, et al: Pregnancy-associated plasma protein A as a marker of acute coronary syndromes. N Engl J Med 2001;345:1022-1029.

127. El-Khairy L, Ueland PM, Refsum H, et al: Plasma total cysteine as a risk factor for vascular disease. The European Concerted Action Project. Circulation 2001;103:2544.

128. Roivainen M, Viik-Kajander M, Palosuo T, et al: Infections, inflammation, and the risk of coronary heart disease. Circulation 2000;101:252.

129. Volpato S, Guralnik JM, Ferrucci L, et al: Cardiovascular disease, interleukin-6, and risk of mortality in older women. Circulation 2001;103:947.

130. Ridker PM, Kundsin RB, Stampfer MJ, et al: Prospective study of chlamydia pneumoniae IgG seropositivity and risks of future myocardial infarction. Circulation 1999;99:1161-1164.

131. Whincup P, Danesh J, Walker M, et al: Prospective study of potentially virulent strains of helicobacter pylori and coronary heart disease in middle-aged men. Circulation 2000;101:1647.

132. Strong JP, Malcom GT, McMahan CA, et al: Prevalence and extent of atherosclerosis in adolescents and young adults. Implications for prevention from the pathobiological determinants of atherosclerosis in youth study. JAMA 1999;281:727-735.

chapter 10

What Cardiologists Need to Know on Depression in Acute Coronary Syndromes

François Lespérance
Nancy Frasure-Smith

In an era when the popular press and the Internet rapidly communicate health care information to patients and families, cardiologists are increasingly called upon to answer questions about the importance of psychosocial factors, both as causes and as complications of cardiac disease. Recent decades have seen a rapid growth of evidence suggesting that a variety of psychosocial factors, including depression, lack of social support, anger, and job stress, may influence prognosis in cardiac patients. More recently, an increasing number of well-designed studies, published in first-line medical and cardiology journals, have focused additional attention on depression as the major psychosocial risk. The strength of the current epidemiologic evidence makes depression something that all cardiologists need to know about. In this chapter, we hope to provide some practical information to help cardiologists understand depression and to cope more efficiently with this major health issue.

WHAT IS DEPRESSION?

The specific diagnostic criteria for depression and the issues surrounding diagnosis in patients with cardiac disease are reviewed later in this chapter, but it is important to realize that some level of negative emotional reaction is expected in response to the threats and losses associated with an acute coronary syndrome. Clinicians have to deal daily with their patients' anxiety, irritability, and sadness. In response to these negative emotions, clinicians provide reassurance, calm patients, and provide them with hope. Usually, these basic emotions improve adaptation and are beneficial. For example, fear of a future heart attack may stimulate medication compliance. However, for some patients the fear is disproportionate to the threat and is not adaptive, as is the case when the intense fear leads to insomnia, atypical chest pain, and avoidance of low-risk activities.

In contrast to sudden fear, which is usually a short-lived reaction, dealing with the grief induced by the losses associated with heart disease is a healing process that takes time. Some sadness or withdrawal from activities may be part of the normal adjustment process, but for some patients, with insufficient resources to accept and cope with the loss, the emotional healing process stalls like a wound that gets infected. This unresolved grief may signal the beginning of a depression. Long stays in the intensive care unit or multiple consecutive hospitalizations can also trigger a depression. Patients start to feel exhausted by fighting for their lives, feel no hope for the future, helpless to change anything in their environment, and eventually they give up. Grief and chronic inescapable stress may be useful in understanding depression in many patients, but these concepts are not always applicable. For particularly susceptible patients, the loss seems trivial and the stresses seem more like daily hassles. In such patients, it is important to look for prior exposures to more significant losses or more intense threats and to consider the importance of strong genetic factors.

PREVALENCE OF DEPRESSION IN PATIENTS WITH CORONARY ARTERY DISEASE

The Global Burden of Disease study found that depression is second only to ischemic heart disease as a cause of disability and early death in industrialized countries.[1] In fact, when cardiac disease and depression coexist, both conditions are adversely affected. Although rates of depression are high in the general community, with 1-month prevalence estimates of 2% to 3% and lifetime prevalences of 6% to 9%,[2] the prevalence of depression in cardiac patients is even higher. Epidemiologic data suggests that in a 25-bed ward, a cardiologist will probably see four patients with major depression and five with a more minor form of depression.[3-10] The numbers are similar for hospitalized patients who have experienced myocardial infarction (MI), unstable angina, congestive heart failure (CHF), coronary bypass, and angioplasty (Table 10-1).

PROGNOSTIC CORRELATES OF DEPRESSION IN CORONARY ARTERY DISEASE

Evidence shows that a variety of psychosocial variables, including depression, low social support, anger and hostility, job strain, and anxiety, may be risk factors both for

TABLE 10–1   PREVALENCE OF DEPRESSION IN HOSPITALIZED PATIENTS WITH CORONARY HEART DISEASE

		MAJOR DEPRESSION	ELEVATED DEPRESSION SYMPTOMS/MINOR DEPRESSION
Myocardial infarction (Frasure-Smith et al, 1995[6])	N=222	16%	17%
Unstable angina (Lespérance et al, 2000[8])	N=430	15%	26%
Congestive heart failure (Jiang et al, 2001[9])	N=374	14%	20%
Catheterization (Hance et al, 1996[11])	N=200	17%	17%
Bypass surgery (Connerney et al, 2001[10])	N=309	20%	8%

the development of coronary heart disease in disease-free persons and for prognosis in patients with established coronary disease. This research has been summarized in several recent major literature reviews published in leading medical journals.[11-13,16] All have come to the conclusion that of all the psychosocial variables, the current evidence is strongest for depression. Further, although research indicates that depression may be a primary risk factor for coronary heart disease, the evidence is strongest for the prognostic impact of depression in patients with established cardiac disease.

Our team in Montreal has carried out several studies of the prognostic importance of depression in acute coronary syndrome patients, including two studies of patients who have experienced MI and one of patients hospitalized with unstable angina. In our earliest study,[5] we interviewed 222 hospitalized post-MI patients. We used a modified version of the Diagnostic Interview Schedule (DIS),[17] which allows trained lay interviewers to collect the data necessary to assess the criteria used by psychiatrists to diagnose depression. Results over the first 6 months after discharge from hospital showed a striking prognostic impact of depression, but the relatively small sample size prevented us from being able to adjust for many covariates. However, in addition to the DIS, patients responded to the 21-item Beck Depression Inventory (BDI),[18] a well-validated, widely used, self-reported measure of depressive symptoms. The BDI is not a diagnostic measure, but scores of 10 or greater are considered indicative of at least mild to moderate symptoms of depression. As time passed after the infarct, the impact of major depression became less strong, but the impact of BDI scores increased. In an expanded sample of 896 post-MI patients that included the patients in the first cohort, baseline BDI scores were independently related to 1-year cardiac mortality (adjusted odds ratio, 3.66; 95% CI, 1.68 to 7.99; P = .0011), after statistical adjustment for the multivariate baseline predictors of 1-year cardiac mortality in the data set including age, Killip class, and the interactions between sex and non–Q wave MI, sex and left-ventricular ejection fraction, and sex and smoking.[19] The adjusted survival curves are shown in Figure 10–1.

Our group found similar results in a study of 430 patients with a non–ST-segment elevation acute coro-

nary syndrome.[8] High BDI scores predicted the combined end point of cardiac death or nonfatal MI, with an adjusted odds ratio of 6.73 (95% CI, 2.43 to 18.64; P < .001) after controlling for other significant prognostic factors that included baseline electrocardiographic evidence of ischemia, left-ventricular ejection fraction, and number of diseased coronary vessels. The adjusted survival curves are shown in Figure 10–2.

The impact of depression on prognosis is not limited to patients with acute coronary syndromes. For example, Jiang et al[9] studied 374 hospitalized patients with CHF. They administered a modified version of the DIS, as well as the BDI, and combined them to define both major depression and minor depression (high BDI scores without meeting criteria for depression). Over 1 year, the patients with major depression were at significantly increased risk of mortality, as well as readmission, compared with those who showed no evidence of depression. Patients with milder depression were not at increased risk. After adjustment for age, New York Heart

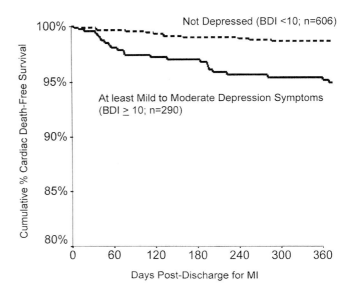

FIGURE 10–1. Adjusted 1-year survival curves in depressed and non-depressed patients after myocardial infarction. BDI, Beck Depression Inventory rating; MI, myocardial infarction.

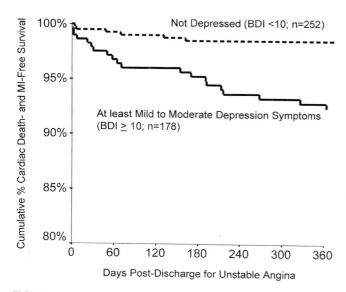

FIGURE 10–2. Adjusted 1-year survival curves in depressed and nondepressed patients with unstable angina. BDI, Beck Depression Inventory rating; MI, myocardial infarction.

Association Class, ejection fraction, and cause of CHF, the impact of major depression on readmissions remained significant (adjusted odds ratio, 2.98; 95% CI, 1.17 to 7.59; P = .03) and its impact on mortality marginally significant (odds ratio, 2.45; 95% CI, 0.78 to 7.48; P = .12).

We recently completed 5-year follow-up of our sample of 896 post-MI patients[20] and found that the risk of cardiac mortality associated with depression symptoms increases in a dose-dependent fashion, with the excess in risk beginning to be apparent at levels below those usually considered to be of clinical significance. Similar results over a much briefer follow-up (4 months) have also been reported by Bush and colleagues[21] in a sample of 144 post-MI patients 65 years and older.

As the results of Jiang et al suggest,[9] the impact of depression is not necessarily limited to mortality and, at least in patients with CHF, includes an increase in risk of readmissions as well. We have observed a similar increase in rates of admission over the first post-MI year.[22] However, in our recent long-term follow-up of post-MI patients,[23] depression's impact on major cardiac events was largely limited to cardiac mortality, suggesting a possible arrhythmic or acute ischemic mechanism. We observed no short- or long-term relationships between depression and revascularization procedures.

Finally, the risks associated with depression are not restricted to cardiac events. Our studies, as well as those of others,[3,10,24] indicate that in cardiac patients, as in patients without physical disease, untreated depression is a condition with a high risk of chronicity. We found that 48% of those patients who had been depressed during hospitalization for an MI, and who survived to 6 months, were still depressed at the 6-month point, and that by 1 year 24% continued to suffer from an episode of major depression.

In summary, depression is common in patients with established cardiac disease. It is associated with increased rates of cardiac death and readmissions, as well as with continuing chronic depression. But what kind of depression increases the risk of cardiac events? Our research among patients with coronary artery disease (CAD), as well as studies by other investigators, suggests that the diagnostic distinction between major and more minor forms of depression may not be relevant in the assessment of cardiac risk. One could suggest that as for cholesterol levels, the less severe the depressive symptoms, the less physically vulnerable the patient. Therefore, the question may not be what a normal level of depressive symptoms is, but at what threshold medical attention is needed. The answer to this question depends on both the outcome of interest and the costs and benefits of available treatment for reducing risk.

EXPLANATORY MODELS OF THE LINKS BETWEEN DEPRESSION AND CORONARY ARTERY DISEASE

Experiments randomly assigning patients to an apparent risk such as depression cannot be performed. Therefore, we are limited to correlational data, which, although prospective, is difficult to interpret in a cause/effect framework. In fact, the link between depression and CAD could reflect at least three different types of relationships (Fig. 10–3). First, depression may directly cause cardiac mortality through biologic or behavioral mechanisms. Second, depression may be a consequence of the systemic complications of cardiovascular disease or its treatment. Finally, both depression and cardiac disease may share a common genetic or pathophysiologic cause and have no causal relationship to each other. These possible models are discussed in the following sections.

Depression As a Cause of Cardiac Mortality

This explanation is supported by cross-sectional evidence that depression is associated with hyperactivity of the sympathoadrenal system, diminished heart rate variability (HRV), and enhanced platelet responsiveness.[16] It is also possible that the worse prognosis in depressed patients is explained by risky behaviors, such as reduced adherence to β-blockers or aspirin and reduced likelihood of stopping smoking or regular exercise.[25]

Research data suggest that major depression, without co-occurrence of CAD, is associated with an elevation of plasma norepinephrine and its metabolites[26] as well as with increased norepinephrine secretion.[27] Increased levels of norepinephrine facilitate the development of ventricular arrhythmias[28] and enhance platelet aggregation though the α_2 receptor.[29] However, increased levels of norepinephrine have not yet been directly demonstrated among depressed patients with CAD.[30]

There is substantial evidence that decreased HRV is a major independent predictor of cardiac mortality after MI.[31] It is thought that decreased HRV reflects increased sympathetic tone or decreased vagal activity, or both. Preliminary studies documenting decreased HRV in

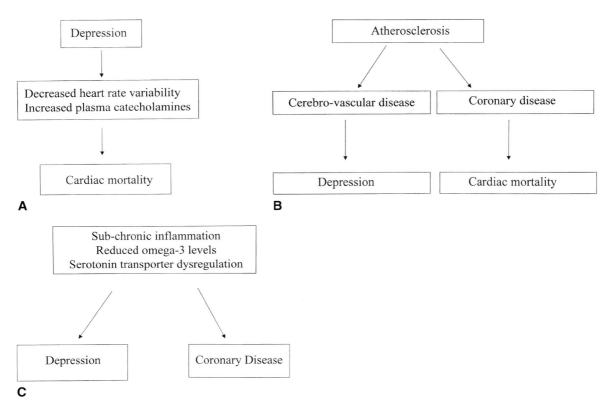

FIGURE 10–3. *A*, Depression as a cause of cardiac mortality. *B*, Cardiovascular disease as a cause of depression. *C*, Depression and coronary artery disease as results of a common cause.

depressed, as compared with nondepressed, patients with CAD[32] were recently confirmed in a larger study.[33] Based on a cross-sectional analysis of data from 500 post-MI patients, Carney et al found that both major and minor depression were associated with reduced 24-hour HRV indices in all spectral analysis frequency bands. Further, all but the high-frequency band remained lower among the depressed after adjustment for potential medical and demographic confounders. Although survival data are not yet available, the Multicenter Post Infarction Project[34] shows that the difference in the very-low-frequency band between depressed and nondepressed patients was great enough to have more than doubled the risk of cardiac mortality. These data support the idea that an arrhythmic mechanism may link depression to cardiac mortality.

In fact, our team documented that depression's impact on 18-month post-MI cardiac mortality was particularly strong among patients with more that 10 premature ventricular complexes per hour during 24-hour Holter monitoring during hospitalization.[6] This suggests a synergistic effect between depression and signs of ventricular irritability in promoting future arrhythmic events. Also of interest is a small study (N = 27) by McFarlane et al,[35] suggesting that in depressed post-MI patients, 6 months of treatment with sertraline, an antidepressant that blocks the reuptake of serotonin, may result in more improvement in the autonomic control of the heart than treatment with placebo. Carney et al[36] also carried out a small (N = 30) uncontrolled study of cognitive-behavioral therapy (CBT) in moderately to severely depressed

patients with CAD. After 8 to 16 CBT sessions, the authors observed a reduction in the mean heart rate and an increase in short-term HRV in the severely depressed, but not in the moderately depressed, patients.

Thrombus formation is a key factor in the rapid progression of CAD and the occurrence of acute MI and episodes of unstable angina. Thus, the hypothesis of an association between depression and increased platelet reactivity is particularly appealing as an explanation of the link between depression and cardiac mortality. Although serotonin is itself a weak agonist of platelet activation, serotonin can potentiate the effect of other agonists in inducing platelet aggregation. Serotonin may also facilitate thrombus formation by inducing coronary vasoconstriction in damaged vessels. For many years, platelets have been used in psychiatry research as a model of serotonin's pre- and post-synaptic function in the brain. This research suggests that an association between depression and increased platelet activation may be mediated through modifications in the regulation of platelet 5HT2 receptors[37] and the serotonin transporter responsible for its reuptake.[38] However, to our knowledge, the relationship between depression and regulation of the 5HT2 receptors on the coronary wall muscles responsible for vasoconstriction has not yet been studied.

A small study using flow cytometric measures of the monoclonal markers of GIIaIIIb expression documented an increase in platelet activation in depressed subjects without cardiac disease,[39] and similar results were found in patients with CAD.[40] Another small preliminary study also documented that plasma levels of markers of platelet activation, such as platelet factor 4 and β-thromboglobulin, were increased in patients with stable CAD.[41] There is also some suggestion that treatment with an antidepressant serotonin reuptake inhibitor (SSRI) may reduce the observed increase in activation.[42-44] Interestingly, Serebruany et al[45] reported that both sertraline and its neurologically inactive metabolite N-desmethylsertraline exhibit significant dose-dependent inhibition of activation in platelets from depressed post-MI patients.

In terms of the potential behavioral explanations of the link between depression and prognosis, it makes sense to think that the reduced interest, self-esteem, sense of control, and hope found in depression translate into poorer compliance with risk-factor modification and medications.[46,47] Recent evidence also suggests that either because of their motivation or the reactions of their physicians, depressed patients may have reduced access to revascularization procedures.[48] The role of smoking cessation in depressed patients is particularly complex. In some ways, nicotine is a self-administered antidepressant for many patients.[49,50] Patients with prior depression are less likely to succeed in smoking cessation programs and may experience a relapse or recurrence of episodes of depression when trying to quit smoking. However, only three antidepressants—bupropion,[51] nortryptiline,[52] and moclobemide[53]—have been documented to facilitate smoking cessation. It is important, therefore, not to consider SSRIs as treatments to help patients quit smoking.[54] In this regard, nondepressed patients with prior episodes of depression who try to stop smoking should be monitored closely to evaluate symptoms suggestive of relapse or recurrence of depression.

Depressed patients are usually less physically active than the nondepressed. In fact, regular physical activity may have intrinsic antidepressant properties and is a potentially useful treatment approach for some patients. Blumenthal et al[55] enrolled 56 depressed patients, at least 50 years old, without known cardiac disease in a 16-week, randomized clinical trial of exercise training (three supervised exercise sessions per week), sertraline (50 to 200 mg), or both exercise and sertraline. The authors found that all treatments were equally efficacious in reducing the severity of depressive symptoms. However, patients randomized to exercise training experienced a significant improvement in aerobic capacity, whereas patients treated only with sertraline did not. Thus, although as yet untested in cardiac patients, regular physical activity may be an adequate alternative to antidepressant medication as a first-line treatment for major depression in patients who are both willing and able to exercise.

Cardiovascular Disease As a Cause of Depression

In this interpretation of the link between depression and cardiac prognosis, cardiovascular disease causes depression-like symptoms, which could be false-positive cases of depression. Most epidemiologic research relies on self-report measures or on structured interview guides administered by research assistants, with little attempt to differentiate symptoms attributable to depression from those associated with the patient's medical condition. Even in clinical practice, clinicians often wonder if some of the apparent symptoms of depression, particularly tiredness or fatigue, are better accounted for by cardiac disease or the side effects of its treatment than by depression. However, there are a few tips that may help to differentiate fatigue due to depression from fatigue due to cardiac disease.

First, although patients with CHF complain of tiredness during or after physical activity, even mental activities, such as watching television or reading books, also tire depressed patients. So, in addition to having a low level of physical energy, depressed patients are mentally exhausted. Emotionally demanding tasks, even when they are usually pleasurable (e.g., seeing friends or family), are particularly difficult for people with depression. They lack the motivation to initiate any activity and have lower satisfaction when they have accomplished a task. Depressed patients have difficulty before (lack of motivation), during (tiredness), and after (lack of satisfaction) activities. Further, our research suggests that there is little correlation between complaints of fatigue and ventricular dysfunction among post-MI patients. Even more intriguing, Skotzko et al[56] reported that among CHF patients, the depressed patients tend to report greater functional impairment and show less effort during a treadmill test despite equivalent Vo_2 max capacity, suggesting that depressed patients tend to underestimate their physical capacity. Other causes of chronic fatigue include subchronic inflammation (discussed more later), reduced flow of blood to the brain due to cerebrovascular disease or low cardiac output, β-blockers, and hypothyroidism. Thyroid function tests should be performed routinely in all patients and, if results are abnormal, depression should be reevaluated after thyroid function has been normalized.

Another issue related to fatigue concerns the clinical impression that β-blockers cause depression. Side effects of β-blockers include sedation, nightmares, impotence, and fatigue. This is not the equivalent of sadness, reduced interest, or low self-esteem. Furthermore, the Beta-Blocker Heart Attack Trial reported no difference between treatment and placebo groups in the percentage of patients who reported "frequent depression that interfered with work, recreation, or sleep" during 30 months of follow-up.[57] Unfortunately, it is likely that depressed cardiac patients are commonly deprived of the potential survival benefits of β-blockers. In our opinion, these patients would be more likely to benefit from antidepressant treatment than from the withdrawal of β-blockade.

An additional example of the possibility that cardiovascular disease causes depression involves the concept of vascular depression, the term introduced to describe late-onset depression associated with cerebrovascular disease.[58] Compared with elderly patients who experienced their first episode of depression earlier in their lives, the elderly with late-onset depression are less likely to have a family history of depression, more likely to show neuropsychological and neuroradiologic abnormalities, and to be at high risk for mortality. Hypertensive and diabetic patients are particularly at risk for neurovascular disease. However, it is difficult to document whether their depression is due to cerebrovascular disease. The routine use of magnetic resonance imaging and neuropsychological testing would be prohibitively expensive. These modalities should be reserved for patients with strong indications of vascular difficulties or for those with treatment-resistant depression.

In summary, teasing out the multiple possible causes of the somatic symptoms of depression, and particularly of fatigue, is difficult. In some patients, antidepressant challenges may provide crucial information. For example, if fatigue does not respond to an antidepressant, whereas other symptoms such as lack of interest do respond, then the contribution of the medical condition becomes clearer. However, without very strong evidence for a specific medical cause explaining a patient's reports of fatigue, we suggest an "inclusive approach" to the diagnosis of depression[59]—that is, to consider fatigue as secondary to depression itself until proven otherwise.

DEPRESSION AND CAD AS RESULTS OF A COMMON CAUSE

In trying to understand the potential links between depression and CAD, we also need to consider the possibility that depression is neither the cause nor the effect of CAD, but that the two may occur together frequently in the same individuals because of a common pathophysiologic mechanism. For example, suppose that a genetically determined dysfunction of the serotonin receptor or transporter in some region of the brain is associated with an increased risk of depression and that the same defect in platelets increases the risk of thrombotic events. In this paradigm, the regulatory state of serotonin in the brain does not need to have a direct influence on serotonin regulation in platelets for there to be an association between depression and CAD. Common genetic defects, with the proper contribution of environmental factors, may lead to two different phenotypic expressions in the same patient.

Two other potential common pathophysiologic mechanisms causing both depression and cardiac disease are subchronic inflammation and reduced intake of omega-3 fatty acids. Subchronic inflammation is an integral part of CAD.[60] For instance, serum markers of inflammation, such as C-reactive protein, interleukin-6, and soluble intercellular adhesion molecule, are increased in patients with CAD and associated with worse prognosis. These markers are also predictive of future CAD in healthy persons with no evidence of disease.

Interesting links also exist between depression and the regulation of immune function and the inflammatory process.[61] A recent meta-analysis of studies of patients without CAD[62] concluded that major depression is associated with leukocytosis, increased CD4/CD8 ratios, increased levels of haptoglobin, prostaglandin E$_2$, interleukin-6, reduced natural killer cell cytotoxity, and reduced lymphocyte proliferative responses to mitogens.

The authors concluded that there is some evidence that major depression is associated with an immune activation reminiscent of an acute-phase response.

The clinical data on inflammation has parallels in experimental studies. Animal research suggests that immune activation can induce depression-like behavior and, conversely, that inescapable chronic stress induces pro-inflammatory cytokines in the brain with subsequent systemic effects. How does this work?[61,63] The pro-inflammatory cytokines interleukin-6 and tumor necrosis factor α, produced by activated immune cells, promote the production of interleukin-6 by the leukocytes, the adipocytes, or the endothelium. Interleukin-6 induces widespread systemic effects, including liver production of the acute-phase proteins (such as C-reactive protein), inhibition of lipoprotein lipase activity, and enhanced platelet aggregation in response to ADP and epinephrine. Interestingly, the systemic pro-inflammatory cytokines circulating in the blood also induce interleukin-1 activity in the hippocampus and hypothalamus, which act as stress messengers and stimulate serotonin and norepinephrine neurotransmission and the release of corticotropin-releasing factor. These changes are probably responsible for the sickness behavior associated with immune activation in animals[64] and may play a role in some depression in human beings. Sickness behavior includes anhedonia-like symptoms, anorexia, weight loss, hypersomnia, fatigue, reduced exploratory behavior (anxiety), impaired memory, impaired social behavior, and altered pain perception, a pattern that parallels depressive symptoms in human beings.

One possible explanation of the higher prevalence and prognostic impact of depressive symptoms in patients with CAD is that the immune activation associated with the recent progression of CAD induces a depressive episode in susceptible patients. The psychological concept of "vital exhaustion," defined as the combination of excess fatigue, irritability, and low morale, may be particularly relevant to understanding links between immune activation and the symptoms of depression. An interesting review paper by Appels et al[65] discusses these issues and reports data linking vital exhaustion to immune activation in a small sample of patients who underwent percutaneous transluminal coronary angioplasty. A large epidemiologic study of the elderly without CAD (N = 4268)[66] found that although C-reactive protein was associated with symptoms of depression as well as symptoms of fatigue, the relationship remained independent of cardiovascular covariates and measures of physical frailty only for fatigue symptoms. It appears that patients reporting the symptoms of vital exhaustion may be more likely to have concomitant immune activation than those with more typical symptoms of depression. Finally, there have been reports of a normalization of inflammatory markers following antidepressant treatment.[61]

It has been hypothesized that a relative deficiency of omega-3 fatty acids may explain the link between depression and heart disease.[67,68] Population-based studies have shown that reduced dietary intake of omega-3 relative to omega-6 fatty acids is associated with increases in the incidence of cardiovascular disease as well as depres-

■ ■ ■

TABLE 10–2   DIAGNOSTIC CRITERIA FOR A MAJOR DEPRESSIVE EPISODE

DEPRESSION SYMPTOMS	CRITERIA FOR MAJOR DEPRESSION
1. Sadness most of the day 2. Loss of interest most of the day 3. Changes in weight or appetite 4. Sleep pattern changes 5. Psychomotor agitation or retardation 6. Fatigue or loss of energy 7. Poor self-esteem, feelings of guilt 8. Inability to concentrate or make decisions 9. Thoughts of suicide or that life is not worth living	• Symptoms 1 or 2 • Total of 5 symptoms • Daily for at least 2 weeks • Impairment in daily functioning

sion. Although it has been documented that red blood cell levels of omega-3 tend to be reduced in depressed patients compared with normal controls, this has yet to be confirmed in depressed cardiovascular patients.[69] Further, in addition to its antiplatelet, anti-arrhythmic, anti-inflammatory, and antitriglyceride properties, it seems that omega-3 may have antidepressant effects, especially in depressed bipolar patients.[70,71]

DIAGNOSIS OF DEPRESSION

Because no laboratory tests exist to diagnose depression, the physician is confronted with the challenge of drawing the line that divides the continuum of human experience into what is and what is not normal. To facilitate diagnosis, clinicians can use the diagnostic criteria of the American Psychiatric Association (DSM-IV).[72] According to these criteria, listed in Table 10–2, the diagnosis of major depression requires at least one of two core symptoms (sadness, or loss of interest or pleasure in most usual activities), with a number of other symptoms, so that a minimum of five or more out of nine DSM clusters of symptoms are present (sadness, loss of interest, sleep difficulties, lost of appetite or weight, fatigue, difficulty concentrating, psychomotor agitation or retardation, low self-esteem or guilt, and thoughts of death or suicide). The diagnosis requires that the symptoms be present most of the day and almost everyday for at least 2 weeks (preferably for at least 1 month) and that they have resulted in some change in function or some impairment in daily activities (see Table 10–2).

Although the DSM has been a valuable tool to improve the reliability of psychiatric diagnoses for epidemiologic and treatment research in mental disorders, it is not a substitute for sound clinical judgment. The diagnosis of depression depends on good interviewing skills and the ability to communicate with the patient to obtain accurate information on his or her current and past emotional, interpersonal, and vocational functioning. It also requires experience to judge whether there has been a significant change in the patient's functioning that is likely to be due to the emotional condition.

In contrast with psychiatric patients, who may experience most of the typical symptoms of depression and acknowledge them easily, patients with cardiac disease tend to have less typical symptoms and to report them less directly (they tend to deny them) (Table 10–3).[73,74] They tend to attribute somatic symptoms of depression to their heart disease and are less likely to consider emotional causes. Their pattern of symptoms may also be different from that of the usual psychiatric patient. Patients with heart disease are more likely to complain of unusual tiredness or lack of energy; unexplained somatic symptoms, including atypical chest pain, dyspnea, and palpitations; anxiety (chronic worries, hypervigilance, multiple somatic complaints); and irritability (sudden bursts of anger and hostility, frequent negative and unpleasant comments to others, hypersensitivity to noise).[75] For these reasons, patients with less than five of the typical clusters of depressive symptoms, but who report other less typical symptoms (see Table 10–2), are probably suffering from a clinically significant depression.

TREATMENT OF DEPRESSION

It is premature to say that treating depression can improve cardiovascular morbidity or mortality. Even the documentation of the cardiovascular safety and efficacy

■ ■ ■

TABLE 10–3   WHEN TO SUSPECT DEPRESSION IN CARDIAC PATIENTS

COMMON SYMPTOMS	SIGNS OF FUNCTIONAL IMPAIRMENT	HEALTH-RELATED BEHAVIORS
Lack of energy	Decreased social contact	Over-reliance on fast food
Easily irritable	Reduced interest in hobbies	Difficulty stopping smoking
Feeling under stress	Not taking care of bills	Avoidance of physical activity
Difficulty sleeping	Poor productivity at work Poor grooming	Frequent visits for unexplained symptoms

of available treatments in reducing the severity of depressive symptoms is quite limited. One comparative trial in patients with stable CAD found that paroxetine is better tolerated and probably as efficacious as nortriptyline.[76] Following a small–open label study,[77] a large randomized (n = 369) placebo-controlled trial, Sertraline Antidepressant Heart Attack Trial (SADHART), evaluated the safety and efficacy of sertraline.[78] Results suggest that these Selective Serotonin Reuptake Inhibitors (SSRI) are safe for the treatment of major depression in recently hospitalized acute coronary syndrome patients. After 16 weeks of treatment, no difference was found between sertraline and placebo in left ventricular ejection fraction, QTc, and other ECG indices, as well as percent of ventricular and supraventricular premature complexes and runs of VPCs on 24-hour Holter monitoring, 24-hour heart rate variability, and the rate of the combined composite endpoint of mortality or urgent cardiac rehospitalization. However, although sertraline was more efficacious than placebo in improving the severity of depressive symptoms among patients who were experiencing a recurrent episode of major depression, the evidence of efficacy for other patients was at best equivocal. In conclusion, more clinical trials among CAD patients are needed to properly guide cardiologists, psychiatrists, and general practitioners. Until more research results are available, the treatment of depression in these patients has to be primarily based on the studies conducted in patients without significant physical disease.

Should We Screen for Depression in Patients with Coronary Artery Disease?

Given the lack of evidence that currently available treatments for depression provide substantial benefits in patients with CAD, we do not recommend systematic screening for depression. Self-report questionnaires like the BDI[18] are rapid and easy but are too sensitive, and they result in many false-positive diagnoses. An interesting alternative may be the recently developed Patient Health Questionnaire.[79] However, systematic screening can overload already scarce mental health resources available for patients seeking help on their own. Instead, we think that cardiologists should include a few questions inquiring about emotional difficulties during patients' regular visits. It is important not to underestimate how important it can be for patients to have their cardiologists demonstrate concern about their global well-being by inquiring about depression symptoms. It may also facilitate patient acceptance of referral to mental health professionals when needed. Some simple questions can be used to open the issue of emotional distress without using the word "depression," which often leads to denial. For example, the following kinds of questions can be particularly useful:

- How have you been coping with your heart disease lately?
- Have you had any difficulty sleeping?
- Have you been more tired or less active than usual?
- Have you felt more stressed than usual?
- Have you been less interested in interacting with others (children, friends)?

Indicators of Depressive Episode Severity

The seriousness of a depressive episode is based on the evaluation of the following factors: duration, number of symptoms and level of impairment during the current episode, and intensity and frequency of past depressions. Although rare in our experience with cardiac patients, any persons with suicidal thoughts or who express a wish to die must be referred for psychiatric evaluation as soon as possible.

Duration of Current Episode

The 2-week duration criteria for a major depressive episode should be applied with caution. Two weeks of multiple symptoms of depression may not be long enough after MI or another acute cardiac condition to justify a diagnosis of major depression. In particular, our post-MI data suggest that many patients experiencing a first episode of major depression remit spontaneously within the following 3 months.[3] Therefore, a reevaluation of depressive symptoms is suggested 1 to 2 months after discharge for patients experiencing their first lifetime episode of major depression during or soon after hospitalization for an acute coronary syndrome. Allowing some time for "daily life psychotherapy" to do its work is usually appropriate in patients with no previous history of depression. However, early psychiatric referral is indicated after a few weeks of depressive symptoms for patients with prior episodes of major depression.

Number of Symptoms

Obviously, the presence of multiple new and severe symptoms of depression usually implies a major depressive episode. However, because some patients tend to exaggerate symptoms and others to deny them, cross-validation by family members is recommended. Furthermore, depression fluctuates over time, and one visit is usually not sufficient to adequately assess the persistence of any particular symptom.

Level of Impairment

The diagnosis of depression depends on evidence that there is some degree of impairment in the patient's usual activities. For example, reduced productivity at work, reduced frequency of social contacts with friends, increasing conflicts with the spouse and family members, and difficulty meeting deadlines or demands provide some evidence that the symptoms of depression have real and concrete consequences in a patient's life. The more spheres of activity affected by depression, the more likely that the patient needs intervention.

Past Depression

As was stated previously, depression is a chronic illness with a clinical presentation that fluctuates over time.[80] Many patients with a minor depression eventually experience a major depressive episode, and the majority of patients with a major depressive episode continue to have residual symptoms for months and years. Furthermore, the number of previous episodes of depression predicts the risk of recurrence. In fact, the risk of recurrence after a first episode of major depression in patients without cardiac disease is 50%; after two episodes it is 70%; and after 3 or more previous episodes it is 90%.[81] Therefore, even mild depressive symptoms in an individual with a past history of major depression need to be considered as serious. They can be the early symptoms of relapse or recurrence.

When to Treat Depression

We think that patients with severe depression or recurrent depression, those expressing suicidal thoughts, and those with comorbid psychiatric disorders such as alcoholism, personality disorders, and anxiety disorders should be referred to psychiatric specialists. For this type of patient, the diagnosis is complicated, long-term care is needed, and treatment usually requires the combination of multiple psychotropic medications and psychotherapy. In contrast, it may be appropriate for a cardiologist to prescribe an antidepressant for patients with a first episode of major depression of moderate severity. However, it is important to have reasonable expectations in terms of success. Data on outpatient treatment in patients without cardiac disease show that, with adequate dosage, some 55% to 65% of depressed patients experience a drop of at least 50% in their scores on scales evaluating the severity of the depression after 6 to 8 weeks of treatment.[82,83] Thus, most patients improve with treatment and a minority experience a complete remission by 2 months. For patients experiencing a complete remission, the antidepressant should be continued for at least 6 months at the same dosage. When patients do not completely respond to a recommended dose of antidepressants taken regularly for at least 6 weeks, diverse supplemental pharmacologic or psychotherapeutic strategies may be tried. Also, the diagnosis of depression needs to be reexamined, including more careful assessment of the consumption of alcohol and the possibility of bipolar disorder, as well as the presence of comorbid anxiety or personality disorders. However, we suggest that treatment-resistant patients be referred to a psychiatrist.

Choice of Antidepressant

Tricyclic antidepressants should be avoided in cardiac patients.[84] The newer antidepressants have more favorable safety profiles and, among them, the SSRIs are the most widely used first-line medications. SSRIs do not have significant effects on heart rate, blood pressure, and cardiac conduction, but they do have side effects, leading some 15% of patients to drop out of treatment. For these reasons, antidepressants should be started at a low dose and with the dosage increased slowly to facilitate tolerance of side effects. The most frequent side effects are nausea, insomnia, sexual dysfunction, drowsiness, and tremor. When patients experience nausea, they should be advised to take medication with meals, and if there is insomnia, the SSRI should be taken in the morning.

However, more important than these side effects is the possibility of drug interactions. Many of the newer antidepressants inhibit one or more of the cytochrome P450 liver isoenzymes involved in the metabolism of other drugs.[85,86] Although most of these interactions are not clinically important, some may be serious. Antidepressants that significantly inhibit the P450 2D6 liver enzyme (paroxetine, fluoxetine, and possibly sertraline) should not be used in combination with the type IC antiarrhythmics, encainide, flecainide, mexiletine, and propafenone. Also, closer monitoring of most β-blockers is suggested because augmentation of β-blockade is possible. Nefazodone, fluvoxamine, and fluoxetine are inhibitors of the P450 3A3/4 isoenzyme that is responsible for the metabolism of calcium channel blockers, most statins, some antiarrhythmics, and cyclosporin, which require additional monitoring, whereas astemizole, terfenadine, and cisapride are contraindicated.

Table 10–4 outlines the risk of interaction and can be used to help avoid drug interactions in the selection of antidepressants. Because antidepressants tend to be

■ ■ ■

TABLE 10–4 RISK OF INTERACTIONS BETWEEN CARDIAC MEDICATIONS AND NEWER ANTIDEPRESSANTS

	P450 2D6 INHIBITORS	P450 3A3/4 INHIBITORS
Antidepressants in order of inhibitory properties	Paroxetine (Paxil) ↓ fluoxetine (Prozac) > sertraline (Zoloft)	Nefazodone (Serzone) >> fluvoxamine (luvox) ↓ fluoxetine (Prozac)
Medications to avoid	Encainide, flecainide, mexiletine, propafenone	Astemizole, cisapride, terfenadine, ketoconazole
Medications requiring extra monitoring	β-blockers: labetolol, metoprolol, pindolol, propranolol, timolol (no known interactions with acebutolol or atenolol)	Anti-arrhythmics: amiodarone, lidocaine, quinidine, propafenone Calcium channel blockers: diltiazem, felodepine, nifedipine, nicardipine, verapamil Statins: atorvastatin, lovastatin, simvastatin (no known interactions with pravastatin) Benzodiazepines: alprazolam, midazolam, triazolam (no known interactions with lorazepam, oxazepam, and clonazepam) Antirejection: cyclosporine

prescribed for long periods, we think that, in order to avoid most major risks of drug interaction, the best choices as a first-line treatment for moderately severe major depression are either citalopram (Celexa), 20 to 40 mg/day, or sertraline (Zoloft), 50 to 200 mg/day. Citalopram has the lowest risk of drug interactions but has not yet been properly evaluated in patients with CAD. In contrast, sertraline (50 to 200 mg/day), thought to probably be without clinically significant risk of drug interactions, is a reasonable alternative given the results of the large SADHART trial.

Besides citalopram and sertraline, two other newer antidepressants have very low risks of drug interactions: venlafaxine (Effexor) and bupropion (Wellbutrin). Bupropion, a non-SSRI antidepressant that blocks reuptake of norepinephrine and dopamine, has been studied in small numbers of patients with congestive heart failure and cardiac arrhythmias and was not found to exacerbate these conditions in these uncontrolled studies.[87] However, it is also an activating antidepressant with insufficient anti-anxiety properties to be a first-line treatment for major depression with predominant anxiety symptoms,[82] which is frequently the case for patients with CAD. Finally, although venlafaxine may be a good choice for patients with CAD, in terms of the risk of drug interactions and being found to be particularly efficacious in psychiatric samples, the SSRIs remain the treatment of reference for depression. Also, the norepinephrine reuptake blocking activity of venlafaxine may be associated with chronic increases in norepinephrine turnover, as seen with desipramine, a potentially negative cardiovascular effect.[88]

If cardiologists are interested in treating major depressive episodes in their patients, they should see them regularly until remission is adequate (minimally monthly). These visits have the goal of assessing side effects and encouraging compliance, social activity, and physical exercise; they also ensure the reevaluation of the severity of depressive symptoms and suicidal ideation, along with provision of some minimal psychological support. It is also important to add that patients who report difficulties in doing their jobs because of depression need to be prescribed sick leave. Patients who experience relapse or do not improve after 8 weeks of this type of treatment should be referred to a psychiatrist.

Psychotherapeutic Intervention

For patients with less severe major depression and those who are unwilling to take antidepressants, two short-term, well-defined forms of psychotherapy are good alternative first-line treatments: CBT[89] and interpersonal psychotherapy (IPT).[90] The primary goal of CBT is to modify the dysfunctional thought patterns that lead to negative emotional reactions. CBT involves structured questioning of patient perceptions and the way they evaluate the meaning of events in everyday life. A large-scale, multisite trial of CBT for post-MI patients aiming at improving cardiac prognosis (Enhancing Recovery in Coronary Heart Disease [ENRICHD]) was recently completed in the United States with funding from the National Heart, Lung, and Blood Institute.[91] The trial

involved 6 months of treatment for patients who were depressed or socially isolated, or both. Preliminary results were presented at the 2001 AHA Scientific Sessions.[92] Although the intervention did not improve 3-year cardiac prognosis, there was some evidence of a mild improvement in the level of depressive symptoms. Thus, although CBT may result in a degree of improvement in depression symptoms, there is no evidence that this improvement translates into improved prognosis.

In contrast with CBT, which emphasizes the importance of dysfunctional thinking patterns, IPT emphasizes the current interpersonal context associated with the onset and persistence of the depressive episode but recognizes the etiologic contribution of genetic, biochemical, developmental, and personality factors. Although IPT has not yet been evaluated as an approach to the treatment of depression in cardiac patients, it deals with problems common to patients with CAD, such as interpersonal conflicts (that lead to hostility, anger, and distress), life transitions, grief, and loss. In addition to depression, IPT addresses the problem of social isolation that has been linked to increased mortality and morbidity in some studies of patients with CAD.[93-95] In fact, a recent secondary analysis of post-MI data collected in Montreal showed that among the depressed patients who survived the first year, those with better baseline support were more likely to experience improvements in depression symptoms than the depressed with lower support.[96] However, overall rates of depression at 1 year remained high, indicating a need for appropriate intervention strategies beyond naturally occurring support for many patients. Thus, IPT may prove to be particularly useful.

Psychosocial Intervention

Patients with acute coronary syndromes face a major life threat during the acute phase of their illness. Although most do not become depressed, many experience difficulties in psychosocial adjustment. Numerous small studies of psychosocial interventions have focused on improving adjustment in cardiac patients. In 1996, Linden and colleagues[97] published a meta-analytic review of the impact of psychosocial interventions on psychological distress (depression and anxiety) and prognosis. With the evidence available at that time, they concluded that psychosocial treatments were better than standard care, and they pointed out that "the common element of all treatments is the underlying assumption that psychological stress contributes to the cardiac disease process, and that stress reduction with psychologically based interventions may be beneficial." However, since the work by Linden et al, two very large trials failed to demonstrate a significant impact of psychosocial treatment on survival.[98,99] Although both targeted psychosocial distress rather than depression, their results echo the outcome of the ENRICHD trial described earlier.

Jones and West[99] studied 2328 post-MI patients randomly assigned to a brief program of psychological intervention or usual care. The program involved seven 2-hour sessions with a clinical psychologist or health visitor who used a variety of approaches including education, counseling, supportive therapy, and teaching of relaxation and stress-management techniques. There was no evidence of program impact on either psychological outcomes or prognosis over both a 6-month and 1-year follow-up period.

We conducted the Montreal Heart Attack Readjustment Trial (M-HART)[98] with the hope of preventing some of the cardiac deaths thought to be provoked by psychological distress. However, it is important to realize that the M-HART program was not designed to treat major depression or high levels of depression symptoms. M-HART was a large (N = 1376), randomized, controlled trial of a multifactorial, case management–type approach to help patients deal with their current sources of distress. Treatment group patients took part in a 1-year program of monthly telephone calls to monitor their psychological symptoms of distress using a standardized questionnaire. Those with high levels of distress at any call received home visits from a project nurse with experience in cardiac care. These visits involved an individually tailored approach in which nurses developed a plan of care to help reduce psychological distress. Although interventions were largely teaching- and advice-oriented, they included support and consultation or referral to other parts of the health care system. Some 83% of the patients in the treatment group received nursing interventions, and on average each patient received five to six home visits and 12 to 13 clinical care phone calls from the project nurse.

Despite the large amount of clinical care that was provided, results at 1 year were disappointing. There was no evidence of any positive or negative impact of the M-HART program on cardiac mortality in men (odds ratio, 0.97; 95% CI, 0.42 to 2.26; $P = .94$), but there was a marginally negative impact in women (odds ratio, 1.96; 95% CI, 0.95 to 4.06; $P = .064$). One of the hypotheses about the failure of the program was that because interventions were provided to such a high percentage of patients, it was likely that interventions took place in some patients who would have coped well on their own. The program may have interfered with the normal post-MI coping process in some patients and thereby paradoxically increased distress. In fact, recently completed 5-year follow-up of the M-HART patients[100] suggests that men with high levels of psychological distress during hospitalization probably experienced a long-term survival benefit associated with the treatment program, but that both men and women whose usual coping style involved avoidance of threatening information (repression) may have experienced increased stress associated with the repeated telephone calls and attempts at education about cardiac disease. Therefore, we think that, to be effective, psychosocial interventions need to match patient needs and that it is important to avoid intervening in patients with mild levels of psychological distress, many of whom will spontaneously improve without professional help.

CONCLUSIONS

Depression is a chronic condition that complicates the course of CAD. We have tried to provide clinical cardiol-ogists with the knowledge necessary to deal with it. Epidemiologic data suggest that depression may not only be a risk factor for the incidence of CAD but also a prognostic factor in patients with established CAD. Pathophysiologic and behavioral hypotheses may explain these epidemiologic findings and may serve as potential targets for psychological and pharmacologic interventions to improve cardiac prognosis. However, depression is more than a cardiac risk factor in search of an effective secondary prevention strategy. Depression has an immense personal and familial toll. The associated levels of intense and chronic psychological pain, interpersonal conflicts, and reduced productivity at work make it all the more imperative that we rapidly identify psychotherapeutic and pharmacologic interventions that are appropriate and effective for depressed cardiac patients. In the interim, cardiologists striving to provide good mental as well as physical care for their patients must rely on knowledge based on the study of treatments for depressed patients without comorbid cardiac conditions, combined with the clinical wisdom of those who have worked with depressed cardiac patients.

REFERENCES

1. Murray CJL, Lopez AD: Global mortality, disability, and the contribution of risk factors: Global burden of disease study. Lancet 1997;349:1436–1442.
2. Murphy JM, Laird NM, Monson RR, et al: A 40-year perspective on the prevalence of depression. Arch Gen Psychiatry 2000;57:209–215.
3. Lespérance F, Frasure-Smith N, Talajic M: Major depression before and after myocardial infarction: Its nature and consequences. Psychosom Med 1996;58:99–110.
4. Ladwig KH, Kieser M, König M, et al: Affective disorders and survival after acute myocardial infarction: Results from the post-infarction late potential study. Eur Heart J 1991;12:959–964.
5. Frasure-Smith N, Lespérance F, Talajic M: Depression following myocardial infarction: Impact on 6-month survival. JAMA 1993;270:1819–1825.
6. Frasure-Smith N, Lespérance F, Talajic M: Depression and 18-month prognosis after myocardial infarction. Circulation 1995;91:999–1005.
7. Koenig HG: Depression in hospitalized older patients with congestive heart failure. Gen Hosp Psychiatry 1998;20:29–43.
8. Lespérance F, Frasure-Smith N, Juneau M, et al: Depression and 1-year prognosis in unstable angina. Arch Intern Med 2000;160:1354–1360.
9. Jiang W, Alexander J, Christopher E, et al: Relationship of depression to increased risk of mortality and rehospitalization in patients with congestive heart failure. Arch Intern Med 2001;161:1849–1856.
10. Connerney I, Shapiro PA, McLaughlin JS, et al: Relation between depression after coronary artery bypass surgery and 12-month outcome: A prospective study. Lancet 2001;358:1766–1771.
11. Hance M, Carney RM, Freedland KE, et al: Depression in patients with coronary heart disease: A 12-month follow-up. Gen Hosp Psychiatry 1996;18:61–65.
12. Hemingway H, Marmot M: Psychosocial factors in the aetiology and prognosis of coronary heart disease: Systematic review of prospective cohort studies. BMJ 1999;318:1460–1467.
13. Glassman AH, Shapiro PA: Depression and the course of coronary artery disease. Am J Psychiatry 1998;155:4–11.
14. Rozanski A, Blumenthal JA, Kaplan J: Impact of psychological factors on the pathogenesis of cardiovascular disease and implications for therapy. Circulation 1999;99:2192–2217.
15. Januzzi JL, Stern TA, Pasternak RC, et al: The influence of anxiety and depression on outcomes of patients with coronary artery disease. Arch Intern Med 2000;160:1913–1921.

16. Musselman DL, Evans DL, Nemeroff CB: The relationship of depression to cardiovascular disease: Epidemiology, biology and treatment. Arch Gen Psychiatry 1998;55:580-592.

17. Robins LN, Helzer JE, Croughan J, et al: National Institute of Mental Health Diagnostic Interview Schedule: Its history, characteristics, and validity. Arch Gen Psychiatry 1981;38:381-389.

18. Beck AT, Ward CH, Mendelson M, et al: An inventory for measuring depression. Arch Gen Psychiatry 1961;4:561-571.

19. Frasure-Smith N, Lespérance F, Juneau M, et al: Gender, depression and one year prognosis after myocardial infarction. Psychosom Med 1999;61:26-37.

20. Lespérance F, Frasure-Smith N, Talajic M, et al: Five-year risk of cardiac mortality in relation to initial severity and one-year changes in depression symptoms after myocardial infarction. Circulation 2002;105:1049-1053.

21. Bush DE, Ziegelstein RC, Tayback M, et al: Even minimal symptoms of depression increase mortality risk after acute myocardial infarction. Am J Cardiol 2001;5:341.

22. Frasure-Smith N, Lespérance F, Gravel G, et al: Depression and health-care costs during the first year following myocardial infarction. J Psychosom Res 2000;48:471-478.

23. Lespérance F, Frasure-Smith N, Talajic M, et al: Five-year risk of cardiac mortality in relation to initial severity and one-year changes in depression symptoms after myocardial infarction. Circulation 2002;105:1049-1053.

24. Schleifer SJ, Macari-Hinson MM, Coyle DA, et al: The nature and course of depression following myocardial infarction. Arch Intern Med 1989;149:1785-1789.

25. Ziegelstein RC: Depression in patients recovering from a myocardial infarction. JAMA 2001;286:1621-1627.

26. Roy A, Pickar D, de Jong J, et al: Norepinephrine and its metabolites in cerebrospinal fluid, plasma, and urine: Relationship to hypothalamic-pituitary-adrenal axis function in depression. Arch Gen Psychiatry 1988;45:849-857.

27. Veith RC, Lewis N, Linares OA, et al: Sympathetic nervous system activity in major depression—basal and desipramine-induced alterations in plasma norepinephrine kinetics. Arch Gen Psychiatry 1993;50:1-12.

28. Podrid PJ, Fuchs T, Candinas R: Role of the sympathetic nervous system in the genesis of ventricular arrhythmia. Circulation 1990;82(Suppl I):103-113.

29. Tofler GH, Brezinski D, Schafer AI, et al: Concurrent morning increase in platelet aggregability and the risk of myocardial infarction and sudden cardiac death. N Engl J Med 1987;316:1514-1518.

30. Carney RM, Freedland KE, Veith RC, et al: Major depression, heart rate, and plasma norepinephrine in patients with coronary heart disease. Biol Psychiatry 1999;45:458-463.

31. Kleiger RE, Stein PK, Bosner MS, et al: Time domain measurements of heart rate variability. Cardiol Clin 1992;10:487-498.

32. Carney RM, Saunders RD, Freedland KE, et al: Association of depression with reduced heart rate variability in coronary artery disease. Am J Cardiol 1995;76:562-564.

33. Carney RM, Blumenthal JA, Stein PK, et al: Depression, heart rate variability, and acute myocardial infarction. Circulation 2001;104:2024-2028.

34. Bigger JT Jr, Fleiss JL, Steinman RC, et al: Frequency domain measures of heart period variability and mortality after myocardial infarction. Circulation 1992;85:164-171.

35. McFarlane A, Kamath MV, Fallen EL, et al: Effects of sertraline on the recovery rate of cardiac autonomic function in depressed patients after acute myocardial infarction. Am Heart J 2001;142:617-623.

36. Carney RM, Freedland KE, Stein PK, et al: Change in heart rate and heart rate variability during treatment for depression in patients with coronary heart disease. Psychosom Med 2000;62:639-647.

37. Arora RC, Meltzer HY: Increased serotonin$_2$ (5-HT$_2$) receptor binding as measured by ^{3}H-lysergic acid diethylamide (^{3}H-LSD) in the blood platelets of depressed patients. Life Sci 1989;44:725-734.

38. Nemeroff CB, Knight DL, Franks J, et al: Further studies on platelet serotonin transporter binding in depression. Am J Psychiatry 1994;151:1623-1625.

39. Musselman DL, Tomer A, Manatunga AK, et al: Exaggerated platelet reactivity in major depression. Am J Psychiatry 1996;153:1313-1317.

40. Pollock BG, Laghrissi-Thode F, Wagner WR: Evaluation of platelet activation in depressed patients with ischemic heart disease after paroxetine or nortriptyline treatment. J Clin Psychopharmacol 2000;20:137-140.

41. Laghrissi-Thode F, Finkel MS, Johnson PC, et al: Elevated platelet factor 4 and ß-thromboglobulin plasma levels in depressed patients with ischemic heart disease. Biol Psychiatry 1997;42:290-295.

42. Markovitz JH, Shuster JL, Chitwood WS, et al: Platelet activation in depression and effects of sertraline treatment: An open-label study. Am J Psychiatry 2000;157:1006-1008.

43. Musselman DL, Marzec UM, Manatunga A, et al: Platelet reactivity in depressed patients treated with paroxetine. Arch Gen Psychiatry 2000;57:875-882.

44. Delisi SM, Konopka LM, O'Connor L, et al: Platelet cytosolic calcium responses to serotonin in depressed patients and controls: Relationship to symptomatology and medication. Biol Psychiatry 1998;43:327-334.

45. Serebruany VL, Gurbel PA, O'Connor CM: Platelet inhibition by sertraline and n-desmethylsertraline: A possible missing link between depression, coronary events, and mortality benefits of selective serotonin reuptake inhibitors. Pharmacol Res 2001;43:453-461.

46. Carney RM, Freedland KE, Eisen SA, et al: Major depression and medication adherence in elderly patients with coronary artery disease. Health Psychol 1995;14:88-90.

47. Ziegelstein RC: Depression, adherence behavior, and coronary disease outcomes. Arch Intern Med 1998;158:808-809.

48. Druss BG, Bradford DW, Rosenheck RA, et al: Mental disorders and use of cardiovascular procedures after myocardial infarction. JAMA 2000;283:506-511.

49. Glassman AH: Cigarette smoking: Implications for psychiatric illness. Am J Psychiatry 1993;150:546-553.

50. Breslau N, Peterson EL, Schultz LR, et al: Major depression and stages of smoking: A longitudinal investigation. Arch Gen Psychiatry 1998;55:161-166.

51. Hurt RD, Sachs DP, Glover ED, et al: A comparison of sustained-release bupropion and placebo for smoking. N Engl J Med 1997;337:1195-1202.

52. Hall SM, Reus VI, Munoz RF, et al: Nortriptyline and cognitive-behavioral therapy in the treatment of cigarette smoking. Arch Gen Psychiatry 1998;55:683-690.

53. Berlin I, Said S, Spreux-Varoqiaux O, et al: A reversible monoamine oxidase A inhibitor (moclobemide) facilities smoking cessation and abstinence in heavy, dependent smokers. Clin Pharmacol Ther 1995;58:444-452.

54. Glassman AH: Psychiatry and cigarettes. Arch Gen Psychiatry 1998;55:692-693.

55. Blumenthal JA, Babyak MA, Moore KA, et al: Effects of exercise training on older patients with major depression. Arch Intern Med 1999;159:2349-2356.

56. Skotzko CE, Krichten C, Zietowski G, et al: Depression is common and precludes accurate assessment of functional status in elderly patients with congestive heart failure. J Cardiac Failure 2000;6:300-305.

57. Davis BR, Furberg C, Williams CB: Survival analysis of adverse effects data in the Beta-Blocker Heart Attack Trial. Clin Pharmacol Ther 1987;41:611-615.

58. Alexopoulos GS, Meyers BS, Young RC, et al: "Vascular depression" hypothesis. Arch Gen Psychiatry 1997;54:915-922.

59. Cohen-Cole SA, Harpe C: Diagnostic assessment of depression in the medically ill. In: Principles of Medical Psychiatry. New York, Grune & Stratton, 1987, pp 23-36.

60. Libby P: Coronary artery injury and the biology of atherosclerosis: Inflammation, thrombosis, and stabilization. Am J Cardiol 2000;86:3J-9J.

61. Connor TJ, Leonard BE: Depression, stress and immunological activation: The role of cytokines in depressive disorders. Life Sci 1998;62:583-606.

62. Zorrilla EP, Luborsky L, McKay JR, et al: The relationship of depression and stressors to immunological assays: A meta-analytic review. Brain Behav Immun 2001;15:199-226.

63. Woods A, Brull DJ, Humphries SE, et al: Genetics of inflammation and risk of coronary artery disease: The central role of interleukin-6. Eur Heart J 2000;21:1574-1583.

64. Dantzer R, Bluthe R-M, Kent S, et al: Behavioral effects of cytokines: An insight into mechanisms of sickness behavior. Methods Neurosci 1993;17:130-150.

65. Appels A: Depression and coronary heart disease: Observations and questions. J Psychosom Res 1997;43:443-452.

66. Kop WJ, Gottdiener JS, Tangen CM, et al: Inflammation and coagulation factors in persons > 65 years of age with symptoms of

depression but without evidence of myocardial ischemia. Am J Cardiol 2002;89:419–424.

67. Maes M, Smith R: Fatty acids, cytokines and major depression. Biol Psychiatry 1998;43:313–314.

68. Severus WE, Littman AB, Stoll AL: Omega-3 fatty acids, homocysteine, and the increased risk of cardiovascular mortality in major depressive disorder. Harvard Rev Psychiatry 2001;9:280–293.

69. Maes M, Christophe A, Delanghe J, et al: Lowered ω3 polyunsaturated fatty acids in serum phospholipids and cholesteryl esters of depressed patients. Psychiatr Res 1999;85:275–291.

70. Edwards R, Peet M, Shay J, et al: Omega-3 polyunsaturated fatty acid levels in the diet and in red blood cell membranes of depressed patients. J Affect Disord 1998;48:149–155.

71. Stoll AL, Severus WE, Freeman MP, et al: Omega 3 fatty acids in bipolar disorder. Arch Gen Psychiatry 1999;56:407–412.

72. American Psychiatric Association CoNaS: Diagnostic and Statistical Manual of Mental Disorders, 4th ed. Washington, D.C., American Psychiatric Association, 1994.

73. Freedland KE, Lustman PJ, Carney RM, et al: Underdiagnosis of depression in patients with coronary artery disease: The role of nonspecific symptoms. Int J Psychiatry Med 1992;22:221–229.

74. Ketterer MW, Kenyon L, Foley BA, et al: Denial of depression as an independent correlate of coronary artery disease. J Health Psychol 1996;1:93–105.

75. Fava M, Abraham M, Pava J, et al: Cardiovascular risk factors in depression: The role of anxiety and anger. Psychosomatics 1996;37:31–37.

76. Roose SP, Laghrissi-Thode F, Kennedy JS, et al: Comparison of paroxetine and nortryptyline in depressed patients with ischemic heart disease. JAMA 1998;279:287–291.

77. Shapiro PA, Lespérance F, Frasure-Smith N, et al: An open-label preliminary trial of sertraline for treatment of major depression after acute myocardial infarction (the SADHAT Trial). Am Heart J 1999;137:1100–1106.

78. Glassman AH, O'Connor CM, Califf R, et al for the SADHART Group. Sertraline treatment of major depression in patients with acute MI or unstable angina. JAMA 2002;288:701–709.

79. Kroenke K, Spitzer RL, Williams JBW: The PHQ-9: Validity of a brief depression severity measure. J Gen Intern Med 2001;16:606–613.

80. Winokur G: All roads lead to depression: clinically homogeneous, etiologically heterogeneous. J Affect Disord 1997;45:97–108.

81. Solomon DA, Keller MB, Leon AC, et al: Recovery from major depression: A 10-year prospective follow-up across multiple episodes. Arch Gen Psychiatry 1997;54:1001–1006.

82. Canadian Network for Mood and Anxiety Treatments (CANMAT): Guidelines for the Diagnosis and Pharmacological Treatment of Depression, 1st ed revised. Toronto, 1999, pp 1–76.

83. Schulberg HC, Katon W, Simon GE, et al: Treating major depression in primary care practice: An update of the agency for health care policy and research practice guidelines. Arch Gen Psychiatry 1998;55:1121–1127.

84. Glassman AH, Preud'homme XA: Review of the cardiovascular effects of heterocyclic antidepressants. J Clin Psychiatry 1993;54:16–22.

85. Harvey AT, Preskorn SH: Cytochrome P450 enzymes: interpretation of their interactions with selective serotonin reuptake inhibitors. Part I. J Clin Psychopharmacol 1996;16:273–285.

86. Nemeroff CB, DeVane L, Pollock BG: Newer antidepressants and the cytochrome P450 system. Am J Psychiatry 1996;153:311–320.

87. Roose SP, Dalack GW, Glassman AH, et al: Cardiovascular effects of bupropion in depressed patients with heart disease. Am J Psychiatry 1991;148:512–516.

88. Veith RC, Lewis N, Linares OA, et al: Sympathetic nervous system activity in major depression—basal and desipramine-induced alterations in plasma norepinephrine kinetics. Arch Gen Psychiatry 1993;50:1–12.

89. Evans MD, Hollon SD, DeRubeis RJ, et al: Differential relapse following cognitive therapy and pharmacotherapy for depression. Arch Gen Psychiatry 1992;49:802–808.

90. Klerman GL, Weissman MM, Rounsaville BJ, et al: Interpersonal Psychotherapy of Depression. Northvale, N.J., Jason Aronsin, 1984.

91. The ENRICHD Investigators: Enhancing recovery in coronary heart disease (ENRICHD) study intervention: Rationale and design. Psychosom Med 2001;63:747–755.

92. Berkman LF, Jaffe AS, for the ENRICHD investigators: The effects of treating depression and low social support on clinical events after a myocardial infarction. Circulation 2001;104:2.

93. Case RB, Moss AJ, Case N, McDermott M, et al: Living alone after myocardial infarction: impact on prognosis. JAMA 1992;267:515–519.

94. Berkman LF, Leo-Summers L, Horwitz RI: Emotional support and survival after myocardial infarction: A prospective, population-based study of the elderly. Ann Intern Med 1992;117:1003–1009.

95. Williams RB, Barefoot JC, Califf RM, et al: Prognostic importance of social and economic resources among medically treated patients with angiographically documented coronary artery disease. JAMA 1992;267:520–524.

96. Frasure-Smith N, Lespérance F, Gravel G, et al: Social support, depression and mortality during the first year after myocardial infarction. Circulation 2000;101:1919–1924.

97. Linden W, Stossel C, Maurice J: Psychosocial interventions for patients with coronary artery disease—A meta-analysis. Arch Intern Med 1996;156:745–752.

98. Frasure-Smith N, Lespérance F, Prince RH, et al: Randomised trial of home-based psychological nursing intervention for patients recovering from myocardial infarction. Lancet 1997;350:473–479.

99. Jones DA, West RR: Psychological rehabilitation after myocardial infarction: Multicenter randomised controlled trial. BMJ 1996;313:1517–1521.

100. Frasure-Smith N, Lespérance F, Gravel G, et al: Long-term survival differences among low-anxious, high-anxious and repressive copers enrolled in the Montreal heart attack readjustment trial. Psychosom Med 2002;64:571–579.

■ ■ ■ chapter**11**

Clinical Recognition of Acute Coronary Syndromes

Howard A. Cooper
Eugene Braunwald

The acute coronary syndromes comprise a spectrum of conditions that includes unstable angina, myocardial infarction (MI) without ST-segment elevation (non–ST-elevation myocardial infarction [NSTEMI]), and MI with ST-segment elevation on the electrocardiogram (ST-elevation MI [STEMI]) (Fig. 11–1). The most common pathophysiologic process that underlies the acute coronary syndromes is rupture or erosion of an unstable atherosclerotic plaque, with subsequent formation of a platelet-fibrin thrombus. The degree to which this thrombus impairs coronary blood flow, the level of myocardial oxygen demand, the presence or absence of collateral flow, and other patient-specific factors combine to determine the clinical presentation. Coronary vasospasm and vasoconstriction, progression of atherosclerosis, and increased myocardial oxygen demand in the presence of a fixed, limited supply may also play pathogenetic roles (Fig. 11–2).[1]

Clinical recognition of acute coronary syndromes involves a detailed history, focused physical examination, the 12-lead electrocardiogram (ECG), and measurement of serum markers of myocardial necrosis. Timely and accurate clinical recognition of acute coronary syndromes is essential to allow for the rapid and appropriate treatment of this potentially life-threatening condition.

HISTORICAL PERSPECTIVE

Angina pectoris literally translates as "strangling in the chest." William Heberden presented one of the earliest descriptions of angina pectoris in 1768 in a lecture to the Royal College of Physicians. In it, he described the classic symptoms of angina, as well as the spectrum of presentations, from stable exertional angina, to angina at rest, to acute MI:

This is a disorder of the breast, marked with strong and peculiar symptoms, considerable for the kind of danger belonging to it.... The seat of it, and sense of strangling and anxiety with which it is attended, may make it not improperly called angina pectoris.... Those who are afflicted with it are seized... with a painful and most disagreeable sensation in the breast, which seems as if it would take their life away, if it were to increase or continue.... When a fit of this sort comes on by walking, its duration is very short, as it goes off almost immediately upon stopping. If it comes on in the night, it will last an hour or two; and I have met with one, in whom it once continued for several days, during all which time the patient seemed to be in imminent danger of death.[2]

In 1937, Sampson and Eliaser[3] and Feil[4] published separate but remarkably similar case series describing a syndrome intermediate between chronic stable angina and acute MI, which they called *impending acute coronary occlusion*. Sampson and Eliaser wrote: "The character of the premonitory attack of precordial pain observed in these patients...rarely differed from their former pain either in its nature—i.e. squeezing, crushing, etc.—or in radiation. The effect of nitroglycerin on the premonitory attack was definitely transient, with failure of complete relief even on repeated doses..."[3] Feil summarized the symptoms of 15 patients as follows: "Substernal or epigastric...pain is complained of—mild, not related to effort or emotional strain...The pain is more or less constant, of a burning and oppressive character and is not relieved by rest or by nitrites. The pain lasts from a few hours to 4 weeks. If the patient has had pre-existing angina of effort and of emotion, he realizes that the attack is unlike the usual picture, that the pain is constant and is not relieved by rest or the accustomed therapy."[4]

Multiple terms for this syndrome proliferated in the literature, including *preinfarction angina, accelerated angina, acute coronary insufficiency,* and *intermediate coronary syndrome.*[5] In 1971, Fowler first used the term *unstable angina,* which he defined as the "sudden onset of one or more anginal attacks a day from a previous background of good health or...a dramatic change in the symptomatic pattern of previously recognized coronary disease... In patients with unstable angina, the attacks, in addition to being more frequent, are also often of longer duration and may occur at rest without an apparent precipitating event... The electrocardiogram shows no evidence of recent infarction, and such serum enzymes as the glutamic oxaloacetic transaminase or the creatine phosphokinase show no diagnostic alterations. For scientific study, however, it is desirable to define the syndrome further by requiring that selective coronary arteriography demonstrate 50% or greater narrowing of one or more of the major coronary arteries."[6]

The term *acute coronary syndromes* (see Fig. 11-1) was first used by Fuster et al in 1985 in order to highlight the common pathophysiologic link that distinguishes unstable angina and acute myocardial from chronic stable angina. The important distinction was made between the fact that "the early and some of the advanced coronary atherosclerotic lesions progress very slowly, probably by means of a complex stepwise biologic process...[whereas] some of the advanced coronary atherosclerotic lesions progress very rapidly, probably by means of complicating anatomic events, one of which is related to a thrombogenic process... These complicated processes appear to be of paramount importance in the pathogenesis of some of the acute coronary syndromes including unstable angina, MI, and sudden coronary death."[7]

In 1989, one of us proposed a clinical classification of unstable angina in order to "separate patients with unstable angina into a manageable number of meaningful and easily understood subgroups based on the severity, the presumed precipitating cause, and the presence of electrocardiographic changes..." (Table 11-1)[5] Patients are divided into three groups based on the severity of angina (I to III) and three groups according to the clinical circumstances of the acute ischemic episode (A to C).

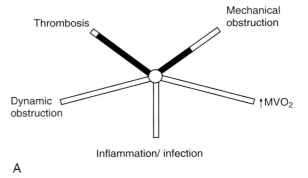

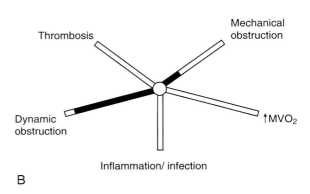

FIGURE 11–2. Schematic of the causes of unstable angina. Each of the five bars (*A* and *B*) represents one of the etiologic mechanisms, and the filled portion of the bar represents the extent to which the mechanism is operative. *A*, This is the most common form of unstable angina, in which atherosclerotic plaque causes moderate (60% diameter) obstruction and acute thrombus overlying plaque causes severe (90% diameter) narrowing. *B*, Most common form of Prinzmetal angina with mild (30% diameter) atherosclerotic obstruction, adjacent to intense (90% diameter) vasoconstriction. MV̇o₂, myocardial oxygen consumption. (From Braunwald E: Unstable angina: An etiologic approach to management. Circulation 1998;98:2219–2222.)

Additional stratification is based on the presence or absence of transient electrocardiographic changes during pain (see Table 1-3).

CLINICAL SETTING

The majority of patients who present with an acute coronary syndrome have an antecedent history of angina, and approximately 80% have a prior history of coronary artery disease. Approximately 55% of patients with unstable angina and 75% of patients with NSTEMI are male. However, women predominate among the rapidly expanding elderly population with unstable angina.[8-11]

Acute coronary syndromes have been found to have a circadian periodicity, with the peak incidence occurring between 6 AM and 12 PM (Fig. 11-3).[12] Acute coronary syndromes can be precipitated by vigorous exercise, particularly in previously sedentary patients. Emotional stress, including that created by natural disasters, may lead to plaque rupture, acute coronary syndromes, and sudden cardiac death.[13] However, the majority of acute coronary syndromes occur in patients with no identifiable trigger.

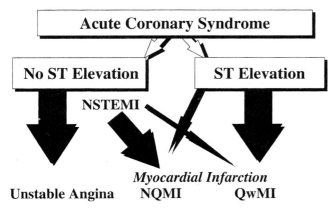

FIGURE 11–1. Nomenclature of acute coronary syndromes. Patients with ischemic discomfort may present with or without ST-segment elevation on the ECG. The majority of patients with ST-segment elevation *(large arrows)* ultimately experience a Q-wave acute myocardial infarction (QwMI), whereas a minority *(small arrow)* experience a non–Q-wave acute myocardial infarction (NQMI). Patients who present without ST-segment elevation are experiencing either unstable angina or a non–ST-elevation myocardial infarction (NSTEMI). The distinction between these two diagnoses is ultimately based on the presence or absence of a cardiac marker detected in the blood. Most patients with NSTEMI do not evolve a Q wave on the 12-lead ECG and are subsequently referred to as having sustained an NQMI; only a minority of patients with NSTEMI show a Q wave and are later said to have sustained a Q-wave MI. The spectrum of clinical conditions that range from unstable angina to non–Q-wave acute myocardial infarction and Q-wave acute myocardial infarction is called acute coronary syndrome. (Adapted from Antman EM, Braunwald E: Acute myocardial infarction. In: Braunwald E, Zipes DP, Libby P, eds: Heart Disease, A Textbook of Cardiovascular Medicine. Philadelphia, WB Saunders, 2001.)

■ ■ ■

TABLE 11–1   CLASSIFICATION OF UNSTABLE ANGINA

| Severity | CLINICAL CIRCUMSTANCES | | |
	A. Develops in presence of extracardiac condition that intensifies myocardial ischemia (secondary UA)	B. Develops in absence of extracardiac condition (primary UA)	C. Develops within 2 wk after AMI (postinfarction UA)
I. New onset of severe angina or accelerated angina; no rest pain	IA	IB	IC
II. Angina at rest within past month but not within preceding 48 hr (Angina at rest, subacute)	IIA	IIB	IIC
III. Angina at rest within 48 hr (Angina at rest, acute)	IIIA	IIIB	IIIC

Patients with UA may also be divided into three groups depending on whether UA occurs 1) in the absence of treatment for chronic stable angina, 2) during treatment for chronic stable angina, or 3) despite maximal anti-ischemic drug therapy. These three groups may be designated by subscripts 1, 2, or 3, respectively. Patients with UA may be further divided into those with and without transient ST-T wave changes during pain.
UA, unstable angina; AMI, acute myocardial infarction.

HISTORY

The hallmark of an acute coronary syndrome is ischemic chest pain. Ischemic pain is typically gradual in onset and may not reach its peak intensity for several minutes. In STEMI this pain characteristically is steady and lasts for more than 30 minutes.[14] In contrast, in unstable angina the pain frequently waxes and wanes, lasting from a few minutes to as long as 20 to 30 minutes.[15] Fleeting chest pain is rarely due to an acute coronary syndrome; the same is true for pain that persists for days. Pain due to ischemia is exacerbated by exertion and may diminish with rest. It is rarely positional or pleuritic, and such a description should suggest the diagnosis of pericarditis.

Ischemic chest pain is visceral. Patients frequently describe such pain using terms such as *pressure, burning, gnawing, tightness*, and *heaviness*. However, ischemic chest pain may also be described as *stabbing, sharp*, or *knifelike*. All of these descriptions, however, suggest a visceral rather than a superficial origin. Palpation of the chest wall does not reproduce the pain. The pain may be mild or severe, depending on patient perception, but is typically severe in STEMI.

The pain in an acute coronary syndrome is most commonly located in the center/left of the chest, with radiation to the left shoulder and arm, neck, and jaw (Fig. 11–4). Less commonly, the pain is epigastric, leading the patient (or physician) to mistake it for indigestion.

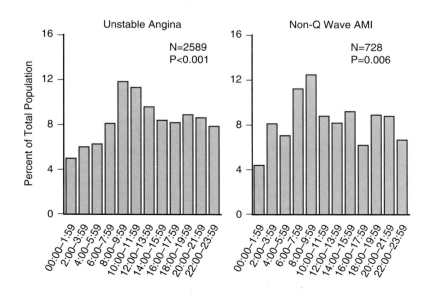

TIMI III Registry

FIGURE 11–3. Circadian variation in the onset of pain in patients with unstable angina and non–Q-wave myocardial infarction (AMI) in the Thrombolysis in Myocardial Ischemia (TIMI) III registry. (From Cannon CP, McCabe CH, Stone PH, et al: Circadian variation in the onset of unstable angina and non–Q-wave acute myocardial infarction [the TIMI III Registry and TIMI IIIB]. Am J Cardiol 1997;79:253–258.)

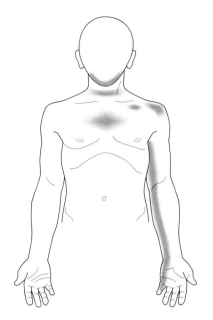

FIGURE 11–4. The "pain" of myocardial infarction commonly radiates to the areas of the body shown here. (From Morris DC: "Chest pain" in patients with myocardial infarction. In: Hurst JW, Morris DC, eds: Chest Pain. Armonk, N.Y., Futura, 2001, pp 275–285.)

Rarely, ischemic chest pain may be perceived on the right side of the chest or the interscapular region. Severe pain that radiates through the chest into the back is highly suggestive of aortic dissection.

Pain that the patient can localize by pointing with one finger is rarely ischemic; rather, ischemic pain usually occupies a substantially larger area. The Levine sign (named for Dr. Samuel A. Levine), in which a patient places a clenched fist over the chest while describing the pain, is classic in acute MI and approximates the size of the painful area (Fig. 11–5).

Patients with acute coronary syndromes, and particularly acute MI (both STEMI and NSTEMI), may have other symptoms, most commonly dyspnea, diaphoresis, nausea, vomiting, and palpitations. Gastrointestinal symptoms are most common with ischemia of the inferior wall. Other atypical symptoms include apprehension or

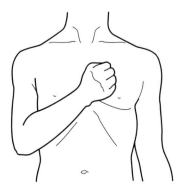

FIGURE 11–5. The Levine sign of acute myocardial ischemia. The clenched fist approximates the area of ischemic discomfort.

anxiety, syncope, acute heart failure, generalized weakness, and acute mental status changes. Atypical symptoms are more common among elderly patients.[16]

Acute coronary syndromes, including MI, also may be clinically silent. Episodes of silent ischemia may be detected by ambulatory ST-segment monitoring.[17] Episodes of silent ischemia, many at rest, have been estimated to occur in up to half of all patients with exertional angina.[18]

PHYSICAL EXAMINATION

The physical examination of patients suffering an acute coronary syndrome can vary from completely unremarkable to dramatic, depending on the degree and location of the ischemia as well as individual patient factors. The more severe signs described later frequently accompany acute MI, including NSTEMI, rather than unstable angina. In addition, many signs of acute ischemia may be transient, occurring only during the ischemia and resolving quickly thereafter.

Patients with an acute coronary syndrome frequently appear anxious, and many restlessly attempt to find a comfortable position. Patients may massage their chest or demonstrate the Levine sign. Diaphoresis, occasionally profound, is common, particularly in inferior infarction. Skin pallor may be evident.

The heart rate can be highly varied, depending on the degree of anxiety, hemodynamic status, location of ischemia, and underlying cardiac rhythm. Commonly, it is elevated and ventricular premature beats are present. However, inferior ischemia is frequently accompanied by bradycardia. Patients with unstable angina are frequently normotensive. With more severe ischemia, the blood pressure may be elevated as a consequence of adrenergic discharge. In inferior ischemia, hypotension due to excess parasympathetic stimulation is common. The administration of nitrates may exacerbate this, particularly in the subset of patients with right-ventricular involvement.

The temperature is usually normal in patients with unstable angina. In NSTEMI, fever frequently develops as a nonspecific response to myocardial necrosis. The fever is usually low-grade, begins within 4 to 8 hours of infarction, and resolves within 4 to 5 days.

In unstable angina, the respiratory rate is most often normal. The respiratory rate may be elevated in acute MI (NSTEMI or STEMI), either from pain and anxiety or from left-ventricular dysfunction. The jugular venous pressure is normal or slightly elevated in the majority of patients with acute coronary syndromes. The lungs are usually clear in patients with unstable angina. Moist rales or wheezing may be heard in the setting of acute NSTEMI complicated by acute left-ventricular dysfunction.

Cardiac Examination

Despite severe symptoms and extensive ischemia, cardiac examination results are often normal in patients with acute coronary syndromes. Abnormalities are more common in those with STEMI/NSTEMI than in those with unstable angina, but abnormalities may occur transiently in any of these syndromes (Table 11-2).

Palpation of the precordium may reveal an abnormal systolic pulsation to the left of the sternum, reflecting a dyskinetic segment of the left ventricle. A palpable presystolic impulse at the apex corresponds to an audible fourth heart sound (S_4), both of which usually occur transiently in patients with unstable angina.

A soft first heart sound may reflect acute left-ventricular dysfunction or may be heard in the presence of a first-degree AV block. An S_4, frequently audible in patients with acute coronary syndromes, is best heard between the left sternal border and the apex and reflects the reduction in left-ventricular compliance associated with ischemia. A third heart sound (S_3) is caused by rapid deceleration of transmitral blood flow during early diastolic filling of the left ventricle and suggests left-ventricular systolic dysfunction.

Systolic murmurs are common among patients with acute coronary syndromes. An apical holosystolic murmur usually results from mitral regurgitation, which can be caused by ischemic dysfunction and displacement of the mitral valve apparatus. This murmur may occur transiently during episodes of ischemia. The systolic murmur of tricuspid regurgitation caused by right-ventricular ischemia or infarction is heard along the left sternal border but is accentuated by inspiration.

Electrocardiogram

The 12-lead ECG is the most important test in patients with a suspected acute coronary syndrome (Fig. 11-6). The ECG provides essential diagnostic and prognostic information and therefore should be performed as soon as possible, preferably within 10 minutes of presentation.[19]

The presence of persistent ST-segment elevation on the ECG by definition distinguishes STEMI from unstable angina and NSTEMI. ST-segment elevation results from epicardial injury, which is usually caused by complete (or near-complete) thrombotic occlusion of an epicardial vessel. The ST-segment vector points toward the region of injury and can frequently identify the infarct-related artery. ST-segment depression can occur either in isolation or in the presence of ST-segment elevation elsewhere on the ECG. In the latter case, ST-segment depression may be due to true ischemia in another vascular territory ("ischemia at a distance") or may be due to reciprocal electrical phenomena. Occasionally, isolated ST-segment depression in the right precordial leads may occur in true posterior infarction.

In the absence of ST-segment elevation elsewhere on the ECG, ST-segment depression is usually associated with subendocardial ischemia. In patients with this finding, the distinction between unstable angina and NSTEMI is based on whether the ST-segment depression is transient or persistent, but ultimately on the detection of serum markers of myocardial necrosis. Acute reperfusion therapy is contraindicated in these patients.[19] In UA/NSTEMI, ST-segment depression is associated with a significantly worse prognosis than isolated T-wave changes (or a normal ECG).[20,21] The location of ST-segment depression on the ECG is less specific for determining the culprit coronary artery than ST-segment elevation.

T-wave inversion is a less specific sign of ischemia. However, in patients suspected to have an acute coronary syndrome, marked (≥ 2 mm) symmetric T-wave inversion strongly suggests acute ischemia. When present in the anterior precordial leads, these indicators are frequently associated with severe stenosis in the proximal left anterior descending coronary artery

■ ▩ ■

TABLE 11–2   LIKELIHOOD THAT SIGNS AND SYMPTOMS REPRESENT AN ACS SECONDARY TO CAD

FEATURE	HIGH LIKELIHOOD (Any of the following)	INTERMEDIATE LIKELIHOOD (Absence of high-likelihood features and presence of any of the following)	LOW LIKELIHOOD (Absence of high- or intermediate-likelihood features but may have)
History	Chest or left arm pain or discomfort as chief symptom reproducing prior documented angina Known history of CAD, including MI	Chest or left arm pain or discomfort as chief symptom Age >70 years Male sex Diabetes mellitus	Probable ischemic symptoms in absence of any of the intermediate likelihood characteristics Recent cocaine use
Examination	Transient MR, hypotension, diaphoresis, pulmonary edema, or rales	Extracardiac vascular disease	Chest discomfort reproduced by palpation
ECG	New, or presumably new, transient ST-segment deviation ($\geq$0.05 mV) or T-wave inversion ($\geq$0.2 mV) with symptoms	Fixed Q waves Abnormal ST segments or T waves not documented to be new	T-wave flattening or inversion in leads with dominant R waves Normal ECG
Cardiac markers	Elevated cardiac TnI, TnT, or CK-MB	Normal	Normal

Braunwald E, Mark DB, Jones RH, et al. Unstable angina: diagnosis and management. Rockville, MD: Agency for Health Care Policy and Research and the National Heart, Lung, and Blood Institute, US Public Health Service, US Department of Health and Human Services; 1994; AHCPR Publication No. 94–0602.

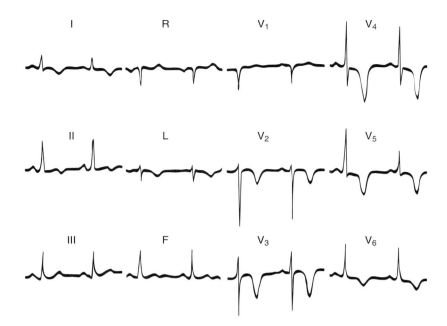

FIGURE 11–6. Electrocardiogram showing deep symmetrical anterolateral T-wave inversion without ST-segment deviation. Such findings are frequently associated with critical stenosis of the left anterior descending coronary artery and are a useful marker of a patient at high risk for subsequent death or myocardial infarction. (From Haines DE, Raabe DS, Gundel WD, Wackers FJ: Anatomic and prognostic significance of new T-wave inversion in unstable angina. Am J Cardiol 1983;52:14-18.)

(see Fig. 11–6). An important alternative cause of deep anterior T-wave inversions is severe central nervous system injury.

The presence of a normal-appearing ECG does not exclude an acute coronary syndrome. Of patients with symptoms consistent with ischemia who have a normal ECG, approximately 4% will be found to have unstable angina and 1% to 6% will have evidence of myocardial necrosis (i.e., NSTEMI).[22,23]

Biochemical Cardiac Markers

The loss of membrane integrity in myocardial cells undergoing necrosis allows intracellular macromolecules to diffuse into the cardiac interstitium. From there, these molecules enter the lymphatics and eventually the cardiac microcirculation. These biochemical cardiac markers can subsequently be detected in the peripheral circulation. In the proper clinical setting, detection of a sufficient concentration of a cardiac marker in the circulation allows the diagnosis of acute MI. This can be particularly helpful in patients who present without ST-segment elevation or with atypical symptoms, in whom the diagnosis of an acute coronary syndrome might otherwise be unclear. In addition, the distinction between unstable angina and acute MI carries important prognostic information (see Chapter 14).

A consensus panel has redefined the diagnosis of MI based on an elevation of cardiac-specific troponin.[24,25] The highly sensitive nature of the cardiac troponins has led to a dramatic increase in the number of patients with acute coronary syndromes who are found to have myocardial necrosis. Approximately 30% of patients who would previously have been diagnosed with unstable angina using a CK-MB standard actually have NSTEMI based on the troponin standard.

OTHER DIAGNOSTIC MODALITIES

Occasionally, the diagnosis of an acute coronary syndrome remains uncertain despite the history, physical examination, ECG, and cardiac markers. In these unusual circumstances, other diagnostic modalities may be used. In the setting of an acute coronary syndrome, the region of the myocardium that is ischemic becomes dysfunctional. If the dysfunctional region is large enough, a wall-motion abnormality may be detected by two-dimensional echocardiography or magnetic resonance imaging (MRI). Myocardial perfusion can be evaluated using nuclear cardiac imaging techniques and MRI. The absence of a perfusion abnormality makes the diagnosis of acute ischemia very unlikely. Finally, in patients in whom reperfusion therapy is being considered but the diagnosis remains uncertain, emergency coronary angiography can identify an occluded coronary artery and allow for immediate percutaneous coronary intervention.

CLINICAL RECOGNITION OF ACUTE CORONARY SYNDROMES

The clinical recognition of an acute coronary syndrome involves the careful integration of the components described earlier. Often, the repetition of certain aspects of the evaluation, such as the clinical examination, ECG, and troponin assessment, can reveal previously undetected and telling abnormalities. This information should be used to categorize patients as having a noncardiac diagnosis, chronic stable angina, possible acute coronary syndrome, or definite acute coronary syndrome. Appropriate triage and specific therapy can then be applied rationally in order to optimize patient outcomes.[19]

REFERENCES

1. Braunwald E: Unstable angina: An etiologic approach to management. Circulation 1998;98:2219-2222.

2. Heberden W: Some account of disorders of the breast. Med Trans R Col Physicians (London) 1772;2:59-67.

3. Sampson JJ, Eliaser M: The diagnosis of impending acute coronary artery occlusion. Am Heart J 1937;13:675-686.

4. Feil H: Preliminary pain in coronary thrombosis. Am J Med Sci 1937;193:42-48.

5. Braunwald E: Unstable angina. A classification. Circulation 1989;80:410-414.

6. Fowler NO: "Preinfarctional" angina: A need for an objective definition and for a controlled clinical trial of its management. Circulation 1971;44:755-758.

7. Fuster V, Steele PM, Chesebro JH: Role of platelets and thrombosis in coronary atherosclerotic disease and sudden death. J Am Coll Cardiol 1985;5:175B-184B.

8. Hochman JS, McCabe CH, Stone PH, et al: Outcome and profile of women and men presenting with acute coronary syndromes: a report from TIMI IIIB. TIMI Investigators. Thrombolysis in Myocardial Infarction. J Am Coll Cardiol 1997;30:141-148.

9. Hochman JS, Tamis JE, Thompson TD, et al: Sex, clinical presentation, and outcome in patients with acute coronary syndromes. Global Use of Strategies to Open Occluded Coronary Arteries in Acute Coronary Syndromes IIb Investigators. N Engl J Med 1999;341:226-232.

10. A comparison of recombinant hirudin with heparin for the treatment of acute coronary syndromes. The Global Use of Strategies to Open Occluded Coronary Arteries (GUSTO) IIb investigators. N Engl J Med 1996;335:775-782.

11. Cannon CP, Braunwald E: Unstable Angina. In: Braunwald E, Zipes D, Libby P, eds: Heart Disease, 6th ed. Philadelphia, WB Saunders, 2001, pp 1232-1271.

12. Cannon CP, McCabe CH, Stone PH, et al: Circadian variation in the onset of unstable angina and non-Q-wave acute myocardial infarction (the TIMI III Registry and TIMI IIIB). Am J Cardiol 1997;79: 253-258.

13. Leor J, Poole WK, Kloner RA: Sudden cardiac death triggered by an earthquake. N Engl J Med 1996;334:413-419.

14. Morris DC: Chest pain in patients with myocardial infarction. In: Hurst JW, Morris DC, eds: Chest Pain. Armonk, NY, Futura, 2001, pp 275-285.

15. Hurst JW: Chest pain in patients with angina pectoris. In: Hurst JW, Morris DC, eds: Chest Pain. Armonk, NY, Futura, 2001, pp 249-274.

16. Sheifer SE, Gersh BJ, Yanez ND III, et al: Prevalence, predisposing factors, and prognosis of clinically unrecognized myocardial infarction in the elderly. J Am Coll Cardiol 2000;35:119-126.

17. Krantz DS, Hedges SM, Gabbay FH, et al: Triggers of angina and ST-segment depression in ambulatory patients with coronary artery disease: evidence for an uncoupling of angina and ischemia. Am Heart J 1994;128:703-712.

18. Cohn PF: Silent myocardial ischemia: Classification, prevalence, and prognosis. Am J Med 1985;79:2-6.

19. Braunwald E, Antman EM, Beasley JW, et al: ACC/AHA guidelines for the management of patients with unstable angina and non-ST-segment elevation myocardial infarction. A report of the American College of Cardiology/American Heart Association Task Force on Practice Guidelines (Committee on the Management of Patients With Unstable Angina). J Am Coll Cardiol 2000;36:970-1062.

20. Cannon CP, McCabe CH, Stone PH, et al: The electrocardiogram predicts one-year outcome of patients with unstable angina and non-Q wave myocardial infarction: Results of the TIMI III Registry ECG Ancillary Study. Thrombolysis in Myocardial Ischemia. J Am Coll Cardiol 1997;30: 133-140.

21. Savonitto S, Ardissino D, Granger CB, et al: Prognostic value of the admission electrocardiogram in acute coronary syndromes. JAMA 1999;281:707-713.

22. Rouan GW, Lee TH, Cook EF, et al: Clinical characteristics and outcome of acute myocardial infarction in patients with initially normal or nonspecific electrocardiograms (a report from the Multicenter Chest Pain Study). Am J Cardiol 1989;64: 1087-1092.

23. Slater DK, Hlatky MA, Mark DB, et al: Outcome in suspected acute myocardial infarction with normal or minimally abnormal admission electrocardiographic findings. Am J Cardiol 1987;60:766-770.

24. Myocardial infarction redefined—a consensus document of The Joint European Society of Cardiology/American College of Cardiology Committee for the redefinition of myocardial infarction. J Am Coll Cardiol 2000;36:959-969.

25. Jaffe AS, Ravkilde J, Roberts R, et al: It's time for a change to a troponin standard. Circulation 2000;102:1216-1220.

■ ▨ ■ chapter **1 2**

Acute Coronary Syndrome in the Emergency Department: Diagnosis, Risk Stratification, and Management

Judd E. Hollander

Potential ischemic heart disease is the third most common cause of emergency department (ED) visits, after trauma and upper respiratory infections. In 1997, 14 million electrocardiograms (ECGs) were obtained on patients in EDs in the United States. There were more than 3 million ED visits with a primary diagnosis of acute chest pain. International consensus guidelines have focused largely on the identification and optimal treatment of patients with acute coronary syndromes (ACS).[1,2] One role of the ED physician is to expedite care of patients with ACS. Another is to identify patients at such low risk for ACS that they can be released safely from the ED without an extended and costly evaluation. This chapter focuses on the specific role of the ED physician in identification, risk stratification, and timely treatment of patients at low risk and high risk of ACS.

Studies evaluating clinical presentation, ECG data, cardiac markers, computer modeling, and imaging modalities have provided insight into identification of high-risk and low-risk patients. Most of these studies have failed to achieve sufficient predictive properties, however, such that patients can be released rapidly from the ED with a less than 1% risk of acute myocardial infarction (MI) or death. Despite the rapid growth of knowledge in this area, the missed acute MI rates have not changed greatly since the 1980s. Incremental decreases in admission rate are inversely related to increases in the missed acute MI rate (Fig. 12–1). There are few broadly accepted consensus guidelines or pathways to allow the rapid release of patients at low risk for ACS.

CLINICAL IDENTIFICATION AND RISK STRATIFICATION OF ACUTE CORONARY SYNDROMES

History and Physical Examination

A carefully conducted history and physical examination comprise the initial assessment of patients presenting with suspected ACS. ACS represent a disease spectrum from chronic stable angina to acute MI. The Canadian Cardiovascular Society divides angina into four classes (Table 12–1). Class I comprises patients in whom ordinary physical activity does not cause angina. Class IV comprises patients who develop anginal symptoms at minimal activity and sometimes at rest. Unstable angina

has been divided into three principal presentations by the Agency for Health Care Policy and Research Clinical Practice guidelines: rest angina, new-onset angina, and increasing angina (Table 12–2).

The use of these classifications and definitions in the ED is problematic. When patients present with acute chest pain syndromes, it often is not clear whether the pain is cardiac or noncardiac in origin. The proper application of the Canadian Cardiovascular Society Classification and the Agency for Health Care Policy and Research Clinical Practice guidelines assumes a diagnosis of ischemic chest pain. These guidelines can be difficult to incorporate into emergency practices, in which the diagnosis is often uncertain. At the time of ED presentation, the most immediate concern is the identification of patients who have ACS from the larger cohort of patients with non-ACS chest pain. Although some risk stratification studies conducted in the ED have an incidence of acute MI of 15% to 20%, these numbers reflect the selection and ascertainment biases of the clinical investigations. More broad-based studies that included all patients who received an ECG for the evaluation of chest pain

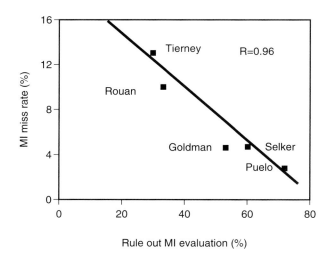

FIGURE 12–1. There is an inverse relationship between the proportion of patients admitted for "rule out acute myocardial infarction (MI)" protocols and the proportion of patients discharged from the emergency department with acute MI (missed acute MI). (From Kontos MC, Jesse RL: Evaluation of the emergency department of chest pain patient. Am J Cardiol 2000;85:32B–39B.)

■■■

TABLE 12–1   CANADIAN CARDIOVASCULAR SOCIETY CLASSIFICATION OF ANGINA

Class I	Angina occurs only with strenuous, rapid, or prolonged exertion. Ordinary physical activity does not cause angina
Class II	Slight limitation of ordinary activity. Angina occurs with climbing stairs rapidly, walking uphill, walking after meals, in cold, in wind, or under emotional stress
Class III	Marked limitations of ordinary physical activity. Angina occurs on walking 1–2 blocks on level ground or climbing one flight of stairs at usual pace
Class IV	Inability to carry on physical activity without discomfort, anginal symptoms may be present at rest

Source: Campsou L. Grading of angina pectoris (letter). Circulation 1976;54: 522–3

syndromes found that 5% of these patients ultimately were diagnosed with acute MI, and an additional 10% had non–acute MI ACS. Of patients, 85% have non-ACS causes for their symptoms. From the ED perspective, it is important to distinguish expeditiously between these two groups of patients (Table 12–3).

The precision of clinical features for the evaluation of chest pain is variable.[3-5] Hickan and colleagues[3] found that features associated with a lower probability of acute MI, such as pleuritic, positional, and sharp chest pain, showed poor-to-fair interphysician reliability (κ 0.27 to 0.44). High-risk features (radiation to left arm, substernal location, and history of acute MI) were more reliable (κ 0.74 to 0.89).[3] History is most reliable in "ruling in" high-risk patients but is less reliable when being used to "rule out" ACS. Likelihood ratios for several clinical features are shown in Table 12–4.

Traditional cardiac risk factors are predictive of coronary artery disease in asymptomatic patients. In the ED, cardiac risk factors are poor predictors of risk for MI or ACS.[6] Traditional cardiac risk factors, such as hypertension, diabetes mellitus, tobacco use, family history of coronary artery disease at an early age, and hypercholesterolemia, are not predictive of the cardiac risk in female ED patients with chest pain. In male patients, only

■■■

TABLE 12–2   MAIN PRESENTATIONS OF UNSTABLE ANGINA

Rest angina	Angina occurring at rest and usually prolonged >20 minutes occurring within 1 week of presentation
New-onset angina	Angina of at least CCSC III severity with onset within 2 months of presentation
Increasing angina	Previously diagnosed angina that is distinctly more frequent, longer in duration, or lower in threshold (increased by at least one CCSC class to at least CCSC III severity)

CCSC, Canadian Cardiovascular Society Classification. Braunwald E, Mark DB, Jones RH, et al: Unstable Angina: Diagnosis and Management. Clinical Practice Guideline No. 10 (amended). AHCPR Publication No. 94-0602. Rockville, MD, Agency for Health Care Policy and Research and the National Health, Lung and Blood Institute, Public Health Service, U.S. Department of Health and Human Services, May 1994.

diabetes and family history are weakly predictive.[6] The distinction between the utility of cardiac risk factors in asymptomatic patients and the relative lack of utility in the ED patients with chest pain is logical. Traditional cardiac risk factors were derived from population-based longitudinal cohort studies of asymptomatic patients. In contrast, ED chest pain patients already have been identified as being at increased risk by the fact that they have symptoms. The presence of symptoms outweighs the predictive abilities of cardiac risk factors. A lack of cardiac risk factors does not decrease cardiac risk in ED patients sufficiently such that they can be released expeditiously from the ED.

Atypical presentations and silent myocardial ischemia are common. Of patients with Q-wave MI identified in large longitudinal studies, 22% to 40% are clinically unrecognized.[7] Women and the elderly are more likely to have atypical presentations. It is unclear whether these patients had atypical symptoms for which they did not pursue medical advice or whether they were truly asymptomatic. The prognosis for patients who have atypical symptoms at the time of MI is worse than that of patients who had more typical symptoms.

Likewise, the use of the physical examination to distinguish conclusively patients with ACS from patients with noncardiac chest pain is suboptimal. Patients with ACS may appear deceptively well without any clinical signs of distress or may be uncomfortable, pale, cyanotic, and in respiratory distress. The first and second heart sounds often are diminished because of poor myocardial contractility. An S_3 is present in 15% to 20% of patients with acute MI. An S_4 is common in patients with long-standing hypertension or myocardial dysfunction. The presence of a murmur can be an ominous sign of flail leaflet of the mitral valve or a ventricular septal defect, or it can reflect long-standing valvular heart disease. In the ED, knowledge about the patient's baseline condition can help establish which signs and symptoms are chronic; however, this information is often not available.

Heavy reliance on individual physical examination findings is not wise. Signs and symptoms of congestive heart failure have poor interrater reliability (S_3 gallop, κ 0.14 to 0.37; rales, κ 0.12 to 0.31; neck vein distention, κ 0.31 to 0.51; hepatomegaly, κ 0.00 to 0.16; and dependent edema, κ 0.27 to 0.64).[5] The heavy use of these individual signs and symptoms to guide management can be misleading in the ED setting.

Electrocardiogram

The standard 12-lead ECG is the best test to identify patients with acute MI on ED presentation.[8] National guidelines call for an ECG to be obtained and interpreted within 10 minutes of presentation.[9] Although it is the best test available to ED physicians, the ECG still has relatively low sensitivity for detection of acute MI. The sensitivity of ST-segment elevation for the detection of acute MI is 35% to 50%, leaving more than half of all acute MI patients unidentified.[8,9] Even among patients with ST-segment elevation MI, ECG variables can risk stratify further the likelihood of 30-day mortality (Table 12–5).[10] The standard 12-lead ECG is useful for cardiovascular

■ ▩ ■

TABLE 12–3 LIKELIHOOD OF SIGNS AND SYMPTOMS REPRESENTING ACUTE CORONARY SYNDROMES SECONDARY TO CORONARY ARTERY DISEASE

CHARACTERISTIC	HIGH LIKELIHOOD (*Any of the following features*)	INTERMEDIATE LIKELIHOOD (*Absence of high likelihood features and any of the following*)	LOW LIKELIHOOD (*Absence of high or intermediate likelihood features but may have the following*)
History	Typical symptoms reproducing prior angina History of prior acute myocardial infarction or known history of coronary artery disease	Chest or left arm discomfort as chief symptom Male sex Diabetes mellitus Multiple cardiac risk factors	Probable ischemic symptoms in absence of any of intermediate likelihood characteristics Recent cocaine use Chest discomfort reproduced by palpation
Examination	Transient mitral regurgitation, hypotension, diaphoresis, pulmonary edema, or rales	Extracardiac vascular disease Fixed Q waves	
ECG	New transient ST-segment deviation (>0.05 mV) or T-wave inversions (>0.2 mV) with symptoms	Abnormal ST segments or T waves not known to new	T-wave flattening or inversion < 1 mm in leads with dominant R waves Normal ECG
Cardiac markers	Elevated cardiac troponin I, troponin T, or CK-MB	Normal	Normal

ECG, electrocardiogram.
From Braunwald E, Mark DB, Jones RH, et al: Unstable Angina: Diagnosis and Management. Clinical Practice Guideline No. 10 (amended). AHCPR Publication No. 94-0602. Rockville, MD, Agency for Health Care Policy and Research and the National Health, Lung and Blood Institute, Public Health Service, U.S. Department of Health and Human Services, May 1994.

risk stratification of patients with potential ACS. Individual ECG features that increase the risk of acute MI in ED patients with chest pain are shown in Table 12-6.[5]

■ ▩ ■

TABLE 12–4 LIKELIHOOD RATIOS FOR CLINICAL FEATURES THAT INCREASE OR DECREASE RISK OF ACUTE MYOCARDIAL INFARCTION IN PATIENTS PRESENTING WITH CHEST PAIN

CLINICAL FEATURE	LIKELIHOOD RATIO (95% CI)
Increased likelihood of acute MI	
Pain in chest or left arm	2.7*
Chest pain radiation	
To right shoulder	2.9(1.4–6.0)
To left arm	2.3 (1.7–3.1)
To left and right arm	7.1 (3.6–14.2)
Chest pain most important symptom	2.0*
History of MI	1.5–3.0†
Nausea or vomiting	1.9 (1.7–2.3)
Diaphoresis	2.0 (1.9–2.2)
Third heart sound	3.2 (1.6–6.5)
Hypotension (systolic BP < 80 mm Hg)	3.1 (1.8–5.2)
Pulmonary crackles	2.1 (1.4–3.1)
Decreased likelihood of acute MI	
Pleuritic chest pain	0.2 (0.2–0.3)
Chest pain sharp or stabbing	0.3 (0.2–0.5)
Positional chest pain	0.3 (0.2–0.4)
Chest pain reproduced by palpation	0.2–0.4†

*Data not available to calculate confidence intervals.
†In heterogeneous studies the likelihood ratios are reported as ranges.
CI, confidence interval; MI, myocardial infarction.
From Panju AA, Hemmelgarm BR, Guyatt GH, Simel DL: Is this patient having a myocardial infarction. JAMA 1998;280:1256–1263.

Patients with normal or nonspecific ECGs have a 1% to 5% incidence of acute MI and a 4% to 23% incidence of having unstable angina.[8,9,11,12] Patients with nondiagnostic ECGs or with ischemia that is not known to be old have a 4% to 7% incidence of acute MI and a 21% to 48% incidence of unstable angina. Demonstration of new ischemia increases the risk of acute MI to 25% to 73% and the risk of unstable angina to 14% to 43%.[8] Diagnostic 12-lead ECGs can dictate treatment pathways, such as fibrinolytic or glycoprotein IIb/IIIa inhibitor use, but a normal ECG does not have sufficient sensitivity to exclude ACS conclusively. The ECG should be used with clinical history and cardiac markers to determine admission location and treatment for patients with ACS.

Because of the relatively poor sensitivity of the standard 12-lead ECG to detect patients with ACS, additional ECG strategies have been proposed. Continuous 12-lead ECG monitors and records new ECGs every 20 seconds. When the ST-segment baseline is altered, the continuous ECG alarms and prints a copy of the new ECG. This technology is employed most often in chest pain observation units, where it might be useful for monitoring patients who present with non–acute MI ACS for ECG evidence of injury.[9] Because of costs, concerns regarding labile ST-segment and T-wave changes from hyperventilation or patient movement, and a lack of ED-based prospective studies, continuous 12-lead ECGs have not been recommended for routine use.[9]

There have been studies of 15-lead, 18-lead, and 22-lead ECGs.[9,13] The addition of V_4R, V_8, and V_9 increased the sensitivity to detect ST-segment elevation to 59% without a loss of specificity in one study.[13] The addition of V_4R-V_6R and V_7-V_9 as posterior leads led to an 8% increase in sensitivity for acute MI relative to a standard 12-lead ECG but at the cost of a 7% decrease in speci-

■ ■ ■

TABLE 12–5 MULTIVARIATE SIGNIFICANCE OF THE ELECTROCARDIOGRAM IN PATIENTS WITH ST-SEGMENT ELEVATION MYOCARDIAL INFARCTION ENROLLED IN GUSTO-1

ELECTROCARDIOGRAM FEATURE	Odds Ratio (95% CI)
Sum of ST-segment deviation (19 mm versus 8 mm)	1.53 (1.38–1.69)
Sum of ST-segment decrease (–1 mm versus – 7 mm)	0.77 (0.72–0.83)
Heart rate (84 versus 60 beats/min)	1.49 (1.41–1.59)
Sum ST-segment increase in II, III, and aVF (6 mm versus 0 mm)	0.79 (0.71–0.89)
QRS duration (100 msec versus 80 msec)	
Anterior infarct	1.55 (1.43–1.68)
Other location	1.08 (1.03–1.13)
Anterior infarction	
QRS duration 100 msec	1.08 (1.03–1.13)
QRS duration 50 msec	0.61 (0.43–0.86)
Inferior infarction	
No prior acute MI	0.67 (0.50–0.90)
Prior acute MI	1.41 (0.98–2.02)
Prior infarction	
Inferior infarction	2.47 (2.02–3.00)
Other location	1.17 (0.98–1.41)

CI, confidence interval; MI, myocardial infarction.
From Hathaway WR, Peterson ED, Wagner GS, et al: Prognostic significance of the initial electrocardiogram in patients with acute myocardial infarction. JAMA 1998;279:387–391.

ficity.[14] The 22-lead and body surface mapping ECGs have not been studied sufficiently to recommend their use. In general, 12-lead ECGs are sufficient. Right-sided leads should be used in the setting of inferior wall infarction to assess possible right ventricular involvement, and V_8 and V_9 leads should be used when the chest pain suggests MI or some abnormalities are observed in the inferior or lateral leads.[9]

■ ■ ■

TABLE 12–6 ELECTROCARDIOGRAM FEATURES PREDICTIVE OF ACUTE MYOCARDIAL INFARCTION IN ACUTE CHEST PAIN PATIENTS

ELECTROCARDIOGRAM FEATURE	LIKELIHOOD RATIO (95% CI)
New ST-segment elevation ≥ 1 mm	5.7–53.9*
New Q wave	5.3–24.8*
Any ST-segment elevation	11.2 (7.1–17.8)
New conduction defect	6.3 (2.5–15.7)
New ST-segment depression	3.0–5.2*
Any Q wave	3.9 (2.7–5.7)
Any ST-segment depression	3.2 (2.5–4.1)
T-wave peaking and/or inversion ≥ 1 mm	3.1†
New T-wave inversion	2.4–2.8*
Any conduction defect	2.7 (1.4–5.4)

*In heterogeneous studies, the likelihood ratios are reported as ranges.
†Data not available to calculate CI.
CI, confidence interval.
From Panju AA, Hemmelgarm BR, Guyatt GH, Simel DL: Is this patient having a myocardial infarction. JAMA 1998;280:1256–1263.

There are several clinical conditions in which ECG interpretation of ACS is difficult, particularly paced rhythms and left bundle-branch blocks. In the setting of a left bundle-branch block, the presence of ST-segment elevation of greater than or equal to 1 mm and concordant with the QRS complex or ST-segment depression greater than or equal to 1 mm in leads V_1, V_2, or V_3 suggests acute MI.[15] ST-segment elevation greater than or equal to 5 mm and discordant with the QRS complex increases the likelihood of acute MI but has poor specificity.

Uncomplicated right ventricular pacing causes secondary repolarization changes of opposing polarity to that of the predominant QRS complex. Most leads have predominant negative QRS complexes followed by ST-segment elevation and positive T waves. ST-segment elevation greater than or equal to 5 mm is most indicative of acute MI in leads with predominantly negative QRS complexes. Any ST-segment elevation concordant to the QRS complex in a predominantly positive QRS complex is highly specific for acute MI. The QRS complex is predominantly negative in leads V_1 to V_3. ST-segment depression in these leads had 80% specificity for acute MI.[16]

Risk Stratification Algorithms

Goldman Risk Score

The Goldman risk score was derived through analysis of clinical data on a large cohort of patients presenting to the ED with chest pain. This algorithm has been prospectively validated and is useful as an initial risk stratification tool.[17] The final algorithm is based heavily on ECG findings and chest pain characteristics (Fig. 12–2). This tool was derived without the assistance of cardiac marker determinations in the ED. The Goldman algorithm stratifies patients into groups with risks of acute MI that vary from 1% to 77%. The sensitivity of the Goldman chest pain protocol for predicting acute MI is 88% to 91%, specificity is 78% to 92%.[18] It does not identify any group with less than 1% risk. It does identify patients safe for a 12-hour observation protocol but has not been able to identify any group of patients safe for ED release. Goldman and colleagues[19] also derived a rule to predict the need for intensive care unit (ICU) admission and development of cardiovascular complications. ST-segment elevation or Q waves on the ECG, other ECG findings indicating myocardial ischemia, low systolic blood pressure, pulmonary rales above the bases, and an exacerbation of known ischemic heart disease all predicted complications. This algorithm has been independently validated, and strict adherence to the protocol would reduce ICU admission by 16%, resulting in potentially large cost savings.[20]

ACI-TIPI

The ACI-TIPI (acute cardiac ischemia time insensitive predictive instrument) is a computer-generated method to determine the likelihood of ACS at the time of initial clinical evaluation. The ACI-TIPI ECG incorporates age, sex, presence of chest or left arm pain, a chief symptom

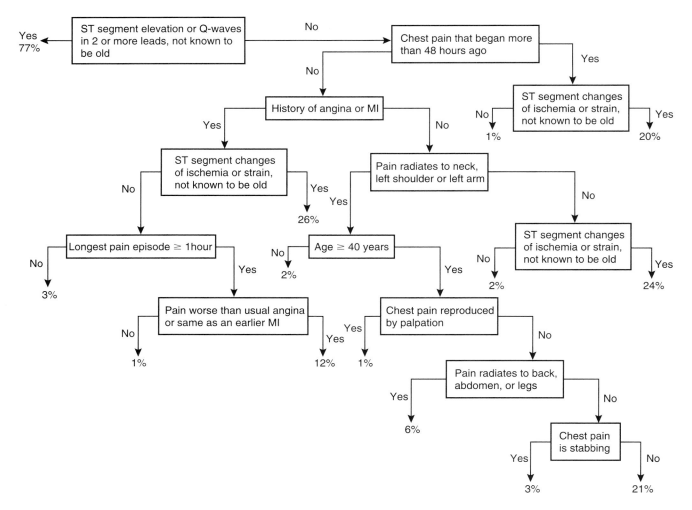

FIGURE 12–2. The Goldman risk stratification algorithm for prediction of acute myocardial infarction. (From Lee TH, Juarez G, Cook EF, et al: Ruling out acute myocardial infarction: A perspective multicenter validation of a 12 hour strategy for patients at low risk. N Engl J Med 1991;324:1239-1246.)

of chest or left arm pain, pathologic Q waves, and the presence and degree of ST-segment elevation or depression and T-wave elevation or inversion. It reports the percent likelihood of *acute cardiac ischemia* on the ECG record. Four studies including 5496 patients found that when combined with physician impression, the ACI-TIPI has a sensitivity of 86% to 95% and a specificity of 78% to 92% for prediction of ACS.[18] When house staff without prior emergency medicine training use the ACI-TIPI, it can speed the time until a disposition decision is made.[21] In a study of more than 10,000 patients with potential ACS, in the subset of patients ultimately not believed to have cardiac ischemia, use of the ACI-TIPI was associated with a non–statistically significant reduction in coronary care unit admissions from 15% to 12% and slight increase in ED discharges to home from 49% to 52%.[22] The ACI-TIPI has not been shown to make a clinically relevant difference in diagnostic accuracy compared with physician judgment alone. As a result, it has not been incorporated widely into clinical practice in EDs.

Artificial Neural Networks

The artificial neural network is a nonlinear statistical paradigm shown to be a powerful modality for the recognition of complex patterns that can maintain accuracy when some input data are missing. The network maps a complex three-dimensional space defined by the constellation of input information characterizing patterns that is provided during training. During testing, the network determines the goodness of fit of unknown patterns to that mapped space. Network function allows for an infinite variability of input information weighting. It is thought that the network's ability to allow variable weighting to input information, as opposed to the fixed weighting of other statistical approaches, allows it to perform more accurately than these other approaches. Additionally the artificial neural network does not require complete and accurate data to maintain optimal performance. This is a distinct advantage for use in real time, when some clinical information may not be readily available.

The artificial neural network can identify accurately the presence of MI in patients with anterior chest pain.[23-25] When initial cardiac troponin I and CK-MB determinations were added to the variables used by the network, the network had a sensitivity of 95% and a specificity of 96% despite the fact that an average of 5% of the input data required by the network were missing on all patients.[24] For prediction of acute MI, the neural network has better sensitivity and specificity than the Goldman risk score and ACI-TIPI. In the same data set, a Goldman risk of greater than or equal to 7% had a sensitivity of 74% and specificity of 68%. An ACI-TIPI greater than or equal to 25% had a sensitivity of 62% and specificity of 73%.[25] The artificial neural network achieved these predictive properties using only data available at the time of ED arrival. It incorporates more clinical information than either the Goldman score or the ACI-TIPI (Table 12-7). It is expected that ongoing prospective studies will define better the impact of artificial neural networks on triage and cost efficiency.

TIMI Risk Score

Although risk stratification is useful for allowing clinicians to triage patients to an optimal location for medical care, it also can be used to identify patients who may be served best by certain costly but efficacious therapies. The Thrombolysis in Myocardial Infarction (TIMI) risk score was derived to enhance treatment decisions by identifying patients most likely to benefit from certain therapies. These scores are useful only in patients already known to have ACS. The TIMI risk score for patients with unstable angina can predict at least one component of a primary end point comprising death, new or recurrent MI, or severe recurrent ischemia requiring urgent revascularization through 14 days after index presentation. The seven TIMI risk score predictor variables are shown in Table 12-8; the total score is the number of these individual risk factors. Event rates increase significantly as the TIMI risk score increases: 4.7% for a score of 0/1, 8.3% for 2, 13.2% for 3, 19.9% for 4, 26.2% for 5, and 40.9% for 6/7.[26]

There is a separate TIMI risk score for ST-elevation MI. It is a simple integer score (Table 12-9). The risk score was evaluated in 84,029 patients with ST-elevation MI from the National Registry of Myocardial Infarction 3.[27] The TIMI risk score correctly predicted risk of death. There was a significant graded increase in mortality with rising score (range, 1.1% to 30%). The risk score showed strong prognostic capacity overall among patients receiving acute reperfusion therapy whether or not they were treated with fibrinolytic therapy or primary percutaneous coronary intervention. Among patients not receiving reperfusion therapy, however, the risk score underestimated death rates.[27]

Markers of Myocardial Injury

The utility of cardiac markers depends on their ability to detect and risk stratify patients with ACS. In the ED, the ideal marker allows early detection of patients with ACS, enables optimal treatment pathways to be initiated, and assists with rapid determination of patient disposition. The optimal use of cardiac markers for ED physicians is different than that of cardiologists. Because 85% of patients who present to the ED with potential ACS do not ultimately have a cardiac cause for their symptoms, a marker with a high negative predictive value would be particularly useful to allow rapid evaluation and release from the ED (Table 12-10). Markers with high positive predictive values are ideal to mobilize more costly evaluations and treatments for patients at high risk of cardiovascular complications. Most patients with acute MI, even patients with nondiagnostic ECGs, can be diagnosed within 3 hours of ED presentation.[28]

Creatine Kinase-MB

In the setting of acute MI, creatine kinase (CK)-MB levels rise to twice the normal levels at 6 hours and peak within approximately 24 hours. Serial CK-MB mass measurements have sensitivity near 90% 3 hours after ED presentation (approximately 6 hours after symptom onset) but are only 36% to 48% sensitive when used at or shortly after presentation.[18, 29] Single CK-MB measurements cannot be used safely to assist in the admission/discharge decision because they do not attain adequate negative predictive values for ACS and would result in an unacceptable rate of missed acute MI and cardiovascular complications. Serial CK-MB measurements over 6 to 9 hours have been used widely in chest pain observation units and are considered sufficient, if negative, to exclude safely acute MI, allowing further diagnostic testing or ED release depending on the clinical scenario. An alternative strategy is to examine the change in CK-MB values within 2 hours of ED presentation. A rise in CK-MB greater than or equal to 1.6 ng/mL over the 2-hour period after presentation achieves a sensitivity for detection of acute MI of 94%, which is better than using the 2-hour CK-MB value alone (75%).[30]

Patients with skeletal muscle disease, acute muscle exertion, chronic renal failure, and cocaine use can have elevations in levels of CK-MB in the absence of infarction.[31-33] To distinguish CK elevations resulting from myocardial injury from those resulting from skeletal muscle injury, the measurement of CK-MB as a percentage of total CK has been used (relative index). There is no clear consensus on whether absolute CK-MB or the CK-MB relative index is the preferred test for patients with potential ACS. The international diagnostic criteria, World Health Organization criteria, and several other consensus conferences recommend use of absolute CK-MB.[34, 35] Many major clinical trials also have used the absolute CK-MB as the diagnostic test for acute MI. Individual institutions vary in their preference for either the absolute CK-MB or the relative index. In the only ED-based study to examine this issue, the use of relative index, rather than absolute CK-MB, at the time of ED presentation to detect acute MI improved specificity (96% versus 93%) and positive predictive value (46% versus 36%) but decreased sensitivity (52% versus 47%) without significantly affecting negative predictive value (96% versus 96%).[36] In skeletal muscle damage, the large amount of total CK may reduce the percentage value of CK-MB by obscuring a

■ ▪ ■

TABLE 12–7   CLINICAL CRITERIA INCLUDED IN SEVERAL EMERGENCY DEPARTMENT RISK STRATIFICATION SCHEMES

	GOLDMAN SCORE	ACI-TIPI	BAXT NEURAL NETWORK
Demographics			
	Age ≥ 40 years	Age Gender	Age Gender Race
Presentation characteristics			
	Chest pain duration ≥ 48 hours	Presence of chest or left arm pain	Left anterior chest pain Left arm pain
	Longest pain episode >1 hour	Chief symptom of chest or left arm pain	
	History of angina or MI		History of prior coronary disease, acute MI, angina, or congestive heart failure
	Pain worse than usual angina or same as prior MI		Pain pressing in nature
	Pain radiates to neck, left shoulder, or left arm		Pain crushing in nature Pain radiating to neck
	Pain radiates to back, abdomen, or legs		Pain radiating to left arm
	Chest pain reproduced by palpation		
	Chest pain is stabbing		Shortness of breath Diaphoresis Nausea and vomiting
Past history			
			Hypertension Diabetes mellitus Elevated cholesterol Family history of coronary artery disease
Electrocardiogram criteria			
	ST-segment elevation or Q waves in ≥2 leads, not known to be old	Pathologic Q waves	Q waves old Q waves not known to be old
	ST-segment changes of ischemia or strain, not known to be old	Presence and degree of ST-segment elevation or depression	ST-segment elevation old ST-segment elevation not known to be old
		T-wave elevation or inversion	T-wave inversion old T-wave inversion not known to be old
			ST-segment depression old ST-segment depression not known to be old
			Left bundle-branch block old Left bundle-branch block not known to be old
			Hyperacute T waves old Hyperacute T waves not known to be old
Cardiac marker determination			
			Including presentation CK, CK-MB, and troponin I

MI, myocardial infarction.

small, but significant, elevated source of CK-MB from the heart, resulting in a loss of sensitivity for detecting concurrent myocardial injury. This loss may affect the ability to diagnose acute MI in the setting of cocaine use, in which ACS and rhabdomyolysis may occur.

CK-MB2 is the subform that is released from the myocardium. After release, it is cleaved by lysine carboxypeptidase, producing a more negatively charged molecule, CK-MB1. Both subforms are in equilibrium. When CK-MB2 is greater than 1.0 U/L or the MB2-to-MB1

■ ■ ■

TABLE 12–8   ELEMENTS OF THE TIMI SCORE FOR UNSTABLE ANGINA*

Age ≥65 years
≥3 traditional risk factors for coronary artery disease
Prior coronary stenosis of ≥50%
ST-segment deviation on presenting electrocardiogram
≥2 anginal events in prior 24 hours
Aspirin use within the 7 days before presentation
Elevated cardiac markers

*The presence of each is assigned 1 point. The maximal possible score is 7

ratio is greater than 1.5, the sensitivity and specificity for the diagnosis of acute MI are improved. In a study using serial sampling every 30 to 60 minutes, the sensitivity for detection of acute MI was 96% and the specificity was 93% to 96%.[37] Other investigators using more common, less frequent, sampling times had less impressive results. The main advantage of CK-MB subforms is that they can identify patients with acute MI earlier than CK-MB when intensive serial sampling strategies are used. These serial sampling techniques are unlikely to be incorporated widely into ED practice because of practical time and staffing constraints.

Cardiac Troponins

Elevations of cardiac troponins I and T are more specific than other markers of myocardial injury. After acute MI, cardiac troponins I and T become elevated after approximately 6 hours, peak at 12 to 24 hours, and remain elevated for 7 to 10 days. Troponins I and T have a higher specificity for myocardial necrosis than CK-MB in selected subsets of patients with ACS, such as patients

■ ■ ■

TABLE 12–9   ELEMENTS OF THE TIMI SCORE FOR ST-SEGMENT ELEVATION ACUTE MYOCERDIAL INFARCTION

CLINICAL RISK INDICATORS	POINTS
Historical	
Age > 75 years	3
Age 65–74 years	2
History of diabetes, hypertension, or angina	1
Physical examination	
Systolic blood pressure < 100 mm Hg	3
Heart rate > 100 beat/min	2
Killip class II–IV	2
Weight < 67 kg	1
Presentation	
Anterior ST-segment elevation or left bundle-branch block	1
Time to reperfusion > 4 hours	1
Total points possible	14

From Morrow DA, Antman EM, Parsons L, et al: Application of the TIMI risk score for ST-elevation MI in the National Registry of Myocardial Infarction 3. JAMA 2001;286:1356–1359.

with recent surgery, cocaine use, chronic renal failure, and skeletal muscle disease.[31, 33] In ED patients with symptoms of ACS, cardiac troponin I has been shown to have similar sensitivity and specificity as CK-MB for detection of acute MI.[32, 38, 39] In ED patients with unselected chest pain syndromes and patients with definite ACS, elevations in cardiac troponin I predict cardiovascular complications independent of CK-MB and the ECG.[38, 39] Minor elevations in cardiac troponin T and I also can identify patients more likely to benefit from an early invasive treatment strategy.[40]

■ ■ ■

TABLE 12–10   SUMMARY OF PREDICTIVE PROPERTIES OF CARDIAC MARKERS OF DIAGNOSIS OF ACUTE MYOCARDIAL INFARCTION

MARKER	NO. STUDIES	NO. SUBJECTS	SENSITIVITY (95% CI)	SPECIFICITY (95% CI)	DIAGNOSTIC ODDS RATIO (95% CI)
At time of presentation					
Creatine kinase	12	3195	37 (31–44)	87 (80–91)	3.9 (2.7–5.7)
CK-MB	19	6425	42 (36–48)	97 (95–98)	25 (18–36)
Myoglobin	18	4172	49 (53–55)	91 (87–94)	11 (8–15)
Troponin I	4	1149	39 (10–78)	93 (88–97)	11 (3.4–34)
Troponin T	6	1348	39 (26–53)	93 (90–96)	9.5 (5.7–16)
CK-MB and myoglobin	3	2283	83 (51–96)	82 (68–90)	17 (7.6–40)
Serial markers					
Creatine kinase	2	786	69–99	68–84	12
CK-MB	14	11,625	79 (71–86)	96 (95–97)	140 (65–310)
Myoglobin	10	1277	89 (80–94)	87 (80–92)	84 (44–160)
Troponin I	2	1393	90–100	83–96	230–460
Troponin T	3	904	93 (85–97)	83–96	83 (33–210)
CK-MB and myoglobin	2	291	100	85 (76–91)	4.3–14
				75–91	

Source: Lau J, Ioannidis JPA, Balk EM, et al: Diagnosing acute cardiac ischemia in the Emergency Department: A systematic review of the accuracy and clinical effect of current technologies. Ann Emerg Med 2001;37:453–460.

The cytosolic component of cardiac troponin T is released from the cell within 3 to 6 hours after symptom onset. Its diagnostic sensitivity for acute MI approaches 100% 10 hours after symptom onset; cardiac troponin T remains elevated for 7 to 10 days after injury. This extended period of elevation results from disintegration of the contractile apparatus and the continued release of cardiac troponin T. Cardiac troponin T is an independent marker of cardiovascular risk in patients with ACS.[38,41] It can stratify risk further when combined with the ECG and CK-MB. In patients admitted to chest pain observation units, cardiac troponin T has higher sensitivity for detection of myocardial necrosis and multivessel coronary artery disease than CK-MB.[42] In unselected ED patient populations with chest pain syndromes, cardiac troponin T elevations increase the risk of 60-day adverse cardiovascular events 3.5-fold.[43] Combined analysis of four studies assessing the predictive properties of single cardiac troponin I values at the time of presentation for acute MI found a sensitivity of 39% and specificity of 93%.[19] A similar analysis of six cardiac troponin T studies found the same results.[18] Serial sampling increases sensitivities to 90% to 100% with specificities of 83% to 96% for cardiac troponin I and 76% to 91% for cardiac troponin T.[18] Elevated values of cardiac troponins in patients with non–ST-segment elevation acute MI increase the short-term risk of death 3.1-fold (1.6% versus 5.2%).[44] Although cardiac troponins are useful for diagnosis and risk stratification of patients with chest pain,[45] ACS, and acute MI, cardiac marker testing in the ED does not identify most ED patients who subsequently have adverse events.[46, 47] Patients with negative markers still require evaluation and testing, as dictated by their clinical presentation.

Most of the data from megatrial subgroup analyses regarding the prognostic importance of troponin measurements are based on central laboratory testing. It is difficult to generalize these results to individual institutions because standardization between individual commercial assays is poor. Measurements of troponin T can vary 20-fold.[48] The coefficient of variation, a measure of precision for an assay, is in the range of 10% to 20% for cardiac troponins.[40] Although biologic "false-positive" cardiac troponin measurements should be exceedingly rare, analytical "false positives" are common as a result of problems with standardization and precision for the current commercial assays.

Patients with jaundice and patients taking heparin have been noted to have falsely low levels of troponin. Falsely positive levels of troponin I have been noted in the presence of sepsis, fibrin clots, and heterophil antibodies.[49] Elevations in cardiac troponin T (and less so cardiac troponin I) have been noted in patients with renal failure.[50] Falsely elevated values are less frequent with third generation tests. Although these measurements have been considered false positive for the diagnosis of acute myocardial infarction, they have been shown to be related to a worse outcome, possibly by marking myocardial cell necrosis, and must be taken seriously.

Myoglobin

Myoglobin has a lower molecular weight and is released more rapidly than CK-MB and cardiac troponins during acute MI. As a result, serum myoglobin levels rise faster than CK-MB, reaching twice-normal values within 2 hours and peaking within 4 hours of acute MI symptom onset. Myoglobin achieves its maximal diagnostic sensitivity within 5 hours of symptom onset.[51] Sensitivity of older assays was poor. Newer monoclonal immunoassay techniques show higher sensitivity and specificity of myoglobin for acute MI in patients presenting within 3 hours of symptom onset. The sensitivity of myoglobin at the time of ED presentation is 49%, exceeding that of CK-MB or troponins, but the specificity is only 87%.[18] Serial quantitative testing over 1 hour, evaluating absolute values and a change of 40 ng/mL, has 91% sensitivity and 99% negative predictive value for acute MI within 1 hour of ED presentation (approximately 3 to 4 hours after symptom onset).[52] One study evaluated the ability of myoglobin to risk stratify ED patients with potential ACS and found that an elevated myoglobin predicted a 3.4-fold risk of adverse cardiovascular events and identified some high-risk patients not otherwise identified by clinical characteristics, CK-MB, or cardiac troponin T.[53]

The main advantage of myoglobin is early detection of patients with acute MI. The disadvantage is that it has poor specificity for acute MI in patients with concurrent trauma or renal failure.

Evaluation of the myoglobin-to-carbonic anhydrase III ratio can enhance the specificity of myoglobin.[54] Carbonic anhydrase III is released from skeletal muscle in a fixed ratio with myoglobin. Combined assays can help determine whether myoglobin is of skeletal or cardiac origin. Using these dual assays, the high early sensitivity of myoglobin is maintained, and specificity is improved. These assays are not yet commercially available. The use of the myoglobin-to-carbonic anhydrase III ratio for risk stratification has not yet been well evaluated.

Markers of Inflammation and Prothrombotic States

Markers of inflammation and markers of platelet activation are still in the relatively early stages of evaluation, but it is suggested they may not be useful in the ED evaluation of patients with potential ACS. Markers of platelet activation, such as P-selectin and other integrins, are theoretically attractive because they can detect platelet activation before myocardial injury. A soluble form of P-selectin, an integral membrane glycoprotein, is elevated in the plasma of patients with ACS compared with normal healthy controls. When P-selectin was evaluated in the ED setting, however, it was not able to risk stratify patients with acute MI and ACS relative to patients with nonischemic chest pain syndromes. The initial sensitivity was 46% and specificity was 76% for acute MI. The predictive properties and area under the curve for acute MI, ACS, and serious cardiac events were not better than the initial CK-MB.[55] Similar results have been found with some inflammatory markers. The favorable predictive properties observed with inflammatory markers in longitudinal cohort studies of patients with potential coronary artery disease may not generalize to the ED, where most patients with potential ACS have confounding medical conditions likely to increase the prevalence of inflammatory markers.

Combinations of Markers

Markers of myocardial injury when used individually at the time of ED presentation do not attain sufficient negative predictive value to allow immediate ED discharge safely. Combinations of two or more cardiac markers increase the early predictive value of these types of strategies, however. Although troponin T and CK-MB have approximately the same rate of rise, there seems to be a benefit to using more than one of the markers to predict adverse cardiovascular events. At the time of ED presentation, the use of both markers rather than either alone increases diagnostic sensitivity greater than 25%.[53] The Diagnostic Cooperative Study found that MB subforms and myoglobin were the most sensitive early indicators for acute MI, and CK-MB and troponins were the most sensitive after 8 to 12 hours.[56] The combination of myoglobin and CK-MB mass has a sensitivity of 85% at the time of presentation and in one study attained 100% sensitivity, specificity, and negative predictive value within 4 hours of ED presentation.[57] When patients with diagnostic ECGs were excluded, the sensitivity of this combination strategy was 80% with a specificity of 84% at the time of presentation. Sensitivity and specificity were 100% within 4 hours of ED arrival.[57] A combination of myoglobin and troponin I can achieve a diagnostic sensitivity of 97% with a 99% negative predictive value within 90 minutes of ED presentation.[58] The addition of CK-MB did not improve diagnostic accuracy within this time frame, but the CK-MB and myoglobin combination had a 92% sensitivity and 99% negative predictive value within this same time frame.

IMAGING MODALITIES

The use of cardiac imaging for risk stratification of ED patients with chest pain has the theoretical advantage that abnormalities can be detected before irreversible myocardial damage.

Echocardiography

Echocardiography, when used to assess wall motion, has a sensitivity for detection of acute MI of approximately 93% but a specificity of only 53% to 57%.[59] It cannot distinguish old from new infarcts. As a result, echocardiography is more useful in patients without a past history of coronary artery disease. Larger areas of infarction and more depressed left ventricular function predict a higher likelihood of cardiovascular complications and an increased mortality.[60] The addition of echocardiography to baseline clinical variables and the initial ECG seems to have independent predictive value.[61] Paventi and colleagues,[62] in a study of 665 ED chest pain patients, found that the predictive properties of echocardiography and myocardial perfusion imaging were similar with respect to acute MI, need for percutaneous transluminal coronary angioplasty, and presence of coronary artery disease.

Rest Sestamibi Imaging

Sestamibi imaging has been studied extensively and is useful for ED risk stratification of patients with chest pain. Technetium sestamibi is a radioisotope that is taken up by the myocardium in proportion to myocardial blood flow. It has prolonged retention in the myocardium and redistributes minimally after injection; this allows injection during symptomatic episodes but enables imaging after patient stabilization. This is an ideal characteristic for use in the ED. Varetto and associates[63] examined the role of ED sestamibi imaging in 64 patients with chest pain syndromes and a nondiagnostic ECG who were admitted to the coronary care unit. Of the 34 patients with a normal perfusion scan, none had a major cardiac event in the ensuing 18 months. Hilton and coworkers[64] studied 102 ED patients with angina with normal or nondiagnostic ECGs who did not have known coronary artery disease and found that sestamibi imaging was the only independent predictor of adverse cardiovascular events during hospitalization. Tatum and colleagues[65] reported results of 338 ED patients with chest pain with normal scans. None of these patients sustained acute MI or cardiac death within the 12-month follow-up period. The high negative predictive values of resting sestamibi imaging can allow early ED discharge of low-risk patients. An abnormal sestamibi scan was associated with a 50-fold increased risk of acute MI and a 14.5-fold increased risk of revascularization over the next 30 days. There was a 30-fold increased risk of death over the ensuing 12 months.[65] Early perfusion imaging was as sensitive as serial troponin I measurements and considerably more sensitive than initial cardiac troponin I determinations.[66]

There are significant practical implementation problems that have prevented widespread adoption of this technology in the ED. The radioisotope is prepared in "batches." The cost of preparation for single-patient use is prohibitive. The increased accuracy of sestamibi imaging when injection occurs during pain warrants rapid technician arrival. The rapid preparation of isotope and timely patient injection can be accomplished only with in-house nuclear medicine services. In the absence of a high volume of ED chest pain patients and cooperative nuclear medicine specialists, this is unlikely to occur 24 hours a day 7 days a week. These issues are practical concerns that make the widespread implementation of this technology difficult.

Electron-Beam Computed Tomography

Electron-beam computed tomography (CT) (see Chapter 20) is useful for detection of high-grade stenosis and occlusion with a sensitivity of 92% and specificity of 94%.[67] McLaughlin and coworkers[68] used electron-beam CT to stratify ED chest pain patients without known coronary artery disease. Only 1 of 48 patients with a negative test had a cardiac event.[68] Laudon and associates[69] found a 100% negative predictive value in 53 patients compared with other assessments for coronary artery disease. Raggi and colleagues[70] studied 207 low-risk to intermediate-risk patients and found that electron-beam

CT had a sensitivity of 74% and a specificity of 89% for the presence of obstructive coronary artery disease. In their bayesian analysis, electron-beam CT provided a cost savings of 45% to 65% over a pathway including treadmill testing. Georgiou and associates[71] performed a prospective observational study of ED chest pain patients. They found the cardiovascular event rate to be 0.6% for the 76 subjects with a calcium score of 0 compared with 14% for the subjects with calcium scores greater than 400. These studies suggest that electron-beam CT can provide some prognostic information for ED chest pain patients, but, as yet, they have not shown the safety of this test to allow early ED release of low-risk patients. Falsely low calcium scores are most common in young patients or patients without long-standing coronary artery disease. These are the patients most likely to be discharged from the ED. The role of electron-beam CT for ED assessment of chest pain patients is unclear.

Immediate Provocative Testing

Stress testing has become commonplace in EDs with chest pain observation units despite a paucity of evidence to show that they are cost-effective tools for risk stratification of ED patients with chest pain. No large studies show the sensitivity and specificity for detection of coronary artery disease in this patient population, and some studies had more false-positive than true-positive tests.[72] Provocative testing to exclude ACS in ED patients with chest pain might have reduced sensitivity and specificity. Patients often are treated with therapeutic agents for potential ACS (β antagonists) while in the ED or observation unit setting. By comparison, optimal testing in the elective outpatient setting involves withholding of therapy before test performance.

Exercise treadmill or pharmacologic testing with or without nuclear imaging and stress echocardiography are safe and can assist cardiovascular risk stratification in the ED.[73-75] Patients with an uneventful observation period, negative cardiac markers, and a normal stress test can be discharged safely with a referral for follow-up. Stress testing usually is used on patients at low risk for ACS or patients who have been "ruled out" for acute MI.

Some evidence supports the use of immediate exercise testing in low-risk ED chest pain patients. Kirk and associates[76] showed the safety of this approach in patients without known ventricular dysfunction who had normal or nonspecific ECGs, even before cardiac markers determination. They found that more than 50% of patients in chest pain observation units met these criteria for immediate exercise testing. All patients with negative tests were discharged from the ED, and none had an adverse cardiovascular event within 30 days.[76]

Interpretation of Previous Diagnostic Testing for Coronary Artery Disease

Prior cardiac catheterization results are useful for risk stratification. Patients who previously have been documented to have minimal (<25%) stenosis or normal coronary arteriograms have an excellent long-term prognosis,

with greater than 98% free from MI 10 years later.[77] Repeat cardiac catheterizations an average of 9 years later found that approximately 90% of patients did not develop even single-vessel coronary artery disease.[78] A recent cardiac catheterization with normal or minimally diseased vessels almost eliminates the possibility of ACS. Most such patients do not require admission for evaluation of potential ACS. If the patient does not have another serious medical condition warranting admission (aortic dissection or pulmonary embolism, acute trauma, Prinzmetal's variant angina), ED discharge or a brief observation period would be appropriate.

Prior exercise and pharmacologic stress tests have not been shown to be useful in the ED. ED physicians do not rely heavily on them for several reasons. Patients often had provocative testing when they were less symptomatic or had more stable anginal patterns. It has not been well established how the results of these tests can be applied to newly symptomatic patients in the ED. Precise results of tests often are not available to the ED physician. When patients complete all stages of the protocol and have no ECG changes and normal imaging studies, exercise treadmill testing can "rule out" acute ischemic syndromes with sensitivities and specificities of 68% to 88% and 73% to 88%.[79] When patients do not meet their target heart rate, exercise testing is less sensitive. Often detailed information about these tests is not available to the ED physician. "On-call" primary care physicians or cardiologists do not have this information immediately available at night. Unless the ED physician can confirm that the patient reached his or her maximal heart rate, had no ECG changes, and had normal imaging or echocardiography (when done), these tests cannot provide a sufficient margin of safety to allow safe release of the patient from the ED without an unacceptable "miss rate."

Chest Pain Observation Units

The difficulty in rapid diagnosis of the ED patient with chest pain with ACS has led to the development of chest pain evaluation units. In general, these units were formed to allow brief periods of observation (6 to 12 hours) while obviating the need for more costly hospital admission in a large cohort of patients with nonspecific chest pain syndromes. A variety of different protocols exist, but most observation protocols incorporate frequent serial marker testing (at 1- to 4-hour intervals) for at least 6 to 12 hours, telemetry monitoring (with continuous single- or 12-lead ECGs) and some form of provocative testing for patients who "rule out" for MI and do not have cardiovascular complications during the observation period. Multiple studies have shown the safety of this approach for low-risk to intermediate-risk patients with or without known coronary artery disease. These units are usually in close proximity to the ED, allowing 24-hour physician intervention, if necessary, but often are staffed with ancillary health care providers to facilitate care. Chest pain observation units are often protocol driven, with strict adherence to clinical pathways.

The number of chest pain units is constantly growing and it was recently estimated that 30% of US hospitals have a CPC, which total 1200 in the country.[80] The CHEPER (Chest Pain Evaluation Registry) study, a multi-site registry of chest pain observation units, found that most patients (76%) are discharged home, avoiding hospital admission.[81] The use of an observation unit increased the proportion of patients receiving a "rule out MI" evaluation from 57% to 67%, reduced the "missed" MI rate from 4.5% to 0.4%, reduced the hospitalization rate from 57% to 47%, and reduced overall hospital costs.[81] The Chest Pain Evaluation in the Emergency Room (CHEER) study, a randomized controlled trial of a chest pain observation unit versus usual care, found that ED observation units are safe, effective, and cost-saving for intermediate-risk patients.[82] It also found reduced overall resource use during the 6 months after the index visit.[82] Roberts and colleagues[83] found a saving of $567 in total hospital cost using an accelerated diagnostic protocol compared with standard care. Additionally, patient satisfaction is increased with the use of chest pain observation units relative to hospitalization.[84]

The ideal chest pain observation unit protocol would have clear criteria for entrance to the unit, be driven by an evidence-based clinical protocol, and facilitate some form of provocative testing either before or shortly after discharge. Close linkage with primary care physicians can facilitate outpatient evaluation further for the many patients with noncardiac causes of chest pain. These units generally are best located in close proximity to the ED, allowing 24-hour attending physician presence for the rare cardiovascular emergency that can occur. Ongoing studies should define better the optimal time period for observation before safe release home.

EMERGENCY DEPARTMENT DISPOSITION

All patients with acute chest pain need to be risk stratified based on the likelihood that they have an ACS. The best tool for initial risk stratification of chest pain patients is the ECG,[8] despite the fact that it does not identify all patients with acute MI. Patients with ST-segment elevation should receive reperfusion therapy and be triaged to the cardiac care unit. Other patients should be evaluated further for their risk of ACS, preferably using validated tools (Goldman score, consensus guidelines, or computerized algorithms) rather than simply clinical impression.

Patients with nonischemic causes of chest pain and patients with a less than 1% risk of 30-day adverse events can be released home from the ED. Patients with stable anginal patterns do not require inpatient evaluation. Patients younger than age 40 years without any cardiac risk factors and without a prior cardiac history have a less than 1% risk of ACS and less than 1% risk of 30-day death, acute MI, or revascularization. Likewise, patients younger than age 40 with a normal ECG and no prior cardiac history have a less than 1% risk of ACS or adverse 30-day cardiovascular events.[85] These groups would be considered very low risk for ACS and are reasonable to discharge without further evaluation. Sestamibi imaging during acute chest pain can exclude ACS sufficiently such that some patients can be discharged safely from the ED without further observation or cardiac marker testing.[65]

Most patients at low risk (1% to 7%) should be treated in an ED observation unit or inpatient setting. ED observation units are safe and cost-effective for patients with nondiagnostic ECGs and other low-risk to intermediate-risk clinical features. Serial cardiac marker determinations, usually over 6 to 9 hours from presentation, can stratify patients further. Patients without recurrent symptoms or cardiovascular complications with negative cardiac marker determinations and a normal stress test are safe for release from the ED. If released without provocative testing, low-risk patients should have close follow-up arranged. ED observation units are available in only 20% of EDs, so most low-risk chest pain patients are still hospitalized. The duration of observation for low-risk patients is not entirely well delineated. Aggressive multiple marker strategies, including serial CK-MB, myoglobin, and cardiac troponin I values, over 90 minutes for low-risk chest pain patients also may allow safe rapid release of some of these patients.[86]

Some data suggest that low-risk chest pain patients with normal or nonspecific ECGs who are admitted to the hospital may not require continuous telemetry monitoring, but this strategy has not been prospectively validated.[87-89] The timing of provocative testing in low-risk patients admitted to non-ICU monitored beds has not been well delineated. Patients admitted to telemetry beds who "rule out" for acute MI have similar 30-day outcomes of patients whether or not they receive inpatient stress testing.[90] This finding suggests that diagnostic stress testing can be accomplished electively as an outpatient for many of these patients.

Intermediate-risk patients should be admitted to a non-ICU monitored setting for serial cardiac markers and provocative testing. Elevated cardiac markers on initial determination may warrant "upgrading" of some patients originally triaged to non-ICU telemetry settings because it increases risk of adverse events. Patients with abnormal but nondiagnostic ECGs may benefit from more intensive observation and monitoring in the cardiac care unit, when initial cardiac markers are elevated. Patients with normal or nonspecific ECGs are low risk for complications and do not automatically warrant more than a non-ICU telemetry setting unless dictated by other clinical parameters (ECG changes, continued chest pain, or cardiovascular complications). Initial cardiac marker determinations should not be used to make the admission/discharge decision. Even when an undetectable troponin I on presentation is combined with a Goldman acute MI risk of less than 4%, there is an unacceptable rate of adverse events at 30 days (1% death, 2% acute MI, and 2% revascularization).[91]

Important premorbid factors related to short-term and long-term prognosis in patients with ACS are the severity of coronary artery disease, left ventricular function, age, and comorbid diseases. For this reason, prior invasive and noninvasive assessments of cardiac function should be taken into account when making ED disposition decisions.

TREATMENT CONSIDERATIONS SPECIFIC TO THE EMERGENCY DEPARTMENT

The treatment of patients with ACS is heavily evidence based and driven by large multicenter international trials. Current management strategies for patients with ACS are discussed extensively in Section 4 of this text. After demonstration of safety and efficacy of treatment strategies, other issues must be considered to optimize incorporation of new treatments into the ED setting, including ease of administration, time required for drug administration, individual institutional and physician preferences, and balancing the needs of multiple patients simultaneously.

From an emergency medicine perspective, the ideal treatment would be one that would be obtained easily (stored in the ED); initiated rapidly (does not require preparation); administered in a single intravenous bolus (or orally); does not require continued intravenous infusion, titration, or monitoring of therapeutic levels; and would be a component of an agreed-on treatment pathway. Although these treatment characteristics would be ideal for treatment of all patients in all hospital locations, they are paramount in the ED, where physicians and nurses are actively caring for multiple critically ill patients simultaneously. There is the added challenge of integrating ED care of ACS patients with multiple primary care providers and cardiologists, each of whom may have their own personal preference on how to care for their patients.

For the treatment of patients with ST-segment elevation acute MI, the decision regarding which patients will be treated with percutaneous interventions, fibrinolytic therapy, or facilitated angioplasty should be protocolized and not addressed anew for each patient who arrives in the ED. Likewise the choice of fibrinolytic agent should be decided in advance and should take into account relative efficacy and safety, ease of administration, and need for concurrent medications. Assuming equivalent efficacy and safety, bolus fibrinolytics would be preferred over agents requiring more complicated intravenous infusions. Concurrent administration of antithrombotic agents that can be given in bolus form would be preferable, especially if the institutional choice of fibrinolytic agent is an agent shown to have improved outcomes with its use.

There is good evidence and widespread consensus that patients with ST-segment elevation acute MI should have fibrinolytic therapy initiated in the ED without delaying care to obtain consultation. For this protocol to optimize patient treatment, it is essential that the care of these patients also not be delayed to determine whether the patient will go to the cardiac catheterization laboratory instead. Protocols to ensure rapid treatment and to enable adherence to treatment guidelines require clear local a priori definitions of which patients will receive primary percutaneous interventions.

For the treatment of non–ST-segment elevation acute MI, the choice of antithrombotic and glycoprotein IIb/IIIa inhibitor agents should be decided before patient arrival and dictated by a clinical pathway. With increased use of an early invasive strategy for patients with acute MI, these decisions become more complicated, in that often the first decision that must be made is whether or not the patient will receive early invasive therapy rather than conservative therapy. For some physicians, the choice of which antithrombotic agent and glycoprotein IIb/IIIa inhibitor agent is used depends on this decision. Although the data regarding time urgency for initiation of treatment in patients with non–ST-segment elevation acute MI or unstable angina is not as compelling as that of ST-segment elevation acute MI, the care of these patients also should be expedited. To this end, the decision on how to manage these patients is handled best via a clinical pathway that requires a minimum of consultation for each new patient.

COCAINE-INDUCED ACUTE CORONARY SYNDROME

The risk of MI is increased 24-fold in the hour after cocaine use.[92] Most MIs occur within 24 hours of cocaine use; however, reports of acute MI several weeks after last use of cocaine exist.[93] Approximately 6% of patients with cocaine-associated chest pain syndromes have acute MI.[94] An additional 14% suffer from transient myocardial ischemia.

Cocaine causes myocardial ischemia through a complex pathophysiology resulting from its acute and chronic effects.[95] Acutely, cocaine results in coronary artery vasoconstriction, tachycardia, systemic arterial hypertension, increased myocardial oxygen demand, platelet aggregation, and in situ thrombus formation. Chronic cocaine users develop accelerated atherosclerosis and left ventricular hypertrophy, which can exacerbate further the oxygen supply/demand mismatch. Myocardial ischemia and infarction have occurred in patients without any underlying atherosclerotic disease or other evidence of preexisting heart disease. Although cocaine can cause myocardial ischemia in patients without coronary artery disease, most patients with cocaine-associated acute MI have atherosclerotic coronary artery disease.[95] Patients with cocaine-associated MI have impaired epicardial and microvascular blood flow.[96]

Risk stratification of patients with cocaine-associated ACS is difficult. Patients with cocaine-associated ACS frequently have atypical chest pain or chest pain delayed for hours to days after their most recent use of cocaine. Acute MI can occur after use of only small amounts of cocaine. Clinical criteria have not been useful. ECGs reveal abnormalities consisting of ST-segment elevation and T-wave inversions that often persist during hospitalization; however, the ECG is less sensitive and less specific for MI in patients who have used cocaine recently. CK-MB assays have diminished specificity for acute MI in cocaine users. Cardiac troponin I or T seems to be more useful.[33]

Resting sestamibi scans can help risk stratify patients with cocaine-associated chest pain syndromes.[97] Patients with normal resting images after injection during pain or patients with normal cardiac markers, normal or nonspecific ECGs, and an uneventful 9- to 12-hour period of observation can be released safely from the ED with follow-up arrangements.[97,98]

The treatment of the cardiovascular effects of cocaine must ensure that the central nervous system effects are not enhanced. Management of patients with cocaine-associated myocardial ischemia should focus on reversal of coronary vasoconstriction, hypertension, tachycardia, and predisposition to thrombus formation.[95] Central nervous system protection and decreased sympathetic outflow should be accomplished with the administration of benzodiazepines. Multiple animal experiments and widespread experience in humans support the use of diazepam as the initial agent for the management of cocaine-intoxicated patients.[1,95,99] Reduction in hypertension and tachycardia decreases the myocardial oxygen demand.

Aspirin or heparin or both should be used as they would be in patients with myocardial ischemia unrelated to cocaine. The success with platelet inhibitors and anticoagulants in traditional MI patients and the propensity of cocaine to induce platelet aggregation support their use, despite a lack of studies in patients with cocaine-associated myocardial ischemia.

Specific anti-ischemic therapy begins with nitroglycerin. Nitroglycerin reverses cocaine-induced coronary artery vasoconstriction and often relieves cocaine-associated chest pain. It should therefore be used although the effects on infarct size and mortality reduction have not been studied.[95]

Patients with continued myocardial ischemia after the use of nitroglycerin should be treated with phentolamine, calcium channel blockers, or thrombolytic agents depending on the clinical circumstances.[1,95] Phentolamine blocks the α-adrenergic effects of cocaine and reverses the coronary vasoconstrictive effects of cocaine. Low doses (1 mg every 2.5 minutes) have been used multiple times without any adverse consequences. The administration of phentolamine is considered a class IIb recommendation.[1]

Verapamil, a calcium channel antagonist, reverses cocaine-induced coronary artery vasoconstriction. Animal studies have shown enhanced central nervous system toxicity from concurrent administration of cocaine and any one of several calcium antagonists (verapamil, diltiazem, and nifedipine). The potentiation of cocaine-associated central nervous system toxicity combined with the limited success of calcium antagonists in traditional MI patients makes them less attractive for use in patients with cocaine-associated MI.[95]

Fibrinolytic therapy is standard for patients with MI unrelated to cocaine; however, the use of these agents in cocaine-associated myocardial ischemia is less clear. There has been no demonstrated efficacy in this patient population. Of patients with cocaine-associated chest pain without MI, 43% meet TIMI criteria for the administration of fibrinolytic agents despite the fact they did not have infarction. The potential administration to patients who are not having an infarction coupled with a low mortality from cocaine-associated MI limits the utility of fibrinolytic agents. Percutaneous interventions might be more appropriate in this group of patients.

Despite the overwhelming success of β-adrenergic antagonists in patients with MI unrelated to cocaine, they should be avoided in patients who have used cocaine recently.[1,95,99] β-Adrenergic antagonists were shown to increase central nervous system toxicity and exacerbate coronary artery vasospasm in several animal models of cocaine toxicity. Clinical series showed that they fail to reverse the hypertensive and tachycardic effects of cocaine. The α-adrenergic agonist effects of cocaine on the coronary vasculature are enhanced by β-adrenergic antagonists, which worsens the severity of cocaine-induced coronary vasoconstriction. Calcium antagonists are therefore preferred over beta blockers.

REFERENCES

1. American Heart Association in Collaboration with the International Liaison Committee on Resuscitation (ILCOR): Guidelines for cardiopulmonary resuscitation and emergency cardiovascular care. Circulation 2000;102:172.
2. Braunwald E, Antman EM, Beasley JW, et al: ACC/AHA guidelines for the management of patients with unstable angina and non-ST segment elevation myocardial infarction: A report of the American College of Cardiology/American Heart Association Task Force on Practice Guidelines (Committee on the Management of Patients with Unstable Angina). J Am Coll Cardiol 2000;36:970–1062.
3. Hickan DH, Sox HC, Sox CH: Systematic bias in recording history in patients with chest pain. J Chronic Dis 1985;38:91–100.
4. Gadsboll N, Hoiland-Carlsen PF, Nielsen GG, et al: Symptoms and signs of heart failure in patients with myocardial infarction: Reproducibility and relationship to chest x-ray, radionuclide ventriculography and right heart catheterization. Eur Heart J 1989;10:1017–1028.
5. Panju AA, Hemmelgarm BR, Guyatt GH, Simel DL: Is this patient having a myocardial infarction? JAMA 1998;280:1256–1263.
6. Jayes RL, Beshansky JR, D'Agostino RB, Selker HP: Do patients' coronary risk factor reports predict acute cardiac ischemia in the emergency department? A multicenter study. J Clin Epidemiol 1992;45:621–626.
7. Sheifer SE, Manolio TA, Gersh BJ: Unrecognized myocardial infarction. Ann Intern Med 2001;135:801–811.
8. Lee T, Cook F, Weisberg M, et al: Acute chest pain in the emergency room: Identification and examination of low risk patients. Arch Intern Med 1985;145:65–69.
9. Selker HP, Zalenski RJ, Antman EM, et al: An evaluation of technologies for identification of acute cardiac ischemia in the emergency department: A report from a National Heart Attack Alert Program Working Group. Ann Emerg Med 1997;29:13–87.
10. Hathaway WR, Peterson ED, Wagner GS, et al: Prognostic significance of the initial electrocardiogram in patients with acute myocardial infarction. JAMA 1998;279:387–391.
11. Slater DK, Hlatky MA, Mark DB, et al: Outcome in suspected acute myocardial infarction with normal or minimally abnormal admission electrocardiographic findings. Am J Cardiol 1987;60:766–770.
12. Brush JE, Brand DA, Acampora D, et al: Use of the initial electrocardiogram to predict in-hospital complications of acute myocardial infarction. N Engl J Med 1985;312:1137–1141.
13. Zalenski RJ, Cooke D, Rydman R, et al: Assessing the diagnostic value of an ECG containing leads V4R, V8 and V9: The 15 lead ECG. Ann Emerg Med 1993;22:786–793.
14. Zalenski RJ, Rydman RJ, Sloan EP, et al: Value of posterior and right ventricular leads in comparison to standard 12 lead electrocardiogram in evaluation of ST segment elevation in suspected acute myocardial infarction. Am J Cardiol 1997;79:1579–1585.
15. Sgarbossa EB, Pinski SL, Barbagelata A, et al: Electrocardiographic diagnosis of evolving acute myocardial infarction in the presence of left bundle branch block. N Engl J Med 1996;334:481–487.
16. Sgarbossa EB, Pinski SL, Gates KB, Wagner GS, for GUSTO-1 Investigators: Early electrocardiographic diagnosis of acute myocardial infarction in the presence of ventricular paced rhythm. Am J Cardiol 1996;77:423–424.
17. Lee TH, Juarez G, Cook EF, et al: Ruling out myocardial infarction: A prospective multicenter validation of a 12 hour strategy for patients at low risk. N Engl J Med 1991;324:1239–1246.

18. Lau J, Ioannidis JPA, Balk EM, et al: Diagnosing acute cardiac ischemia in the emergency department: A systematic review of the accuracy and clinical effect of current technologies. Ann Emerg Med 2001;37:453–460.

19. Goldman L, Cook EF, Johnson PA, et al: Prediction of the need for intensive care in patients who come to emergency departments with chest pain. N Engl J Med 1996;334:1498–1508.

20. Qamar A, McPherson C, Babb J, et al: The Goldman algorithm revisited: Prospective evaluation of a computer-derived algorithm versus unaided physician judgment in suspected acute myocardial infarction. Am Heart J 1999;138:705–709.

21. Sarasin FP, Reymond JM, Griffith JL, et al: Impact of the acute cardiac ischemia time insensitive predictive instrument (ACI-TIPI) on the speed of triage decision making for emergency department patients presenting with chest pain: A controlled clinical trial. J Gen Intern Med 1994;9:187–194.

22. Selker HP, Beshanski JR, Griffith JL, et al: Use of the acute cardiac ischemia time-insensitive predictive instrument (ACI-TIPI) to assist with triage of patients with chest pain or other symptoms suggestive of acute cardiac ischemia: A multicenter, controlled clinical trial. Ann Intern Med 1998;129:845–855.

23. Kennedy RL, Harrison RF, Burton AM, et al: An artificial neural network system for diagnosis of acute myocardial infarction (AMI) in the accident and emergency department: Evaluation and comparison with serum myoglobin measurements. Comput Methods Programs Biomed 1997;52:93–103.

24. Baxt WG, Shofer FS, Sites FD, Hollander JE: A neural computational aid to the diagnosis of acute myocardial infarction. Ann Emerg Med 2002;40:575–583.

25. Baxt WG: Neural computational aid to the diagnosis of acute myocardial infarction. Presented at Society of Academic Emergency Medicine annual meeting, Atlanta, May 2001.

26. Antman EM, Cohen M, Bernink PJ, et al: The TIMI risk score for unstable angina/non-ST elevation MI: A method for prognostication and therapeutic decision making. JAMA 2000;284:835–842.

27. Morrow DA, Antman EM, Parsons L, et al: Application of the TIMI risk score for ST-elevation MI in the National Registry of Myocardial Infarction 3. JAMA 2001;286:1356–1359.

28. Kontos MC, Anderson FP, Schmidt KA, et al: Early diagnosis of acute myocardial infarction in patients without ST segment elevation. Am J Cardiol 1999;83:155–158.

29. Gibler WB, Lewis LM, Erb RE, et al: Early detection of acute myocardial infarction in patients presenting with chest pain and nondiagnostic ECGs: Serial CK-MB sampling in the emergency department. Ann Emerg Med 1990;19:1359–1366.

30. Fesmire FM, Percy RF, Bardoner JB, et al: Serial creatinine kinase MB testing during emergency department evaluation of chest pain: Utility of a 2 hour delta CK-MB of + 1.6 ng.ml. Am Heart J 1998;136:237–244.

31. Adams JE III, Bodor GS, Davila-Roman VG, et al: Cardiac troponin I: A marker with high specificity for cardiac injury. Circulation 1993;88:101–106.

32. Brogan GX Jr, Hollander JE, McCuskey CF, et al: Evaluation of a new assay for cardiac troponin I vs creatine kinase-MB for the diagnosis of acute myocardial infarction. Acad Emerg Med 1997;4:6–12.

33. Hollander JE, Levitt MA, Young GP, et al: Effect of recent cocaine use on the specificity of cardiac markers for diagnosis of acute myocardial infarction. Am Heart J 1998;135:245–252.

34. Tunstall-Pedoe H, Kuulasmaa K, Annouyel P, et al: The WHO MONICA project: Myocardial infarction and coronary deaths in the World Health Organization MONICA project. Circulation 1994;90:588–612.

35. ACC/AHA guidelines for the management of patients with acute myocardial infarction. J Am Coll Cardiol 1996;28:1328–1428.

36. Capellan O, Sites F, Shofer FS, Hollander JE: Risk stratification of ED patients with ACS using initial absolute CK-MB vs. CK-MB RI [abstract]. Acad Emerg Med 2001;8:503–504.

37. Puleo PR, Meyer D, Wathen C, et al: Use of a rapid assay of subforms of creatine kinase MB to diagnose or rule out acute myocardial infarction. N Engl J Med 1994;331:561–566.

38. Green GB, Li DJ, Bessman ES, et al: The prognostic significance of troponin I and troponin T. Acad Emerg Med 1998;5:758–767.

39. Antman EM, Tanasijevic MJ, Thompson B, et al: Cardiac specific troponin I levels predict the risk of mortality in patients with acute coronary syndromes. N Engl J Med 1996;335:1342–1349.

40. Morrow DA, Cannon CP, Rifai N, et al: Ability of minor elevations of troponins I and T to predict benefit from an early invasive strategy in patients with unstable angina and non ST segment elevation myocardial infarction. JAMA 2001;286:2405–2412.

41. Ohman EM, Armstrong PW, Christenson RH, et al: Cardiac troponin-T levels for risk stratification in acute myocardial ischemia. N Engl J Med 1996;335:1333–1341.

42. Newby LK, Kaplan AL, Granger BB, et al: Comparison of cardiac troponin T versus creatine kinase-MB for risk stratification in a chest pain evaluation unit. Am J Cardiol 2000;85:801–805.

43. Sayre MR, Kaufmann KH, Chen IW, et al: Measurement of cardiac troponin T is an effective method for predicting complications among emergency department patients with chest pain. Ann Emerg Med 1998;31:539–549.

44. Heidenreich PA, Alloggiamento T, Melsop K, et al: The prognostic value of troponin in patients with non-ST elevation acute coronary syndromes: A meta-analysis. J Am Coll Cardiol 2001;38:478–485.

45. Hamm CW, Goldmann BU, Heeschen C, et al: Emergency room triage of patients with acute chest pain by means of rapid testing for cardiac troponin T or troponin I. N Engl J Med 1997;337:1648–1653.

46. McErlean ES, Deluca SA, van Lente F, et al: Comparison of troponin T versus creatine kinase MB in suspected acute coronary syndromes. Am J Cardiol 2000;85:421–426.

47. Kontos MC, Anderson FP, Alimard R, et al: Ability of troponin I to predict cardiac events in patients admitted from the emergency department. J Am Coll Cardiol 2000;36:1818–1823.

48. Datta P, Foster K, Dasgupta A: Comparison of immunoreactivity of five human cardiac troponin I assays toward free and complexed forms of the antigen: Implications for assay discordance. Clin Chem 1999;45:1002–1008.

49. Quinn MJ, Moliterno DJ: Troponins in acute coronary syndromes: More TACTICS for an early invasive strategy. JAMA 2001;286:2461–2462.

50. Wayand D, Baum M, Schatzle G, et al: Cardiac troponin T and I in end stage renal failure. Clin Chem 2000;46:1345–1350.

51. DeWinter RJ, Lijmer JG, Koster RW, et al: Diagnostic accuracy of myoglobin concentration for the early diagnosis of acute myocardial infarction. Ann Emerg Med 2000;35:113–120.

52. Brogan GX Jr, Friedman S, McCuskey C, et al: Evaluation of a new rapid quantitative immunoassay for serum myoglobin versus CK-MB for ruling out acute myocardial infarction in the emergency department. Ann Emerg Med 1994;24:665–671.

53. Green GB, Beaudreau RW, Chan DW, et al: Use of troponin T and creatine kinase MB subunit levels for risk stratification of emergency department patients with possible myocardial ischemia. Ann Emerg Med 1998;31:19–29.

54. Brogan GX, Vuori J, Freidman S, et al: Improved specificity of myoglobin plus carbonic anhydrase versus that of creatine kinase-MB for the early diagnosis of acute myocardial infarction. Ann Emerg Med 1996;27:22–28.

55. Hollander JE, Muttreja MR, Dalesandro MR, Shofer FS: Risk stratification of ED patients with acute coronary syndromes using P-Selectin. J Am Coll Cardiol 1999;34:95–105.

56. Zimmerman J, Fromm R, Meyer D, et al: Diagnostic marker cooperative study for the diagnosis of myocardial infarction. Circulation 1999;99:1671–1677.

57. Kontos MC, Anderson FP, Hanbury CM, et al: Use of the combination of myoglobin and CKMB mass for the rapid diagnosis of acute myocardial infarction. Am J Emerg Med 1997;15:14–19.

58. McCord J, Nowak RM, McCullough PA, et al: Ninety-minute exclusion of acute myocardial infarction by use of quantitative point-of-care testing of myoglobin and troponin I. Circulation 2001;104:1483–1488.

59. Selker HP, Zalenski RJ, Antman EM, et al: An evaluation of technologies for identification of acute cardiac ischemia in the emergency department: A report from a National Heart Attack Alert Program Working Group. Ann Emerg Med 1997;29:13–87.

60. Fleischmann KE, Lee TH, Come PC, et al: Echocardiographic prediction of complications in patients with chest pain. Am J Cardiol 1997;79:292–298.

61. Kontos MC, Arrowood JA, Paulsen WHJ, Nixon JV: Early echocardiography can predict cardiac events in emergency department patients with chest pain. Ann Emerg Med 1998;31:550–557.

62. Paventi S, Parafati MA, DiLuzio E, Pelligrino CA. Usefulness of two dimensional echocardiography and myocardial perfusion imaging for immediate evaluation of chest pain in the emergency department. Resuscitation 2001;49:47-51.

63. Varetto T, Cantalupi D, Altieri A, Orlandi C: Emergency room technetium-99m sestamibi imaging to rule out acute myocardial ischemia events in patients with nondiagnostic electrocardiograms. J Am Coll Cardiol 1993;22:1804-1808.

64. Hilton TC, Thompson RC, Williams HJ, et al: Technetium-99m sestamibi myocardial perfusion imaging in the emergency room evaluation of chest pain. J Am Coll Cardiol 1994;23:1016-1022.

65. Tatum JL, Jesse RL, Kontos MC, et al: Comprehensive strategy for the evaluation and triage of the chest pain patient. Ann Emerg Med 1997;29:116-125.

66. Kontos MC, Jesse RL, Anderson FA, et al: Comparison of myocardial perfusion imaging and cardiac troponin I in patients admitted to the emergency department with chest pain. Circulation 1999;99:2073-2078.

67. Achenbach S, Moshage W, Ropers D, et al: Value of electron beam computed tomography for the noninvasive detection of high grade coronary artery stenosis and occlusions. N Engl J Med 1998;339:1964-1971.

68. McLaughlin VV, Balogh T, Rich S. Utility of electron beam computed tomography to stratify patients presenting to the emergency room with chest pain. Am J Cardiol 1999;84:327-328.

69. Laudon DA, Vukov LF, Breen JF, et al: Use of electron beam computed tomography in the evaluation of chest pain patients in the emergency department. Ann Emerg Med 1998;33:15-21.

70. Raggi P, Callister TQ, Cooil B, et al: Evaluation of chest pain in patients with low to intermediate pretest probability of coronary artery disease by electron beam computed tomography. Am J Cardiol 2000;85:283-288.

71. Georgiou D, Budoff MJ, Kaufer E, et al: Screening patients with chest pain in the emergency department using electron beam tomography: A follow-up study. J Am Coll Cardiol 2001;38:105-110.

72. Lindsay J Jr, Bonnet YD, Pinnow EE: Routine stress testing for triage of patients with chest pain: Is it worth the candle? Ann Emerg Med 1998;32:600-603.

73. Diercks DB, Gibler WB, Liu T, et al: Identification of patients at risk by graded exercise testing in an emergency department chest pain center. Am J Cardiol 2000;86:289-292.

74. Trippi JA, Lee KS, Kopp G, et al: Dobutamine stress tele-echocardiography for evaluation of emergency department patients with chest pain. J Am Coll Cardiol 1997;30:627-632.

75. Colon PJ 3rd, Guarisco JS, Murgo J, Cheirif J: Utility of stress echocardiography in the triage of patients with atypical chest pain from the emergency department. Am J Cardiol 1998;82:1282-1284.

76. Kirk JD, Turnipseed S, Lewis WR, Amsterdam EA: Evaluation of chest pain in low risk patients presenting to the emergency department: The role of immediate exercise testing. Ann Emerg Med 1998;32:1-7.

77. Pitts WR, Lange RA, Cigarroa JE, Hillis LD: Repeat coronary angiography in patients with chest pain and previously normal coronary angiogram. Am J Cardiol 1997;80:1086-1087.

78. Papanicolaou MN, Califf RM, Hlatky MA, et al: Prognostic implications of angiographically normal and insignificantly narrowed coronary arteries. Am J Cardiol 1986;58:1181-1187.

79. Lee TH, Boucher CA: Noninvasive tests in patients with stable coronary artery disease. N Engl J Med 2001;344:1840-1845.

80. Chest pain centers: concepts, information, function. http://www.scpep.org/cpc/index.htlm

81. Graff LG, Dallara J, Ross MA, et al: Impact on the care of the emergency department chest pain patients from the Chest Pain Evaluation Registry (CHEPER) study. Am J Cardiol 1997;80:563-568.

82. Farkouh ME, Smars PA, Reeder GS, et al: A clinical trial of a chest pain observation unit for patients with unstable angina. N Engl J Med 1998;339:1882-1888.

83. Roberts RR, Zalenski RJ, Mensah EK, et al: Costs of an emergency department based accelerated diagnostic protocol vs hospitalization in patients with chest pain. JAMA 1997;278:1670-1676.

84. Rydman RJ, Zalenski RJ, Roberts RR, et al: Patient satisfaction with an emergency department chest pain observation unit. Ann Emerg Med 1997;29:109-115.

85. Walker NJ, Sites FD, Shofer FS, Hollander JE: Characteristics and outcomes of young adults who present to the emergency department with chest pain. Acad Emerg Med 2001;8:703-708.

86. Ng SM, Krishnaswamy P, Morissey R, et al: Ninety minute accelerated critical pathway for chest pain evaluation. Am J Cardiol 2001;88:611-617.

87. Hollander JE, Valentine SM, McCuskey C, Brogan GX: Are monitored telemetry beds necessary for patients with nontraumatic chest pain and normal or nonspecific electrocardiograms? Am J Cardiol 1997;79:1110-1111.

88. Estrada CA, Prasad NK, Rosman HS, Young MJ: Outcomes of patients hospitalized to a telemetry unit. Am J Cardiol 1994;74:357-362.

89. Estrada CA, Rosman HS, Prasad NK, et al: Role of telemetry monitoring in the non-intensive care unit. Am J Cardiol 1995;76:960-965.

90. Wu GM, Sites FD, Shofer FS, Hollander JE: Does stress testing impact 30-day CV outcomes for patients admitted to non-ICU telemetry beds? [abstract]. Acad Emerg Med 2001;8:507.

91. Limkakeng A Jr, Gibler WB, Pollack C, et al: Combination of Goldman risk and initial cardiac troponin I for emergency department chest pain patient risk stratification. Acad Emerg Med 2001;8:696-702.

92. Mittleman MA, Mintzer D, Maclure M, et al: Triggering of myocardial infarction by cocaine. Circulation 1999;99:2737-2741.

93. Hollander JE, Hoffman RS: Cocaine induced myocardial infarction: An analysis and review of the literature. J Emerg Med 1992;10:169-177.

94. Hollander JE, Hoffman RS, Gennis P, et al: Prospective multicenter evaluation of cocaine associated chest pain. Acad Emerg Med 1994;1:330-339.

95. Hollander JE: Management of cocaine associated myocardial ischemia. N Engl J Med 1995;333:1267-1272.

96. Weber JE, Gibson CM, Hynes C, et al: Quantitative comparison of coronary artery flow and myocardial perfusion in patients with acute myocardial infarction in the presence vs absence of recent cocaine use. Acad Emerg Med 2001;8:539-540.

97. Kontos MC, Schmidt KL, Nicholson CS, et al: Myocardial perfusion imaging with technetium-99m sestamibi in patients with cocaine associated chest pain. Ann Emerg Med 1999;33:639-645.

98. Kushman SO, Storrow AB, Liu T, Gibler WB: Cocaine associated chest pain in a chest pain center. Am J Cardiol 2000;85:394-396.

99. Lange RA, Hillis LD: Cardiovascular complications of cocaine use. N Engl J Med 2001;345:351-358.

Electrocardiogram, ECG Monitoring, and Provocative Stress Testing in Acute Coronary Syndromes

Brian Y. L. Wong
Yuling Fu
Paul W. Armstrong

The electrocardiogram (ECG) is not only the oldest but continues to be the most widely used cardiovascular diagnostic procedure. It has evolved to become an indispensable tool in the initial evaluation of a variety of cardiac symptoms, partly because of simplicity in recording, ready and wide accessibility, ease of repeated assessment, and low cost. This renaissance has been further stimulated by recent pathophysiologic and outcome studies of acute coronary syndromes (ACSs).

Patients who present to hospital with acute chest pain constitute a diagnostically and prognostically heterogeneous group: Only 17% of these patients actually have evidence of acute cardiac ischemia (8% acute myocardial infarction [AMI], 9% unstable angina) according to a recent prospective study of over 10,000 patients.[5] The initial (first, or admission) ECG is a simple but powerful prognostic tool that allows patients with acute chest pain to be instantly stratified into three subgroups that have diverse short-[12] and long-term prognosis (Fig. 13–1),[13-15] namely those presenting with (1) ST elevation (with or without concomitant ST depression), (2) ST depression or T-wave inversion, or both (without concomitant ST elevation), and (3) nondiagnostic ST-T changes or a normal-appearing ECG. This classification thus provides a framework with which subsequent diagnostic and therapeutic strategies can be aligned.

In recent years, the traditional role of cardiac monitoring for arrhythmia detection has expanded to include the online recording and analysis of quantitative ST-segment information. This forms the basis for continuous ischemia monitoring, whose role in the evaluation of patients with ACS is still being actively defined. Exercise testing continues to play a major role in risk stratification following an episode of acute chest pain. However, optimal timing and intensity of stress testing remain controversial.

In line with the main theme of the textbook, this chapter primarily addresses the role of the initial (and serial) 12-lead ECGs, continuous ST-segment monitoring, and exercise stress testing at various stages of evaluation among patients presenting with non–ST-elevation (NSTE) ACS. Given the magnitude and clinical significance of ST-elevation ACS, however, its distinction from NSTE ACS is highlighted and the roles of various electrocardiographic modalities in this setting are surveyed.

ST-ELEVATION VERSUS NON–ST-ELEVATION ACUTE CORONARY SYNDROMES: PRACTICAL TERMINOLOGY WITH IMPORTANT PATHOPHYSIOLOGIC, CLINICAL, AND PROGNOSTIC DISTINCTIONS

The contemporary approach to ACS lies in the fundamental distinction between presence and absence of ST-segment elevation on the presenting ECG. The presence of regional ST-segment elevation represents epicardial injury and is associated with a high prevalence of total thrombotic coronary occlusion and subsequent new pathologic Q-wave formation (80%),[21] thus encompassing the clinical syndrome of "ST elevation ACS," "Q-wave myocardial infarction (MI)," or "transmural MI." Rapid, complete, and sustained macro- and micro-vascular reperfusion, either by mechanical or pharmacologic means, are definitive therapeutic goals in this setting. (Rarely, transient ST elevation related to vasospasm in an angiographically normal coronary artery, as in the Prinzmetal variant, may be abolished by coronary vasodilator therapy.) As distinguished from ST elevation ACS, the occurrence of such ST-T changes as ST depression, T-wave inversion, nondiagnostic ST-T changes, or a normal-appearing ECG in ACS are thought to represent subendocardial ischemia due to the presence of subocclusive thrombus or unfavorable coronary blood supply/demand condition, or both, thus encompassing the clinical syndrome of NSTE ACS.

The prevalence of different presenting ECG patterns varies substantially among large clinical trials of patients with ACS owing to heterogeneous inclusion criteria. In a single-center study of 440 unselected patients admitted for suspected ACS,[19] ST elevation (>1 mm in more than two contiguous leads, with or without concomitant ST depression or T-wave inversion) was present on the

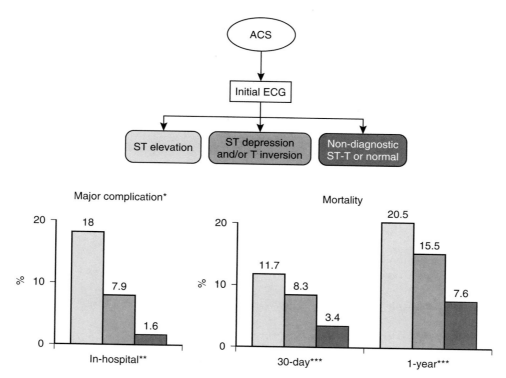

FIGURE 13–1. The central role of the initial ECG in the evaluation of acute coronary syndromes (ACS). The initial ECG allows instantaneous stratification of patients with ACS into three prognostic subgroups based on their presenting ST-T features and their respective association with in-hospital major complications *(lower left panel)* and postdischarge mortality at 30 days and 1 year *(lower right panel)*. See text for definitions of ECG subgroups. *, *Major complication* refers to ventricular fibrillation, cardiac arrest, complete heart block, insertion of a temporary pacemaker, emergency cardioversion, cardiogenic shock, use of an intra-aortic balloon pump, intubation, recurrent ischemia, or urgent revascularization. Numerical data adapted from Goldman L, Cook EF, Johnson PA, et al: Prediction of the need for intensive care in patients who come to emergency departments with acute chest pain. N Engl J Med 334:1498–1504, 1996; and Nyman I, Areskog M, Areskog NH, et al: Very early risk stratification by electrocardiogram at rest in men with suspected unstable coronary heart disease. J Intern Med 234:293–301, 1993**, *P* value not reported. ***, *P* < .05.

initial 12-lead ECG in 13% of all patients; ST depression (>1 mm in more than two contiguous leads) or T-wave inversion (>1 mm in more than two contiguous leads), or both in 9%; nondiagnostic ST-T changes in 14%; and a normal-appearing ECG in 15%. Noteworthy was that a substantial proportion (27%) of patients had uninterpretable ST-T changes (e.g., left bundle branch block, left-ventricular hypertrophy with or without strain, paced rhythm) at presentation. Although such patients were traditionally excluded from large clinical trials, recent data from the *P*latelet IIb/IIIb *A*ntagonism for the *R*eduction of *A*cute coronary syndrome events in a *G*lobal *O*rganization *N*etwork (PARAGON)-A study[18] suggests an almost doubled 1-year mortality rate among patients with NSTE ACS presenting with these ECG confounders (12.6% vs. 6.5% in those without ECG confounders). This increased rate might be explained by the increased age and incidence of previous MI and revascularization among those presenting with ECG confounders.

Notwithstanding the pathophysiologic significance of the STE versus NSTE ACS classification, further ECG subcategorization under this broad scheme enables more-precise risk definition in both the short and the long term, as was shown in the Global Utilization of Streptokinase and t-PA (alteplase) for Occluded coronary arteries (GUSTO)-IIb study.[13] Table 13–1 summarizes the rates of enrollment MI, short- and long-term reinfarction, and death for patients presenting with STE ACS (namely those with STE alone or with concomitant ST depression on the initial ECG) versus those presenting with NSTE ACS (i.e., ST depression with or without concomitant T-wave inversion), isolated T-wave inversion, or a nondiagnostic or normal-appearing ECG, respectively. Figure 13–2 illustrates the diverse natural history of these ECG subgroups.

The higher rates of early events (during the first 30 days) in STE ACS (vs. NSTE ACS) may be explained by the higher incidence of enrollment MI (>80%) (see Table 13–1), which carries an immediate risk of fatal ventricular arrhythmia, left-ventricular pump failure, and cardiac rupture. Compared with patients with STE alone, patients with both ST elevation and ST depression tended to have larger infarcts, more symptoms of congestive heart failure, and worse left-ventricular function[50]—and thus even higher event rates in both the short and the long term. In contrast, patients with ST depression were less likely to evolve MI at presentation (48%), which corresponded to a lower short-term event rate (see Table 13–1). However, the incidence of both

TABLE 13–1 SHORT- AND LONG-TERM PROGNOSIS ACCORDING TO ST-T ABNORMALITIES ON THE ADMISSION ELECTROCARDIOGRAM

	ST-ELEVATION ACS		NON–ST-ELEVATION ACS		
	ST Elevation Alone	ST Elevation and Depression	ST Depression ± T Inversion	Isolated T Inversion	Nondiagnostic or Normal ECG
Enrollment MI (%)	81.0	89.0	48.0	32.0	< 10
Death (%)					
30 days	5.1	6.6	5.1	1.7	
6 months	6.8	9.1	8.9	3.4	
Re-MI (%)					
30 days	5.0	7.1	7.0	4.2	
6 months	6.8	8.9	9.2	5.4	
Death/re-MI (%)					
30 days	9.4	12.4	10.5	5.5	3.4
6 months	12.3	15.7	15.4	8.1	
1 year	16.0	26.0	18.0	14.0	8.0

ACS, acute coronary syndrome; ECG, electrocardiogram; MI, myocardial infarction.
Data from references 13, 14, 65.

death and reinfarction continued to increase during follow-up in this subgroup, exceeding that of patients with STE alone by 1 month and approaching that of patients with both ST elevation and ST depression by 6 months (see Fig. 13–2).

Patients with isolated T-wave inversion had a relatively benign prognosis compared with the other groups, likely because of a less severe coronary disease burden at angiography.[13] Patients with nondiagnostic or normal-appearing ECGs at presentation exhibited the lowest rates of enrollment MI[65] and adverse events during both short- and long-term follow-up (see Table 13–1).[14]

In view of the fact that this ECG subcategorization enhances the prognostic utility of the classic STE versus the NSTE binary scheme, it thus provides the framework for subsequent discussion on the role of various electrocardiographic modalities.

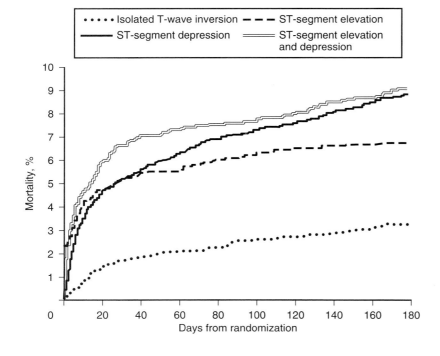

FIGURE 13–2. Kaplan-Meier estimates of probability of death. (From Savonitto S, Ardissino D, Granger CB, et al: Prognostic significance of the admission electrocardiogram in acute coronary syndromes. JAMA 1999;281:707–713. Copyright 1999, American Medical Association.)

PRESENTATION WITH ST DEPRESSION OR T-WAVE INVERSION, OR BOTH (WITHOUT CONCOMITANT ST ELEVATION) ON THE INITIAL ECG

Clinical Utility of the Initial and Serial 12-Lead ECGs

Estimation of Myocardium at Risk and Location of Coronary Artery Disease

Angiographic features such as the extent of coronary artery disease (CAD) has traditionally been used to estimate the amount of myocardium at risk. Because of the invasive nature of angiography, such admission ECG features as the presence, magnitude, and extent of ST shift had been examined in relation to their ability to predict unfavorable angiographic features. Langer et al[74] and more recently Diderholm and colleagues[27] in the Fragmin and Fast Revascularization during Instability in Coronary artery disease (FRISC) II investigations found a significantly higher prevalence of multivessel and left main disease among patients with unstable angina who had ST depression on the admission ECG. Papapietro et al[22] observed a correlation between the maximal magnitude of transient ST-segment shifts, and three- versus one- or two-vessel CAD among patients presenting with unstable angina. Furthermore, in an angioplasty model of acute transient ischemia, Cohen et al[23] found that both the sum of ST shifts and the total number of leads with ST shifts correlated well with the percentage of left-ventricular perimeter in jeopardy.

The jeopardy score, developed as an instrument to estimate the amount of myocardium at risk based on the particular location of coronary artery stenoses, has been shown to have superior prognostic value than the number of diseased vessels.[24] Applying this score in patients with NSTE ACS, Cohen et al[25] found that the extent of myocardium in jeopardy had the strongest correlation with total number of leads bearing new ST deviation on the admission ECG and to a lesser degree with maximal or sum of ST deviation.

In the absence of regional ST-segment elevation, the admission ECG generally is only of limited value in localizing the culprit lesion. Perhaps the most important exception to this rule relates to the presence of a specific pattern of ST-T abnormalities first described by de Zwaan et al.[26] This pattern consisted of an isoelectric or minimally elevated takeoff of the ST segment, followed by a concave or straight ST segment passing into a symmetrically inverted T wave in leads V_2 and V_3. Similar patterns may be present in V_1 and V_4. Occasionally, the takeoff of the ST segment may be below the isoelectric line with a convex ST segment passing into a deeply inverted T wave in V_5 and V_6. This pattern has a sensitivity of 69% and specificity of 89% in predicting significant proximal left anterior descending stenosis.[63]

Assessment of Short- and Long-Term Prognosis

Numerous studies[13-18,25,27-29] have demonstrated the prognostic value of new-onset, or presumably new-onset, ST-segment depression on the admission ECG in the form of both univariate and multivariate predictors of short- and long-term adverse clinical outcome (Table 13-2). Noteworthy is that the event rates differ widely among different studies of patients with NSTE ACS, owing to such factors as patient inclusion criteria, treatment received, clinical end-point definition, and duration of follow-up. Accordingly, the absolute event rates associated with any given degree of ST depression also differed among these studies. Nevertheless, several clinically relevant statements about the prognostic value of new or presumably new ST depression on the admission ECG can be made in more general terms:

- Because less than half of patients with NSTE ACS experience MI at presentation (see Table 13-1), ST depression on admission is relatively insensitive for the detection of MI (sensitivity ranges from 15% to 40%).[13,19] Although deeper or more extensive ST depression is associated with increased specificity,[17] this occurs at the expense of further loss in sensitivity without improving the overall diagnostic accuracy.
- The traditional 1 mm cutoff for defining clinically significant ST depression should now be revised to 0.5 mm in view of its consistently demonstrated prognostic value in several large-scale studies.[13,15-16,28-29]
- Notwithstanding its limited value in detecting MI at presentation, ST depression on admission significantly predicts re-infarction and mortality up to 4 years following hospital discharge, even after adjustment for important baseline characteristics.[16]

Recent evidence from the PARAGON-A study[18] showed that ST depression on admission was more than simply a qualitative predictor by demonstrating a quantitative relationship between both magnitude and distribution of ST depression and short- and longer-term outcomes. In particular, patients with no ST depression, greater than 1 mm of ST depression, greater than 2 mm of ST depression, and greater than 2 mm of ST depression in more than two contiguous leads on admission exhibited progressively higher rates of MI at presentation, re-infarction, and death up to 1 year (Table 13-3; Fig. 13-3). Furthermore, preliminary data from the PARAGON-B study[64] suggested that persistence of early ST depression or emergence of late ST depression in hospital tended to adversely affect prognosis, whereas normalization of baseline ST depression by hospital discharge conferred a better outcome. The potential additive value of the discharge ECG is currently under investigation.

The prognostic value of a new-onset isolated T wave on admission is less well-defined owing to the conflicting evidence in the literature. One important exception are patients presenting with the characteristic anterior ST-T pattern described by de Zwaan et al[26] (see previous discussion for details), of whom 42% went on to experience an extensive anterior MI along with a 12% mortality rate within 6 weeks of the initial NSTE presentation. Longer-term (up to 4 years) follow-up revealed a substantial risk of cardiac mortality and re-infarction

TABLE 13–2 SUMMARY OF MAJOR STUDIES ON PROGNOSTIC VALUE OF ST-T ABNORMALITIES IN NSTE ACS*

STUDIES (REF.)	SAMPLE SIZE	ST-T CRITERIA ON THE ADMISSION ECG (PREVALENCE)	MAJOR FINDINGS	SIGNIFICANT COVARIATE PREDICTORS
ST-T Abnormalities as Univariate Predictor				
Cohen et al. (25)	90†	ST deviation ≥ 1 mm in ≥ 2 leads (63%)	Higher 3-month rates of death, MI, recurrent ischemia, revascularization in the presence of ST changes (77% vs. 36% without ST changes)	N/A
Lee et al. (17)	136‡	ST depression ≥ 1 mm any lead (100%)	Mortality gradient at 1 year according to degree of baseline ST depression: 14% (1 mm) vs. 39% (2 mm) vs. 30% (≥ 3 mm)	N/A
RISC study (14)	911§	ST depression (±T↓) ≥ 1 mm any lead (24%); isolated T↓ (31%)	Death/MI at 1 year: 7.6% (no ST-T changes) vs. 13.6% (isolated T↓) vs. 18.1% (ST depression)	N/A
ST-T Abnormalities as Multivariate Predictor				
Hyde et al. (16)	367§	ST depression ≥ 0.5 mm any lead (47%); isolated T↓ ≥ 1 mm any lead (16%)	ST depression ≥ 0.5 mm but not isolated T↓ significantly predicted lower 4-year survival	Age, CHF, revascularization
TIMI 3 Registry (15)	1416§	ST deviation ≥ 0.5 mm any lead (27%); isolated T↓ ≥ 1 mm any lead (22%)	ST deviation ≥ 0.5 mm but not isolated T↓ significantly predicted death/MI at 1 year	Age, fibrinolysis within past week, nitrate within past week, LBBB, other major illnesses, poor compliance with follow-up
PARAGON A study (18)	1588‡	ST depression ≥ 1 mm any lead (43%)	Mortality gradient at 1 year according to degree of baseline ST depression: 2% (no depression) vs. 7.8% (1 mm) vs. 13.4% (≥ 2 mm)	Age, COPD, previous MI, CHF, PVD, diabetes, previous PTCA, cerebrovascular disease
TIMI-11B study (28)	1957†	ST deviation ≥ 0.5 mm any lead (72%)	Risk of death, MI, or urgent revascularization in the presence of ST deviation was 1.5 times that without ST deviation	Age, ≥3 cardiac risk factors, prior CAD ≥ 50% stenosis, ≥2 anginal events in prior 24 hours, use of aspirin in prior week, elevated biomarkers‖
FRISC II (27)	2457†	ST depression ≥ 0.5 mm any lead (46%); isolated T↓ ≥ 1 mm any lead (36%)	ST depression ≥ 0.5 mm but not isolated T↓ significantly predicted higher death/MI at 1 year	Age, diabetes, ≥ 2 antianginal medications, TnT ≥ 0.06 μg/L, CHF (or LVEF < 45%), early invasive strategy
GUSTO-2B Study (13)	6986‡	ST depression ≥ 0.5 mm any lead (35%); isolated T↓ ≥ 1 mm any lead (22%)	Death/MI at 6 months: 3.4% (isolated T↓) vs. 8.9% (ST depression), $P < 0.02$	Age, Killip class, tachycardia, PVD diabetes, previous angina, hypertension, elevated CK on admission
PURSUIT (29)	9461†	ST depression ≥ 0.5 mm any lead (50%); isolated T↓ ≥ 1 mm any lead (NR)	ST depression, but not T↓ was associated with near-doubling of 30-day mortality	Age, heart rate, systolic BP, CHF elevated CK on admission, prior CABG, diabetes, CCS III/IV angina in past 6 weeks, region of enrollment, prior use of β-blocker or CCB

CABG, coronary artery bypass graft; CAD, coronary artery disease; CCB, calcium channel blocker; CHF, congestive heart failure; COPD, chronic obstructive pulmonary disease; LVEF, left-ventricular endometrial failure; N/A, not available; TT, troponin T.

*NSTE ACS encompasses the clinical syndromes of unstable angina and non-ST-elevation myocardial infarction. ST-T changes are described in individual footnotes.

†Part of composite inclusion criteria.

‡Necessary inclusion criteria.

§Not an inclusion criterion.

‖Biomarkers included CK and/or troponin.

TABLE 13–3   DEGREE OF ST-SEGMENT DEPRESSION ON ADMISSION ELECTROCARDIOGRAM AND PROGNOSIS

	NO ST↓	ST ↓ = 1 MM	ST ↓ ≥ 2 MM
Enrollment MI (%)	28.2	38.8	55.1
Death (%)			
30 days	0.7	2.8	6.3
6 months	1.1	6.2	12.0
Re-infarction (%)			
30 days	6.8	11.2	14.1
6 months	8.4	14.1	16.3
Death/re-infarction (%)			
30 days	7.2	12.1	17.1
6 months	9.2	16.7	23.9

↓, depression; MI; myocardial infarction.
Data from reference 18.

associated with this ECG pattern when such patients were treated medically.[30,63]

Significance of ST Deviation Recorded During Chest Pain

The classic natural history studies of unstable angina in 1970s and early 1980s[31-33] provided the first clue on the utility of ECG recorded during chest pain. Among patients admitted for NSTE ACS who subsequently experienced recurrent chest pain in the hospital, approximately 55% exhibited transient ST depression or T-wave inversion, or both, during recurrent pain.[22,32] This phenomenon was shown to correlate with the presence of multivessel disease[22] and higher rates of death or re-infarction up to 3 years after discharge.[31,33] Although ST depression during chest pain is a less important prognostic factor than such predictors as left-ventricular ejection fraction, left main CAD, or triple vessel CAD,[34-35] such depression can be combined with other clinical features, such as the nature of the presenting event,[36] continuing angina in hospital,[31,33] or technetium-99m pyrophosphate scintigraphy[33] to enhance risk stratification.

The superior prognostic value of ST deviation recorded during chest pain as compared with that recorded irrespective of pain status was shown in a study of 90 patients admitted for NSTE ACS.[25] Considering all patients, an admission ECG with ST deviation had a 79% positive predictive value for adverse clinical events at 3 months and a 64% negative predictive value. These values improved to 89% and 72%, respectively, in the subset of patients whose admission ECG was recorded during chest pain. Furthermore, in the GUSTO-2b study,[37] refractory ischemia defined as recurrent ischemic symptom with ST-T changes greater than 10 minutes despite medical therapy was associated with a near tripling of adjusted 1-year mortality among those presenting with NSTE ACS, thus highlighting the prognostic significance of ST deviation recorded during chest pain in this patient subgroup.

Integration of ST-T Information into Patient Care

Contemporary management of NSTE ACS emphasizes early identification of high-risk patient subgroups in whom intensive anticoagulant therapy, an early invasive strategy, or both may be used to maximize the benefit/risk ratio. In line with this guiding principle, recent data from the Efficacy and Safety of Subcutaneous Enoxaparin in Non-Q Wave Coronary Events (ESSENCE) study[38] suggest that the greatest benefit of enoxaparin over unfractionated heparin is achieved in the highest-risk ECG subgroup, i.e., patients with ST-segment depression on the admission ECG. Furthermore, an early invasive strategy in the FRISC II study substantially decreased death and re-infarction at 1 year in the presence of ST depression on the admission ECG; however, no benefit was seen in the absence of such changes.[27]

Nevertheless, given the heterogeneous nature of this clinical syndrome, a predictive instrument that simultaneously accounts for the admission ECG features and other clinically relevant factors should enable more-precise risk quantification at the time of presentation, thus forming the basis for selection of subsequent therapy. Table 13–2 outlines the multivariate models derived from several major clinical trials in NSTE ACS. Collectively, they have demonstrated the independent and additive prognostic value of ST-segment depression and T-wave inversion among other clinically important variables. The Thrombolysis in Myocardial Infarction (TIMI) risk score[28] for NSTE ACS is probably the most widely adopted scheme for prognostication and therapeutic decision-making to date. This seven-point score, originally derived from baseline clinical data in the TIMI-IIB study, allowed discrimination of as much as a tenfold difference in risk of death, nonfatal MI, or recurrent ischemia through 14 days after initiation of anticoagulant

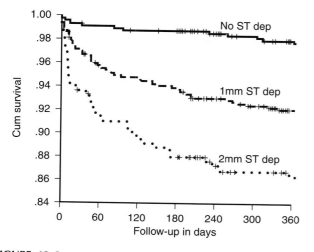

FIGURE 13–3. Survival curves corresponding to the categories of no ST-segment depression (dep), 1 mm ST-segment depression, and >2 mm ST-segment depression in the PARAGON-A study. (From Kaul P, Fu Y, Chang WC, et al: Prognostic value of ST-segment depression in acute coronary syndromes: Insights from PARAGON-A applied to GUSTO-IIb. J Am Coll Cardiol 38:64–71, 2001. Copyright 2001, Elsevier Science.)

therapy. Importantly, the efficacy of enoxaparin in this study was positively related to the patient's baseline risk as indicated by the TIMI risk score. Thus, this instrument allows optimal selection of patients for intensive anticoagulation as early as at the time of presentation. In addition, recent application of this[39] and another similar[40] risk score in the TIMI-18 and FRISC II studies, respectively, shows that the benefit of an early invasive strategy is limited to those with intermediate- or high-risk score, irrespective of whether upstream glycoprotein IIb/IIIa antagonist was initiated[39] or not.[40]

Clinical Utility of Continuous ST-Segment Monitoring

As noted previously, several clinical (e.g., recurrent ischemia) and angiographic features (e.g., multivessel CAD and intracoronary thrombus) serve as major determinants of adverse clinical outcomes in NSTE ACS. Because over 90% of episodes of recurrent ischemia following unstable angina are silent,[76] relying on symptoms alone misses most of such events. Continuous ST-segment monitoring, now commercially available in its three most popular techniques (two- or three-lead Holter ST-segment monitor, the continuously updated 12-lead system, and the continuous vectorcardiographic monitor based on the Frank (x, y, z) orthogonal leads system), is an attractive tool that allows online display of continuously updated quantitative ST-segment information (except for the Holter ST monitor, which only allows retrospective playback and analysis). At present, continuous ST-segment monitoring is the only objective means for documenting the presence, frequency, duration, and intensity of silent ischemia as well as its relationship with high-risk angiographic features (such as multivessel CAD and intracoronary thrombus) and adverse clinical outcome.

Relationship Between Myocardial Ischemia Detected by ST Monitoring and Angiographic Findings

In a study[76] of 135 patients with unstable angina who underwent 24-hour Holter monitoring (initiated 6.5 hours after onset of chest pain) and subsequently coronary angiography (at a mean of 4 days after admission), 36% were found to have intracoronary thrombus, whereas 66% of patients had Holter-detected transient ST-segment deviation (elevation or depression). Compared with patients without thrombus, the presence of thrombus marked a significantly higher incidence of Holter-detected ST-segment deviation (80% vs. 58%, $P < .025$), longer duration of ST deviation (110 minutes vs. 60 minutes, $P < .05$), and greater number of episodes of ST deviation (6 vs. 4, $P < .01$) over the 24-hour monitoring period. In addition, significantly more patients with Holter-detected ST-segment deviation had left main (18% vs. 4%, $P < .05$) or severe three-vessel CAD (76% vs. 54%, $P < .01$).

Relationship Between Myocardial Ischemia Detected by ST Monitoring and Clinical Outcome

In the era prior to the general use of low-molecular-weight heparin and glycoprotein IIb/IIIa inhibitors, inter-mittent ST-segment deviation (ST elevation or depression detected by continuous ST-segment monitoring) occurred in 50% to 66% of patients with NSTE ACS.[74-75] When accompanied by angina, these symptomatic ischemic episodes were associated with a near tripling of the mortality rate at 1 year.[37] However, symptomatic ischemia in this setting only accounts for less than 10% of all recurrent ischemic episodes as defined by intermittent ST deviation[74-75]; the remaining majority are silent. Even though silent ischemia generally tends to be of shorter duration and is associated with less ST deviation than symptomatic ischemia,[74] it has been correlated with transient abnormalities in myocardial perfusion and function,[12] higher rates of in-hospital adverse events (death, nonfatal MI, or urgent revascularization),[74] and 30-day death,[75] nonfatal MI,[77] and urgent revascularization.[75]

A fundamentally important question is whether continuous ST-segment monitoring (of any kind) provides additional prognostic information to the more conventional means of risk stratification, such as ECG and markers of myocardial injury. Overall, Holter monitoring was more sensitive than the initial ECG in identifying patients with unfavorable hospital outcome.[74] However, this added benefit occurred primarily among those with a normal-appearing baseline ECG, whereas the presence of ST deviation on the baseline ECG attenuated the usefulness of continuous ST monitoring. In another study[80] of 212 patients with unstable angina who underwent continuous ST-segment monitoring 48 hours after admission, both initial ECG ST depression and ST deviation detected by continuous ST monitoring were significant univariate predictors of adverse hospital events (death, nonfatal MI, urgent revascularization). However, ECG ST depression lost, whereas ST deviation maintained, prognostic significance in the multivariate analysis.

The additive prognostic role of continuous ST vector-cardiographic monitoring to that of biochemical markers was further shown in a study of 232 patients with NSTE ACS,[77] in which both cardiac troponin T and ST vector deviation (by 24-hour continuous ST vectorcardio-graphic monitoring) were significant independent predictors of 30-day death or nonfatal MI. By adding ST vector deviation to cardiac troponin T, subgroups of patients at high (presence of both markers), intermediate (presence of either marker), and low (no marker present) risk could be further identified.

In addition, continuous ST-segment monitoring allows examination of the impact of antithrombotic therapy or its withdrawal on ischemia burden among patients with NSTE ACS. During three-lead ST-segment monitoring in the ESSENCE study,[81] enoxaparin treatment delayed time to first ischemic episode whereas its discontinuation was associated with less rebound ischemia compared with unfractionated heparin therapy. Thus, appropriate use of this tool to evaluate ischemia and its response to treatment in both clinical and research settings should further advance our ability to stratify risk and potentially alter prognosis.

The prognostic utility of both Holter monitoring[74-75] and continuous ST vectorcardiography[77] in NSTE ACS have been separately shown. However, few studies have directly compared their predictive performances. An

■■■

TABLE 13–4   UTILITY OF EXERCISE STRESS TESTING IN ACUTE CORONARY SYNDROMES

	OBJECTIVES OF EST	TIMING OF EST	TYPE OF EST	POTENTIAL OUTCOMES
ST elevation	1°: determine prognosis 2°: functional assessment	3-5 days after uncomplicated MI	Symptom-limited	Inducible ST ↓ predicts higher cardiac mortality[87-90]
ST depression and/or T-wave inversion	1°: diagnose CAD : determine prognosis 2°: functional assessment	After 2-3 days of no symptoms	Symptom-limited	Inducible ST ↓ predicts higher rates of death and nonfatal MI[91-94]
Nondiagnostic ST-T changes	1°: diagnose CAD 2°: determine prognosis	After 6-12 hours of no symptoms	Symptom-limited	Inducible ST ↓ predicts higher risk of three-vessel disease[98]

For definition of ST elevation, ST depression and/or T-wave inversion, and nondiagnostic ST-T changes, see Fig. 13–1 legend. 1° denotes primary; 2° denotes secondary. CAD, coronary artery disease; EST, exercise stress test; MI, myocardial infarction.

inherent limitation of these studies relates to the absence of a true gold standard for defining silent ischemia, against which other modalities can be compared. Dellborg et al[79] found that continuous vectorcardiography seemed to be more sensitive than two-channel Holter monitoring in detecting symptomatic ST depression, but it remains difficult to judge their relative abilities in detecting silent ischemia. Other factors that may influence the choice of monitoring modality include such considerations as online versus offline ST-segment analysis and the number of leads available for monitoring: It has been shown that 12-lead recordings had a better sensitivity for detection of ST deviations than 3-lead recordings in patients with unstable angina,[78] possibly related to the nonlocalizable nature of subendocardial ischemia in this population.

Role of Exercise Stress Testing in Patients with Acute Chest Pain and ST Depression, T-Wave Inversion (Without Concomitant ST Elevation), or Both on the Initial ECG

Exercise stress testing is traditionally used to detect significant obstructive CAD among patients with stable patterns of chest pain. The prognostic value of such testing has been well established. Using data from 2842 inpatients with known or suspected CAD who underwent exercise stress test before coronary angiography, Mark et al[84] incorporated markers of exercise capacity (exercise time [minutes]), exercise-induced ischemia (maximal ST deviation [millimeters]), and exercise-induced angina (grade 0 to 2) in a multivariate model to develop and subsequently validate[85] the Duke treadmill score for the prediction of annual mortality rate in patients with stable CAD.

Among patients presenting with NSTE ACS, the primary objectives of exercise stress testing are to confirm the diagnosis of CAD and assess prognosis (Table 13-4). Analogous end points are generally found to be predictive of future cardiac events in this setting as among patients with stable CAD. These end points can be summarized as either the inability to exercise or achievement of low maximal workload or the development of inducible ischemia, especially at low workload (Table 13-5). Indicators of persistently reduced vagal activity after stress testing, manifested as delayed heart rate recovery during the first minute after graded exercise, has

emerged as an independent prognostic indicator[86] of mortality among patients with stable chest pain. This feature, however, has not been formally evaluated among patients with NSTE ACS.

The American College of Cardiology/American Heart Association (ACC/AHA) guidelines for the management of unstable angina and NSTE MI[2] recommend that a low-level exercise stress test may be carried out in low-risk patients who have been asymptomatic for 12 to 24 hours, whereas a symptom-limited test can be conducted in patients without recurrent ischemia at 7 to 10 days. Numerous recent studies consistently demonstrate that it is safe to perform a symptom-limited exercise test as early as after 2[94] to 3 days[91-93] of an event-free observation period among medically stable patients. The precise timing and choice of stress intensity in this patient population will likely continue to vary according to regional practice patterns, but it should be emphasized that a predischarge stress test is still generally preferred over a postdischarge test for risk

■■■

TABLE 13–5   ADVERSE PROGNOSTIC FEATURES IN EXERCISE STRESS TESTING

Exercise-Induced Ischemia

Inducible angina
Inducible ST-segment depression ≥ 1 mm (horizontal or down-sloping), especially at <5 METs
Inducible ST-segment depression ≥ 2 mm (horizontal or down-sloping)
Sustained ST depression > 3 minutes after cessation of exercise

Limited Exercise Capacity

Unable to exercise
Maximal exercise capacity < 6 METs

Hemodynamic Compromise

Failure of SBP to increase by ≥ 10 mmHg; or SBP decrease by ≥ 10 mmHg during exercise
Sustained or symptomatic ventricular tachyarrhythmia

Autonomic Dysfunction or Chronotropic Incompetence

Failure of HR to decrease by more than 12 BPM (from the HR at peak exercise) during the first minute after exercise
Unable to achieve a peak HR > 120 BPM, without the influence of heart rate–slowing agents

HR, heart rate; BPM, beats per minute; METs, metabolic equivalents; SBP, systolic blood pressure.

■ ▪ ■

TABLE 13–6 BASELINE ECG FEATURES CONFOUNDING INTERPRETATION OF ISCHEMIA DURING EXERCISE ECG TESTING

Baseline ECG features that preclude its usefulness in detecting ischemia (alternative imaging modality is essential):
- Complete left bundle branch block
- Pre-excitation syndrome
- Electronically paced or other ventricular rhythm
- Resting ST depression >1 mm

Baseline ECG features that may limit its usefulness in detecting ischemia (alternative imaging modality may be considered but not essential):
- Resting ST depression <1 mm (e.g., digitalis effect, left-ventricular hypertrophy)

stratification: The latter approach fails to predict any recurrent cardiac events that occur early after discharge. Approximately 50% of all events in the first year occur during the first month after discharge.[95]

Patients in whom baseline ECG abnormalities confound ST-segment interpretation (Table 13–6) should undergo exercise stress imaging (myocardial perfusion or echocardiography) whenever possible. Pharmacologic stress should replace exercise stress for those who are unable to exercise. Because none of these modalities is clearly superior to the others, the choice of test in any given institution should depend on availability, local expertise, and cost.

An emerging strategy in the early risk stratification of patients with medically stable unstable angina is the combination of myocardial necrosis markers and ECG indicators of residual myocardial ischemia. Lindahl et al[91] evaluated such a strategy in 766 patients with unstable angina. The strategy combined the predictive utilities of a peak troponin T during first 24 hours of admission and a predischarge symptom-limited bicycle test performed at a median of 5 days after admission. Both measures were shown to be independent predictors of death or nonfatal MI at 5 months. Moreover, the combination approach allowed better risk discrimination than either measure alone. The advantages of this approach are:

- Ability to identify a larger proportion of similarly high-risk patients compared with either measure alone (i.e., 20% risk at 5 months in about one third of all patients)

- Ability to identify a subgroup at extremely low risk (i.e., 1% risk at 5 months) in whom continued medical therapy is most appropriate and avoidance of hospital admission may be feasible

PRESENTATION WITH NONDIAGNOSTIC ST-T CHANGES OR NORMAL-APPEARING INITIAL ECG

Clinical Utility of the Initial and Serial 12-Lead ECGs

Patients in this category are at low risk of MI at presentation (see Table 13–1), and even should MI occur at presentation they tend to have a more favorable short-term outcome than those with more typical ECG changes of AMI.[66] Notwithstanding this low risk profile, however, missed diagnoses of AMI are most likely when the initial ECG either appears normal or is nondiagnostic.[5] Even though about 40% of all patients with AMI have nondiagnostic ST-T changes on their initial ECGs, only 2.1% of all patients with AMI were mistakenly discharged from the emergency department,[5] possibly related to the supplementary use of other noninvasive measures such as biochemical markers of myocardial injury.

There are several possible explanations for the apparent absence of diagnostic ST-T changes among patients with AMI. The well-established phenomenon of an "electrically silent" zone referable to the vascular territory of the LCx artery was described earlier. Furthermore, cancellation of electrical forces due to ischemia in opposite ventricular walls ("balanced ischemia"), a condition that may occur with underlying severe three-vessel or left main CAD, is another possible reason accounting for the absence of ST-T changes despite ongoing myocardial ischemia. It is now clear that coronary artery reperfusion is a dynamic process, with intermittent occlusion and re-opening, thus creating a time-dependent current of injury that may be missed by serial static ECGs. The presence of significant collateral circulation may further attenuate the severity of ischemia and thus the magnitude of ST elevation on the ECG.

In view of the inherent limitations of the standard ECG and the potential consequences of missed diagnoses of AMI, other strategies have been attempted to maximize the sensitivity of MI detection on the initial ECG. Performing serial 12-lead ECGs increases the overall sensitivity of MI detection.[41] In addition, approximately 8% of patients with acute cardiac chest pain and nondiagnostic initial 12-lead ECG display ST elevation only in posterior (V_7 to V_9) or right precordial (V_3R to V_6R) leads.[42] It has been shown that the systematic performance of 15-lead ECG (i.e., standard limb leads, V_1 to V_3, V_4R, V_8 to V_9) increases the probability of detecting ST elevation from 47% to 59% without loss of specificity.[42]

Clinical Utility of Continuous ST-Segment Monitoring

Jernberg et al[82] examined the prognostic role of 12-hour continuous 12-lead ST-segment monitoring in 630 consecutive patients with suspected ACS without diagnostic ST elevation on their initial ECGs, in whom 53% had either nondiagnostic ST-T changes or a normal-appearing initial ECG. Overall, about 16% of patients experienced transient ST deviations, the majority of which (74%) occurred among those with baseline ECG ST-T changes; only 22% of these transient ischemic episodes occurred in patients with nondiagnostic or normal-appearing initial ECG. In a multivariate analysis, however, only elevated baseline troponin T and the presence of ST deviation by continuous monitoring, but not initial ECG ST depression, remained significant independent predictors of 30-day death or nonfatal MI. The addition of ST deviation (by continuous ST monitoring for 6 hours) to troponin T allowed further stratification of patients into high (positive troponin T and ST deviation), intermediate (either positive troponin T or ST deviation), or low (negative troponin T and ST deviation) risk subgroups.[110] Importantly, a more prolonged ST monitoring period of up to 12 hours or an additional troponin T measurement at 12-hours, or both did not significantly add to the prognostic value to the 6-hour evaluation in the low-risk population.

Role of Exercise Stress Testing in Patients with Acute Chest Pain and Nondiagnostic or Normal-Appearing Initial ECG

Not infrequently, the diagnosis of CAD remains questionable among patients in this category even after the initial clinical and laboratory evaluation. In these circumstances, the physician should first address the likelihood of underlying CAD based on the patient's age, gender, and characteristics of chest pain.[1] Patients with known or suspected CAD (moderate to high likelihood) who do not demonstrate any biochemical evidence of myocardial necrosis, recurrent ischemia, or further electrocardiographic evolution are suitable for subsequent exercise stress testing; those who are unlikely to have underlying CAD and continue to be stable during observation may be discharged directly from the emergency room. The primary objective of stress testing in this setting is diagnosing significant CAD. Other practical aspects of stress testing are summarized in Tables 13–4 through 13–6.

In view of the low overall event rate and the established safety of early exercise testing in this clinical setting, the concept of an emergency room–based accelerated risk-stratification strategy utilizing a systematic, protocol-driven approach directed at the early separation of patients into high- and low-risk categories becomes attractive. Several emergency room–based chest pain unit protocols have been reported and are well-summarized elsewhere.[4] Collectively, these units have proved safe, efficient (by allowing earlier identification of low-risk patients for discharge), and cost-effective (by avoiding unnecessary hospitalizations).[100] Another potential advantage of this strategy is improved treatment effectiveness and patient outcomes by virtue of earlier identification of high-risk patients, allowing for more-rapid delivery of proven therapy.

PRESENTATION WITH ST ELEVATION ON THE INITIAL ECG

Clinical Utility of the Initial 12-Lead ECG

Infarct Location and Correlation with the Infarct-Related Artery

Infarct location is traditionally classified according to the presence and location of ST-segment elevation or pathologic Q waves, or both. However, the presence, location, extent, and magnitude of ST deviation in any given region can be influenced by a variety of non–infarct-related factors, thus resulting in the electrocardiographic representation of certain anatomic regions (anterior and inferior walls) better than others (apical, posterior, basal, lateral, and septal regions). For example, ST elevation in V_1 to V_3, frequently known as septal MI, is in fact significantly associated with apical wall-motion abnormalities.[43] Alternatively, the most frequent ECG correlate of septal hypokinesis is ST elevation in V_3 to V_4.[43]

A complete account of the ECG correlates of infarct-related artery (IRA) site and location is beyond the scope of this chapter. However, some of the key observations are highlighted in Table 13–7. An excellent recent review of this topic can be found elsewhere.[3]

Assessment of Prognosis

In the setting of ST-elevation ACS, anterior MI is generally associated with higher mortality rate than inferior MI,

■ ▪ ■

TABLE 13–7 ELECTROCARDIOGRAPHIC PREDICTION OF THE LOCATION AND SITE OF CULPRIT LESION IN ST-ELEVATION MYOCARDIAL INFARCTION

INFARCT LOCATION	CULPRIT VESSEL LOCATION	SITE	SUGGESTIVE ECG FEATURES*
Anterior	LAD	Proximal to D_1	ST↑aVL; ST ↓ III, aVF (3)
		Proximal to S_1	ST ↑ aVR; new RBBB; ST ↓V_5 (3)
	D_1	Proximal	ST ↑ I, aVL, V_2; isoelectric/depressed ST V_4-V_6; ST ↓ II, III, aVF (44)
Inferior	LCx	Proximal	Absence of ST ↓ aVL; ST ↑ aVL (45)
		Any	ST ↑ II > ST ↑ III (3)
		Any	ST ↓ V_1-V_3 (3)
		Any	ST ↓ V_3 / ST ↑ III ratio > 1.2 (46)
	RCA	Proximal	ST ↓ V_3 / ST ↑ III ratio < 0.5 (3)
		Mid	ST ↓ V_3 / ST ↑ III ratio > 0.5 but < 1.2 (46)
		Any	Reciprocal ST ↓ aVL (45)
		Any	ST ↑ III > ST ↑ II (3)

*These features are suggestive but not all-inclusive of ECG changes that may occur in any given myocardial infarction pattern. LAD, left anterior descending; LCx, left circumflex; RCA, right coronary artery; D_1, first diagonal branch; S_1, first septal branch; ST ↑, ST elevation; ST ↓, ST depression. Reference number is given in parentheses.

even when adjusted for infarct size.[6] Acute inferior MI accompanied by right-ventricular involvement,[7] concomitant anterior ST depression (V_1 to V_3),[50] posterior ST elevation (V_7 to V_9),[51] or a combination thereof confers significantly worse in-hospital[7,50-51] and long-term[50] clinical outcomes than uncomplicated inferior MI. Development of either new left (LBBB) or right bundle branch block (RBBB) nearly doubles the in-hospital mortality rate compared with no bundle branch block (BBB) (23% vs. 13%; $P < .001$).[48]

Given the myriad of prognostic information that can be acquired from the initial ECG in patients with ST-elevation ACS, physicians may find it difficult to (1) integrate the various ECG features into a unified approach and (2) combine the prognostic information derived from ECG and clinical variables because there may be significant interaction among these features. Hathaway et al[47] performed an important retrospective analysis aimed at evaluating the independent prognostic value associated with various baseline clinical predictors and initial ECG variables, based on data from 34,166 patients enrolled in the GUSTO-1 trial who presented within 6 hours of pain onset without confounding variables on the initial ECG before fibrinolysis. In this multivariate analysis, which adjusted for other independent clinical predictors, the sum of ST deviation (both elevation or depression; odds ratio, 1.53), heart rate (odds ratio, 1.49), QRS duration (odds ratio, 1.55 for anterior MI, 1.08 for nonanterior MI), and evidence of prior MI during acute inferior MI (odds ratio, 2.47) constituted the strongest independent ECG predictors of 30-day mortality.

---

1. Find Points for Each Risk Marker

Systolic Blood Pressure mm Hg	Points	Pulse bpm	Points	Sum of Absolute ST-Segment Deviation mm	Points	QRS Duration, milliseconds Nonanterior MI	Points	Anterior MI	Points
40	46	40	0	0	0	60	22	60	16
50	40	60	0	10	7	80	23	80	21
60	34	80	6	20	15	100	25	100	26
70	28	100	11	30	19	120	26	120	31
80	23	120	17	40	19	140	27	140	36
90	17	140	23	50	19	160	29	160	41
100	11	160	28	60	19	180	30	180	47
110	6	180	34	70	19	200	32	200	52
120	0	200	40	80	18				
130	0								
140	0								
150	0								
160	0								

Age y	Points	Height cm	Points	Diabetes	Points	Killip class	Points	ECG Prior MI	Points
20	0	140	30	No	0	I	0	Yes	10
30	13	150	27	Yes	6	II	8		
40	25	160	23			III	18	No	
50	38	170	19			IV	30	Inferior Mi	0
60	50	180	15					Noninferior Mi	10
70	62	190	11	Prior					
80	75	200	8	CABG	Points				
90	87	210	4	No	0				
100	100	220	0	Yes	10				

2. Sum Points for All Risk Markers

Systolic Blood Pressure	___
Pulse	___
Sum of Absolute ST Segment Deviation	___
QRS Duration	___
Age	___
Height	___
Diabetes	___
Prior CABG	___
Killip class	___
ECG prior MI	___
Total	___

3. Look up Risk Corresponding to Point Total

Total Points	Probability of 30-Day Mortality
61	0.001
87	0.005
98	0.01
110	0.02
117	0.03
122	0.04
125	0.05
129	0.06
131	0.07
134	0.08
136	0.09
138	0.10
151	0.20
167	0.40
180	0.60
196	0.80

FIGURE 13–4. Nomogram for estimating 30-day mortality from initial clinical and electrocardiographic variables. bpm, beats per minute; CABG, coronary artery bypass graft; ECG, electrocardiogram; MI, myocardial infarction. (From Hathaway WR, Peterson ED, Wagner GS, et al: Prognostic significance of the initial electrocardiogram in patients with acute myocardial infarction. The GUSTO-1 Investigators. JAMA 279:387–391, 1998. Copyright 1998, American Medical Association.)

A nomogram derived from this multivariate model provided excellent discrimination of 30-day mortality (C-index, 0.83) and is shown in Figure 13–4. Of interest, the number of leads with ST elevation, new right bundle branch block, or left anterior or posterior hemiblock were significant univariate, but not multivariate, predictors. Also, the prognostic value of ischemia grade on the initial ECG was not evaluated in this model. Nevertheless, this simple tool should greatly assist physicians in more accurately predicting 30-day mortality.

Therapeutic Decision Regarding Prehospitalization Fibrinolysis

Reduction in the time to reperfusion may have major impact on patient outcome after AMI. In this light, an ECG recorded during the prehospital phase offers several potential advantages

- Earlier diagnosis of AMI
- Appropriate triage to institution best suited to the needs of any given patient
- Potential to trigger a more rapid in-hospital response by minimizing the "door-to-needle" or "door-to-balloon" time
- Facilitation of appropriate prehospital administration of a fibrinolytic agent

Prehospital ECG has therefore been promoted as a means of minimizing total time from symptom onset to initiation of reperfusion therapy.

The feasibility of prehospital ECG recording and transmission by trained personnel was established by various groups in the early 1990s. A systematic review of eight controlled studies of prehospital 12-lead ECG recording among patients with AMI showed a consistent reduction (by 10 to 30 minutes) in the door-to-needle time.[52] The total time from symptom onset to fibrinolysis can be further shortened by prehospital initiation of fibrinolytic therapy, as shown in another meta-analysis of six randomized controlled trials.[53] Compared with in-hospital fibrinolysis, prehospital fibrinolysis resulted in an average reduction of time to fibrinolysis by 58 minutes (range, 30 to 130 minutes). This translates into a 17% relative reduction in hospital mortality, or an absolute gain of 16 lives per thousand patients treated for each hour saved by prehospital initiation of fibrinolytic therapy.

Clinical Utility of Serial 12-Lead ECGs

Assessment of the Patency of the Infarct-Related Artery After Fibrinolysis

Perhaps one of the most important chapters in modern clinical electrocardiography relates to the recognition of the utility of serial ECGs as bedside marker of reperfusion. During acute ischemia, the ST segment becomes elevated because of the loss of resting membrane potential and shortening of the plateau phase (phase 2) of the action potential in the ischemic myocardium. Both changes are mediated by an increase in extracellular potassium concentration. Successful reperfusion allows for rapid washout of tissue potassium; therefore, rapid resolution of ST elevation following fibrinolysis has been proposed as a marker of reperfusion. Its clinical significance is underscored by the need for timely decisions about appropriate rescue mechanical reperfusion therapy in order to improve patient outcome.

In the TIMI-14 study,[54] angiographic patency rates (assessed by extent of ST-segment resolution) were as follows:

- TIMI 2/3 flow: complete (>70%), 94%; partial (30% to 69%), 72%; no ST resolution (<30%), 68%; $P < .0001$
- TIMI 3 flow: complete, 79%; partial, 50%; no ST resolution, 44%; $P < .0001$

In general, the high prevalence of IRA patency associated with modern pharmacologic reperfusion regimens[54-56] results in high positive predictive values (80% to 95%), despite the relatively low specificities (40% to 80%) of ST-segment resolution for predicting vessel patency.

Table 13–8 illustrates the impact of various ST-segment resolution thresholds (i.e., 30% vs. 50% vs. 70%) and angiographic patency definition (i.e., TIMI 2/3 vs. TIMI 3 flow) on the diagnostic performances of a widely accepted ST-resolution algorithm (Schröder et al[57]: complete ST resolution, >70%; partial resolution, 30% to 69%; no resolution, <30%). Noteworthy is that although most patients who experienced complete ST-segment resolution following fibrinolysis also had TIMI 3 flow, the reverse was not true. The clinical significance of this observation is discussed later in the discussion of ECG assessment of myocardial reperfusion.

Because complete ST-segment resolution after fibrinolysis significantly predicts IRA patency, it can be

■ ▩ ■

TABLE 13–8   OPERATING CHARACTERISTICS OF ST-SEGMENT RESOLUTION FOR PATENCY ASSESSMENT AS A FUNCTION OF DEGREE OF RESOLUTION AND TIMI FLOW

THRESHOLD	SENSITIVITY	SPECIFICITY	PPV	NPV
TIMI-2 or -3 flow at 90 minutes				
ST resolution ≥ 70%	54%	85%	94%	30%
ST resolution ≥ 50%	69%	67%	90%	33%
ST resolution ≥ 30%	78%	45%	86%	32%
TIMI-3 flow at 90 minutes				
ST resolution ≥ 70%	59%	74%	79%	53%
ST resolution ≥ 50%	71%	54%	72%	54%
ST resolution ≥ 30%	81%	39%	68%	56%

NPV, negative predictive value; PPV, positive predictive value.
From de Lemos JA, et al: ST-segment resolution and infarct-related artery patency and flow after thrombolytic therapy. Am J Cardiol 85: 299–304, 2000.

expected that the degree of ST-segment resolution also carries prognostically useful information. Indeed, a mortality gradient over both the short and the long term among AMI survivors, inversely related to the extent of ST-segment resolution up to 24 hours following fibrinolysis, has been consistently observed in several large fibrinolytic trials (Table 13–9).[54-55,57-59] Adding to these observations, the Assessment of the Safety and Efficacy of a New Thrombolytic (ASSENT)-2 ECG substudies[21,59-60] provide further insights into the time dependence of the prognostic value associated with different degrees of ST-segment resolution. Among 13,100 patients presenting with AMI within 6 hours of symptom onset who were free from any confounders on the initial ECG or in-hospital re-infarction,[59] the proportion of patients who experienced complete (>70%) ST-segment resolution 24 to 36 hours following fibrinolysis was highest if they presented within 2 hours of onset (55.6% vs. 43% among those who presented 4 to 6 hours of onset) (Fig. 13–5A). Importantly, even among the 51% of patients who ultimately experienced complete ST-segment resolution, a gradient of risk existed such that the time to treatment was positively related to 1-year mortality rates (time to treatment < 2 hours, 3.8%; 2 to 4 hours, 5.2%; 4 to 6 hours, 6.5%; $P < .002$) (Fig. 13–5B).

The current understanding of the prognostic significance of new pathologic Q waves after acute MI is still evolving. Early studies were generally small and have adopted heterogeneous Q-wave definitions and timings of ascertainment. In the more recent GUSTO-1 angiographic substudy,[20] lack of Q-wave formation 24 hours following fibrinolytic therapy, when compared with Q-wave MI, was more likely to be associated with early, complete, and sustained IRA patency (typically in a distal location of a non–left anterior descending (LAD) coronary artery), with resultant limitation of myocardial territory at risk (i.e., lesser ST-segment elevation or nonanterior location, or both), better global and regional left-ventricular function, and improved short-term (in-hospital) and long-term (2-year) survival. Adding to this observation, the ASSENT-2 investigators[21] showed that the extent of ST-segment resolution 24 to 36 hours following fibrinolysis remained predictive of 1-year mortality, irrespective of the presence or absence of new pathologic Q-wave formation. Furthermore, by comparing ECGs obtained 24 to 36 hours after fibrinolysis and at discharge, patients with no Q-wave formation or Q-wave regression experienced better 1-year survival than those with either delayed Q-wave formation or persistent Q wave after 36 hours.[60]

Aside from the utility of the ST segment and Q wave, data from the GUSTO-1 angiographic substudy[61] suggested that an inverted T wave in the infarct zone found at a median of 8 days following fibrinolysis was an independent negative predictor of 30-day mortality (adjusted odds ratio, 0.38; 95% CI, 0.18 to 0.78), although its presence did not significantly predict IRA patency (TIMI 3 flow). Because T-wave inversion is a common evolutionary ECG feature during and after ST-segment resolution post AMI, it remains to be seen whether this feature provides additional prognostic value to that of ST-segment resolution in future studies.

Assessment of Myocardial Reperfusion

Contemporary regimens of fibrinolytic therapy, on average, resulted in a 60% TIMI 3 flow rate or 80% TIMI 2/3 flow rate among patients presenting with ST-elevation ACS. In contrast, the prevalence of complete ST-segment resolution post fibrinolysis was substantially lower, averaging 47% to <70% (see Table 13–8). This mismatch between angiographic patency and ST-segment resolution is reminiscent of the discrepancy between epicardial and microvascular flow, in which 16% to 23% of

■ ▪ ■

TABLE 13–9   PROGNOSTIC VALUE OF ST-SEGMENT RESOLUTION ON SERIAL ECGS FOLLOWING FIBRINOLYSIS

STUDY	N	NO. ECGS, TIME APART	CALCULATION OF ST-SEGMENT DEVIATION	DEFINITION OF ST RESOLUTION (% OF TOTAL POPULATION)	MORTALITY	
					30-Day	
TIMI-14[54]	444	2, 90 minutes	Schröder's method*	ST resolution ≥ 70% (47%) ST resolution 30–69% (27%) ST resolution < 30% (27%)	0.6% 2.1% 3.8%	
					35-Day	
INJECT[57]	1398	2, 180 minutes	Schröder's method	ST resolution ≥ 70% (49%) ST resolution 30–69% (30%) ST resolution < 30% (21%)	2.5% 4.3% 17.5%	
					30-Day	**1-Year**
ASSENT-2[59]	13,100	2, 24 hours	Schröder's method	ST resolution ≥ 70% (51%) ST resolution 30–69% (35%) ST resolution < 30% (14%)	2.5% 4.1% 6.3%	5.1% 8.0% 9.7%
					30-Day	**6-Month**
GISSI-2[58]	7426	2, 4 hours	ΣST ↑ all leads	ST resolution ≥ 50% (67%) ST resolution < 50% (33%)	3.5% 5.7%	7.4% 9.9%

*Schröder's criteria (Ref. 57): Anterior MI: $\Sigma ST\uparrow V_1-V_6$, I, aVL + $\Sigma ST\downarrow$ II, III, aVF; Inferior MI: $\Sigma ST\uparrow$ II, III, aVF (I, aVL, V_5, V_6 if present) + $\Sigma ST\downarrow V_1-V_4$.

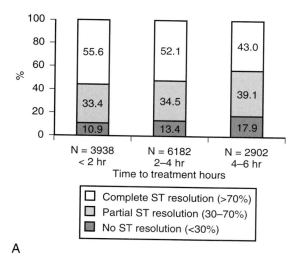

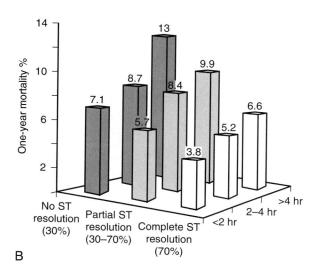

FIGURE 13–5. *A,* Distribution of ST-segment resolution according to time to fibrinolytic therapy. *B,* One-year mortality rate by degree of ST-segment resolution and time from symptom onset to fibrinolytic therapy. (Reprinted from Fu Y, Goodman SG, Chang WC, et al: Time to treatment influences the impact of ST segment resolution on one-year prognosis: Insights from the ASSENT-2 trial. Circulation 104:2653–2659, 2001. Copyright 2001, Lippincott Williams & Wilkins.)

patients developed microvascular no reflow (by myocardial contrast echocardiography) following successful coronary reperfusion (TIMI 3 flow) by either primary angioplasty[8] or intracoronary fibrinolysis[9] within 12 hours of onset of a first anterior AMI. Furthermore, using the angiographic blush to grade myocardial perfusion, Gibson et al[10] demonstrated a mortality gradient across a spectrum of myocardial perfusion grades that is independent of flow in the epicardial IRA. In particular, absence of myocardial perfusion (i.e., microvascular lack of reflow) following fibrinolysis was related to a higher mortality despite normal epicardial (TIMI 3) flow.

This epicardial-microvascular flow discordance mirrors that between ST-segment resolution and epicardial flow, thus setting the stage for exploring the relationship between ST-segment resolution and microvascular integrity after epicardial vessel patency has been

achieved. Thirty-seven patients with AMI underwent myocardial contrast echocardiography before and immediately after successful primary angioplasty to TIMI-3 flow in a prospective study.[62] Eleven patients (30%) experienced no reflow by myocardial contrast echocardiography. Using a 50% cutoff point for ST-segment resolution, ST-segment resolution was complete in 77% of those who experienced reflow but in only 9% of those with no reflow (*P* = .0002): ST resolution represented a highly specific (91%) predictive instrument with a reasonable sensitivity (77%) and an overall diagnostic accuracy of 81%.

Clinical Utility of Continuous ST-Segment Monitoring

Coronary artery reperfusion in the early phase of MI was often unstable and was characterized by intermittent ST reelevation in approximately one third of patients with AMI following successful fibrinolysis. Thus, the conventional approach of comparing serial static ECGs may only capture a snapshot, rather than the entire process, of reperfusion. In contrast, continuous ST-segment monitoring can provide a graphical representation of the entire process of reperfusion, characterized by the occurrence, speed, and stability of reperfusion during and following the administration of fibrinolytic therapy. This potentially allows more accurate bedside assessment of IRA patency and detection of silent ischemia and re-occlusion following initial successful reperfusion.

Assessment of IRA Patency

The GUSTO-1 ECG ischemia monitoring substudy[69] provided the largest prospective head-to-head comparison among the three available ST-monitoring techniques. In this study, 302 patients underwent one of three methods of continuous ST-segment monitoring for more than 18 hours from the start of fibrinolytic therapy and angiographic patency (TIMI 2/3 flow) assessment at either 90 or 180 minutes following fibrinolytic therapy. All three methods showed remarkably similar overall accuracy in detecting coronary reperfusion (68% to 71%), with some variation in relation to patency predictive value (vector vs. 12-lead vs. Holter: 76% vs. 74% vs. 67%) and occlusion predictive value (vector vs. 12-lead vs. Holter: 52% vs. 63% vs. 71%).

A more fundamental question directly relevant to our daily practice is whether continuous ST-segment monitoring (of any kind) provides more accurate assessment of IRA patency than serial ECGs. In the TAMI-7 study,[71] continuous 12-lead ST-segment monitoring was compared against five serial static ECG methods for their ability to predict IRA patency in 82 patients with AMI who underwent angiography at a median of 124 minutes after initiation of fibrinolytic therapy. At the time of angiography, the best static ECG method (sensitivity for reperfusion, 93%; specificity, 60%; accuracy, 83%) and continuous ST monitoring (sensitivity, 93%; specificity, 64%; accuracy, 85%) had almost identical predictive performances and as high as 90% agreement in patency assessment.

Evaluation of Recurrent Ischemia After Initial Reperfusion

Using Holter ST-segment monitoring on either day 4 or day 7 after fibrinolytic therapy for AMI, 32% of patients were found to have transient ST depression, a marker of higher-grade IRA luminal stenosis; less recovery of left-ventricular function at discharge; and higher rates of death and re-infarction at 18 months compared with those without ST depression during Holter monitoring.[72] This finding was corroborated by results from the GUSTO-1 ST-segment monitoring substudy,[73] which found a strikingly similar 33% incidence of new ST-segment shift (ST depression in 38%, ST elevation in remaining 62%) by continuous ST-segment monitoring initiated 6 to 24 hours after fibrinolytic therapy. In addition, both presence and duration of ST-segment shift significantly predicted higher 1-year mortality rates.

Role of Exercise Stress Testing After ST Elevation Acute Coronary Syndrome

The primary objectives, patient eligibility, and interpretation of exercise stress testing in this setting are similar to that in NSTE ACS and are summarized in Tables 13–4 through 13–6. Major secondary objectives after MI include the provision of functional data important for activity counseling, exercise prescription as part of formal cardiac rehabilitation, and evaluation of symptomatic response to pharmacologic or revascularization measures.

The ACC/AHA guidelines on exercise stress testing[1] recommend submaximal testing at 4 to 7 days; if results are negative, this test should be followed by a symptom-limited stress test at 3 to 6 weeks. Alternatively, symptom-limited stress testing may be conducted earlier, i.e., prior to or soon after discharge. A negative stress test result identifies patients at very low risk for a cardiac event in the next year, whereas the presence of exercise-induced ST depression increases the risk of cardiac mortality post MI, irrespective of the use of fibrinolytic therapy.[87-90] Both predischarge submaximal and postdischarge symptom-limited stress testing have been shown to be safe in both the prethrombolytic and the thrombolytic era.[1] Because more than 50% of fatal cardiac events in the first year following AMI occur within the first month after discharge, a predischarge stress test is desirable and should be incorporated into routine management.

Because of concern about patient safety, exercise stress testing is generally avoided during the first 3 days of an uncomplicated AMI.[1] This view had been challenged as early as in the 1980s. Topol et al[88] randomized 80 patients following an uncomplicated reperfused AMI to either an early exercise thallium test on day 3 or conventional risk stratification on days 7 to 10. Early stress testing was not complicated by any major cardiac event. At 6 months of follow-up, no deaths occurred and both groups had similar reinfarction rates. Of note, a substantial proportion of enrolled patients have undergone primary or rescue angioplasty during the acute phase of MI, and thus the generalizability of this study result to patients who received fibrinolytic therapy alone can be questioned. A more recent observational study examined the short- and long-term safety of early symptom-limited exercise stress testing after an uncomplicated AMI.[89] At the discretion of the attending physicians, 216 patients (most patients received fibrinolytic therapy alone) were selected to undergo predischarge stress testing using the Bruce protocol on day 3 following AMI; 74% were discharged within 1 day of the stress test. No fatal or major nonfatal cardiac complication resulted from the early stress testing. At 1 year of follow-up, patients who underwent early stress testing continued to have a low mortality rate (4%). These safety data on early stress testing should stimulate the systematic implementation of an early discharge policy among carefully selected patients with uncomplicated AMI.

A PERSPECTIVE ON THE COMBINED USE OF DIFFERENT ELECTROCARDIOGRAPHIC MODALITIES IN ACUTE CORONARY SYNDROMES—PRESENT AND FUTURE

At present, the initial ECG plays a central role in the initial evaluation of ACS. It allows instant risk stratification and thereby expedites delivery of optimal treatment, appropriate intensity of monitoring during observation, and predischarge work-up (Fig. 13–6). In addition to the electrocardiographic recognition of *magnitude, distribution,* and *resolution* of ST shift and their quantitative relation with such factors as time to treatment, before/after treatment, and nature of treatment, the initial ECG further enhances a physician's ability to stratify risk, select therapy, and assess treatment response across the entire ACS spectrum. Continuous ST-segment monitoring adds the extra dimensions of *frequency* and *duration* to the process of ischemia detection across the entire ACS spectrum, thereby providing additive prognostic information to that of ECG and cardiac markers. Exercise stress testing is safe, efficient, and cost-effective and remains the cornerstone of predischarge risk stratification among patients with medically stabilized ACS.

In the coming years, early and continuous risk stratification will be key emphases in the overall management of patients with ACS. This process can be expected to begin very early during the hospital course, or even before hospital arrival, via routine prehospital computerized ECG transmission. Incorporation of quantitative ST-segment data obtained both on admission and during hospitalization into clinical risk scores should refine our ability to stratify risk and select appropriate treatment strategies across the entire ACS spectrum. An ongoing challenge for the practicing physician is to effectively integrate the myriad of invasive and noninvasive prognostic information emerging at different stages of evaluation into the master care plan.

The limited sensitivity in AMI detection remains the Achilles heel of the standard 12-lead ECG. Potential strategies to circumvent this shortcoming include:

- Simple but reliable measures to optimize the capability of existing ECG technique; for example, the routine per-

PARADIGM FOR ELECTROCARDIOGRAPHIC ASSESSMENT IN ACUTE CORONARY SYNDROMES

Initial ECG	Admission (Emergency room or hospital unit)	Observation (Emergency room or hospital unit)	Discharge
ST elevation	Comparing the initial ECG against repeat ECG 60–90 minutes following fibrinolysis allows: • Assessment of IRA patency status • Assessment of myocardial perfusion status • Assessment of prognosis	Ascertainment of pathologic Q wave(s) at 24-36 hours has additional prognostic value Repeat ECG(s) with recurrent symptom Consider continuous ST-segment monitoring following fibrinolysis for at least 24 hours: • Detection of transient (both silent or symptomatic) ST-segment deviation	Ascertainment of pathologic Q wave(s) at discharge allows assessment of Q wave evolution which provides incremental prognostic information Pre-discharge symptom-limited exercise stress test: • Day 3-5 after uncomplicated MI • Use pharmacologic stress or imaging studies as indicated
ST depression and/or T wave inversion	Initial ECG provides short- and long-term prognostic information based on: • Presence of ST depression or T wave inversion • Extent and magnitude of ST depression	Repeat ECG(s) with recurrent symptom Consider continuous ST-segment monitoring for at least 24 hours: • Detection of transient (both silent or symptomatic) ST-segment deviation	Evaluation of ST segment status at discharge allows assessment of ST segment evolution which may be prognostically important Pre-discharge symptom-limited exercise stress test: • After 2-3 days of symptom-free period
Non-diagnostic ST/T or normal	Initial ECG non-diagnostic 15-lead ECG (including posterior and right precordial leads) should be performed to rule out isolated posterior or right ventricular MI	At least one follow-up ECG within 1 hour Repeat ECG(s) with recurrent symptom Role of continuous ST-segment monitoring in this low-risk setting is less well established.	Pre-discharge symptom-limited exercise stress test should be performed after 6-12 hours of symptom-free period among patients at moderate to high risk of underlying coronary artery disease Patients who remained stable after 6-12 hours of observation and are deemed to be at low risk of underlying coronary artery disease may be directly discharged

FIGURE 13–6. Paradigm for electrocardiographic assessment in acute coronary syndromes. MI, myocardial infarction.

formance of right precordial or posterior chest leads or simply obtaining serial or previous ECGs for comparison

• Efforts to integrate such features as high resolution, additional leads, and three-dimensional vectorcardiography into computerized algorithms to improve the intrinsic diagnostic capability of the surface ECG
• Efforts to supplement the ECG with other highly sensitive markers of injury, such as myoglobin, CK MB isoforms, and cardiac troponins to optimize the overall accuracy in the diagnosis of AMI

Ultimately, enhanced understanding of the pathophysiology of ACS as well as its electrocardiographic manifestations may improve our ability to recognize, evaluate, and stratify risk, thus favorably altering the clinical course of patients presenting with ACS.

REFERENCES

1. Gibbons RJ, Balady GJ, Beasley JW, et al: ACC/AHA guidelines for exercise testing: A report of the American College of Cardiology/American Heart Association Task Force on Practice Guidelines (Committee on Exercise Testing). J Am Coll Cardiol 1997;30: 260–315.
2. Braunwald E, Antman EM, Beasley JW, et al: ACC/AHA guidelines for the management of patients with unstable angina and non-ST-segment elevation myocardial infarction: A report of the American College of Cardiology/American Heart Association Task Force on Practice Guidelines (Committee on the Management of Patients With Unstable Angina). J Am Coll Cardiol 2000;36:970–1062.
3. Sgarbossa EB, Birnbaum Y, Parrillo JE: Electrocardiographic diagnosis of acute myocardial infarction: Current concepts for the clinician. Am Heart J 2001;141:507–517.
4. Storrow AB, Gibler WB: Chest pain centers: Diagnosis of acute coronary syndromes. Ann Emerg Med 35:449–461, 2000.

5. Pope JH, Aufderheide TP, Ruthazer R, et al: Missed diagnoses of acute cardiac ischemia in the emergency department. N Engl J Med 2000;342:1163–1170.

6. Lee KL, Woodlief LH, Topol EJ, et al: Predictors of 30-day mortality in the era of reperfusion for acute myocardial infarction. Results from an international trial of 41,021 patients. GUSTO-1 Investigators. Circulation 1995;91:1659–1668.

7. Zehender M, Kasper W, Kauder E, et al: Right ventricular infarction as an independent predictor of prognosis after acute inferior myocardial infarction. N Engl J Med 1993;328:981–988.

8. Ito H, Okamura A, Iwakura K, et al: Myocardial perfusion patterns related to thrombolysis in myocardial infarction perfusion grades after coronary angioplasty in patients with acute anterior wall myocardial infarction. Circulation 1996;93:1993–1999.

9. Ito H, Tomooka T, Sakai N, et al: Lack of myocardial perfusion immediately after successful thrombolysis. A predictor of poor recovery of left ventricular function in anterior myocardial infarction. Circulation 1992;85:1699–1705.

10. Gibson CM, Cannon CP, Murphy SA, et al: Relationship of TIMI myocardial perfusion grade to mortality after administration of thrombolytic drugs. Circulation 2000;101:125–130.

11. Chierchia S, Lazzari M, Freedman B, et al: Impairment of myocardial perfusion and function during painless myocardial ischemia. J Am Coll Cardiol 1983;1:924–930.

12. Goldman L, Cook EF, Johnson PA, et al: Prediction of the need for intensive care in patients who come to emergency departments with acute chest pain. N Engl J Med 1996;334:1498–1504.

13. Savonitto S, Ardissino D, Granger CB, et al: Prognostic significance of the admission electrocardiogram in acute coronary syndromes. JAMA 1999;281:707–713.

14. Nyman I, Areskog M, Areskog NH, et al: Very early risk stratification by electrocardiogram at rest in men with suspected unstable coronary heart disease. J Intern Med 1993;234:293–301.

15. Cannon CP, McCabe CH, Stone PH, et al: The electrocardiogram predicts one-year outcome of patients with unstable angina and non-Q-wave myocardial infarction: Results of the TIMI III registry ECG ancillary study. J Am Coll Cardiol 1997;30:133–140.

16. Hyde TA, French JK, Wong CK, et al: Four-year survival of patients with acute coronary syndromes without ST segment elevation and prognostic significance of 0.5-mm ST segment depression. Am J Cardiol 1999;84:379–385.

17. Lee HS, Cross SJ, Rawles JM, et al: Patients with suspected myocardial infarction who present with ST depression. Lancet 1993;342:1204–1207.

18. Kaul P, Fu Y, Chang WC, et al: Prognostic value of ST-segment depression in acute coronary syndromes: Insights from PARAGON-A applied to GUSTO-IIb. J Am Coll Cardiol 2001;38:64–71.

19. Fesmire FM, Percy RF, Wears RL, et al: Initial ECG in Q wave and non-Q wave myocardial infarction. Ann Emerg Med 1989;18:741–746.

20. Goodman SG, Langer A, Ross AM, et al: Non-Q-wave versus Q-wave myocardial infarction after thrombolytic therapy: Angiographic and prognostic insights from the global utilization of streptokinase and tissue plasminogen activator for occluded coronary arteries-I angiographic substudy. GUSTO-I Angiographic Investigators. Circulation 1998;97:444–450.

21. Lockwood E, Fu Y, Wong B, et al: Does 24-hour ST segment resolution post-fibrinolysis add prognostic value to a Q wave? ASSENT-2 electrocardiographic sub-study. Can J Cardiol 2001;17(Suppl C):A318.

22. Papapietro SE, Niess GS, Paine TD, et al: Transient electrocardiographic changes in patients with unstable angina: relation to coronary artery anatomy. Am J Cardiol 1980;46:28–33.

23. Cohen M, Scharpf SJ, Rentrop KP: Prospective analysis of electrocardiographic variables as markers for extent and location of acute wall motion abnormalities observed during coronary angioplasty in human subjects. J Am Coll Cardiol 1987;10:17–24.

24. Califf RM, Phillips III HR, Hindman MC, et al: Prognostic value of a coronary artery jeopardy score. J Am Coll Cardiol 1985;5:1055–1063.

25. Cohen M, Hawkins L, Greenberg S, Fuster V: Usefulness of ST-segment changes in > 2 leads on the emergency room electrocardiogram in either unstable angina pectoris or non-Q-wave myocardial infarction in predicting outcome. Am J Cardiol 1991;67:1368–1367.

26. de Zwaan C, Bär FWHM, Wellens HJJ: Characteristic electrocardiographic pattern indicating a critical stenosis high in left anterior descending coronary artery in patients admitted because of impending myocardial infarction. Am Heart J 1982;103:730–736.

27. Diderholm E, Andrén B, Frostfeldt G, et al: ST depression in ECG at entry indicates severe coronary lesions and large benefits of an early invasive treatment strategy in unstable coronary artery disease. The FRISC II ECG substudy. Eur Heart J 2002;23:41–49.

28. Antman EM, Cohen M, Bernink PJ, et al: The TIMI risk score for unstable angina/non-ST elevation MI: A method for prognostication and therapeutic decision making. JAMA 2000;284:835–842.

29. Boersma E, Pieper KS, Steyerberg EW, et al: Predictors of outcome in patients with acute coronary syndromes without persistent ST-segment elevation. Results from an international trial of 9461 patients. Circulation 2000;101:2557–2567.

30. de Zwaan C, Bär FW, Janssen JHA, et al: Angiographic and clinical characteristics of patients with unstable angina showing an ECG pattern indicating critical narrowing of the proximal LAD coronary artery. Am Heart J 1989;117:657–665.

31. Gazes PC, Mobley EM, Faris HM, et al: Preinfarctional (unstable) angina—a prospective study—ten year follow-up. Circulation 1973;48:331–337.

32. Demoulin TC, Bertholet M, Chevigne M, et al: Prognostic significance of electrocardiographic findings in angina at rest: Therapeutic implications. Br Heart J 1981;46:320–324.

33. Olson HG, Lyons KP, Aronow WS, et al: The high-risk angina patient: identification by clinical features, hospital course, electrocardiography and technetium-99m stannous pyrophosphate scintigraphy. Circulation 1981;64:674–684.

34. De Servi S, Berzuini C, Poma E, et al: Long-term survival and risk stratification in patients with angina at rest undergoing medical treatment. Int J Cardiol 1989;22:43–50.

35. Severi S, Orsini E, Marraccini P, et al: The basal electrocardiogram and the exercise stress test in assessing prognosis in patients with unstable angina. Eur Heart J 1988;9:441–446.

36. Rizik DG, Healy S, Margulis A, et al: A new clinical classification for hospital prognosis of unstable angina pectoris. Am J Cardiol 1995;75:993–997.

37. Armstrong PW, Fu Y, Chang WC, et al: Acute coronary syndromes in the GUSTO-IIb trial. Prognostic insights and impact of recurrent ischemia. Circulation 1998;98:1860–1868.

38. Goodman SG, Bozovich G, Tan M, et al: The greatest benefit of enoxaparin (low molecular weight heparin) over unfractionated heparin in acute coronary syndromes is achieved in patients presenting with ST segment depression. Circulation 2001;104:A2598.

39. Sabatine MS, Morrow DA, Giugliano RP, et al: Implications of upstream GP IIb/IIIa inhibition and stenting in the invasive management of UA/NSTEMI: A comparison of TIMI IIIB and TACTICS-TIMI 18. Circulation 2001;104:A2595.

40. Lagerqvist B, Diderholm E, Lindahl B, Wallentin L: High risk score predicts bad outcome in patients with unstable coronary artery disease: FRISC II sub-study. Circulation 2001;104:A3065.

41. Gibler WB, Sayre MR, Levy RC, et al: Serial 12-lead electrocardiographic monitoring in patients presenting to the emergency department with chest pain. J Electrocardiol 1993;26(Suppl):238–243.

42. Zalenski RI, Rydman RI, Sloan EP, et al: Value of posterior and right ventricular leads in comparison to the standard 12-lead electrocardiogram in evaluation of ST-segment elevation in suspected acute myocardial infarction. Am J Cardiol 1997;79:1579–1585.

43. Shalev Y, Fogelman R, Oettinger M, et al: Does the electrocardiographic pattern of "anteroseptal" myocardial infarction correlate with the anatomic location of myocardial injury? Am J Cardiol 1995;75:763–766.

44. Sclarovsky S, Birnbaum Y, Solodky A, et al: Isolated midanterior myocardial infarction: A special electrocardiographic sub-type of acute myocardial infarction consisting of ST elevation in nonconsecutive leads and two different morphologic types of ST depression. Int J Cardiol 1994;46:37–47.

45. Hasdai D, Birnbaum Y, Herz I, et al: ST segment depression in lateral limb leads in inferior wall acute myocardial infarction: Implications regarding the culprit artery and the site of obstruction. Eur Heart J 1995;16:1549–1553.

46. Kosuge M, Kimura K, Ishikawa T, et al: New electrocardiographic criteria for predicting the site of coronary artery occlusion in infe-

rior wall acute myocardial infarction. Am J Cardiol 1998;82: 1318-1322.

47. Hathaway WR, Peterson ED, Wagner GS, et al: Prognostic significance of the initial electrocardiogram in patients with acute myocardial infarction. The GUSTO-1 Investigators. JAMA 1998;279:387-391.

48. Go AS, Barron HV, Rundle AC, et al: Bundle-branch block and in-hospital mortality in acute myocardial infarction. National Registry of Myocardial Infarction 2 Investigators. Ann Intern Med 1998;129:690-697.

49. Hasdai D, Sclarovsky S, Solodky A, et al: Prognostic significance of the initial electrocardiographic pattern in patients with inferior wall acute myocardial infarction. Clin Cardiol 1996;19:31-36.

50. Peterson ED, Hathaway WR, Zabel KM, et al: Prognostic significance of precordial ST segment depression during inferior myocardial infarction in the thrombolytic era: Results in 16,521 patients. J Am Coll Cardiol 1996;28:305-312.

51. Matetzky S, Freimark D, Chouraqui P, et al: Significance of ST segment elevations in posterior chest leads (V7-V9) in patients with acute inferior myocardial infarction: Application for thrombolytic therapy. J Am Coll Cardiol 1998;31:506-511.

52. Brown SGA, Galloway DM: Effect of ambulance 12-lead ECG recording on times to hospital reperfusion in acute myocardial infarction. MJA 2000;172:81-84.

53. Morrison LJ, Verbeek PR, McDonald AC, et al: Mortality and prehospital thrombolysis for acute myocardial infarction. JAMA 2000;283:2686-2692.

54. de Lemos JA, Antman EM, Giugliano RP, et al: ST-segment resolution and infarct-related artery patency and flow after thrombolytic therapy. Am J Cardiol 2000;85:299-304.

55. Barbash GI, Roth A, Hod H, et al: Rapid resolution of ST elevation and prediction of clinical outcome in patients undergoing thrombolysis with alteplase (recombinant tissue-type plasminogen activator): Results of the Israeli Study of Early Intervention in Myocardial Infarction. Br Heart J 1990;64:241-247.

56. Clemmensen P, Ohman M, Sevilla DC, et al: Changes in standard electrocardiographic ST-segment elevation predictive of successful reperfusion in acute myocardial infarction. Am J Cardiol 1990;66:1407-1411.

57. Schröder R, Wegscheider K, Schröder K, et al: Extent of early ST segment elevation resolution: A strong predictor of outcome in patients with acute myocardial infarction and a sensitive measure to compare thrombolytic regimens. J Am Coll Cardiol 1995;26:1657-1664.

58. Mauri F, Maggioni AP, Franzosi MG, et al: A simple electrocardiographic predictor of the outcome of patients with acute myocardial infarction treated with a thrombolytic agent. A Gruppo Italiano per lo Studio della Sopravvivenza nell'Infarto Miocardico (GISSI-2)-Derived analysis. J Am Coll Cardiol 1994;24:600-607.

59. Fu Y, Goodman SG, Chang WC, et al: Time to treatment influences the impact of ST segment resolution on one-year prognosis: Insights from the ASSENT-2 trial. Circulation 2001;104:2653-2659.

60. Fu Y, Goodman SG, Chang WC, et al: Incidence and prognosis of non-Q-wave MI in the thrombolytic era: Insights from ASSENT-2 study. J Am Coll Cardiol 2000;35(Suppl A):390A.

61. Sgarbossa EB, Meyer PM, Pinski SL, et al: Negative T waves shortly after ST-elevation acute myocardial infarction are a powerful marker for improved survival rate. Am Heart J 2000;140:385-394.

62. Santoro GM, Valenti R, Buonamici P, et al: Relation between ST-segment changes and myocardial perfusion evaluated by myocardial contrast echocardiography in patients with acute myocardial infarction treated with direct angioplasty. Am J Cardiol 1998;82:932-937.

63. Haines DE, Raabe DS, Gundel WD, et al: Anatomic and prognostic significance of new T wave inversion in unstable angina. Am J Cardiol 1983;52:14-18.

64. Hersi A, Fu Y, Wong B, et al: Does the discharge ECG provide additional prognostic insight(s) from that acquired on admission? Can J Cardiol 2001;17(Suppl C):A482.

65. Rouan GW, Lee TH, Cook EF, et al: Clincial characteristics and outcome of acute myocardial infarction in patients with initially normal or nonspecific electrocardiograms (a report from the Multicenter Chest Pain Study). Am J Cardiol 1989;64:1087-1092.

66. Welch RD, Zalenski RJ, Frederick PD, et al: Prognostic value of a normal or nonspecific initial electrocardiogram in acute myocardial infarction. JAMA 2001;286:1977-1984.

67. Slater DK, Hlatky MA, Mark DB, et al: Outcome in suspected acute myocardial infarction with normal or minimally abnormal admission electrocardiographic findings. Am J Cardiol 1987;60:766-770.

68. Singh N, Mironov D, Armstrong PW, et al: Heart rate variability assessment early after acute myocardial infarction. Pathophysiological and prognostic correlates. Circulation 1996;93:1388-1395.

69. Klootwijk P, Langer A, Meij S, et al: Non-invasive prediction of reperfusion and coronary artery patency by continuous ST-segment monitoring in the GUSTO-1 trial. Eur Heart J 1996;17:689-698.

70. Krucoff MW, Croll MA, Pope JE, et al: Continuously updated 12-lead ST-segment recovery analysis for myocardial infarct artery patency assessment and its correlation with multiple simultaneous early angiographic observations. Am J Cardiol 1993;71:145-151.

71. Veldkamp RF, Green CL, Wilkins ML, et al: Comparison of continuous ST-segment recovery analysis with methods using static electrocardiograms for noninvasive patency assessment during acute myocardial infarction. Am J Cardiol 1994;73:1069-1074.

72. Langer A, Minkowitz J, Dorian P, et al: Pathophysiology and prognostic significance of Holter-detected ST segment depression after myocardial infarction. J Am Coll Cardiol 1992;20:1313-1317.

73. Langer A, Krucoff MW, Klootwijk P, et al: Prognostic significance of ST segment shift early after resolution of ST elevation in patients with myocardial infarction treated with thrombolytic therapy: The GUSTO-1 ST segment monitoring substudy. J Am Coll Cardiol 1998;31:783-789.

74. Langer A, Freeman MR, Armstrong PW: ST segment shift in unstable angina: Pathophysiology and association with coronary anatomy and hospital outcome. J Am Coll Cardiol 1989;13:1495-1502.

75. Gottlieb SO, Weisfeldt ML, Ouyang P, et al: Silent ischemia as a marker for early unfavorable outcomes in patients with unstable angina. N Engl J Med 1986;314:1214-1219.

76. Langer A, Freeman MR, Armstrong PW: Relation of angiographically detected intracoronary thrombus and silent myocardial ischemia in unstable angina pectoris. Am J Cardiol 1990;66:1381-1382.

77. Norgaard BL, Andersen K, Dellborg M, et al: Admission risk assessment by cardiac troponin T in unstable coronary artery disease: Additional prognostic information from continuous ST segment monitoring. J Am Coll Cardiol 1999;33:1519-1527.

78. Klootwijk P, Meij S, Es GA, et al: Comparison of usefulness of computer assisted continuous 48-hour 3-lead with 12-lead ECG ischemia monitoring for detection and quantification of ischemia in patients with unstable angina. Eur Heart J 1997;18:931-940.

79. Dellborg M, Malmberg K, Rydén L, et al: Dynamic on-line vectorcardiography improves and simplifies in-hospital ischemia monitoring of patients with unstable angina. J Am Coll Cardiol 1995;26:1501-1507.

80. Patel DJ, Holdright DR, Knight CJ, et al: Early continuous ST segment monitoring in unstable angina: Prognostic value additional to the clinical characteristics and the admission electrocardiogram. Heart 1996;75:222-228.

81. Goodman SG, Barr A, Sobtchouk A, et al: Low molecular weight heparin decreases rebound ischemia in unstable angina or non-Q-wave myocardial infarction: The Canadian ESSENCE ST segment monitoring substudy. J Am Coll Cardiol 2000;36:1507-1513.

82. Jernberg T, Lindahl B, Wallentin L: ST-segment monitoring with continuous 12-lead ECG improves early risk stratification in patients with chest pain and ECG nondiagnostic of acute myocardial infarction. J Am Coll Cardiol 1999;34:1413-1419.

83. Jernberg T, Lindahl B, Wallentin L: The combination of a continuous 12-lead ECG and troponin T. A valuable tool for risk stratification during the first 6 hours in patients with chest pain and a nondiagnostic ECG. Eur Heart J 2000;21:1464-1472.

84. Mark DB, Hlatky MA, Harrell FE Jr, et al: Exercise treadmill score for predicting prognosis in coronary artery disease. Ann Intern Med 1987;106:793-800.

85. Mark DB, Shaw L, Harrell FE Jr, et al: Prognostic value of a treadmill exercise score in outpatients with suspected coronary artery disease. N Engl J Med 1991;325:849-853.

86. Cole CR, Blackstone EH, Pashkow FJ, et al: Heart-rate recovery immediately after exercise as a predictor of mortality. N Engl J Med 1999;341:1351-1357.

87. Theroux P, Waters DD, Halphen C, et al: Prognostic value of exercise testing soon after myocardial infarction. N Engl J Med 1979;301:341-345.

88. Topol EJ, Burek K, O'Neill WW, et al: A randomized controlled trial of hospital discharge three days after myocardial infarction in the era of reperfusion. N Engl J Med 1988;318:1083–1088.

89. Senaratne MPJ, Smith G, Gulamhusein SS: Feasibility and safety of early exercise testing using the Bruce protocol after acute myocardial infarction. J Am Coll Cardiol 2000;35:1212–1220.

90. Ekstrand K, Bostrom PA, Lilja B, et al: Submaximal early exercise test compared to clinical findings for evaluation of short- and long-term prognosis after the first myocardial infarction. Result from the MONICA Projects in Augsburg and Toulouse. Eur Heart J 1997;18:822–834.

91. Lindahl B, Andrén B, Ohlsson J, et al: Risk stratification in unstable coronary artery disease. Additive value of troponin T determinations and pre-discharge exercise tests. Eur Heart J 1997;18:762–770.

92. Nyman I, Wallentin L, Areskog M, et al: Risk stratification by early exercise testing after an episode of unstable coronary artery disease. The RISC study group. Int J Cardiol 1993;39:131–142.

93. Wilcox I, Freedman SB, Allman KC, et al: Prognostic significance of a predischarge exercise test in risk stratification after unstable angina pectoris. J Am Coll Cardiol 1991;18:677–683.

94. Nyman I, Larsson H, Areskog M, et al: The predictive value of silent ischemia at an exercise test before discharge after an episode of unstable coronary artery disease. Am Heart J 1992;123:324–331.

95. Larsson H, Areskog M, Areskog NH, et al: Should the exercise test (ET) be performed at discharge or one month later after an episode of unstable angina or non-Q-wave myocardial infarction?. Int J Cardiol 1991;7:7–14.

96. Gaspoz JM, Lee TH, Weinstein MC, et al: Cost-effectiveness of a new short-stay unit to "rule out" acute myocardial infarction in low risk patients. J Am Coll Cardiol 1994;24:1249–1259.

97. Zalenski RJ, McCarren M, Roberts R, et al: An evaluation of a chest pain diagnostic protocol to exclude acute cardiac ischemia in the emergency department. Arch Intern Med 1997;157:1085–1091.

98. Butman SM, Olson HG, Butman LK: Early exercise testing after stabilization of unstable angina: Correlation with coronary angiographic findings and subsequent cardiac events. Am Heart J 1986;111:11–18.

99. Polanczyk CA, Johnson PA, Hartley LH, et al: Clinical correlates and prognostic significance of early negative exercise tolerance test in patients with acute chest pain seen in the hospital emergency department. Am J Cardiol 1998;81:288–292.

100. Farkouh ME, Smars PA, Reeder GS, et al: A clinical trial of a chest-pain observation unit for patients with unstable angina. N Engl J Med 1998;339:1882–1888.

Biochemical Markers of Myocardial Necrosis

Christian W. Hamm
Christopher Heeschen

Biochemical markers have been routinely used for decades to clinically assess myocardial cell damage in patients with suspected acute coronary syndromes. Today, biochemical markers are pivotal for diagnosis, risk stratification, and guidance of treatment (Fig. 14-1).[1-3] Accordingly, such markers have obtained a central role in the clinical guidelines for acute coronary syndromes in the United States as well as in Europe.[4-6]

In recent years, biomarkers have bettered our understanding of the underlying pathophysiology of acute coronary syndromes. Convincing evidence shows that both inflammatory and thrombotic mechanisms are involved.[7] Inflammatory mechanisms promote plaque fissuring or erosion, which exposes thrombogenic contents such as collagen to the circulation, followed by platelet activation and platelet adhesion. Further platelet activation results in thrombus formation. If this thrombus is occlusive, a typical myocardial infarction usually results, in most cases followed by the release of cardiac biomarkers. If the thrombus does not or only transiently occludes the artery, the patient commonly has unstable angina. Because of distal embolization from the liable thrombus formation, focal cell necroses in the myocardium supplied by the culprit artery may occur, but this is more difficult to detect.[8,9]

BIOCHEMICAL MARKERS IN THE PERIPHERAL BLOOD

In clinical routine, three biochemical markers for detecting myocardial cell injury are currently established: creatine kinase MB, myoglobin, and the troponins (Table 14-1).

Creatine kinase MB (CK-MB) has for many years been the gold standard for the detection of myocardial cell necrosis despite its limiting shortcomings related to diagnostic accuracy and sensitivity. Patients were once considered to have non–ST-elevation myocardial infarctions when CK release was greater than twice the upper limit of normal. With improved treatment strategies, the demand for advanced diagnostic parameters has grown. New assay generations for the immunologic determination of CK-MB mass have improved the analytical accuracy but have not considerably increased the sensitivity for detecting minimal myocardial injury. Another limitation of CK-MB measurements is the late rise in the set-

ting of acute myocardial infarction, reducing the value of this measurement for guiding rapid therapeutic decision-making. Accordingly, new markers have been introduced to overcome the biochemical limitations of CK-MB measurements.

Myoglobin appears to be the best available routine marker for the early detection of acute myocardial infarction.[10,11] After the onset of pain, myoglobin reaches elevated serum concentrations within 2 hours and peaks within 4 to 6 hours. This results in a high sensitivity for the detection of myocardial infarctions when patients with trauma or renal insufficiency are excluded. However, specificity is low because elevated levels are often observed in noncardiac conditions and the negative predictive value declines rapidly after the onset of symptoms because of myoglobin's short half-life.

Cardiac troponins have been introduced, overcoming the limitations of both CK-MB and myoglobin measurements.[12,13] Troponin C, T, and I are structural proteins that modulate the interaction between actin and myosin in both skeletal and cardiac myocytes. Although expressed in skeletal muscle, troponin I and troponin T (but not troponin C) have isoforms that are unique to cardiac myocytes. Accordingly, several immunoassays for the determination of either cardiac troponin T or troponin I have been developed.[14-19] In contrast with CK-MB and myoglobin, cardiac troponin I and troponin T are usually not detectable in the peripheral blood of healthy persons and thus demonstrate a greater proportional rise above the reference value in the setting of myocardial necrosis. As such, troponins enable detection of a very faint "signal" of release from cardiac myocytes against minimal background "noise" in the peripheral circulation and are more sensitive for detecting myocardial necrosis than the traditional CK-MB or myoglobin measurements. In about one third of patients with acute coronary syndromes without persistent ST elevations, troponins are found to be elevated (Table 14-2). Cardiac troponins remain elevated after myocardial infarction for up to 10 to 14 days after cardiac injury.[20]

Although the CK-MB isoform is present as 1% to 3% of total skeletal muscle CK, the cardiac-specific isoforms of troponin I and T do not exist in normal skeletal myocytes. Therefore, troponins are more specific for

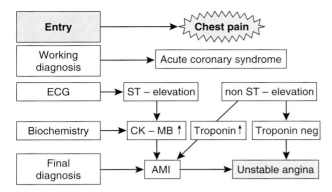

FIGURE 14–1. Terminology of acute coronary syndrome based on cardiac biomarkers. AMI, acute myocardial infarction; CK-MB, creatinine kinase B; ECG, electrocardiogram; neg, negative; ST, ST segment.

cardiac injury than traditional markers (Fig. 14–2). In conditions of "false-positive" elevated CK-MB or myoglobin, as with skeletal muscle trauma, troponins accurately identify any cardiac involvement. On the basis of these

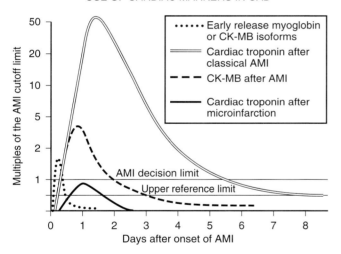

USE OF CARDIAC MARKERS IN CAD

FIGURE 14–2. Release kinetics of cardiac biomarkers. AMI, acute myocardial infarction; CK-MB, creatinine kinase B. (After Wu AH, Apple FS, Gibler WB, et al: National Academy of Clinical Biochemistry Standards of Laboratory Practice: Recommendations for the use of cardiac markers in coronary artery diseases. Clin Chem 45:1104–1121, 1999.)

TABLE 14–2   TROPONIN ELEVATION IN PATIENTS WITH ACUTE CORONARY SYNDROMES WITHOUT PERSISTENT ST ELEVATIONS

	STUDY	N	% POSITIVE
Troponin T	Hamm, 1992[32]	84	40
	Ravkilde, 1993[33]	127	35
	Wu, 1995[34]	131	21
	Lindahl, 1996[35]	593	51
	Hamm, 1997[56]	315	29
	Luescher, 1997[39]	516	48
	CAPTURE, 1998[74]	890	24
	PRISM 1999[75]	2222	29
Troponin I	Galvani, 1996[38]	91	24
	Antman, 1996[37]	948	25
	Hamm, 1997[56]	315	36
	Luescher, 1997[39]	516	41
	PRISM study 1999[75]	2222	28

properties, troponin T and troponin I have proven to compare favorably to CK-MB for the initial diagnosis of myocardial infarction and to offer additional diagnostic information in the case of normal or borderline elevation of CK-MB or concomitant skeletal muscle injury (e.g., in the setting of trauma or surgery).

Elevation of cardiac troponins may occur in the setting of nonischemic myocardial injury, e.g., myocarditis, severe congestive heart failure, pulmonary embolism, or cardiotoxic chemotherapeutic agents.[21-24] This should not be labeled as a false-positive result but rather reflect the sensitivity of the marker. True false-positive results have been documented for troponin T in the setting of skeletal myopathies or chronic renal failure and for troponin I related to interaction of the immunoassays with fibrin strands or heterophilic antibodies.[25-27] Although current assay generations have largely overcome these deficiencies, infrequent false-positive results may still occur.

BIOCHEMICAL MARKERS FOR EMERGENT RISK STRATIFICATION

Physicians caring for patients with acute chest pain constantly maneuver between unnecessary admissions

TABLE 14–1   CHARACTERISTICS OF CARDIAC BIOMARKERS

CARDIAC MARKER	CARDIAC SPECIFICITY	MOLECULAR WEIGHT (D)	FIRST RISE (HOURS)	PEAK OCCLUSION (HOURS)	PEAK REPERFUSION (HOURS)	RETURN TO NORMAL
Myoglobin	–	17.800	2	?	?	24–48 hours
CK-MB mass	+	86.000	4	24	16	48–72 hours
Troponin T	++	33.000	2–4	38	14	10 days
Troponin I	++	22.500	2–4	16	12	7 days

and premature discharges of high-risk patients. The ECG is the most readily available tool for identifying patients with ST-segment elevation, who are likely to have myocardial infarction and who should receive immediate reperfusion therapy.[28] Establishing the correct diagnosis in the patients without ST-segment elevations, however, can be much more challenging. Unidentified myocardial infarctions remain a serious public health problem and are the leading cause of malpractice cases in the emergency room setting.[29] Prematurely discharged patients more often have been seen by physicians with less professional experience, frequently presented with atypical symptoms and nondiagnostic ECG findings, were younger, and subsequently were at higher risk than admitted patients.[29,30] According to today's standards, however, ruling out acute myocardial infarction in these patients is an incomplete strategy. The target has moved to risk stratification, with the objective being not only to detect evolving myocardial infarctions but also to identify patients who are at risk for a life-threatening cardiac event in the near future. In this setting, biochemical markers play a central role.

Markers of inflammation, such as C-reactive protein, have been found helpful in predicting long-term prognosis, whereas improved markers of cell necrosis, mainly cardiac troponins, have become a valuable tool in the acute-phase assessment.[31] Numerous studies provide convincing evidence that cardiac troponins are powerful tools for risk stratification of non–ST-elevation acute coronary syndromes.[32-39] CK-MB and myoglobin are much less powerful predictors of risk. A meta-analysis of 14 trials examining either troponin T or troponin I in different settings showed that troponin T and I are

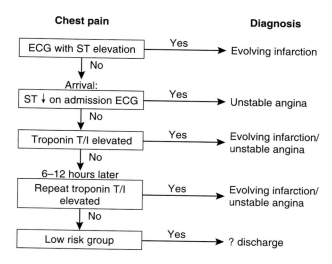

FIGURE 14–4. Diagnostic algorithm for patients with acute coronary syndromes based on the American College of Cardiology/American Heart Association guidelines[4] as well as the European Society of Cardiology Task Force Report.[5] ECG, electrocardiogram.

highly predictive for the risk of death or acute myocardial infarction during 30-day follow-up, with a cumulative odds ratio of 2.7 (95% CI, 2.1 to 3.4) in patients with unstable angina and elevated troponin T and 4.2 (95% CI, 2.7 to 6.4) with elevated troponin I.[40] This predictive capacity of the troponins is independent of important clinical risk factors including age, ST-segment deviation, and presence of heart failure. Another meta-analysis calculated a more than 9-fold increase in the risk for death and myocardial infarction in patients with elevated troponins (Fig. 14–3).[41] Consequently, the American College of Cardiology/American Heart Association guidelines[4] as well as the European Society of Cardiology Task Force Report[5] included troponin measurements in their diagnostic algorithms for patients with acute coronary syndromes (Fig. 14–4).

POINT-OF-CARE TESTING

In patients with acute coronary syndromes without ST elevations who are clinically stable, minor time delays may not be as critical as in ST-elevation myocardial infarction. However, to establish the correct diagnosis for prompt triage, point-of-care or bedside testing for biochemical markers may become advantageous in acute coronary syndromes. Point-of-care tests are characterized as assays to be performed either directly at the bedside or at "near patient" locations such as the emergency department, chest pain evaluation center, or intensive care unit. Therefore, the rationale behind point-of-care testing is the improvement in analytical turnaround time. Suspected acute coronary syndromes present a possibly life-threatening condition in which time savings for therapeutic decision-making and further management may be decisive. The American College of Cardiology/American Heart Association guidelines require a turnaround

TROPONINS IN UNSTABLE ANGINA: METAANALYSIS
DEATH/ AMI 30 DAYS FOLLOW-UP

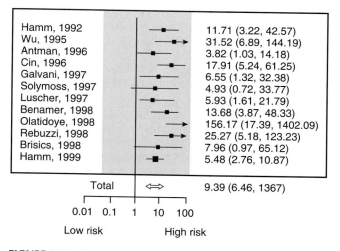

FIGURE 14–3. Meta-analysis of the predictive value of troponin elevation in patients with acute coronary syndromes (relative risk and 95% confidence intervals). Compared with troponin-negative patients, patients with at least one positive troponin test result experienced a more than ninefold increase in the risk of death and myocardial infarction.[41]

time of 30 to 60 minutes.[4] The National Academy of Clinical Biochemistry advises implementation of point-of-care test systems if the hospital logistics cannot consistently deliver cardiac marker results within 1 hour.[42] Necessarily, point-of-care techniques have to be analytically accurate and equivalent to centralized laboratory methods.

Point-of-care assays are available for the determination of CK-MB, myoglobin, and troponins.[43-50] These handheld disposable assays utilize small quantities of anticoagulated blood to detect abnormal concentrations of cardiac proteins within 15 to 20 minutes. Based on immunochromatic methods, these assays allow qualitative determination of myocardial proteins by using monoclonal or polyclonal antibodies directed against the target protein. Application of a defined amount of whole blood or plasma onto the test strip initiates the assay process. From whole-blood samples, cellular blood components are separated by a permeable membrane. If concentrations of cardiac markers are abnormal, color-labeled antibodies bind to the proteins. By means of solid-phase technology, the antibody-protein complex adheres to an immobilized ligand as part of the test kit and the process of antibody binding and migration finally results in an identifiable color development at a specified region of the test kit (Fig. 14–5).

Point-of-care tests read visually and are therefore observer-dependent. A further major limitation is that visual assessment only allows a yes-or-no statement without definitive information regarding the concentration of the marker in the blood. In general, a darker or earlier developing signal line indicates a higher concentration of the marker in the sample, but this reading remains subjective. Careful reading exactly at the assay's indicated time, under good illumination, is essential to avoid observer misinterpretation, especially in case of marginal antibody binding. Even the faintest coloring should be read as a positive test result. No special skill or prolonged training is required to read these assays. Accordingly, these tests can be performed by various members of the health care team.[51] Numerous studies have shown that point-of-care test systems are reliable, provided the precautions are observed.[52-58] A time to signal appearance of less than 10 minutes has been shown to identify patients at particular risk.[59] For troponin T, an optical reading system is offered, which also provides a printout of a quantitative result.[60]

HOW MANY MARKERS TO MEASURE?

Another frequently discussed issue relates to the question of whether we gain diagnostic accuracy by using multiple markers. The National Academy of Clinical Biochemistry recommends the use of an early (rise within 6 hours) and definite marker for establishing the diagnosis of myocardial infarction.[42] As the gold standard for detecting myocardial cell necrosis, troponins are part of all recent recommendations.[4,5]

Myoglobin is released earlier in acute myocardial infarction but lacks cardiac specificity. The combination of both markers may seem appealing. A recent large study including patients who presented relatively early to the hospital (median, < 3 hours) suggests that the

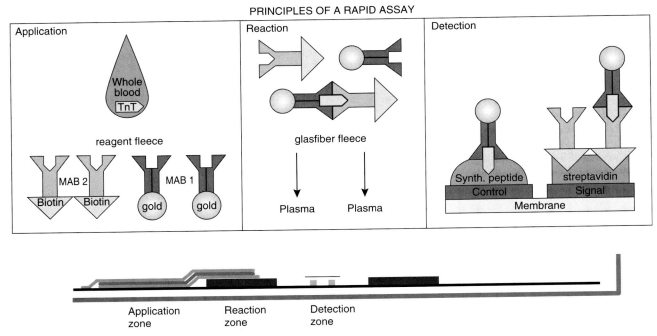

PRINCIPLES OF A RAPID ASSAY

FIGURE 14–5. In qualitative bedside tests, a solid-phase technology is employed. The color-labeled antibody-protein complex adheres to an immobilized ligand. In case of significant antigen concentration in the blood sample, the accumulation of those color-labeled complexes leads to an identifiable color development at a specified region of the test kit. MAB, monoclonal antibody.

value of adding myoglobin to diagnostic work-up programs is greatest in the time window of 4 to 6 hours after the onset of pain.[61] Elevated myoglobin levels might be helpful for early triage at the level of care but, in contrast with troponins, such levels have yet to show a proven implication for treatment. There is no indication for fibrinolytic therapy in the absence of ST-segment elevations or new left bundle branch block. A patient with elevated myoglobin levels may be a candidate for immediate coronary angiography as part of the diagnostic work-up; however, invasive facilities are neither available everywhere nor available around the clock, and apparently such facilities are not often used in this scenario. Therefore, patients generally have to wait 6 hours for the troponin results to complete the risk-stratification protocol. Myoglobin, however, can be helpful for detecting reinfarction in patients with postinfarction angina when troponins are still elevated.

CK-MB may be measured because it still provides a kind of familiar backup safety. United States guidelines, however, state that CK-MB will be replaced after a transition phase by troponin measurements.[4] Though no longer critical to the initial evaluation of patients with suspected acute coronary syndromes, serial determination of CK-MB may still offer useful clinical information in specific situations at low cost. Among patients admitted with myocardial infarction, the magnitude and time course of CK-MB elevation and decline correlates strongly with infarct size and provides a noninvasive marker of reperfusion. Although the troponins may provide comparable data regarding infarct size and reperfusion, the clinical meaning of peak values remains less familiar to clinicians and the prolonged decline relative to CK-MB confounds the ability to detect reinfarction. Similarly, among patients undergoing percutaneous coronary intervention, the clinical interpretation of specific levels of CK-MB elevation after procedures remains on firmer ground, being established by greater clinical and research experience. Finally, when the timing of a myocardial event is unclear or a nonischemic source of myocardial injury is being considered, the absence or presence of the characteristic rise and fall of CK-MB may represent useful diagnostic information. Thus, CK-MB will likely continue to play a role in the monitoring of patients hospitalized with acute coronary syndromes. For risk stratification, however, CK-MB and myoglobin will not play a relevant role.

Combined test devices that increase diagnostic capability include myoglobin as early marker, troponin I as the cardiac-specific marker, and CK-MB as the traditional marker. A one-step handheld device (Biosite Diagnostics, San Diego, CA) automatically detects myoglobin, CK-MB mass, and troponin I in about 15 minutes from whole-blood and plasma samples through a combination of photochemical signaling and microcapillary technology.[48] In these assays, blood cells are separated from plasma via filters and subsequent incubation of the antigen with fluorescent antibody conjugates. If abnormal concentrations of the markers are detected, conjugates specific for each marker are produced and the intensity of the fluorescent signal is determined. Another panel system is available for rapid quantitative determination of myoglo-

bin, CK mass, and troponin I in whole-blood samples (First Medical, Mountain View, CA). This system uses a test disk and analyzer to perform solid phase fluorescence immunoassays at a turnaround time of 19 minutes. A fluorometric analyzer (Stratus CS STAT, Dade Behring) for rapid whole-blood measurement of CK-MB, myoglobin, and troponin I has also been shown to provide high diagnostic accuracy and reliable quantitative troponin I results from whole blood samples within 15 minutes.[62]

MYOCARDIAL INFARCTION REDEFINED

A key point is the fact that the gold standard for myocardial damage has changed and myocardial infarction therefore has been redefined. The consensus document of the Joint European Society of Cardiology/American College of Cardiology Committee has refined the contemporary diagnosis of myocardial infarction according to biochemical grounds.[63] The committee's recommendations specify a diagnostic limit for myocardial infarction using cardiac troponins based on the 99th percentile of levels among healthy controls rather than comparison with CK-MB. Acceptable imprecision (coefficient of variation) at the 99th percentile for each assay should be defined as 10%. Each laboratory has to confirm the range of reference values in their specific setting.

This change in definition will increase the frequency of the diagnosis of myocardial infarction and will have important implications for the interpretation of epidemiologic research and clinical trials as well as for clinical care. Although many physicians currently have conceptual difficulties with the translation of this paradigm change into clinical practice, the increased risk in patients with elevated troponin levels justifies this new perception. Consequently, our procedures for ruling out myocardial infarction need to be based on troponins representing the more sensitive and specific cardiac markers and which may be elevated when all other markers are still within the normal range.

However, widespread consensus has not yet been achieved regarding appropriate thresholds for the troponins in the diagnosis of myocardial infarction. Central to this problem is the fact that the cardiac troponins offer higher sensitivity than the established gold standard, CK-MB. To date, reported diagnostic thresholds have been based on analysis of receiver operating characteristics compared with World Health Organization criteria for acute myocardial infarction using CK-MB. However, troponin T and troponin I levels have been elevated in 25% to 50% of patients presenting with non–ST-elevation ischemic syndromes without elevation of CK-MB. Whether all such elevations represent irreversible myocyte injury remains an issue of significant scientific and clinical interest.[66] Although there is substantial evidence that even mild elevation of the cardiac troponins is important to prognosis, the possibility that low-level increases may occur in the setting of reversible ischemic injury raises some question as to whether such increases should be embraced by the diagnostic limits for myocardial infarction. Whether related to reversible or irreversible myocardial injury, the prognostic importance of detectable levels of cardiac troponins among patients with normal CK-MB has shifted the traditional boundaries between unstable angina and non–ST-elevation myocardial infarction. Nevertheless, supported by a substantial body of data, the cardiac troponins are the preferred primary markers for risk stratification of suspected acute coronary syndromes.

The conceptual difficulty with defining the appropriate diagnostic threshold for troponins is further compounded by the availability of multiple assays for troponin I for which different reference ranges have been developed. For troponin I, many manufacturers report two decision limits: a "diagnostic" limit for the definitive diagnosis of myocardial infarction based on prior comparisons to CK-MB and a lower limit "suggestive" of myocardial injury that is important to prognosis. Though the challenge of developing terminology and diagnostic thresholds around low-level troponin elevation has been debated, the clinical importance of increased troponin levels in suspected acute coronary syndromes is firmly established.

There is no fundamental clinical difference between troponin T and troponin I. Differences between study results are predominantly explained by varying inclusion criteria, differences in sampling patterns, and use of assays with different diagnostic cut-offs. The decision limits must be based on carefully conducted clinical studies for individual troponin I assays and should not be generalized among different troponin I assays. For troponin T, levels as low as 0.01 μg/L have been shown to be associated with adverse cardiac outcomes in acute coronary syndromes.[64] According to the FRagmin and Fast Revascularisation during InStability in Coronary artery disease (FRISC) studies, a troponin T level of 0.03 μg/L appears to be the appropriate threshold.[65] Low levels of troponins appear to carry the highest risk in patients with acute coronary syndromes.[67] However, the application of this threshold among more heterogeneous populations of patients presenting to the emergency department requires prospective evaluation. Currently,

the diagnostic threshold for troponin T may be maintained at 0.1 μg/L.

HOW TO APPLY TROPONIN MEASUREMENTS IN CLINICAL ROUTINE?

Diagnostic strategies for the evaluation of acute chest pain have to be reliable and simple. The objective is to reduce mortality and morbidity by initiating the best therapy. Common diagnostic sense is necessary to detect other noncoronary but critical conditions such as dissecting aortic aneurysms. The ECG allows the exclusion of acute myocardial infarctions requiring immediate therapeutic response. Troponins can best identify high-risk coronary patients. However, several practical aspects for optimizing the sampling protocols in emergency units and for combining troponin measurements with other markers in the clinical routine setting still need to be clarified. Troponins can be understood only in concert with other parameters. The admission ECG does not only serve to exclude ST-elevation acute myocardial infarction but can also be used as a powerful predictor of future risk.[68,69] However, troponins seem to better discriminate between low- and high-risk patients (Fig. 14–6).[56] Risk stratification was also improved by combining a treadmill test with the troponin result.[70]

There is general consent that testing for troponins only on admission to the hospital is insufficient because a single test misses 10% to 15% of high-risk patients.[56,71] Timing for the second test has not yet been clearly defined. The European Society of Cardiology recommends repeating troponin testing between 6 and 12 hours after arrival in the emergency unit.[5] The American version[4] asks for a repeat test 8 to 12 hours after the onset of pain, a minor but sometimes decisive difference in the perception in the work-up of the individual patient. Previous studies before the troponins era had suggested a 12-hour rule-out strategy.[72] A prospective study using troponin T and troponin I bedside tests proposed an interval of 6 hours to identify high-risk

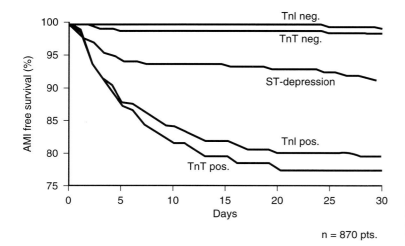

FIGURE 14–6. Troponins and the electrocardiogram. Acute myocardial infarction (AMI)-free survival based on troponins compared with ST depression.[2] neg, negative; TnI, troponin I; TnT, troponin T.

n = 870 pts.

patients[56] or a 6-hour work-up program to exclude myocardial infarction.[73]

CONCLUSIONS AND PERSPECTIVES

Biochemical markers for detecting myocardial injury are essential to the assessment and treatment of patients with acute coronary syndromes. When clinicians have to base triage, treatment, and monitoring on time-sensitive test results, point-of-care testing offers a rapid and convenient diagnostic option complementary to centralized laboratory testing. This is particularly true when the choice of effective therapy depends on cardiac biomarkers. Studies have demonstrated the link between the troponin result and effectiveness of glycoprotein IIb/IIIa antagonists or low-molecular-weight heparin has been demonstrated (Figs. 14–7 and 14–8).[74-78] In this scenario, troponins are a surrogate marker of the active thrombotic processes (Fig. 14–9).

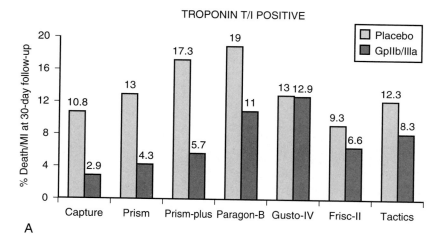

FIGURE 14–7A. Treatment effect of glycoprotein (Gp) IIb/IIIa inhibitors, low-molecular-weight heparin, and early intervention in troponin-positive patients. (Modified from Bertrand ME, Simoons ML, Fox KA, et al: Management of acute coronary syndromes: Acute coronary syndromes without persistent ST segment elevation. Recommendations of the Task Force of the European Society of Cardiology. Eur Heart J 21:1406–1432, 2000.)

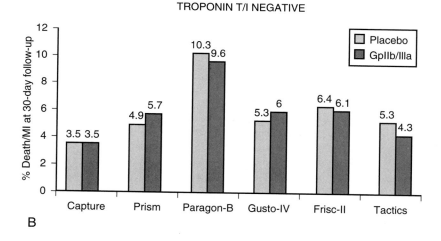

FIGURE 14–7B. Treatment effect of glycoprotein (Gp) IIb/IIIa inhibitors, low-molecular-weight heparin, and early intervention in troponin-negative patients. (Modified from Bertrand ME, Simoons ML, Fox KA, et al: Management of acute coronary syndromes: Acute coronary syndromes without persistent ST segment elevation. Recommendations of the Task Force of the European Society of Cardiology. Eur Heart J 21:1406–1432, 2000.)

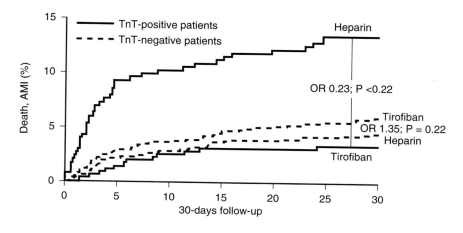

FIGURE 14–8. Treatment effect of tirofiban compared with placebo in the PRISM study in troponin-positive and troponin-negative patients. OR, odds ratio; TnT, troponin T. (Modified from Heeschen C, Hamm CW, Goldmann B, et al: Troponin concentrations for stratification of patients with acute coronary syndromes in relation to therapeutic efficacy of tirofiban. PRISM Study Investigators. Platelet Receptor Inhibition in Ischemic Syndrome Management. Lancet 354:1757–1762, 1999.)

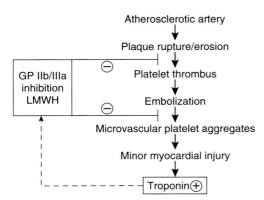

FIGURE 14–9. Link between platelets, troponin, and treatment benefit. Troponins appear to represent a surrogate marker for active thrombotic processes. Microembolization from liable thrombus formation leads to focal cell necroses in the myocardium supplied by the culprit artery that can be detected by troponin determination. LMWH, low-molecular-weight heparin.

Biomarkers should not be understood as mutually exclusive methods. Used in conjunction with information from the history, physical examination, and 12-lead electrocardiogram, cardiac markers aid in establishing the diagnosis of myocardial infarction, assessing the risk of subsequent cardiac events, and formulating plans for further evaluation and treatment. Moreover, biomarkers have the potential to provide insight into the specific pathophysiology of coronary ischemia for the individual patient. Meeting each of these objectives, the cardiac troponins have been established as highly specific and sensitive markers of myocardial injury that function as powerful tools for defining prognosis and guiding therapy for patients with acute coronary syndromes. Inflammatory markers such as highly sensitive C-reactive protein may provide a complementary tool for risk assessment before cellular damage occurs.[79]

REFERENCES

1. Hamm CW, Bertrand M, Braunwald E: Acute coronary syndrome without ST elevation: Implementation of new guidelines. Lancet 2001;358:1533-1538.
2. Hamm CW, Braunwald E: A classification of unstable angina revisited. Circulation 2000;102:118-122.
3. Klootwijk P, Hamm C: Acute coronary syndromes: Diagnosis. Lancet 1999;353:SII10-SII15.
4. Braunwald E, Antman EM, Beasley JW, et al: ACC/AHA guidelines for the management of patients with unstable angina and non-ST-segment elevation myocardial infarction: Executive summary and recommendations. A report of the American College of Cardiology/American Heart Association Task Force on pPractice Guidelines (Committee on the Management of Patients with Unstable Angina). Circulation 2000;102:1193-1209.
5. Bertrand ME, Simoons ML, Fox KA, et al: Management of acute coronary syndromes: acute coronary syndromes without persistent ST segment elevation: Recommendations of the Task Force of the European Society of Cardiology. Eur Heart J 2000;21:1406-1432.
6. Guideline for the management of patients with acute coronary syndromes without persistent ECG ST segment elevation. British Cardiac Society Guidelines and Medical Practice Committee and Royal College of Physicians Clinical Effectiveness and Evaluation Unit. Heart 85:133-142, 2001.
7. Braunwald E: Unstable angina: An etiologic approach to management. Circulation 1998;98:2219-2222.
8. Davies MJ, Thomas AC, Knapman PA, Hangartner JR: Intramyocardial platelet aggregation in patients with unstable angina suffering sudden ischemic cardiac death. Circulation 1986;73:418-427.
9. Falk E: Unstable angina with fatal outcome: Dynamic coronary thrombosis leading to infarction and/or sudden death. Autopsy evidence of recurrent mural thrombosis with peripheral embolization culminating in total vascular occlusion. Circulation 1985;71:699-708.
10. Brogan GX Jr, Friedman S, McCuskey C, et al: Evaluation of a new rapid quantitative immunoassay for serum myoglobin versus CK-MB for ruling out acute myocardial infarction in the emergency department. Ann Emerg Med 1994;24:665-671.
11. de Winter RJ, Koster RW, Sturk A, Sanders GT: Value of myoglobin, troponin T, and CK-MBmass in ruling out an acute myocardial infarction in the emergency room. Circulation 1995;92:3401-3407.
12. Gerhardt W, Nordin G, Ljungdahl L: Can troponin T replace CK MBmass as "gold standard" for acute myocardial infarction ("AMI")? Scand J Clin Lab Invest Suppl 230:83-89, 1999.
13. Jaffe AS, Ravkilde J, Roberts R, et al: It's time for a change to a troponin standard. Circulation 2000;102:1216-1220.
14. Katus HA, Looser S, Hallermayer K, et al: Development and in vitro characterization of a new immunoassay of cardiac troponin T. Clin Chem 1992;38:386-393.
15. Bodor GS, Porter S, Landt Y, Ladenson JH: Development of monoclonal antibodies for an assay of cardiac troponin-I and preliminary results in suspected cases of myocardial infarction. Clin Chem 1992;38:2203-2214.
16. Larue C, Ferrieres G, Laprade M, et al: Antigenic definition of cardiac troponin I. Clin Chem Lab Med 1998;36:361-365.
17. Apple FS, Maturen AJ, Mullins RE, et al: Multicenter clinical and analytical evaluation of the AxSYM troponin-I immunoassay to assist in the diagnosis of myocardial infarction. Clin Chem 1999;45:206-212.
18. Christenson RH, Apple FS, Morgan DL, et al: Cardiac troponin I measurement with the ACCESS immunoassay system: Analytical and clinical performance characteristics. Clin Chem 1998;44:52-60.
19. Davies E, Gawad Y, Takahashi M, et al: Analytical performance and clinical utility of a sensitive immunoassay for determination of human cardiac troponin I. Clin Biochem 1997;30:479-490.
20. Katus HA, Remppis A, Neumann FJ, et al: Diagnostic efficiency of troponin T measurements in acute myocardial infarction. Circulation 1991;83:902-912.
21. Giannitsis E, Muller-Bardorff M, Kurowski V, et al: Independent prognostic value of cardiac troponin T in patients with confirmed pulmonary embolism. Circulation 2000;102:211-217.
22. Missov E, Calzolari C, Pau B: Circulating cardiac troponin I in severe congestive heart failure. Circulation 1997;96:2953-2958.
23. Lauer B, Niederau C, Kuhl U, et al: Cardiac troponin T in patients with clinically suspected myocarditis. J Am Coll Cardiol 1997;30:1354-1359.
24. Smith SC, Ladenson JH, Mason JW, Jaffe AS: Elevations of cardiac troponin I associated with myocarditis. Experimental and clinical correlates. Circulation 1997;95:163-168.
25. McLaurin MD, Apple FS, Voss EM, et al: Cardiac troponin I, cardiac troponin T, and creatine kinase MB in dialysis patients without ischemic heart disease: Evidence of cardiac troponin T expression in skeletal muscle. Clin Chem 1997;43:976-982.
26. Frankel WL, Herold DA, Ziegler TW, Fitzgerald RL: Cardiac troponin T is elevated in asymptomatic patients with chronic renal failure. Am J Clin Pathol 1996;106:118-123.
27. Labugger R, Organ L, Collier C, et al: Extensive troponin I and T modification detected in serum from patients with acute myocardial infarction. Circulation 2000;102:1221-1226.
28. Indications for fibrinolytic therapy in suspected acute myocardial infarction: Collaborative overview of early mortality and major morbidity results from all randomised trials of more than 1000 patients. Fibrinolytic Therapy Trialists' (FTT) Collaborative Group. Lancet 1994;343:311-322.
29. Rusnak RA, Stair TO, Hansen K, Fastow JS: Litigation against the emergency physician: Common features in cases of missed myocardial infarction. Ann Emerg Med 18:1029-1034, 1989.
30. Pope JH, Aufderheide TP, Ruthazer R, et al: Missed diagnoses of acute cardiac ischemia in the emergency department. N Engl J Med 2000;342:1163-1170.

31. Heeschen C, Hamm CW, Bruemmer J, Simoons ML: Predictive value of C-reactive protein and troponin T in patients with unstable angina: a comparative analysis. CAPTURE Investigators. Chimeric c7E3 AntiPlatelet Therapy in Unstable angina REfractory to standard treatment trial. J Am Coll Cardiol 2000;35:1535-1542.

32. Hamm CW, Ravkilde J, Gerhardt W, et al: The prognostic value of serum troponin T in unstable angina. N Engl J Med 1992;327:146-150.

33. Ravkilde J, Horder M, Gerhardt W, et al: Diagnostic performance and prognostic value of serum troponin T in suspected acute myocardial infarction. Scand J Clin Lab Invest 1993;53:677-685.

34. Wu AH, Abbas SA, Green S, et al: Prognostic value of cardiac troponin T in unstable angina pectoris. Am J Cardiol 1995;76:970-972.

35. Lindahl B, Venge P, Wallentin L: Relation between troponin T and the risk of subsequent cardiac events in unstable coronary artery disease. The FRISC study group. Circulation 1996;93:1651-1657.

36. Ohman EM, Armstrong PW, Christenson RH, et al: Cardiac troponin T levels for risk stratification in acute myocardial ischemia. GUSTO IIA Investigators. N Engl J Med 1996;335:1333-1341.

37. Antman EM, Tanasijevic MJ, Thompson B, et al: Cardiac-specific troponin I levels to predict the risk of mortality in patients with acute coronary syndromes. N Engl J Med 1996;335:1342-1349.

38. Galvani M, Ottani F, Ferrini D, et al: Prognostic influence of elevated values of cardiac troponin I in patients with unstable angina. Circulation 1997;95:2053-2059.

39. Luescher MS, Thygesen K, Ravkilde J, Heickendorff L: Applicability of cardiac troponin T and I for early risk stratification in unstable coronary artery disease. TRIM Study Group. Thrombin Inhibition in Myocardial ischemia. Circulation 1997;96:2578-2585.

40. Olatidoye AG, Wu AH, Feng YJ, Waters D: Prognostic role of troponin T versus troponin I in unstable angina pectoris for cardiac events with meta-analysis comparing published studies. Am J Cardiol 1998;81:1405-1410.

41. Ottani F, Galvani M, Nicolini FA, et al: Elevated cardiac troponin levels predict the risk of adverse outcome in patients with acute coronary syndromes. Am Heart J 2000;140:917-927.

42. Wu AH, Apple FS, Gibler WB, et al: National Academy of Clinical Biochemistry Standards of Laboratory Practice: Recommendations for the use of cardiac markers in coronary artery diseases. Clin Chem 1999;45:1104-1121.

43. Muller-Bardorff M, Freitag H, Scheffold T, et al: Development and characterization of a rapid assay for bedside determinations of cardiac troponin T. Circulation 1995;92:2869-2875.

44. Antman EM, Grudzien C, Sacks DB: Evaluation of a rapid bedside assay for detection of serum cardiac troponin T. JAMA 1995;273:1279-1282.

45. Heeschen C, Goldmann BU, Moeller RH, Hamm CW: Analytical performance and clinical application of a new rapid bedside assay for the detection of serum cardiac troponin I. Clin Chem 1998;44:1925-1930.

46. Brogan GX Jr, Bock JL, McCuskey CF, et al: Evaluation of cardiac STATus CK-MB/myoglobin device for rapidly ruling out acute myocardial infarction. Clin Lab Med 1997;17:655-668.

47. Muller-Bardorff M, Hallermayer K, Schroder A, et al: Improved troponin T ELISA specific for cardiac troponin T isoform: Assay development and analytical validation. Clin Chem 1997;43:458-466.

48. Apple FS, Christenson RH, Valdes R Jr, et al: Simultaneous rapid measurement of whole blood myoglobin, creatine kinase MB, and cardiac troponin I by the triage cardiac panel for detection of myocardial infarction. Clin Chem 1999;45:199-205.

49. Luscher MS, Ravkilde J, Thygesen K: Clinical application of two novel rapid bedside tests for the detection of cardiac troponin T and creatine kinase-MB mass/myoglobin in whole blood in acute myocardial infarction. Cardiology 1998;89:222-228.

50. Panteghini M, Pagani F: Characterization of a rapid immunochromatographic assay for simultaneous detection of high concentrations of myoglobin and CK-MB in whole blood. Clin Chem 1996;42:1292-1293.

51. Sylven C, Lindahl S, Hellkvist K, et al: Excellent reliability of nurse-based bedside diagnosis of acute myocardial infarction by rapid dry-strip creatine kinase MB, myoglobin, and troponin T. Am Heart J 1998;135:677-683.

52. Gerhardt W, Ljungdahl L, Collinson PO, et al: An improved rapid troponin T test with a decreased detection limit: A multicentre study of the analytical and clinical performance in suspected myocardial damage. Scand J Clin Lab Invest 1997;57:549-557.

53. Azzazy HM, Duh SH, Fitzgerald RL, et al: Multisite study of a second generation whole blood rapid assay for cardiac troponin T. Ann Clin Biochem 1999;36:438-446.

54. Collinson PO, Thomas S, Siu L, et al: Rapid troponin T measurement in whole blood for detection of myocardial damage. Ann Clin Biochem 1995;32:454-458.

55. Christenson RH, Fitzgerald RL, Ochs L, et al: Characteristics of a 20-minute whole blood rapid assay for cardiac troponin T. Clin Biochem 1997;30:27-33.

56. Hamm CW, Goldmann BU, Heeschen C, et al: Emergency room triage of patients with acute chest pain by means of rapid testing for cardiac troponin T or troponin I. N Engl J Med 1997;337:1648-1653.

57. Evaluation of a bedside whole-blood rapid troponin T assay in the emergency department. Rapid Evaluation by Assay of Cardiac Troponin T (REACTT) Investigators Study Group. Acad Emerg Med 1997;4:1018-1024.

58. Ohman EM, Armstrong PW, White HD, et al: Risk stratification with a point-of-care cardiac troponin T test in acute myocardial infarction. GUSTOIII Investigators. Global Use of Strategies To Open Occluded Coronary Arteries. Am J Cardiol 1999;84:1281-1286.

59. Antman EM, Sacks DB, Rifai N, et al: Time to positivity of a rapid bedside assay for cardiac-specific troponin T predicts prognosis in acute coronary syndromes: A Thrombolysis in Myocardial Infarction (TIMI) 11A substudy. J Am Coll Cardiol 1998;31:326-330.

60. Muller-Bardorff M, Rauscher T, Kampmann M, et al: Quantitative bedside assay for cardiac troponin T: A complementary method to centralized laboratory testing. Clin Chem 1999;45:1002-1008.

61. Gibler WB, Hoekstra JW, Weaver WD, et al: A randomized trial of the effects of early cardiac serum marker availability on reperfusion therapy in patients with acute myocardial infarction: The serial markers, acute myocardial infarction and rapid treatment trial (SMARTT). J Am Coll Cardiol 2000;36:1500-1506.

62. Heeschen C, Goldmann BU, Langenbrink L, et al: Evaluation of a rapid whole blood ELISA for quantification of troponin I in patients with acute chest pain. Clin Chem 1999;45:1789-1796.

63. Myocardial infarction redefined—a consensus document of The Joint European Society of Cardiology/American College of Cardiology Committee for the redefinition of myocardial infarction. Eur Heart J 2000;21:1502-1513.

64. Cannon CP, Weintraub WS, Demopoulos LA, et al: Comparison of early invasive and conservative strategies in patients with unstable coronary syndromes treated with the glycoprotein IIb/IIIa inhibitor tirofiban. N Engl J Med 2001;344:1879-1887.

65. Long-term low-molecular-mass heparin in unstable coronary-artery disease: FRISC II prospective randomised multicentre study. FRagmin and Fast Revascularisation during InStability in Coronary artery disease Investigators. Lancet 1999;354:701-707.

66. Antman EM, Grudzien C, Mitchell RN Sacks DB: Detection of unsuspected myocardial necrosis by rapid bedside assay for cardiac troponin T. Am Heart J 1997;133:596-598.

67. Lindahl B, Diderholm E, Lagerqvist B, et al: Mechanisms behind the prognostic value of troponin T in unstable coronary artery disease: A FRISC II substudy. J Am Coll Cardiol 2001;38:979-986.

68. Kaul P, Fu Y, Chang WC, et al: Prognostic value of ST segment depression in acute coronary syndromes: Insights from PARAGON-A applied to GUSTO-IIb. PARAGON-A and GUSTO IIb Investigators. Platelet IIb/IIIa Antagonism for the Reduction of Acute Global Organization Network. J Am Coll Cardiol 2001;38:64-71.

69. Savonitto S, Ardissino D, Granger CB, et al: Prognostic value of the admission electrocardiogram in acute coronary syndromes. JAMA 1999;281:707-713.

70. Lindahl B, Andren B, Ohlsson J, et al: Risk stratification in unstable coronary artery disease. Additive value of troponin T determinations and pre-discharge exercise tests. FRISK Study Group. Eur Heart J 1997;18:762-770.

71. van Domburg RT, Cobbaert C, Kimman GJ, et al: Long-term prognostic value of serial troponin T bedside tests in patients with acute coronary syndromes. Am J Cardiol 2000;86:623-627.

72. Lee TH, Juarez G, Cook EF et al: Ruling out acute myocardial infarction. A prospective multicenter validation of a 12-hour strategy for patients at low risk. N Engl J Med 1991;324:1239-1246.

73. McCord J, Nowak RM, McCullough PA, et al: Ninety- minute exclusion of acute myocardial infarction by use of quantitative point-of-care testing of myoglobin and troponin I. Circulation 2001;104:1483–1488.

74. Hamm CW, Heeschen C, Goldmann B, et al: Benefit of abciximab in patients with refractory unstable angina in relation to serum troponin T levels. c7E3 Fab Antiplatelet Therapy in Unstable Refractory Angina (CAPTURE) Study Investigators. N Engl J Med 1999;340:1623–1629.

75. Heeschen C, Hamm CW, Goldmann B, et al: Troponin concentrations for stratification of patients with acute coronary syndromes in relation to therapeutic efficacy of tirofiban. PRISM Study Investigators. Platelet Receptor Inhibition in Ischemic Syndrome Management. Lancet 1999;354:1757–1762.

76. Newby LK, Ohman EM, Christenson RH, et al: Benefit of glycoprotein IIb/IIIa inhibition in patients with acute coronary syndromes and troponin t-positive status: The paragon-B troponin T substudy. Circulation 2001;103:2891–2896.

77. Lindahl B, Venge P, Wallentin L: Troponin T identifies patients with unstable coronary artery disease who benefit from long-term antithrombotic protection. Fragmin in Unstable Coronary Artery Disease (FRISC) Study Group. J Am Coll Cardiol 1997;29: 43–48.

78. Morrow DA, Antman EM, Tanasijevic M, et al: Cardiac troponin I for stratification of early outcomes and the efficacy of enoxaparin in unstable angina: A TIMI-11B substudy. J Am Coll Cardiol 2000;36:1812–1817.

79. Ridker PM: High-sensitivity C-reactive protein: potential adjunct for global risk assessment in the primary prevention of cardiovascular disease. Circulation 2001;103:1813–1818.

Markers of a Thrombotic State

Jane A. Leopold
Joseph Loscalzo

The acute coronary syndromes encompass the spectrum of unstable angina, non–ST-segment myocardial infarction, and acute ST-elevation myocardial infarction. These syndromes may be recognized clinically by symptoms, electrocardiographic abnormalities, and changes in serum markers. The creatine kinase MB isoenzyme (CK-MB)[1] and, more recently, cardiac troponins T and I[2,3] have been held as the gold standard for the diagnosis of myocardial infarction; however, these markers signal that myocardial injury has already occurred. Thus, in order to identify patients early in the course of an acute coronary event, the pathobiology of vascular injury or plaque rupture that promotes thrombosis in situ has been examined with an eye toward identifying unique circulating markers. Recognition of the integral role of platelets and coagulation factors in acute coronary events has facilitated the identification of novel serum markers that reflect thrombus formation. These novel markers may be used clinically to identify patients with acute coronary syndromes and myocardial ischemia early in their course to allow therapeutic intervention before myocardial necrosis occurs.

DETERMINANTS OF THROMBUS FORMATION

Thrombus Formation

In order to designate clinically useful serum markers of a thrombotic state, it is first necessary to examine the highly integrated and regulated sequence of events that results in thrombus formation. Under basal conditions, platelets circulate in an unactivated state and do not adhere to the endothelium owing to endothelial cell products that maintain a nonthrombogenic milieu. For example, endothelial cells metabolize arachidonate and endoperoxides to prostacyclin to inhibit platelet aggregation by activating platelet adenylyl cyclase, thereby increasing levels of cyclic adenosine monophosphate.[4] Endothelium-derived nitric oxide diffuses across platelet membranes to activate guanylyl cyclase and increase cyclic guanosine monophosphate levels to prevent platelet adhesion and activation.[5] The endothelium constitutively expresses the surface receptor thrombomodulin, which binds thrombin with high affinity and facilitates its ability to activate protein C, and the enzyme ecto-ADPase, which converts adenosine diphosphate (ADP) to adenosine monophosphate to confer anticoagulant properties on the cell surface.[6,7] Endothelial cell dysfunction significantly perturbs these homeostatic mechanisms and promotes platelet adhesion.

Vascular injury exposes the subendothelial matrix to circulating platelets, which adhere to collagen via the surface receptors glycoprotein Ia/IIa and to von Willebrand factor, and thereby collagen, via glycoprotein Ib/IX.[8] In areas of pathologic shear stress (>30 dynes/cm^2), platelet aggregation may occur independent of adhesion.[9] Once collagen and thrombin bind to their respective receptors, phospholipase C–dependent hydrolysis of membrane phospholipids ensues to produce inositol 1,4,5-bisphosphate and diacylglycerol.[10] 1,4,5-Bisphosphate increases levels of intraplatelet calcium, resulting in phosphorylation of the myosin light chain. These events have been implicated in platelet shape change, contraction, and secretion.[11] Diacylglycerol, in turn, activates protein kinase C to phosphorylate pleckstrin and promote secretion of platelet granules to release ADP and serotonin.[12] Weak platelet agonists, such as ADP and serotonin, activate phospholipase A$_2$ to release arachidonic acid, which is metabolized to form prostaglandin endoperoxides and thromboxane A$_2$. These compounds, in turn, feed back to activate phospholipase C and increase 1,4,5-bisphosphate and diacylglycerol generation.[12]

These intraplatelet signaling events result in platelet shape change from the characteristic discoid shape to one with finger-like projections (pseudopodia).[13] Granule secretion occurs concomitant with shape change, and additional platelets are recruited, undergo shape change, and aggregate on the initial layer of adherent platelets to form a hemostatic plug. Platelet-specific proteins of a-granule origin released from activated platelets have been identified as platelet-derived markers of a thrombotic state that may be measured in plasma. Activated platelets additionally promote the generation of insoluble fibrin by exposing negatively charged phospholipid sites to support assembly of procoagulant factors ("tenase" assembly) on their surface membrane.[14]

Coagulation Cascade

Concomitant with formation of the primary hemostatic plug is a series of reactions aimed at the generation and amplification of thrombin. Tissue factor, a membrane-bound protein exposed after vascular injury, binds both inactive and active factor VII. This action promotes the conversion of factors IX and X to their active forms (IXa and Xa, respectively) that, together with factor VIIa, feed back to amplify factor VII bound to tissue factor. Factors IXa and Xa may either associate with the tissue factor-VIIa complex or bind to the surface of nearby activated platelets.[15] Prothrombin, factor Xa, and factor Va make up the prothrombinase complex that converts prothrombin to thrombin, thereby releasing prothrombin fragment 1.2 (F1.2). In addition, several amplification loops increase the generation of thrombin such that maximum thrombin generation occurs after the formation of the fibrin clot. Thrombin, in turn, cleaves fibrinogen to yield fibrin and fibrinopeptides A and B. This process is regulated by thrombin binding antithrombin III to form the thrombin-antithrombin III complex (TAT). Thrombin-catalyzed activation of factor XIII importantly stabilizes the growing thrombus by covalently cross-linking fibrin.[16]

MARKERS THAT ORIGINATE FROM FIBRIN FORMATION

Markers of fibrin formation and degradation have demonstrated clinical promise for the early detection of

coronary thrombosis associated with acute coronary syndromes (Fig. 15-1). Assays have been developed to measure several markers of fibrin formation, including F1.2, TAT, fibrinopeptides A and B, and soluble fibrin (Table 15-1).

F1.2 is formed by cleavage of prothrombin by the factor Xa/Va complex. This degradation results in the formation of α-thrombin and the 32-amino acid F1.2. Because factor Xa-mediated activation of prothrombin requires the formation of factor Xa/Va complex in the presence of calcium on the platelet membrane surface, F1.2 may be a sensitive marker of prothrombin activation and is therefore a useful marker of thrombin generation. TAT also monitors the generation of thrombin and, owing to its rapid turnover, is thought to be a useful plasma marker of thrombosis.[17]

Fibrinopeptides A and B are released by the proteolytic action of thrombin on fibrinogen. Fibrinopeptide A is a 16-amino-acid peptide that is cleaved from the amino terminus of the fibrinogen a-chain and has a 3- to 5-minute half-life in plasma. Fibrinopeptide A is detectable in plasma earlier than fibrinopeptide B because it is released more rapidly from fibrinogen, resulting in the

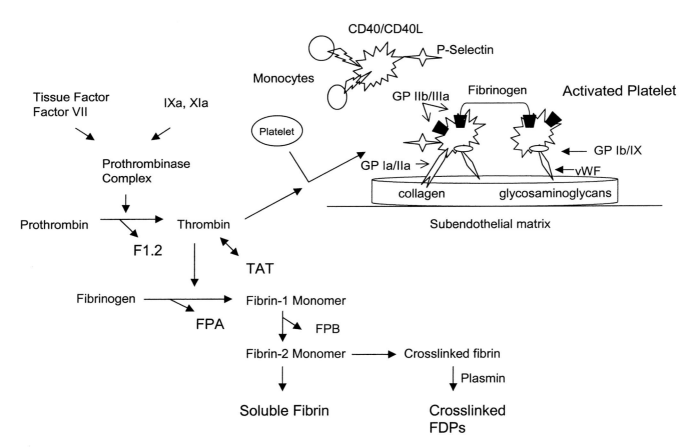

FIGURE 15–1. Fibrin formation, degradation, and thrombus formation. Tissue factor, factor VII, and factors IXa, XIa, and XIIIa form the prothrombinase complex, which converts prothrombin to thrombin and the prothrombin fragment 1.2 (F1.2). Thrombin may also be inactivated by binding to antithrombin III via heparan catalysis to form the thrombin-antithrombin III complex (TAT). Thrombin cleaves fibrinogen to fibrin-1 monomer and fibrinopeptide A (FPA) and subsequently cleaves fibrinopeptide B (FPB) to yield the fibrin-2 monomer. The fibrin-2 monomer may form soluble or cross-linked fibrin. Cross-linked fibrin is degraded by the action of plasmin to form fibrin degradation products (FDPs). Thrombin additionally promotes thrombosis. Platelets become activated, adhere to sites of vessel injury by glycoprotein (GP) Ib/IX receptor–mediated binding to von Willebrand factor as well as glycoprotein Ia/IIa receptor–mediated binding to collagen, and platelets expose surface markers of activation, including the glycoprotein IIb/IIIa receptor, P-selectin, and negatively charged phosphatidylserine residues as well as ligands such as CD40/CD40L, which bind circulating monocytes and form monocyte-platelet aggregates.[17,39]

. . .

TABLE 15–1   MARKERS OF FIBRIN FORMATION

Thrombin Activity

Fibrinopeptide A
Fibrinopeptide B
Soluble fibrin

Thrombin Elaboration

Thrombin–antithrombin III complex
Prothrombin fragment 1.2

---

formation of the intermediate fibrin I peptide. Fibrinopeptide B is cleaved from the amino terminus of the β-chain of fibrinogen or fibrin I and is a 14-amino-acid peptide. The sequential cleavage of fibrinopeptide A and B results in the formation of fibrin II monomer. Fibrinopeptide A levels have been used extensively as a measure of thrombosis, and levels may be determined from 24-hour urine collections or plasma.[17]

Owing to the short plasma half-life of F1.2, TAT, and fibrinopeptides A and B, soluble fibrin, which has a longer half-life in plasma, may be a more useful measurement in certain situations. Soluble fibrin is formed when fibrinopeptide A is cleaved and circulating fibrinogen in plasma associates with the intermediate fibrin I. Elevated levels of soluble fibrin, as a marker of thrombosis, have been measured in patients with acute coronary syndromes.[17]

Markers of Fibrin Formation Are Associated with Acute Coronary Syndromes

Prothrombin fragment 1.2, TAT, and fibrinopeptide A were identified as markers of acute coronary syndromes in 36 consecutive patients with unstable angina and non–ST-segment myocardial infarction in the Thrombolysis in Myocardial Infarction (TIMI) IIIB trial. Compared with healthy, age-matched controls, thrombin generation as measured by F1.2 (0.12 ± 0.8 vs. 0.19 ± 0.14 nmol/L), TAT formation (3.4 ± 1.0 vs. 12.1 ± 17.8 ng/mL), and fibrin formation as determined by fibrinopeptide A generation (7.5 ± 2.3 vs. 15.8 ± 23.5 ng/mL) were increased significantly in patients with acute coronary syndromes. In addition, platelet activation was enhanced in patients with unstable symptoms (2.5% ± 2.0% vs. 10.6% ± 2.4%), suggesting that these markers of fibrin formation correlate well with platelet activation.[18]

Although these markers are increased in patients with active symptoms, it is useful to note that F1.2 and fibrinopeptide A levels persist in plasma for different times. In one study, F1.2 and fibrinopeptide A levels were measured at the time of admission and at 6-month follow-up in patients with unstable angina or an acute myocardial infarction. On admission, the plasma levels of both plasma F1.2 and fibrinopeptide A were elevated, suggesting ongoing thrombosis. Among patients with an uneventful clinical course after 6 months, the median plasma levels of plasma F1.2 were unchanged whereas those of fibrinopeptide A had decreased significantly.

These observations suggest that F1.2 either remains elevated for a prolonged period or, more likely, identifies a group of patients with a persistent hypercoagulable state characterized by minimal but ongoing generation of fibrin.[19]

Fibrinopeptide A levels have been used to localize cases along the spectrum of coronary syndromes. In fact, fibrinopeptide A levels were found to be significantly higher in patients with acute coronary syndromes than in patients with stable anginal symptoms and were as much as five times higher in patients who suffered sudden cardiac death. Furthermore, levels of fibrinopeptide A were shown to be elevated in patients with an acute myocardial infarction compared with those with unstable angina, suggesting that fibrinopeptide A levels may be useful clinically to distinguish patients with stable from unstable coronary syndromes.[20]

Elevated levels of fibrinopeptide A may additionally predict outcome in patients with acute coronary syndromes. In a prospective study of patients with unstable angina, markedly elevated levels of fibrinopeptide A were associated with an increased risk of an adverse event during hospitalization. In multivariate analysis, persistent myocardial ischemia, visible thrombus at coronary angiography, and high plasma levels of fibrinopeptide A were the only independent predictors of in-hospital myocardial infarction or death.[21] In addition, fibrinopeptide A levels may predict outcome following percutaneous revascularization procedures. In 54 patients with acute coronary syndromes who underwent angioplasty, an elevated level of fibrinopeptide A measured before the procedure correlated significantly with an increased likelihood of an adverse event over the ensuing 6 months. After percutaneous revascularization, fibrinopeptide A levels were decreased markedly compared with preprocedure levels.[22]

Markers of Fibrin Formation Are Associated with Coronary Thrombosis

Elevated levels of fibrinopeptide A have been demonstrated in patients with acute coronary syndromes and angiographic evidence of intracoronary thrombus, suggesting the association between activation markers and ongoing thrombosis. This observation was confirmed in 29 patients with unstable angina and fluctuating ST-segment abnormalities on EKG who had higher fibrinopeptide A plasma levels than patients with stable T-wave inversion alone. At catheterization, coronary angiography revealed that 55% of patients with ST-segment shifts had lesions with morphologic characteristics consistent with plaque complicated by thrombosis compared with 22% of those with T-wave inversion. Fibrinopeptide A concentrations were significantly increased in 64% of patients in whom complex lesions were noted on angiographic examination.[17]

In a second study, fibrinopeptide A levels were correlated further with TIMI thrombus grade (0 to 4) in 42 patients with unstable angina. Elevated levels of urinary fibrinopeptide A were related to the presence of a filling defect (grade 4) or contrast staining (grade 3). All patients with marked increases in urinary fibrinopeptide

A levels showed grade 3 or 4 thrombus. Patients with reversible ST-segment abnormalities had significantly higher levels of fibrinopeptide A, and, in turn, ST-segment changes correlated significantly with the angiographic presence of thrombus. Despite these striking correlations, there remained a small group of patients who had no elevation in fibrinopeptide A levels with angiographically visible thrombus, and, conversely, other patients with increased fibrinopeptide A levels in the absence of visible thrombus. These findings may be explained by the observation that coronary thrombosis is a dynamic process, fibrinopeptide A is a marker of ongoing thrombosis released only during active clot formation, and the coronary angiogram is less sensitive than angioscopy for visualization of mural thrombi.[17]

Markers of Fibrin Formation and Anticoagulation Therapy

Anticoagulant therapy improves the prognosis of patients with unstable angina and acute myocardial infarction by decreasing the incidence of refractory angina, infarction, and death such that anticoagulant agents have become a fundamental component in the management of acute coronary syndromes (Table 15–2). Fibrinopeptide A levels have been shown to decrease after the administration of heparin owing to the greater inhibition of thrombin exerted by the antithrombin III/heparin complex. Persistently elevated levels of fibrinopeptide A in patients receiving heparin may therefore be used to identify patients who are resistant to heparin.[17] In contrast with what is observed for fibrinopeptide A, levels of F1.2 are not reduced by heparin therapy, even at doses that achieve a therapeutic activated partial thromboplastin time and decrease fibrinopeptide A levels. Furthermore, when patients treated with heparin who had recurrent angina or reinfarction or who had died were examined, they had persistently elevated levels of F1.2 and fibrinopeptide A, suggesting inadequate suppression of thrombin generation.[23] Among patients treated with heparin or hirudin prior to percutaneous coronary intervention, persons with fibrinopeptide A levels of less than 5 ng/mL showed significant improvement in luminal cross-sectional area and TIMI flow grade on serial angiograms over a 24-hour period compared with patients who had higher fibrinopeptide A levels.[24]

To examine the effects of thrombolytic therapy for ST-segment elevation myocardial infarction on markers of thrombin generation and clinical outcome, patients enrolled in the Global Utilization of Streptokinase and TPA for Occluded Coronary Arteries (GUSTO) I study underwent measurement of plasma F1.2 and fibrinopeptide A levels at baseline and at different time points after thrombolytic therapy was initiated. Fibrinopeptide A levels were elevated at baseline and increased 90 minutes after the administration of streptokinase and heparin. Despite adjunctive heparin therapy, F1.2 levels remained elevated, suggesting a continued hypercoagulable state. Interestingly, levels of F1.2 at study entry were significantly related to the risk of reinfarction or death at 30 days, and levels measured 12 hours after the initiation of therapy remained an independent predictor of 30-day mortality.[25]

Although intracoronary thrombus formation is a common pathophysiologic finding associated with acute ST-segment elevation myocardial infarction and unstable angina, thrombolytic therapy has not demonstrated efficacy, and may even be harmful, when administered to patients with unstable angina. When patients with unstable angina were randomized to receive a 60-minute or 48-hour infusion of streptokinase or placebo in addition to heparin, there was no detectable change (from baseline) in thrombin generation in patients who received the placebo. In contrast, an early increase in thrombin production was measured in patients who received either the acute or the prolonged streptokinase infusion. In the later group, higher levels of F1.2 persisted throughout the 48 hours of streptokinase infusion. In addition, patients treated with prolonged thrombolytic infusion were more likely to experience myocardial infarction that tended to occur when thrombolysis was initiated. Among patients treated with heparin alone, events occurred throughout the 72-hour study period.[26]

To examine the effect of platelet inhibition with a glycoprotein IIb/IIIa receptor antagonist on thrombin generation and activity, investigators measured fibrinopeptide A and F1.2 levels in 32 patients with acute coronary syndromes undergoing percutaneous revascularization and treated with aspirin, heparin, and abciximab. After a successful coronary revascularization, there was a significant decrease in fibrinopeptide A (1.46 ± 1.16 ng/mL) and F1.2 levels (0.59 ± 0.22 nmol/L) compared with levels measured prior to intervention. In patients who did not receive a glycoprotein IIb/IIIa

■ ▪ ■

TABLE 15–2   INFLUENCE OF ANTICOAGULANT THERAPY ON MARKERS OF THROMBIN ACTIVITY

	FIBRINOPEPTIDE A	PROTHROMBIN FRAGMENT 1.2
Heparin	↓	No change
Hirudin	↓	↓
Streptokinase	↓	↑
Recombinant tissue-type plasminogen activator	↓	↑
Glycoprotein IIb/III antagonists	↓	↓

Data from references 27, 59, 60.

antagonist as adjunctive therapy, there was a slight increase in fibrinopeptide A levels (2.25 ± 1.58 ng/mL) and an increase in F1.2 levels (0.22 ± 0.3 nmol/L), suggesting that the addition of abciximab to standard anticoagulant therapy with aspirin and heparin is associated with a significant decrease in thrombin generation.[27]

Markers of Fibrin Formation As Predictors of Acute Coronary Syndromes

Although increases in circulating activation markers have been associated with acute coronary syndromes, activation markers indicate the presence of thrombosis in any vascular bed. It is also recognized that circulating levels of markers may increase in the absence of overt thrombosis, reflecting a "prethrombotic state." Therefore, in patients with acute coronary syndromes, the specificity and positive predictive value of the various markers for the presence of coronary thrombus remains low. Several studies have been conducted to examine the utility of markers of fibrin formation as predictors of acute coronary syndromes and have yielded conflicting results.[17]

In an initial study of 150 patients with unstable angina, patients with increased fibrinopeptide A levels had a higher incidence of nonfatal myocardial infarction or death than patients with normal levels, suggesting that fibrinopeptide A levels may predict outcome; however, these findings were disputed in the GUSTO-I substudy that failed to relate plasma fibrinopeptide A levels at admission to the outcome of death or reinfarction at 30 days.[17]

The predictive value of fibrinopeptide A was examined in a heterogeneous population of patients who presented to the emergency department for evaluation of chest pain. In 247 patients, fibrinopeptide A levels were measured from urine samples; to validate the findings, troponin I, myoglobin, and myosin light chains were also measured in serum. By multivariate analysis, patients with elevated fibrinopeptide A levels were 4.82 times as likely to have a major adverse cardiac event, including death, myocardial infarction, recurrent angina, or revascularization, at 1 week (P = .002; 95% CI, 1.78 to 13.03), whereas those with an elevated troponin I were 9.41 times as likely to have an event (P < .001; 95% CI, 2.84 to 31.17) during this period. At 6 months following the initial presentation, an elevated fibrinopeptide A level was the only independent predictor of events during the interim period, with an odds ratio of 9.57 (P < .001; 95% CI, 3.29 to 27.8) and was the only marker to predict a shorter event-free survival. All other markers failed to correlate independently with cardiac events (Fig. 15-2).[28]

No compelling data ascertain the prognostic value of increased F1.2 or TAT levels in patients with unstable angina or non–ST-segment elevation myocardial infarction. Increased F1.2 levels have been documented for up to 6 months after the first episode of unstable angina or acute myocardial infarction; however, F1.2 levels have not been associated with the risk of cardiac events. In patients with acute myocardial infarction who received thrombolytic agents, baseline F1.2 concentrations were

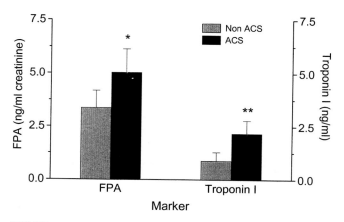

FIGURE 15–2. Fibrinopeptide A and acute coronary syndromes. Fibrinopeptide A levels were measured in patients who presented to the emergency department for the evaluation of chest pain. Fibrinopeptide A, a marker of thrombus formation, was determined and compared with troponin I, a measure of myocardial injury, in patients with chest pain. Patients who were admitted with the diagnosis of acute coronary syndrome had significantly higher levels of fibrinopeptide A and troponin I than patients with noncardiac chest pain. ACS, acute coronary syndrome; FPA, fibrinopeptide A; *, P < .04 vs. non-ACS; **, P < .003 vs. non-ACS.[28]

higher in patients who experienced an adverse outcome than in those who experienced no complications after the infarction. In this study population, TAT levels were not significantly different between the two patient groups.[17]

Moreover, one study of patients who presented to the emergency department for the evaluation of chest pain failed to demonstrate the diagnostic utility of F1.2 and TAT levels. In this study, 80 patients with chest pain were compared with 20 healthy controls. There was no difference in F1.2 and TAT levels between patients with noncardiac chest pain and healthy volunteers, but patients with an acute coronary syndrome had higher TAT levels than control patients; however, patients with an acute ST-segment myocardial infarction had F1.2 and TAT levels well below that observed for patients with unstable angina and congestive heart failure. These findings suggest that F1.2 and TAT may not be useful in the triage of patients with chest pain in the emergency department.[29]

In recent studies, soluble fibrin has been shown to predict outcome in patients with acute coronary syndromes. When 159 patients with electrocardiographic evidence of myocardial ischemia were evaluated within 24 hours of symptom onset, 103 patients were found to have evidence consistent with myocardial infarction and 56 were classified as having unstable angina. Pretreatment soluble fibrin levels were measured on admission, and patients were observed for adverse clinical events during the hospital course. Approximately 11.9% of patients reached the clinical end point of myocardial infarction or death during hospitalization. Patients who experienced an adverse outcome were found to have higher initial soluble fibrin levels than those patients with an uncomplicated course. When patients were evaluated by tercile of soluble fibrin levels, event rates increased proportionally with soluble fibrin concentrations (7.5% in the lower, 7.5% in the middle, and 20.7% in the highest tercile; P = .036). In the highest tercile, the relative risk of death or myocardial infarction was 1.92 (95% CI, 1.21 to 3.06).[17]

MARKERS THAT ORIGINATE FROM FIBRIN DEGRADATION

Indices of fibrinolytic activity and fibrin degradation, including endogenous tissue-type plasminogen activator (t-PA), plasminogen activator inhibitor type-1 (PAI-1), plasmin-α_2-antiplasmin complexes, and cross-linked fibrinogen degradation products (FDPs), have also been suggested as markers of a thrombotic state with clinical value in the assessment of patients with acute coronary syndromes (Table 15–3).

The vascular endothelium synthesizes and releases t-PA to facilitate local fibrinolysis of fibrin-based clots. Impaired t-PA release has been associated with systemic disorders characterized by endothelial dysfunction, such as diabetes mellitus, and may promote thrombotic complications in these patients.[30] In a series of 38 patients with confirmed acute coronary syndromes, t-PA levels were determined before and after the administration of heparin. At hospital admission, patients with unstable angina had significantly higher levels of plasma t-PA than healthy age-matched controls. Furthermore, heparin infusion was associated with an increase in t-PA release in patients with an acute coronary syndrome.[31] Among 31 patients with unstable coronary syndromes, plasma t-PA mass concentrations, a more sensitive measure of t-PA levels, were positively correlated with complexity of culprit coronary artery lesion morphology.[32]

PAI-1 is also released from endothelial cells and complexes with t-PA to neutralize its actions. In fact, it is the formation of these complexes that may render t-PA a less useful marker of thrombosis because concentrations of t-PA and PAI-1 measured by standard activity assays may be inaccurate. Nevertheless, elevated PAI-1 levels have been measured in patients with coronary heart disease risk factors, hypertriglyceridemia, insulin resistance, and an activated renin-angiotensin-aldosterone system.[33] Therefore, it is not surprising that increased levels of PAI-1 have been detected in patients with active unstable angina as compared with healthy subjects.[31,32]

Plasmin-α_2-antiplasmin complexes are formed during fibrinolytic activation and have been measured as evidence of plasmin generation. In fact, in one study of 85 patients with post-infarction angina, new-onset angina, or crescendo angina, plasmin-α_2-antiplasmin levels were significantly higher than at hospital admission compared with healthy subjects; however, increased levels of this marker of a thrombotic state did not correlate with in-hospital adverse events, nor did they predict outcome 6 months after hospitalization. Thus, the clinical utility of plasmin-α_2-antiplasmin levels remains unclear.[34]

Cross-linked FDPs are a heterogeneous group of polypeptides that formed by the degradation of fibrinogen, fibrin monomer I, fibrin II monomer, or cross-linked fibrin polymers by plasmin. Proteolysis of fibrinogen yields fragments X, Y, D, and E, which are recognized as FDPs. Digestion of cross-linked fibrin results in the release of numerous cleavage products, including XY, DD, and DY. Of these, the D-dimer fragment, which contains D regions cross-linked at the γ-chains, is the best characterized. The plasma concentrations of FDPs reflect plasmin-mediated fibrin turnover and, therefore, are a sensitive marker of ongoing thrombosis.[17,30]

Increased plasma levels of FDPs are a marker of increased risk for major adverse events following hospital admission with an acute myocardial infarction. The prognostic value of increased cross-linked FDPs was evaluated in 109 patients with unstable angina or acute myocardial infarction not eligible for thrombolytic therapy (Fig. 15–3). In this cohort, 24.4% of patients with a positive FDP result reached the primary end point of in-hospital death or infarction compared with 7.9% of patients with a negative result (relative risk, 2.2; 95% CI, 1.2 to 3.8), suggesting that early measurement of FDPs predicts in-hospital outcome.[35]

To examine the diagnostic value of D-dimer measurements in patients with chest pain, investigators obtained levels in 257 consecutive patients with chest pain who presented to the emergency department for evaluation. D-dimer and fibrinogen levels were significantly higher in patients with ischemic cardiac events than in patients with noncardiac chest pain. D-dimer levels greater than 500 μg/L were found to have an independent diagnostic value for myocardial infarction and improved the diagnostic sensitivity of the electrocardiogram and history from 73% to 92%. Thus, D-dimer levels may add independent information to the clinical assessment for myocardial infarction.[34]

D-dimer levels may also be elevated in patients with stable coronary disease. This issue was examined in 312 patients with angiographically proven coronary artery disease and 477 age-matched healthy subjects. Median D-dimer levels were significantly higher in patients with established coronary disease than in controls (11.2 vs. 2.8 ng/mL; $P < .001$). Furthermore, the odds ratio for presence of coronary artery disease was found to be 2.6 (95% CI, 1.9 to 3.5) based on D-dimer levels in the highest quartile compared with the lower three quartiles. These observations suggest that plasma D-dimer levels correlate with the presence of coronary artery disease in patients with stable angina.[36]

■ ▪ ■

TABLE 15–3   MARKERS OF FIBRINOLYTIC ACTIVITY AND FIBRIN FORMATION

Tissue-type plasminogen activator
Plaminogen activator inhibitor type 1
Plasmin-α_2-antiplasmin complex
Fibrin degradation products

FACTORS IX AND XI

In acute coronary syndromes, thrombus formation is initiated by the activation of soluble clotting factors to form

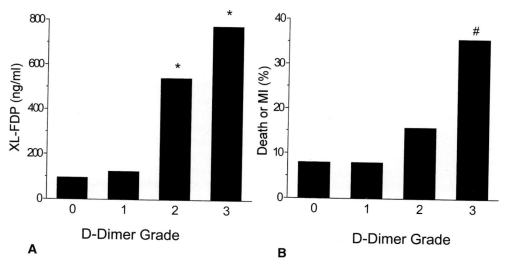

FIGURE 15–3. The prognostic value of cross-linked fibrin degradation product levels. Cross-linked fibrin degradation products (XL-FDP) and D-dimer levels were measured in 109 patients with acute coronary syndromes. *A*, D-dimer levels were graded as 0 = negative (n = 63), 1 = trace (n = 13), 2 = positive (n = 19), and 3 = strongly positive (n = 14), and these levels were found to correlate with XL-FDP levels as determined by enzyme-linked immunosorbent assay. *B*, Elevated D-dimer levels were associated with a higher incidence of death or myocardial infarction (MI), suggesting that a subgroup of patients may benefit from more aggressive antiplatelet therapy. ACS, acute coronary syndrome; *, *P* < .001 vs. grade 0; #, *P* < .01 vs. grade 0.[35]

the catalytic tissue factor–factor VIIa complex. This complex, in turn, activates factors X and IX to generate thrombin. Thrombin-dependent activation of factor XI serves as an amplification pathway to form additional thrombin. This pathway is regulated further by inactivation of factor XIa by the circulating inhibitors, C1-inhibitor and α_2-antiplasmin. Factor XIa–inhibitor complexes are detectable in plasma; in fact, it has been demonstrated that approximately 47% of factor XIa is inactivated by C1 inhibitor whereas 24.5% is inactivated by α_2-antiplasmin. The remaining 28.5% of factor XIa complexes with antithrombin III or α_1-antitrypsin to render it inactive.[37]

To determine whether factors XI and IX may serve as a marker of thrombosis in acute coronary syndromes, 150 patients with acute myocardial infarction, unstable angina, or stable angina were evaluated. Interestingly, factor XIa–C1 inhibitor complexes, which may only be measured within hours of initiation of the clotting cascade, were detected in 24% of patients who presented with an acute myocardial infarction compared with 8% of patients with unstable angina and 4% of patients with stable angina. In contrast, factor XIa–α_1-antitrypsin complexes, which may be measured up to 10 days after the index event, were equally elevated among the patient groups. Similarly, factor IX peptide levels were higher in patients with an acute myocardial infarction or unstable angina than in patients with stable angina, suggesting that activation of these clotting factors may be a useful diagnostic marker in patients with acute coronary syndromes.[38]

PLATELET-DERIVED MARKERS OF THROMBOSIS

Intracoronary plaque disruption due to spontaneous rupture or mechanical intervention serves as a nidus for local platelet activation and aggregation. This pathophysiologic process may progress until an occlusive thrombus is formed, resulting in symptoms recognized clinically as an acute coronary syndrome.

Owing to the wide spectrum of outcomes in patients with acute coronary syndromes and the dynamic nature of thrombus formation and lysis, markers of platelet activation have significant clinical utility. At present, several markers of platelet activation have been identified and validated to assess platelet activation in vivo by ex vivo measures in patients with acute coronary syndromes (Table 15–4).

Platelet Factor 4 and β-Thromboglobulin

One method to assess platelet activation is to measure platelet-release products in platelet-poor plasma. In fact, platelet factor 4 and β-thromboglobulin, proteins released from α-granules after platelet activation, may be measured by radioimmunoassay or enzyme-linked immunoadsorbent assays and provide a simple method to evaluate platelet activation.[39] Levels of platelet factor 4 and β-thromboglobulin were shown to be elevated in patients with unstable angina for up to 2 days after the index event, falling gradually thereafter.[40] Furthermore, in patients with an acute myocardial infarction, levels of β-thromboglobulin were increased significantly compared with healthy control subjects (105 ± 27 IU/mL vs. 35 ± 9 IU/mL; *P* < .001), decreased after successful reperfusion therapy with streptokinase, and elevated again only in patients who experienced postinfarction angina, thereby demonstrating that activated platelets modulate acute coronary syndromes.[41] In contrast, the Angina Prognosis Study in Stockholm (APSIS), which measured platelet counts and β-thromboglobulin levels in 809 patients with stable angina, failed to relate these markers to cardiovascular outcomes.[42] This may be due

■ ▨ ■

TABLE 15–4   PLATELET MARKERS OF THOMBOSIS DETECTED BY FLOW CYTOMETRY

Exposure of granule membrane markers
   CD62p (P-selectin)
   CD63
   LAMP-1
   CD40L
Glycoprotein IIb/IIIa activation–dependent changes
Binding of secreted proteins
   Thrombospondin
   Multimerin
Exposure of phosphatidylserine on exofacial plasma membrane
Monocyte–platelet aggregates
   CD40L/CD40
   CD62p-PSGL1
   CD36-TSP-CD36
   Macl-Fg-glycoprotein IIb/IIIa
Platelet microparticles

in part to the fact that patients enrolled in the study had stable rather than unstable symptoms.

P-Selectin

Whole blood flow cytometry has been developed for clinical application to analyze activated platelets, platelet hyperreactivity, platelet-leukocyte aggregates, and circulating platelet microparticles. The platelet activation markers that are commonly measured include exposure of granule membrane markers, including P-selectin (also known as CD62p), CD63, LAMP-1, and CD40L; activation-dependent changes in the conformation of the GP IIb/IIIa complex; binding of secreted proteins such as multimerin; and exposure of the negatively charged phospholipid phosphatidylserine, which is involved in binding of coagulation factors and assembly of enzyme-cofactor complexes.[39]

Soluble P-selectin derived from activated platelets has additionally been shown to be a useful marker of platelet activation. P-selectin is a membrane protein that is expressed only on the surface of activated platelets and is detectable by flow cytometry. After enzymatic cleavage of membrane-bound P-selectin, soluble P-selectin is released, circulates in plasma, and may be measured as an index of platelet activation. In vivo studies have demonstrated that degranulated platelets rapidly lose surface P-selectin while they continue to circulate and function normally. Therefore, accurate determination of P-selectin requires measurement of both surface expression and plasma levels. In healthy control subjects, soluble P-selectin has been validated as a marker specific for platelet activation; however, in patients with acute coronary syndromes it is possible that endothelial injury may contribute to measurable P-selectin levels.[39] Utilizing these markers, investigators have evaluated platelet activation and the influence of anticoagulant therapies in patients with acute coronary syndromes and during percutaneous revascularization procedures.

The utility of P-selectin as a marker to follow the time course of platelet activation in patients with acute coronary syndromes was evaluated in the TIMI 12 trial (Fig.

15–4). In this phase II trial of sibrafiban, an oral selective antagonist of the platelet glycoprotein IIb/IIIa receptor, P-selectin levels were measured at several time points over a 28-day period in a subset of 90 patients. At baseline, P-selectin levels in patients with active symptoms were significantly increased compared with stable patients (27.6% ± 18.7% vs. 10.9% ± 7.1%; P < .005), suggesting that enhanced platelet activation was associated with unstable patients. Although P-selectin levels declined significantly over the 28-day period in both patient groups, at day 28, those patients who initially presented with active chest pain continued to demonstrate evidence of platelet activation when compared with patients in stable condition.[43]

The sensitivity of P-selectin as a marker of platelet activation was examined by determining the threshold of α-granule degranulation and fibrinogen binding in patients with acute coronary syndromes using flow cytometry in whole blood samples. Compared with the case in normal volunteers, ADP-induced fibrinogen binding was found to be a low-threshold activation event, with 40% of platelets binding fibrinogen in response to 0.2 μmol/L of ADP. Degranulation of α-granules was a higher threshold event with 33% of platelets expressing P-selectin in response to 1 μmol/L ADP. Interestingly, ADP-mediated P-selectin expression was increased in patients with acute coronary syndromes compared with healthy subjects, but no difference in ADP-induced fibrinogen binding was observed.[44]

Clinically, increased P-selectin levels, reflecting platelet activation, have been found on platelets obtained proximal to a ruptured coronary plaque. Among patients undergoing percutaneous coronary revascularization procedures, blood samples were acquired from a guiding catheter placed in to the culprit vessel immediately proximal to a ruptured plaque. When aortic blood sam-

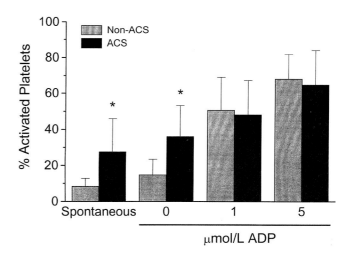

FIGURE 15–4. Acute coronary syndromes and platelet activation. Patients who present with an acute coronary syndrome demonstrated enhanced baseline platelet activation compared with healthy volunteers; however, there was no significant difference in platelet activation after stimulation with increasing concentrations of adenosine diphosphate (ADP). Platelet activation was measured by analysis of P-selectin as detected by flow cytometry. ACS, acute coronary syndrome; *, P < .005 vs. non-ACS.[43]

ples were collected from 23 patients with acute coronary syndromes and compared with those from 22 patients with stable angina and no angiographic evidence of plaque rupture, the groups showed no significant difference in P-selectin expression in response to 0.2 µM ADP (6.1% ± 1% vs. 6.9% ± 1.4%); however, P-selectin expression was increased in platelets obtained from samples taken immediately proximal to the lesion (8.8% ± 1.6% vs. 6.5% ± 1.4%), suggesting increased local platelet reactivity.[45]

Owing to the observed differences in P-selectin levels, and, therefore to platelet reactivity, among patients with acute coronary syndromes compared with those with stable symptoms, there has been some speculation that P-selectin levels may differ between patients who present with an acute myocardial infarction and patients who present with unstable angina. As expected, the percentage of platelets expressing P-selectin was higher in patients with an acute myocardial infarction than in patients with unstable angina (9.1% vs. 4.2%; P = .03), suggesting that enhanced platelet activation is associated with myocardial infarction.[46]

Measurement of platelet and soluble P-selectin levels, when compared with traditional markers of myocardial necrosis, has been used to triage patients who present to the emergency department with chest pain. In 122 patients who presented to the emergency department for evaluation, P-selectin levels were shown to correlate strongly with CK-MB isoenzyme levels. Furthermore, platelet P-selectin and CK-MB were found to be independent predictors of acute myocardial infarction. Interestingly, the diagnostic value of P-selectin was increased by concomitant myoglobin and cardiac troponin I measurements.[47]

CD40L/CD40

One limitation associated with measurement of surface markers on circulating activated platelets is that fully activated platelets may be localized in thrombi and thereby immobilized. It has been previously demonstrated that activated platelets bind both monocytes and neutrophils by a number of different receptor-ligand pairs or associations, including platelet P-selectin–leukocyte P-selectin glycoprotein ligand-1 (CD62p-PSGL1); platelet CD36–thrombospondin-1–macrophage CD36 (CD36-TSP-1-CD36); and platelet CD40L–monocyte/macrophage CD40. For example, activated platelets express the surface marker P-selectin, which binds PSGL-1 on the plasma membrane of neutrophils or monocytes and facilitates rolling of leukocytes on adherent, activated platelets.[48] CD36, formerly known as glycoprotein IV, has been identified in monocytes and macrophages in addition to platelets. CD36 binds thrombospondin-1, released from platelet α-granules or present in the extracellular membrane, myeloperoxidase-oxidized LDL, and long-chain fatty acids and thereby forms a bridge between activated platelets and monocytes/macrophages.[49] CD40L is found preformed in platelets and rapidly recycled to the surface membrane after exposure to thrombin and platelet activation. CD40L binds CD40 that is constitutively expressed on monocytes and macrophages, thereby recruiting leukocytes to areas of thrombus formation.[50] Thus, platelet-leukocyte complexes may be a more sensitive marker of in vivo platelet activation; in fact, increased numbers of circulating platelet-leukocyte complexes have been demonstrated in patients with acute coronary syndromes.[39] In addition, these associations suggest a mechanism by which thrombosis and inflammation may be linked.

CD40L/CD40 expression on platelets has been shown to be two times higher in patients with an acute myocardial infarction and three times higher in patients with unstable angina than in healthy volunteers. In addition, levels of soluble CD40L/CD40 was found to be approximately 1.5 times higher in patients with acute coronary syndromes than in controls. At 6 months after the index event, CD40L/CD40 expression levels were significantly reduced in patients with acute coronary syndromes and had in fact returned to baseline levels comparable to those observed in normal volunteers. Interestingly, patients who required evaluation during the interim for recurrent angina or requiring revascularization procedures were found to have elevated levels of CD40L/CD40 concordant with their symptoms compared with the rest of the study group.[51]

Monocyte–Platelet Aggregates

Circulating monocyte–platelet aggregates have additionally been suggested to be a more sensitive marker of in vivo platelet activation than surface P-selectin. In a baboon model infused with autologous, biotinylated platelets, flow-cytometric analysis demonstrated that infused degranulated platelets rapidly formed circulating aggregates with monocytes and neutrophils in vivo. Approximately 30 minutes after the infusion, the percentage of circulating monocytes aggregated with infused platelets persisted at high levels; on the other hand, the percentage of circulating neutrophils aggregated with infused platelets, as well as platelet surface P-selectin of nonaggregated infused platelets, returned toward baseline. These observations were confirmed in patients with acute coronary syndromes who underwent percutaneous revascularization. Blood samples obtained at the time of catheterization revealed an increased number of circulating monocyte–platelet aggregates and, to a lesser extent, neutrophil–platelet aggregates, but not P-selectin–positive platelets, suggesting that circulating monocyte–platelet aggregates are a more sensitive marker of in vivo platelet activation than platelet surface P-selectin.[52]

Monocyte-platelet aggregates have also been shown to predict acute myocardial infarction. In one study of 93 patients who presented to the emergency department for the evaluation of chest pain, 9 patients with documented acute myocardial infarction were found to have a higher level of circulating monocyte–platelet aggregates than patients without a myocardial infarction or normal controls; the percentage of P-selectin–positive platelets was not significantly different.[52] These observations were confirmed in a larger study of 211 consecutive patients who presented to the emergency department with chest pain. In this group, 61 patients were deemed to have suffered acute myocardial infarction. These patients, compared with those without infarction, had increased numbers of circulating monocyte-platelet aggregates. After adjusting for age, the odds ratio of acute myocardial infarction for patients in the highest quartile compared with those in the lowest quartile of monocyte-platelet aggregate numbers was 10.8 (95% CI, 3.6 to 32.0). Of note, circulating monocyte-platelet aggregate levels were highest in patients who presented to the emergency department within 4 hours of symptom onset. In addition, 57% of patients with an elevated level of monocyte-platelet aggregates had normal creatine kinase levels at the time of evaluation, demonstrating that circulating monocyte-platelet aggregates are an early marker of myocardial infarction.[53]

The influence of anticoagulant therapy with heparin and glycoprotein IIb/IIIa antagonists on platelet activation as measured by monocyte-platelet aggregates, neutrophil platelet aggregates, and P-selectin levels was examined by whole blood flow cytometry in 40 patients with unstable angina. Patients were treated with either unfractionated or low-molecular-weight heparin and abciximab before a planned percutaneous coronary revascularization procedure. Patients who received unfractionated, but not low-molecular-weight, heparin had increased numbers of P-selectin-positive platelets, a finding that was reversed with abciximab administration. At 8 to 10 and 16 to 24 hours after the initiation of anticoagulant therapy, the number of P-selectin-positive platelets and platelet degranulation in response to thrombin receptor-activating peptide was decreased by approximately 50%. Interestingly, heparin administration increased the number of monocyte-platelet aggregates and neutrophil-platelet aggregates, whereas the abciximab bolus decreased aggregate formation and monocyte-platelet aggregate levels fell below baseline and remained there for up to 16 to 24 hours. These observations suggest that unfractionated heparin, but not low-molecular-weight heparin, degranulates platelets in patients with unstable angina, whereas both types of heparin increase the number of circulating monocyte-platelet aggregates that may be reversed with glycoprotein IIb/IIIa receptor blockade.[54]

Microparticle Shedding

Aminophospholipid exposure and microparticle shedding are also markers of platelet activation. Flow cytometry was used to measure platelet procoagulant activity by annexin V binding and platelet microparticle shedding in venous and coronary blood samples from 30 patients with unstable angina before and after percutaneous revascularization procedures. Compared with control subjects, baseline levels of platelet procoagulant activity and microparticle shedding were significantly increased. Microparticle shedding was found to be greater (1) in the coronary arterial blood than in venous samples and (2) in the coronary blood of patients with proximal, as opposed to distal, lesions. GP IIb/IIIa receptor and P-selectin expression declined 24 to 48 hours after the procedure, but platelet procoagulant activity

and microparticle shedding were not significantly altered.[55]

ENDOTHELIUM-DERIVED MICROPARTICLES AS MARKERS OF THROMBOSIS

Tissue factor activity is highly dependent on the negatively charged phosphatidylserine that is redistributed to the cell surface during apoptotic cell death. Interestingly, shed membrane apoptotic microparticles rich in phosphatidylserine are produced in considerable amounts within human atherosclerotic plaque and have been shown to contain almost all of the tissue factor activity. These cell-derived microparticles with procoagulant activity may additionally be released into the peripheral circulation and therefore serve as a thrombotic marker in acute coronary syndromes. This mechanism was confirmed in a study of 39 patients with established coronary heart disease, including 27 patients with unstable symptoms. Levels of procoagulant microparticles of endothelial origin were determined by isolation with annexin V and assayed with a prothrombinase assay for procoagulant activity. Levels of procoagulant microparticles were found to be significantly elevated in patients with acute coronary syndromes compared with patients with noncardiac chest pain or stable angina. Therefore, elevated levels of endothelial microparticles serve as a marker of a thrombotic state associated with acute coronary syndromes and contribute further to the initiation and perpetuation of coronary thrombosis.[56]

CONCLUSIONS

The clinical symptoms associated with acute coronary syndromes arise from spontaneous plaque rupture, resulting in platelet activation and thrombus formation. These pathobiologic events are common across the spectrum of unstable coronary syndromes and, owing to the degree of intracoronary thrombus formation (i.e., occlusive vs. nonocclusive), determine clinical presentation and outcome.[57, 58] The current diagnostic markers reflect myocardial necrosis. Measurement of markers that indicate ongoing thrombosis, fibrin formation, or degradation offer promise as novel diagnostic indicators for patients with acute coronary syndromes. Such markers may serve to identify patients for therapeutic intervention earlier in their clinical course.

REFERENCES

1. Lee TH, Rouan GW, Weisberg MC, et al: Sensitivity of routine clinical criteria for diagnosing myocardial infarction within 24 hours of hospitalization. Ann Intern Med 1987;106:181–186.
2. Collinson PO, Wiggins N, Gaze DC: Clinical evaluation of the ACS:180 cardiac troponin I assay. Ann Clin Biochem 2001;38:509–519.
3. Collinson PO, Boa FG, Gaze DC: Measurement of cardiac troponins. Ann Clin Biochem 2001;38:423–449.
4. Best LC, Marten J, Russell RG, et al: Prostacyclin increases cyclic AMP levels and adenylate cyclase activity in platelets. Nature 1977;267:850–852.

5. Radomski MW, Palmer RM, Moncada S: Endogenous nitric oxide inhibits human platelet adhesion to vascular endothelium. Lancet 1987;2:1057-1058.

6. Hourani SM, Cusack NJ: Pharmacological receptors on blood platelets. Pharmacol Rev 1991;43:243-298.

7. Ware JA, Heistad DD: Seminars in medicine of the Beth Israel Hospital, Boston. Platelet-endothelium interactions. N Engl J Med 1993;328:628-635.

8. Kroll MH, Harris TS, Moake JL, et al: von Willebrand factor binding to platelet GpIb initiates signals for platelet activation. J Clin Invest 1991;88:1568-1573.

9. Chow TW, Hellums JD, Moake JL, et al: Shear stress-induced von Willebrand factor binding to platelet glycoprotein Ib initiates calcium influx associated with aggregation. Blood 1992;80:113-120.

10. Karniguian A, Grelac F, Levy-Toledano S, et al: Collagen-induced platelet activation mainly involves the protein kinase C pathway. Biochem J 1990;268:325-331.

11. Daniel JL, Molish IR, Rigmaiden M, et al: Evidence for a role of myosin phosphorylation in the initiation of the platelet shape change response. J Biol Chem 1984;259:9826-9831.

12. Kroll MH, Schafer AI: Biochemical mechanisms of platelet activation. Blood 1989;74:1181-1195.

13. Janmey PA, Lamb JA, Ezzell RM, et al: Effects of actin filaments on fibrin clot structure and lysis. Blood 1992;80:928-936.

14. Zwaal RF, Comfurius P, Bevers EM: Lipid-protein interactions in blood coagulation. Biochim Biophys Acta 1998;1376:433-453.

15. Mann KG, van't Neer C, Cawthern K, et al: The role of the tissue factor pathway in initiation of coagulation. Blood Coagul Fibrinolysis 1998;9(Suppl 1):S3-S7.

16. Dahlback B: Blood coagulation. Lancet 2000;355:1627-1632.

17. Ottani F, Galvani M: Prognostic role of hemostatic markers in acute coronary syndromes patients. Clin Chim Acta 2001;311:33-39.

18. Becker RC, Bovill EG, Corrao JM, et al: Dynamic nature of thrombin generation, fibrin formation, and platelet activation in unstable angina and non-q-wave myocardial infarction. J Thromb Thrombolysis 1995;2:57-64.

19. Merlini PA, Bauer KA, Oltrona L, et al: Persistent activation of coagulation mechanism in unstable angina and myocardial infarction. Circulation 1994;90:61-68.

20. Manten A, de Winter RJ, Minnema MC, et al: Procoagulant and proinflammatory activity in acute coronary syndromes. Cardiovasc Res 1998;40:389-395.

21. Ardissino D, Merlini PA, Gamba T, et al: Thrombin activity and early outcome in unstable angina pectoris. Circulation 1996;93:1634-1639.

22. Wilensky RL, Pyles JM, Fineberg N: Increased thrombin activity correlates with increased ischemic event rate after percutaneous transluminal coronary angioplasty: Lack of efficacy of locally delivered urokinase. Am Heart J 1999;138(2 Part 1):319-325.

23. Merlini PA, Ardissino D, Bauer KA, et al: Persistent thrombin generation during heparin therapy in patients with acute coronary syndromes. Arterioscler Thromb Vasc Biol 1997;17:1325-1330.

24. Rao AK, Sun L, Chesebro JH, et al: Distinct effects of recombinant desulfatohirudin (Revasc) and heparin on plasma levels of fibrinopeptide A and prothrombin fragment F1.2 in unstable angina. A multicenter trial. Circulation 1996;94:2389-2395.

25. Granger CB, Becker R, Tracy RD, et al: Thrombin generation, inhibition and clinical outcomes in patients with acute myocardial infarction treated with thrombolytic therapy and heparin: Results from the GUSTO-I Trial. GUSTO-I Hemostasis Substudy Group. Global Utilization of Streptokinase and TPA for Occluded Coronary Arteries. J Am Coll Cardiol 1998;31:497-505.

26. Merlini PA, Ardissino D, Bauer KA, et al: Activation of the hemostatic mechanism during thrombolysis in patients with unstable angina pectoris. Blood 1995;86:3327-3332.

27. Dangas G, Marmur JD, King TE, et al: Effects of platelet glycoprotein IIb/IIIa inhibition with abciximab on thrombin generation and activity during percutaneous coronary intervention. Am Heart J 1999;138(1 Part 1):49-54.

28. Sonel A, Sasseen BM, Fineberg N, et al: Prospective study correlating fibrinopeptide A, troponin I, myoglobin, and myosin light chain levels with early and late ischemic events in consecutive patients presenting to the emergency department with chest pain. Circulation 2000;102:1107-1113.

29. McKenzie ME, Pothula A, Gurbel PA, et al: Failure of thrombin generation markers to triage patients presenting with chest pain. Cardiology 1999;92:53-58.

30. Fareed J, Hoppensteadt DA, Leya F, et al: Useful laboratory tests for studying thrombogenesis in acute cardiac syndromes. Clin Chem 1998;44:1845-1853.

31. Olivotti L, Spallarossa P, Piana A, et al: Maximal endothelial tissue plasminogen activator release is not impaired in patients with acute coronary syndromes before heparin treatment. Blood Coagul Fibrinolysis 2001;12:261-267.

32. Hoffmeister HM, Jur M, Helbur U, et al: Correlation between coronary morphology and molecular markers of fibrinolysis in unstable angina pectoris. Atherosclerosis 1999;144:151-157.

33. Huber K: Defective fibrinolytic states as triggers of myocardial infarction: The cardiologist's view. Ital Heart J 2001;2:646-651.

34. Bayes-Genis A, Guindo J, Oliver A, et al: Elevated levels of plasmin-alpha2 antiplasmin complexes in unstable angina. Thromb Haemost 1999;81:865-868.

35. Galvani M, Ottani F, Puggioni R, et al: Value of a new bedside D-dimer assay for early risk stratification of patients with acute coronary syndromes. Circulation 1996;94:I-133.

36. Koenig W, Rothenbacher D, Hoffmeister A, et al: Plasma fibrin D-dimer levels and risk of stable coronary artery disease: results of a large case-control study. Arterioscler Thromb Vasc Biol 2001;21:1701-1705.

37. Wuillemin WA, Minnema M, Meijers JC, et al: Inactivation of factor XIa in human plasma assessed by measuring factor XIa-protease inhibitor complexes: Major role for C1-inhibitor. Blood 1995;85:1517-1526.

38. Minnema MC, Peters RJ, de Winter R, et al: Activation of clotting factors XI and IX in patients with acute myocardial infarction. Arterioscler Thromb Vasc Biol 2000;20:2489-2493.

39. Harrison P: Progress in the assessment of platelet function. Br J Haematol 2000;111:733-744.

40. al-Nozha M, Gader AM, al-Momen AK, et al: Haemostatic variables in patients with unstable angina. Int J Cardiol 1994;43:269-277.

41. Salvioni A, Marenzi G, Lauri G, et al: Beta-thromboglobulin plasma levels in the first week after myocardial infarction: Influence of thrombolytic therapy. Am Heart J 1994;128:472-476.

42. Held C, Hjemdahl P, Hakan Wallen N, et al: Inflammatory and hemostatic markers in relation to cardiovascular prognosis in patients with stable angina pectoris. Results from the APSIS study. The Angina Prognosis Study in Stockholm. Atherosclerosis 2000;148:179-188.

43. Ault KA, Cannon CP, Mitchell J, et al: Platelet activation in patients after an acute coronary syndrome: Results from the TIMI-12 trial. Thrombolysis in Myocardial Infarction. J Am Coll Cardiol 1999;33:634-639.

44. Holmes MB, Sobel BE, Howard DB, et al: Differences between activation thresholds for platelet P-selectin glycoprotein IIb-IIIa expression and their clinical implications. Thromb Res 1999;95:75-82.

45. Kabbani SS, Watkins MW, Holoch PA, et al: Platelet reactivity in coronary ostial blood: A reflection of the thrombotic state accompanying plaque rupture and of the adequacy of anti-thrombotic therapy. J Thromb Thrombolysis 2001;12:171-176.

46. Mathur A, Robinson MS, Cotton J, et al: Platelet reactivity in acute coronary syndromes: Evidence for differences in platelet behaviour between unstable angina and myocardial infarction. Thromb Haemost 2001;85:989-994.

47. Serebruany VL, Levine DJ, Nair GV, et al: Usefulness of combining necrosis and platelet markers in triaging patients presenting with chest pain to the emergency department. J Thromb Thrombolysis 2001;11:155-162.

48. Zimmerman GA: Two by two: The pairings of P-selectin and P-selectin glycoprotein ligand 1. Proc Natl Acad Sci U S A 2001;98:10023-10024.

49. Febbraio M, Hajjar DP, Silverstein RL: CD36: A class B scavenger receptor involved in angiogenesis, atherosclerosis, inflammation, and lipid metabolism. J Clin Invest 2001;108:785-791.

50. Henn V, Steinbach S, Buchner K, et al: The inflammatory action of CD40 ligand (CD154) expressed on activated human platelets is temporally limited by coexpressed CD40. Blood 2001;98:1047-1054.

51. Garlichs CD, Eskafi S, Raaz D, et al: Patients with acute coronary syndromes express enhanced CD40 ligand/CD154 on platelets. Heart 2001;86:649-655.

52. Michelson AD, Barnard MR, Krueger LA, et al: Circulating monocyte-platelet aggregates are a more sensitive marker of in vivo platelet activation than platelet surface P-selectin: Studies in baboons, human coronary intervention, and human acute myocardial infarction. Circulation 2001;104:1533–1537.

53. Furman MI, Barnard MR, Krueger LA, et al: Circulating monocyte-platelet aggregates are an early marker of acute myocardial infarction. J Am Coll Cardiol 2001;38:1002–1006.

54. Furman MI, Kereiakes DJ, Krueger LA, et al: Leukocyte-platelet aggregation, platelet surface P-selectin, and platelet surface glycoprotein IIIa after percutaneous coronary intervention: Effects of dalteparin or unfractionated heparin in combination with abciximab. Am Heart J 2001;142:790–798.

55. Vidal C, Spaulding C, Picard F, et al: Flow cytometry detection of platelet procoagulation activity and microparticles in patients with unstable angina treated by percutaneous coronary angioplasty and stent implantation. Thromb Haemost 2001;86:784–790.

56. Mallat Z, Benamer H, Hugel B, et al: Elevated levels of shed membrane microparticles with procoagulant potential in the peripheral circulating blood of patients with acute coronary syndromes. Circulation 2000;101:841–843.

57. Mizuno K, Satomura K, Miyamoto A, et al: Angioscopic evaluation of coronary-artery thrombi in acute coronary syndromes. N Engl J Med 1992;326:287–291.

58. Chesebro JH, Fuster V: Thrombosis in unstable angina. N Engl J Med 1992;327:192–194.

59. Reganon E, Ferrando F, Vila V, et al: Increase in thrombin generation after coronary thrombolysis with rt-PA or streptokinase with simultaneous heparin versus heparin alone. Haemostasis 1998;28:99–105.

60. Merlini PA, Ardissino D, Rosenberg RD, et al: In vivo thrombin generation and activity during and after intravenous infusion of heparin or recombinant hirudin in patients with unstable angina pectoris. Arterioscler Thromb Vasc Biol 2000;20:2162–2166.

chapter 16

Markers of Inflammation

Giovanna Liuzzo
Luigi M. Biasucci

The idea that inflammation plays a key role in atherosclerosis and its complications has received considerable attention.[1] Inflammatory cell infiltration is observed in atherosclerotic plaques at virtually all stages, from the fatty streak to the advanced atheromatous lesions.[1] Although all of the potential triggers of inflammation are not fully known, cytokines, oxidized lipoproteins, and local (coronary) and distant (dental, gastric, pulmonary) infections have been implicated.[2,3] Inflammatory cells also may play a key role in promoting plaque disruption by stimulating matrix degradation, inhibiting smooth muscle cell function or survival, and promoting thrombosis by producing tissue factor and inducing vasocontriction.[2-4] Similarly the protective effects of a variety of interventions, such as statins, aspirin, and fibrates, are often associated with the evidence of reduced inflammation, further strengthening the notion that inflammation and the acute complications of atherosclerosis are causally related.

In view of the persuasive evidence implicating inflammation in atherosclerosis and in acute coronary syndromes (ACS), several investigators examined a variety of circulating markers of inflammation to predict either the presence of vascular disease or the risk of vascular events in a variety of clinical settings.[5] These markers included C-reactive protein (CRP), serum amyloid A protein (SAA), heat-shock proteins, proinflammatory cytokines, and many leukocyte adhesion molecules. Of the variety of circulating markers, CRP, an acute-phase reactant produced by the liver in response to interleukin (IL)-6, has been the best studied, with the most consistent relationship to future risk under different clinical settings (i.e., asymptomatic, otherwise healthy subjects; patients with peripheral and stable coronary artery disease; and patients with unstable angina).[5,6] The availability of a reliable, reproducible assay with a high sensitivity for CRP adds to its attractiveness as a circulating marker of risk. The focus on inflammation as a crucial player in atherothrombosis is likely to lead to novel anti-inflammatory strategies against vascular disease in the near future.

INFLAMMATORY INFILTRATES OF UNSTABLE PLAQUES

Early insight into the role of inflammation in cardiovascular disease came from the seminal observations of pathologists (see Chapter 5). Careful studies of unstable atherosclerotic plaques led to the recognition of inflammatory cell infiltrates underneath acute coronary thrombi with or without an associated plaque fissure (Table 16-1).[7-10] Inflammatory cells, including macrophages, B and T lymphocytes, and mast cells, were found in the intima and in the surrounding adventitial nerves. Macrophages and, to a lesser extent, T lymphocytes are the dominant cells at the immediate site of either plaque rupture or superficial erosion. These rupture-related inflammatory cells are activated, indicating ongoing inflammation at the site of plaque disruption. The shoulder regions of the eccentric plaques are sites of predilection for active inflammation (endothelial activation, macrophages, and mast cell infiltration) and disruption.[7-10]

T Lymphocytes

T lymphocytes have been shown to be $CD4^+$ helper and $CD8^+$ cytotoxic cells approximately in a similar amount and to be memory $CD45RO^+$ cells expressing HLA-DR antigen and IL-2 receptor (sign of recent activation) in large proportion.[2,3,9,11] Plaque-related lymphocytes mainly produce interferon (IFN)-γ, a pleiotropic cytokine that activates macrophages, with subsequent synthesis of

■ ■ ■

TABLE 16–1 LOCAL SIGNS OF INFLAMMATION IN ACUTE CORONARY SYNDROMES

INFLAMMATORY INFILTRATES OF UNSTABLE CORONARY PLAQUES

Lymphocytes: $CD4^+$ and $CD8^+$ T cells, with memory $CD45RO^+$ phenotype; expression of markers of recent activation (HLA-DR$^+$, CD25$^+$); production of proinflammatory cytokines (INF-γ)
Macrophages: expression of markers of recent activation (HLA-DR$^+$); production of matrix-degrading proteinases and proinflammatory cytokines; expression of procoagulant molecules (tissue factors)
Mast cells: production of matrix-degrading proteinases
Localized to the culprit lesion
Diffused to multiple coronary sites

INFLAMMATORY RESPONSES FROM VASCULAR CELLS

Endothelial cells: endothelial cell activation; expression of adhesion molecules; production of cytokines and chemokines; acquisition of procoagulant and vasoconstrictor properties
Smooth muscle cells: inhibition of smooth muscle cell function or survival with inhibition of de novo synthesis of interstitial collagen; cytokine production

INF, interferon.

matrix-degrading proteases and expression of procoagulant molecules, and inhibits collagen secretion by smooth muscle cells.[12,13]

Macrophages

Macrophages, expressing frequently HLA-DR antigens, and mast cells are particularly abundant in the shoulder regions of the plaque, which are the regions more prone to rupture, and may contribute, through the synthesis of their proteases, to its rupture.[7-10] Macrophages and circulating monocytes also produce proinflammatory cytokines, such as IL-1, IL-6, and tumor necrosis factor (TNF)-α, which activate the endothelium, have procoagulant properties, and may activate neutrophils.[2,3]

Incomplete Specificity for Acute Coronary Syndromes of Plaque Inflammation

Because coronary plaques with inflammatory cell infiltrates are also found in autopsy studies of stable angina patients[14,15] and of individuals without ischemic symptoms dying accidentally,[16] they are insufficient on their own to explain the development of the instability. Inflammation, under some conditions, may contribute to the development of atherosclerosis; in other circumstances, it may cause acute activation of the vascular wall with consequent local thrombosis and vasoconstriction (with or without plaque fissure).[17]

Widespread Inflammatory Involvement of the Coronary Arterial Bed

The hypothesis that inflammation of a vulnerable plaque may be responsible for the development of ACS is stimulating a variety of technologic developments for vulnerable plaque detection[18,19] and for "passivation."[20] It is still unclear, however, whether the inflammatory process is confined to a single vulnerable plaque or is more widespread in the coronary vasculature.

The possibility of widespread rather than isolated plaque inflammatory involvement of the coronary arterial bed is suggested by the report of multiple complex coronary plaques in patients with acute myocardial infarction (MI)[21] and by previous postmortem findings of multiple fissured plaques with superimposed thrombosis.[22] An intriguing observation was made at the time of bypass surgery: the report of red streaks with perivascular inflammatory infiltrates along one or more coronary artery branches in 21 of 200 patients with unstable angina.[23] Patients with the red streaks were indistinguishable clinically from patients without the red streaks. In some patients, the involvement of long segments of coronary artery and of multiple coronary arteries, including arteries that were angiographically normal, suggests a diffuse process, rather than localized to the site of a single coronary plaque. A widespread acute inflammatory process in the coronary arterial bed would have important implications for a clearer understanding of the pathogenesis and eventually for the treatment and prevention of ACS.

From the observations of pathologists, a picture emerges of atherosclerosis as a chronic disease that, from its origin to its ultimate complications, involves inflammatory cells (T cells, monocytes, macrophages), inflammatory proteins (cytokines, chemokines), and inflammatory responses from the vascular cells (endothelial cell expression of adhesion molecules). Cytokines, adhesion molecules, and other inflammatory mediators typical of immune interactions have been found also in the peripheral circulation of patients with atherosclerosis, suggesting that the described mechanism is systemic or, at least, is not confined to the arterial wall but may have a systemic "reverberation."

SYSTEMIC MARKERS OF INFLAMMATION

In many patients with unstable angina and acute MI, systemic signs of inflammation are detectable (Table 16-2). In ACS, the inflammatory process is not confined to the coronary plaque but is systemic or at least has a systemic component. Systemic inflammatory markers, such as CRP, have an independent prognostic value supporting the pathogenetic role of inflammation.[24]

Activated Circulating Leukocytes

The existence of an acute inflammatory state in unstable angina and MI is supported by clinical studies showing activation of circulating neutrophils,[25-29] lymphocytes,[30-36] and monocytes (see Table 16-2).[27,37,38]

Neutrophils

Mehta and colleagues[25] and Dinerman and colleagues[26] showed 15-fold higher levels of a neutrophil elastase–derived fibrinopeptide B in patients with unstable angina compared with controls and patients with stable angina. Increased expression of neutrophil and monocyte adhesion molecules was observed during the passage of these cells through the coronary circulation by Mazzone and associates,[27] possibly as a result of endothelial activation. Circulating neutrophils in patients with acute MI and unstable angina were found to have reduced myeloperoxidase content, indicative of a significant release of myeloperoxidase from neutrophils and of their activation.[28] Buffon and coworkers[29] confirmed previous reports that in unstable angina, leukocytes become activated as they traverse the coronary vascular bed and that such activation also may be detectable systemically. These authors also found that in unstable angina, a widespread inflammatory neutrophil activation occurs across the coronary vascular bed, independent of culprit stenosis location and of ischemia. These findings carry important pathophysiologic implications and challenge the concept of a single coronary vulnerable plaque in unstable coronary syndromes.[29]

Lymphocytes

Activation of monocytes by lymphocytes in unstable, but not stable, patients and limited to the acute phase

■ ■ ■

TABLE 16–2   SYSTEMIC SIGNS OF INFLAMMATION IN ACUTE CORONARY SYNDROMES

ACTIVATED CIRCULATING LEUKOCYTES

Lymphocytes: HLA-DR$^+$, CD25$^+$, IFN-γ^+, $\uparrow\uparrow$ IL-2 soluble receptor
Monocytes: integrin up-regulation, tissue factor expression
Neutrophils: integrin up-regulation, $\uparrow\uparrow$ elastase, neutrophil degranulation, reduced intracellular myeloperoxidase content

ELEVATED LEVELS OF SOLUBLE INFLAMMATORY MARKERS

Acute-phase proteins: fibrinogen, CRP, SAA
Cytokines: IL-6, IL-1 receptor antagonist, TNF-α
Adhesion molecules: sVCAM-1, sICAM-1, sE-selectin, sP-selectin
Others: ceruloplasmin, neopterin, heat-shock proteins

CRP, C-reactive protein; IFN, interferon; IL, interleukin; SAA, serum anyloid A protein; TNF, tumor mecrosis factor.

of the instability was reported by Neri Serneri and colleagues,[30] who proposed that unstable angina is associated with an acute transient burst of inflammation, with lymphocyte activation triggered by unknown factors (see later). These findings are supported by an increased procoagulant activity in circulating monocytes[37] and by the elevation of circulating monocytes/macrophages and T lymphocytes expressing DR major histocompatibility complex class II antigens.[31] They also are compatible with the abundant expression of HLA-DR antigens on inflammatory cells and adjacent smooth muscle cells in plaques beneath thrombi.[7,9]

More recently, Neri Serneri and colleagues[31] provided direct evidence that circulating T lymphocytes from patients with unstable angina, but not from patients with stable effort angina, are activated and that enhanced lymphocyte activation is associated with a worst prognosis. At variance with Neri Serneri and colleagues, Caligiuri and coworkers[32] found that in unstable angina, lymphocyte activation is inversely related to the intensity of inflammation as indicated by plasma levels of CRP and that lymphocyte activation increases during the following 2 weeks in patients with waning of symptoms. These findings may be in keeping with the elevation of IL-2 soluble receptor, a marker of lymphocyte activation, in patients with stable angina and lower restenosis rate after percutaneous transluminal coronary angioplasty[33] and may suggest that lymphocyte activation may be protective, possibly by secretion of anti-inflammatory cytokines, such as IL-4 and IL-10.

The presence of activated T lymphocytes in unstable angina patients implies antigenic stimulation, but the nature of such antigens remains to be investigated. Several autoantigens expressed in the atherosclerotic plaque are able to elicit an immune response, including oxidized low-density lipoprotein (LDL) and heat-shock proteins.[2,3] Infectious agents, such as *Chlamydia pneumoniae*, cytomegalovirus, and *Helicobacter pylori*, have been associated to ischemic heart disease in several epidemiologic studies.[39] Cytomegalovirus and *C. pneumoniae* have been detected frequently in advanced coronary atherosclerotic lesions and could be the target for activated lymphocytes within the plaques.[40] The encouraging results of early studies are not confirmed, however, by more recent trials using antibiotic therapy to reduce the risk of acute coronary events.

Liuzzo and associates[34] found that patients with unstable angina are characterized by the expansion of an unusual subset of circulating T cells, expressing the CD4$^+$CD28^{null} phenotype. These unusual T cells are committed to the production of IFN-γ. The chronic up-regulation of IFN-γ in unstable angina patients could lead to subsequent activation of monocytes/macrophages in the circulation and in tissue lesions. The finding that CD28-deficient T cells have cytolytic capability suggests that immune reactions in individuals with such T cells are deviated toward a high risk for tissue damage. Environmental and genetic mechanisms could underlie the perturbation of the T-cell repertoire. In particular, because the defect in CD28 cell surface expression may result from chronic exposure to antigen, the expansion of CD4$^+$CD28^{null} T cells may reflect a persistent immune response to microorganisms or autoantigens contained in atherosclerotic plaques. The report of T lymphocytes circulating in the peripheral blood and infiltrating coronary artery wall that undergo clonal expansion and produce large quantities of IFN-γ[35] and consequently of proinflammatory cytokines, in response to restricted antigenic stimulation,[35,36] suggests the possibility that these lymphocytes may initiate the cascade of events and in turn may effect or modulate the inflammatory response. Why these lymphocytes localize in the coronary vasculature is unknown but may be related to antigenic epitopes, which influence their distribution and clustering in coronary artery segments.

Monocytes

In patients with unstable angina in whom platelet production of thromboxane A$_2$ was blocked by low-dose aspirin, Vejar and associates[41] found that urinary excretion of the thromboxane A$_2$ metabolite, 11-dehydro-thromboxane B$_2$, was often much higher than that found during coronary angioplasty in stable patients who were on a similar dose of aspirin. This observation suggests the possible origin of this metabolite from monocytes in which thromboxane A$_2$ production by the inducible cyclooxygenase 2 is not inhibited by low-dose aspirin (which was sufficient to block irreversibly platelet cyclooxygenase and platelet thromboxane production). The thromboxane A$_2$ biosynthesis in unstable angina was examined as modified by two cyclooxygenase inhibitors differentially affecting cyclooxygenase 2 despite comparable impact on platelet cyclooxygenase 1. Indobufen, which largely suppresses monocyte cyclooxygenase 2 activity at therapeutic plasma concentration, is more efficient in reducing urinary excretion of 11-dehydro-thromboxane B$_2$ than aspirin in patients with unstable angina.[42] Circulating monocyte activation in patients with ACS also is supported by the up-regulation of adhesion molecule expression during the passage of these cells through the coronary circulation,[27] by the increased expression of the procoagulant tissue factor,[37] and by the enhanced response of blood monocytes to in vitro lipopolysaccharide challenge shown in patients with recurrent unstable angina.[38]

Elevated Levels of Soluble Markers of Inflammation

Increased concentrations of the highly sensitive acute-phase proteins, CRP and SAA[43,44]; of proinflammatory cytokines, IL-6 and IL-1 receptor antagonist (a member of the IL-1 gene family)[45,46]; and of many soluble leukocyte adhesion molecules were reported in patients with unstable angina (see Table 16–2). The intensity of the acute-phase response was shown to be closely related to the short-term and long-term outcome.[5,6,24,47]

The prevalence of systemically detectable inflammatory markers in ACS varies. CRP and IL-6 are elevated in about 70% of patients with severe unstable angina on admission,[43-45] in 50% at discharge, and in 45% at 6 months,[48] and such elevation is associated with recurrent instability and recurrent MI. Accordingly, elevated CRP and IL-6 levels are found before the appearance of markers of myocardial necrosis in nearly all patients with MI preceded by unstable angina but in less than 50% of patients with MI not preceded by unstable angina.[49] The triggers of coronary thrombosis are likely to be multiple and not the same in all patients with ACS.

CLINICAL USE OF MARKERS OF INFLAMMATION FOR PROGNOSTIC STRATIFICATION OF PATIENTS WITH ACUTE CORONARY SYNDROMES

Role of C-Reactive Protein

Accumulating data suggest that markers of inflammation may be reliable markers of risk of cardiovascular events in the short term and long term and may have an incremental value in addition to the other risk markers. This is particularly true for CRP, the prototypic acute-phase reactant, whose level increases rapidly after an inflammatory stimulus and may rise 100-fold according to the intensity of the stimulus. CRP is not consumed to a significant extent in any process, and its clearance is not affected in any known situation; its concentration depends only on its rate of production and excretion. The half-life of 19 hours makes CRP a protein of easy detection in the circulation but rapidly adjusting after a stimulus.[50] In humans, the major inducer of CRP is IL-6, which in turn is induced by TNF-α, IL-1, platelet-derived growth factor, antigens, and endotoxins. CRP is a molecule involved in defense mechanisms, and it is part of the so-called innate defense.[51,52] CRP not only binds selectively to LDL, especially oxidized and modified LDL as found in atheromatous plaques,[53] but also it is deposited in most of such plaques,[54,55] and it has a range of proinflammatory properties that potentially could contribute to the pathogenesis, progression, and complications of atheroma.[51,52]

The presence of CRP within the plaque and its binding to LDL may have many effects. First, the capacity of aggregated and ligand-complexed human CRP to activate the classic complement pathway has long been known.[51,53] CRP is particularly potent in activating C3 and can express the major opsonic and chemotactic functions of the complement system. Second, bound CRP may be recognized by a subset of cellular Fc(γ) receptors and directly activate phagocytic cells.[51,54] Third, CRP has been reported to stimulate tissue factor production by peripheral blood monocytes and could have important procoagulant effects.[51,56] Fourth, CRP directly induces the expression of leukocyte adhesion molecules and of monocyte chemoattractant protein 1 by human endothelial cells, an inflammatory effect that can be inhibited by statins and PPAR-α activators.[57,58] The known CRP properties are not unique to this molecule but are shared with other molecules or systems. The variety of its functions makes CRP an important modulator of the inflammatory response, however, and suggests that its role (also in cardiovascular disease) may be more than that of a marker of inflammation. CRP is an almost ideal marker of disease activity in many inflammatory and infective diseases; it is a protein that is not released or degraded ex vivo, being stable in blood samples after prolonged storage at ambient temperature and delayed treatment of the samples. Finally, high sensitivity assays are now commercially available that make CRP measurement easy, inexpensive, precise, and reproducible (a World Health Organization standard for CRP exists).

Short-Term Prognostic Stratification of Patients with Acute Coronary Syndromes

In 1994, Liuzzo and coworkers[44] reported on the prognostic value of CRP and SAA in patients with severe unstable angina and normal troponin levels. A value of CRP greater than 0.3 mg/dL on admission in patients with unstable angina had a sensitivity of 90% and a specificity of 82% for predicting subsequent in-hospital cardiac events (cardiac death, MI, or the urgent need for coronary revascularization). The sensitivity increased to 100% in patients with a CRP value greater than 1.0 mg/dL on admission and in patients who had any increase in CRP levels during the study. In the same study, patients presenting with an acute MI with symptom onset less than 3 hours and a history of preceding unstable angina also had elevated levels of CRP.[44] These data show that two different populations can be discerned: one with high CRP and high risk and one with low CRP and low risk. In the first population, an inflammatory reaction is likely to play an important role in altering the stable course of disease. A third population also exists, in which a severe course of disease is unrelated to inflammation, as in most patients with unheralded MI[49]; in these patients, other components, such as mechanical plaque rupture, hypercoagulable state, or vasoconstriction, can trigger plaque instability.

Although a trend was present, because of the small number of patients, an association with the hard end point death and MI was not shown in the aforementioned study. Such an association was present in a larger population of 251 patients with unstable angina, in which CRP levels were independently associated with the combined in-hospital end point of death and MI.[59] In this study, a CRP level greater than 19 mg/L (or 1.9 mg/dL) was associated with a fivefold increase in risk of death and MI. In the TIMI IIA study, Morrow and colleagues[60] observed a significant association between CRP levels and risk of death at 14 days. In this study of 437 patients with unstable angina and non–Q wave MI, a CRP level greater than 1.55 mg/dL showed a sensitivity of 86% and a specificity of 76% for death at 14 days. In other studies (see Table 16-2), mainly reanalysis of large multicenter trials, no association was found between CRP levels at entry and risk of death and MI.[61,62] It is possible that the positive results observed in the smaller aforementioned studies were the results of the play of chance because of the smaller number of patients enrolled. More probably, the positive results were due to more careful and strict entry criteria. Studies including large numbers of patients with unstable angina less severe than Braunwald's class IIIB and having a less severe prognosis or, conversely, studies including patients with non–Q wave MI, in which the prognosis largely depends on the amount of myocardial damage, may not be able to detect the prognostic value of CRP. Also the baseline left ventricular function (before the index acute event) should be considered because patients with baseline severe left ventricular dysfunction are likely to have a worse prognosis independent of their inflammatory status. Table 16-3 summarizes the previously discussed studies on the association between CRP levels and short-term prognostic stratification of patients with ACS.[44,60-64]

Long-Term Prognostic Stratification of Patients with Acute Coronary Syndromes

In 1995, the ECAT (European Concerted Action on Thrombosis and Disabilities Angina Pectoris) study was published.[65] In this study, more than 3000 patients with either stable or unstable angina were enrolled and followed for 2 years; major cardiovascular events were significantly associated with levels of fibrinogen and CRP, although with borderline significance. In 1997, the same group published a new study in which CRP measurements were obtained by an ultrasensitive method. In this study, patients in top quintiles of CRP showed a twofold increased risk of major cardiovascular events during the follow-up period.[66]

Toss and colleagues[67] examined 965 patients from the FRISC (Fragmin during Instability in Coronary Artery Disease) study population. They found that elevated levels of CRP (>10 mg/L) were associated with a 7.5% rate of death at 150 days in patients with unstable angina and with non–Q wave MI independent of their troponin status compared with 2.2% rate of death in patients with CRP levels less than 2 mg/L. These data were confirmed in a follow-up study extended to 4 years, in which CRP levels greater than 10 mg/L were associated with a 16.5% risk of death versus 5.7% in patients with CRP less than 2 mg/L, adjusted relative risk 2.6 (1.5 to 4.6).[68] In this study, the increased risk associated with elevated CRP was seen at all levels of troponin T. It remained significant even when the multivariate analysis was restricted to patients with an index diagnosis of unstable angina. Several factors may influence the levels of CRP and act as confounders. In the study of Lindahl and coworkers,[68] however, there were no major changes in the relative risk of death that was associated with CRP levels after adjustment for age, smoking status, body mass index, and sex. Biasucci and associates[69] showed that elevated levels (>3 mg/L) of CRP at discharge are an independent predictor of new ischemic events, including death, MI, and new hospitalization for recurrent unstable angina. An odds ratio of 8.57 was shown in a multivariate analysis also including age, sex, fibrinogen levels, cholesterol

■ ■ ■

TABLE 16–3   C-REACTIVE PROTEIN LEVELS AND SHORT-TERM OUTCOME IN UNSTABLE ANGINA AND NON–Q WAVE MYOCARDIAL INFARCTION

AUTHOR	PATIENTS	PRIMARY END POINT	ASSAY USED	CUT OFF	RESULTS
Liuzzo, 1994[44]	Braunwald IIIB UA (31 patients)	In-hospital cardiac death, MI, urgent revascularization	High sensitivity microparticle enzyme immunoassay	0.3 mg/dL	Significantly higher event rate in patients with CRP >3 mg/L
Oltrona, 1997[61]	Braunwald IIIB UA (140 patients)	In-hospital cardiac death, MI, revascularization	Nephelometry	10 mg/L	No difference in event rate
Morrow, 1998[60]	UA and non–Q wave MI (437 patients of TIMI IIA)	Death at 14 days	Nephelometry	1.55 mg/dL	Increased risk of death for CRP >1.55 mg/dL. Additive value of CRP and troponin T
Rebuzzi, 1998[63]	Braunwald IIIB UA (102 patients)	Death and MI in-hospital and at 3 months	High-sensitivity microparticle enzyme immunoassay	3 mg/L	Higher incidence of MI in CRP >3 mg/L. Additive value of CRP and troponin T
Montalescot, 1998[62]	UA and non–Q wave MI (68 patients of ESSENCE)	Death, MI, recurrent angina, revascularization	Nephelometry	5 mg/L	No significant association at 14 days
Verheggen, 1999[64]	Braunwald IIIB UA (211 patients)	Refractory in-hospital UA	Nephelometry	6 mg/L	CRP higher in refractory angina versus symptom-free

CRP, C-reactive protein; MI, myocardial infarction; UA, unstable angina.

levels, family history, diabetes, cigarette smoking, hypertension, and multivessel disease. This study also showed that CRP remains elevated for at least 12 months after the index events in a large proportion of patients with unstable angina. In patients with high CRP, percutaneous coronary intervention (PCI) or coronary artery bypass graft surgery did not change the 1-year rate of recurrence of ischemic events. This finding is in line with the observations that elevated CRP levels are associated with increased risk of restenosis and of acute complications after balloon angioplasty in stable and unstable angina[70,71] and that CRP is associated with an increased risk of new ischemic events 8 years after coronary artery bypass graft surgery.[72]

Ferreiros and colleagues[73] reported a follow-up study of patients with unstable angina and non–Q wave MI and confirmed that elevated levels of CRP are associated with an elevated risk of coronary events (combined end point of recurrent angina, MI, and death) at 90 days. CRP levels obtained at entry or at discharge were significantly associated with future events, but CRP levels at discharge were better predictors of events (hazard ratio, 3.16). In this study, a cutoff value of 1.5 mg/dL (no high sensitivity method used) was chosen on the basis of a receiver operator characteristic curve; refractory angina, MI, and death were considered as events. Heeschen and coworkers[74] published a retrospective analysis of the data of the CAPTURE (Chimeric c7E3 AntiPlatelet Therapy in Unstable angina REfractory to standard treatment) trial. In this article, CRP greater than 10 mg/L was predictive of cardiac risk (death and MI) at 6 months (18.9% versus 9.5%), independently of troponin T status.[74]

A large prospective study of 1042 consecutive, unselected patients with non–ST-segment elevation ACS treated with an aggressive revascularization strategy confirmed CRP as a strong independent predictor of short-term and long-term mortality. Patients with CRP greater than 10 mg/L have a fourfold increase in in-hospital and long-term mortality (mean follow-up, 20 months). Early revascularization does not ameliorate the negative prognostic impact of elevated CRP. In contrast, CRP seems to be an even more potent predictor of mortality with this strategy. These findings are particularly relevant because they derive from a prospective study of consecutive, unselected patients rather than a randomized trial, eliminating selection bias and allowing extrapolation into clinical practice. The excess risk in patients with CRP greater than 10 mg/L in this study persists despite a strict adherence to current secondary prevention guidelines, including the use of statins.[75] Table 16–4 summarizes the previously discussed studies on the association between CRP levels and long-term prognostic stratification of patients with ACS.[66–69,73–75]

Potential Additive Value of C-Reactive Protein in Risk Assessment

Troponins (T and I) are excellent markers of cardiac risk in unstable angina and non–Q wave MI. This fact raises the question of whether CRP is of additional value for the prognostic stratification of ACS. The first studies addressing the issue of the additional value of CRP over troponins were published in 1998. Morrow and colleagues,[60] in a substudy of the TIMI IIA, showed that CRP and troponin T had additive prognostic value in unstable angina and non–Q wave MI. In particular, low levels of CRP and negative troponin T were associated with less than 1% risk of death at 14 days; high CRP (1.55 mg/dL) and early positive bedside troponin T were associated with a 9% risk. Rebuzzi and associates[63] confirmed in 102 patients with unstable angina that negative troponin T and low levels of CRP (<3 mg/L) are associated with low risk of MI (<2% at 3 months). They also showed that CRP is useful for risk stratification of patients with negative troponin T, 15% of whom, all with elevated CRP, had a MI at 3 months.[63] More recently, other studies investigated the additive role of CRP with troponins. In particular, the large multicenter trials FRISC and CAPTURE in retrospective analyses found that CRP predictive value is independent of troponin T status.[68,74] In the CAPTURE study, admission levels of CRP were independent predictors of cardiac risk (death and MI) and repeated coronary revascularization. In both studies, the association of high CRP plus high troponin T was confirmed as a strong marker of future events; conversely the association of low CRP and low or negative troponin T was a marker of an excellent prognosis.[68,74] Tables 16–3 and 16–4 also summarize the studies showing the potential additive value of CRP in risk assessment.[60,63,68,74]

C-Reactive Protein and Percutaneous Coronary Interventions

PCIs are nowadays the leading treatment for ACS, accounting for more than 50% of all interventional treatments. Despite major advances in the technique and in the additional pharmacologic therapy, such as the use of stents and glycoprotein (GP) IIb/IIIa inhibitors, at least 10% of patients having a PCI are expected to have restenosis within 3 to 6 months. None of the classic risk factors and none of the other procedure-related parameters, with the exception of final lumen gain, have been found to be useful as predictors of restenosis. The availability of a reliable and simple marker of restenosis before the procedure would be of interest to the interventional cardiologist because stents and GPIIb/IIIa inhibitors are expensive, and their use may have limitations, such as in-stent restenosis or bleeding.

CRP has been shown to be an independent marker of late restenosis and of early complications in balloon angioplasty by Buffon and colleagues.[70] In two other studies, CRP levels after stenting also were associated with an increased risk of restenosis.[76,77] In the large CAPTURE trial, CRP levels greater than 10 mg/L were associated with an increased risk of cardiac risk (death and MI) and restenosis at 6 months (but not with early events).[74] No interaction was observed between CRP values and benefit of treatment with abciximab; however, the absolute differences in cardiac risk of about 7% between CRP-positive and CRP-negative patients may be useful in clinical practice to guide more aggressive med-

■ ■ ■

TABLE 16–4 C-REACTIVE PROTEIN LEVELS AND LONG-TERM OUTCOME IN UNSTABLE ANGINA AND NON–Q WAVE MYOCARDIAL INFARCTION

AUTHOR	PATIENTS	PRIMARY END POINT	ASSAY USED	CUT OFF	RESULTS
Haverkate, 1997[66]	2121 outpatients with UA and SA (ECAT)	Sudden death and fatal and nonfatal	Ultrasensitive ELISA	3.6 mg/L	RR = 2, upper quintile of CRP (>3.6 mg/L) versus the first 4
Toss, 1997[67]	UA and non–Q wave MI (965 patients of FRISC)	Death and/or MI at 5 months	Turbidimetric assay	10 mg/L	RR of death = 3.5 upper vs lower tertile. Additive value of CRP and troponin T
Biasucci, 1999[69]	Brauwald IIIB UA (53 patients)	Death, MI, recurrent UA at 1 year	High-sensitivity nephelometry	3 mg/L	Association between CRP at discharge and event rate at 1 year.
Ferreiros, 1999[73]	Braunwald IIIB UA (194 patients)	Total death, MI, refractory angina at 90 days	ELISA	1.5 mg/dL	CRP at entry and at discharge predicts late outcome
Lindahl, 2000[68]	917 patients with UA (FRISC)	Cardiac death during a follow-up of 37 months	Turbidimetric assay	10 mg/L	RR of death = 2.6 upper tertile versus the other 2. Additive value of CRP and troponin T
Heeschen, 2000[74]	Braunwald IIIB UA (447 patients of CAPTURE)	Death, MI at 30 days and 6 months	High-sensitivity nephelometry	10 mg/L	Higher event rate at 30 days and 6 months in CRP-positive patients. Additive value of CRP and troponin T.
Muller, 2002[75]	1042 patients with non–ST-segment elevation ACS treated with early invasive strategy	In-hospital and long-term mortality (mean follow-up, 20 months)	Turbidimetric assay	10 mg/L	CRP is a strong independent predictor of short-term and long-term mortality (odds ratio, 4.1).

ACS, acute coronary syndromes; CRP, C-reactive protein; ELISA, enzyme-linked immunosorbent assay; MI, myocardial infarction; RR, relative risk, SA, stable angina; UA, unstable angina.

ical treatment. All published data but those of Zhou and colleagues,[78] who studied patients undergoing atherectomy, are consistent in indicating that CRP is a powerful marker of late restenosis and that measurement of CRP before PCI may give important information. Within a single-center registry of contemporary percutaneous coronary revascularization strategies including 727 consecutive patients, elevated levels of CRP before the procedure were associated with progressive increase in death or MI at 30 days (lowest quartile, 3.9%, versus highest quartile, 14.2%). Among clinical and procedural characteristics, baseline CRP remained predictive of adverse events, with the highest quartile of CRP associated with an odds ratio for 30-day death or MI of greater than 3.68.[71] The same authors found that among patients with an elevated baseline level of CRP undergoing coronary stenting, pretreatment with clopidogrel was associated with a substantial reduction in 30-day death and acute MI.[79] Tomoda and Aoki[80] observed that high CRP levels (>3 mg/L) are associated with an increased risk of cardiovascular events, including procedural failure, in primary angioplasty, independent of elevation of markers of myocardial damage. In a large prospective study of 1042 patients with non–ST-segment elevation ACS treated with an aggressive revascularization strategy, patients with CRP greater than 10 mg/L had a fourfold increase in in-hospital and long-term mortality.[75] Table 16–5 summarizes the previously discussed studies on the association between CRP levels and cardiovascular events and long-term restenosis after PCI.[70,71,74-77,79]

C-Reactive Protein and Primary Prevention of Ischemic Heart Disease

The most important data relating to CRP and vascular diseases derive from large-scale epidemiologic studies in which minor elevations in CRP among apparently healthy men were associated with future risk of MI, stroke, and peripheral vascular disease. In the Physicians' Health Study, about 22,000 middle-aged healthy men, with no prior history of MI, stroke, or cancer had blood samples drawn at baseline.[81] CRP was measured in 543 apparently healthy men in whom MI, stroke, or venous thrombosis subsequently developed and in 543 matched apparently healthy men who did not report vascular disease during a follow-up period exceeding 8 years. Participants were randomly assigned to receive aspirin or placebo at the beginning of the study. The men in the quartile with the highest CRP values had three times the risk of MI (relative risk, 2.9; $P < .001$) of men in the lowest quartile. Risks were stable over long periods, were not modified by smoking, and were independent of other lipid-related and non–lipid-related risk factors. Aspirin in a dosage of 325 mg on alternate days, which is far below any dosage showing known anti-inflammatory effect, brought a risk reduction of roughly 50% to 55% in the fourth quartile of CRP concentrations, with decreasing effects in the lower CRP quartiles.

Epidemiologic data supporting the role of CRP as a marker for vascular risk are consistent across different study populations, including smokers enrolled in the

■ ■ ■

TABLE 16–5 C-REACTIVE PROTEIN LEVELS AND CARDIOVASCULAR EVENTS AFTER PERCUTANEOUS CORONARY INTERVENTION

AUTHOR	PATIENTS	PRIMARY END POINT	ASSAY USED	CUT OFF	RESULTS
Buffon, 1999[70]	121 patients (57% UA)	Early adverse events; clinical restenosis at 1 year	High-sensitivity nephelometry	3 mg/L	RR = 12.2 and 6.2 for early adverse events and clinical restenosis by tertiles of CRP
Heeschen, 2000[74]	Braunwald IIIB UA (447 patients of CAPTURE)	Death, MI at 30 days and 6 months	High-sensitivity nephelometry	10 mg/L	Higher event rate (and restenosis) at 30 days and 6 months in CRP-positive patients
Versaci, 2000[76]	Brauwald IIIB UA (62 patients)	Death, MI, recurrent UA at 1 year	Immunoturbidimetric assay	5 mg/L	3% of low CRP versus 60% of high CRP patients had an end point
Walter, 2001[77]	276 patients (51% with ACS)	Combined end point: death, MI, restenosis at 6 months	Turbidimetric assay	5 mg/L	RR = 2.0 tertiles II–III of CRP versus I
Chew, 2001[71]	727 patients (>50% with ACS)	30-day rate of death or MI	High-sensitivity nephelometry	0.3 mg/dL	Highest quartile of CRP: odds ratio for excess 30-day death or MI of 3.68
Muller, 2002[75]	1042 patients with non–ST-segment elevation ACS treated with early invasive strategy	In-hospital and long-term mortality (mean follow-up 20 months)	Turbidimetric assay	10 mg/L	CRP is a strong independent predictor of short-term and long-term mortality (odds ratio, 4.1).

ACS, acute coronary syndromes; CRP, C-reactive protein; MI, myocardial infarction; RR, relative risk; UA, unstable angina.

MRFIT (Multiple Risk Factor Intervention Trial)[82]; elderly patients followed in the Cardiovascular Health Study[83]; postmenopausal women in the Women's Health Study[84]; and European populations in three independent cohorts, the MONICA Augsberg cohort,[85] the Helsinki Heart Study,[86] and the British Regional Practice study.[87]

All prospective studies so far published including only individuals without known cardiovascular disease have shown highly consistent results, reporting a relative risk between 3 and 3.5 for levels of CRP still within the normal range. In most of these studies, effect of CRP on vascular risk remained highly significant after adjustment for traditional risk factors typically used in global risk-assessment programs.

Of particular interest is the additive value of CRP with the total cholesterol–to–high-density lipoprotein (HDL) cholesterol ratio, a well-known risk factor for ischemic heart disease. Analysis of the data of the Physicians' Health Study, considering the risk associated with cholesterol ratio and CRP levels expressed in tertiles, showed that the association of CRP and cholesterol ratio in the top tertiles carries a risk much higher than that associated with the top tertile of cholesterol ratio alone. Also, patients in the middle tertile of cholesterol ratio but in the higher tertile of CRP have a risk higher than that associated with being in the top tertile of cholesterol ratio alone.[88]

The observation that the addition of CRP testing to standard lipid screening provides an improved method to determine vascular risk and the accumulating evidence that CRP may have direct inflammatory effects on endothelial cells[57,58] have implications for the use of statins. In the CARE (Cholesterol and Recurrent Events) trial, random allocation to pravastatin attenuated the excess vascular risk associated with low-grade, systemic inflammation[89] and significantly reduced CRP levels over a 5-year follow-up period.[90] In that study, the change in

CRP attributable to pravastatin was unrelated to changes in LDL cholesterol, an observation supporting the hypothesis that statin therapy may have important non-lipid anti-inflammatory effects. These data have been confirmed in randomized trials of cerivastatin and of lovastatin. In a cohort of 785 patients with primary hypercholesterolemia, CRP levels were significantly reduced within 8 weeks of therapy with cerivastatin in a lipid-independent manner.[91] In the AFCAPS/TexCAPS (Air Force/Texas Coronary Atherosclerosis Prevention Study), lovastatin therapy prevented coronary events in participants with higher values of CRP (but still within the normal range) whose baseline levels of LDL cholesterol were lower than 149.1 mg/dL, the median value in a population selected for average levels of LDL cholesterol.[92] In contrast, in participants whose levels of CRP and LDL cholesterol were below the median levels in the population, statin therapy did not significantly reduce the risk of coronary events. Because primary prevention studies consistently have found that individuals with low LDL cholesterol but high CRP levels are at high vascular risk, these data also support the hypothesis that statin therapy might be effective in the absence of overt hyperlipidemia, an issue in need of direct testing in future clinical trials.

Other Soluble Markers of Inflammation

Cytokines

Because CRP gene transcription in the liver is stimulated by IL-6, a pleiotropic cytokine, CRP levels are generally well correlated with circulating levels of IL-6. It is not surprising that similar to CRP, circulating IL-6 also provides prognostic information in ischemic heart disease (Table 16–6). This idea first was suggested by Biasucci and colleagues[45,46] and was established further by

TABLE 16–6   OTHER SOLUBLE MARKERS OF INFLAMMATION

CYTOKINES

Interleukin-6: elevated levels are common in unstable angina, correlate with CRP, and are related to prognosis and to the benefit of an early invasive strategy; increased risk of future cardiac events in apparently healthy people

Interleukin-1Ra: elevated levels are common in unstable angina, correlate with CRP, and are related to prognosis

Tumor necrosis factor-α: increased risk of recurrent coronary events after myocardial infarction

SOLUBLE CELLULAR ADHESION MOLECULES

Soluble ICAM-1: increased risk of cardiac death in stable and unstable angina; increased risk of future cardiac events in apparently healthy people

Soluble VCAM-1: increased risk of cardiac death in stable and unstable angina and in diabetes; no relation with future cardiac events in initially healthy people

Soluble E-selectin: increased risk of cardiac death in stable and unstable angina

Soluble P-selectin: increased risk of future cardiac events in apparently healthy people

---

Ridker and associates.[93] Biasucci and colleagues[45,46] provided direct evidence that proinflammatory cytokines are involved in the mechanisms leading to instability. These authors showed that elevated serum levels of IL-6 and IL-1 receptor antagonist are common in unstable angina, correlate with CRP, and are related to prognosis, strengthening the importance of inflammation in unstable angina. Ridker and associates[93] showed that serum levels of IL-6 were predictive of the risk of MI, and although IL-6 levels were correlated with CRP levels, the association between IL-6 and the risk of MI remained significant even after adjustment for CRP levels.

In the population of the CARE study, plasma concentration of TNF-α, a multifunctional cytokine with diverse systemic effects, was found to be elevated many months after MI among individuals at increased risk for recurrent coronary events. Specifically, individuals with the highest levels of TNF-α were found to have a three-fold increase in the risk of recurrent MI or coronary death. The elevated risk associated with elevation of TNF-α was independent of other traditional risk factors and was independent of CRP levels, although a strong correlation between TNF-α and CRP levels was observed.[94]

Lindmark and coworkers[95] measured circulating levels of IL-6 among patients enrolled in the prospective FRISC II trial comparing invasive versus conservative management of patients with ACS. Elevated IL-6 levels were a strong and independent predictor of mortality for patients treated with the invasive and the conservative arms. Among patients with elevated IL-6 levels, assignment to the early invasive strategy strongly reduced mortality at 12 months (5.1% absolute risk reduction). Although IL-6 levels correlated with mortality, high levels of IL-6 were not predictive of the composite end point of death and MI at 6 to 12 months.[95]

Soluble Cellular Adhesion Molecules

Leukocyte infiltration of the vascular wall plays a key role in atherosclerotic plaque formation, development, and acute complication. The adhesion and transendothelial migration of circulating leukocytes is mediated largely by cellular adhesion molecules (CAMs)—a diverse group of integrin, immunoglobulin, and selectin proteins involved in the binding of cell to cell and cell to extracellular matrix. Clinical interest in the CAMs has grown with the observation that concentrations of soluble CAMs are high among individuals with dyslipidemia and that plasma concentrations of certain CAMs are associated with an increased risk of future events (see Table 16–6). Prospective data of soluble adhesion molecules are sparse.[96]

Although a prolonged elevation of soluble adhesion molecules in unstable angina and MI for 6 months is described[97] and levels of sVCAM-1 are associated with death in diabetic patients, those were not related to future cardiac events in initially healthy individuals.[98] An association between levels of sICAM-1 or P-selectin and future cardiac events in apparently healthy individuals could be shown, however.[99,100] In a prospective study deriving from a large cohort of patients with angiographically documented coronary artery disease, baseline sVCAM-1, sICAM-1, and E-selectin concentrations were elevated among patients with future fatal cardiovascular events, with sVCAM-1 revealing the strongest association with future death from cardiovascular causes in patients with stable and with unstable angina. sVCAM-1 added to the predictive value of CRP.[101]

In the torrent of reports on the predictive value of markers of inflammation, it is unclear whether one marker of inflammation is superior to another (i.e., CRP, SAA, IL-6, soluble adhesion molecules, or others) and whether the same inflammatory marker should be used to predict risk in acute and chronic phases of coronary disease. Based on data from the Women's Health Study, the magnitude of predictive value for CRP seems substantially greater than that for ICAM-1, VCAM-1, IL-6, and P-selectin (Table 16–7).[84] In part, the greater prognostic utility of CRP reflects the long half-life and stability of this molecule, coupled with a lack of circadian variation and low coefficients of variation when measured with high sensitivity assays.

The meaning of diverse markers of inflammation could be different. The risk of future MI associated with raised concentrations of sICAM-1 seems to increase with length of follow-up. In the Physicians' Health Study, a nonsignificant increase in risk was seen for events occurring in the first 2 years of follow-up, whereas among events occurring after 2 years, a significant twofold increase in risk was observed.[99] Although this difference may have been due to chance, such a time-dependent effect may implicate a role for sICAM-1 early in the atherosclerotic process, at least compared with CRP, for which risks remain stable over time. CRP may have a role as marker and mediator of enhanced inflammatory responses toward a variety of potential, infectious and noninfectious stimuli that may influence the development of ACS.

■ ■ ■

TABLE 16–7 PROGNOSTIC VALUE OF VARIOUS BIOLOGIC MARKERS IN HEALTHY WOMEN

BIOLOGIC MARKER	RELATIVE RISK (95% CI) OF FUTURE CARDIOVASCULAR EVENTS*
sVCAM-1	1.1 (0.6–2.0)
Lipoprotein(a)	1.3 (0.7–2.4)
Homocysteine	2.0 (1.1–3.8)
Interleukin-6	2.2 (1.1–4.3)
sP-selectin	2.2 (1.1–4.3)
LDL cholesterol	2.4 (1.3–4.6)
Total cholesterol	2.4 (1.3–4.7)
sICAM-1	2.6 (1.3–5.1)
Serum amyloid A protein	3.0 (1.5–6.0)
Ratio total cholesterol to HDL cholesterol	3.4 (1.8–5.9)
C-reactive protein	4.4 (2.2–8.9)

*Top versus bottom quartile after adjustment for age and smoking.
CI, confidence interval; HDL, high-density lipoprotein; LDL, low-density lipoprotein.
Data modified from Ridker PM, Hennekens CH, Buring JE, et al: C-reactive protein and other markers of inflammation in the prediction of cardiovascular disease in women. N Engl J Med 2000;342:836–843.

Practical Considerations

The available data strongly recommend the use of CRP as a prognostic marker in patients with unstable angina and non–Q wave MI (see Tables 16–3 and 16–4). The data are strong and consistent for midterm to long-term prognosis; a relative risk between 2.3 and 20 has been found in different studies. The data are less consistent for the in-hospital prognostic stratification of these patients. When studying patients with ACS, values higher than 10 mg/L could be found easily because CRP can increase 1000-fold after a stimulus, and there is evidence that in some patients an enhanced responsiveness might lead to high CRP levels in response to mild stimuli.[38,49,102] In the presence of overt inflammatory and infective disease, the data should be taken cautiously, and CRP values possibly (long-term stratification) should be repeated at least two times after the underlying disease has disappeared.

When to Sample

The data available in the literature in the clinical setting of ACS are based mainly on samples taken on admission, and this is the best sample for in-hospital risk stratification of such patients. In the studies in which samples were taken also at discharge, the discharge samples seem to predict midterm to long-term prognosis better than the samples on admission.[69,73] This is probably due to the fact that discharge levels more closely represent the baseline inflammatory status of the patients and their intrinsic risk secondary to the inflammatory activity. Conversely, samples taken at entry may reflect the acute-phase reaction associated with the index ischemic or necrotic event. The increasingly common policy of treat-

ing invasively patients with severe unstable angina and discharging them soon after PCI may induce the same acute-phase reaction in the predischarge samples, however, making it reasonable to assess CRP levels at entry for all aims. When possible, a sample at discharge and 1 to 3 months after discharge may be useful because it is likely that the highest risk of future events is confined to patients with sustained levels of CRP over time.

To determine the habitual level of CRP in healthy individuals or in individuals with stable coronary artery disease, one blood sample is sufficient if CRP is less than the decision limit (i.e., <3 mg/L); otherwise a second blood sample should be taken after 2 weeks or later. If CRP levels are greater than the decision limit in both determinations, and all the other diseases or conditions known to determine an acute-phase response are excluded, the subject should be considered as at high risk for future cardiovascular events. The within-person biologic variability of CRP is low over a long period, leading further support to the fact that CRP is a good and biologically stable predictor of future cardiovascular events despite the fact that is an acute-phase reactant, proving that the patient is not suffering from an active infection or using a drug that affects CRP concentration. CRP values greater than 15 mg/L (99th percentile of the general population) indicate active inflammation; patients should be advised to have a repeated measurement in 2 to 3 weeks or after the infection is resolved.

Cutoff Levels

A major problem with the clinical use of CRP for prognostic stratification of patients with ongoing, stable or unstable coronary heart disease is the choice of the appropriate cutoff levels to differentiate between low-risk and high-risk patients. Because patients with different clinical presentations have been studied using different assays, the data in the literature are not comparable. Few studies have used the high-sensitivity CRP assay in patients with ACS. Because CRP levels in this condition are usually elevated, a high-sensitivity CRP assay may not be as crucial as in primary prevention. The many data suggesting a low risk for low levels of CRP in patients with ACS are in favor, however, of the use of a high-sensitivity CRP assay also in these patients. In general, the discriminating cutoff CRP values that best separate low-risk and high-risk groups seem to be higher in patients (>3 mg/L or >10 mg/L) than in individuals without known cardiovascular diseases (>1 mg/L) and seem to vary in different syndromes and according to the end points (recurrent instability, MI, or death) considered. On the basis of the data so far available in literature, it seems reasonable to consider different cutoff levels. A CRP level of 3 mg/L should be used for midterm and long-term stratification of stable and unstable patients, if samples are taken at discharge, and is probably a good marker of the combined end point death, MI, new coronary events, and restenosis after PCI. A CRP level of 10 mg/L can be proposed for the stratification of risk of death (and, to a lesser extent, MI). Levels less than 3 mg/L are associated in all studies with a low risk of events.

For the purpose of assessing risk of future first coronary events, CRP concentration should be interpreted using cutoff points established by prospective clinical studies. Each patient should be classified into quintile of risk, depending on the CRP concentration. Models containing CRP and total cholesterol (or the total cholesterol-to-HDL cholesterol ratio) are better able to predict future risk of first coronary events than those containing CRP alone.[81,84] The relative risks of future first coronary events for men and women were computed in quintiles from the Physicians' Health Study and Women's Health Study databases. Overall, for each quintile increase in CRP, the adjusted relative risk of having a future cardiovascular event increased 26% for men and 33% for women. Because risk estimates seem to be linear across the spectrum of inflammation, these sequential quintiles can be considered in clinical terms to represent individuals with low, mild, moderate, high, and highest relative risks of future cardiovascular events (Table 16-8).[47]

Collectively the data available so far suggest that low CRP blood levels, possibly less than 1 mg/L for primary prevention and less than 3 mg/L for secondary prevention, are predictive of a low cardiovascular risk. At one end of the spectrum, a single high sensitivity measurement could be sufficient to reassure many patients when they are found to have low CRP levels. At the other end of the spectrum, patients with known cardiovascular diseases and persistently elevated CRP values are at high risk and should be followed carefully with appropriate risk reduction strategies. Above which cutoff value individuals without known disease should be considered at elevated risk and below which cutoff value patients with various atherothrombotic syndromes should be considered at low risk require further evaluation and consensus because the available evidence suggests that in normal individuals and in patients, the gradient of risk is continuous.

Standard and High-Sensitivity Assays for C-Reactive Protein Determination

Historically, CRP has been measured in clinical laboratories by immunoturbidimetric and immunonephelo-metric assays designed to detect active inflammation and infection. The dynamic range of these assays spans from 3 mg/L (the 90th percentile of the general population) to greater than 100 mg/L. Such traditional assays do not have appropriate sensitivity in the range required, however, for the determination of cardiovascular risk in apparently healthy individuals and in patients with known ischemic heart disease. In recognition of this limitation, initial epidemiologic studies used research-based assays designed to determine CRP levels with excellent fidelity and reproducibility across the normal range. The high-sensitivity methods initially developed used enzyme-linked immunosorbent assay (ELISA) methodology, and a single in-house ELISA assay was used for population studies.[79-81] More recently, automated immunonephelometric, immunoturbidimetric, and immunoluminometric high-sensitivity CRP assays have been developed and are commercially available. These assays have improved sensitivity and precision at low concentration of CRP and seem to have acceptable test characteristics for vascular risk prediction. These methods are standardized against the International Federation of Clinical Chemistry Certified Reference Material (CRM) 470 standard rather than against the older World Health Organization International Reference Standard for CRP Immunoassay 85/506. Currently, CRP concentrations of 0.15 mg/L (<2.5th percentile in the general population) can be measured reliably. Not all high-sensitivity CRP assays have a similar sensitivity or lower limit of quantification (Table 16-9).[103] Because the CRP value of an individual patient is interpreted in the context of cutoff points established by prospective clinical studies, standardization of CRP assays is crucial. Poor agreement among methods will lead to misclassification and mismanagement of patients. The analytical performance and clinical efficacy of the in-house ELISA assay used in earlier population studies[81-83] were compared with those of an automated and commercially available latex-enhanced method (Dade Behring, Marberg, Germany) used at present in several prospective studies.[84,92] Excellent analytical agreement between the two methods was reported, linking the earlier and the present

■ ■ ■

TABLE 16–8   RELATIVE RISK ESTIMATES FOR FUTURE CORONARY EVENTS IN MEN AND WOMEN ASSOCIATED WITH QUINTILES OF C-REACTIVE PROTEIN AND TOTAL CHOLESTEROL-TO-HDL CHOLESTEROL RATIO*

QUINTILE OF TC/HDL-C RATIO	RISK ESTIMATE		QUINTILES OF CRP (MG/L)				
	Men	Women	1 (<0.7) Low	2 (0.7–1.1) Mild	3 (1.2–1.9) Moderate	4 (2.0–3.8) High	5 (3.9–15.0) Highest
1	<3.4	<3.4	1	1.2	1.4	1.7	2.2
2	3.4–4.0	3.4–4.1	1.4	1.7	2.1	2.5	3
3	4.1–4.7	4.2–4.7	2	2.5	2.9	3.5	4.2
4	4.8–5.5	4.8–5.8	2.9	3.5	4.2	5.1	6
5	>5.5	>5.8	4.2	5	6	7.2	8.7

CRP, C-reactive protein; TC/HDL-C, total cholesterol–to–high-density lipoprotein cholesterol.
*Relative risk estimates and TC/HDL-C ratio were derived from the Physician's Health Study and Women's Health Study databases.[81,84] CRP concentrations were derived from population-based surveys.[47]

■ ■ ■

TABLE 16–9 SUMMARY INFORMATION FOR NINE AUTOMATED HIGH-SENSITIVITY CRP METHODS

REAGENT MANUFACTURER	REAGENT DESCRIPTION	METHODOLOGY	ANALYZER	ASSAY RANGE (MG/L)	LIMIT OF DETECTION (MG/L)	PRECISION AT CONCENTRATION OF 0.2 MG/L (CV, %)
Dade Behring	N high-Sensitivity CRP	IN	BN II	0.175–11	0.02	4.9
Daiichi	Pure Auto S CRP	IT	Hitachi 911	0.2–60	0.04	6.1
Denka Seiken	CRP-Latex (II) high-sensitive application	IT	Hitachi 911	0.05–10	0.03	5.1
Diagnostic Products Corporation	CRP	IL	IMMUNO-LITE 2000	0.1–250	0.02	12
Iatron	HS-CRP	IT	Hitachi 911	0.05–4	0.005	3.4
Kamiya	K-Assay CRP (I)	IT	Hitachi 917	0.1–20	0.32	13
Olympus	CRP (Latex) Sensitive Application	IT	Olympus AU640	0.5–20	0.08	44
Roche	Tina-quant CRP (Latex) US	IT	Hitachi 917	0.1–20	0.21	7.2
Wako	CRP-UL	IT	Hitachi 917	0.05–10	0.06	11

CV, coefficient of variation; IN, immunonephelometric; IT, immunoturbidimetric; IL, immunoluminometric.
Data modified from Roberts WL, Moulton L, Law TC, et al: Evaluation of nine automated high-sensitivity C-reactive protein methods: Implications for clinical and epidemiological applications. Clin Chem 2001, 47:418–425.

data and ensuring consistency among reported high-sensitivity CRP values.[47] On the basis of these reports, the U.S. Food and Drug Administration approved the use of this latex-enhanced method in the risk assessment of cardiovascular disease. This latex-enhanced method usually is used as the reference procedure when comparison studies of various high-sensitivity CRP assays are conducted (see Table 16–9).[103]

Management of Patients with Elevated Levels of C-Reactive Protein

Specific therapies have not been evaluated for their ability to reduce CRP levels, and there is no direct evidence to indicate that reduction of CRP results in reduced risk of cardiovascular events. Data derived from randomized clinical trials of statin therapy suggest, however, that the risk reduction achieved by these agents is greater in the presence of elevated CRP levels. Patients with high levels of CRP, especially when associated with high or borderline cholesterol levels, should be treated with statins in the long term and probably in the short term. This is also likely to be true, although not yet shown, for patients undergoing PCI. High CRP levels, carrying a higher risk, not only suggest more aggressive medical therapy in the long term, but also, although there are no data to confirm this hypothesis, aggressive and invasive therapy in the short term, including use of GPIIb/IIIa inhibitors; high doses of statins; and, when PCI is requested, provisional stenting. It was shown that the periprocedural administration of the GPIIb/IIIa inhibitor abciximab reduces the rise in levels of circulating inflammatory markers after percutaneous coronary revascularization.[104] Emerging

evidence suggests that the striking reduction of cardiovascular events obtained with angiotensin-converting enzyme inhibitor therapy might be related to anti-inflammatory effects.[3,105] The use of biochemical markers as a guide to therapy is an uncontroversial issue in the future, and there is no doubt that CRP has all the characteristics to be an ideal marker. Whether new therapies, such as IL antagonists or inhibitors of the inflammatory pathway, will be beneficial in the future cannot be anticipated. In this case, the role of CRP as a guide to specific therapy would be enhanced greatly (Table 16-10).

■ ■ ■

TABLE 16–10 CLINICAL UTILITY OF MEASURING INFLAMMATORY MARKERS IN PATIENTS WITH ACUTE CORONARY SYNDROMES

For a novel inflammatory marker to have a clinical role there must be:
A widely available diagnostic test with high reproducibility
  (This is the case for CRP as measured by high-sensitive assays)
Prospective prognostic studies
  (Several studies are available for CRP and fibrinogen)
Additive information on top of traditional prognostic indicators and risk factors
  (No conclusive data; some studies suggest an incremental prognostic value of CRP)
Treatments able to modify the inflammatory marker by itself
  (No conclusive data; statins? ACE inhibitors? PPAR activators? GPIIb/IIIa inhibitors? antibiotics?)

ACE, angiotensin-converting enzyme; CRP, C-reactive protein; GP, glycoprotein; PPAR, peroxisome proliferator-activated receptors

INFLAMMATION IN ACUTE CORONARY SYNDROMES: A PRIMARY OR SECONDARY PHENOMENON?

It is well known that many biologic changes, distant from the sites of inflammation and involving many systems, may accompany inflammation. These systemic changes have been referred as the *acute-phase response*, even though they accompany acute and chronic inflammatory disorders, and they involve all the systemic markers of inflammation discussed in this chapter. The question arises about the specificity of systemic markers of inflammation for ACS and about their role in the pathogenesis of ACS. The acute-phase response that commonly is observed in patients with unstable angina might be only a marker of instability and represent the vascular response to endothelial disruption and thrombus formation or the consequence of myocardial cell damage. On the other side of the spectrum, inflammation might be a primary pathogenetic process in which lymphocyte and monocyte/macrophage activation causes myocardial ischemia and the occurrence of unstable angina and acute MI via the formation of a variety of inflammatory mediators that can cause plaque destabilization, vasoconstriction, and activation of the hemostatic system (Table 16–11).

Studies have shown that the inflammatory response in unstable angina is not an epiphenomenon. It cannot be attributed to minor degrees of myocardial cell necrosis, a potent stimulus for acute-phase reactants, as ruled out by normal levels of troponin T, a highly sensitive marker of minimal myocardial cell damage, in strictly selected patients with raised concentrations of CRP and severe unstable angina.[44] It cannot be attributed to the severity of atherosclerosis because there is no correlation between the degree of atherosclerosis and the acute-phase response in patients with chronic stable angina or peripheral vascular disease, despite much more extensive atherosclerotic involvement.[44,70] It cannot be attributed to episodic activation of the hemostatic system

because the systemic elevation of markers of thrombin production is not followed by further elevation of acute-phase proteins.[106] Finally, it cannot be attributed to ischemia-reperfusion injury because circulating neutrophils were not activated and CRP levels were not increased in patients with variant angina (a "human model" of transmural myocardial ischemia not associated with plaque instability or thrombus formation but caused by occlusive epicardial coronary artery spasm) despite a significantly larger number of ischemic episodes and a greater total ischemic burden during Holter monitoring.[28,107]

Most patients with unstable angina have concentrations of CRP above the normal range at discharge and at 3 months.[69] Available data converge to suggest that the elevation of inflammatory markers in ACS is mediated by an ongoing inflammatory process not confined to the plaque and exclude the possibility that acute ischemia, thrombosis, or an undetected acute illness is solely responsible for the acute-phase response in ACS.

MECHANISMS OF THE ACUTE-PHASE RESPONSE

Although there is a torrent of reports on the predictive value of CRP, the stimuli that trigger the low-grade up-regulation of CRP production that predicts coronary events in general populations or the more substantial CRP values associated with poor prognosis in severe unstable angina or after angioplasty have not been clearly identified. Atherosclerosis by itself shares many characteristics of a chronic inflammatory process. Many stimuli may incite the ongoing reaction found in atherosclerosis, including chronic infection of the vessels with microorganisms such as cytomegalovirus and *C. pneumoniae* (see Chapter 7). Several autoantigens expressed in the atherosclerotic plaque can elicit an immune response, including oxidized LDL and heat-shock proteins.[2,3] The causes of the acute exacerbation or activation of an until then chronic, quiet inflammatory process resulting in the expression of adhesion molecules and production of inflammatory cytokines and lytic proteases and leading to endothelial dysfunction and platelet aggregation with subsequent thrombosis are incompletely understood (Fig. 16–1; see Table 16–11).

Although chronic infections may lead to low-grade inflammatory conditions, CRP levels were found to be more closely associated with adverse long-term prognosis than seropositivity to infectious agents.[108,109] The correlation between elevated CRP levels and prognosis may be mediated by the vascular effects of proinflammatory cytokines, IL-1, TNF-α, and in particular IL-6, produced by activated circulating monocytes, resident macrophages, and activated endothelium, which also are the major inducers of the hepatic production of CRP.[2,3,24] In the low-risk individuals enrolled in the Physicians' Health Study[81] and in the Women's Health Study,[84] a gradient of risk for MI at 2, 4, and 6 years of follow-up also was observed for CRP levels within the normal range. As

---

■ ■ ■

TABLE 16–11   POSSIBLE CAUSES OF INFLAMMATION IN ACUTE CORONARY SYNDROMES

Systemic signs of inflammation in acute coronary syndromes may be:
  Part of the inflammatory response to atherosclerosis
  Consequence of acute ischemia
  Consequence of hemostatic system activation
  A pathogenetic component associated with prognosis

Possible causes of inflammation are:
  Oxidized LDL
  Infections
    Cytomegalovirus
    Chlamydia pneumoniae
    Helicobacter pylori
  Altered immune and/or inflammatory responses

LDL, low-density lipoprotein.

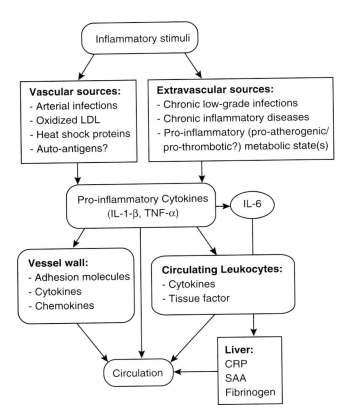

FIGURE 16–1. Circulating levels of inflammatory markers provide a reflection of the underlying inflammatory response. Systemic or local inflammation, either in the blood vessel itself or elsewhere, triggers the production of proinflammatory cytokines (e.g., interleukin [IL]-1β or tumor necrosis factor [TNF]-α). These cytokines can directly elicit production by endothelial cells, leukocytes, and other cells of adhesion molecules; procoagulants; and other mediators that may be released in soluble form into circulating blood. Cytokines such as IL-1β or TNF-α also stimulate the production of IL-6, which induces expression of hepatic genes encoding acute-phase reactants found in blood, including C-reactive protein (CRP), serum amyloid A protein (SAA), and fibrinogen. These markers in serum can provide a window on the inflammatory status of the individual. They might derive from inflammatory pathways arising from atheroma and reflect the degree of inflammatory activity within coronary lesions. They also might derive from nonvascular sources and reflect inflammatory states, such as chronic infections, that may accelerate atherogenesis and its manifestations. Regardless of the source of inflammation, prospective epidemiologic studies showed that measurements of serum inflammatory markers at each level of this pathway are associated with increased coronary risk. LDL, low-density lipoprotein. (Modified from Libby P, Ridker PM: Novel inflammatory markers of coronary risk: Theory versus practice. Circulation 1999;100:1148–1150.)

CRP levels within the normal range seem unlikely to indicate subclinical inflammatory states capable of affecting coronary arteries in the long term, they might represent a marker of circulating inflammatory cell susceptibility to develop enhanced inflammatory responses toward a variety of potential, infectious and noninfectious stimuli.

This possibility is supported by two studies from Liuzzo and colleagues[49,102] showing that during unstable phases of angina, patients with CRP elevation exhibit an enhanced in vivo acute-phase response to the stimuli elicited by coronary angioplasty and angiogra-

phy[102] and to acute myocardial necrosis,[49] which is unrelated to plaque disruption and to the extent of myocardial tissue damage but correlated with baseline CRP levels. These findings agree with the observation that the monocytes of patients with recurrent phases of unstable angina and persistent elevation of acute-phase reactants exhibit a greatly enhanced production of IL-6 in response to lipopolysaccharide challenge 6 months after the last acute event.[38] The magnitude of this response is linearly related to circulating levels of CRP also within the normal range. These in vitro findings confirm the hypothesis that the individual response to stimuli of different origin, possibly including the infectious ones, may play a major role in determining the magnitude of the inflammatory reaction and clinical outcome.

An enhanced acute-phase responsiveness of circulating monocytes to low-grade inflammatory stimuli, which may be genetically determined, may contribute to explain the greater predictive value of CRP than that of seropositivity to chronic infectious agents, oxidized LDL antibodies, and homocysteine. It also may contribute to explain the long-term predictive value of CRP levels within the accepted normal range in low-risk individuals. At the other pole of interpretation of these important observations is the possibility that CRP itself may have a significant pathogenetic role in atherogenesis and plaque destabilization (see earlier) (Fig. 16–2).

CONCLUSIONS

Inflammation is a major feature of atherothrombosis, and there is growing evidence of an association between systemic inflammation and the occurrence of stroke, peripheral artery disease, unstable angina, and MI. Such an inflammatory component may be the final common result of a variety of infectious and noninfectious inflammatory stimuli and of the individual immunologic and inflammatory response.

Among the many inflammatory markers that have been associated with ACS, CRP seems to be the most useful for clinical purposes, as it has been shown to have a powerful predictive relationship, even within the range previously considered to be normal, with major cardiovascular events. Although CRP values correlate closely with other diverse markers of inflammation, some of which also may have a predictive value, albeit generally less significant, CRP itself is particularly interesting because not only does it bind selectively to LDL, especially oxidized and modified LDL as found in atheromatous plaques, but also it is deposited in most such plaques, and it has a range of proinflammatory properties that potentially could contribute to the pathogenesis, progression, and complications of atheroma.

So far, systemic markers of inflammation have been found to be useful for the prognostic stratification of patients with ACS and have contributed significantly to the knowledge of the mechanisms involved in the pathogenesis of these syndromes. Whether these markers also may be used as a guide to therapy is not clear. The

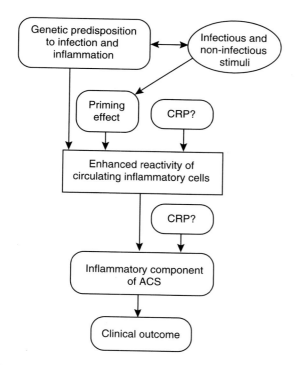

FIGURE 16–2. Role of inflammation in the pathogenesis of acute coronary syndromes (ACS). The genetically determined individual response to stimuli of different origin, possibly including the infectious ones, may play a major role in determining the magnitude of the inflammatory reaction and clinical outcome in ACS. Inflammation may cause local endothelial activation and, possibly, plaque fissure, leading to episodic thrombogenic and vasoconstrictor stimuli, which could be important components of the onset, waxing, and waning of unstable angina and of its evolution toward infarction. C-reactive protein (CRP) itself may have a significant pathogenetic role in atherogenesis and plaque destabilization.

availability of specific anti-inflammatory drugs, able to block selectively CRP or other inflammatory pathways, might represent a new option for ACS therapy in the future and, if effective, may prove the primary role of inflammation in the pathogenesis of these syndromes.

REFERENCES

1. Ross R: Atherosclerosis: An inflammatory disease. N Engl J Med 1999;340:115–126.
2. Libby P: Molecular bases of the acute coronary syndromes. Circulation 1995;91:2844–2850.
3. Libby P: Current concepts of the pathogenesis of the acute coronary syndromes. Circulation 2001;104:365–372.
4. Shah PK: Plaque disruption and thrombosis: Potential role of inflammation and infection. Cardiol Clin 1999;17:271–281.
5. Ridker PM: Evaluating novel cardiovascular risk factors: Can we do better predicting heart attacks? Ann Intern Med 1999;130:933–937.
6. Biasucci LM, Liuzzo G, Colizzi C, et al: Clinical use of C-reactive protein for the prognostic stratification of patients with ischemic heart disease. Ital Heart J 2001;2:164–171.
7. van der Wal AC, Becker AE, van der Loos CM, et al: Site of intimal rupture or erosion of thrombosed coronary atherosclerotic plaques is characterized by an inflammatory process irrespective of the dominant plaque morphology. Circulation 1994;89:36–44.
8. Moreno PR, Falk E, Palacios IF, et al: Macrophage infiltration in acute coronary syndromes: Implications for plaque rupture. Circulation 1994;90:775–778.
9. van der Wal AC, Piek JJ, de Boer OJ, et al: Recent activation of the plaque immune response in coronary lesions underlying acute coronary syndromes. Heart 1998;80:14–18.
10. Kaartinen M, Penttilä A, Kovanen PT: Accumulation of activated mast cells in the shoulder region of human coronary atheroma, the predilection site of atheromatous rupture. Circulation 1994;90:1669–1678.
11. Stemme S, Holm J, Hansson GK: T lymphocytes in human atherosclerotic plaques are memory cells expressing CD45RO and the integrin VLA-1. Arterioscler Thromb Vasc Biol 1992;12:206–211.
12. Gallis Z, Sukhova G, Lark M, et al: Increased expression of matrix metalloproteinases and matrix degrading activity in vulnerable regions of human atherosclerotic plaques. J Clin Invest 1994;94:2493–2503.
13. Shah PK, Falk E, Badimon JJ, et al: Human monocyte-derived macrophages induce collagen breakdown in fibrous caps of atherosclerotic plaques: Potential role of matrix-degrading metalloproteinases and implication for plaque rupture. Circulation 1995;92:1565–1569.
14. van der Wal AC, Becker AE, Koch KT, et al: Clinically stable angina pectoris is not necessarily associated with histologically stable atherosclerotic plaques. Heart 1996;76:312–316.
15. Arbustini E, Grasso M, Diegoli M, et al: Coronary atherosclerosis plaques with and without thrombus in ischemic heart syndromes: A morphologic immunohistochemical and biochemical study. Am J Cardiol 1991;68:36B–50B.
16. van der Wal AC, Das PK, van de Berg DB, et al: Atherosclerotic lesions in humans—in situ immunophenotypic analysis suggesting an immune mediated response. Lab Invest 1989;61:166–170.
17. Maseri A: Ischemic Heart Disease: A Rational Basis for Clinical Practice and Clinical Research. New York, Churchill Livingstone, 1995, pp 237–301.
18. Casscells W, Hathorn B, David M, et al: Thermal detection of cellular infiltrates in living atherosclerotic plaques: Possible implications for plaque rupture and thrombosis. Lancet 1996;347:1447–1451.
19. Fayad ZA, Fuster V, Fallon JT, et al: Noninvasive in vivo human coronary artery lumen and wall imaging using black-blood magnetic resonance imaging. Circulation 2000;102:506–510.
20. Rabbani R, Topol EJ: Strategies to achieve coronary arterial plaque stabilization. Cardiovasc Res 1999;41:402–417.
21. Goldstein JA, Demetriou D, Grines CL, et al: Multiple complex coronary plaques in patients with acute myocardial infarction. N Engl J Med 2000;343:915–922.
22. Falk E, Shah PK, Fuster V: Coronary plaque disruption. Circulation 1995;92:657–671.
23. Wallsh E, Weinstein GS, Franzone A, et al: Inflammation of the coronary arteries in patients with unstable angina. Tex Heart Inst J 1986;16:105–113.
24. Libby P, Ridker PM: Novel inflammatory markers of coronary risk: Theory versus practice. Circulation 1999;100:1148–1150.
25. Mehta J, Dinerman J, Mehta P, et al: Neutrophil function in ischemic heart disease. Circulation 1989;79:549–556.
26. Dinerman JL, Mehta JL, Saldeen TGP, et al: Increased neutrophil elastase release in unstable angina pectoris and acute myocardial infarction. J Am Coll Cardiol 1990;15:1559–1563.
27. Mazzone A, De Servi S, Ricevuti G, et al: Increased expression of neutrophil and monocyte adhesion molecules in unstable coronary artery disease. Circulation 1993;88:358–363.
28. Biasucci LM, D'Onofrio G, Liuzzo G, et al: Intracellular neutrophil myeloperoxidase is reduced in unstable angina and myocardial infarction, but its reduction is not related to ischemia. J Am Coll Cardiol 1996;27:611–616.
29. Buffon A, Biasucci LM, Liuzzo G, et al: Widespread coronary inflammation in patients with unstable angina. N Engl J Med 2002;347:5–12.
30. Neri Serneri GG, Abbate R, Gori AM, et al: Transient intermittent lymphocyte activation is responsible for the instability of angina. Circulation 1992;86:790–797.
31. Neri Serneri GG, Prisco D, Martini F, et al: Acute T-cell activation is detectable in unstable angina. Circulation 1997;95:1806–1812.
32. Caligiuri G, Liuzzo G, Biasucci LM, et al: Immune system activation follows inflammation in unstable angina: Pathogenetic implications. J Am Coll Cardiol 1998;32:1295–1304.
33. Blum A, Sclarovsky S, Shohat B: T lymphocyte activation in stable angina pectoris and after percutaneous transluminal coronary angioplasty. Circulation 1995;91:20–22.

34. Liuzzo G, Kopecky SL, O'Fallon MW, et al: Perturbation of the T cell repertoire in patients with unstable angina. Circulation 1999;100:2135-2139.

35. Liuzzo G, Goronzy JJ, Yang H, et al: Monoclonal T-cell proliferation and plaque instability in acute coronary syndromes. Circulation 2000;101:2883-2888.

36. Caligiuri G, Paulsson G, Nicoletti A, et al: Evidence for antigen-driven T-cell response in unstable angina. Circulation 2000;102:1114-1119.

37. Jude B, Agraou B, McFadden EP, et al: Evidence for time-dependent activation of monocytes in the systemic circulation in unstable angina but not in acute myocardial infarction or in stable angina. Circulation 1994;90:1662-1668.

38. Liuzzo G, Angiolillo DJ, Buffon A, et al: Enhanced response of blood monocytes to in vitro lipopolysaccharide-challenge in patients with recurrent unstable angina. Circulation 2001;103:2236-2241.

39. Danesh J, Collins R, Peto R: Chronic infections and coronary artery disease: Is there a link? Lancet 1997;350:430-436.

40. Kol A, Bourcier T, Lichtman AH, et al: Chlamydial and human heat shock protein 60s activate human vascular endothelium, smooth muscle cells, and macrophages. J Clin Invest 1999;103:571-577.

41. Vejar M, Fragasso G, Hackett D, et al: Dissociation of platelet activation and spontaneous myocardial ischemia in unstable angina. Thromb Haemost 1990;63:163-168.

42. Cipollone F, Patrignani P, Greco A, et al: Differential suppression of thromboxane biosynthesis by indobufen and aspirin in patients with unstable angina. Circulation 1997;96:1109-1116.

43. Berk BC, Weintraub WS, Alexander RW: Elevation of C-reactive protein in active coronary disease. Am J Cardiol 1990;65:168-172.

44. Liuzzo G, Biasucci LM, Gallimore JR, et al: The prognostic value of C-reactive protein and serum amyloid A protein in severe unstable angina. N Engl J Med 1994;331:417-424.

45. Biasucci LM, Vitelli A, Liuzzo G, et al: Elevated levels of IL-6 in unstable angina. Circulation 1996;94:874-877.

46. Biasucci LM, Liuzzo G, Fantuzzi G, et al: Increasing levels of IL-1Ra and of IL-6 during the first two days of hospitalization in unstable angina are associated with increased risk of in-hospital coronary events. Circulation 1999;99:2079-2084.

47. Ridker P: High sensitivity C-reactive protein: Potential adjunct for global risk assessment in primary prevention of cardiovascular disease. Circulation 2001;103:1813-1818.

48. Biasucci LM, Liuzzo G, Grillo RL, et al: Elevated levels of C-reactive protein at discharge in patients with unstable angina predict recurrent instability. Circulation 1999;99:855-860.

49. Liuzzo G, Biasucci LM, Gallimore JR, et al: Enhanced inflammatory response in patients with pre-infarction unstable angina. J Am Coll Cardiol 1999;34:1696-1703.

50. Pepys MB, Baltz ML: Acute phase proteins with special reference to C-reactive protein and related proteins (pentaxins) and serum amyloid A protein. Adv Immunol 1983;34:141-212.

51. Lagrand WK, Visser CA, et al: C-reactive protein as a cardiovascular risk factor: More than an epiphenomenon? Circulation 1999;100:96-102.

52. Pepys MB, Hirschfield GM: C-reactive protein and atherothrombosis. Ital Heart J 2001;2:196-199.

53. Bhakdi S, Torzewski M, Klouche M, et al: Complement and atherogenesis: Binding of CRP to degraded, nonoxidized LDL enhances complement activation. Arterioscler Thromb Vasc Biol 1999;19:2348-2354.

54. Torzewski M, Rist C, Mortensen RF, et al: C-reactive protein in the arterial intima: Role of C-reactive protein receptor-dependent monocyte recruitment in atherogenesis. Arterioscler Thromb Vasc Biol 2000;20:2094-2098.

55. Zhang YX, Cliff WJ, Schoefl GI, et al: Coronary C-reactive protein distribution: Its relation to development of atherosclerosis. Atherosclerosis 1999;145:375-379.

56. Nakagomi A, Freedman SB, Geczy CL: Interferon-γ and lipopolysaccharide potentiate monocyte tissue factor induction by C-reactive protein: Relationship with age, sex, and hormone replacement treatment. Circulation 2000;101:1785-1791.

57. Pasceri V, Willerson JT, Yeh ET: Direct proinflammatory effect of C-reactive protein on human endothelial cells. Circulation 2000;102:2165-2168.

58. Pasceri V, Chang J, Willerson JT, et al: Modulation of C-reactive protein-mediated monocyte chemoattractant protein-1 induction in human endothelial cells by anti-atherosclerosis drugs. Circulation 2001;103:2531-2534.

59. Biasucci LM, Meo A, Buffon A, et al: Independent prognostic value of CRP levels for in-hospital death and myocardial infarction in unstable angina [abstract]. Circulation 2000;102(Suppl):499.

60. Morrow DA, Rifai N, Antman EM, et al: C-reactive protein is a potent predictor of mortality independently of and in combination with troponin T in acute coronary syndromes: A TIMI IIA substudy. Thrombolysis in Myocardial Infarction. J Am Coll Cardiol 1998;31:1460-1465.

61. Oltrona L, Ardissino D, Merlini PA, et al: C-reactive protein elevation and early outcome in patients with unstable angina pectoris. Am J Cardiol 1997;80:1002-1006.

62. Montalescot G, Philippe F, Ankri A, et al: Early increase of von Willebrand factor predicts adverse outcome in unstable coronary artery disease: Beneficial effects of enoxaparin. French Investigators of the ESSENCE Trial. Circulation 1998;98:294-299.

63. Rebuzzi AG, Quaranta G, Liuzzo G, et al: Incremental prognostic value of serum levels of troponin T and C-reactive protein on admission in patients with unstable angina pectoris. Am J Cardiol 1998;82:715-719.

64. Verheggen PW, de Maat MP, Cats VM, et al: Inflammatory status as a main determinant of outcome in patients with unstable angina, independent of coagulation activation and endothelial cell function. Eur Heart J 1999;20:567-574.

65. Thompson SG, Kienast J, Pyke SD, et al: Hemostatic factors and the risk of myocardial infarction or sudden death in patients with angina pectoris. European Concerted Action on Thrombosis and Disabilities Angina Pectoris Study Group. N Engl J Med 1995;332:635-641.

66. Haverkate F, Thompson SG, Pyke SD, et al: Production of C-reactive protein and risk of coronary events in stable and unstable angina. European Concerted Action on Thrombosis and Disabilities Angina Pectoris Study Group. Lancet 1997;349:462-466.

67. Toss H, Lindahl B, Siegbahn A, et al: Prognostic influence of increased fibrinogen and C-reactive protein levels in unstable coronary artery disease. FRISC Study Group. Fragmin during Instability in Coronary Artery Disease. Circulation 1997;96:4204-4210.

68. Lindahl B, Toss H, Siegbahn A, et al: Markers of myocardial damage and inflammation in relation to long-term mortality in unstable coronary artery disease. FRISC Study Group. Fragmin during Instability in Coronary Artery Disease. N Engl J Med 2000;343:1139-1147.

69. Biasucci LM, Liuzzo G, Grillo RL, et al: Elevated levels of C-reactive protein at discharge in patients with unstable angina predict recurrent instability. Circulation 1999;99:855-860.

70. Buffon A, Liuzzo G, Biasucci LM, et al: Preprocedural serum levels of C-reactive protein predict early complications and late restenosis after coronary angioplasty. J Am Coll Cardiol 1999;34:1512-1521.

71. Chew DP, Bhatt DL, Robbins MA, et al: Incremental prognostic value of elevated baseline C-reactive protein among established markers of risk in percutaneous coronary intervention. Circulation 2001;104:992-997.

72. Milazzo D, Biasucci LM, Luciani N, et al: Elevated levels of C-reactive protein before coronary artery bypass grafting predict recurrence of ischemic events. Am J Cardiol 1999;84:459-461, A9.

73. Ferreiros ER, Boissonnet CP, Pizarro R, et al: Independent prognostic value of elevated C-reactive protein in unstable angina. Circulation 1999;100:1958-1963.

74. Heeschen C, Hamm CW, Bruemmer J, et al: Predictive value of C-reactive protein and troponin T in patients with unstable angina: A comparative analysis. CAPTURE Investigators. Chimeric c7E3 AntiPlatelet Therapy in Unstable angina REfractory to standard treatment trial. J Am Coll Cardiol 2000;35:1535-1542.

75. Muller C, Buetter HJ, Hodgson JM, et al: Inflammation and long-term mortality after non-ST elevation acute coronary syndromes treated with a very early invasive strategy in 1042 consecutive patients. Circulation 2002;105:1412-1415.

76. Versaci F, Gaspardone A, Tomai F, et al: Predictive value of C-reactive protein in patients with unstable angina pectoris undergoing coronary artery stent implantation. Am J Cardiol 2000;85:92-95, A8.

77. Walter DH, Fichtlscherer S, Sellwig M, et al: Preprocedural C-reactive protein levels and cardiovascular events after coronary stent implantation. J Am Coll Cardiol 2001;37:839-846.

78. Zhou YF, Csako G, Grayston JT, et al: Lack of association of restenosis following coronary angioplasty with elevated C-reactive protein levels or seropositivity to *Chlamydia pneumoniae*. Am J Cardiol 1999;84:595–598, A8.

79. Chew DP, Bhatt DL, Robbins MA, et al: Effect of clopidogrel added to aspirin before percutaneous coronary intervention on the risk associated with C-reactive protein. Am J Cardiol 2001; 88:672–674.

80. Tomoda H, Aoki N: Prognostic value of C-reactive protein levels within six hours after the onset of acute myocardial infarction. Am Heart J 2000;140:324–328.

81. Ridker PM, Cushman M, Stampfer MJ, et al: Inflammation, aspirin, and the risk of cardiovascular disease in apparently healthy men. N Engl J Med 1997;336:973–979.

82. Kuller LH, Russel PT, Shaten J, et al, for the MRFIT Research Group: Relation of C-reactive Protein and Coronary Heart Disease in the MRFIT Nested Case-Control Study. Am J Epidemiol 1996;144: 537–547.

83. Tracy RP, Lemaitre RN, Psaty BM, et al: Relationship of C-reactive protein to risk of cardiovascular disease in elderly: Results from the Cardiovascular Health Study and the Rural Health Promotion Project. Arterioscler Thromb Vasc Biol 1997;17:1121–1127.

84. Ridker PM, Hennekens CH, Buring JE, et al: C-reactive protein and other markers of inflammation in the prediction of cardiovascular disease in women. N Engl J Med 2000;342:836–843.

85. Koening W, Sund M, Froelich M, et al: C-reactive protein, a sensitive marker of inflammation, predicts future risk of coronary heart disease in initially healthy middle-aged men: Results from the MONICA Augsberg Cohort Study, 1984 to 1992. Circulation 1999;99: 237–242.

86. Roivainen M, Viik-Kajander M, Palouso T, et al: Infections, inflammation and the risk of coronary heart disease. Circulation 2000;101: 252–257.

87. Danesh J, Whincup P, Walker M, et al: Low grade inflammation and coronary heart disease: Prospective study and updated meta-analyses. BMJ 2000;321:199–201.

88. Ridker PM, Glynn RJ, Hennekens CH: C-reactive protein adds to the predictive value of total and HDL cholesterol in determining risk of first myocardial infarction. Circulation 1998;97: 2007–2011.

89. Ridker PM, Rifai N, Pfeffer MA, et al: Inflammation, pravastatin, and the risk of coronary events after myocardial infarction in patients with average cholesterol levels. Cholesterol and Recurrent Events (CARE) Investigators. Circulation 1998;98: 839–844.

90. Ridker PM, Rifai N, Pfeffer M, et al: Long-term effects of pravastatin on plasma concentration of C-reactive protein. Circulation 1999;100:230–235.

91. Ridker PM, Rifai N, Lowenthal SP: Rapid reduction in C-reactive protein with cerivastatin among 785 patients with primary hypercholesterolemia. Circulation 2001;103:1191–1193.

92. Ridker PM, Rifai N, Clearfield M, et al, for the Air Force/Texas Coronary Atherosclerosis Prevention Study Investigators: Measurement of C-reactive protein for the targeting of statin therapy in the primary prevention of acute coronary events. N Engl J Med 2001;344:1959–1965.

93. Ridker PM, Rifai N, Stampfer M, et al: Plasma concentration of interleukin-6 and the risk of future myocardial infarction among apparently healthy men. Circulation 2000;101:1767–1772.

94. Ridker PM, Rifai N, Pfeffer M, et al: Elevation of tumor necrosis factor-α and increased risk of recurrent coronary events after myocardial infarction. Circulation 2000;101:2149–2153.

95. Lindmark E, Diderholm E, Wallentin L, et al: Relationship between interleukin 6 and mortality in patients with unstable coronary artery disease: Effects of an early invasive or noninvasive strategy. JAMA 2001;286:2107–2113.

96. Malik I, Danesh J, Whincup P, et al: Soluble adhesion molecules and prediction of coronary heart disease: A prospective study and meta-analysis. Lancet 2001;358:971–975.

97. Mulvihill NT, Foley JB, Murphy R, et al: Evidence of prolonged inflammation in unstable angina and non-Q wave myocardial infarction. J Am Coll Cardiol 2000;36:1210–1216.

98. de Lemos JA, Hennekens CH, Ridker PM: Plasma concentration of soluble vascular cell adhesion molecule-1 and subsequent cardiovascular risk. J Am Coll Cardiol 2000;36:423–426.

99. Ridker PM, Hennekens CH, Roitman-Johnson B, et al: Plasma concentration of soluble intercellular adhesion molecule 1 and risk of future myocardial infarction in apparently healthy men. Lancet 1998;351:88–92.

100. Ridker PM, Buring JE, Rifai N: Soluble P-selectin and the risk of future cardiovascular events. Circulation 2001;103:491–495.

101. Blankenberg S, Rupprecht HJ, Bickel C, et al: Circulating cell adhesion molecules and death in patients with coronary artery disease. Circulation 2001;104:1336–1342.

102. Liuzzo G, Buffon A, Biasucci LM, et al: Enhanced inflammatory response to coronary angioplasty in patients with severe unstable angina. Circulation 1998;98:2370–2376.

103. Roberts WL, Moulton L, Law TC, et al: Evaluation of nine automated high-sensitivity C-reactive protein methods: Implications for clinical and epidemiological applications. Clin Chem 2001;47:418–425.

104. Lincoff AM, Kereiakes DJ, Mascelli MA, et al: Abciximab suppresses the rise in levels of circulating inflammatory markers after percutaneous coronary revascularization. Circulation 2001;104: 163–167.

105. Hernandez-Presa M, Buston C, Ortego M, et al: Angiotensin converting enzyme inhibition prevents arterial nuclear factor-kappa B activation, monocyte chemoattractant protein-1 expression, and macrophage infiltration in a rabbit model of early accelerated atherosclerosis. Circulation 1997;95:1532–1541.

106. Biasucci LM, Liuzzo G, Caligiuri G, et al: Activation of the coagulation system doesn't elicit a detectable acute phase reaction in unstable angina. Am J Cardiol 1996;77:85–87.

107. Liuzzo G, Biasucci LM, Rebuzzi AG, et al: The plasma protein acute phase response in unstable angina is not induced by ischemic injury. Circulation 1996;94:874–877.

108. Ridker PM, Kundsin RB, Stampfer MJ, et al: Prospective study of *Chlamydia pneumoniae* IgG seropositivity and risks of future myocardial infarction. Circulation 1999;99:1161–1164.

109. Hoffmeister A, Rothenbacher D, Wanner P, et al: Seropositivity to chlamydial lipopolysaccharide and *Chlamydia pneumoniae*, systemic inflammation and stable coronary artery disease: Negative results of a case-control study. J Am Coll Cardiol 2000;35:112–118.

Coronary Angiography and the Culprit Lesion in Acute Coronary Syndromes

François Ledru
Johan H. C. Reiber
Joan C. Tuinenburg
Gerhard Koning
Jacques Lespérance

Since the first reports of the use of contrast coronary arteriography in the late 1950s and early 1960s, coronary angiography has become the gold standard to explore in patients the correlation between coronary anatomy, clinical presentation, and natural history of coronary artery disease (CAD),[1] and options for revascularization. Miniaturization, improvements in radiographic equipment and image quality, and quantitative angiography coupled with growing experience opened the eras of coronary bypass surgery in the early 1960s and of percutaneous coronary interventions in the 1970s.[2,3] More recently, coronary angiography has been applied in the acute phase of acute ischemic syndromes, first in unstable angina and later in myocardial infarction (MI). The work of DeWood and colleagues[4] published in 1980 provided the first descriptions of coronary anatomy during the early hours of an evolving acute MI. Since the 1980s, the ability to characterize the angiographic anatomy in acute coronary events has had a major impact on improving quality of care of patients with acute coronary syndromes (ACS). This chapter first reviews the basics for image acquisition and quantitative coronary arteriography (QCA) and second the clinical use of the various descriptors of the culprit lesion in patients with an ACS.

TECHNIQUE OF ANGIOGRAPHIC ACQUISITION

This description is limited to digital image acquisition and treatment, which has now replaced the analog 35-mm cinefilm acquisition (Fig. 17–1). In the digital approach, the output image of the image intensifier is projected onto the input target of a video camera or CCD (charge-coupled device) camera.[5] The analog video output signal is modified electronically in the so-called white compression unit, to enhance the contrast difference that is attenuated by x-ray absorption (e.g., vertebrae and contrast-filled arteries or ventricle) and reduce the contrast differences in areas with low x-ray absorption (e.g., lungs). The approach has markedly improved image resolution. The video signal is digitized

at a resolution of 512×512 pixels $\times 8$ bits on most x-ray systems and 1024×1024 pixels $\times 12$ bits on some other x-ray systems and is stored on high-speed and high-capacity disks (RAID system) for subsequent analysis. This resolution in the standard 512×512 pixels $\times 8$ bits mode is associated with a typically relatively large pixel size of about 0.2 mm compared with that achievable with cinefilm that was typically 0.08 to 0.10 mm following optical magnification. A complete patient study can be stored in DICOM format on CD-ROM after the procedure.

New developments in image intensifier technology will lead to replacement of the conventional vacuum tube by a completely digital flat panel image intensifier or digital detector. First-generation systems are currently available. Typical matrix size of the flat panel for the General Electric system is 1000×1000 pixels, but the actual image matrix size ranges from 600×600 pixels for a 12-cm field-of-view to 836×836 pixels for a 17-cm field-of-view with 12 bits depth for cardiac acquisitions. These flat panels are characterized by linear responses and the absence of geometric distortions, such as that caused by pincushion.

METHODS FOR ANGIOGRAPHIC CHARACTERIZATION

History of Quantitative Coronary Arteriography

QCA was developed in the 1970s to study vessel vasomotion and the influence of drugs on the regression and progression of CAD.[6,7] Vessel contours were first traced manually on optic x-ray frames. Later, semiautomated algorithms for edge detection were developed.[8-10] In the early 1980s, the introduction of coronary revascularization procedures and the growing interest in drug effects on stabilization and regression of existing CAD and on the prevention of new lesions regenerated interest in QCA.[11] The first-generation QCA systems developed in the 1980s were based on 35-mm cinefilm analysis. In the mid-1980s, digital systems were

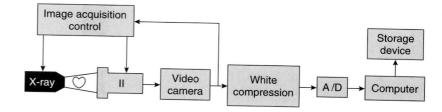

FIGURE 17–1. Block diagram of digital angiographic x-ray system.

introduced into the catheterization laboratory to support the angiographer during interventional procedures, first with single digital frames displayed for road map purposes and later with cineloops and on-line QCA.[12] The second-generation systems introduced between 1990 and 1994 were further improved for more precise edge detection of digital images and for corrections of the overestimation of vessels smaller than 1.2 mm.[13] Third-generation QCA systems developed between 1995 and 1998 provided solutions for the quantitative analysis of complex lesion morphology using the gradient field transform (GFT)[14] and an improved diameter function analysis.[15] The establishment of DICOM for digital image exchange and HL7 for data administration led to the integration of QCA systems in the complex hospital environment. In 1999, the enhanced capabilities of modern workstations led to the introduction of fourth-generation QCA systems, characterized by simplified portability for digital DICOM viewers, network connectivity, improved software for data reporting and database manipulation, and new options for specialized QCA applications, such as in brachytherapy.[16] Although most modern QCA packages are based on a linear programming approach (i.e., a minimal cost algorithm) for contour detection, differences still exist in the qualities of the various packages, which need to be validated.[17]

Basic Principles of Quantitative Coronary Arteriography

The requirements for application of a QCA package in a routine clinical or research environment are as follows:

- Minimal user interaction for the selection and processing of the coronary segment to be analyzed.
- Minimal editing of the automatically determined results and a rare need to edit the findings, such as the detected contours of the arterial segments.
- A short analysis time (≤10 seconds).
- Highly accurate and precise results with minimal systematic and random errors in the assessment of the morphologic data. This needs to be validated with phantoms and angiographic results.

The QCA-CMS (Clinical Measurement Solutions; MEDIS medical imaging systems, Leiden, The Netherlands) algorithms were designed to respond to these requirements.[9,12,18] Figure 17–2 summarizes the operational procedures. The operator first selects with a mouse the start and end of the coronary segment to be analyzed. The analysis follows automatically resulting in a display of the detected contours (see Fig. 17–2D). The intermediate steps shown in Figure 17–2B and C are not usually displayed. However, an option is available to the operator for editing the contours with minimal cost algorithm (MCA) iterations to preserve the brightness information. This MCA approach is fast and generally valid for images of variable quality. However, some highly complex morphology, such as post procedure dissection, may not be analyzed properly. A more complex algorithm, the GFT,[14] has been developed to circumvent these limitations. It is applied by a third iteration[14] of the contour detection procedure. An example of the GFT is shown in Figure 17–3.

Calibration Procedure

To provide absolute numbers on vessel sizes, a calibration factor expressed in mm/pixel is needed. This is achieved by applying the MCA edge-detection procedure for parallel boundaries on a non-tapering section of the contrast-filled catheter. The calibration can be a weak part of the analysis chain because the quality of the display of the catheter images is often variable. When a calibration factor cannot be obtained for any reason, only the percentage diameter narrowing of the obstruction can be measured.

It is recommended to use catheters of the same type (size, material, and manufacturer) for repeated QCA measures in the same patient. Catheter sizes should be 6F or more to limit the variability of the calibration factor. Further information on QCA calibration standardization can be found elsewhere in the literature.[19]

Coronary Segment Analysis

The diameter function is determined from the left-hand and right-hand contours of the arterial segment (Fig. 17–4).[15] The percent diameter reduction is the most widely assessed parameter. Calculation of this parameter requires a reference diameter value. A user-defined reference diameter at a so-called normal portion of the vessel or an automated or interpolated reference diameter serves this purpose. In the interpolated approach, the reference diameter is reconstructed at the exact site of the obstruction of interest. This approach is usually preferred because it requires no user interaction, takes into account vessel tapering, and minimizes overestimation or underestimation by calculating the reference value in the stenotic segment analyzed (see Fig. 17–4).

Other parameters that can be derived automatically from the diameter function include the obstruction diameter (mm), the length of obstruction (mm),[12] the area of the atherosclerotic plaque (mm²), the plaque

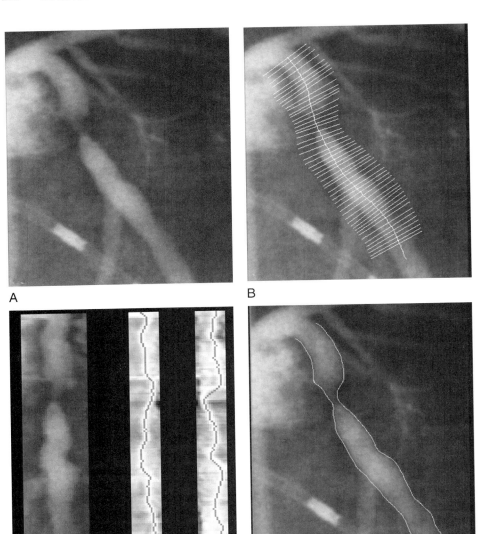

A

B

C

D

FIGURE 17–2. Basic principles of the minimum cost algorithm contour-detection algorithm as shown in digitized cinefilm images. *A,* Image shows the segment to be analyzed. *B,* After the pathline has been detected, scanlines are defined perpendicular to this first model (i.e., the pathline). *C,* The image is resampled along the scanlines, and corresponding gray-level values are stored in a rectangular matrix (see straightened vessel segment at *left*). Next, the changes in gray-level values (edge-strength values) along the horizontal lines are calculated in this rectangular matrix and stored in separate "cost" matrices for the left-hand and the right-hand contours (at *right*). The minimum cost algorithm searches for optimal contour paths in these cost matrices *(curves).* A similar procedure is followed in the second iteration, using these contours as models. *D,* The detected contours are transformed back to the original image, and the diameter measurements can be performed.

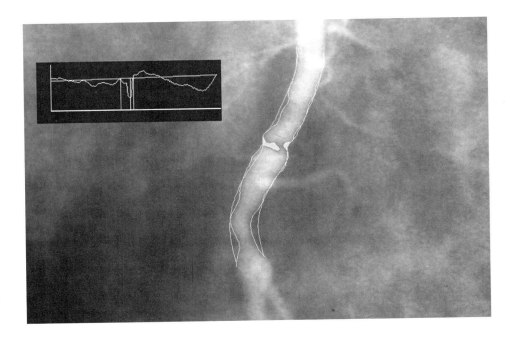

FIGURE 17–3. Example of the outcome of gradient field transform analysis on a vessel segment with a severe complex stenosis. Conventional approaches with the minimum cost algorithm are not able to follow automatically the abrupt changes in morphology.

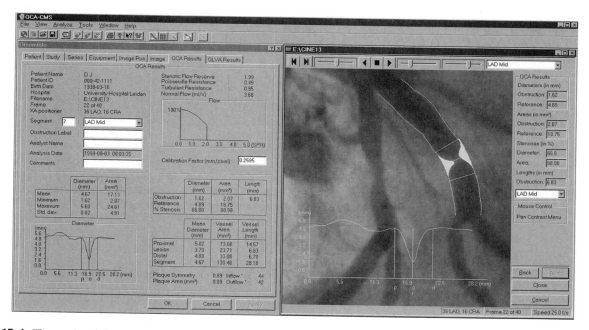

FIGURE 17–4. The results of the minimum cost algorithm, including the reconstructed original vessel contours, plaque area *(shaded)*, and the diameter function, are presented for QCA-CMS V4.0. All the derived absolute and relative quantitative coronary arteriography (QCA) parameters are presented in the QCA DICOM-box *(left)*.

symmetry (value between 0 and 1, no unit), the inflow and outflow angles,[20] and the functional stenotic flow reserve.[21] Figure 17–5 illustrates how the symmetry index and the inflow and outflow angles are calculated.

A stenotic flow reserve index can be derived from a mathematical/physiologic model, by assessing the maximal hyperemic flow through a single obstruction. It corresponds to a wind tunnel test of the stenosis under standardized conditions.[22] The stenotic flow reserve is 4 or 5 in disease-free segments, and decreases in correlation with the severity of the obstruction.

We introduced and validated the diffuse index, which allows objective assessment of the extent of a plaque within a stent or an obstruction.[22-26] This index is derived from the diameter function (Fig. 17–6). Its value to characterize the culprit lesions in ACS remains to be studied.

Densitometry

Because the x-ray arteriogram is a two-dimensional projection of a three-dimensional structure, the measured

FIGURE 17–5. Calculation of the symmetry index and inflow/outflow angles. *A,* The symmetry index is measured as the ratio of the area of each border of the stenosis in the two-dimensional representation (a and b, b being conventionally greater than a). It ranges from 0% (asymmetry) to 100% (symmetry). *B,* The inflow/outflow angles are calculated from the diameter function. The stenosis inlet corresponds to the distance between the proximal boundary of the stenosis (P) and maximal obstruction (O) and the stenosis outlet to the area between the maximal obstruction and the distal boundary of the stenosis (D). The inflow and outflow geometric angles are calculated as the angles of lines drawn between P and O and between O and D. The average angles correspond to the angles of the linear regressions of the diameter function between P and O and between O and D. The maximal angles are calculated at the maximal slopes of the inflow and outflow diameter function. All angles are corrected for the tapering (β) of the analyzed segment.[20] (From Ledru F, Théroux T, Lespérance J, et al: Geometric features of coronary artery lesions favoring acute occlusion and myocardial infarction: A quantitative angiographic study. J Am Coll Cardiol 1999;33:1353–1361.)

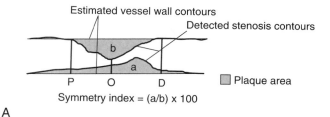

Symmetry Index

Symmetry index = (a/b) × 100

A

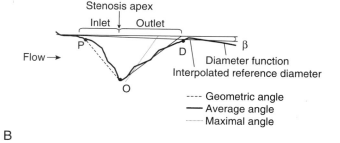

Diameter Function and Derived Angles

B

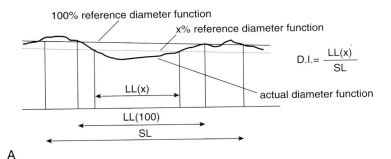

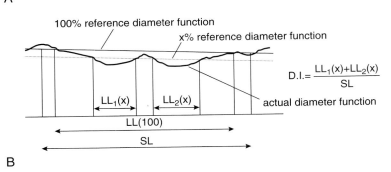

A

B

FIGURE 17-6. Schema of calculation of diffuse index (DI). *A,* Usually lesion length (LL) of a coronary narrowing is derived from the 100% reference diameter function (LL(100)). By shifting the reference diameter function downward in a parallel pattern through the diameter function, the modified LL at a percentage *x* of the reference diameter function (LL(x)) becomes smaller. Dividing this length (LL(x)) within the stent by the total stent length (SL) provides a measure of the DI at a percentage x of the reference diameter function (*A,* DI = LL(x)/SL). *B,* In case the reference diameter function intersects the actual diameter function several times within the stent, the summation of the segments where the reference diameter function runs above the actual diameter function is divided by the total stent length (*B,* DI = (LL₁(x) + LL₂(x))/ SL).[25] (From Ishii Y, van Weert A, Hekking E, et al: A novel quantitative method for evaluating diffuse in-stent narrowing at follow-up angiography. Cathet Cardiovasc Intervent 2001;54:309-317. Used by permission of Wiley-Liss, Inc, a subsidiary of John Wiley & Sons, Inc. Copyright © 2001 Cathet Cardiovasc Intervent.)

values may be of limited value in vessels with irregular cross sections. For this reason, much effort has been invested to derive information on the path lengths of the x-rays through vessels based on brightness levels.[10] With such information, cross-sectional areas could be calculated from a single angiographic view. This approach is called the *densitometric measurement technique.*

Theoretically, densitometry could be the solution for computing the vessel's cross-sectional area from a single angiographic view. So far, however, densitometry failed to provide reliable results,[27] reducing the enthusiasm for the approach. It may be of interest to revisit the densitometric approaches on digital systems, which control better the entire transfer function of the x-ray system.

Requirements for the Appropriate Use of Quantitative Coronary Arteriography in the Clinical Setting

The primary objective of QCA measurements in clinical research is to quantify accurately the impact of interventions on changes in the diameter functions, such as acute lumen gain and late lumen loss. This quantification is best achieved by applying exactly the same settings in the baseline and follow-up studies, by replicating the same views, the same doses of vasodilator and the same contrast media, and by using the same catheter type and material, and, if possible, the same catheterization laboratory.[28]

Quantitative Coronary Arteriography Validation

All QCA analytical software packages generate numbers describing the morphology of the coronary segment ana-

lyzed. It is crucial to validate the strengths and weaknesses of the various packages.

Validation is described in terms of the systematic error or accuracy, defined as the average signed difference between repeated measurements (i.e., measurement 1 minus measurement 2), and the random error or precision, calculated as the standard deviation of these signed differences. Guidelines for standards for systematic and random error values of absolute vessel dimensions have been established and are shown in Table 17-1.[12,13,19,29]

Plexiglas Phantom Studies

The QCA-CMS V4.0 analytical package was validated using a Plexiglas phantom with tube sizes of 0.80 to 5.00 mm. The tubes were filled with 100% contrast medium,

■ ▓ ■

TABLE 17-1 GUIDELINES FOR SYSTEMATIC AND RANDOM ERRORS OF A STATE-OF-THE-ART QUANTITATIVE CORONARY ARTERIOGRAPHY SYSTEM*

TYPE OF STUDY	SYSTEMATIC ERROR (MM)	RANDOM ERROR (MM)
Plexiglas phantom, off patient	<0.10	0.10-0.13
Plexiglas phantom, on patient	<0.10	0.10-0.13
Intraobserver variabilities		0.10-0.15
Interobserver variabilities		0.10-0.15
Short-term variabilities		0.15-0.25
Medium-term variabilities		0.20-0.30
Inter-core laboratory variability		0.10-0.15

*The systematic error values for the Plexiglas phantom apply to each of the individual measurements.

■ ■ ■

TABLE 17–2   QUANTITATIVE CORONARY ARTERIOGRAPHY RESULTS FOR A PLEXIGLAS PHANTOM ACQUIRED ON A HOMOGENEOUS BACKGROUND

II-SIZE	KV-LEVEL	DIGITAL 512[2] SE ± RE	ON-LINE SE ± RE	CINEFILM V4.0 SE ± RE
5-inch	60 kV	0.00 ± 0.04	–0.02 ± 0.05	0.03 ± 0.03
	75 kV	0.00 ± 0.07	–0.02 ± 0.07	–0.02 ± 0.07
	90 kV	–0.01 ± 0.09	–0.04 ± 0.11	–0.04 ± 0.11
7-inch	60 kV	0.01 ± 0.05	0.00 ± 0.05	0.05 ± 0.05
	75 kV	0.01 ± 0.07	–0.02 ± 0.08	0.00 ± 0.08
	90 kV	–0.01 ± 0.10	0.00 ± 0.10	–0.03 ± 0.10

RE, random error; SE, systematic error.

and the data were obtained at 60, 75, and 90 kV, using 5-inch and 7-inch image intensifier sizes. Three different analyses were carried out: (1) off-line from 35-mm cinefilm, (2) off-line from DICOM-CD, and (3) on-line from video digitized frames. The off-patient results are presented in Table 17–2. They show that the systematic and random errors were within the guidelines for all three acquisition modes. Variability or random errors increased with increasing kilovoltage level because of loss of image contrast levels. The lowest variability was obtained with the digital 5122 images, although the differences are small. The overall variability was slightly higher when the phantom was positioned on a nonhomogeneous background (patient's chest) compared with a homogeneous background.[13]

In Vivo Plugs

The ultimate test for a QCA system validation is the analysis of angiograms with known dimensions of the obstructions. For this purpose, small plastic plugs (outer diameters of 2.5 to 3.5 mm, inner diameters of 0.5 to 1.57 mm, length of approximately 7.5 mm) are introduced with a catheter into the coronary arteries of dogs. Images are acquired on cinefilm and in digital format. The comparison of mean diameters and standard deviations of these obstructions with the true inner diameter of the plugs has provided systematic and random errors in the range observed with the coronary Plexiglas phantom models.[13]

Interobserver and Intraobserver and Short-Term and Medium-Term Variabilities

Extensive data on interobservers and intraobservers and on short-term and medium-term variability are available. A summary of these results using the ACA/DCI V1.0 (Phillips Medical Systems, Best, The Netherlands) analytical software package[12] is presented in Table 17–3. The interobserver and intraobserver variability studies on routinely obtained digital coronary arteriograms showed a systematic error close to 0. The random errors for obstruction diameters were less than 0.11 mm and for the interpolated reference diameters less than 0.13 mm. Larger variabilities were observed, however, between short-term acquisitions repeated 5 minutes apart and at

the end of the catheterization procedure. These could be explained by variations in the procedures for repeated catheter calibration.

Interlaboratory Variability

The widespread use of QCA raises the question of the validity of comparing data obtained in different laboratories. This is important when data from various core laboratories are pooled. It is likely that systematic differences will exist between laboratories in the measurements of absolute dimensions. Trends in the same direction would support but not prove data validity. Objective validation of the reproducibility of these data is needed. The sources of variability between laboratories are multiple, including the equipment used, quality of the image, selection of coronary segments, frame selection, frame digitization (for cinefilm), and local experience of technicians in image analyses. Significant differences have been observed between different angiographic core laboratories, particularly when different QCA systems were used.[30]

We compared the results obtained in two core laboratories (Heart Core B.V., Leiden, the Netherlands, and the Montreal Heart Institute, Montreal, Canada) that have standardized their entire QCA procedure by implementing and validating common standard operating procedures.

■ ■ ■

TABLE 17–3   INTEROBSERVER AND INTRAOBSERVER AND SHORT-TERM AND MEDIUM-TERM VARIABILITIES USING THE ACA/DCI V1.0 ANALYTICAL SOFTWARE PACKAGE

VARIABILITIES	OBSTRUCTION DIAMETER (MM) SE ± RE	REFERENCE DIAMETER (MM) SE ± RE
Interobserver	–0.02 ± 0.11	–0.01 ± 0.13
Intraobserver	0.03 ± 0.10	0.03 ± 0.13
Short-term	0.00 ± 0.19	–0.02 ± 0.22
Medium-term	0.03 ± 0.18	–0.02 ± 0.34

RE, random error; SE, systematic error.

The most common differences observed between the two sites for the most important QCA parameters are presented in Table 17-4. Systematic errors were small between the two sites, and random errors were within the ranges previously reported for interobserver variability (see Table 17-1). Some of the data variations could have been introduced by the different video systems on the cinefilm digitizers (PAL and NTSC) used by the two sites. It can be concluded from this study that the interlaboratory variabilities can be minimal and within the range of that reported for interobserver and intraobserver variabilities when all procedures are carefully standardized.[29] Validation of the entire analysis procedure is required on a regular basis to ensure maintenance of high-quality standards.

Qualitative Descriptors of Lesion Complexity

Plaque morphology has received a great deal of attention since the original description by Levin and colleagues in 1981 of a correlation between complex plaques observed on a postmortem angiogram and the histologic findings.[31] Complex plaques at angiography are characterized by various degrees of eccentricity, irregularity, ulceration, filling defects, or haziness. These features have been described extensively elsewhere[32] and are summarized here.

Eccentricity

The term *eccentricity* describes lesions that have a lumen that lies in the outer quarter of the artery lumen diameter. Ambrose and colleagues[33] subdivided eccentric lesions into lesions with smooth borders and a broad neck (type I eccentric) and lesions with a narrow neck or irregular borders or both (type II eccentric).

Irregularities

The endoluminal edges of coronary lesions may be smooth and regular or coarse and irregular with a saw-tooth appearance (Fig. 17-7). These irregular lesions are not drawn easily because their borders may be hazy (Fig. 17-8). They may represent ruptured plaques, lesions with superimposed microthrombi, or recanalized thrombi (see Fig. 17-8).[31] Because irregularity is a highly subjective descriptor, Kalbfleisch and coworkers[34] attempted quantification with a contour edge detection technique using curvature and fractal analyses applied to each arterial border. Five morphometric parameters added information on plaque that was independent of the degree of lumen narrowing.

Ulcerations

Ulcerations are craters within a stenosis that are opacified by contrast medium. They presumably represent sequela of a ruptured plaque (Figs. 17-9 and 17-10). Ulcerations observed during acute MI may represent a mixture of plaque debris and thrombi that disappear following spontaneous or pharmacologic fibrinolysis with plaque healing. Wilson and associates[35] defined an index of ulceration assessed as the ratio of the diameter at the site of the least severe stenosis to the maximal intralesional diameter (Fig. 17-11). The ratio was independent

TABLE 17-4 INTERLABORATORY SYSTEMATIC AND RANDOM ERRORS IN THE INDIVIDUAL MEASUREMENTS FOR TWO HIGHLY STANDARDIZED AND COLLABORATING CORE LABORATORIES

N = 63	SYSTEMATIC ERROR	RANDOM ERROR
Obstruction diameter (mm)	-0.06	0.14
Reference diameter (mm)	-0.02	0.15
Percentage diameter stenosis (%)	1.83	4.96
Mean segment diameter (mm)	0.00	0.10

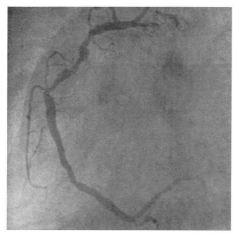
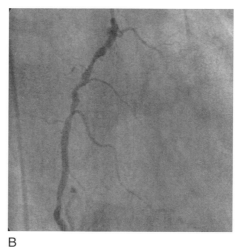

FIGURE 17-7. Complex lesion of the right coronary artery. Long plaque of the proximal right coronary artery with multiple irregularities and abrupt extremities discovered 8 days after a non–Q-wave myocardial infarction in a middle-aged man who had been treated conservatively. It is associated with a TIMI 2 grade flow.[61] *A*, 45-degree left anterior oblique view. *B*, 90-degree left anterior oblique view.

A

B

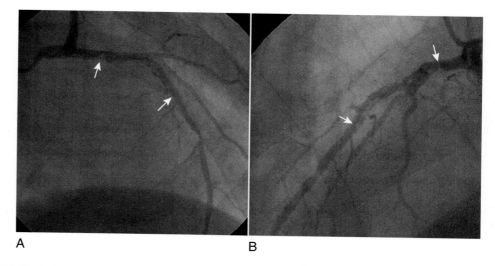

FIGURE 17–8. Recanalized thrombus of the left anterior descending artery. A 60-year-old woman presenting with symptoms of heart failure related to a dilated cardiomyopathy, a history of myocardial infarction, and a left bundle-branch block. The angiogram (cranial right anterior oblique view in *A;* left lateral view in *B*) shows multiple hazy intraluminal filling defects (extending between *arrows*) without any well-delineated lumen. The clinical history and angiographic aspect suggest recanalized thrombus. The antegrade blood flow was almost normal, but no viability of the anterior left ventricular myocardium could be shown.

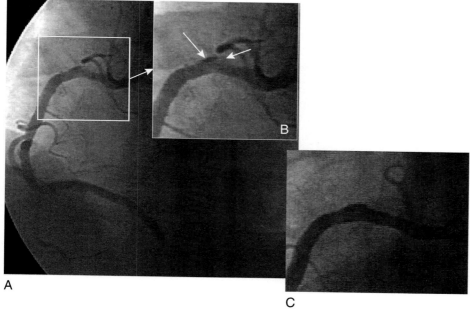

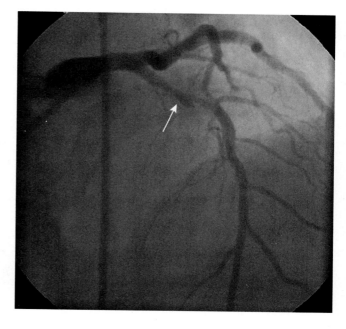

FIGURE 17–9. Ruptured plaque of the proximal right coronary artery. A 71-year-old man presenting with prolonged chest discomfort and a non–ST-segment elevation inferior myocardial infarction. *A,* Early (<4 hours) catheterization shows a patent right coronary artery with TIMI 3 grade flow and an ulcer in the proximal portion. *B,* Magnification reveals a well-delineated ulceration *(plain arrow)* with a linear horizontal filling defect *(dashed arrow)* suggestive of a ruptured fibrous cap. *C,* Control angiogram after 2 months shows a healed ulceration, with smooth borders and no remaining intraluminal defect. The plaque developed within the vessel wall without any deformation of the lumen itself.

FIGURE 17–10. Healed ulceration of the left anterior descending artery. Typical aspect of ulceration within a large atheromatous plaque of the proximal left anterior descending artery. The ulcer is deep with a sharp distal edge. An anterior Q-wave myocardial infarction occurred 3 months before, treated by thombolytics and conventional medications.

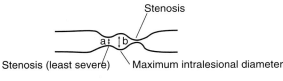

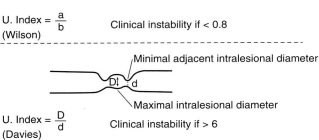

Stenosis

Stenosis (least severe)   Maximum intralesional diameter

U. Index = $\dfrac{a}{b}$ Clinical instability if < 0.8
(Wilson)

Minimal adjacent intralesional diameter

Maximal intralesional diameter

U. Index = $\dfrac{D}{d}$ Clinical instability if > 6
(Davies)

FIGURE 17–11. Ulceration indices. This scheme describes two methods to evaluate the degree of ulceration within a plaque, proposed by Wilson and colleagues[34] *(top panel)* and Davies and colleagues[35] *(bottom panel).* (From Lespérance J, Théroux P, Hudon G, et al: A new look at coronary angiograms: Plaque morphology as a help to diagnosis and to evaluate outcome. Int J Card Imaging 1994;10:75–94. Reprinted with permission from Kluwer Academic Publishers.)

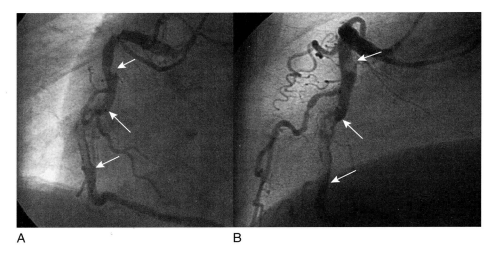

FIGURE 17–12. Intraluminal filling defects in the mid right coronary artery. Typical aspects of intracoronary thrombus with well-defined intraluminal lucencies, surrounded by contrast medium (*A,* 45-degree left anterior oblique projection; *B,* 90-degree left anterior oblique projection) in a 65-year-old patient admitted for refractory non–ST-segment elevation infarction in the inferior wall. The first thrombus in the proximal mid right coronary artery *(dashed arrows)* appears adherent to the vessel wall, whereas the second and longer thrombus in the distal mid right coronary artery *(plain arrows)* partially occludes the vessel lumen.

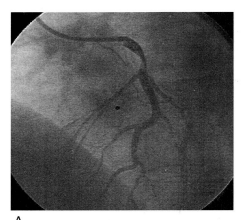

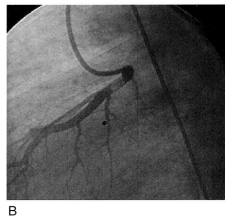

FIGURE 17–13. Intraluminal filling defect in the proximal left anterior descending artery in a young man. This 31-year-old patient was admitted for sustained and refractory chest pain with 5-mm ST-segment depression in the anterior electrocardiogram leads. Emergency (<2 hour) catheterization (*A,* 30-degree left anterior oblique view; *B,* 90-degree left anterior oblique view) showed an occlusive well-defined, oblong-shaped thrombus of the proximal left anterior descending artery. The coronary vessel walls appear otherwise smooth. The patient was treated by heparin and discharged on aspirin and clopidogrel for 6 months. The 6-month

FIGURE 17–13. *Continued*
catheterization (*C* and *D* in the same respective views as in *A* and *B*) showed complete spontaneous lysis of the thrombus and normal underlying vessel wall. A few hours before chest pain, the patient had been drunk, which could have triggered increased thrombogenicity and acute coronary thrombosis.

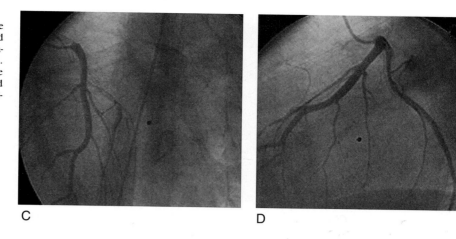

of stenosis severity and could discriminate culprit lesions in unstable angina from lesions in stable angina.[35] Davies and colleagues[36] redefined this index as the ratio of maximal to minimal intralesional diameter (see Fig. 17–11) and used it to predict clinical instability after thrombolysis in acute MI.

Intraluminal Filling Defects and Occlusions

Intraluminal filling defects are defined as intraluminal radiotransparent images, adherent or not to the underlying plaque with contrast medium surrounding the defect (Figs. 17–12, 17–13, and 17–14*C* and *D*). A filling defect is highly specific for a thrombus when smooth and well delineated by the contrast medium. Less typical aspects are frequent and are defined as probable thrombus.[37–39]

Using angioscopy as the reference detection method of thrombus in vivo, Franzen and associates[40] showed that the presence of an intraluminal filling defect in at least two projections had 36% sensitivity and 86% specificity for the presence of thrombus. These figures are consistent with earlier findings.[41,42] Coronary angiograms frequently underestimate and sometimes misinterpret the true presence of a thrombus. Occlusive thrombi usually show a squared-off or a convex-shaped termination creating a stump (Fig. 17–15). Stagnation of the contrast medium may indicate a fresh thrombotic occlusion. Old coronary occlusions usually taper from a proximal side branch that provides runoff, preventing blood stasis and contrast-medium stagnation. In old occlusion, the homolateral or contralateral collaterals are usually well developed.

FIGURE 17–14. Unexpected acute thrombosis of the proximal left anterior descending artery. This 51-year-old patient was admitted for exertional angina 3 years after a previous coronary angioplasty of an ostial lesion of the first obtuse marginal branch. Opacification of the left main artery (*A*, right anterior oblique view; *B*, left anterior oblique view) showed a less than 50% restenosis of the marginal branch ostium and irregularities of the proximal left anterior descending artery without any lumen narrowing *(arrows)*. The patient was readmitted 6 months later for refractory rest chest pain with transient ST-segment elevation in the anterior electrocardiogram leads. Urgent catheterization (*C* and *D* in the same projection as in *A* and *B*) showed an intraluminal filling defect *(arrows)* at the location of the former irregular plaque of the proximal left anterior descending artery. This case illustrates how acute thrombosis may complicate mild but irregular coronary plaques often considered benign.

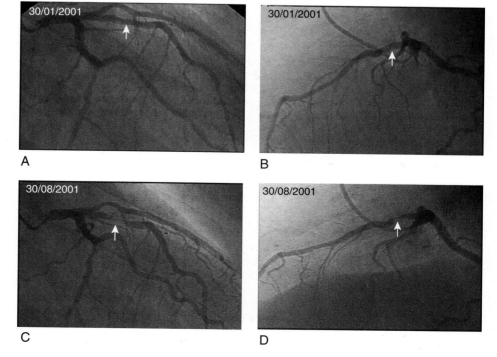

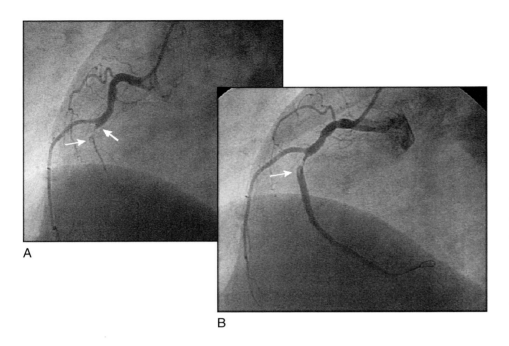

A

B

FIGURE 17–15. Acute thrombotic occlusion of the right coronary artery. *A,* Acute ST-segment elevation myocardial infarction in a 67-year-old patient who underwent immediate angioplasty. An acute occlusion of the mid right coronary artery with a stump shape is seen *(smaller arrow).* Slow antegrade flow allows identification of an intraluminal filling defect suggestive of a tiny thrombus *(larger arrow).* *B,* After balloon predilation, a mobile clot adherent to the plaque is seen *(arrow).*

CLINICAL APPLICATIONS

Angiographic characterization of lesions in ACS is particularly useful in the early hours or days that follow the acute event. It helps identify the culprit lesion and permit target pharmacologic treatment or revascularization or both. It also can be useful to identify the lesions at risk before they become clinically manifest.

Non–ST-Segment Elevation Acute Coronary Syndrome

Culprit Lesion Morphology During Acute Coronary Syndromes

After the first descriptions of ischemia-related coronary lesions by Ambrose and colleagues in 1985,[33] coronary angiography emerged as an invaluable tool to understand better the pathophysiology of ACS, identify possible therapeutic targets, and develop new treatment strategies. Culprit lesions responsible for non–ST-segment elevation ACS are remarkable for their diverse morphology, likely reflecting different mechanisms or various stages of ischemia. The typical ischemia-related lesion is characterized by a complex morphology with an intravascular or mural thrombus or a (sub)total fresh coronary occlusion with reduced TIMI (Thrombolysis In Myocardial Ischemia) flow grade.

How to Identify the Culprit Lesion. The culprit lesion usually is readily identifiable in patients with single-vessel disease. Of the 5546 patients who had angiography in the Platelet Glycoprotein II Gl IIIa in Unstable Angina: Receptor Suppression Using Integrilin Therapy (PURSUIT) trial, 29% had single-vessel disease, and 59% had multivessel disease.[43] In the Veterans Affairs Non–Q-Wave Infarction Strategies in Hospital (VANQWISH)

Study, 77% of the 920 patients with a non–ST-segment elevation enrolled had multivessel disease.[44] In patients with multivessel disease, the culprit lesion usually is identified by comparing coronary anatomy with the sites of the ischemia on the 12-lead electrocardiogram or of regional dysfunction on a ventriculogram. In the absence of electrocardiogram changes and wall motion abnormalities, the culprit lesion is identified by its complex morphology and the presence of an intracoronary thrombus. In the absence of these diagnostic features, the most severe lesion with some anatomic importance is usually considered the culprit lesion.[42,45] The criterion of severity by itself can be misleading at times, as discussed in the section on the identification of lesions at risk of complications. The concept of a single culprit lesion also may be misleading because multiple complex lesions are found in 30% of patients with an acute coronary syndrome.[45-48]

An absence of stenoses greater than or equal to 50% lumen diameter reduction has been reported in 6% to 20% of patients with unstable angina,[43,49-53] more frequently in nonwhite populations, women, and in patients with a normal electrocardiogram.[49]

Complex Morphology. As shown in Table 17-5, complex lesions are found in 27% to 84% of ACS patients and are 1.5 to 9 times more frequent in unstable angina than in stable chronic angina.[42,45,50,51,54-60,61] The timing of angiography after the last chest pain episode does not influence complexity. It was described in 42% of the patients catheterized within 24 hours, 42% of patients catheterized urgently after 3.9 ± 2.2 days, and in 38% of patients undergoing angiography after 6.6 ± 1.5 days.[50] The TIMI flow is often delayed when the borders are irregular but not when they are smooth,[45,62] suggesting that complex morphology could influence the hemorheology of obstructive plaques or yield distal embolization and reduced tissue perfusion.

TABLE 17–5 CULPRIT LESION MORPHOLOGY IN NON–ST-SEGMENT ELEVATION ACUTE CORONARY SYNDROMES*

STUDY REFERENCE	NO. PATIENTS	INCLUSION CRITERIA	TIME DELAY OF ANGIOGRAPHY	COMPLEX MORPHOLOGY			INTRALUMINAL FILLING DEFECTS (NONOCCLUSIVE, POSSIBLE OR DEFINITE THROMBUS)			TOTAL OCCLUSION		
				ACS	SA	P value	ACS	SA	P value	ACS	SA	P value
Zack et al, 1984[119]	120	Unstable angina	NA				12%	0%	<.05			
Ambrose et al, 1985[33]	110	Unstable angina	NA	71%	20%	<.001	35%	3%	<.0001			
Bresnahan et al, 1985[120]	268	Unstable angina	NA				37%	0%	<.0001			
Capone et al, 1985[63]	154	Rest angina	<14 days									
Kranjec et al, 1987[54]	104	Unstable angina	NA	27%	3%	<.01						
Haft et al, 1987[55]	109	Unstable angina	NA	73%	47%	<.01						
Williams et al, 1988[56]	101	Rest or crescendo angina	5 ± 2 days	61%			27%					
Cowley et al, 1989[57]	89	Prolonged or rest pain	24 ± 18 hours	84%	15%	<.0001	45%	5%	<.005	13%	0	NS
Freeman et al, 1989[50]	78	Crescendo or rest angina within 24 hours	Early (≤ 24 hr) and late (> 24 hr)	54%			40.5					
Rehr et al, 1989[58]	92	Prolonged rest angina	26 ± 22 hours	70%	21%	<.001	42%	17%	<.02			
Bugiardini et al, 1991[59]	116	Unstable angina	< 8 days	71%	25%	<.001	22%					
Cools et al, 1992[60]	138	Unstable angina	NA	59%			34%	2%	<.001			
TIMI IIIA trial, 1993[37]	306	Non–ST-segment elevation acute syndrome	< 24 hours†				35%					
Ahmed et al, 1993[65]	288	Unstable angina	NA	70%	38%	<.01	16%	2%	.01	22%	24%	NS
Rupprecht et al, 1995[51]	400	Unstable angina	NA	61%	34%	<.0001	7%	1%	.006	18%	25%	NS
De Servi et al, 1996[61]	58	Braunwald class B angina	4 ± 2 days	53%								
Dangas et al, 1997[45]	200	Unstable angina	NA	49%			14%			15%		
Calton et al, 1998[52]	100	Unstable angina	NA	50%			17%			24%		
Zhao et al, 1999[39]	1491	Non–ST-segment elevation acute syndrome	< 5 days†				39%			9%		

*Definition of unstable angina was crescendo angina, rest angina, de novo or postinfarction angina, unless restricted to subclasses as stated. Myocardial infarctions (either Q-wave or non–Q-wave) were excluded except in the TIMI IIIA[36] and PRISM-PLUS[38] trials, in which non–Q-wave infarctions represented 32% and 44% of the population. Time delay accounts for the delay between the last chest pain episode and coronary angiography. Complex morphology is defined as ulceration, irregular or overhanging borders, intraluminal filling defects, or total occlusion.
†Per protocol. ACS, acute coronary syndrome; NA, not available; NS, not significant for P > .05; SA, stable chronic angina.

Intracoronary Thrombus. Intraluminal or mural filling defects of various shapes and congruity are present in 7% to 45% of patients with non–ST-segment elevation ACS (see Table 17-5 and Figs. 17-12, 17-13C and D, and 17-14C and D). Contrasting with the irregular morphology, the earlier the angiography is performed after the last episode of rest angina, the more frequently intraluminal filling defects can be seen: 52% of patients catheterized within 24 hours and 28% of patients catheterized after 48 hours (p < 0.008) in one study [63] and 43% versus 38% respectively (p = 0.07) in another.[64] It was shown that angiography underestimates the true incidence of thrombus compared with angioscopy.[41,42] In rest angina, two thirds of thrombi are grayish white at angioscopy, and in ST-segment elevation acute MI, they are red or mixed red and white.[64] The former represent platelet rich thrombi and the latter fibrin rich thrombi. Thrombosis can rarely occur on apparently smooth lesions (Fig. 17-13C and D), but are most often associated with complex lesions (Fig. 17-14C and D).

Quantitative Characteristics. The presence of thrombi or of occlusions limits proper QCA of unstable coronary lesions. When quantification is possible, percent diameter stenosis, minimum lumen diameter or area, or lengths of nonthrombotic ischemia-related lesions are in general in the same range as in stable angina patients.[33,35,42,65] The severity of the underlying stenosis of the culprit lesion was measured after excluding the thrombotic component in a large cohort of 1491 ACS patients treated with antithrombin and antiplatelet agents who had coronary angiography within 4 days after admission in the PRISM-PLUS (Platelet Receptor Inhibition for Ischemic Syndrome Management in Patients Limited by Unstable Signs and Symptoms) trial: 24% of culprit stenoses had less than 50% diameter stenosis, 23% had stenoses between 51% and 70%, and 45% had stenoses between 71% and 99%.[39] Total occlusion (TIMI flow grade 0 or 1) was seen in less than 15% (see Table 17-5), half of them associated with a fresh thrombus (convex shape and contrast retention or stump).[39]

Many investigators looked at collateral filling evaluated by the Rentrop classification. Grade II or III, representing incomplete or complete filling of the distal coronary vasculature downstream the occlusion,[66] was equally frequent in ACS and in stable angina patients: 10% versus 8% in one study[33] and 23% versus 27% in another.[51]

The QCA indices of plaque irregularity have been validated in cohorts of unstable angina patients. Wilson and associates[35] described a lower ulceration index, meaning deeper ulcerations in unstable angina patients compared with stable angina patients (0.62 ± 0.05 versus 0.96 ± 0.01, P < .05). A cutoff value of 0.78 could discriminate in one study all unstable from stable lesions independently of the percent diameter stenosis. Kalbfleisch and coworkers[34] also showed that morphometric parameters based on curvature peaks quantification and fractal analyses of the stenosis borders differed significantly between unstable and stable culprit lesions, indicating greater complexity and irregularity in the former lesions.

Other Mechanisms or Culprit Lesion Features. Although complex morphology is the most common and specific feature of culprit lesions in ACS, other findings can occasionally account for acute or recurrent ischemia. ACS may develop on a noncomplex and nonprogressive stenosis or downstream an old occlusion with reduced oxygen transport (anemia, hypoxia) or increased oxygen demand (arrhythmia, uncontrolled hypertension, infectious disease, anxious states). This

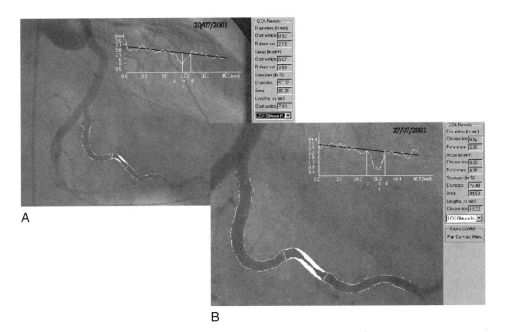

A

B

FIGURE 17–16. Recurrent rest angina resulting from a rapidly progressing coronary plaque. This 51-year-old man had episodic rest angina. *A,* Initial catheterization (after intracoronary nitrates) showed a single short stenosis of intermediate severity of the first obtuse marginal branch (57% diameter stenosis), with a smooth and regular shape. He was discharged under medical treatment to be rehospitalized a week later for recurrent rest chest pain episodes and transient ST-segment depression in the apical ECG leads. Cardiac markers were normal. *B,* Urgent catheterization showed that the culprit lesion had progressed to 77% diameter stenosis with no change in shape and morphology. This case illustrates how rapidly progressing plaques—otherwise of simple morphology and shape—may be responsible for acute coronary syndromes.

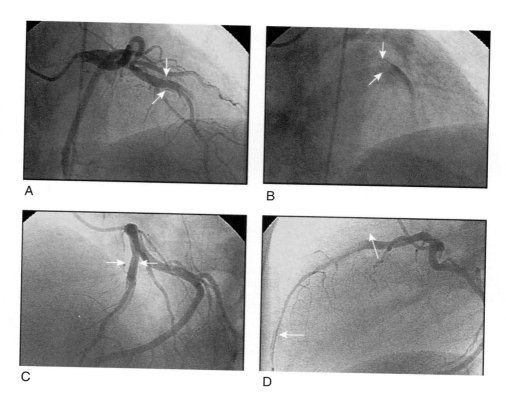

FIGURE 17-17. Spontaneous dissection in apparently normal coronary arteries. This 42-year-old woman, free from any significant medical history, was admitted for recurrent angina within hours associated with ST-segment elevation during the chest pain episodes. *A–D,* Urgent catheterization showed a spontaneous dissection of the mid left anterior descending artery (*A* and *C, plain arrows*) with contrast retention in the false lumen (*B*). The dissection was long and extended toward the distal left anterior descending artery (*D, dashed arrow*) with oscillating antegrade TIMI flow grade. The coronary arteries appeared otherwise normal. No precipitating factors were identified. The patient had many stents implanted that did not prevent evolution to a Q-wave anterior myocardial infarction. After 1-year follow-up, she had no recurrence of coronary artery dissection.

corresponds to the clinical diagnosis of secondary unstable angina. The unstable state also can be a consequence of a rapid progression in the severity of a moderately obstructive stenosis, as illustrated in Figure 17-16. In this case, a simple and symmetric plaque located in the obtuse marginal branch progressed during a 1-week interval from 57% to 77% diameter stenosis, with no evidence of a plaque complexity. Rapid plaque progression has been described as a hallmark of unstable angina.[67]

There also are reports on nontraumatic spontaneous dissections of coronary arteries. Such dissections usually are associated with some degree of myocardial necrosis or with sudden cardiac death. These dissections may involve one or the two coronary arteries simultaneously. Little is known about this entity.[68-71] Most cases have occurred in women with no evidence of CAD, often in the peripartum period (Fig. 17-17). One third of cases occur in men, usually in association with CAD and a dissected obstructive plaque. Inflammation and eosinophilic infiltrates have been described in association with rupture in the absence of CAD. Spontaneous dissections can occur in genetic diseases, such as Marfan and Ehlers-Danlos syndromes, representing most often retrograde dissection originating from the ascending aorta.

The mechanisms accounting for myocardial ischemia in the 6% to 20% of patients with no stenoses greater than 50% stenosis can be multiple but remain often imprecise. Ischemia in these patients can be explained by recurrent episodes of vasospasm, as illustrated in Figure 17-18; distal microembolization[72]; myocardial bridging[73]; impaired myocardial microcir-

culation; myocardial hypertrophy; and a low pain threshold (see Chapter 41). In the TIMI IIIA trial, 14% of the 391 patients who had angiography within 24 hours after the last chest pain had no stenoses greater than or equal to 60% stenosis, and 6% had no stenoses greater than or equal to 20%[49]; 7% of these patients had irregular plaques, but none had a complex plaque or a thrombus. A slow filling, as determined by a TIMI flow grade less than or equal to 2 or by an increased opacification time was noted, however, in 32% of the patients, the slow filling frequently involving more than one vessel. Severe complications are infrequent in patients with less than 50% lesion stenosis,[53] but recurrence of chest pain on treatment is frequent (see Chapter 41).

Correlation Between Clinical Presentation and Culprit Lesion Morphology in Acute Coronary Syndromes. To date, six studies have correlated the angiographic characteristics of the culprit lesion with the clinical presentation and severity of ACS, usually using the Braunwald classification.[74] Dangas and colleagues[45] showed associations between rest angina and a complex lesion with total occlusion and reduced TIMI grade flow; postinfarction angina with intraluminal thrombi, total occlusion, and reduced TIMI grade flow; and refractory angina with intraluminal thrombi. Two other studies showed a correlation between the presence of transient or persistent ST-segment depression or T-wave inversion or both and a complex or thrombotic culprit lesion.[50,51] No such correlations were observed, however, in other large cohorts of patients.[52,61,65]

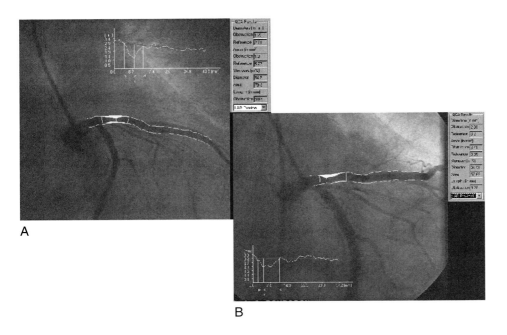

FIGURE 17–18. Recurrent rest angina cuased by diffuse spasm of the left anterior descending artery. This 51-year-old woman with fibrodysplasia of the renal arteries was admitted for multiple morning episodes of chest pain resistant to medical therapy (β-blocker, calcium blocker, and aspirin). After administration of glyco-protein IIbIIIa platelet inhibitors and heparin with discontinuation of the vasoactive drugs, early catheterization was performed. *A,* Before injection of intracoronary nitrates, the angiogram showed an intermediate stenosis of the proximal left anterior descending artery and a diffusely spastic artery (reference vessel diameter 2.7 mm). *B,* After injection of nitrates, it showed only a mildly severe proximal stenosis and spasm resolution (reference vessel diameter 3.2 mm).

Histopathologic Correlations and Pathophysiologic Implications.

In a study of 111 patients undergoing atherectomy for stenoses greater than 75% diameter, Haft and colleagues[75] showed that thrombus was present in 81% of complex plaques compared with 10% of plaques with smooth borders. Inflammatory cells were as frequent in smooth as in complex plaques. Angiographic, angioscopic, and histologic findings in ACS all concur to suggest similar pathophysiologic processes in ACS and ST-segment elevation MI. It is unclear, however, why destabilized coronary plaques can cause such a wide spectrum of clinical presentations from accelerated angina and reversible ischemia to complete thrombotic occlusion and acute MI. Local factors, such as endothelium dysfunction,[76] stenosis geometry and rheology disturbances,[21,77] and systemic factors, such as platelet hyperaggregability[78] and impaired fibrinolytic activity,[79] may have some influence. Further studies are needed to understand better the interactions between these various contributing factors. Angiography shows that a more severe clinical presentation and symptoms that are more refractory are associated with more extensive underlying CAD and complex plaque with a thrombus.

Culprit Lesion Morphology and Response to Treatment

Coronary angiography provides useful surrogate markers of treatment efficacy in ST-segment elevation MI and improvement in TIMI grade flow from 0 and 1 to grade 2 and from grade 2 to grade 3 correlates with improved survival. Such is not always the case in non–ST-segment elevation ACS. In the TIMI IIIA trial that included 306 patients, thrombolysis improved flow after 90 minutes, but not the clinical evolution. In the PRISM-PLUS trial, patients who received the combination of tirofiban and heparin compared with heparin alone had a reduced thrombus burden after 48 hours ($P = 0.22$) and a better TIMI grade flow ($P = 0.002$), whereas the severity of the underlying plaque was unchanged.[39]

Culprit Lesion Morphology and Prognosis

Most studies relating outcome to angiographic morphology of the culprit lesion had a short 30-day follow-up. In all but one[80] of these studies,[39,50,59] the presence of a thrombus, of complex culprit morphology, or of reduced TIMI flow grade strongly predicted death, MI, or recurrent angina requiring an urgent revascularization. In the C7E3 Antiplatelet Therapy in Unstable Refractory angina (CAPTURE) trial, angiographic morphology, however, was not as potent a predictor as troponin T levels.[81]

Long-term data in patients with medically stabilized unstable angina were obtained from a small cohort of 85 highly selected patients from the United Kingdom who had been waiting for CABG for 8 months. Adverse events occurred in 31% of these patients, including death in one patient, nonfatal MI in 25 patients, and recurrent ACS. The repeated angiography in these patients showed progression by 20% or more in the severity of one coronary obstruction in 72% of patients. The progression involved the culprit lesion in 56% of cases, 80% of them to complete occlusion. Complex culprit lesions had a threefold to fourfold increase in the risk of progression, resulting in more coronary events compared with smooth lesions (37% versus 19%, $P = .09$). Lesions greater than 50% diameter stenosis progressed and occluded more frequently than less severe lesions. This study shows that complex lesions are at risk of accelerated progression and of an adverse clinical outcome.

■ ■ ■

TABLE 17–6 STENOSIS SEVERITY BY QUANTITATIVE CORONARY ANGIOGRAPHY AND OCCURRENCE OF ACUTE MYOCARDIAL INFARCTION[*]

STUDY REFERENCE	TIME INTERVAL BETWEEN ANGIOGRAMS (mos)	NO. OF PATIENTS	CULPRIT % STENOSIS (MEAN ± SD)	NONCULPRIT % STENOSIS (MEAN ± SD)	UNIVARIATE P VALUE
Little et al, 1988[86]	0–75 (median 11)	29	44 ± 15	NA	
Taeymans et al, 1992[93]	<36 (mean 10 ± 11)	38	47.5 ± 17.8	41.0 ± 12.5	<.05
Ledru et al, 1999[20]	<36 (mean 15 ± 10)	84	45.3 ± 14.9	40.1 ± 13.3	.0011[†]

[*] All studies are retrospective and selected medically treated patients with a documented acute myocardial infarction and coronary angiography performed before the acute myocardial infarction without any coronary procedure or event in the meantime. Quantitative coronary angiography was performed by automatic edge contour detection systems. Acute myocardial infarction is defined by an acute coronary syndrome with ST-segment elevation or creatine kinase rise and includes Q-wave and non–Q-wave infarctions.
[†]Conditional regression analysis (the patient is his or her own control).
NA, not applicable.

The Lesion at Risk of ST-Segment Elevation Myocardial Infarction

Following the pioneer work of DeWood and colleagues,[4] coronary angiography has been used increasingly in acute MI for diagnostic, research, and therapeutic purposes. It is now performed acutely whenever possible for the purpose of angioplasty and stent implantation.

Many studies have attempted to characterize the lesion at risk of a myocardial infarction by looking at angiograms of MI patients who had a previous angiogram.

Stenosis Severity

Stenosis severity historically has received the greatest attention. Ellis and coworkers[83] showed in 259 medically treated patients from the Coronary Artery Surgery Study (CASS) registry followed up for at least 3 years that the risk of occlusion of the left anterior descending artery and its branches increased in relation to the severity of the previous stenosis risk by 2%, 6.6%, 8.2%, and 15.3% of lesions with <50%, 50% to 69%, 70% to 89%, and 90% to 98% diameter stenosis, respectively. No postinfarct angiography was, however, performed in these patients to confirm the exact location of the acute thrombosis. Subsequent studies confirmed this finding (Table 17–6) but also showed that, in more than 50% of cases, the initial stenosis was less than 50% lumen diameter reduction (Table 17–7). Similar findings were obtained with caliper methods of quantification,[84,85] with 8% to 29% of lesions responsible for an acute MI being almost unnoticeable (diameter stenosis <20%) on a previous angiogram. Figures 17–13 and 17–14 illustrate cases of acute thrombosis on prior non-severe lesions.[20,86] The CASS study[87] shed some light on the significance of the initial stenosis by showing that the rate of occlusion with or without symptoms increases with increasing severity of the stenosis, from 0.7% with no stenosis to 23.6% with severe stenosis (Fig. 17–19). The number of non-severe lesions, however, exceeded by one third the number of severe stenoses, resulting in a higher percent frequency in non-severe lesions. A European study reported similar findings among 246 patients followed up for an average of 46 months.[88] When analyzing these data, it should be remembered that only 15% to 20% of new coronary

■ ▪ ■

TABLE 17–7 DISTRIBUTION OF CULPRIT LESION SEVERITY AT PREINFARCTION CORONARY ANGIOGRAPHY[*]

STUDY REFERENCE	NO. OF PATIENTS	NO OR <25% STENOSIS	<50% STENOSIS[†]	≥50% STENOSIS
Little et al, 1988[86]	29	14%	66%	34%
Taeymans et al, 1992[93]	38	—	47%	53%
Tousoulis et al, 1998[90]	24	29%	58%	42%
Ledru et al, 1999[20]	84	8%	59%	41%
Total	175	11%	57%	43%

[*] All studies are retrospective and used a computer-assisted method for the quantification of diameter stenosis. Caliper methods—not shown here—provided similar data.[83,84]
All patients were selected by the index acute myocardial infarction (either Q-wave or non–Q-wave) defined as an acute chest pain syndrome with transient ST-segment elevation and creatine kinase rise.
[†]Including coronary segments with < 25% diameter stenosis.

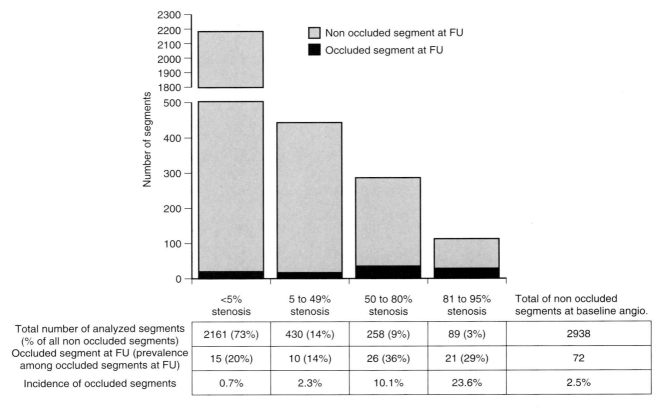

	<5% stenosis	5 to 49% stenosis	50 to 80% stenosis	81 to 95% stenosis	Total of non occluded segments at baseline angio.
Total number of analyzed segments (% of all non occluded segments)	2161 (73%)	430 (14%)	258 (9%)	89 (3%)	2938
Occluded segment at FU (prevalence among occluded segments at FU)	15 (20%)	10 (14%)	26 (36%)	21 (29%)	72
Incidence of occluded segments	0.7%	2.3%	10.1%	23.6%	2.5%

FIGURE 17–19. Relation between initial coronary segment narrowing and future occlusion (recalculated from Alderman and colleagues[86]). The coronary anatomy of 298 CASS randomized patients was compared on the baseline angiography and on the protocol-required angiography 60 months later. A total of 2938 patent coronary artery segments not occluded at baseline angiography were visually analyzed. The table displays the absolute number of occluded coronary segments at follow-up categorized by initial percent severity and recalculated from the publication. The last row of the table shows that the incidence of occlusion at follow-up was increasing with the initial percent narrowing of the diseased segments. When looking at the 72 occluded segments at follow-up, however, more than a third were initially less than 50% diameter stenosis. This figure illustrates how the most severe stenoses may have the highest risk of thrombotic occlusion, although they may not be the more prevalent category of occlusion-prone lesions.

occlusions are symptomatic or associated with new Q waves.[89]

One study that correlated stenosis severity, new coronary occlusion, and concomitant symptoms, showed that symptomatic MI occurred more frequently in less severe stenosis (48% diameter reduction) and asymptomatic occlusion more frequently in more severe stenosis (74% reduction, $P < 0.005$).[84] It also was reported, although not consistently, that lesions leading to non–Q-wave acute MI were on average more severe than lesions leading to a Q-wave acute MI (Table 17–8).[84,90,91] Dacanay and colleagues[91] described two categories of stenoses associated with non–Q-wave acute MI, the first being mild stenoses less than 20% diameter stenosis and the second severe stenoses greater than 75% diameter stenosis. The mechanisms leading to Q-wave MI appear more

■ ▦ ■

TABLE 17–8 COMPARED PREINFARCTION DIAMETER SEVERITY OF CORONARY LESIONS RESPONSIBLE FOR Q-WAVE AND NON–Q-WAVE ACUTE MYOCARDIAL INFARCTION*

STUDY REFERENCE	NO. OF PATIENTS	Q-WAVE INFARCTION	NON–Q-WAVE INFARCTION	p VALUE
Dacanay et al, 1994[91]	70	44 ± 25%	23 ± 35%	< 0.01
		50% with > 50% stenosis	36% with > 50% stenosis	NS
Tousoulis et al, 1998[90]	24	53 ± 6%	58 ± 6%	NS
		50% with >50% stenosis	71% with > 50% stenosis	< 0.05

* The stenosis diameter severity of the preinfarction culprit lesions is compared between Q-wave and non–Q-wave myocardial infarctions. The studies are retrospective and used a caliper[91] or a computer-assisted[90] method for quantification of diameter stenosis. All patients were selected by the index acute myocardial infarction (either Q-wave or non–Q-wave) defined as an acute chest pain syndrome with transient ST-segment elevation and creatine kinase rise. Results are given with mean ± SD. For further comments, see text.
NS, not significant for univariate p value > .05.

stereotyped and those leading to non–Q-wave MI more variable with influence of various factors, such as the collateral circulation or ischemic preconditioning.

Other Quantitative Stenosis Predictive of Acute Myocardial Infarction

Stenosis Length. The CASS registry correlated stenosis length with risk of thrombotic occlusion using a semi-quantitative method[92] to show that the longer the stenosis, the higher the odds of an acute MI within the following 3 years. In another study, the odds of occlusion were twice as high in long lesions (>5 mm by visual analysis) than in short lesions (≤5 mm) after correction for stenosis severity.[88] QCA did not confirm these findings, however (Table 17–9).[20,93] Altogether, the data show only a weak association between stenosis length and future occlusion.

Symmetry Index. Two studies looked at the predictive value of the symmetry index (see Table 17–9). The study by Ledru and associates[20] challenged the empirical concept that the eccentricity of a stenosis defined as type I or type II eccentric lesion is a marker of unstable atheromatous plaque.[94] In this study, a greater symmetry index was the most powerful predictor of future occlusion and acute MI by univariate and multivariate conditional analyses,[20] ahead of stenosis severity. More remains to be learned on the correlations that exist between in-vivo symmetry and symmetry assessed by histology or intravascular ultrasound.

Inflow and Outflow Angles. Vascular stenoses influence flow rheology with convergence and divergence, in flow, downstream pressure recovery, and turbulence generation. The effects have been extensively studied in flow chambers but less so in vivo.[77] Two studies examined the clinical significance of steepness of inflow and outflow angles (see Table 17–9 and Fig. 17–5 for definition). In the study by Ledru and coworkers,[20] the abruptness of the outflow angle assessed by average or maximal outflow angles, but not the inflow angle, consistently predicted future occlusion and acute MI. This finding strongly supports a contribution of plaque geometry to rupture and thrombus formation. Abrupt stenosis expansion increases flow separation and vortices generation that favor wall vibration, fatigue, and plaque disruption. Low shear conditions in vortices and secondary flows can promote platelet aggregation and thrombus growth.[95] These measurements have limited applicability in patient management because they require QCA and may not be discriminative in individual patients.

Qualitative Descriptors

Lesion Complexity. Lesion irregularity or complexity (type II eccentric lesions) are associated with coronary occlusion and acute MI (Table 17–10). Lesion complexity in one study was the strongest predictor of a future anterior MI infarction (odds ratio, 6.64; $P = .001$).[92] In another study complex plaques predicted more often a

Q-wave acute MI than non–Q-wave acute MI (56% versus 13%; $P < .001$).[91] These data, added to a high rate of progression reported in patients with ACS on a waiting list for CABG,[82] show that complex morphology is specific of unstable plaques at risk of acute events or rapid disease progression.

Vessel Bifurcation. The rheologic conditions found in the vicinity of division branches contribute to early atherosclerosis formation and may promote plaque fissuration, platelet deposition, and thrombosis. The occlusions in acute MI often are located at branching points in the left or right coronary arteries. Studies that have looked at specific aspects of plaques located at bifurcations have provided little information, however, on plaques prone to rupture (see Table 17–10).

Inducible Spasm. Vasospasm has long been implicated as a potential cause of plaque formation, progression, and rupture. In a review of 239 patients who had an ergonovine testing during a previous angiogram, Nobuyoshi and colleagues[85] reported that a positive test was a strong predictor of new MI (see Table 17–10) and disease progression. The study, however, did not correlate the site of spasm to the site of progression, leaving uncertainties on the exact role of spasm.

Risk Scores. The more extensive the underlying CAD, the greater is the risk of progression. A score has been designed as the sum of coronary artery segment showing presence of the disease, independently of the severity of the obstruction. This extent score was a strong predictor of progression of the disease.[96] Progression to MI could be more frequent in proximal or mid artery position, or in the right coronary artery.[97]

Natural History of Plaque Progression

Progression by quantitative angiography criteria is defined as a reduction of 15% or more of lumen diameter, corresponding to 2 SDs or more repeated measurements obtained over time for a given stenosis.[98] The significance of this definition has been validated in clinical studies. Progression is associated with an increased risk of major cardiac events, including sudden death and acute MI. In a prospective progression-regression angiographic trial, Waters and associates[99] showed that such progression on two iterative angiograms obtained 2 years apart was associated with a 7.3-fold increase in the risk of cardiac death and a 2.3-fold increase in the risk of cardiac death or acute MI within the next 44 months, compared with patients with no such progression.

The relationship between progression, coronary occlusion, and a future acute coronary event is complex and nonlinear. From the prospective progression-regression angiographic International Nifedipine Trial on Antiatherosclerotic Therapy (INTACT) study of patients with stable angina followed for 3 years, Lichtlen and colleagues[89] described stenosis progression in 56% of 230 patients; the progression involved preexisting stenoses in

TABLE 17–9 QUANTITATIVE CHARACTERISTICS DERIVED FROM AUTOMATED QUANTITATIVE ANGIOGRAPHY OTHER THAN PERCENT SEVERITY ASSOCIATED WITH ONSET OF OCCLUSION WITH ACUTE MYOCARDIAL INFARCTION

STUDY REFERENCE	NO. OF PATIENTS	STENOSIS LENGTH (MM)			GEOMETRIC INFLOW ANGLE (°)[†]			GEOMETRIC OUTFLOW ANGLE (°)[†]			SYMMETRY INDEX (%)[†]		
		Culprit	Non culprit	P value	Culprit	Non culprit	P value	Culprit	Non culprit	P value	Culprit	Non culprit	P value
Taeymans et al, 1992[93]	38	7.2 ± 3.1	7.1 ± 3.1	NS	21 ± 10	16 ± 7	<.05	20 ± 10	16 ± 8	<.05	46 ± 28	44 ± 29	NS
Ledru et al, 1999[20]	84	10.3 ± 4.9	8.7 ± 4.8	.01	16 ± 10	17 ± 9	NS	16 ± 10	14 ± 8	.05	64 ± 27	49 ± 28	<.0001

*Both studies are retrospective and used a computer-assisted method for delineation of the arterial borders and quantification of stenosis characteristics. All patients were selected by the index acute myocardial infarction (either Q-wave or non–Q-wave) defined as an acute chest pain syndrome with transient ST-segment segment elevation and creative kinase rise. Time delay between angiograms was less than 36 months (10 ± 11 months in Taeymans et al[93] and 15 ± 10 months in Ledru et al[20].

Figures are expressed as mean ± SD.

†See Figure 18–5 for definition and description.

NS, not significant for P value >.05.

■ ■ ■

TABLE 17–10   QUALITATIVE CHARACTERISTICS ASSOCIATED WITH ONSET OF OCCLUSION WITH ACUTE MYOCARDIAL INFARCTION*

STENOSIS CHARACTERISTIC ASSOCIATED WITH MYOCARDIAL INFARCTION	STUDY REFERENCE	TIME INTERVAL BETWEEN ANGIOGRAMS (MO)	NO. OF PATIENTS	PREVALENCE OF FACTOR IN		UNIVARIATE *P* VALUE
				Culprit Lesions	Nonculprit Lesions	
Lesion complexity/ irregularity	Little et al, 1988[86]	0–75 (median 11)	29	100%	NA	
	Ellis et al, 1989[92]	36	259	16%	3.5%	.001
	Taeymans et al, 1992[93]	<36 (mean [SD] 10 [11])	38	47%	67%	.05
Division branch	Tousoulis et al, 1998[90]	mean (SD) 26 (4)	24	50%	21%	<.01
	Ellis et al, 1989[92]	36	259	61%	55%	NS
	Taeymans et al, 1992[93]	<36 (mean [SD] 10 [11])	38	76%	52%	<.05
Provocable spasm with ergonovine	Nobuyoshi et al, 1991[85]	0–120	239	39%	8%	<.05

*All studies are retrospective. Lesion complexity was defined as type II eccentric lesions.[33] Division branch within the stenosis was considered significant if its diameter was at least 25% of the stenosed artery.[92] Provocable spasm was induced by intra-aortic injection of ergonovine maleate during coronary angiography.[85] NA, not applicable; NS, not significant for *P* value > .05.

approximately 10% (82 of 838 preexisting stenoses >20% diameter reduction) and 144 initially disease-free segments. A total of 25 new occlusions occurred, 40% of them in initially normal segments; less than one fifth of the occlusions were associated with overt MI. Additional insights on patterns of progression were provided by a small but unique study of 36 patients with progression (≥ 15% diameter reduction) over a one-year period and with four angiograms performed within the same year, one every four months. Marked progression was observed in 14 patients with stenosis of 44%, 46%, 46%, and 48% at first, second, third, and last angiogram, and slow progression in 22 patients with stenosis of 44%, 50%, 59%, and 69% respectively. Marked progression was associated with angina or myocardial infarction in 71% of patients and Ambrose type 2 eccentric lesions in 57%. Slow progression was associated with angina in 14% of patients. The levels of C-reactive protein were elevated in patients with slow progression but not in patients with abrupt progression. The study was retrospective and involved only few and selected patients, and the observation period could have underestimated the risk of an acute event. Nevertheless, it suggests that the mechanisms involved in disease progression could vary between patients.

Influence of Timing of Angiography

Angiography provides only a one-time look into a disease that is dynamic. The findings on plaque severity and morphology are influenced by the clinical situation when angiography is performed. The sooner angiography is obtained during the acute phase, the more severe will be the lesion.[91,93,101] Similar observations were made for the inflow[93] and outflow angles.[20] The symmetry index, on the other hand, is relatively independent of time from the index infarction, suggesting that it is more related to plaque structure, composition, and stability.[20]

LIMITATIONS OF ANGIOGRAPHY AND ANGIOGRAPHIC STUDIES

Although coronary angiography is closely linked to modern cardiology, angiographic data in ACS needs to be interpreted critically. The belief that angiograms could inform on the risk of ACS is based on only small selected series of patients catheterized at various times before the index event. These studies have provided information on the state of the plaque at one time point with no perspective on serial or dynamic changes that have preceded the syndrome. Longitudinal prospective studies on disease progression have been obtained in progression-regression trials in relatively low-risk populations, with an annual event rate of approximately 3%.[89,90]

Studies during the early phase of ACS are confounded by numerous factors, including the acute and secondary distortion of the culprit lesion by rupture, intraplaque hemorrhage, intravascular thrombus formation, and treatment modalities.[20] Similar difficulties are encountered when the culprit lesion is studied after the acute phase during the healing and remodeling processes that can be influenced by the severity of the initial injury and medications and interventions applied.

More general limitations of angiography also need to be considered. Luminography provides information on the lining of the plaque but not on atherosclerosis, which is basically a disease of the arterial wall. Angiography underestimates early atheroma, the true size of the underlying plaque and its lipid content, because of the compensatory enlargement that accommodates young atheromatous lesions.[102-104] It also may underestimate the true dimension of the control vessel, atherosclerosis being a diffuse process, particularly in diabetic[105] and elderly patients. Visual analysis even with expert eyes remains highly subjective, as attested by the interindividual variability observed in describing complex lesions in ACS (see Table 17-5) and the various classifications that have been developed for the diagnosis of intraluminal thrombus. Although some attempt has been made to quantify *complexity* objectively, the work is still preliminary.[34,35] Modern QCA packages provide reproducible measures of stenosis dimensions when the angiograms are adequate, which may not be the case in retrospective studies of angiograms performed by various operators and in nonstandardized conditions.[106]

FUTURE PERSPECTIVES

Identification of the lesion at risk of rupture is a challenge of modern cardiology. Development in automated segmentation of parts of or the entire coronary tree from two (preferably orthogonal) views is anticipated. Three-dimensional reconstruction would be another step forward to allow calculation of shear stress based on computational fluid dynamics and stress and strain of the vessels in relation to plaque formation.[107] One of the major challenges in QCA is the reproducible quantification of the lesion complexity. The development of the diffuse index represents a first step in that direction. Further improvements in image acquisition techniques and image resolution would facilitate more accurate detection and quantification of small irregularities of the endoluminal boundaries that indicate surface erosion or endothelial tears. Quantification of the extent and degree of myocardial blush in the x-ray images may allow studies of angiogenesis and of collateral circulation.

The ability to obtain insight into the components of the plaque and its dynamic pathology would help knowledge of the mechanisms of plaque rupture and thrombosis and of the influence of preventive management strategies. Intravascular ultrasound already provides useful information in that direction (see Chapter 18).[40,108-112] Noninvasive imaging by multislice spiral computed tomography coronary angiography[113,114] and magnetic resonance angiography[115,116] is even more promising (see Chapter 20).

Because of the inherent limitations of iodine-contrast angiography, the future will likely integrate other imaging techniques and a new imaging technology. QCA will be integrated with quantitative intravascular ultrasound to help guide the best interventional procedure, based on lesion and wall morphology, and the location in the coronary tree. Other approaches under development are intravascular ultrasound elastography, thermography,[117] optical coherence tomography,[118] and Raman spectroscopy (see Chapter 21). A few strategies eventually will emerge that will be clinically relevant and cost-effective. Until that time, coronary angiography remains an essential tool in the management, risk stratification, and therapy of patients with ACS. The limitations are counterbalanced by a widespread availability, access, and an excellent cost-effectiveness ratio. Complementary imaging modalities of the vessel wall and surface are already emerging.

REFERENCES

1. Mueller RL, Sanborn TA: The history of interventional cardiology: Cardiac catheterization, angioplasty, and related interventions. Am Heart J 1995;129:146-172.
2. Gruentzig A, Turina M, Schneider J: Experimental percutaneous dilatation of coronary artery stenosis. Circulation 1976;54:81.
3. Gruentzig AR, Senning A, Siegenthaler WE: Nonoperative dilation of coronary artery stenosis: Percutaneous transluminal coronary angioplasty. N Engl J Med 1979;301:61-68.
4. DeWood MA, Spores J, Notske R, et al: Prevalence of total coronary occlusion during the early hours of transmural myocardial infarction. N Engl J Med 1980;303:897-902.
5. Bashore T: Fundamentals of X-ray imaging and radiation safety. Cathet Cardiovasc Interv 2001;54:126-135.
6. Brown BG, Bolson E, Frimer M, et al: Quantitative coronary arteriography: Estimation of dimensions, hemodynamic resistance, and atheroma mass of coronary artery lesions using the arteriogram and digital computation. Circulation 1977;55:329-337.
7. Gensini G, Kelly A, Da Costa B, et al: Quantitative angiography: The measurement of coronary vaso-motility in the intact animal and man. Chest 1971;60:522-530.
8. Reiber J, Booman F, Tan H, et al: A cardiac imaging analysis system: Objective quantitative processing of angiocardiograms. In Proceedings of Computers in Cardiology. Stanford, CA, IEEE, 1978, pp 239-242.
9. Reiber JHC, Serruys PW, Kooijman CJ, et al: Assessment of short-, medium-, and long-term variations in arterial dimensions from computer-assisted quantitation of coronary cineangiograms. Circulation 1985;71:280-288.
10. Reiber J, Serruys P: Quantitative coronary angiography. In Marcus M, Schelbert H, Skorton D, Wolf G (eds): Cardiac Imaging: A Companion to Braunwald's Heart Disease. Philadelphia, WB Saunders, 1991, pp 211-281.
11. Lipid-lowering therapy and progression of coronary atherosclerosis. In Bruschke A, Reiber J, Lie K, and Wellens H (eds): Developments in Cardiovascular Medicine. Dordrecht, Kluwer Academic Publishers, 1996;18:15-210.
12. Reiber JH, van der Zwet PM, Koning G, et al: Accuracy and precision of quantitative digital coronary arteriography: Observer-, short-, and medium-term variabilities. Cathet Cardiovasc Diagn 1993;28: 187-198.
13. Reiber JHC, Von Land CD, Koning G, et al: Comparison of accuracy and precision of quantitative coronary arterial analysis between cinefilm and digital systems. In Reiber JHC, Serruys PW (eds): Progress in Quantitative Coronary Arteriography. Dordrecht, Kluwer Academic Publishers, 1994, pp 67-87.
14. van der Zwet PM, Reiber JH: A new approach for the quantification of complex lesion morphology: The gradient field transform: Basic principles and validation results. J Am Coll Cardiol 1994;24: 216-224.
15. Reiber J, Schiemanck L, van der Zwet P, et al: State-of-the-art in quantitative coronary arteriography as of 1996. In Reiber J and van der Wall E (eds): Cardiovascular Imaging. Dordrecht, Kluwer Academic Publishers, 1996, pp 39-56.
16. Lansky AJ, Desai KJ, Bonan R, et al: Quantitative coronary angiography methodology in vascular brachytherapy II. In Waksman R (ed): Vascular Brachytherapy, 3rd ed. Armonk, NY, Futura, 2002, pp 543-563.
17. Reiber JHC, Koning G, von Land CD, et al: Why and how should QCA systems be validated? In Reiber JHC, Serruys PW (eds): Progress in Quantitative Coronary Arteriography. Dordrecht, Kluwer Academic Publishers, 1994, pp 33-48.
18. Reiber J, Koning G, Dijkstra J, et al: Angiography and intravascular ultrasound. In Sonka M, Fitzpatrick J (eds): Handbook of Medical Imaging. Belligham, WA, SPIE Press, 2001, pp 711-808.
19. Lespérance J, Bilodeau L, Reiber J, et al: Issues in the performance of quantitative coronary angiography in clinical research trials. In Reiber J, van der Wall E (eds): What's New in Cardiovascular Imaging? Dordrecht, Kluwer Academic Publishers, 1998, pp 31-46.
20. Ledru F, Théroux T, Lespérance J, et al: Geometric features of coronary artery lesions favoring acute occlusion and myocardial infarction: A quantitative angiographic study. J Am Coll Cardiol 1999;33:1353-1361.

21. Danzi GB, Pirelli S, Mauri L, et al: Which variable of stenosis severity best describes the significance of an isolated left anterior descending coronary artery lesion? Correlation between quantitative coronary angiography, intercoronary Doppler measurements and high dose dipyridamole echocardiography. J Am Coll Cardiol 1998;31:526-533.

22. Kirkeeide R: Coronary obstructions, morphology and physiologic significance. In Reiber J, Serruys P (eds): Quantitative Coronary Arteriography. Dordrecht, Kluwer Academic Publishers, 1991, pp 229-244.

23. Strauss BH, Umans VA, van Suylen RJ, et al: Directional atherectomy for treatment of restenosis within coronary stents: Clinical, angiographic and histologic results. J Am Coll Cardiol 1992;20: 1465-1473.

24. Mudra H, Regar E, Klauss V, et al: Serial follow-up after optimized ultrasound-guided deployment of Palmaz-Schatz stents: In-stent neointimal proliferation without significant reference segment response. Circulation 1997;95:363-370.

25. Dussaillant G, Mintz G, Pichard A, et al: Small stent size and intimal hyperplasia contribute to restenosis: A volumetric intravascular ultrasound analysis. J Am Coll Cardiol 1995;26:720-724.

26. Ishii Y, van Weert A, Hekking E, et al: A novel quantitative method for evaluating diffuse in-stent narrowing at follow-up angiography. Cathet Cardiovasc Intervent 2001;54:309-317.

27. Reiber J: An overview of coronary quantitation techniques as of 1989. In Reiber J, Serruys P (eds): Quantitative Coronary Arteriography. Dordrecht, Kluwer Academic Publishers, 1991, pp 55-132.

28. Reiber J, Jukema J, Koning G, et al: Quality control in quantitative coronary arteriography. In Bruschke A, Reiber J, Lie K, Wellens H (eds): Lipid Lowering Therapy and Progression of Coronary Atherosclerosis. Dordrecht, Kluwer Academic Publishers, 1996, pp 45-63.

29. Tuinenburg JC, Koning G, Hekking E, et al: One core lab at two international sites, is that feasible? An inter-core lab and intra-observer variability study. Catheter Cardiovasc Interv 2002;56: 333-340.

30. Beauman G, Reiber J, Koning G, et al: Angiographic core laboratories analyses of arterial phantom images: Comparative evaluations of accuracy and precision. In Reiber J, Serruys P (eds): Progress in Quantitative Coronary Arteriography. Dordrecht, Kluwer Academic Publishers, 1994, pp 87-104.

31. Levin DC, Fallon JT: Significance of the angiographic morphology of localized coronary stenoses: Histopathologic correlations. Circulation 1982;66:316-320.

32. Lespérance J, Théroux P, Hudon G, et al: A new look at coronary angiograms: Plaque morphology as a help to diagnosis and to evaluate outcome. Int J Card Imaging 1994;10:75-94.

33. Ambrose J, Winters S, Stern A, et al: Angiographic morphology and the pathogenesis of unstable angina pectoris. J Am Coll Cardiol 1985;5:609-616.

34. Kalbfleisch SJ, Mc Guillem MJ, Simon S, et al: Automated quantitation of indexes of coronary lesion complexity: Comparison between patients with stable and unstable angina. Circulation 1990;82:439-447.

35. Wilson R, Holida M, White C: Quantitative angiographic morphology of coronary stenoses leading to myocardial infarction or unstable angina. Circulation 1986;73:286-293.

36. Davies SW, Marchant B, Lyons JP, et al: Irregular coronary lesion morphology after thrombolysis predicts early clinical instability. J Am Coll Cardiol 1991;18:669-674.

37. Early effects of tissue-type plasminogen activator added to conventional therapy on the culprit coronary lesion in patients presenting with ischemic cardiac pain at rest: Results of the Thrombolysis in Myocardial Ischemia (TIMI IIIA) Trial. Circulation 1993;87:38-52.

38. Gurbel PA, Navetta FI, Bates ER, et al: Lesion-directed administration of alteplase with intracoronary heparin in patients with unstable angina and coronary thrombus undergoing angioplasty. Cathet Cardiovasc Diagn 1996;37:382-391.

39. Zhao XQ, Theroux P, Snapinn SM, et al: Intracoronary thrombus and platelet glycoprotein IIb/IIIa receptor blockade with tirofiban in unstable angina or non-Q-wave myocardial infarction: Angiographic results from the PRISM-PLUS trial (Platelet Receptor Inhibition for Ischemic Syndrome Management in Patients Limited by Unstable Signs and Symptoms). PRISM-PLUS Investigators. Circulation 1999;100:1609-1615.

40. Franzen D, Sechtem U, Hopp HW: Comparison of angioscopic, intravascular ultrasonic, and angiographic detection of thrombus in coronary stenosis. Am J Cardiol 1998;82:1273-1275.

41. Sherman CT, Litvack F, Grundfest W, et al: Coronary angioscopy in patients with unstable angina pectoris. N Engl J Med 1986;315: 913-919.

42. de Feyter P, Ozaki Y, Baptista J, et al: Ischemia-related lesion characteristics in patients with stable and unstable angina: A study with intracoronary angioscopy and ultrasound. Circulation 1995;92: 1408-1413.

43. Kleiman N, Lincoff A, Flaker G, et al: Early percutaneous coronary intervention, platelet inhibition with Eptifibatide, and clinical outcomes in patients with acute coronary syndromes. Circulation 2000;101:751-757.

44. Boden W, O'Rourke R, Crawford M, et al: Outcomes in patients with acute non-Q wave myocardial infarction randomly assigned to an invasive as compared with a conservative management strategy. N Engl J Med 1998;338:1785-1792.

45. Dangas G, Mehran R, Wallenstein S, et al: Correlation of angiographic morphology and clinical presentation in unstable angina. J Am Coll Cardiol 1997;29:519-525.

46. Falk E: Unstable angina with fatal outcome: Dynamic coronary thrombosis leading to infarction and/or sudden death: Autopsy evidence of recurrent mural thrombosis with peripheral embolization culminating in total vascular occlusion. Circulation 1985;71: 699-708.

47. Garcia-Moll X, Coccolo F, Cole D, et al: Serum neopterin and complex stenosis morphology in patients with unstable angina. J Am Coll Cardiol 2000;35:956-962.

48. Goldstein JA, Demetriou D, Grines CL, et al: Multiple complex coronary plaques in patients with acute myocardial infarction. N Engl J Med 2000;343:915-922.

49. Diver DJ, Bier JD, Ferreira PE, et al: Clinical and arteriographic characterization of patients with unstable angina without critical coronary arterial narrowing (from the TIMI-IIIA Trial). Am J Cardiol 1994;74:531-537.

50. Freeman MR, Williams AE, Chisholm RJ, et al: Intracoronary thrombus and complex morphology in unstable angina: Relation to timing of angiography and in-hospital cardiac events. Circulation 1989;80:17-23.

51. Rupprecht H, Sohn H, Kearney P, et al: Clinical predictors of unstable coronary lesion morphology. Eur Heart J 1995;16:1526-1534.

52. Calton R, Satija T, Dhanoa J, et al: Correlation of Braunwald's clinical classification of unstable angina pectoris with angiographic extent of disease, lesion morphology and intra-luminal thrombus. Indian Heart J 1998;50:300-306.

53. Roe M, Harrington R, Prosper D, et al: Clinical and therapeutic profile of patients with acute coronary syndromes who do not have significant coronary artery disease. The Platelet Glycoprotein IIb/IIIa in Unstable Angina: Receptor Suppression Using Integrilin Therapy (PURSUIT) Trial investigators. Circulation 2000;102: 1101-1116.

54. Kranjec I, Delaye J, Didier B, et al: Angiographic morphology and intraluminal coronary artery thrombus in patients with angina pectoris: Clinical correlations. Eur Heart J 1987;8:106-115.

55. Haft J, Goldstein J, Niemiera M: Coronary angiographic lesion of unstable angina. Chest 1987;92:609-612.

56. Williams A, Freeman M, Chisholm R, et al: Angiographic morphology in unstable angina pectoris. Am J Cardiol 1988;62:1024-1027.

57. Cowley M, DiSciascio G, Rehr R, et al: Angiographic observations and clinical relevance of coronary thrombus in unstable angina pectoris. Am J Cardiol 1989;63:108E-113E.

58. Rehr R, Disciascio G, Vetrovec G, et al: Angiographic morphology of coronary artery stenoses in prolonged rest angina: Evidence of intracoronary thrombosis. J Am Coll Cardiol 1989;14: 1429-1437.

59. Bugiardini R, Pozzati A, Borghi A, et al: Angiographic morphology in unstable angina and its relation to transient myocardial ischemia and hospital outcome. Am J Cardiol 1991;67:460-464.

60. Cools F, Vrints C, Snoeck J: Angiographic coronary artery lesion morphology and pathogenetic mechanisms of myocardial ischemia

in stable and unstable coronary artery disease syndromes. Acta Cardiol 1992;47:13-30.

61. De Servi S, Arbustini E, Marsico F, et al: Correlation between clinical and morphologic findings in unstable angina. Am J Cardiol 1996; 77:128-132.

62. Thrombolysis in Myocardial Infarction (TIMI) Trial: Phase I findings. TIMI Study Group. N Engl J Med 1985;312:932-936.

63. Capone G, Wolf N, Meyer B, et al: Frequency of intracoronary filling defects by angiography in angina pectoris. Am J Cardiol 1985;56:403-406.

64. Mizuno K, Satomura K, Miyamoto A, et al: Angioscopic evaluation of coronary-artery thrombi in acute coronary syndromes. N Engl J Med 1992;326:287-291.

65. Ahmed W, Bittl J, Braunwald E: Relation between clinical presentation and angiographic findings in unstable angina pectoris, and comparison with that in stable angina. Am J Cardiol 1993;72: 544-550.

66. Rentrop KP, Feit F, Sherman W, et al: Serial angiographic assessment of coronary artery obstruction and collateral flow in acute myocardial infarction: Report from the second Mount Sinai-New York University Reperfusion Trial. Circulation 1989;80:1166-1175.

67. Moise A, Theroux P, Taeymans Y, et al: Unstable angina and progression of coronary atherosclerosis. N Engl J Med 1983;309:685-689.

68. DeMaio S, Kinsella S, Silverman M: Clinical course and long term prognosis of spontaneous coronary artery dissection. Am J Cardiol 1989;64:471-474.

69. Kay J, Wilkins G, Williams M: Spontaneous coronary artery dissection presenting with unstable angina. J Invasive Cardiol 1998; 10:274-276.

70. Mulvany N, Ranson D, Pilbeam M: Isolated dissection of the coronary artery: A post-mortem study of seven cases. Pathology 2001;33:307-311.

71. Celik S, Sagcan A, Altintig A, et al: Primary spontaneous coronary artery dissection in atherosclerotic patients: Reports of nine cases with review of the pertinent literature. Eur J Cardiothorac Surg 2001;20:573-576.

72. Topol EJ, Yadav JS: Recognition of the importance of embolization in atherosclerotic vascular disease. Circulation 2000;101:570-580.

73. Bauters C, Chmait A, Tricot O, et al: Coronary thrombosis and myocardial bridging. Circulation 2002;105:130.

74. Braunwald E, Jones RH, Mark DB, et al: Diagnosing and managing unstable angina. Agency for Health Care Policy and Research. Circulation 1994;90:613-622.

75. Haft J, Christou C, Goldstein J, et al: Correlation of atherectomy specimen histology with coronary arteriographic lesion morphologic appearance in patients with stable and unstable angina. Am Heart J 1995;130:420-424.

76. Falk E, Fernandez-Ortiz A: Role of thrombosis in atherosclerosis and its complications. Am J Cardiol 1995;75:3B-11B.

77. Baumgartner H, Schima H, Tulzer G, et al: Effect of stenosis geometry on the Doppler-Catheter gradient relation in vitro: A manifestation of pressure recovery. J Am Coll Cardiol 1993;21:1018-1025.

78. Chakhtoura EY, Shamoon FE, Haft JI, et al: Comparison of platelet activation in unstable and stable angina pectoris and correlation with coronary angiographic findings. Am J Cardiol 2000;86:835-839.

79. Juhan-Vague I: Haemostatic parameters and vascular risk. Atherosclerosis 1996;124(Suppl):S49-S55.

80. Bar FW, Raynaud P, Renkin JP, et al: Coronary angiographic findings do not predict clinical outcome in patients with unstable angina. J Am Coll Cardiol 1994;24:1453-1459.

81. Heeschen C, van Den Brand MJ, Hamm CW, et al: Angiographic findings in patients with refractory unstable angina according to troponin T status. Circulation 1999;100:1509-1514.

82. Chen L, Chester MR, Redwood S, et al: Angiographic stenosis progression and coronary events in patients with 'stabilized' unstable angina. Circulation 1995;91:2319-2324.

83. Ellis S, Alderman E, Cain K, et al: Prediction of risk of anterior myocardial infarction by lesion severity and measurement method of stenoses in the left anterior descending coronary distribution: A CASS registry study. J Am Coll Cardiol 1988;11:908-916.

84. Ambrose JA, Tannenbaum MA, Alexopoulos D, et al: Angiographic progression of coronary artery disease and the development of myocardial infarction. J Am Coll Cardiol 1988;12:56-62.

85. Nobuyoshi M, Tanaka M, Nosaka H, et al: Progression of coronary atherosclerosis: Is coronary spasm related to progression? J Am Coll Cardiol 1991;18:904-910.

86. Little WC, Constantinescu M, Applegate RJ, et al: Can coronary angiography predict the site of a subsequent myocardial infarction in patients with mild-to-moderate coronary artery disease? Circulation 1988;78:1157-1166.

87. Alderman EL, Corley SD, Fisher LD, et al: Five-year angiographic follow-up of factors associated with progression of coronary artery disease in the Coronary Artery Surgery Study (CASS). CASS participating investigators and staff. J Am Coll Cardiol 1993;22: 1141-1154.

88. Petursson MK, Jonmundsson EH, Brekkan A, et al: Angiographic predictors of new coronary occlusions. Am Heart J 1995; 129:515-520.

89. Lichtlen PR, Nikutta P, Jost S, et al: Anatomical progression of coronary artery disease in humans as seen by prospective, repeated, quantitated coronary angiography: Relation to clinical events and risk factors. The INTACT Study Group. Circulation 1992;86: 828-838.

90. Tousoulis D, Davies G, Crake T, et al: Angiographic characteristics of infarct-related and non-infarct-related stenoses in patients in whom stable angina progressed to acute myocardial infarction. Am Heart J 1998;136:382-388.

91. Dacanay S, Kennedy HL, Uretz E, et al: Morphological and quantitative angiographic analyses of progression of coronary stenoses: A comparison of Q-wave and non-Q-wave myocardial infarction. Circulation 1994;90:1739-1746.

92. Ellis S, Alderman EL, Cain K, et al: Morphology of left descending coronary territory lesions as a predictor of anterior myocardial infarction: A CASS registry study. J Am Coll Cardiol 1989;13: 1481-1491.

93. Taeymans Y, Théroux P, Lespérance J, et al: Quantitative angiographic morphology of the coronary artery lesion at risk of thrombotic occlusion. Circulation 1992;85:78-85.

94. Ambrose JA, Winters SL, Arora RR, et al: Angiographic evolution of coronary artery morphology in unstable angina. J Am Coll Cardiol 1986;7:472-478.

95. Koenig W, Ernst E: The possible role of hemorheology in atherothrombogenesis. Atherosclerosis 1992;94:93-107.

96. Moise A, Lesperance J, Théroux P, et al: Clinical and angiographic predictors of new total coronary occlusion in coronary artery disease: Analysis of 313 nonoperated patients. Am J Cardiol 1984;54:1176-1181.

97. Jost S, Deckers JW, Nikutta P, et al: Progression of coronary artery disease is dependent on anatomic location and diameter. J Am Coll Cardiol 1993;21:1339-1346.

98. Lespérance J, Waters D: Measuring progression and regression of coronary atherosclerosis in clinical trials: Problems and progress. Int J Card Imaging 1992;8:165-173.

99. Waters D, Craven T, Lespérance J: Prognosis significance of progression of coronary atherosclerosis. Circulation 1993;87: 1067-1075.

100. Yokoya K, Takatsu H, Suzuki T, et al: Process of progression of coronary artery lesions from mild or moderate stenosis to moderate or severe stenosis: A study based on four serial coronary arteriograms per year. Circulation 1999;100:903-909.

101. Giroud D, Li JM, Urban P, et al: Relation of the site of acute myocardial infarction to the most severe coronary arterial stenosis at prior angiography. Am J Cardiol 1992;69:729-732.

102. Glagov S, Weisenberg E, Zarins CK, et al: Compensatory enlargement of human atherosclerotic coronary arteries. N Engl J Med 1987;316:1371-1375.

103. Porter TR, Sears T, Xie F, et al: Intravascular ultrasound study of angiographically mildly diseased coronary arteries. J Am Coll Cardiol 1993;22:1858-1865.

104. Mann JM, Davies MJ: Vulnerable plaque: Relation of characteristics to degree of stenosis in human coronary arteries. Circulation 1996;94:928-931.

105. Ledru F, Ducimetiere P, Battaglia S, et al: New diagnostic criteria for diabetes and coronary artery disease: Insights from an angiographic study. J Am Coll Cardiol 2001;37:1543-1550.

106. Hermiller JB, Cusma JT, Spero LA, et al: Quantitative and qualitative coronary angiographic analysis: Review of methods, utility, and limitations. Cathet Cardiovasc Diagn 1992;25: 110-131.

107. Reiber JH: Is the time of 3D representation of the coronary system by X-ray angiography for interventional cardiology almost there? Int J Card Imaging 2000;16:428.

108. Nissen SE, Gurley JC: Application of intravascular ultrasound for detection and quantitation of coronary atherosclerosis. Int J Card Imaging 1991;6:165-177.

109. Nissen SE, Gurley JC, Grines CL, et al: Intravascular ultrasound assessment of lumen size and wall morphology in normal subjects and patients with coronary artery disease. Circulation 1991;84:1087-1099.

110. Tobis JM, Mallery J, Mahon D, et al: Intravascular ultrasound imaging of human coronary arteries in vivo: Analysis of tissue characterizations with comparison to in vitro histological specimens. Circulation 1991;83:913-926.

111. Kimura BJ, Bhargava V, De Maria AN: Value and limitations of intravascular ultrasound imaging in characterizing coronary atherosclerotic plaque. Am Heart J 1995;130:386-396.

112. Maheswaran B, Leung CY, Gutfinger DE, et al: Intravascular ultrasound appearance of normal and mildly diseased coronary arteries: Correlation with histologic specimens. Am Heart J 1995;130:976-986.

113. Achenbach S, Giesler T, Ropers D, et al: Detection of coronary artery stenoses by contrast-enhanced, retrospectively electrocardiographically-gated, multislice spiral computed tomography. Circulation 2001;103:2535-2538.

114. Nieman K, Oudkerk M, Rensing BJ, et al: Coronary angiography with multi-slice computed tomography. Lancet 2001;357:599-603.

115. Kim WY, Danias PG, Stuber M, et al: Coronary magnetic resonance angiography for the detection of coronary stenoses. N Engl J Med 2001;345:1863-1869.

116. Yuan C, Mitsumori LM, Beach KW, et al: Carotid atherosclerotic plaque: Noninvasive MR characterization and identification of vulnerable lesions. Radiology 2001;221:285-299.

117. Stefanadis C, Diamantopoulos L, Vlachopoulos C, et al: Thermal heterogeneity within human atherosclerotic coronary arteries detected in vivo: A new method of detection by application of a special thermography catheter. Circulation 1999;99:1965-1971.

118. Patwari P, Weissman NJ, Boppart SA, et al: Assessment of coronary plaque with optical coherence tomography and high-frequency ultrasound. Am J Cardiol 2000;85:641-644.

119. Zack P, Ischinger T, Aker U, et al: The occurrence of angiographically detected intracoronary thrombus in patients with unstable angina pectoris. Am Heart J 1984;108:1408-1412.

120. Bresnahan D, Davis J, Holmes DJ, et al: Angiographic occurrence and clinical correlates of intraluminal coronary artery thrombus: Role of unstable angina. J Am Coll Cardiol 1985;6:285-289.

■ ■ ■ c h a p t e r **1 8**

Echocardiography in Acute Coronary Syndromes

Ady Butnaru
Anique Ducharme
Jean-Claude Tardif

Given the high prevalence of coronary artery disease (CAD), evaluation of patients with suspected or documented ischemic heart disease is one of the most common indications for echocardiography. History taking and physical examination in a patient suspected of having CAD remain central to the diagnostic process. Echocardiography, as a rapid, noninvasive, ambulatory, and nonexpensive modality, has a unique role, however, in diagnosing CAD, assessing the extent and severity of the disease and providing important prognostic information that can decisively affect the therapeutic approach. The echocardiographic evaluation focuses on the functional outcome of CAD, the global and segmental wall function, and the complications of myocardial infarction (MI). This chapter focuses on the use of echocardiography for the diagnosis and management of suspected or proven acute coronary syndromes (ACS).

SEQUENCE OF EVENTS IN ISCHEMIA

Ischemia results from an abnormal myocardial oxygen supply-to-demand ratio. Blood flow is usually adequate for myocardial oxygen demands at rest, unless there is critical (>90% diameter stenosis) coronary artery narrowing. Imbalance occurs in the presence of a physiologically significant stenosis when oxygen demand is increased, as with exercise, mental stress, or pharmacologic interventions, or when myocardial perfusion is reduced by subtotal or total coronary occlusion secondary to atherothrombosis.[1] The first abnormalities to take place (Fig. 18-1) when coronary blood flow is insufficient to meet myocardial demand are cellular biochemical changes; followed by a perfusion defect (detected by radionuclide techniques); then diastolic dysfunction characterized by abnormalities of relaxation or compliance; and shortly afterward, impairment of regional systolic wall thickening and motion. The ischemic electrocardiogram (ECG) changes and clinical symptoms of angina (if they appear) are late manifestations of ischemia.[2] Given this sequence of events, echocardiography represents a unique and sensitive tool for early detection of myocardial ischemia, particularly by its ability to identify regional wall motion abnormalities.

EVALUATION OF SYSTOLIC FUNCTION IN ACUTE CORONARY SYNDROMES

Qualitative and Semiquantitative Evaluation of Regional and Global Systolic Function

Global and regional ventricular function can be evaluated with two-dimensional echocardiography. With ventricular contraction, a target point chosen along the endocardial interface moves inward, toward the center of the ventricle (endocardial excursion); the cavity area decreases (area shrinkage), and the distance between the endocardial and epicardial interfaces increases (wall thickening). A few seconds after coronary occlusion, a decrease in the amplitude of endocardial excursion and wall thickening becomes apparent in the area supplied by the obstructed artery.[3] The abnormality is defined as *hypokinesis* when contraction is normally directed but reduced in magnitude, *akinesis* when it is absent, or *dyskinesis* when there is systolic bulging.

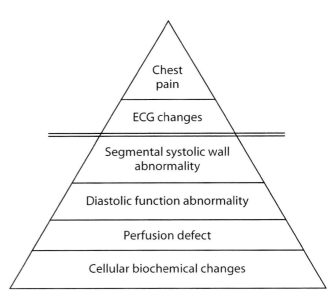

FIGURE 18-1. The sequence of events during myocardial ischemia. ECG, electrocardiogram.

Semiquantitative assessment of regional left ventricular contraction is provided by the *wall motion score index* (WMSI). The left ventricle is divided into 16 segments (Fig. 18–2), as suggested by the American Society of Echocardiography, and a score is assigned to each segment according to its contractility. A score of 1 is given to a normally contracting or hyperkinetic segment; 2, for a hypokinetic segment; 3, for akinesis; and 4, in the presence of a dyskinetic segment. There is no specific score for compensatory hyperkinesis. The WMSI is equal to the sum of the regional scores divided by the number of evaluable segments and can vary between 1 (for normal ventricular contraction) and 3.9 (for severe systolic dysfunction) (Fig. 18–3). Because CAD causes segmental dysfunction, which can be accompanied by compensatory hyperkinesis of nonischemic segments, regional assessment of systolic function is more sensitive for the detection of ischemia than global approaches. The prognostic value of the motion score has been shown in clinical studies. Among a group of patients admitted with acute MI, patients with favorable indices (best quintile) had an incidence of cardiovascular death of 8% at 1 year. In contrast, patients with motion indices in the worst quintile

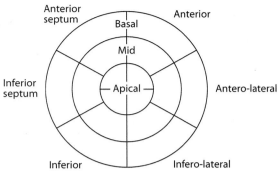

Wall motion score index

a) **Bull's eye target diagram of the 16 LV segments**

b) **Wall motion score**
   1. Normal/Hyperkinesia
   2. Hypokinesia
   3. Akinesia
   4. Dyskinesia

c) **WMSI** = $\dfrac{\text{Sum of wall motion scores}}{\text{Number of segments evaluated}}$

FIGURE 18–3. *a,* The 16 segments of the left ventricle displayed as a bull's eye. *b,* The wall motion score, which assigns a number according to the contractile function of each segment. *c,* The wall motion score index (WMSI) is obtained by dividing the sum of the scores of evaluable segments by the number of segments evaluated.

had a mortality of 51% at 1 year.[4] Kan and associates[5] examined the value of WMSI in patients with acute MI and found a significantly higher mortality rate in the group with the most abnormal score indices compared with patients with favorable ones (61% versus 3%). In another study in post-MI patients, a good correlation was observed between the echocardiographic WMSI and the ejection fraction measured by radionuclide ventriculography.[6]

Global systolic function can be qualitatively classified as normal or mildly, moderately, or severely reduced, but this information is considered incomplete by most clinicians. In contrast, determination of the left ventricular ejection fraction has major prognostic significance in patients with CAD. In the clinical setting, visual estimation of the left ventricular ejection fraction has become a common practice. The correlation between the visual echocardiographic estimation and the radionuclide determination is good, especially in patients with impaired ejection fraction.[7] The *eyeball method* requires experience, however, and clinicians should validate their own performance with quantitative methods. All echocardiographic approaches for the assessment of regional and global ventricular function also need to take into account the quality of endocardial border definition, the asynchronous contraction patterns observed with pacemakers or conduction defects, the abnormal postoperative septal motion, and the heterogeneity of normal ventricular function.

The *mitral annulus motion* toward the apex also can be used as an indirect measure of left ventricular systolic

a) **Parasternal long axis view**

b) **Parasternal short axis views**

Basal — Mid — Apical

c) **Apical views**

Apical 4-chamber — Apical 2-chamber — Apical long-axis

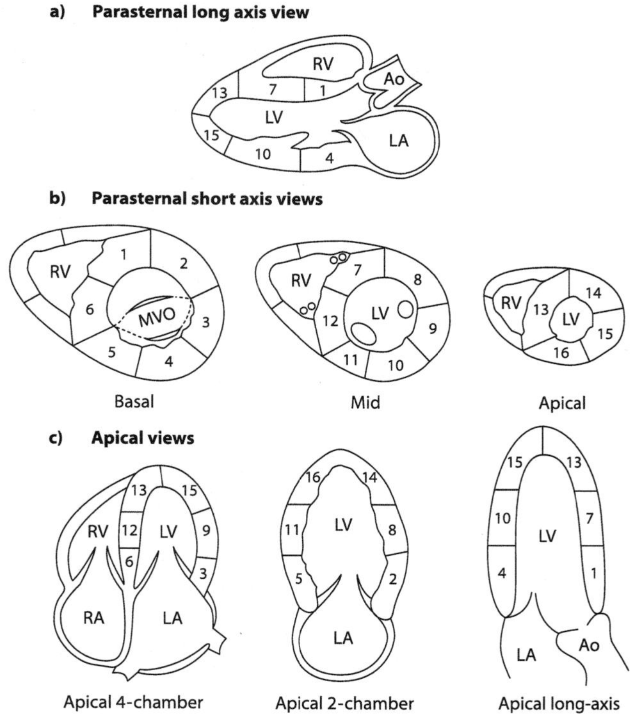

FIGURE 18–2. Schematic of the 16 segments of the left ventricle, as described by the American Society of Echocardiography. *a,* Parasternal long-axis view. *b,* Parasternal short-axis views. *c,* Apical views. The numbers in the diagram correspond to the following segments: 1, basal anteroseptum; 2, basal anterior wall; 3, basal anterolateral wall; 4, basal inferolateral wall; 5, basal inferior wall; 6, basal inferior septum; 7, mid anterior septum; 8, mid anterior wall; 9, mid anterolateral wall; 10, mid inferolateral wall; 11, mid inferior wall; 12, mid inferior septum; 13, septal apex; 14, anterior apex; 15, lateral apex; 16, inferior apex. Ao, aorta; LA, left atrium; LV, left ventricle, MVO, mitral valve orifice; RA, right atrium; RV, right ventricle.

function. It usually is measured in the apical four-chamber view, where the movement of the mitral annulus is parallel to the ultrasound beam and is normally 12 ± 2 mm. A motion of less than 8 mm has been reported to have a sensitivity of 98% and a specificity of 82% for the identification of an ejection fraction less than 50%.[8] Pai and colleagues[9] examined the mitral annular systolic excursion in 57 patients with a wide range of left ventricular ejection function (13% to 84%) and found a good correlation ($r = .95, P < .001$) with the ejection fraction measured by the radionuclide approach.

Quantitative Evaluation of Left Ventricular Systolic Function

Quantitative evaluation of left ventricular systolic function is based on endocardial border tracing, with or without epicardial border tracing, at end diastole and end systole in one or preferably several views.[10-13] Assessment is based on either analysis of wall motion (endocardial excursion) or wall thickening (interface separation). Evaluation of regional wall thickening is not influenced by cardiac translation or rotation, as opposed to wall motion, but requires excellent definition and tracing of the endocardial and the epicardial borders, which constitutes its major limitation. Most quantitative methods are based on the evaluation of wall motion. The *centerline method* is a quantitative approach to assess regional ventricular function, which first involves the construction of a line halfway between the end-diastolic and end-systolic endocardial perimeters.[14] The endocardial excursion is determined along 100 equally spaced chords perpendicular to this centerline. Motion is normalized for heart size by dividing by the length of the end-diastolic perimeter. The normalized length of each line is converted into units of standard deviations from the normal excursion along a given chord, which allows the regional heterogeneity of ventricular contraction to be taken into account. By convention, negative and positive values indicate hypokinetic and hyperkinetic chords. The extent of abnormal wall motion is calculated as the number of chords with hypokinesis equal to or more severe than 2 standard deviations. The severity of wall motion abnormalities is calculated as the area under the curve below the 0 standard deviation line.

Quantitative assessment of global systolic function requires determination of the left ventricular cavity dimensions. Volume estimations are based on geometric assumptions about ventricular shape, which range from a simple ellipsoid to a complex hemicylindrical, hemiellipsoid shape.[15] Descriptions of each geometric shape and the corresponding formula and requirements are beyond the scope of this chapter. Nevertheless, the *biplane modified Simpson's formula* is the most commonly used approach in clinical practice to assess left ventricular volumes and global function and involves tracing of the endocardial borders in the apical four-chamber and two-chamber views, at end systole and end diastole. Determination of the left ventricular end-diastolic volume (EDV) and end-systolic volume (ESV) allows calculation of the stroke volume (EDV - ESV = SV),

cardiac output (SV × heart rate), and ejection fraction ([SV/EDV] × 100).[16,17]

Evaluation of Diastolic Function in Acute Coronary Syndromes

Studies have shown changes in the transmitral flow profile after balloon inflation–induced coronary occlusion, which are secondary to impaired left ventricular relaxation.[18] There is a decrease in the peak rate of early filling (E wave) resulting in a reduced proportion of total left ventricular filling during the rapid filling phase, an increased rate of filling secondary to atrial contraction (A wave) and a reduced E/A ratio with a prolonged deceleration time (Fig. 18–4).[19] These changes parallel the worsening of diastolic function measured invasively by the peak negative dp/dt, the left ventricular end-diastolic pressure, and the time constant of isovolumic relaxation[20] and may be present even when systolic function remains normal. In ACS, most patients present with the typical abnormal relaxation pattern (E/A ratio <1, prolonged mitral deceleration time [>250 ms]). A large infarct size or severe systolic dysfunction can result,

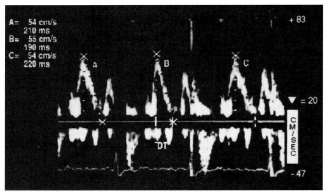

A

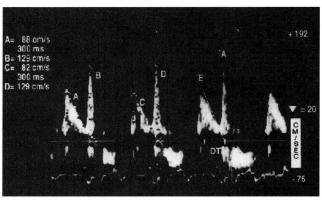

B

FIGURE 18–4. *A*, Example of a normal Doppler mitral profile. E wave is 54 cm/s, deceleration time (DT) is 210 mg, and E/A ratio is greater than 1. *B*, Mitral flow velocity recording shows abnormal relaxation. E/A ratio is 0.7, and DT is prolonged (300 ms). (From Tardif JC, Rouleau JL: Diastolic dysfunction. Can J Cardiol 1996;12:389-398.)

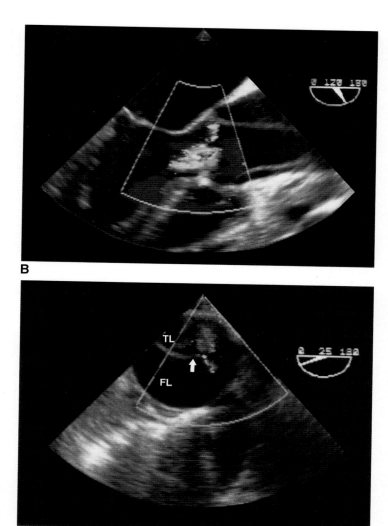

B

C

FIGURE 18–5. *B,* Color-flow Doppler revealed the associated aortic regurgitation. *C,* Short-axis view of the descending thoracic aorta shows communication between the true lumen (TL) and the false lumen (FL), which are separated by the intimal flap *(arrow).* (See text page 254 for Figure 18–5*A.*)

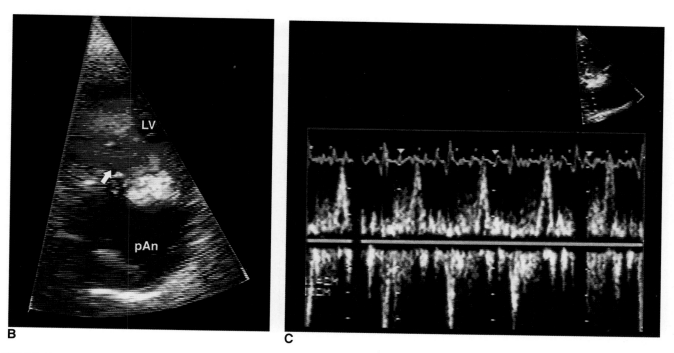

B

C

FIGURE 18–7. *B,* By color Doppler, flow is seen from the LV toward the pseudoaneurysmal cavity *(arrow). C,* Pulsed-wave Doppler showed to-and-fro velocities. Ao, aorta; LA, left atrium; MV, mitral valve, pAn, pseudoaneurysm. (See text page 257 for Figure 18–7*A.*)

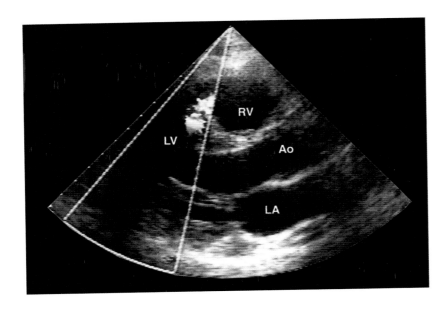

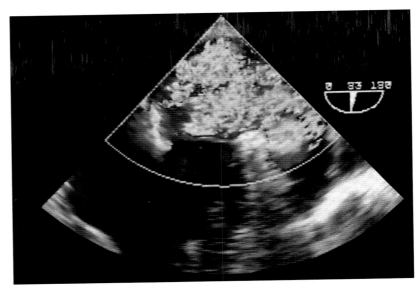

FIGURE 18–8. Three days after an acute anterior myocardial infarction, clinical deterioration and a new systolic murmur were observed in this patient. Parasternal long-axis view with color Doppler showed a shunt from the left to the right ventricle, consistent with a ventricular septal defect. Ao, aorta; LA, left atrium; LV, left ventricle; RV, right ventricle.

FIGURE 18–9. *A*, Transesophageal echocardiography in a two-chamber view (83 degrees) shows severe mitral regurgitation after acute myocardial infarction, secondary to a ruptured papillary muscle. (See text page 258 for Figure 18–9*B*.)

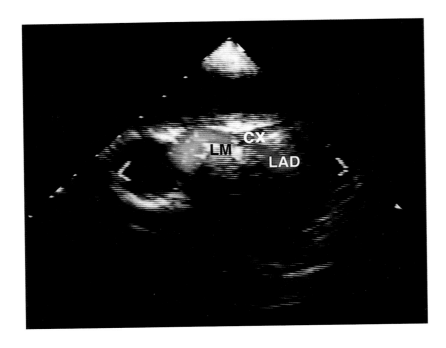

FIGURE 18–12. Transesophageal echocardiography shows flow in the left main (LM) coronary artery and its bifurcation, the left anterior descending (LAD) artery, and circumflex (CX) artery.

however, in a restrictive pattern (high peak E wave velocity, E/A >2, and deceleration time <150 ms), which reflects abnormal ventricular compliance with elevated filling pressures.[19] A third Doppler pattern also can be seen, which is constituted by a E/A ratio between 1 and 2 and a deceleration time between 150 and 250 ms. This pseudonormal pattern can be differentiated from a truly normal Doppler profile by determining the isovolumic relaxation time using the mitral and aortic Doppler profiles or by analyzing pulmonary venous flow.[19] The Valsalva maneuver also can be used to establish the distinction because the decrease in venous return induces abnormalities in the mitral E/A ratio (<1) and deceleration time (>250 ms) in patients with the pseudonormal pattern, but these indices remain normal in patients without diastolic dysfunction. Emerging echocardiographic approaches for the assessment of diastolic function exist and include tissue Doppler imaging,[21] diastolic color kinesis,[22] and color M-mode.[23]

In experimental models, restoration of normal coronary flow causes the Doppler changes to return to baseline within 15 seconds. Normalization of the Doppler velocity profile can be delayed, however, in the clinical setting. After successful coronary angioplasty, improvement in the transmitral flow velocity profile may take 48 hours or sometimes several days,[24,25] depending on the duration and the severity of the ischemic insult before revascularization. This delayed normalization may reflect improvement in diastolic function of the myocardial segments that previously were chronically ischemic or that were stunned.

ROLE OF ECHOCARDIOGRAPHY IN THE EMERGENCY DEPARTMENT

Patients with chest pain in the emergency department can present an important diagnostic dilemma. Chest pain may be the manifestation of several cardiac and noncardiac disorders, one of the most important being acute MI. The early treatment of acute MI is crucial to improve myocardial perfusion, limit cell necrosis, and ultimately save the patient's life. Since early treatment leads to better results, a method that accurately and rapidly diagnoses these patients is of great clinical utility. Classically the diagnosis of acute MI is based on the triad of the clinical history, ECG, and serum enzyme levels. The clinical history is frequently neither classic nor specific. Levels of cardiac enzymes are often normal on initial sampling and can take many hours to become elevated.[26] A typical injury pattern on the ECG is helpful when present but provides a specific diagnosis in only 40% to 50% of patients with ACS.[27] This problem is particularly evident in patients with an occlusion of the circumflex artery.

The early diagnosis of an acute MI from this classic triad is not always possible. Fewer than one third of patients presenting to the emergency department with chest pain are eventually proved to have ACS,[28] whereas 5% to 10% of patients who do have acute MI are mistakenly discharged from the emergency department.[29] The accurate distinction between the two groups of patients is challenging and important. Alternate diagnostic strategies have been suggested and include serial enzyme assessment with new isoforms, ST-segment monitoring, and early exercise testing. Because echocardiography allows rapid bedside assessment, it may be the optimal method for early diagnosis of acute ischemia and MI in patients with suggestive symptoms but nondiagnostic ECGs.[30] The presence of a regional wall motion abnormality on echocardiography has a high sensitivity (88% to 93%) but relatively low specificity (41% to 53%) for the diagnosis of acute MI.[31-33] The absence of such wall motion abnormalities during or immediately after chest pain identifies a subset of patients, however, unlikely to have MI, with a negative predictive value of approximately 95%.[34] Kontos and associates[35] compared two-dimensional echocardiography with scintigraphic perfusion imaging and found a good correlation in this setting with a concordance of 89% between both modalities. Some clinical centers use exercise echocardiography after a normal standard echocardiogram to evaluate patients with suspected myocardial ischemia in the emergency department and to allow an early discharge.[36]

Echocardiography can be a useful tool in the emergency department for the triage of patients with chest pain. It can help in the diagnosis of ACS, the evaluation of the myocardial area at risk and global ventricular function, and the rapid and precise identification of complications in unstable patients. Echocardiography also can be useful in excluding other possible causes of chest pain, such as aortic dissection (Fig. 18–5), massive pulmonary embolus, acute pericarditis with pericardial effusion, aortic stenosis, hypertrophic cardiomyopathy, and mitral valve prolapse. In addition, echocardiography can provide important prognostic information in patients with chest pain by identifying patients at risk of early or late cardiac events, in addition to clinical and ECG variables.[37] The incidence of these cardiac events (death, urgent revascularization, MI) is increased significantly in patients with chest pain, wall motion abnormalities, and impaired systolic function compared with patients without left ventricular dysfunction on echocardiography.[38]

ECHOCARDIOGRAPHY IN ACUTE MYOCARDIAL INFARCTION

Using correlative studies with coronary angiography and echocardiography in patients with acute MI, the specific coronary artery perfusing each left ventricular segment was determined (Fig. 18–6). In the parasternal long-axis view, the anterior interventricular septum is perfused by the left anterior descending artery, the first 1 to 2 cm being perfused by the first septal perforator, allowing determination of whether the obstruction is proximal or distal to this left anterior descending branch. The inferolateral wall usually is perfused by the circumflex artery. In the parasternal short-axis view, the left anterior descending artery supplies the anterior wall and the anterior septum, the circumflex artery supplies the lateral wall, and the right coronary artery supplies the inferior septum and inferior wall. In the apical two-chamber view, the anterior wall is perfused by the left anterior descending artery, the inferior wall is supplied by the

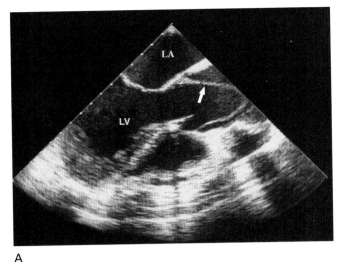

A

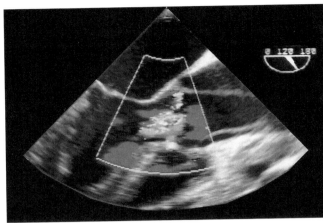

B

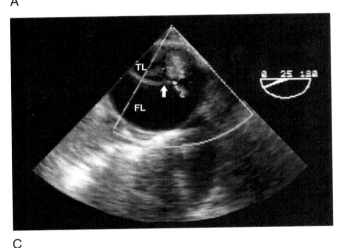

C

FIGURE 18–5. *A,* Transesophageal echocardiography shows a typical dissection of the ascending aorta, observed in the long-axis view (120 degrees), with the intimal flap *(arrow)* identified. LA, left atrium; LV, left ventricle. *B,* Color-flow Doppler revealed the associated aortic regurgitation. *C,* Short-axis view of the descending thoracic aorta shows communication between the true lumen (TL) and the false lumen (FL), which are separated by the intimal flap *(arrow).* (*B* and *C,* see color plates.)

right coronary artery, and the apex often has a dual coronary support. In the apical four-chamber view, the mid septum is perfused by the left anterior descending artery, whereas the basal portion is usually part of the right coronary artery territory, with the basal and mid-lateral walls being supplied by the circumflex artery.

The early stage of an acute transmural MI is characterized on echocardiography by a decreased amplitude of regional endocardial excursion with normal wall thickness, followed in 4 to 6 weeks by wall thinning in the affected region and often increased echogenicity secondary to a fibrotic response. A transmural infarction generally produces profound changes in regional left ventricular function, most of the affected segments being akinetic or dyskinetic and the others being severely hypokinetic. In contrast, a nontransmural infarction results in a lesser degree of hypokinesis and better global ventricular function.[39,40] Studies have found a good correlation between histologic evidence of infarction and the presence of segmental dysfunction on echocardiography in more than 90% of cases.[41] Experimentally, necrosis of 20% or less of the wall thickness results in a decrease in systolic thickening of approximately 50%, whereas necrosis of more than 20% of the thickness of

the myocardium is uniformly associated with systolic thinning.[42,43] The presence or absence of wall motion abnormalities may be more related to the extent of transmural involvement rather than the circumferential extent of an infarct.[44] Shortly after coronary occlusion (<2 days), experimental and clinical studies also have shown that the extent of wall motion abnormalities as shown by echocardiography correlates well with actual infarct size.[45] Echocardiography can overestimate infarct size, however, because of contractile abnormalities ("tethering") in the noninfarcted myocardium immediately adjacent to the severely ischemic regions.[41,42] The mechanism responsible for this phenomenon may be that the vulnerable myocardium is metabolically abnormal (adenosine triphosphate depletion) and placed under unfavorable regional loading conditions, leading to apparent dysfunction. This myocardium contiguous to the infarcted area also may exhibit reversible postischemic dysfunction (stunning).[46] The stunned myocardium has had, by definition, flow restored (by angioplasty, thrombolysis, or spontaneously) yet remains temporarily dysfunctional because gradual improvement in left ventricular function may take 10 to 14 days. Echocardiography combined with dobutamine infusion

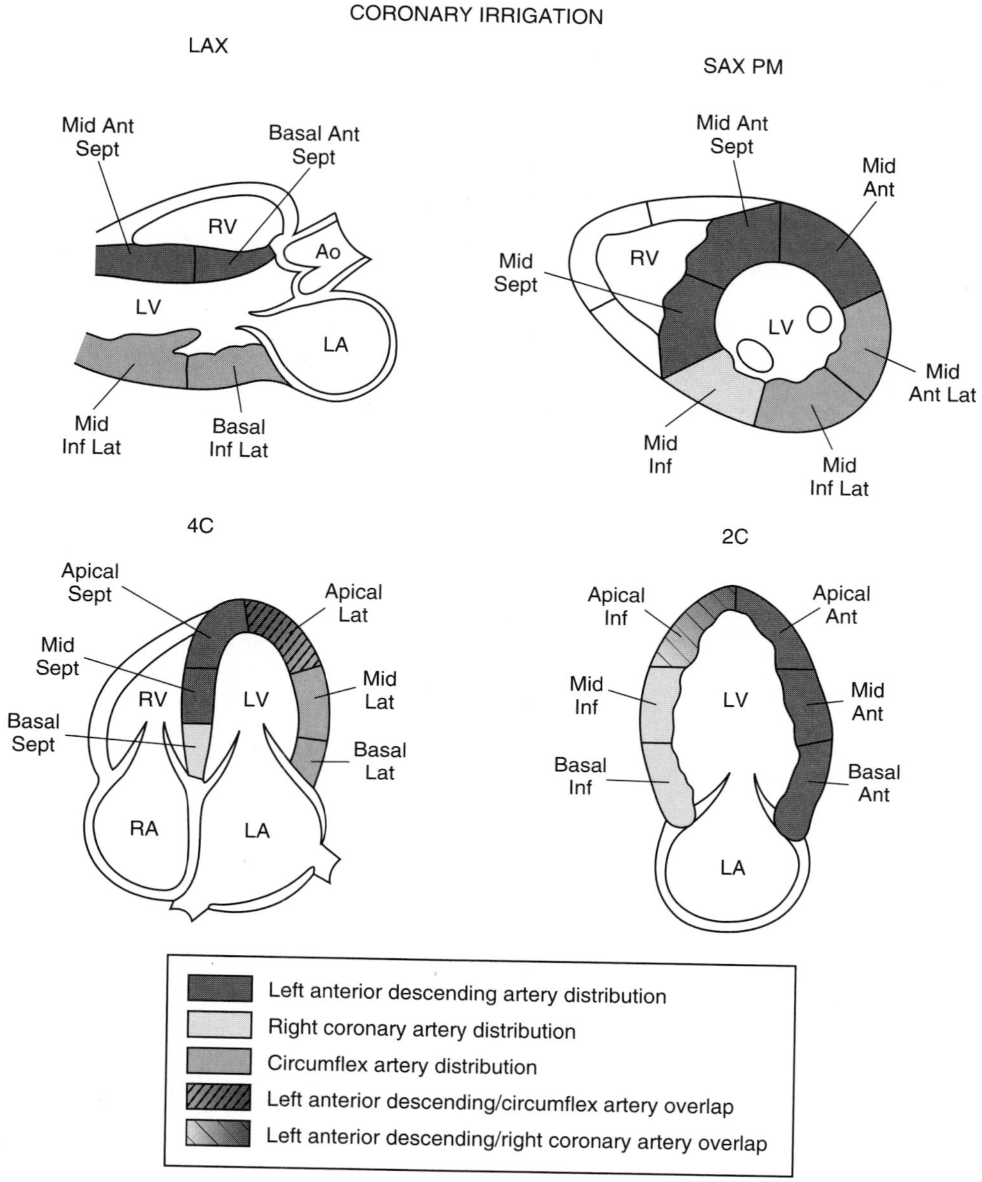

FIGURE 18–6. Diagram shows coronary perfusion of the 16 left ventricular segments. The apical lateral segment may be supplied by either the left anterior descending artery or the circumflex artery. The apical inferior segment may be supplied by either the left anterior descending artery or the right coronary artery. LAX, parasternal long-axis view; SAX PM, parasternal short-axis view at the papillary muscle level; 4C, apical four-chamber view; 2C, apical two-chamber view.

(5 to 10 µg/kg/min) (see later) can be used to distinguish stunned myocardium after thrombolytic therapy from nonviable myocardium, the former responding to low-dose inotropic stimulation.[47]

Relationship Between Abnormal Wall Motion and Electrocardiographic Infarct Location

Heger and colleagues[3] reported that 95% of patients with ECG evidence of Q waves in leads II, III, and aVF have wall motion abnormalities involving at least one of the *inferior* segments. When the inferior wall myocardial infarction was complicated by a ventricular septal defect, echocardiography identified involvement of the inferior portion of the interventricular septum[3] despite the absence of ECG evidence of septal involvement in any of these patients. The echocardiographically defined wall motion abnormalities were a better predictor of the extent and location of infarction, especially because the inferior septum cannot be assessed accurately by the ECG. Lateral wall involvement often is associated with inferoposterior infarction. Patients with inferoposterior infarction and lateral wall involvement on the ECG have wall motion abnormalities that usually extend to the basal segments.[48]

When an *anterior wall* infarction is identified on the ECG, at least one of the anterior segments presents a regional wall motion abnormality on echocardiography.[3] The extent of wall motion abnormalities is influenced by the location of the obstruction in the left anterior descending coronary artery.[49] All the segments of the anterior septum and anterior wall and the apex are affected if the obstruction occurs proximal to the first septal perforator artery, whereas obstruction distal to the first septal perforator characteristically spares the basal segments of the anterior septum and anterior wall. The sensitivity and specificity of the 12-lead ECG for the detection of an apical infarction are low despite several ECG criteria.[50,51] In contrast, apical dysfunction is identified and quantified clearly by echocardiography.[52] One potential pitfall of transthoracic imaging is incorrect positioning in the apical views, which truncates the true left ventricular apex, but the experienced echocardiographer ensures that the transducer is sufficiently low and lateral on the chest to avoid this problem. No Q waves were found on ECG in more than a third of 64 patients with apical akinesis by echocardiography.[53] When abnormal Q waves were present and apical asynergy was identified by echocardiography, the ECG correctly localized the infarct at the apex in only 10% of patients.[51] The presence of Q waves nevertheless is associated with a larger and more severe degree of apical dysfunction, and persistent ST-segment elevations may suggest the presence of a left ventricular aneurysm on the echocardiogram.

Echocardiography After Reperfusion Therapy

Multiple prospective randomized trials showed that the restoration of antegrade flow after pharmacologic or mechanical reperfusion is usually associated with improved wall motion, fewer complications, and decreased mortality. The extent of systolic function recovery is related to the duration of the occlusion (a prompt treatment begun in the first 2 hours after the onset of the chest pain gives the best results), the extent of the ischemic zone, and the success of reperfusion.[2] The time to achieve complete functional recovery after reperfusion varies from patient to patient and from segment to segment in the same patient. Studies with sequential echocardiograms suggest, however, that recovery usually occurs 24 hours to 10 days after reperfusion but may take 3 to 4 weeks if stunning is present.[54] The value of contrast echocardiography to determine microvascular integrity and myocardial reperfusion is discussed in another section.

The role of echocardiography in the assessment of left ventricular remodeling goes beyond the short-term evaluation during the course of ACS. In successfully reperfused patients, left ventricular dimensions remain stable and tend to regress 3 months after acute MI, whereas left ventricular dimensions continue to increase in patients without successful reperfusion.[55] Late reperfusion with thrombolytic therapy may prevent acute and chronic infarct expansion regardless of myocardial salvage.[56,57] Patency of the infarct-related coronary artery (either by spontaneous reperfusion or by angioplasty), occurring within days of the acute MI, also has been associated with an improvement in regional function and an attenuation of left ventricular dilation 1 to 6 months after the initial event.[58,59]

Complications of Myocardial Infarction

Echocardiography is a sensitive, rapid, and useful tool for the diagnosis of complications after MI. In the few cases in which the transthoracic approach does not allow adequate assessment, transesophageal echocardiography (TEE) can lead to the correct diagnosis or to a more precise evaluation of the complication.

Left Ventricular Aneurysm

Most left ventricular aneurysms are complications of MI, and they are classified as true or false aneurysms.

True Aneurysm. This is the most common type of ventricular aneurysm, which occurred in approximately one fifth of all cases of transmural MI before the routine use of reperfusion therapy. In 1986, in a prospective echocardiographic study, Visser and coworkers[60] reported that a left ventricular aneurysm was found in 22% of patients with nonreperfused transmural MI—32% and 9% in anterior and posterior infarcts. The aneurysm results from expansion of the infarct area and thinning of the myocardium and contains all three layers of the ventricular wall. Echocardiographically the aneurysmal segments are dyskinetic or akinetic, and the distortion of the left ventricular shape (with a wide neck) persists in diastole. Almost 90% of true left ventricular aneurysms involve the apex, but extension to the anterior wall is common. The remaining cases generally involve the inferobasal region. Detection of an aneurysm within the first 5 days of hospitalization has been associated with high mortality rates at 3 months and 1 year after MI, probably reflecting the larger infarct size and the more depressed global systolic function.[60,61] It is also a site of predilection for thrombus formation.

False or Pseudoaneurysm. This rare and potentially life-threatening entity results from a rupture into the myocardium, the extravasated blood being contained by the parietal pericardium. Pathologically a small channel connects the left ventricle with a large blood and thrombus–filled cavity lined by fibrous pericardial tissue, and a tear in the myocardium can be identified. Echocardiographically an echo-free area outside the left ventricular cavity is seen connected to it by a narrow neck, with an abrupt interruption in the ventricular wall. Bulging also can be observed in the false aneurysm during each systole (Fig. 18-7).[62] Since a ventricular pseudoaneurysm is a contained rupture, mortality is high, and urgent surgery is warranted as soon as the diagnosis is made with echocardiography.

Ventricular Septal Defect

Ventricular septal defect is an uncommon complication of MI (<1%), which is associated with high mortality rates of 54% in the first week and 87% within 2 months if left untreated.[63] Most ischemic ventricular septal defects are associated with extensive MI and multivessel CAD. Rupture of the interventricular septum is more common with anterior than inferior infarcts. The perforation may be a direct through-and-through hole or may be more irregular and serpiginous with a variable defect size but usually less than 4 cm in diameter. The time from

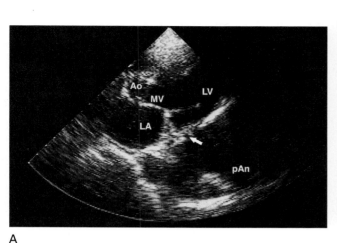

A

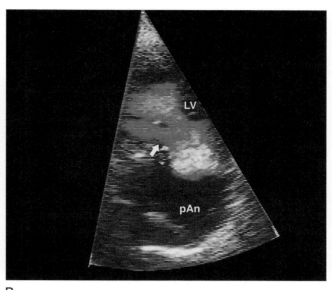

B

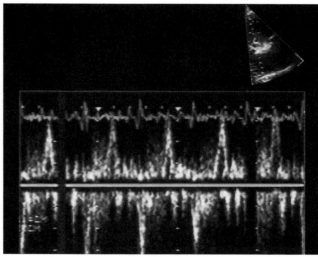

C

FIGURE 18–7. *A,* Parasternal long-axis view (with the apex of the left ventricle [LV] on the right side) shows abrupt discontinuity of the basal inferolateral wall *(arrow)* resulting in a communication between the LV and a large cavity that appeared to be a pseudoaneurysm. The "aneurysmal" cavity was pulsatile during real-time imaging. *B,* By color Doppler, flow is seen from the LV toward the pseudoaneurysmal cavity *(arrow). C,* Pulsed-wave Doppler showed to-and-fro velocities. Ao, aorta; LA, left atrium; MV, mitral valve; pAn, pseudoaneurysm. (*B* and *C,* see color plates.)

the onset of pain until septal perforation can vary from a few hours to 9 days after MI but is on average 3 to 4 days. Echocardiography often detects directly the septal defect as an interruption in the myocardium in an akinetic region, often at the junction with normal or hyperkinetic tissue (Fig. 18–8). Kishon and colleagues[64] reported that two-dimensional echocardiography identified 68% of ventricular septal defects after MI, but the sensitivity was increased to 95% when two-dimensional imaging was combined with Doppler evaluation.

As a complication of anterior infarction, the septal defect usually is located distally near the apex, in association with anterior akinesis. Careful two-dimensional and color Doppler scanning of the ventricular septum is required during the echocardiographic examination, particularly in the apical four-chamber and five-chamber views. When a ventricular septal defect occurs with an inferior infarction, the apex generally is spared, and the

defect is in the basal septum, generally associated with an extensive area of inferior wall dyskinesis. Commonly the ventricular septal defect in the basal inferior septum is identified using an off-axis position, with an intermediate rotation between the apical four-chamber and two-chamber views. Pulsed, continuous-wave and color Doppler confirm the left-to-right shunt across the septal defect. The defect size determined by color Doppler echocardiography has been shown to correlate closely with that determined at surgery or autopsy and with the pulmonic-to-systemic flow ratio measured at cardiac catheterization.[65]

Papillary Muscle Rupture

Papillary muscle rupture is a rare but dramatic complication of an acute transmural MI. Because of its more limited blood supply, the posteromedial papillary muscle is

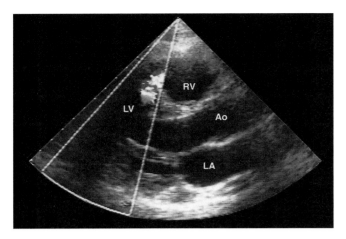

FIGURE 18–8. Three days after an acute anterior myocardial infarction, clinical deterioration and a new systolic murmur were observed in this patient. Parasternal long-axis view with color Doppler showed a shunt from the left to the right ventricle, consistent with a ventricular septal defect. Ao, aorta; LA, left atrium; LV, left ventricle; RV, right ventricle. (See color plates.)

more frequently involved. For that reason, papillary muscle rupture occurs more commonly in the setting of an inferior wall MI. Clinically, partial rupture of a papillary muscle head is seen more frequently, as complete rupture generally is rapidly fatal. Two-dimensional echocardiography can show accurately the structural abnormality of the mitral apparatus, which usually includes a flail leaflet or prolapse and partial or complete rupture of one of the papillary muscle heads, and excludes the presence of a ventricular septal defect (Fig. 18-9).[66] Because chordae tendinae originating from the posteromedial papillary muscle are connected to both mitral leaflets, it is important to realize that a flail anterior leaflet can complicate an acute inferior wall infarct. The left ventricle is often hyperdynamic in the presence of papillary muscle rupture, and this frequently

renders difficult the identification of a regional wall motion abnormality in the inferior wall. The addition of color flow Doppler permits the identification of mitral regurgitation and assessment of its severity in nearly all patients, with excellent correlation with angiography.[67] In the presence of an eccentric jet or a noncompliant left atrium (as commonly encountered in this setting), color Doppler occasionally may underestimate the severity of mitral regurgitation, however, and a thorough echocardiographic assessment is required, using TEE when needed (see Fig. 18-9).

Ventricular Free Wall Rupture

Rupture of the left ventricular free wall is usually a sudden event, which accounts for 10% to 15% of all in-hospital deaths after acute MI, generally in older hypertensive patients with Q wave infarcts. Impending cardiac rupture may be suspected in the setting of post-MI pericarditis, repetitive emesis, restlessness, and agitation or if there is a deviation from the expected pattern of T wave evolution on ECG.[68] Echocardiographic recognition of free wall rupture, although unusual because of rapid hemodynamic deterioration, occasionally has been shown, allowing rapid intervention.[68]

Left Ventricular Thrombus

A relatively frequent complication of acute MI before the era of thrombolytic therapy, left ventricular thrombi are found more often after anterior wall and large infarcts,[69] as is the case of ventricular aneurysms. Echocardiographically a left ventricular thrombus appears as a focal mass on the endocardial contour of an akinetic or dyskinetic segment. It may be fixed, may be pedunculated and freely mobile, or may have a fixed base with mobile filaments extending from its surface (Fig. 18-10). A newly formed ventricular thrombus is often only mildly echogenic, but its appearance may be speckled or

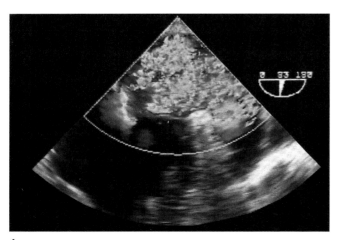

A

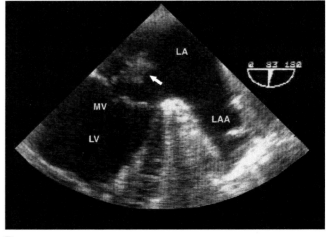

B

FIGURE 18–9. *A,* Transesophageal echocardiography in a two-chamber view (83 degrees) shows severe mitral regurgitation after acute myocardial infarction, secondary to a ruptured papillary muscle. *B,* The papillary muscle prolapsed freely into the left atrium (LA) during systole *(arrow).* This patient required emergency mitral valve (MV) repair. LAA, left atrial appendage; LV, left ventricle. *(A,* see color plates.)

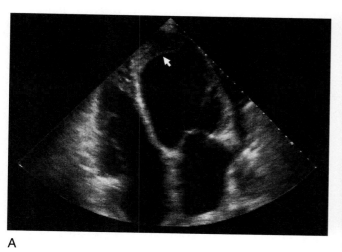

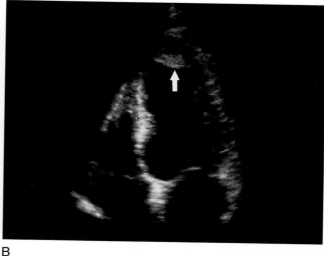

A

B

FIGURE 18–10. *A* and *B,* Left ventricular thrombi in the apical four-chamber view from two different patients. An organized and nonmobile thrombus *(arrow in A)* and a mobile thrombus *(arrow in B)* in a region of akinesia and apical aneurysm. The latter patient suffered a stroke within hours of this echocardiographic examination.

contain areas brighter than the surrounding myocardium. The echogenicity can increase, however, and calcification may be found when the thrombus is organized. Because most left ventricular thrombi are in the apical region, standard and off-axis apical views (with optimized imaging of the region of interest) often are required to confirm their presence and to distinguish them from a near-field artifact or a fibrous band. Before thrombolysis and routine anticoagulation of the high-risk patients, thrombi generally became echocardiographically detectable 5 to 10 days after MI. Echocardiographic detection of a left ventricular thrombus within 48 to 72 hours after MI has been reported to be associated with a poor prognosis probably because it indicates extensive regional dysfunction.[70] Several prospective studies reported that thrombi that are mobile, protrude into the ventricular cavity, or are adjacent to zones of hyperkinetic wall motion are more likely to result in an embolic event.[70,71] The natural course of left ventricular thrombi is variable—in several series, little change took place in the first few months after MI, although regression and ultimate disappearance is also possible.[71]

Right Ventricular Infarction

The clinical diagnosis of a right ventricular infarction requires a high level of suspicion because the sensitivity and specificity of clinical and ECG signs are imperfect.[72] Diagnosis of right-sided involvement in the setting of an acute inferior infarct can change significantly the clinical management of these patients, since "intractable cardiogenic shock" may become easily reversible with volume repletion. Transthoracic echocardiography is an excellent modality to identify right ventricular infarction. Findings include right ventricular regional hypokinesis or akinesis or global dysfunction, usually with left ventricular inferior wall involvement. Because infarction of

the right ventricle sometimes may be revealed only by dysfunction of its inferior wall, attention should be paid to this region in optimized parasternal short-axis views. Right ventricular dilation, interventricular diastolic septal flattening, tricuspid regurgitation, reduced systolic excursion of the tricuspid annulus, and dilation of the inferior vena cavae also can be found and point toward the correct diagnosis.

Prognosis After Myocardial Infarction

The prognosis after MI is determined in part by the severity of systolic dysfunction (infarct size) and the presence and extent of ischemic myocardium.[73] Large MIs (infarct areas covering >35% of the left ventricular perimeter) carry a bad prognosis with a mortality exceeding 50%, whereas smaller infarcts are associated with a better prognosis.[74] The WMSI and the left ventricular ejection fraction are powerful predictors of prognosis after MI and permit risk stratification. In multivariate analysis, the WMSI has been found to be a stronger predictor than most clinical and hemodynamic parameters.[4-6,75,76] A high WMSI value identifies patients at risk for in-hospital mortality, heart failure, malignant arrhythmias, and cardiogenic shock.[33] Sabia and colleagues[33] reported that all patients with in-hospital complications (cardiogenic shock, life-threatening arrhythmias, and recurrent angina) had regional segmental wall motion abnormalities on their initial echocardiogram. In contrast, a low WMSI can prospectively identify patients at low risk after MI. The WMSI has important therapeutic implications because early interventions are recommended in high-risk patients, and medical treatment and early hospital discharge are considered in low-risk patients.[77] A resting transthoracic echocardiogram also has been shown to be a better tool than the ECG to distinguish infarct extension from recurrent ischemia and to quantify the amount of myocardium at risk.[73,78] During MI, the nonaffected segments are usually hyperdynamic as a compensatory mechanism. The absence of such compensatory hyperkinesis suggests multivessel coronary disease[32,33,79] and is associated with an increased incidence of death, cardiogenic shock, progression to a worse Killip class, and reinfarction.[80] The echocardiographic assessment of left ventricular systolic function also predicts long-term prognosis after the infarct.[81] In a study of 512 post-MI patients who were followed with echocardiograms at 11 days and 1 year, the left ventricular end-systolic area and systolic function were strong predictors of death and cardiac events, and prevention of ventricular enlargement with an angiotensin-converting enzyme inhibitor improved clinical outcome with a relative risk reduction of 35%.[81] The prognostic role of stress echocardiography is discussed subsequently.

ECHOCARDIOGRAPHY AND MYOCARDIAL ISCHEMIA

Diagnosis of Acute Coronary Syndromes Using Resting Echocardiography

Transthoracic echocardiography performed during ongoing chest pain, early in the diagnostic pathway, is useful in the evaluation of patients with a moderately high probability of ACS, a nondiagnostic ECG, and a normal cardiac enzyme profile. When two-dimensional echocardiography is performed during an episode of chest pain, segmental wall motion abnormalities may be detected in 90% to 95% of cases of transmural infarction and in 80% to 90% of subendocardial infarctions, with a specificity between 80% and 90%.[2] The incidence of regional wall motion abnormalities decreases to 47%, however, when echocardiography is performed later in the diagnostic pathway.[34] The detection of a segmental wall motion abnormality suggests an acute ischemic event, but in patients with preexisting CAD, it may be difficult to differentiate the acute event from an old infarct. Nevertheless, the absence of segmental wall motion abnormalities early in the diagnostic work-up carries a high negative predictive value.[77] In patients with unstable angina and no prior MI, the presence of regional wall motion abnormalities predicted significant CAD with a sensitivity of 88%, a specificity of 78%, and a positive predictive value of 85%.[32]

Exercise Stress Echocardiography

Exercise stress echocardiography is a well-established technique to detect the presence and severity of CAD, which may be particularly useful in patients with an inconclusive standard stress test. Its accuracy has been shown to be superior to that of exercise ECG.[82] Stress echocardiography is not recommended in the acute phase of a suspected coronary event. In patients without ongoing symptoms or with atypical chest pain, with normal serial cardiac enzymes and ECGs, and a normal resting echocardiogram, exercise echocardiography can be performed within 24 hours. In a study of 95 patients without prior MI, the sensitivity of exercise echocardiography and exercise ECG was 80% and 42% ($P < .001$) and the specificity was 87% and 74% to identify CAD.[83] Armstrong and colleagues[84] reported in a similar patient population a sensitivity of 80% for detecting CAD with exercise echocardiography compared with only 43% with exercise ECG. After MI, stress echocardiography is performed to document the presence, extent, and severity of wall motion abnormalities in an effort to identify a subset of patients at high risk for recurrent ischemia, MI, and death.[85-87] When compared with the exercise test alone, exercise echocardiography increased the sensitivity from 55% to 80% and the specificity from 65% to 95% for identifying patients at risk of new ischemic events shortly after infarction was documented.[86] A study after uncomplicated MI showed a fivefold increase in risk in patients with positive stress echocardiography despite a high-threshold positive exercise ECG.[88]

Exercise echocardiography also can be used to assess the long-term prognosis after MI. In one study, evidence of new or worsened wall motion abnormality on stress echocardiography was associated with a relative risk of 5.1 for cardiac events or revascularization at 44 ± 11 months.[89] Krivokapich and associates[90] found that an inducible wall motion abnormality on exercise echocardiography predicted cardiac events (MI, revascularization, or death) over the next 12 months with a specificity of 86%.[90] Most patients (80% to 95%) without major events over a long-term follow-up period did not present new regional abnormalities during the initial stress echocardiography.[88,89,91] A normal exercise echocardiogram is associated with a low (4%) rate of cardiac events and an excellent prognosis over the next 28 months despite an abnormal exercise ECG.[86] In patients with prior MI, development of stress-induced regional wall motion abnormalities remote from the area of infarction has been shown to be predictive of multivessel CAD with a sensitivity of 77% and specificity of 95%, identifying a population with a worse prognosis.[85] A meta-analysis by Fleischmann and coworkers[92] that compared exercise echocardiography with exercise single-photon emission computed tomography (SPECT) imaging in the diagnosis of CAD showed that echocardiography had a sensitivity similar to that of exercise SPECT imaging (85% versus 87%) but a higher specificity (77% versus 65%).[92] The long-term prognostic value (3.7 years) of exercise echocardiography and nuclear perfusion imaging also has been compared and shown to be similar.[93]

Pharmacologic Stress Echocardiography

In patients who cannot perform exercise, a pharmacologic approach can be used to perform a stress echocardiogram.

Dobutamine Stress Echocardiography

Dobutamine has a positive inotropic effect at low doses (5 to 10 µg/kg/min), with additional inotropic and chronotropic effects at higher doses. The increase in systolic blood pressure during the infusion can be more pronounced in hypertensive patients when compared with normotensive patients. A paradoxic hypotension occasionally can be observed and is due to either the vasodilating effect of dobutamine or transient outflow tract obstruction but is rarely caused by ischemia.[94] β-Blockers may attenuate the physiologic response to dobutamine by competing at the receptor level, and it is recommended to withhold them 24 hours before the examination, when clinically possible.

There are two possible indications for dobutamine stress echocardiography after ACS. The first indication is demonstration of myocardial viability in a hypokinetic or akinetic region, which suggests that regional systolic function would improve either after revascularization in the case of hibernating myocardium[95] or spontaneously after recovery from stunning.[47,96] A biphasic response to increasing dobutamine doses characterized by enhanced thickening at low doses (5 to 10 µg/kg/min) indicating viability and deterioration of thickening at higher doses (>10 µg/kg/min) indicating ischemia is the most accurate echocardiographic criterion to detect viable but hypoperfused myocardium (Fig. 18–11).[97] The sensitivity of low-dose dobutamine stress echocardiography is 88% and the specificity is 87% to identify hibernating myocardium.[98] Arnese and colleagues[99] found that the

specificity of low-dose dobutamine was 95% compared with only 48% for 201-thallium SPECT for predicting the recovery of function after revascularization. The greater the number of viable myocardial segments, the greater is the probability of improvement in regional and global left ventricular function after revascularization. The value of low-dose dobutamine stress echocardiography has been compared with that of positron emission tomography and nuclear perfusion imaging for the assessment of myocardial viability.[97,98,100] Cumulative data from multiple studies suggest that thallium SPECT images provide better sensitivity compared with dobutamine echocardiography for this indication (89% versus 81%), but low-dose dobutamine stress echocardiography has a higher specificity (83% versus 69%).[102] In comparison, positron emission tomography scanning has a positive predictive value of 82% and a negative predictive value of 83% for predicting recovery after revascularization, with an excellent agreement with dobutamine stress echocardiography.[100]

The second indication for dobutamine stress echocardiography in ACS is for the assessment of the presence, severity, and extent of residual ischemia.[101-105] Greco and coworkers[106] showed that an abnormal predischarge dobutamine stress echocardiogram performed

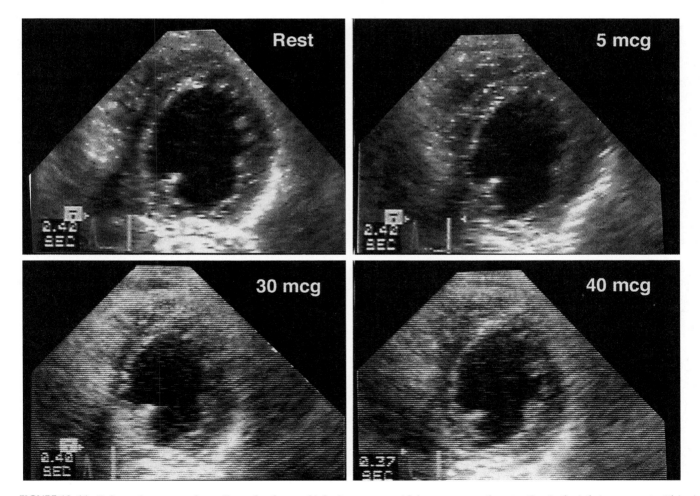

FIGURE 18–11. Dobutamine stress echocardiography shows a biphasic response with improvement of contraction in the inferior segment with a low dose of dobutamine (5 µg/kg/min) and dyskinesis of the same segment at higher doses (30 to 40 µg/kg/min), showing viability and ischemia.

after uncomplicated MI was found to be an independent predictor of outcome in multivariate analysis when other clinical and exercise variables were included and was associated with a relative risk of 5.5 for cardiac death and MI at a mean follow-up of 17 ± 13 months. For this indication, the dobutamine infusion can be increased to 40 µg/kg/min. The overall sensitivity has ranged from 76% to 89% and the specificity from 70% to 95% for the detection of significant stenoses (≥50% narrowing of the arterial diameter) shown at coronary angiography.[79] These values are greater for the detection of multivessel or left main coronary disease. Multivessel disease detected by dobutamine stress echocardiography is a better predictor of an adverse clinical outcome than when it is identified by angiography,[107] a phenomenon that has been shown previously with thallium-201 perfusion imaging.[108]

Dipyridamole Stress Echocardiography

Dipyridamole increases local adenosine levels by inhibiting reuptake into the endothelial cells. The mechanism of action of dipyridamole as an agent to detect ischemia is believed to be a *coronary steal*, in which normal arteries respond by a maximal dilation, whereas arteries with significant stenosis have a reduced response, resulting in flow heterogeneity.[109] The systemic vasodilation induced by dipyridamole and the compensatory increase in heart rate also may lead to a modest increase in myocardial oxygen demand. In post-MI patients, the sensitivity of dipyridamole stress echocardiography is 68% and the specificity 100% for the detection of remote ischemia compared with angiography.[110,111] In one study, dipyridamole stress echocardiography had a higher sensitivity and specificity than exercise stress echocardiography.[110] In another study of 925 patients evaluated with dipyridamole echocardiography in the post-MI setting, the presence of ischemia and its time of onset were important predictors of death and other cardiac events.[109] The use of a higher dose of dipyridamole (0.84 mg/kg) has been reported to increase the sensitivity of the test (74% to 83%) without lowering its specificity[110,112] but was associated with a higher incidence of side effects (nausea, headache, flushing, dyspnea). Finally, small studies with adenosine stress echocardiography have shown an overall sensitivity of 74% for detecting multivessel disease and only 39% for detecting one-vessel disease compared with dobutamine stress echocardiography.[113]

Comparison of Stress Echocardiography Techniques

There is a comparable level of accuracy for identifying CAD with stress echocardiography and with nuclear imaging techniques.[92,101] Echocardiography may be less sensitive to mild degrees of ischemia but is more specific.[92,114] Dobutamine stress echocardiography was more sensitive than high-dose dipyridamole ultrasound imaging in detecting single-vessel CAD in one study, but both methods had the same sensitivity for multivessel

CAD.[115] Although pharmacologic stress echocardiography may seem to be a more elegant approach, treadmill exercise echocardiography provides important clinical information by combining assessment of energy expenditure with the imaging technique. In patients with suboptimal transthoracic images, dobutamine TEE has been performed and seems to be a reliable tool for ischemia detection and viability assessment.[116] The availability of side-by-side comparison of rest and stress images with the development of digitization has enhanced markedly the ability to recognize stress-induced regional wall motion abnormalities. The introduction of tissue harmonics, which provide much better image quality and endocardial definition, especially in patients who are technically difficult to evaluate, has improved further accuracy in identifying wall motion abnormalities.

TRANSESOPHAGEAL ECHOCARDIOGRAPHY AND ACUTE CORONARY SYNDROMES

TEE is a useful alternative when the transthoracic approach is technically difficult and provides suboptimal or nondiagnostic images, as may be the case in obese patients, patients with lung disease, or patients with recent cardiothoracic surgery. Assessment of regional and global ventricular function can be performed with TEE at rest or with stress, either dobutamine infusion or cardiac pacing. Detection and detailed evaluation of mechanical complications of an acute MI, such as a ruptured papillary muscle (see Fig. 18–9) or a ventricular septal defect, also is possible with TEE.[117] Mitral regurgitation secondary to ischemia or infarction is a frequent finding in patients with ACS, but it is occasionally difficult to determine precisely its severity or mechanism with transthoracic echocardiography.[118,119] TEE provides additional information, with important therapeutic implications, especially if mitral valve repair is being considered. TEE also can be useful in patients with ACS and atrial fibrillation (whether the cause or effect of the ischemia), particularly if the duration is unknown, and the ventricular response is difficult to control. Ruling out the presence of an intracardiac thrombus before cardioversion is a reliable and safe method in this setting. Occasionally a suspected embolus during the course of an acute ischemic syndrome may represent an indication for TEE. Finally, TEE also can help to rule out aortic dissection in patients with acute chest pain of uncertain origin (see Fig. 18–5).[120]

DIRECT VISUALIZATION OF CORONARY ARTERIES

Transthoracic echocardiography can visualize only a portion of the left main and proximal left anterior descending coronary arteries in approximately 60% to 70% of adult patients.[121,122] Improved visualization of the coronary arteries is possible with TEE. Yoshida and colleagues[123] reported a sensitivity of 91% and a specificity of 100% for the detection of significant proximal left main coronary narrowing (>50% diameter stenosis) with biplane TEE compared with angiography. Multiplane TEE allows enhanced visualization of extended lengths of the coronary arteries (Fig. 18-12). Tardif and colleagues[124] showed that the left main coronary artery with its bifurcation could be visualized in all patients with a sensitivity of 100% for detection of coronary narrowings compared with angiography. The proximal and mid segments of the left anterior descending coronary artery were visualized in 69% and 31%, the proximal and mid segments of the circumflex artery in 80% and 51%, and the corresponding segments of the right artery in 84% and 16%.

INTRAVASCULAR ULTRASOUND AND ACUTE CORONARY SYNDROMES

Intravascular ultrasound (IVUS) imaging uses miniaturized transducers at the tip of catheters to provide tomographic images of coronary arteries.[125,126] Coronary angiography, the traditional approach used to evaluate CAD, has well-known limitations. It provides a planar perspective of the coronary arterial lumen and not the wall, yet atherosclerosis is primarily a disease of the arterial wall. The stenosis severity may be underestimated with angiography because the reference segment with which the stenosis is compared may be involved in the diffuse atherosclerotic process (Fig. 18-13).[127] In contrast, IVUS provides cross-sectional images of the arterial lumen and wall, allowing not only determination of lumen dimen-

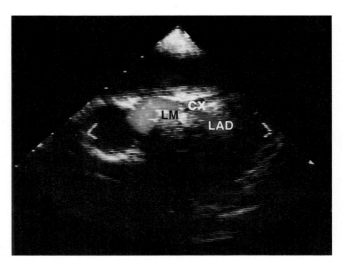

FIGURE 18–12. Transesophageal echocardiography shows flow in the left main (LM) coronary artery and its bifurcation, the left anterior descending (LAD) artery, and circumflex (CX) artery. (See color plates.)

sions and architecture, but also assessment of the composition, morphology, and volume of plaques, which are major determinants of the clinical expression of coronary atherosclerosis. Study of patients with angiographically mildly diseased coronary arteries revealed that half of them had narrowings of 50% or more on IVUS (see Fig. 20-13).[128] IVUS examination has applications in the setting of ACS. One important indication is for the evaluation of suspected left main CAD when doubt persists after angiography.[129] Other ambiguous lesions on

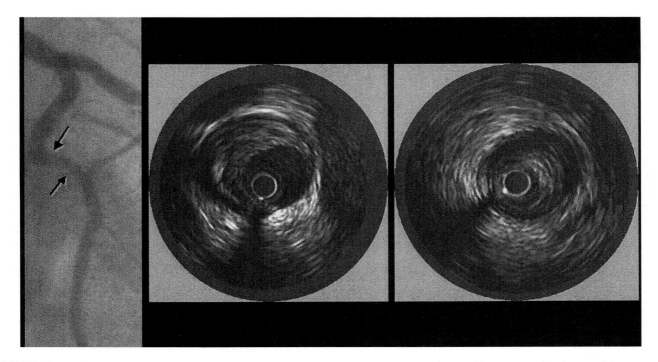

FIGURE 18–13. Angiographic *(left)* underestimation of the severity of coronary artery disease, revealed by intravascular ultrasound *(center and right panels)*. There is mild angiographic luminal narrowing *(distal arrow)* when the lesion is compared with a pseudonormal reference segment *(proximal arrow)*. On intravascular ultrasound, the *reference segment* shows significant plaque burden *(central panel)*, and the severity of the target lesion *(right panel)* is better appreciated.

angiography also can be clarified with IVUS, such as bifurcation lesions of unknown severity and problematic stenoses visualized only in a single angiographic projection. IVUS is useful in patients with recurrent chest pain after percutaneous coronary interventions to determine whether a significant narrowing is present or a technical problem occurred (persistent flow-limiting dissection, stent underdeployment, or stent undersizing) in the dilated vessel.

MYOCARDIAL CONTRAST ECHOCARDIOGRAPHY AND ACUTE CORONARY SYNDROMES

The use of ultrasound for the assessment of myocardial perfusion has generated a lot of interest and promise because echocardiography is readily available, does not result in exposure to radioactive agents, and has better spatial resolution than nuclear medicine approaches. Myocardial contrast echocardiography images the coronary microcirculation and provides insight into its integrity and functional status by using microbubbles as intravascular tracers. Advances such as triggered harmonic imaging have enabled the detection of myocardial perfusion after venous injection of transpulmonary contrast agents.[130] Other technical advances have included the development of second-generation microbubbles containing nondiffusible, high-molecular-weight gases with low solubility.[131]

In patients with suspected ACS, myocardial contrast echocardiography can assist in establishing the diagnosis, which is supported by the presence of a perfusion defect. The risk area also can be determined in this setting and is defined as the myocardial area related to an occluded coronary artery that would undergo necrosis if the occlusion were maintained. Because necrosis occurs at a flow rate less than 0.2 to 0.3 mL/g/min, and microbubbles are not detected in the myocardium under these flow conditions, the risk area during coronary occlusion usually is defined by myocardial contrast echocardiography as the region without enhancement. Good correlations were found between ultrasound-defined perfusion defects and the risk area on technetium autoradiography and myocardial scintigraphy.[132] After reperfusion, myocardial contrast echocardiography can help to determine the success of therapy (tissue reperfusion) and the extent of salvaged myocardium.[133]

Another possible application of myocardial contrast echocardiography during or immediately after ACS is in the evaluation of myocardial viability. Despite successful restoration of epicardial flow during angioplasty, 30% of patients lack myocardial perfusion at the cellular level.[134] These areas of low or no reflow develop because of microvascular disruption, plugging by debris, or myocardial edema. Because the extent of cellular and microvascular injury is directly related, patients with no reflow on myocardial contrast echocardiography have significantly less recovery of regional and global left ventricular function at 1-month follow-up compared with patients with adequate myocardial perfusion[135] and are more likely to have TIMI (Thrombolysis In Myocardial

Infarction) grade 2 epicardial flow. Even among patients with TIMI grade 3 flow, however, a significant functional improvement is observed only in the patients with reflow on contrast echocardiography.[136] It is possible to differentiate infarcted and viable areas with contrast echocardiography because the definitive perfusion defect denotes the extent of cellular damage, and areas with contrast enhancement indicate patients with microvascular integrity and viable myocardium. deFilippi and colleagues[137] compared myocardial contrast and dobutamine stress echocardiography to predict recovery of left ventricular function after revascularization in patients with ischemic heart disease. They showed that these approaches had similar values to predict recovery of hypokinetic segments but that dobutamine echocardiography is better to predict functional improvement of akinetic segments (positive predictive value, 85% versus 55%). Meza and associates[138] reported in a similar patient population a sensitivity of approximately 80% for both approaches and a low specificity (30%), but these values improved to 90% and 50% when both echocardiographic modalities were combined. Myocardial viability also can be determined with contrast echocardiography in patients without an open infarct-related artery because the viable myocardium perfused through collateral flow shows contrast enhancement (on injection in the relevant coronary artery). The demonstration of collateral perfusion is more accurate with myocardial contrast echocardiography than with coronary angiography because the latter can define vessels only greater than 100 μ, whereas most collateral channels are smaller. The correlation between the spatial extent of collateral perfusion within an infarct zone by contrast echocardiography and angiographic collaterals is poor.

It is possible to determine the physiologic significance of a coronary stenosis using an intravenous injection of contrast microbubbles during pharmacologic stress, based on a perfusion mismatch detected between the stenosed and normal bed. Myocardial contrast echocardiography has been found to have a good concordance with nuclear perfusion imaging for this indication in a few studies,[139] although other investigators reported lower diagnostic accuracy with current techniques.[140,141] Myocardial contrast echocardiography presently has several limitations. The main problems are related to inadequate myocardial opacification, contrast shadowing, blooming, and wall motion artifacts. Although great progress has been made in the field of myocardial contrast echocardiography, widespread clinical application of this technique awaits greater availability of newer contrast agents, confirmation of adequate concordance with nuclear perfusion imaging in multicenter studies, and demonstration of good reproducibility and low interobserver variability.

BRACHIAL ULTRASOUND AND ACUTE CORONARY SYNDROMES

The vascular endothelium modulates vessel tone by releasing various active substances, the most important being nitric oxide. Endothelial dysfunction, which results in reduced availability of nitric oxide, disturbs the protective regulatory balance and ultimately contributes to atherogenesis, CAD progression, and possibly acute coronary events.[142] The assessment of endothelial function can be done noninvasively using high-resolution ultrasound examination of the brachial artery or angiographically by directly assessing the coronary arteries. Anderson and colleagues showed that endothelial function measured at the brachial artery level correlates closely with that in coronary arteries.[143] During the brachial artery ultrasound examination, endothelial function is assessed by comparing the arterial diameter at baseline with that during hyperemia induced by the sudden increase in arterial flow on release of cuff-induced occlusion. Esper and coworkers[144] using this technique showed that patients with ACS have endothelial dysfunction that persists after patients are initially stabilized. Numerous studies showed that risk factors for CAD impair endothelial function and that their treatment is associated with an improvement in endothelial-dependent vasodilation. In the Reduction of Cholesterol in Ischemia and Function of the Endothelium (RECIFE) study, cholesterol-lowering therapy initiated early after admission in patients with ACS rapidly improved endothelial function with only 6 weeks of treatment.[145] In patients with ACS, the impairment in endothelial function also was shown to correlate with elevated C-reactive protein levels and to resolve with normalization of markers of systemic inflammation over time.[146]

CONCLUSIONS

Rest and stress echocardiography are useful in the emergency department for the diagnostic work-up of patients with chest pain. Echocardiography also provides important information on systolic and diastolic ventricular function in patients with ACS. Evaluation of residual ischemia and of myocardial viability after ACS can be done with stress echocardiography. IVUS can complement the angiographic evaluation in selected patients, such as patients with ambiguous lesions in the left main coronary artery, at bifurcations, or at other sites. Assessment of myocardial viability and perfusion with contrast echocardiography is another emerging approach that has the potential to expand further the use of cardiac ultrasound. Echocardiography should be an integral part of the diagnostic and prognostic evaluation of patients with ACS.

REFERENCES

1. Théroux P, Ross J, Franklin D, et al: Regional myocardial function in the conscious dog during acute coronary occlusion and responses to morphine, propranolol, nitroglycerin and lidocaine. Circulation 1976;53:302–314.
2. Zabalgoitia M, Ismaeil M: Diagnostic and prognostic use of stress echo in acute coronary syndromes including emergency department imaging. Echocardiography 2000;17:479–493.
3. Heger JJ, Weyman AC, Wann LS, et al: Cross sectional echocardiography in acute myocardial infarction: Detection and localizing of regional left ventricle asynergy. Circulation 1979;60:531–538.
4. Berning J, Steensgaard-Hansen F: Early estimation of risk by echocardiographic determination of wall motion index in an unselected population with acute myocardial infarction. Am J Cardiol 1990;65:567–576.
5. Kan G, Visser CA, Koolen JJ, et al: Short and long term predictive value of admission wall motion score in acute myocardial infarction: A cross echocardiographic study of 345 patients. Br Heart J 1986;56:422–427.
6. Galasko GIW, Basu S, Lahiri A, et al: A prospective comparison of echocardiographic wall motion score index and radionuclide ejection fraction in predicting outcome following acute myocardial infarction. Heart 2001;86:271–276.
7. Rich S, Sheikh A, Gallastegui J: Determination of left ventricular ejection function by visual estimation during real-time two-dimensional echocardiography. Am Heart J 1982;104:603–606.
8. Simonson JS, Schiller NB: Descent of the base of the left ventricle: An echocardiographic index of left ventricular function. J Am Soc Echocardiogr 1989;2:25–35.
9. Pai RG, Bodenheimer MM, Pai SM, et al: Usefulness of systolic excursion of the mitral anulus as an index of left ventricular systolic function. Am J Cardiol 1991;67:222–224.
10. Pandian NG, Kerber RE: Two dimensional echocardiography in experimental coronary stenosis: Sensitivity and specificity in detecting transient myocardial dyskinesis: Comparison with sonomicrometers. Circulation 1982;66:597–602.
11. Haendchen RV, Wyatt HL, Maurer G, et al: Quantitation of regional cardiac function by two dimensional echocardiography: Patterns of contraction in the normal left ventricle. Circulation 1983;67:1234–1245.
12. Ascah KJ, Gillam LD, Davidoff R, et al: Evolution of the temporal contraction sequence after acute experimental myocardial infarction. J Am Coll Cardiol 1989;13:730–736.
13. Gillam LD, Hogan RD, Foale RA, et al: A comparison of quantitative echocardiographic methods for delineating infarct-induced abnormal wall motion. Circulation 1984;70:113–122.
14. Sheehan FH, Bolson EL, Dodge HT, et al: Advantages and applications of the centerline method for characterizing regional ventricular function. Circulation 1986;74:293–305.
15. Folland ED, Parisi AF, Moynihan PF, et al: Assessment of left ventricular ejection fraction and volumes by real-time, two-dimensional echocardiography: A comparison of cineangiographic and radionuclide techniques. Circulation 1979;60:760–766.
16. American Society of Echocardiography Committee on Standards, Subcommittee on Quantitation of Two-dimensional Echocardiograms: Schiller NG, Shah PM, Crawford M, et al: Recommendations for quantitation of the left ventricle by two-dimensional echocardiography. J Am Soc Echocardiogr 1989;2:358–367.
17. Parisi AF, Moynihan PF, Feldman CL, et al: Approaches to determination of left ventricular volume and ejection fraction by real time two-dimensional echocardiography. Clin Cardiol 1979;2:257–263.
18. Labovitz AJ, Lewen MK, Kern M, et al: Evaluation of left ventricular systolic and diastolic dysfunction during transient myocardial ischemia produced by angioplasty. J Am Coll Cardiol 1987;10:748–755.
19. Tardif JC, Rouleau JL: Diastolic dysfunction. Can J Cardiol 1996;12:389–398.
20. Paulsen SH: Clinical aspects of left ventricular diastolic function assessed by Doppler echocardiography. Dan Med Bull 2001;48:199–210.
21. Waggoner AD, Bierig SM: Tissue Doppler imaging: A useful echocardiographic method for the cardiac sonographer to assess systolic and diastolic ventricular function. J Am Soc Echocardiogr 2001;14:1143–1152.
22. Vignon P, Mor-Avi V, Weinert L, et al: Quantitative evaluation of global and regional left ventricular diastolic function with color kinesis. Circulation 1998;97:1053–1061.
23. Kawano Y, Ohmori K, Wada Y, et al: A novel color M-mode Doppler echocardiographic index for left ventricular relaxation: Depth of the maximal velocity point of left ventricular inflow in early diastole. Heart Vessels 2000;15:205–213.
24. Masuyama T, Kodama K, Nakatani S, et al: Effects of changes in coronary stenosis on left ventricular diastolic filling assessed with pulsed Doppler echocardiography. J Am Coll Cardiol 1988;11:744–751.

25. Wind BE, Sneider AR, Buda AJ, et al: Pulsed Doppler assessment of left ventricular diastolic filling in coronary artery disease before and immediately after coronary angioplasty. Am J Cardiol 1987;59:1041-1046.

26. Mohler ER 3rd, Ryan T, Segar DS, et al: Clinical utility of troponin T levels and echocardiography in the emergency department. Am Heart J 1998;135:253-260.

27. Norell M, Lythall D, Coghlan G, et al: Limited value of the resting electrocardiogram in assessing patients with recent onset chest pain: Lessons from a chest pain clinic. Br Heart J 1992;67:53-56.

28. Roberts R, Fromm RE: Management of acute syndromes based on risk stratification by biochemical markers: An idea whose time has come. Circulation 1998;98:1831-1833.

29. McCarthy BD, Beshansky JR, D'Agostino RB, et al: Missed diagnosis of acute myocardial infarction in the emergency department: Results from a multicenter study. Ann Emerg Med 1993;22:579-582.

30. Stewart WJ, Douglas PS, Sagar K, et al: Echocardiography in emergency medicine: A policy by the American Society of Echocardiography and the American College of Cardiology. The task force on Echocardiography in Emergency Medicine of the American Society of Echocardiography and the Echocardiography and Technology and Practice Executive Committees of the American College of Cardiology. J Am Coll Cardiol 1999;33:586-588.

31. Sasaki H, Charuzi Y, Beeder C, et al: Utility of echocardiography for the early assessment of patients with nondiagnostic chest pain. Am Heart J 1986;112:494-497.

32. Peels CH, Visser CA, Kupper AJ, et al: Usefulness of two-dimensional echocardiography for immediate detection of myocardial ischemia in the emergency room. Am J Cardiol 1990;65:687-691.

33. Sabia P, Afrookteh A, Touchstone DA, et al: Value of regional wall motion abnormality in the emergency room diagnosis of acute myocardial infarction: A prospective study using two-dimensional echocardiography. Circulation 1991;84(3 suppl):185-192.

34. Gibler WB, Runyon JP, Levy RC, et al: A rapid diagnostic and treatment center for patients with chest pain in the emergency department. Ann Emerg Med 1995;25:1-8.

35. Kontos MC, Arrowood JA, Jesse RL, et al: Comparison between two-dimensional echocardiography and myocardial perfusion imaging in the emergency department in patients with possible myocardial ischemia. Am Heart J 1998;136:724-733.

36. Colon PJ 3rd, Guarisco JS, Murgo J, et al: Utility of stress echocardiography in the triage of patients with atypical chest pain from the emergency department. Am J Cardiol 1998;82:1282-1284.

37. Kontos MC, Arrowood JA, Paulsen WH, et al: Early echocardiography can predict cardiac events in emergency department patients with chest pain. Ann Emerg Med 1998;31:550-557.

38. Fleischmann KE, Goldman L, Robiolio PA, et al: Echocardiographic correlates of survival in patients with chest pain. J Am Coll Cardiol 1994;23:1390-1396.

39. Romano S, Dagianti A, Penco M, et al: Usefulness of echocardiography in the prognostic evaluation of non-Q wave myocardial infarction. Am J Cardiol 2000;86:43G-45G.

40. Siu SC, Weyman AE, Picard MH: Echo-Doppler in the management of acute non-Q wave myocardial infarction. Am J Card Imaging 1992;6:119-126.

41. Weiss JL, Bulckley BH, Hutchins GM, et al: Two dimensional echocardiographic recognition of myocardial injury in man: Comparison with postmortem studies. Circulation 1981;63:401-408.

42. Lieberman AN, Weiss JL, Jugdutt BI, et al: Two dimensional echocardiography and infarct size: Relationship of regional wall motion and thickening to the extent of myocardial infarction in the dog. Circulation 1981;63:739-746.

43. Pandian NG, Skorton DJ, Collins SM, et al: Myocardial infarct size threshold for 2-dimensional echocardiographic detection: Sensitivity of systolic wall thickening and endocardial motion abnormalities in small versus large infarcts. Am J Cardiol 1985;55:551-555.

44. Pandian NG, Kieso RA, Kerber RE: Two dimensional echocardiography in experimental coronary artery stenosis: Relationship between systolic wall thinning and regional myocardial perfusion in severe coronary stenosis. Circulation 1982;66:603-611.

45. Pandian NG, Koyanagi S, Skorton DJ, et al: Relationships between two dimensional echocardiographic wall thickening abnormalities and myocardial infarct size and coronary risk area in normal and hypertrophied myocardium in dogs. Am J Cardiol 1983;52:1318-1325.

46. Kloner RA, Jennings RB: Consequences of brief ischemia: Stunning, preconditioning, and their clinical implications. Circulation 2001;104:2981-2989.

47. Smart SC, Sewada S, Ryan T, et al: Low dose dobutamine echocardiography detects reversible dysfunction after thrombolytic therapy of acute myocardial infarction. Circulation 1993;88:405-415.

48. Heger JJ, Weyman AE, Wann S, et al: Cross-sectional echocardiographic analysis of the extent of left ventricular asynergy in acute myocardial infarction. Circulation 1980;61:1113-1118.

49. Porter A, Strasberg B, Vaturi M, et al: Correlation between electrocardiographic subtypes of anterior myocardial infarction and regional abnormalities of wall motion. Coron Artery Dis 2000;11:489-493.

50. Young E, Cohn PF, Gorlin R, et al: Vectorcardiographic diagnosis and electrocardiographic correlation in left ventricular asynergy due to coronary artery disease: Severe asynergy of the anterior and apical segments. Circulation 1975;51:467-476.

51. Giannuzzi P, Imparato A, Temporelli PL, et al: Inaccuracy of various proposed electrocardiographic criteria in the diagnosis of apical infarction—a critical review. Eur Heart J 1989;10:880-888.

52. Hickman HO, Weyman AE, Wann LS, et al: Cross sectional echocardiography of the cardiac apex. Circulation 1977;56(suppl 3):589.

53. Errichetti A, Homma S, Guyer DE, et al: Limitations of the 12-lead electrocardiogram in predicting segmental apical dysfunction: comparison with apical dysfunction by 2-D echocardiography. Circulation 1987;76:IV-226.

54. Otto CM, Stratton JR, Maynard C, et al: Echocardiographic evaluation of segmental wall motion early and late after thrombolytic therapy in acute myocardial infarction. The Western Washington Tissue Plasminogen Activator Emergency Room Trial. Am J Cardiol 1990;65:132-138.

55. Picard MH, Wilkins GT, Ray PA, et al: Progressive changes in ventricular structure and function during the year after acute myocardial infarction. Am Heart J 1992;124:24-31.

56. Hochman JS, Choo H: Limitation of myocardial infarct expansion by reperfusion independent of myocardial salvage. Circulation 1987;75:299-306.

57. Force T, Kemper A, Leavitt M, et al: Acute reduction in functional infarct expansion with late coronary reperfusion: Assessment with quantitative two-dimensional echocardiography. J Am Coll Cardiol 1988;11:192-200.

58. Jeremy RW, Hackworthy RA, Bautovich G, et al: Infarct artery perfusion and changes in left ventricular volume in the month after acute myocardial infarction. J Am Coll Cardiol 1987;9:989-995.

59. Siu SC, Nidorf SM, Galambos GS, et al: The effect of late patency of the infarct-related coronary artery on left ventricular morphology and regional function after thrombolysis. Am Heart J 1992;124:265-272.

60. Visser CA, Kan G, Meltzer RS, et al: Incidence, timing, and prognostic value of left ventricular aneurysm formation after myocardial infarction: A prospective, serial echocardiographic study of 158 patients. Am J Cardiol 1986;57:729-732.

61. Meizlish JL, Berger HJ, Plankey M, et al: Functional left ventricular aneurysm formation after acute anterior transmural myocardial infarction: Incidence, natural history, and prognostic complications. N Engl J Med 1984;311:1001-1006.

62. Catherwood E, Mintz GS, Kottler MN, et al: Two dimensional echocardiographic recognition of left ventricular pseudoaneurysm. Circulation 1980;62:294-303.

63. Ammash NM, Warnes CA: Ventricular septal defects in adults. Ann Intern Med 2001;135:812-824.

64. Kishon Y, Iqbal A, Oh JK, et al: Evolution of echocardiographic modalities in detection of post-myocardial infarction ventricular septal defect and papillary muscle rupture. Am Heart J 1993;126:667-675.

65. Helmke F, Mahan EF, Nanda NC, et al: Two-dimensional echocardiography and Doppler color flow mapping in the diagnosis and prognosis of ventricular septal rupture. Circulation 1990;81:1775-1783.

66. Bansal RC, Eng AK, Shakudo M: Role of two-dimensional echocardiography, pulsed, continuous wave and color flow Doppler techniques in the assessment of ventricular septal rupture after myocardial infarction. Am J Cardiol 1990;65:852-860.

67. Smyllie JH, Sutherland GR, Geuskens R, et al: Doppler color flow mapping in the diagnosis of ventricular septal rupture after myocardial infarction. J Am Coll Cardiol 1990;15:1449-1455.

68. Olliva PB, Hammill SC, Edwards WD: Cardiac rupture, a clinical predictable complication of acute myocardial infarction. J Am Coll Cardiol 1993;22:720-726.

69. Asinger RW, Mikell FL, Elsperger J, et al: Incidence of left ventricular thrombosis after acute transmural myocardial infarction. N Engl J Med 1981;305:297-302.

70. Spirito P, Belloti P, Chiarella F, et al: Prognostic significance and natural history of left ventricular thrombi in patients with acute anterior myocardial infarction: A two-dimensional echocardiographic study. Circulation 1985;72:774-780.

71. Neskovic AN, Marinkovic J, Bojic M, et al: Predictors of left ventricular thrombus formation and disappearance after anterior wall myocardial infarction. Eur Heart J 1998;19:908-916.

72. Kinch JW, Ryan TJ: Right ventricular infarction. N Engl J Med 1994;330:1211-1217.

73. Domingo E, Alvarez A, Garcia del Castillo H, et al: Prognostic value of segmental contractility assessed by cross sectional echocardiography in first acute myocardial infarction. Eur Heart J 1989;10:532-537.

74. Picard MH, Wilkins GT, Ray PA, et al: Natural history of left ventricular size and function after acute myocardial infarction: Assessment and prediction by echocardiographic endocardial surface mapping. Circulation 1990;82:484-494.

75. Nishimura RA, Tajik AJ, Shub C, et al: Role of two dimensional echocardiography in the prediction of in hospital complications after acute myocardial infarction. J Am Coll Cardiol 1984;4:1080-1087.

76. Bourdillon PD, Broderick TM, Sawada SG, et al: Regional wall motion index for infarct and noninfarct regions after reperfusion in acute myocardial infarction: Comparison with global wall motion index. J Am Soc Echocardiogr 1989;2:398-407.

77. Launbjerg J, Berning J, Fruergaard P, et al: Sensitivity and specificity of echocardiographic identification of patients eligible for safe early discharge after acute myocardial infarction. Am Heart J 1992;124:846-853.

78. Isaacsohn JL, Earle MG, Kemper AJ, et al: Postmyocardial infarction pain and infarct extension in the coronary care unit: Role of two dimensional echocardiography. J Am Coll Cardiol 1988;11:246-251.

79. Shen WK, Khandheria BK, Edwards WD, et al: Value and limitations of two-dimensional echocardiography in predicting myocardial infarct size. Am J Cardiol 1991;68:1143-1149.

80. Gibson RS, Bishop HL, Stamm RB, et al: Value of early two dimensional echocardiography in patients with acute myocardial infarction. Am J Cardiol 1982;49:1110-1119.

81. St. John Sutton M, Pfeffer MA, Plappert T, et al: Quantitative two dimensional echocardiographic measurements are major predictors of adverse cardiovascular events after acute myocardial infarction. Circulation 1994;89:68-75.

82. Ryan T, Vasey CG, Presity CF, et al: Exercise echocardiography: Detection of coronary artery disease in patients with normal left ventricular wall motion at rest. J Am Coll Cardiol 1988;11:993-999.

83. Marwick TH, Nemec JJ, Pashkow FJ, et al: Accuracy and limitations of exercise echocardiography in a routine clinical setting. J Am Coll Cardiol 1992;19:74-81.

84. Armstrong WF, O'Donnell J, Dillon JC, et al: Complementary value of two-dimensional exercise echocardiography to routine treadmill testing. Ann Intern Med 1986;105:829-835.

85. Jaarsma W, Visser CA, Kupper AJ, et al: Usefulness of two dimensional exercise echocardiography shortly after myocardial infarction. Am J Cardiol 1986;57:86-90.

86. Ryan T, Armstrong WF, O'Donnell JA, et al: Risk stratification after acute myocardial infarction by means of exercise two dimensional echocardiography. Am Heart J 1987;114:1305-1316.

87. Applegate RJ, Dell'Italia LJ, Crawford MH, et al: Usefulness of two-dimensional echocardiography during low-level exercise testing early after uncomplicated acute myocardial infarction. Am J Cardiol 1987;60:10-14.

88. Bigi R, Desideri A, Galati A, et al: Incremental prognostic value of stress echocardiography as an adjunct to exercise electrocardiography after uncomplicated myocardial infarction. Heart 2001;85:417-423.

89. Marwick TH, Mehta R, Arheart K, et al: Use of exercise echocardiography for prognostic evaluation of patients with known or suspected coronary artery disease. J Am Coll Cardiol 1997;30:83-90.

90. Krivokapich J, Child JS, Gerber RS, et al: Prognostic usefulness of positive or negative exercise stress echocardiography for predicting coronary events in ensuing twelve months. Am J Cardiol 1993;71:646-651.

91. Heupler S, Mehta R, Lobo A, et al: Prognostic implications of exercise echocardiography in women with known or suspected coronary artery disease. J Am Coll Cardiol 1997;30:414-420.

92. Fleischmann KE, Hunink MGM, Kuntz KM, et al: Exercise echocardiography or exercise SPECT imaging? A meta-analysis of diagnostic test performance. JAMA 1998;280:913-920.

93. Olmos LI, Dakik J, Gordon R, et al: Long-term prognostic value of exercise echocardiography compared with exercise ^{201}Tl, ECG, and clinical variables in patients evaluated for coronary artery disease. Circulation 1998;98:2679-2686.

94. Marcovitz PA, Bach DS, Mathias W, et al: Paradoxical hypotension during dobutamine stress echocardiography: Clinical and diagnostic implications. J Am Coll Cardiol 1993;21:1080-108693.

95. Cigarroa CG, deFilippi CR, Brickner E, et al: Dobutamine stress echocardiography identifies hibernating myocardium and predicts recovery of left ventricular function after coronary revascularization. Circulation 1993;88:430-436.

96. Previtali M, Fetiveau R, Lanzarini L, et al: Prognostic value of myocardial viability and ischemia detected by dobutamine stress echocardiography early after acute myocardial infarction treated with thrombolysis. J Am Coll Cardiol 1998;32:380-386.

97. Beller GA: Assessment of myocardial viability. Curr Opin Cardiol 1997;12:459-467.

98. Perrone-Filardi P, Pace L, Prastaro M, et al: Assessment of myocardial viability in patients with chronic coronary artery disease: Rest-4hour-24hour ^{201}Tl tomography versus dobutamine echocardiography. Circulation 1996;94:2712-2719.

99. Arnese M, Cornel JH, Salustry A, et al: Prediction of improvement of regional left ventricular function after surgical revascularization: A comparison of low-dose dobutamine echocardiography with 201 Tl single-photon emission computed tomography. Circulation 1995;91:2748-2752.

100. Bonow RO: Identification of viable myocardium. Circulation 1996;94:2674-2680.

101. Pierard LA: Evaluating risk in unstable angina: Role of pharmacological stress echocardiography. Eur Heart J 2000;21:1041-1043.

102. Smart SC, Knickelbine T, Stoiber TR, et al: Safety and accuracy of dobutamine-atropine stress echocardiography for the detection of residual stenosis of the infarct related artery and multivessel disease during first week after acute myocardial infarction. Circulation 1997;95:1394-1401.

103. Carlos ME, Smart SC, Wynsen JC, et al: Dobutamine stress echocardiography for risk stratification after myocardial infarction. Circulation 1997;95:1402-1410.

104. Sitges M, Pare C, Azqueta M, et al: Feasibility and prognostic value of dobutamine-atropine stress echocardiography early in unstable angina. Eur Heart J 2000;21:1063-1071.

105. de la Torre MM, San Roman JA, Bermejo J, et al: Prognostic power of dobutamine echocardiography after uncomplicated acute myocardial infarction in the elderly. Chest 2001;120:1200-1205.

106. Greco CA, Salustri A, Seccareccia F, et al: Prognostic value of dobutamine echocardiography early after uncomplicated acute myocardial infarction: A comparison with exercise electrocardiography. J Am Coll Cardiol 1997;29:261-267.

107. Gleijnse ML, Fioretti PM, Roelandt JR: Methodology, feasibility, safety and diagnostic accuracy of dobutamine stress echocardiography. J Am Coll Cardiol 1997;30:595-606.

108. Gibson RS, Watson DD, Craddock GB, et al: Prediction of cardiac events after uncomplicated myocardial infarction: A prospective study comparing predischarge exercise thallium-201 scintigraphy and coronary angiography. Circulation 1983;68:321-336.

109. Picano E, Marraccini P, Lattanzi F, et al: Dipyridamole-echocardiography test as a clue for assessing the organic "ceiling" of individual coronary reserve. Eur Heart J 1987;8:38-44.

110. Bolognese L, Sarrasso G, Aralda D, et al: High dose dipyridamole echocardiography early after uncomplicated acute myocardial infarction: Correlation with exercise testing and coronary angiography. J Am Coll Cardiol 1989;14:357-363.

111. Bolognese L, Rossi L, Sarasso G, et al: Silent versus symptomatic dipyridamole-induced ischemia after myocardial infarction: Clinical and prognostic significance. J Am Coll Cardiol 1992;19:953-959.

112. Camerieri A, Picano E, Landi P, et al: Prognostic value of dipyridamole echocardiography early after myocardial infarction in elderly patients: Echo Persantine Italian Cooperative (EPIC) Study Group. J Am Coll Cardiol 1993;22:1809-1815.

113. Anthopoulos LP, Bonou MS, Sioras EP, et al: Echocardiographic detection of the extent of coronary artery disease in the elderly using dobutamine and adenosine infusion. Coron Artery Dis 1997;8:633-643.

114. Marwick T, D'Hondt AM, Baudhuin T, et al: Optimal use of dobutamine stress for the detection and evaluation of coronary artery disease: Combination with echocardiography or scintigraphy, or both? J Am Coll Cardiol 1993;22:159-167.

115. Sochowski RA, Yvorchuk KJ, Yang Y, et al: Dobutamine and dipyridamole stress echocardiography in patients with a low incidence of severe coronary artery disease. J Am Soc Echocardiogr 1995;8:482-487.

116. Ismaeil M, Trusevich T, Nottestand SY, et al: Dobutamine esophageal echo in the assessment of coronary artery disease: Comparison with dobutamine transthoracic echo in the same setting. J Am Coll Cardiol 1995;274A.

117. Koenig K, Kasper W, Hofmann T, et al: Transesophageal echocardiography for diagnosis of rupture of the ventricular septum or left ventricular papillary muscle during acute myocardial infarction. Am J Cardiol 1987;59:362.

118. Kaul S, Spotnitz WD, Glasheen WP, et al: Mechanism of ischemic mitral regurgitation: An experimental evaluation. Circulation 1991;84:2167-2180.

119. Kono T, Sabbah HN, Rosman H, et al: Mechanism of functional mitral regurgitation during acute myocardial ischemia. J Am Coll Cardiol 1992;19:1101-1105.

120. Adachi H, Kyo S, Takamoto S, et al: Early diagnosis and surgical intervention of acute aortic dissection by transesophageal color flow mapping. Circulation 1990;82(4 suppl):19-23.

121. Douglas PS, Fiolkoski J, Berko B, et al: Echocardiographic visualization of coronary artery anatomy in the adult. J Am Coll Cardiol 1988;11:565-567.

122. Ryan T, Armstrong WF, Feigenbaum H: Prospective evaluation of left main coronary artery using digital two-dimensional echocardiography. J Am Coll Cardiol 1986;7:807-812.

123. Yoshida K, Yoshikawa J, Hozumi T, et al: Detection of left main coronary artery stenosis by transesophageal color Doppler and two-dimensional echocardiography. Circulation 1990;81:1271-1276.

124. Tardif JC, Vannan MA, Taylor K, et al: Delineation of extended lengths of coronary arteries by multiple transesophageal echocardiography. J Am Coll Cardiol 1994;24:909-914.

125. Tardif JC, Pandian NG: Intravascular and intracardiac ultrasound. Coron Artery Dis 1995;6:35-41.

126. Tardif JC, Pandian NG: Intravascular ultrasound imaging in peripheral arterial and coronary artery disease. Curr Opin Cardiol 1994;9:627-633.

127. Mintz GS, Painter JA, Pichard AD, et al: Atherosclerosis in angiographically "normal" coronary artery reference segments: An intravascular ultrasound study with clinical correlations. J Am Coll Cardiol 1995;25:1479-1485.

128. Porter TR, Sears T, Xie F, et al: Intravascular ultrasound study of angiographically mildly diseased coronary arteries. J Am Coll Cardiol 1993;22:1858-1865.

129. Pande AK, Tardif JC, Doucet S, et al: Intravascular ultrasound for diagnosis of left main coronary artery stenosis. Can J Cardiol 1996;12:757-759.

130. Wei K, Skyba DM, Firschke C, et al: Interactions between microbubbles and ultrasound: In vivo and in vitro observations. J Am Coll Cardiol 1997;29:1081-1088.

131. Firschke C, Lindner JR, Wei K, et al: Myocardial perfusion imaging in the setting of coronary artery stenosis and acute myocardial infarction using venous injection of a second-generation echocardiographic contrast agent. Circulation 1997;96:959-967.

132. Kaul S, Senior R, Dittrich H, et al: Detection of coronary artery disease with myocardial contrast echocardiography: Comparison with 99m-Tc-Sestamibi single photon emission computed tomography. Circulation 1996;96:785-792.

133. Ragosta M, Camarano G, Kaul S, et al: Microvascular integrity indicates myocellular viability in patients with recent myocardial infarction: New insights using myocardial contrast echocardiography. Circulation 1994;89:2562-2569.

134. Iliceto S, Galiuto L, Marshese A, et al: Analysis of microvascular integrity, contractile reserve, and myocardial viability after acute myocardial infarction by dobutamine echocardiography and myocardial contrast echocardiography. Am J Cardiol 1996;77:441-445.

135. Ito H, Tomooka T, Sakai N, et al: Lack of myocardial perfusion immediately after successful thrombolysis: A predictor of poor recovery of left ventricular function in anterior myocardial infarction. Circulation 1992;85:1699-1705.

136. Ito H, Okamura A, Iwakura K, et al: Myocardial perfusion patterns related to thrombolysis in myocardial infarction perfusion grades after coronary angioplasty in patients with acute anterior wall myocardial infarction. Circulation 1996;93:1993-1999.

137. deFilippi CR, Willett DL, Walleed NI, et al: Comparison of myocardial contrast echocardiography and low-dose dobutamine stress echocardiography in predicting recovery of left ventricular function after coronary revascularization in chronic ischemic heart disease. Circulation 1995;92:2863-2868.

138. Meza MF, Ramee S, Collins T, et al: Knowledge of perfusion and contractile reserve improves the predictive value of recovery of regional myocardial function postrevascularization: A study using the combination of myocardial contrast echocardiography and dobutamine echocardiography. Circulation 1997;96:3459-3465.

139. Kaul S, Senior R, Dittrich H, et al: Detection of coronary artery disease with myocardial contrast echocardiography. Circulation 1997;96:785-792.

140. Jucquois I, Nihoyannopoulos P, D'Hondt A-M, et al: Comparison of myocardial contrast echocardiography with NC100100 and 99mTc sestamibi SPECT for detection of resting myocardial perfusion abnormalities in patients with previous myocardial infarction. Heart 2000;83:518-524.

141. Henle SK, Noblin J, Goree-Best P, et al: Assessment of myocardial perfusion by harmonic power Doppler imaging at rest and during adenosine stress: Comparison with 99mTc-sestamibi SPECT imaging. Circulation 2000;102:55-60.

142. Jones CJH, Kuo L, Davis MJ, et al: Role of nitric oxide in coronary microvascular response to adenosine and increased metabolic demands. Circulation 1996;91:1807-1813.

143. Anderson TJ, Uehata A, Gerard MD, et al: Close relation of endothelial function in the human coronary and peripheral circulation. J Am Coll Cardiol 1995;26:1235-1241.

144. Esper RJ, Vilarino G, Cacharron JL, et al: Impaired endothelial function in patients with rapidly stabilized unstable angina: Assessment by noninvasive brachial artery ultrasound. Clin Cardiol 1999;22:699-703.

145. Dupuis J, Tardif JC, Cernacek P, et al: Cholesterol reduction rapidly improves endothelial function after acute coronary syndromes (RECIFE study). Circulation 1999;99:3227-3233.

146. Fichtlscherer S, Zeiher AM: Endothelial dysfunction in acute coronary syndromes: Association with elevated C-reactive protein in endothelial dysfunction. Ann Med 2000;32:515-518.

■ ■ ■ chapter 1 9

Nuclear Cardiology Techniques in Acute Coronary Syndromes

Kenneth A. Brown

The primary goal of physicians with patients presenting with an acute coronary syndrome (ACS) is to choose a treatment strategy that optimizes outcome for each individual patient. Physicians also increasingly are asked to use medical resources in a way that minimizes the economic impact. Such decisions that involve consideration of the *cost-effectiveness* of an approach necessarily involve an understanding of an individual patient's risk for important cardiac events, such as death or myocardial infarction (MI). Interventions that are expensive and that carry their own risk are most beneficial in patients who have the greatest risk of future cardiac events. Conversely, low-risk patients are unlikely to benefit from any intervention, especially one that itself has risks of complications. Knowledge of the determinants of risk in patients presenting with ACS allows physicians to make cost-effective management decisions that most benefit individual patients. In this context, nuclear cardiology techniques offer the physician important tools to help make such decisions because these techniques can assess accurately two of the most important determinants of prognosis in patients with ACS: left ventricular dysfunction and current jeopardized viable myocardium. These factors represent two interactive influences: the extent of permanent damage and the extent of future myocardium at risk. This chapter reviews the current data involving the use of nuclear cardiology techniques to determine cardiac risk in ACS and shows how they can be integrated into a comprehensive, rational management strategy.

LEFT VENTRICULAR FUNCTION

Determination of left ventricular function using radionuclide angiography has been shown to be a powerful predictor of outcome in patients who present with an acute MI.[1-5] Left ventricular ejection fraction measured by radionuclide techniques probably has been the most valuable index of function because of its reproducibility and its consistent predictive value. In the MPRG (Multicenter Post Infarction Research Group) study, patients who had presented with an acute MI underwent predischarge radionuclide angiography.[1] The 1-year cardiac mortality rate was exponentially inversely related to left ventricular ejection fraction (Fig. 19-1). Cardiac mortality increased, especially after ejection fraction decreased to less than 40%.

The influence of left ventricular function on outcome has persisted even as the overall outcome after acute MI improved with the introduction of thrombolysis and percutaneous coronary interventions. In the TIMI (Thrombolysis In Myocardial Infarction) trial, overall cardiac death rate was lower than in the MPRG trial, but the increased relationship between ejection fraction and annual cardiac mortality rate was retained (see Fig 19-1).[2] Similarly the CAMI (Canadian Assessment of Myocardial Infarction) study evaluated the outcome of patients with acute MI in the thrombolytic era of the 1990s.[3] These investigators found an inverse relationship between ejection fraction and 1-year cardiac mortality that matched the MPRG findings closely (Fig. 19-2). The differences were greatest at the low end (ejection fraction <20%), possibly reflecting the ameliorative effects of angiotensin-converting enzyme inhibitor or β-blocker treatment that became the standard of care in the 1990s.

Several other studies confirmed the important prognostic value of ejection fraction in patients receiving thrombolysis. Simoons and colleagues found that 5-year

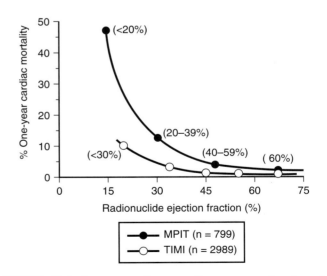

FIGURE 19–1. One-year cardiac mortality rate as a function of radionuclide angiographic ejection fraction in the Multicenter Post-Infarction Research Group Trial (MPIT) and the Thrombolysis in Myocardial Infarction (TIMI) trial. Mortality rate increases as ejection fraction decreases. The overall mortality rate was higher in the MPIT cohort. (From Bonow RO: Prognostic assessment in coronary. J Nucl Cardiol 1:280–291.)

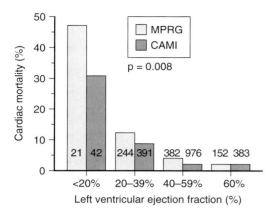

FIGURE 19–2. One-year cardiac mortality as a function of radionuclide left ventricular ejection fraction in the Multicenter Postinfarction Research Group (MPRG) trial and the Canadian Assessment of Myocardial Infarction (CAMI) study. Cardiac mortality in patients with poor function (ejection fraction <20%) was better in the more recent CAMI cohort. (From Rouleau JL, Talajik M, Sussex B, et al: Myocardial infarction patients in the 1990s—their risk factors, stratification and survival in Canada: The Canadian Assessment of Myocardial Infarction [CAMI] Study. J Am Coll Cardiol 1996;27:1119–1127.)

survival was only approximately 40% in patients with left ventricular ejection fraction less than 30% compared with greater than 90% survival when ejection fraction was greater than 40%.[4] Similarly, Dakik and coworkers[5] found the risk of cardiac events increased as ejection fraction decreased in patients receiving thrombolysis for acute MI. Event-free survival was approximately 75% for patients with ejection fraction of 40% compared with less than 25% for patients with ejection fraction less than 40%.

Limitations of Measurement of Left Ventricular Function

Although left ventricular ejection fraction has a powerful ability to predict cardiac mortality after acute MI, it has some limitations. First, although the measurement of ejection fraction itself with radionuclide angiography is highly reproducible and accurate,[6] indices of left ventricular function measured early after MI may change over time even in the short term. This change may reflect evolving post-MI cardiac physiology, including transient stunning and hyperkinesis. Christian and colleagues[7] found that 16% of patients with acute MI showed a rise in ejection fraction of 8% determined by radionuclide angiography between discharge and 6 weeks. At discharge, the ejection fraction in this group was less than predicted based on the size of the MI determined by myocardial perfusion imaging. This suggests that the rise in ejection fraction at 6 weeks reflected a resolution of myocardial stunning. Conversely, 19% of patients showed a fall in ejection fraction of 8% by 6 weeks. Although remodeling can explain a decrease in left ventricular function over time after acute MI, these patients had a discharge ejection fraction that was greater than predicted based on the infarct size, suggesting that the decrease in ejection fraction over 6 weeks more likely

reflected resolution of early hyperkinesis in the noninfarct zone.

Hibernating myocardium is another factor that may affect left ventricular function in the setting of prior MI. To the extent that it is present, hibernating myocardium is important to identify since coronary revascularization can improve left ventricular function and survival.[8] Although hibernating myocardium may be an important factor in determining prognosis and management in chronic ischemic cardiomyopathy, its role in acute MI is likely to be small. Aside from the transient influences of stunning or hyperkinesis, left ventricular ejection fraction probably primarily reflects the *permanent* damage done by acute MI, which accounts for its strong prognostic value. Although it is clear that ejection fraction, reflecting the extent of scar, is a powerful predictor of mortality, however, it reflects the "horses out of the barn." Although β-blockers and angiotensin-converting enzyme inhibitors may increase survival, it is an unproved hypothesis that revascularization alters outcome in this setting in the absence of stunning or hibernation, or of other critical artery stenosis.

Outcome that can be altered by surgical or percutaneous intervention is more likely related to the extent of jeopardized viable myocardium that is present after the insult of the acute MI. As is reviewed subsequently, there are much data to suggest that the presence and extent of jeopardized viable myocardium defined by stress nuclear myocardial perfusion imaging (MPI) is the most important predictor of outcome in patients with acute MI. There is an important interaction between the extent of permanent damage (scar) and the extent of additional viable myocardium at risk.

PROGNOSTIC VALUE OF JEOPARDIZED VIABLE MYOCARDIUM DETERMINED BY STRESS NUCLEAR MYOCARDIAL PERFUSION IMAGING

Because reversible defects on stress MPI accurately identify and quantify jeopardized viable myocardium, this technique can play an important role in assessment of risk after acute MI (Table 19–1). Probably the most consistent observation reported in the literature regarding the prognostic value of stress nuclear MPI is that the presence and extent of transient defects, reflecting jeopardized viable myocardium, predict important cardiac events.[9,10] A direct relationship between myocardium at risk identified by nuclear MPI and patients at risk for cardiac events first was reported by Brown and colleagues in 1983.[11] They compared the prognostic value of exercise thallium-201 imaging, exercise treadmill testing, coronary angiography, and clinical data and found that the best predictor of cardiac death or nonfatal MI was the number of segments with transient thallium-201 defects. These early findings were confirmed and expanded by many investigators.[9,10] Ladenheim and colleagues[12] found that among clinical and scintigraphic indices, the number of reversible perfusion defects on stress thallium-201 images was the best predictor of

■ ■ ■

TABLE 19–1 ADVANTAGES OF NUCLEAR MYOCARDIAL PERFUSION IMAGING FOR EVALUATING PATIENTS AFTER MYOCARDIAL INFARCTION

Increased sensitivity for detecting ischemia and multivessel disease
Increased prognostic value: jeopardized viable myocardium predicts
   death or myocardial infarction
Ability to localize ischemia to individual coronary territories
Distinguish infarct zone from noninfarct zone myocardium at risk
Evaluate left ventricular function and perfusion simultaneously
Can use vasodilator stress as adjuvant allowing earlier risk
   stratification

---

future cardiac events. Similar observations were made in a wide clinical spectrum of patients: patients with suspected coronary artery disease (CAD) or known angiographic CAD; patients undergoing noncardiac surgery; patients with remote prior MI; and, as discussed subsequently, patients presenting with unstable angina or acute MI.[9] The powerful predictive value of nuclear MPI is retained whether the stress agent is exercise, vasodilator stress, or an adrenergic agent[9,10] and regardless of whether the perfusion tracer is thallium-201, technetium 99m (Tc 99m)–based agents such as sestamibi or tetrafosmin, or positron emission tomography imaging agents.[9,10,13–15] For each of these modalities of imaging and patient cohorts, the most consistent finding has been that cardiac risk is related directly to the presence and, more importantly, the *extent* of jeopardized viable myocardium.

Acute ST-Segment Elevation Myocardial Infarction

The prognostic value of exercise MPI in the post-MI setting first was reported by Gibson and colleagues.[16] Predischarge submaximal exercise thallium-201 MPI was compared with clinical, exercise, and coronary angiographic data for predicting subsequent cardiac events. Reversible thallium-201 defects, defects involving multiple coronary territories, and increased lung thallium-201 uptake (reflecting left ventricular dysfunction) were the most important prognostic MPI variables. Compared with clinical or coronary angiography, these indices were significantly more sensitive for detecting patients at risk for cardiac events (Fig. 19–3). The greater sensitivity for detecting the patient at risk translated into a greater ability to identify the low-risk patient who is unlikely to benefit from further invasive or interventional procedures. Subsequently, many studies confirmed the prognostic value of exercise MPI in patients presenting with an acute MI.[9,10] Wilson and colleagues[17] showed that in patients with acute MI and single-vessel CAD, late cardiac events were related to the presence and extent of transient defects on submaximal exercise MPI but not to clinical or exercise electrocardiogram (ECG) data. Travin and associates[18] used regression analysis of clinical, exercise

ECG, and exercise sestamibi single-photon emission computed tomography (SPECT) MPI variables in patients with acute MI and found that only the number of

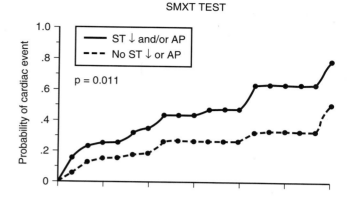

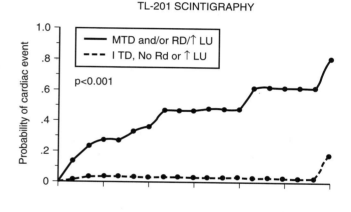

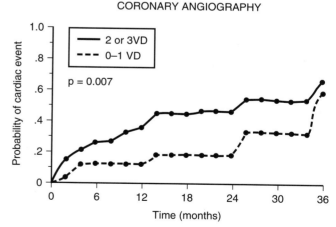

FIGURE 19–3. Cumulative probability of cardiac event over time as a function of high-risk *(solid line)* and low-risk *(dashed line)* criteria for submaximal exercise test (SMXT) *(top panel)*, thallium-201 (TL-201) imaging *(middle panel)*, and coronary angiography *(lower panel)*. Thallium-201 imaging better separated high-risk from low-risk patients. AP, angina pectoris; LU, lung uptake; MTD, multiple vascular territory thallium-201 defects; Rd, redistribution (reversible defects); ST↓, ST-segment depression; VD, vessels diseased. (From Gibson RS, Watson DD, Craddock GB, et al: Prediction of cardiac events after uncomplicated myocardial infarction: A prospective study comparing predischarge exercise thallium-201 scintigraphy and coronary angiography. Circulation 1983;68:321–336.)

reversible defects was a significant predictor of cardiac events (Fig. 19–4). As in patients with chronic stable CAD, there is compelling evidence that the risk of future cardiac events in patients with acute MI is strongly related to the presence and, more importantly, the extent of jeopardized viable myocardium.

Indirect Markers of Ischemia

Several indirect markers of ischemia on stress MPI have been shown to have adverse prognostic implications, although they have been incompletely studied in patients with acute MI. Increased thallium-201 lung uptake on exercise MPI has been shown to reflect stress-induced rises in left ventricular filling pressure[19,20] and has been associated with severe CAD and resting and exercise-induced left ventricular dysfunction.[21–24] It has been shown to predict an increased risk of cardiac events in patients with acute MI and with chronic coronary disease.[16,25,26] Transient left ventricular dilation on stress compared with rest imaging also has been related to extensive CAD and left ventricular dysfunction[27–29] and has been associated with increased risk of cardiac events.[27,30] More data are needed to understand the full clinical implications of these findings, especially in patients with ACS.

Vasodilator Stress Myocardial Perfusion Imaging

Vasodilator stress may have a particular advantage over exercise as an adjunct to MPI in patients with acute MI. It produces a greater hyperemic stimulus compared with submaximal exercise and consequently has been shown to have greater sensitivity for detecting CAD when used with stress MPI,[31] an important issue for risk stratification in the post-MI setting. Leppo and coworkers[32] were the first to show that vasodilator stress, using intravenous dipyridamole, with thallium-201 MPI predicted

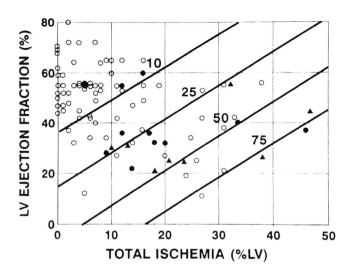

FIGURE 19–5. One-year cardiac risk of death or nonfatal myocardial infarction as a function of left ventricular (LV) ejection fraction and total ischemia on adenosine thallium-201 imaging after myocardial infarction. Diagonal lines represent isobars of percent risk. For a given ejection fraction, risk increases as total ischemia increases. For a given degree of ischemia, risk increases as ejection fraction decreases. (From Mahmarian JJ, Pratt CM, Nishimura S, et al: Quantitative adenosine ^{201}T1 single-photon emission computed tomography for the early assessment of patients surviving acute myocardial infarction. Circulation 1993;87:1197–1210.)

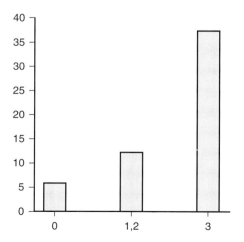

FIGURE 19–4. Cardiac event rate as a function of the number of reversible defects on exercise Tc 99m sestamibi imaging after uncomplicated myocardial infarction. The cardiac event rate rises as the number of reversible defects increases. (Adapted from Travin MI, Dessouki A, Cameron T, Heller GV: Use of exercise technetium-99m sestamibi SPECT imaging to detect residual ischemia and for risk stratification after acute myocardial infarction. Am J Cardiol 1995;74:665–669.)

cardiac events when performed 10 to 16 days after MI. Compared with clinical and radionuclide ventriculographic left ventricular function data, these investigators found that reversible thallium-201 defects were the only significant predictor of late cardiac death or MI and identified 92% of patients at risk for such future cardiac events. Subsequently, other investigators confirmed the predictive value of reversible defects on dipyridamole-MPI reflecting jeopardized viable myocardium in patients with acute MI.[9,10]

Adenosine also has been found to be valuable as a vasodilator adjuvant for stress MPI after MI. Mahmarian and colleagues[33,34] described the early and late prognostic value of adenosine thallium-201 SPECT MPI in patients with acute MI. Imaging detected jeopardized viable myocardium in 59% of infarct zones and in 92% of noninfarct zones supplied by a stenotic artery.[33] Angiographic patency did not predict the presence or extent of jeopardized myocardium. In-hospital cardiac events occurred in 43% of patients with significant reversible defects compared with 9% without significant reversibility. Over a mean 16-month follow-up, the best predictors of cardiac events were extent of reversible thallium-201 defects and ejection fraction.[34] The authors showed that adenosine MPI data had significant incremental prognostic value when added to clinical and angiographic data, improving the ability to predict cardiac events twofold to fivefold. The negative impact of MPI ischemia on outcome was additive to left ventricular ejection fraction (Fig. 19–5), consistent with the paradigm that the extent of residual jeopardized viable myocardium and left ventricular function are the primary determinants of outcome after MI.

Dobutamine Stress Myocardial Perfusion Imaging

Dobutamine adrenergic stimulation offers an alternative to vasodilator stress as an adjunct to MPI in patients unable to exercise. This alternative is particularly useful in patients with contraindications to vasodilators, such as bronchospasm, recent caffeine or methylxanthine exposure, high-degree atrioventricular block, or hypotension. Previous reports described sensitivity and specificity for detecting CAD comparable to exercise or vasodilator stress nuclear imaging.[35] Several studies showed that dobutamine stress MPI has significant prognostic value in patients with stable CAD[36-40] or before noncardiac vascular surgery.[42,43] Data in stable coronary disease suggest that, as with exercise MPI, the risk of death or MI is related directly to the extent of jeopardized viable myocardium on dobutamine stress MPI.[37] Few data are available, however, for dobutamine MPI in the post-MI setting. In contrast to vasodilators, dobutamine produces a much more marked increase in heart rate and blood pressure, leading to induction of true ischemia in the setting of coronary lesions, rather than just heterogeneity of hyperemia. Consequently, although dobutamine stress MPI can be performed safely, it needs to be applied more cautiously in the post-MI setting, especially the early post-MI setting.

Coma-Canella and colleagues[43] performed dobutamine stress thallium-201 SPECT and radionuclide angiography a mean of 16 days after MI. They found that extent of ischemia on SPECT imaging correlated with abnormal dobutamine-induced regional wall motion. No angiographic or prognostic data were reported. Elhendy and coworkers[44] reported a sensitivity of 74% and 71% for detecting remote and infarct-related coronary disease using dobutamine stress thallium-201 SPECT in 71 patients more than 3 months after acute MI. Specificity was 80% to 83%. These authors also reported similar sensitivities, specificities, and predictive values for dobutamine stress MPI and echocardiography in detecting remote and infarct-related coronary disease in patients with prior MI.[45] In this cohort, most of the patients were studied several years after MI. In contrast, Lancellotti and coworkers[46] compared dobutamine stress MPI and echocardiography performed a mean of 5 days after MI. In this small select cohort of 75 patients, there were no serious dobutamine-related complications. MPI was a sensitive and specific predictor of infarct-related stenoses (70% and 83%) and multivessel disease (67% and 93%) and was comparable to stress echocardiography.

Dobutamine stress MPI seems to assess accurately post-MI coronary anatomy, and there is internal consistency between dobutamine-induced perfusion defects and inducible wall motion abnormalities. Determination of the prognostic implications and the safety of dobutamine stress MPI awaits further data, however.

Early Post–Myocardial Infarction Risk Stratification

In addition to its greater sensitivity for detecting CAD, vasodilator stress MPI has other advantages that can allow it to play an important role in the early, in-hospital management of post-MI patients. In contrast to exercise, vasodilator stress induces only modest changes in determinants of myocardial oxygen demand.[47-50] In addition, the hemodynamic effects are brief (adenosine) or rapidly reversible (dipyridamole).[24,25] As a consequence, risk stratification with vasodilator stress MPI can be performed safely potentially much earlier than exercise after acute MI. Management decisions can be made sooner than the standard 5- to 7-day post-MI, predischarge evaluation, potentially shortening hospitalization and reducing costs. In addition, identifying high-risk patients and directing appropriate treatment sooner can prevent early cardiac events. Brown and colleagues[51] first reported a series of 50 patients who underwent dipyridamole thallium-201 MPI 1 to 4 days (mean, 2.6 days) after acute MI. No serious adverse effects occurred with dipyridamole administration. Clinical, ECG, cardiac catheterization, and thallium-201 MPI data were analyzed, and the only significant predictor of in-hospital ischemic cardiac events was the presence of reversible defects in the infarct zone. Nine (45%) of 20 patients with infarct zone reversible defects had in-hospital ischemic cardiac events compared with 0 of 30 patients without ($P = .0001$). Over a mean 12-month follow-up period, there were three additional cardiac events in patients with reversible defects, whereas patients without reversible defects remained free of cardiac events. It seemed that early risk stratification with dipyridamole MPI could identify high-risk patients, who could be referred early to invasive procedures and revascularization, and low-risk patients, who could be discharged early safely without further interventions.

These pilot data led to a much larger multicenter study involving 451 patients that was designed to compare the prognostic value of dipyridamole Tc 99m sestamibi SPECT MPI performed 2 to 4 days after acute MI with standard submaximal exercise MPI obtained at 6 to 12 days.[52] Confirming the pilot safety data, no significant adverse effects were attributable to the dipyridamole infusion. Clinical and stress test data were compared with MPI data, including a summed stress score, reflecting the size and severity of the defect on the stress images; summed rest score, reflecting the size and severity of the defect on the rest image; and summed difference score, reflecting the degree of reversibility between stress and rest images. The dipyridamole MPI summed stress and reversibility scores were significant multivariate predictors of in-hospital cardiac events. Patients were followed for a mean of 2 years. The dipyridamole MPI summed stress, rest, and difference scores were each significant multivariate predictors of future cardiac death or MI. Consistent with the theme emphasized in this review, indices of scar (summed rest score) and ischemia (summed difference score) were significant determinants of outcome after MI. Dipyridamole MPI showed better ability to risk-stratify patients than submaximal exercise MPI. This was manifest as a greater ability to separate low-risk from high-risk patients. Not only was significant prognostic data available earlier with dipyridamole MPI compared with submaximal exercise MPI, but also the information was superior at separating high-risk from low-risk patients.

There was an important interaction between the size of the initial stress defect and the degree of reversibility for determining individual patient risk. For a given size of stress defect, cardiac risk increased as the degree of reversibility, reflecting jeopardized viable myocardium, increased. Patients with a small defect (low summed stress score) had an overall annual cardiac death or MI rate of 2%, but this decreased to 0% in patients with little or no ischemia and increased to 4% in patients whose defect was primarily reversible. The interaction was greatest in patients with intermediate-sized stress defects. The overall annual event rate was 5%, but knowing this degree of jeopardized viable myocardium allowed further risk stratification: 0% with no or small ischemia increasing to 6% with intermediate ischemia and 17% with extensive ischemia. The interaction was least in patients with large stress defects since the event rate remained high in patients with extensive infarction but little or no ischemia.

This study showed that vasodilator stress MPI can be performed safely early in the post-MI period and provides powerful prognostic data not only sooner, but also superior to submaximal exercise MPI data. It allows identification of high-risk patients, who are candidates for early intervention, and low-risk patients, who can be considered for early discharge.

Selective Versus Nonselective Invasive Approach after an Acute Myocardial Infarction (ST-Segment Elevation)

Implicit in an ischemia-guided selective approach to cardiac catheterization and revascularization for the patient with acute MI is the assumption that patient outcome will be at least as good as a nonselective approach, in which every patient is referred for catheterization, and revascularization decisions are based on coronary anatomy. There are now substantial data to support such an assumption (Table 19–2).[53-56] The TIMI IIB trial compared the outcome of 3262 patients presenting with acute ST-segment elevation MI who were randomized to angiography and anatomy-guided revascularization versus a "conservative" or ischemia-guided approach, in which patients were referred to angiography and revascularization only if there was symptomatic or exercise-induced ECG evidence of ischemia.[53] The composite end point of death or MI at 6 weeks occurred in 10.9% of the invasive group compared with 9.7% of the ischemia-guided group (P = not significant). Although the more sensitive nuclear MPI was not used in the conservative ischemia-guided group, the outcome was at least as good as the nonselective invasive group. Similar findings were reported from the SWIFT (Should We Intervene Following Thrombolysis?) trial,[54] which compared outcome of patients with acute ST-seg-

■ ▪ ■

TABLE 19–2 SUMMARY OF RANDOMIZED TRIALS EVALUATING SELECTIVE VERSUS NONSELECTIVE STRATEGY OF CATHETERIZATION AFTER MYOCARDIAL INFARCTION

ST-SEGMENT ELEVATION MI FOLLOWING THROMBOLYSIS

Outcome not different with selective (ischemia-guided) catheterization/revascularization compared with nonselective (anatomy-guided)
  strategies
    TIMI IIB trial
    SWIFT trial
If no provokable ischemia, event-free survival not improved with intervention: 100% event-free survival with Med Rx
    TOPS trial

UNSTABLE ANGINA AND NON–ST-SEGMENT ELEVATION MI

Outcome not different with selective (ischemia-guided) catheterization/revascularization compared with nonselective (anatomy-guided)
  strategies
    TIMI IIIB
Outcome better with selective (ischemia-guided) strategy
    VANQWISH trial
Use of catheterization and revascularization more efficient with ischemia-guided strategy
    TIMI IIIB trial
    VANQWISH trial
      Recent cost-effectiveness data favoring ischemia-guided strategy
    FRISC II trial
      Outcome better with invasive strategy
      Nuclear imaging not used
      High threshold for crossover to catheterization/revascularization (≥ 3 mm ST-segment depression)
    TACTICS-TIMI 18 trial
      Glycoprotein IIb/IIIa platelet inhibitors used in all patients
      Stents used in interventional group
      Overall outcome better with nonselective interventional strategy
      Benefit of nonselective interventional strategy limited to high-risk subgroup (~40% of total cohort)
      Outcome in low-risk subgroups (~60% of total cohort) not different between strategies

MI, myocardial infarction.

ment elevation treated with thrombolysis and randomized to early invasive, anatomy-guided intervention versus conservative, ischemia-guided intervention. The death or MI rate at 1 year was 19.1% versus 16.6% in the invasive and conservative groups (*P* = not significant). The TOPS (Treatment of Post-Thrombolytic Stenoses) study included patients who presented with acute ST-segment elevation MI, received thrombolysis, had angiographically significant infarct vessel disease (>50% stenosis), but had a negative stress functional study (generally thallium-201 MPI).[55] Patients were randomized either to medical treatment without intervention or to delayed coronary angioplasty day 4 to 14. The infarct-free survival at 12 months was 100% in the medical treatment group versus 89% in the angioplasty group (*P* = .07). The infarcts that occurred in the angioplasty group all were procedure related. Functional noninvasive risk stratification was able to identify a population of patients at low risk for cardiac events treated medically that is not benefited (and possibly harmed) by intervention.

A registry study emphasized how a nonselective approach to coronary intervention in patients with acute MI may lead to a poorer outcome even when performed by experts. Dakik and Verani[56] reported the disposition and outcome of a large consecutive series of patients admitted to Baylor Methodist Hospital, a major cardiac tertiary care hospital, with either acute MI or unstable angina. The first diagnostic test was cardiac catheterization in 72% of 1704 patients admitted with acute MI; only 6% had a nuclear MPI, and only 1% had a stress test as the first diagnostic study. The overall revascularization rate was 49%, but it was much higher in patients evaluated solely by angiography (70%) than in patients undergoing stress MPI (29%) (*P* < .001). The higher revascularization rate did not translate into a better outcome, however. The in-hospital mortality rate was significantly higher in patients evaluated with angiography alone (10%) compared with patients evaluated with nuclear MPI (1%). The differences were more striking among patients undergoing coronary revascularization (Fig. 19-6). The mortality was 10% in patients evaluated with angiography alone compared with 0% in patients evaluated with nuclear MPI. These differences could not be explained by a higher clinical risk pattern in the angiography group: There were no differences in the frequency of hypertension, diabetes mellitus, or anterior MI, and patients undergoing angiography were younger (*P* = .05) and tended to have less heart failure. Even in a major cardiac medical center, a nonselective invasive approach does not lead to a better outcome but may be associated with a worse outcome. Performing invasive and interventional procedures only can add risk to patients who already have a low risk of cardiac events. The better outcome of patients undergoing nuclear MPI as part of their post-MI evaluation presumably was related to the ability of this procedure to distinguish such low-risk patients from the high-risk cohort that would benefit from revascularization.

Compelling data exist suggesting that a selective, ischemia-guided strategy of invasive procedures and interventions leads to an equivalent, if not better, outcome compared with a nonselective approach in patients with ST-segment elevation MI who receive thrombolysis. Conversely, there is no convincing evidence that post-MI patients do better with coronary intervention in the absence of provokable ischemia. Whether newer advances in intervention, such as stents, will alter this conclusion is currently unknown and requires further study. Advances in the medical treatment of acute MI patients also have occurred, including the introduction of glycoprotein IIb/IIIa inhibitors, statins, and angiotensin-converting enzyme inhibitors and greater recognition of the benefit of β-blockers.

Unstable Angina and Non–ST-Segment Elevation Myocardial Infarction

Patients with unstable angina or non–ST-segment elevation MI are another ACS cohort for whom traditional management has involved an aggressive invasive approach because of the presumption that the syndrome either is an immediate precursor to MI (unstable angina) or is associated with an incomplete and unstable infarction (non–ST-segment elevation MI).

The unstable angina cohort is heterogeneous, and it is necessary to distinguish truly refractory unstable patients from "stabilizable" patients responsive to medical treatment. Many studies have shown that aspirin, heparin, β-blockers, nifedipine, and glycoprotein IIb/IIIa platelet inhibitors can reduce the death and MI rate in patients presenting with unstable angina.[57] There also are data that intensification of an existing medical regimen can reduce the medically refractory rate.[58] Patients

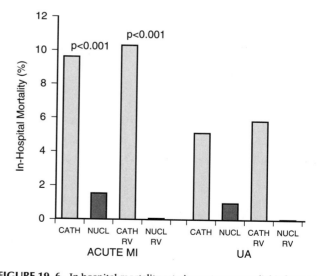

FIGURE 19–6. In-hospital mortality rate in acute myocardial infarction (MI) or unstable angina (UA) patients undergoing cardiac catheterization (CATH) alone as a diagnostic procedure versus patients undergoing nuclear imaging (NUCL). Analogous mortality data are shown for patients undergoing coronary revascularization (RV). In-hospital mortality rate was significantly lower in patients receiving nuclear imaging as part of their evaluation compared with cardiac catheterization alone. Abbreviations as in Figure 10. (Adapted from Dakik HA, Verani MS: Use of invasive and nuclear stress testing in patients with acute ischemic syndromes in a large, urban, university-affiliated hospital. J Nucl Cardiol 2000;7:328–332.)

who present with unstable angina who continue to have recurrent chest pain require coronary revascularization. In patients who are stabilized with institution or intensification of medical treatment, however, it is reasonable to ask whether noninvasive evaluation with stress MPI can distinguish low-risk patients, whose outcome is unlikely to be improved with revascularization, from high-risk patients, who are likely to benefit.

Risk stratification in patients with unstable angina first was evaluated by Hillert and colleagues,[59] who performed submaximal exercise thallium-201 MPI in patients who were stabilized after admission with unstable angina. Over a 12-week follow-up period, 15 of 19 patients with reversible defects developed MI or had class III/IV angina compared with only 2 of 18 patients without reversible defects ($P < .001$). In a larger series of 158 patients admitted with an acute non-MI coronary syndrome, an acute MI or cardiac death occurred in 21% of patients with reversible exercise thallium-201 defects compared with only 3% without reversible defects over a median 14-month follow-up period.[60] When compared with Holter ECG, stress ECG, and cardiac catheterization data, the extent of reversible defects on MPI was the only significant multivariate predictor of cardiac events.[61]

Brown[62] described a series of 52 patients presenting with unstable angina who responded to initial medical treatment and underwent exercise thallium-201 MPI before discharge. The only significant multivariate predictor of cardiac death or MI over a 39-month follow-up period was the presence of reversible defects. Cardiac death or MI occurred in 26% of patients with reversible defects compared with only 3% of patients without reversible defects (<1% annual rate). Stress ECG had no predictive value. These findings were confirmed in a similar cohort of 126 patients.[63] Over a mean 12-month follow-up period, 10 (25%) of 40 patients with reversible defects had cardiac death or MI compared with only 1 (1%) of 86 patients without reversible defects ($P < .001$). Similar to the findings of Brown,[62] neither fixed perfusion defects nor exercise ECG predicted cardiac events.

Although most of these studies involve small cohorts, they are remarkably consistent and are consistent with data in other coronary heart disease patient cohorts. Reversible defects, reflecting jeopardized viable myocardium, predict important cardiac events. Table 19-3 summarizes the data for studies using death and MI as end points. Reversible defects identify a high-risk cohort with a 20% to 26% risk of cardiac death or MI over a 1- to 3-year time frame. Such a cohort would be expected to benefit from coronary revascularization. Patients without reversible defects, especially patients with normal perfusion, have a low risk of cardiac events, however, and are not likely to benefit from intervention.

Similar to unstable angina, patients who present with non–ST-segment elevation (formerly non–Q wave) MI are a heterogeneous population. Not all such infarctions are either subendocardial or incomplete. Pathologic studies showed that although the infarcts tend to be smaller, the transmural distribution is not much different from Q wave or ST-segment elevation MI.[64] The smaller size of the non–Q wave infarction is associated with a higher frequency of residual jeopardized viable myocardium. Gibson and coworkers[65] evaluated clinical and stress MPI results in patients with acute non–Q wave MI and found that infarct zone reversible defects were present in 60% of patients compared with 36% with Q wave MI ($P < .01$).[65] Only 1 of 35 (3%) non–Q wave MI patients without infarct zone reversibility on MPI developed recurrent MI over a mean 27-month follow-up period compared with 15 of 52 (29%) patients with infarct zone reversibility.[65]

As with unstable angina patients, the heterogeneity of the cohort suggests that a routine indiscriminate nonselective approach of invasive procedures and interventions may not lead to a better outcome compared with a selective approach guided by a technique capable of identifying low-risk and high-risk patient subgroups.

Selective Versus Nonselective Invasive Approach to Unstable Angina and Non–ST-Segment Elevation Myocardial Infarction

The TIMI IIIB trial examined the effect of thrombolysis and the possible benefit of an early nonselective invasive strategy in 1473 patients with either unstable angina or non–Q wave MI.[66] Thrombolysis was harmful in this

■ ▓ ■

TABLE 19–3 PREDICTIVE VALUE OF STRESS NUCLEAR MYOCARDIAL PERFUSION IMAGING IN PATIENTS PRESENTING WITH UNSTABLE ANGINA

Study	n	Follow-Up (mo)	CARDIAC DEATH/MI		
			RD n/n (%)	No RD	Normal Study
Madsen et al[60]	158	14	6/29 (21%)	4/129 (3%)	2/97 (2%)
Brown[62]	52	39	6/23 (26%)	1/29 (3%)	0/15 (0%)
Stratmann[AU] et al[63]	126	12	10/40 (25%)	1/86 (1%)	1/52 (2%)
			Annualized Cardiac Death/MI Rate (% per year)		
Madsen et al[60]			18	2.6	1.8
Brown[62]			8	0.9	0
Stratmann et al[63]			25	1.0	1.9
Weighted average	336		19	1.7	1.6

MI, myocardial infarction; RD, reversible defect.

cohort, with a higher incidence of fatal and nonfatal MI (7.4%) compared with placebo (4.9%) ($P < .05$). More germane to the current discussion, the study also randomized patients either to early cardiac catheterization followed by anatomy-guided revascularization or to a "conservative" strategy of selective catheterization and revascularization in response to spontaneous ischemia or ischemia provoked on a predischarge submaximal exercise thallium-201 study. There was no difference in the primary end points of death, nonfatal MI, or a positive 6-week exercise test in the invasive or conservative subgroups ($P = .33$ to $.78$). There was no difference in death or MI at 1 year.[67] As in the TIMI IIB trial, a nonselective invasive approach to this ACS cohort did not lead to a better outcome. The nonselective strategy was associated with a less efficient use of expensive medical resources. By design, nearly all the patients in the invasive group received cardiac catheterization (98%), but only 61% underwent coronary revascularization. Coronary angiography was performed in about 40% of patients without leading to an intervention. In the selective conservative subgroup, cardiac catheterization was performed in 64% of patients because of spontaneous or provoked ischemia; 77% of this group underwent revascularization. Only 15% of the overall conservative group underwent angiography without revascularization. The use of invasive procedures to define who should undergo coronary revascularization was more efficient with a selective ischemia-guided approach.

The VANQWISH (Veterans Affairs Non Q-Wave Infarction Strategies in Hospital) trial results were more striking.[68] Similar to the TIMI IIIB trial, 920 patients with non–Q wave MI were randomized to a nonselective invasive strategy or to a conservative strategy of selective catheterization with recurrent chest pain or ischemia on stress thallium-201 imaging. In this trial, death or MI was greater in the nonselective invasive group at 1 month and 1 year ($P < 0.05$), although this was no longer statistically significant at 2 years. The ischemia-guided conservative patients without angiography had a low 30-day death rate (1%) comparable to the rate with angioplasty (1.3%), indicating that stress MPI could identify low-risk patients who would not benefit from intervention even when intervention can be performed with a low complication rate. As with the TIMI IIIB trial, the resource use was far more efficient in the selective ischemia-guided cohort. Although angioplasty was performed in 96% of the invasive group, only 44% underwent revascularization. More than half of this subgroup underwent angiography without the information leading to revascularization. In contrast, only 15% of the ischemia-guided conservative cohort went to the catheterization laboratory without going on to revascularization.

One of the criticisms of the VANQWISH trial is the high mortality rate in the invasive arm patients who had coronary artery bypass surgery.

Limitations of the TIMI II/IIIB and VANQWISH trials are that the trials were performed before the introduction of glycoprotein IIb/IIIa platelet inhibitors and the use of intracoronary stents, which conceivably improved the outcome of an invasive approach. These issues were addressed in the Treat Angina with Aggrastat and Determine Cost of Therapy with an Invasive or Conservative Strategy—Thrombolysis in Myocardial Infarction (TACTICS-TIMI 18) trial.[69] A total of 2220 patients with unstable angina or non–ST-segment elevation MI were treated with glycoprotein IIb/IIIa inhibitors and randomized to the usual nonselective invasive approach (using stents when clinically indicated) versus an ischemia-guided conservative strategy based on spontaneous ischemia or the results of exercise imaging. In the overall cohort, outcome (death, MI, or rehospitalization for ACS) was better in the invasive subgroup. This benefit was confined, however, to the high-risk subgroup of patients with either ST-segment changes on presentation or serum troponin greater than 0.01 mg/mL. In the approximately 60% of patients without these markers, there was no difference in outcome based on strategy. The invasive strategy showed a borderline benefit in an intermediate risk subgroup based on TIMI risk score.

The TACTICS-TIMI 18 trial suggests that a nonselective invasive approach may have an advantage in high-risk patients. In low-risk patients, an ischemia-guided selective approach to coronary angiography and intervention seems to lead an outcome at least as good as a nonselective strategy. A reanalysis of the TIMI IIIB trial confirms this principle.[70] When TIMI IIIB patients were stratified clinically by age, ECG changes, enzymes, and symptoms, benefit of a nonselective invasive approach at 42 days was seen only in the high-risk or very-high-risk subgroup. Such patients accounted for only 19% of the total group. however. There was a trend for a superior outcome with a selective ischemia-guided conservative approach in low-risk subgroups. By 1 year, the interaction between clinical risk and strategy was not statistically significant.

The FRISC (Fragmin and Fast Revascularization during Instability in Coronary Artery Disease) II trial also compared an invasive and conservative approach in patients presenting with ACS and found an outcome advantage for the invasive strategy (9.4% death or MI versus 12.1% in the conservative group at 6 months).[71] A threshold of greater than 3 mm ST-segment depression on stress testing before referring to angiography and revascularization was used. As a result, although the cohort was fairly high risk (57% with multivessel or left main disease, 58% with elevated troponin, 22% with prior MI, 46% with ST-segment abnormalities on presentation), only 10% of the conservative group was referred for early angiography, and only 9% underwent revascularization. This study does not address the role of a selective approach to angiography in the ACS patient based on using modern, sensitive stress nuclear MPI or echo imaging to identify patients at risk for cardiac events.

The experience at Baylor Methodist Hospital with 2414 patients presenting with unstable angina was similar to their previously described experience with acute MI.[43] Most patients (nearly 80%) had cardiac catheterization as their first diagnostic test, and most had revascularization (see Fig. 19–6). Only 5% were first screened with stress nuclear MPI; an additional 4% underwent MPI after catheterization. Similar to acute MI patients, the invasive approach did not lead to a better outcome in patients admitted with unstable angina. The in-hospital mortality for patients undergoing catheterization without nuclear MPI was 5% compared with 1% in patients who were evaluated with MPI ($P < .001$) (see Fig. 19-11). The mortality was 6% in revascularized patients evaluated only with angiography compared with 0% in patients undergoing nuclear MPI before revascularization ($P < .001$). Although this was not a randomized trial, the difference in outcome between the approaches could not be explained by a higher risk clinical profile in the catheterization group. There was a trend toward a higher incidence of heart failure in the nuclear MPI group ($P = .06$). This study suggests that using nuclear MPI to choose patients for angiography and revascularization may lead to a better outcome and sounds another note of caution about a routine nonselective invasive approach.

EMERGENCY DEPARTMENT TRIAGE OF PATIENTS PRESENTING WITH CHEST PAIN

The identification of ACS in patients who present to the emergency department with nonspecific symptoms and nonischemic ECG changes is problematic because although the true incidence is low, the clinical risk associated with ACS is high and can be reduced with effective treatments when the diagnosis is made correctly. Consequently, physicians tend to have a low threshold for admission of such patients leading to higher costs, although most patients are discharged later without the diagnosis of MI or unstable angina.[72] Despite the best clinical judgment of physicians, the missed MI rate ranges from 2% to 10%.[73-78] This basic dilemma results from the intrinsic nonspecific nature of the presenting complaint and the low sensitivity and specificity of the ECG.[73,74,79-81] Clinical risk factors have been shown to be of little benefit because of their low specificity.[72,82-87] Serum biomarkers of myocardial imaging (troponin, CK-MB) are very helpful to diagnose acute MI when sampled serially over time, but initial levels at the time of emergency department presentation have a low sensitivity for acute MI. Acute injection of a radionuclide MPI agent at the time of presentation followed by early imaging offers a possible technique for detecting myocardial ischemia at the time of emergency department presentation. Such an approach potentially can improve sensitivity and specificity for detecting patients at risk for cardiac events leading to a more cost-effective triage of the problematic patient.

Early Data

In 1976, Wackers and colleagues[88] showed that a single injection of thallium-201 had a high sensitivity for detecting patients with acute MI that appeared to be time dependent: The sensitivity was 100% when injected within 6 hours, 96% when injected within 24 hours, and 79% when injected after 48 hours. Serial imaging in individual patients showed a reduction in the size of the defect over 24 hours, suggesting that early initial imaging reflected infarct plus ischemia that resolved with time. Early studies showed a much lower sensitivity for detect-

ing patients with unstable angina compared with patients with acute MI.[89] Although no patient presenting with acute MI had a normal imaging study, half the patients presenting with unstable angina had normal imaging. This finding probably was related to the wide time-frame of tracer injection after presentation to the emergency department (10 hours), as other studies have shown the sensitivity of rest thallium-201 imaging to be time-dependent in patients presenting with unstable angina.[90] Wackers and colleagues[90] found the sensitivity for unstable angina was 84% when patients were injected within 6 hours of chest pain compared with 19% when injected 12 to 18 hours after chest pain. The frequency of ischemia seen on rest thallium-201 imaging seems to be related to the type of presenting clinical syndrome.[91] After a rest injection of thallium-201, serial initial and delayed imaging showed that 19 of 19 (100%) patients presenting with crescendo exertional unstable angina had transient defects compared with only 3 of 12 (25%) with rest angina alone and 4 of 34 (12%) with stable angina ($P < .0001$). The high frequency of resting ischemia occurred in the crescendo angina group even though no patient had chest pain within 4 hours of injection.

These early studies, which all used planar imaging, showed the potential for using this technique to identify high-risk and low-risk patients. Wackers and colleagues[90] showed that rest thallium-201 injection within 18 hours of chest pain could identify 76% of patients who went on to have a complicated hospital course. Van der Wieken and coworkers[92] showed that 99% of patients presenting with chest pain and nondiagnostic ECG who had normal thallium-201 rest imaging within 12 hours of presentation did not go on to develop an acute MI.[92]

Technetium 99m–Based Single-Photon Emission Computed Tomography Myocardial Perfusion Imaging

The introduction of Tc 99m–based perfusion agents (sestamibi and tetrofosmin) has improved the potential of rest MPI for risk stratification of patients with chest pain presenting to the emergency department. The improved dosimetry makes the agents more suitable for SPECT with improved sensitivity for detecting ischemia and infarction, especially in the left circumflex artery territory.[93-97] The superior dosimetry also makes the agents suitable for evaluation of ventricular function, which can improve the predictive value of the test.[98,99] Finally, because (in contrast to thallium-201) the myocardial distribution remains stable over time, injection of a Tc 99m–based tracer does not need to be closely linked in time with imaging, facilitating the logistics of using this technique.[100-102] Patients can be injected rapidly in the emergency department, and imaging can be arranged when convenient without loss of diagnostic information.

Bilodeau and colleagues[103] evaluated the sensitivity of SPECT imaging after an injection of Tc 99m sestamibi at rest during chest pain and after resolution in 45 patients presenting to the emergency department without known CAD. The sensitivity for detection of CAD was

96% when injection occurred during chest pain and 65% when injection occurred during a pain-free period. This sensitivity was significantly higher than for 12-lead ECG (35% to 38%). The specificity for resting MPI was also fairly high—79% with chest pain and 84% without. The location of the perfusion defect corresponded with the most severe coronary lesion on angiography in 88% of patients, and the size of the perfusion defect correlated to the extent of CAD. Rest Tc 99m sestamibi SPECT imaging showed high promise as a tool for screening patients on presentation to the emergency department with chest pain of unclear origin. Subsequent studies confirmed its potential value.

Varetto and colleagues[104] examined the predictive value of rest Tc 99m sestamibi SPECT imaging in a series of 64 patients presenting to the emergency department with chest pain but nondiagnostic ECG. None of the 34 patients with normal imaging subsequently were found to have CAD, whereas 27 of 30 (90%) patients with perfusion defects either were determined to have unstable angina or were ruled in for acute MI. Of the 14 patients with unstable angina, 11 had defects despite being injected 2 to 8 hours (mean, 5 hours) after the rest pain had resolved. Repeat imaging 12 to 24 hours later showed complete resolution of the defects. Injection of Tc 99m sestamibi at the time of presentation seemed to be highly sensitive (100%) and specific (92%) for detecting patients with CAD, even if injection was done after chest pain had resolved for several hours. Because the defects had normalized by 24 to 48 hours, however, there was a gradual resolution of ischemia; the rate probably reflects the severity of the ischemic insult. It would be expected that the sensitivity for detecting ischemia would be greatest if injection were made when the chest pain was still present.

Hilton and coworkers[105] took the next step and evaluated the ability of rest Tc 99m sestamibi SPECT imaging in the emergency department to predict subsequent cardiac events in 102 patients with anginal symptoms but normal or nondiagnostic ECG. All patients in this series were injected while still having chest pain. Patients without defects had a cardiac event rate of only 1%, whereas 71% of patients with definite perfusion defects had cardiac events. Equivocal imaging results were associated with an intermediate risk (13%). The ability to separate low-risk from high-risk patients was superior for rest Tc 99m sestamibi imaging compared with clinical or ECG data (Figs. 19–7 and 19–8).

Other studies using either Tc 99m sestamibi or Tc 99m tetrofosmin subsequently reported similar findings of a high sensitivity for detecting patients at risk for acute MI and other cardiac events.[106–109] This translates into a high negative predictive value for such cardiac events (Table 19–4). Rest imaging in the emergency department can be a helpful tool for determining whether or not a patient can be sent home safely for additional outpatient evaluation. A comprehensive goal-driven strategy that integrates clinical risk and acute rest Tc 99m sestamibi MPI was introduced at the Medical College of Virginia (Fig. 19–9).[106,110] Level 1 and 2 patients (high to very high

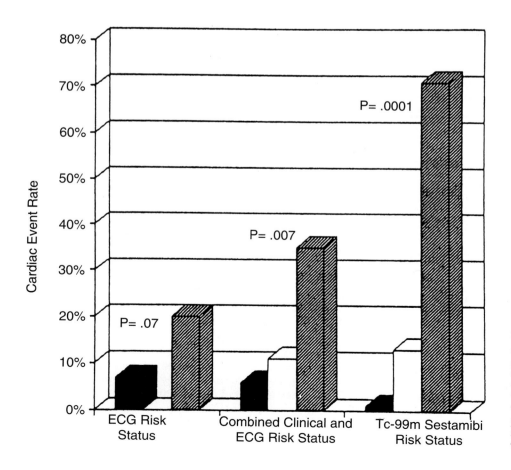

FIGURE 19–7. Risk of cardiac events in patients presenting to the emergency department with chest pain and nondiagnostic electrocardiogram (ECG), using ECG results versus ECG plus clinical data or acute Tc 99m sestamibi imaging results. The ability to separate low-risk and high-risk subgroups was better with Tc 99m sestamibi imaging than ECG alone or with clinical data. (From Hilton TC, Thompson RC, Williams HJ, et al: Technetium-99m sestamibi myocardial perfusion imaging in the emergency room evaluation of chest pain. J Am Coll Cardiol 1994;23:1016–1022.)

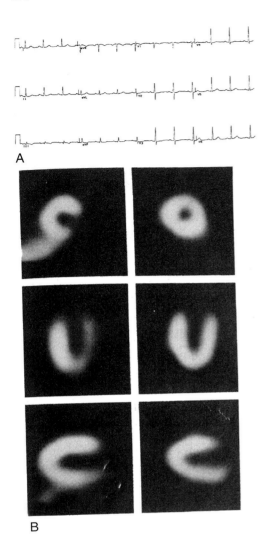

A

B

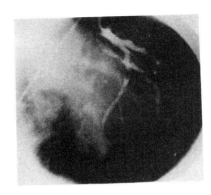

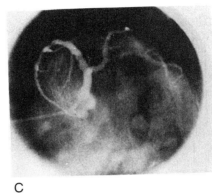

C

FIGURE 19–8. *A,* A 60-year-old man presenting with chest pain but non-specific electrocardiogram. *B,* Acute Tc 99m sestamibi imaging in the short-axis *(top),* horizontal long-axis *(middle),* and vertical long-axis *(bottom)* projection shows a perfusion defect in the lateral wall *(left column).* *C,* Coronary angiography showed a high-grade lesion in the left circumflex artery on right anterior oblique *(upper)* and left anterior oblique *(lower)* projections. After coronary angioplasty, repeat Tc 99m sestamibi imaging showed resolution of the perfusion defect (*B, right column*). (From Hilton TC, Thompson RC, Williams HJ, et al: Technetium-99m sestamibi myocardial perfusion imaging in the emergency room evaluation of chest pain. J Am Coll Cardiol 1994;23:1016–1022.)

■ ▪ ■

TABLE 19–4 NEGATIVE PREDICTIVE VALUE OF NORMAL REST TECHNETIUM 99m SESTAMIBI IMAGING IN PATIENTS WHO PRESENT TO THE EMERGENCY DEPARTMENT WITH CHEST PAIN AND NONDIAGNOSTIC ELECTROCARDIOGRAM

AUTHORS	YEAR	TOTAL PATIENTS	NORMAL PATIENTS (% OF TOTAL)	NPV (%)
Bilodeau et al[103]	1991	45	26 (58%)	94
Varetto et al[104]	1993	64	34 (53%)	100
Hilton et al[105]	1994	102	70 (69%)	99
Tatum et al[106]	1997	438	338 (77%)	100
Kontos et al[107]	1997	532	361 (68%)	99
Heller et al[108]	1998	357	204 (57%)	99
Kontos et al[109]	1998	620	379 (61%)	99

NPV, negative predictive value:

risk) were presumed to have ischemia and were admitted. Level 3 and 4 patients (low to moderate risk) had Tc 99m sestamibi imaging–guided management, whereas level 5 patients (very low risk) were sent home without additional testing. Among 438 patients undergoing acute imaging (level 3 or 4), 338 patients had normal imaging results. Over the next year, no patient with normal imaging had an acute MI, and only 10 (3%) underwent coronary revascularization. In contrast, of the 100 patients with resting perfusion defects, 42 developed an ischemic cardiac event, including 20 (20%) deaths or MIs. Acute rest imaging can play an important role in identifying low-risk patients who can be sent home safely and high-risk patients who require additional study.

ACT Strategy for Chest Pain Evaluation and Triage
Risk Based and Goal-Driven

Level Assignment Based on CP Character, History, and Initial ECG

RISK →

Level	Risk	Goal	Disposition	Diagnostic Strategy
1	Very High	Intervention	Treat and Admit CICU	Presenting ECG
2	High	Intervention	Admit CICU	Serial ECGs and Markers
3	Moderate	R/in ACS	"Fast Track"	Serial ECGs Acute Perfusion Imaging
4	Low	Risk Stratification	ED Workup	Acute Perfusion Imaging
5	Very Low	Alternate Diagnosis	Home	Appropriate Referral

Acute Cardiac Team (ACT) Medical College of Virginia Hospitals / VCU / Richmond, Va.

FIGURE 19–9. Strategy at Medical College of Virginia Hospitals for chest pain evaluation and triage in the emergency department based on assessment of clinical risk and integration of acute nuclear perfusion imaging into decision analysis for low-risk and moderate-risk patients. (From Tatum JL, Jesse RL: Emergency department triage and imaging of patients with acute chest pain. In Zaret BL, Beller GA [eds]: Nuclear Cardiology State of the Art and Future Directions, 2nd ed. St Louis, Mosby, 1999, pp 468–489.)

Cost-Effectiveness

Several studies evaluated the potential cost savings associated with the use of acute emergency department imaging to guide management.[111-113] In a series of patients presenting to the emergency department with unexplained chest pain, Weissman and associates[111] compared the costs of acute Tc 99m sestamibi imaging plus the costs of altered management based on imaging results with the costs of managing patients before imaging was introduced. Using acute imaging to guide management, costs were reduced by almost $800 per patient, and no patient sent home on the basis of normal imaging had an adverse event. Similarly, Radensky and colleagues[112] compared a strategy of using acute Tc 99m sestamibi imaging to guide admission (positive scan) or discharge (normal scan) with a strategy that used only clinical and ECG data. They found that costs were reduced by more than $1000 per patient by using acute imaging to guide triage of patients. The cost savings were due to a much lower admission rate for patients who *did not* have cardiac events with the imaging-guided strategy (14%) versus the clinical and ECG data–guided strategy (54%). At the same time, the sensitivity for detecting patients at risk for cardiac events using imaging was not compromised: 94% versus 88% for the clinical and ECG data strategy.

Stowers and coworkers[113] compared the resource use and outcome of intermediate-risk patients presenting to the emergency department with chest pain and no ECG evidence of acute ischemia who were randomized to either conventional or Tc 99m sestamibi MPI–guided management. In the MPI-guided group, patients were treated according to a predefined protocol based on imaging results. Patients with a positive scan underwent cardiac catheterization, whereas patients with a negative scan underwent exercise treadmill testing. Patients in the conventional treatment group were managed at their physician's discretion. Investigators found that although in-hospital and 30-day event rates were similar, MPI-guided patients had $1843 less median in-hospital costs and 2 days shorter hospitalizations than conventionally treated patients. Cost savings were related to a lower rate of cardiac catheterization and the shorter stay.

Acute rest MPI in the emergency department can be an effective diagnostic and prognostic tool that can help physicians make management decisions for patients with undefined chest pain syndromes, leading to cost savings without compromising patient outcomes. This tool should become increasingly attractive as pressures for cost containment increase at the same time that usage of emergency department resources grows.

CONCLUSIONS

Nuclear cardiology techniques have powerful diagnostic and prognostic value that can help physicians make timely and rational management decisions across a wide spectrum of patients with ACS. By distinguishing the low-risk patient who would not benefit from further testing or intervention from the high-risk patient who would benefit, nuclear techniques can lead to cost-effective use of medical resources and to optimizing patient outcome. It also can help evaluate the presence of viable myocardium in patients with left ventricular dysfunction as an additional guide toward revascularization.

REFERENCES

1. Risk stratification and survival after myocardial infarction. N Engl J Med 1983;309:331–336.

2. Zaret BL, Wackers FJ, Terrin ML, et al: Value of radionuclide rest and exercise left ventricular ejection fraction in assessing survival of patients after thrombolytic therapy for acute myocardial infarction: Results of Thrombolysis in Myocardial Infarction (TIMI) phase II study. The TIMI Study Group. J Am Coll Cardiol 1995;26:73–79.

3. Rouleau JL, Talajik M, Sussex B, et al: Myocardial infarction patients in the 1990s—their risk factors, stratification and survival in Canada: The Canadian Assessment of Myocardial Infarction (CAMI) Study. J Am Coll Cardiol 1996;27:1119–1127.

4. Simoons ML, Vos J, Tijssen JG, et al: Long-term benefit of early thrombolytic therapy in patients with acute myocardial infarction: 5 year follow-up of a trial conducted by the Interuniversity Cardiology Institute of the Netherlands. J Am Coll Cardiol 1989;14:1609–1615.

5. Dakik HA, Mahmarian JJ, Kimball KT, et al: Prognostic value of exercise ^{201}T1 tomography in patients treated with thrombolytic therapy during acute myocardial infarction. Circulation 1996;94: 2735–2742.

6. Beller GA: Clinical Nuclear Cardiology. Philadelphia, WB Saunders, 1995, pp 21–36.

7. Christian TF, Behrenbeck T, Pellikka PA, et al: Mismatch of left ventricular function and infarct size demonstrated by technetium-99m-isonitrile imaging after reperfusion therapy for acute myocardial infarction: Identification of myocardial stunning and hyperkinesias. J Am Coll Cardiol 1990;16:1632–1638.

8. Allman KC, Shaw LJ, Hachamovitch R, Udelson JE: Myocardial viability testing and impact of revascularization on prognosis in patients with coronary artery disease and left ventricular dysfunction: A meta-analysis. J Am Coll Cardiol 2002;39:1151–1158.

9. Brown KA: Prognostic value of thallium-201 myocardial perfusion imaging: A diagnostic tool comes to age. Circulation 1991;83: 363–381.

10. Brown KA: Prognostic value of myocardial perfusion imaging: State of the art and new developments. J Nucl Cardiol 1996;3:516–537.

11. Brown KA, Boucher CA, Okada RD, et al: Prognostic value of exercise thallium-201 imaging in patients presenting for evaluation of chest pain. J Am Coll Cardiol 1983;1:994–1001.

12. Ladenheim ML, Pollack BH, Royanski A, et al: Extent and severity of myocardial reperfusion as predictors of prognosis in patients with suspected coronary artery disease. J Am Coll Cardiol 1986;7: 464–471.

13. Eitzman D, Al-Aour Z, Kanter HL, et al: Clinical outcome of patients with advanced coronary artery disease after viability studies with positron emission tomography. J Am Coll Cardiol 1992; 20:559–565.

14. Lee KS, Marwick TH, Cook SA, et al: Prognosis of patients with left ventricular dysfunction, with and without viable myocardium after myocardial infarction. Circulation 1994;90:2687–2694.

15. Tamaki N, Kawamoto M, Takahashi N, et al: Prognostic value of an increase in fluorine-18 deoxyglucose uptake in patients with myocardial infarction: Comparison with stress thallium imaging. J Am Coll Cardiol 1993;22:1621–1627.

16. Gibson RS, Watson DD, Craddock GB, et al: Prediction of cardiac events after uncomplicated myocardial infarction: A prospective study comparing predischarge exercise thallium-201 scintigraphy and coronary angiography. Circulation 1983;68:321–336.

17. Wilson WW, Gibson RS, Nygaard TW, et al: Acute myocardial infarction associated with single vessel coronary artery disease: An analysis of clinical outcome and the prognostic importance of vessel patency and residual ischemic myocardium. J Am Coll Cardiol 1988;11:223–234.

18. Travin MI, Dessouki A, Cameron T, Heller GV: Use of exercise technetium-99m sestamibi SPECT imaging to detect residual ischemia and for risk stratification after acute myocardial infarction. Am J Cardiol 1995;74:665–669.

19. Boucher CA, Zir LM, Beller GA, et al: Increased lung uptake of thallium-201 during exercise myocardial imaging: Clinical, hemodynamic and angiographic implications in patients with coronary artery disease. Am J Cardiol 1980;46:189–196.

20. Brown KA, McKay R, Heller GV, et al: Hemodynamic determinants of lung thallium-201 uptake in patients during atrial pacing stress. Am Heart J 1986;111:103–107.

21. Bingham JB, McKusick KA, Strauss HW, et al: Influence of coronary artery disease on pulmonary uptake of thallium-201. Am J Cardiol 1980;46:821–826.

22. Bodenheimer MM, Wackers FJTH, Schwartz RG, et al: Prognostic significance of a fixed thallium defect one to six months after onset of acute myocardial infarction or unstable angina. Multicenter Myocardial Ischemia Research Group. Am J Cardiol 1994;74: 1196–1200.

23. Brown KA, Boucher CA, Okada RD, et al: Quantification of pulmonary thallium-201 activity after upright exercise in normal persons: Importance of peak heart rate and propranolol usage in defining normal values. Am J Cardiol 1984;53:1678–1682.

24. Kushner FG, Okada RD, Kirshenbaum HD, et al: Lung thallium-201 uptake after stress testing in patients with coronary artery disease. Circulation 1981;63:341–347.

25. Kaul S, Finkelstein DM, Homma S, et al: Superiority of quantitative exercise thallium-201 variables in determining long-term prognosis in ambulatory patients with chest pain: A comparison with cardiac catheterization. J Am Coll Cardiol 1988;12:25–34.

26. Gill JB, Ruddy TD, Newell JB, et al: Prognostic importance of thallium uptake by the lungs during exercise in coronary artery disease. N Engl J Med 1987;317:1486–1489.

27. Lette J, Lapointe J, Waters D, et al: Transient left ventricular cavity dilation during dipyridamole-thallium imaging as an indicator of severe coronary artery disease. Am J Cardiol 1990;66: 1163–1170.

28. Stolzenberg J: Dilatation of left ventricular cavity on stress thallium scans as an indicator of ischemic disease. Clin Nucl Med 1980;5:289–291.

29. Weiss AT, Berman DS, Lew AS, et al: Transient ischemic dilation of the left ventricle on stress thallium-201 scintigraphy: A marker of severe and extensive coronary artery disease. J Am Coll Cardiol 1987;9:752–759.

30. Krawczynska EG, Weintraub WS, Garcia EV, et al: Left ventricular dilatation and multivessel coronary artery disease on thallium-201 SPECT are important prognostic indicators in patients with large defects in the left anterior descending distribution. Am J Cardiol 1994;74:1233–1239.

31. Young DZ, Guiney TE, McKusick KA, et al: Unmasking potential myocardial ischemia with dipyridamole-thallium imaging in patients with normal submaximal exercise thallium tests. Am J Noninvas Cardiol 1987;1:11–17.

32. Leppo JA, O'Brien J, Rothendler JA, et al: Dipyridamole-thallium-201 scintigraphy in the prediction of future cardiac events after acute myocardial infarction. N Engl J Med 1984;310:1014–1018.

33. Mahmarian JJ, Pratt CM, Nishimura S, et al: Quantitative adenosine ^{201}T1 single-photon emission computed tomography for the early assessment of patients surviving acute myocardial infarction. Circulation 1993;87:1197–1210.

34. Mahmarian JJ, Mahmarian AC, Marks GF, et al: Role of adenosine thallium-201 tomography for defining long-term risk in patients after acute myocardial infarction. J Am Coll Cardiol 1995;25: 1333–1340.

35. Geleijnse ML, Elhendy A, Fioretti PM, Roeland JR: Dobutamine stress myocardial perfusion imaging. J Am Coll Cardiol 2000;36: 2017–2027.

36. Geleijnse ML, Elhendy A, Van Domburg RT, et al: Prognostic significance of normal dobutamine-atropine stress sestamibi scintigraphy in women with chest pain. Am J Cardiol 1996;77:1057–1061.

37. Geleijnse ML, Elhendy A, Van Domburg RT, et al: Prognostic value of dobutamine-atropine stress technetium-99m sestamibi perfusion scintigraphy in patients with chest pain. J Am Coll Cardiol 1996; 28:447–454.

38. Geleijnse ML, Elhendy A, Cornel JH, et al: Cardiac imaging for risk stratification with dobutamine-atropine stress testing in patients with chest pain: Echocardiography, perfusion scintigraphy or both? Circulation 1997;96:137–147.

39. Senior R, Raval U, Lahiri A: Prognostic value of stress dobutamine technetium-99m sestamibi single-photon emission computed tomography (SPECT) in patients with suspected coronary artery disease. Am J Cardiol 1996;78:1092–1096.

40. Calnon DA, McGrath PD, Doss AL, et al: Prognostic value of dobutamine stress technetium-99m sestamibi single-photon emission computed tomography myocardial perfusion imaging: Stratification of a high-risk population. J Am Coll Cardiol 2001;38: 1511–1517.

41. Van Damme H, Piérard L, Gillain D, et al: Cardiac risk assessment before vascular surgery: A prospective study comparing clinical evaluation, dobutamine stress echocardiography and dobutamine Tc-99m sestamibi tomoscintigraphy. Cardiovasc Surg 1997;5:54–64.

42. Elliott BM, Robison JG, Zellner JL, Hendrix GH: Dobutamine-201Tl imaging: Assessing cardiac risk associated with vascular surgery. Circulation 1991;84(Suppl III):III54–III60.

43. Coma-Canella I, Gomez Martinez MV, Rodrigo F, Castro Beiras JM: The dobutamine stress test with thallium-201 single-photon emission computed tomography and radionuclide angiography: Postinfarction study. J Am Coll Cardiol 1993;22:399–406.

44. Elhendy A, Cornel JH, Roelandt JR, et al: Dobutamine thallium-201 SPECT imaging for assessment of peri-infarction and remote myocardial ischemia. J Nucl Med 1996;37:1951–1956.

45. Elhendy A, Geleijnse ML, Roelandt JR, et al: Comparison of dobutamine stress echocardiography and 99m-technetium sestamibi SPECT myocardial perfusion scintigraphy for predicting extent of coronary artery disease in patients with healed myocardial infarction. Am J Cardiol 1997;79:7–12.

46. Lancellotti P, Benoit T, Rigo R, Pierard LA: Dobutamine stress echocardiography versus quantitative technetium-99m sestamibi SPECT for detecting residual stenosis and multivessel disease after myocardial infarction. Heart 2001;86:510–515.

47. Leppo JA, Boucher CA, Okada RD, et al: Serial Tl-201 myocardial imaging after dipyridamole infusion: Diagnostic utility in detecting coronary stenoses and relationship to regional wall motion. Circulation 1982;66:649–656.

48. Iskandrian AS, Heo J, Askenase A, et al: Dipyridamole cardiac imaging. Am Heart J 1988;115:432–443.

49. Homma S, Gilliland Y, Guiney TE, et al: Safety of intravenous dipyridamole for stress testing with thallium imaging. Am J Cardiol 1987;59:152–154.

50. Iskandrian AS, Verani MS: Pharmacologic stress testing and other alternative techniques in the diagnosis of coronary artery disease. In Iskandrian AS, Verani MS (eds): Nuclear Cardiac Imaging: Principles and Applications, 2nd ed. Philadelphia, FA Davis, 1995.

51. Brown KA, O'Meara J, Chambers CE, Plante DA: Ability of dipyridamole-thallium-201 imaging 1 to 4 days after acute myocardial infarction to predict in-hospital and late recurrent myocardial ischemic events. Am J Cardiol 1990;65:160–167.

52. Brown KA, Heller GV, Landin RJ, et al: Early dipyridamole Tc99m-sestamibi SPECT imaging 2–4 days after acute myocardial infarction predicts in-hospital and post-discharge cardiac events: Comparison with submaximal exercise imaging. Circulation 1999;100:2060–2066.

53. Comparison of invasive and conservative strategies after treatment with intravenous tissue plasminogen activator in acute myocardial infarction: Results of the Thrombolysis in Myocardial Infarction (TIMI) phase II trial. The TIMI Study Group. N Engl J Med 1989;320:618–627.

54. SWIFT trial of delayed elective intervention vs conservative treatment after thrombolysis with anistreplase in acute myocardial infarction. SWIFT (Should We Intervene Following Thrombolysis?) Trial Study Group. BMJ 1991;302:555–560.

55. Ellis SG, Mooney MR, George BS, et al: Randomized trial of late elective angioplasty versus conservative management for patients with residual stenoses after thrombolytic treatment of myocardial infarction. Treatment of Post-Thrombolytic Stenoses (TOPS) Study Group. Circulation 1992;86:1400–1406.

56. Dakik HA, Verani MS: Use of invasive and nuclear stress testing in patients with acute ischemic syndromes in a large, urban, university-affiliated hospital. J Nucl Cardiol 2000;7:328–332.

57. Cannon CP, Braunwald E: Unstable angina. In Braunwald E, Zipes DP, Library P (eds): Heart Disease, vol 2, 6th ed. Philadelphia, WB Saunders, 2001, pp 1232–1271.

58. Grambow DW, Topol EJ: Effect of maximal medical therapy on refractoriness of unstable angina pectoris. Am J Cardiol 1992;70:577–581.

59. Hillert MC, Narahara KA, Smitherman TC, et al: Thallium-201 perfusion imaging after the treatment of unstable angina pectoris: Relationship to clinical outcome. West J Med 1986;145:355–340.

60. Madsen JK, Stubgaard M, Utne HE, et al: Prognosis and thallium-201 scintigraphy in patients admitted with chest pain without confirmed acute myocardial infarction. Br Heart J 1988;59:184–189.

61. Marmur JD, Freeman MR, Langer A, et al: Prognosis in medically stabilized unstable angina: Early Holter ST segment monitoring compared with predischarge exercise thallium tomography. Ann Intern Med 1990;113:575–579.

62. Brown KA: Prognostic value of thallium-201 myocardial perfusion imaging in patients with unstable angina who respond to medical treatment. J Am Coll Cardiol 1991;17:1053–1057.

63. Stratmann HG, Younis LT, Wittry MD, et al: Exercise technetium-99m myocardial tomography for the risk stratification of men with medically treated unstable angina pectoris. Am J Cardiol 1995;76:236–240.

64. Phibbs B, Marcus F, Marriott HJ, et al: Q-wave versus non-Q wave myocardial infarction: A meaningless distinction. J Am Coll Cardiol 1999;33:576–582.

65. Gibson RS, Beller GA, Gheorghiade M, et al: The prevalence and clinical significance of residual myocardial ischemia 2 weeks after uncomplicated non-Q-wave myocardial infarction: Prospective natural history study. Circulation 1986;73:1186–1198.

66. TIMI Study Group: Effects of tissue plasminogen activator and a comparison of early invasive and conservative strategies in unstable angina and non-Q-wave myocardial infarction. Results of the TIMI IIIB trial. Circulation 1994;89:1545–1556.

67. Anderson HV, Cannon CP, Stone PH, et al: One-year results of the thrombolysis in myocardial infarction (TIMI) IIIB trial: A randomized comparison of tissue-type plasminogen activator versus placebo and early invasive versus early conservative strategies in unstable angina and non-Q wave myocardial infarction. J Am Coll Cardiol 1995;26:1643–1650.

68. Boden WE, O'Rourke RA, Crawford MH, et al: Outcomes in patients with acute non-Q wave myocardial infarction randomly assigned to an invasive as compared to a conservative management strategy. N Engl J Med 1998;338:1785–1792.

69. Cannon CP, Weintraub WS, Demopoulos LA, et al: Comparison of early invasive and conservative strategies in patients with unstable coronary syndromes treated with the glycoprotein IIb (IIIa) inhibitor tizofiban. N Engl J Med 2001;344:1879–1887.

70. Solomon DH, Stone PH, Glynn RJ, et al: Use of risk stratification to identify patients with unstable angina likeliest to benefit from an invasive versus conservative management strategy. J Am Coll Cardiol 2001;38:969–978.

71. FRagmin and Fast Revascularisation during InStability in Coronary artery disease Investigators. Invasive compared with non-invasive treatment in unstable coronary artery disease: FRISC II prospective randomised multicentre study. Lancet 1999;354:708–715.

72. Lee TH, Cook EF, Weisberg M, et al: Acute chest pain in the emergency room: Identification and examination of low-risk patients. Arch Intern Med 1985;145:65–69.

73. Lee TH, Rouan GW, Weisberg MC, et al: Clinical characteristics and natural history of patients with acute myocardial infarction sent home from the emergency room. Am J Cardiol 1987;60:219–224.

74. McCarthy BD, Beshanky JR, D'Agostino RB, et al: Missed diagnoses of acute myocardial infarction in the emergency department results from a multicenter study. Ann Emerg Med 1993;22:579–582.

75. Pozen MW, D'Agostino RB, Selker HP, et al: A predictive instrument to improve coronary-care-unit admission practices in acute ischemic heart disease: A prospective multicenter trial. N Engl J Med 1984;310:1273–1278.

76. Puleo PR, Meyer D, Wathen C, et al: Use of a rapid assay of subforms of creatine kinase-MB to diagnose or rule out acute myocardial infarction. N Engl J Med 1994;331:561–566.

77. Rouan GW, Hedges JR, Toltzis R, et al: A chest clinic pain to improve the follow-up of patients released from an urban university teaching hospital emergency department. Ann Emerg Med 1987;16:1145–1150.

78. Tierney WM, Fitzgerald J, McHenry R, et al: Physicians' estimates of the probability of myocardial infarction in emergency room patients with chest pain. Med Decis Making 1986;6:12–17.

79. Young GP, Green TR: The role of single ECG, creatine kinase and CKMB in diagnosing patients with acute chest pain. Am J Emerg Med 1993;11:444–449.

80. Zarling EJ, Sexton H, Milnor PJ: Failure to diagnose acute myocardial infarction: The clinicopathologic experience at the large community hospital. JAMA 1983;250:1177–1181.

81. Pope JH, Aufderheide TP, Ruthazer R, Woolard RH, Feldman JA, Beshansky JR, Griffith JL, Selker HP: Missed diagnoses of acute

cardiac ischemia in the emergency department. N Engl J Med 2000;342:1163–1170.

82. Pozen MW, D'Agostino RB, Selker HP, et al: A predictive instrument to improve coronary-care-unit admission practices in acute ischemic heart disease: A prospective multicenter trial. N Engl J Med 1984;310:1273–1278.

83. Goldman L, Weinberg M, Weisberg M, et al: A computer-derived protocol to aid in the diagnosis of emergency room patients with acute chest pain. N Engl J Med 1982;307:588–596.

84. Goldman L, Cook EF, Brand DA, et al: A computer protocol to predict myocardial infarction in emergency department patients with chest pain. N Engl J Med 1988;318:797–803.

85. Tierney WM, Roth BJ, Psaty B, et al: Predictors of myocardial infarction in emergency room patients. Crit Care Med 1985;13:526–531.

86. Jayes RL Jr, Beshansky JR, D'Agostino RB, et al: Do patients' coronary risk factor reports predict acute cardiac ischemia in the emergency department? A multicenter study. J Clin Epidemiol 1992;45:621–626.

87. Rouan GW, Lee TH, Cook EF, et al: Clinical characteristics and outcome of acute myocardial infarction in patients with initially normal or nonspecific electrocardiograms (a report from the Multicenter Chest Pain Study). Am J Cardiol 1989;64:1087–1092.

88. Wackers FJ, Sokole EB, Samson G, et al: Value and limitations of thallium-201 scintigraphy in the acute phase of myocardial infarction. N Engl J Med 1976;295:1–5.

89. Wackers FJ, Lie KI, Liem KL, et al: Potential value of thallium-201 scintigraphy as a means of selecting patients for the coronary care unit. Br Heart J 1979;41:111–117.

90. Wackers FJ, Lie KI, Liem KL, et al: Thallium-201 scintigraphy in unstable angina pectoris. Circulation 1978;57:738–742.

91. Brown KA, Okada RD, Boucher CA, et al: Serial thallium-201 imaging at rest in patients with unstable and stable angina pectoris: Relationship of myocardial perfusion at rest to presenting clinical syndrome. Am Heart J 1983;106:70–77.

92. van der Wieken LR, Kan G, Belfer AJ, et al: Thallium-201 scanning to decide CCU admission in patients with non-diagnostic electrocardiograms. Int J Cardiol 1983;4:285–295.

93. Ritchie JL, Williams DL, Harp G, et al: Transaxial tomography with thallium-201 for detecting remote myocardial infarction: Comparison with planar imaging. Am J Cardiol 1982;50:1236–1241.

94. Tamaki S, Kambara H, Kadota K, et al: Improved detection of myocardial infarction by emission computed tomography with thallium-201: Relation to infarct size. Br Heart J 1984;52:621–627.

95. Whal JM, Hakki A-H, Iskandrian AS, et al: Scintigraphic characterization of Q wave and non-Q-wave acute myocardial infarction. Am Heart J 1985;109:769–775.

96. DePasquale EE, Nody AC, DePuey EG, et al: Quantitative rotational thallium-201 tomography for identifying and localizing coronary artery disease. Circulation 1988;77:316–327.

97. Fintel DJ, Links JM, Brinker JA, et al: Improved diagnostic performance of exercise thallium-201 single photon emission computed tomography over planar imaging in the diagnosis of coronary artery disease: A receiver operating characteristic analysis. J Am Coll Cardiol 1989;13:600–612.

98. DePuey EG, Rozanski A: Using gated technetium-99m-sestamibi SPECT to characterize fixed myocardial defects as infarct or artifact. J Nucl Med 1995;36:952–955.

99. Nicholson CS, Tatum JL, Jesse RL, et al: The value of gated tomographic Tc-99m sestamibi perfusion imaging in acute ischemic syndromes. J Nucl Cardiol 1995;2:S57.

100. Okada RD, Glover D, Gafney T, Williams S: Myocardial kinetics of technetium-99m-hexakis-2-methoxy-2-methylpropyl isonitrile. Circulation 1988;77:491–498.

101. Li QS, Frank TL, Franceschi D, et al: Technetium-99m-methoxy isobutyl isonitrile (RP30) for quantification of myocardial ischemia and reperfusion in dogs. J Nucl Med 1988;29:1539–1548.

102. Christian TF, Clements IP, Gibbons RJ: Noninvasive identification of myocardium at risk in patients with acute myocardial infarction and nondiagnostic electrocardiograms with technetium-99m-sestamibi. Circulation 1991;83:1615–1620.

103. Bilodeau L, Theroux P, Gregoire J, et al: Technetium-99m sestamibi tomography in patients with spontaneous chest pain: Correlations with clinical, electrocardiographic and angiographic findings. J Am Coll Cardiol 1991;18:1684–1691.

104. Varetto T, Cantalupi D, Altieri A, et al: Emergency room technetium-99m sestamibi imaging to rule out acute myocardial ischemic events in patients with nondiagnostic electrocardiograms. J Am Coll Cardiol 1993;22:1804–1808.

105. Hilton TC, Thompson RC, Williams HJ, et al: Technetium-99m sestamibi myocardial perfusion imaging in the emergency room evaluation of chest pain. J Am Coll Cardiol 1994;23:1016–1022.

106. Tatum JL, Jesse RI, Kontos MC, et al: A comprehensive strategy for the evaluation and triage of the chest pain patient. Ann Emerg Med 1997;29:116–125.

107. Kontos MC, Jesse RL, Schmidt KL, et al: Value of acute rest sestamibi perfusion imaging for evaluation of patients admitted to the emergency department with chest pain. J Am Coll Cardiol 1997;30:976–982.

108. Heller GV, Stowers SA, Hendel RC, et al: Clinical value of acute rest technetium-99m tetrofosmin tomographic myocardial perfusion imaging in patients with acute chest pain and nondiagnostic electrocardiograms. J Am Coll Cardiol 1998;31:1011–1017.

109. Kontos MC, Arrowood JA, Jesse RL, et al: Comparison of echocardiography and myocardial perfusion imaging for diagnosing emergency department patients with chest pain. Am Heart J 1998;136:724–733.

110. Tatum JL, Jesse RL: Emergency department triage and imaging of patients with acute chest pain. In Zaret BL, Beller GA (eds): Nuclear Cardiology State of the Art and Future Directions, 2nd ed. St Louis, Mosby, 1999, pp 468–489.

111. Weissman IA, Dickinson CZ, Dworkin HJ, et al: Cost-effectiveness of myocardial perfusion imaging with SPECT in the emergency department evaluation of patients with unexplained chest pain. Radiology 1996;199:353–357.

112. Radensky PW, Hilton TC, Fulmer H, et al: Potential cost effectiveness of initial myocardial perfusion imaging for assessment of emergency department patients with chest pain. Am J Cardiol 1997;79:595–599.

113. Stowers SA, Eisenstein EL, Wackers FJTh, et al: An economic analysis of an aggressive diagnostic strategy with single photon emission computed tomography myocardial perfusion imaging and early exercise stress testing in emergency department patients who present with chest pain but nondiagnostic electrocardiograms: Results from a randomized trial. Ann Emerg Med 2000;35:17–25.

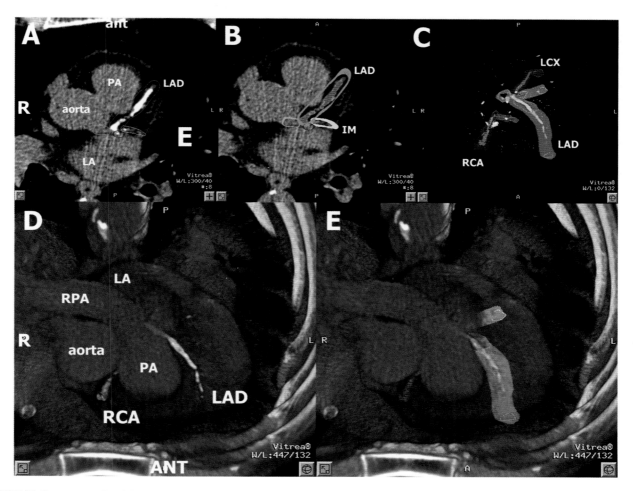

FIGURE 20–3. An example of detection and quantification of coronary calcium. *A*, To selectively quantify coronary calcified deposits, the coronary arteries are manually contoured in the axial slices. *B* and *C*, These contours are then connected and voxels within the boundaries of the segmented volume, which have density values beyond the threshold (130 HU) and are labeled *(red)*. *D* and *E*, In the three-dimensional volume-rendered representations of the nonenhanced MSCT scans, the calcifications in the left anterior descending artery (LAD) and right coronary artery (RCA) are easily spotted. The respective Agatston and volume score of the main branches were: left main 0, 0; LAD 988, 629; left circumflex branch (LCX):673, 445; RCA: 1629, 1061; posterior descending artery: 40, 35. The total score for this patient was 3330 or 2170, respectively, which can be considered high, regardless of his age. ANT, anterior; LA, left atrium; PA, pulmonary artery; R, right; RPA, right pulmonary artery.

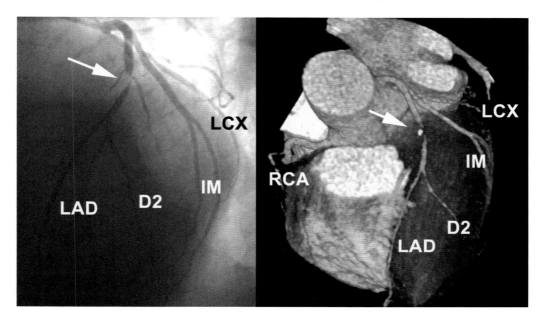

FIGURE 20–6. Conventional CT and MSCT coronary angiograms (three-dimensional volume-rendered) of a patient with a stenotic coronary lesion in the middle left anterior descending branch (LAD), just distal from the small first diagonal branch. The calcified contents of the plaque are visualized on the MSCT angiogram. The left circumflex coronary artery (LCX), right coronary artery (RCA), second diagonal branch (D2), and intermediate branch (IM) can also be appreciated.

Computed Tomography in Coronary Artery Disease

Pim J. de Feyter
Koen Nieman

Coronary artery wall and lumen imaging poses the greatest challenge to any diagnostic technique: The coronary arteries are small and tortuous and course in complex multiple planes around the heart, while cardiac contraction and respiration cause motion artifacts. Therefore, coronary imaging requires high spatial resolution and high-speed acquisition technology. In the mid-1980s, electron beam computed tomography (EBCT) was introduced. This scanner was capable of acquiring tomograms in as little as 50 ms and 100 ms. The high spatial resolution and high-speed acquisition allowed detection and quantification of coronary calcification and, in a substantial number of patients, the contrast-enhanced coronary lumen was adequately imaged.

More recently, another technique of high spatial resolution and fast acquisition has been introduced: multislice spiral computed tomography (MSCT). This technique is also able to detect and quantify coronary calcifications and to visualize coronary arteries.

Both noninvasive coronary imaging techniques are gradually emerging as new diagnostic tools into the cardiology department. The usefulness of both techniques in the diagnosis and management of coronary artery disease, and in particular acute coronary syndromes, is just beginning to evolve.

EBCT AND MSCT SCANNERS

Two types of scanners are used for noninvasive assessment of the coronary arteries. Both scanners can produce nonenhanced scans for calcium quantification and contrast-enhanced scans for luminal assessment of the coronary arteries. Although calcium deposits can be detected in contrast-enhanced scans as well, quantification is regarded as unreliable in the presence of contrast media. Contrast-enhancement is achieved by continuous injection of an iodine-containing medium in a peripheral vein, typically the antecubital vein, throughout the duration of the scan, accounting for the contrast-transit time.

To compensate for cardiac motion and prevent motion artifacts, the data acquisition or image reconstruction needs to be synchronized with the electrocardiogram (ECG). The data acquisition needs to be performed within the time of a single breath hold.

Electron Beam Computed Tomography

The EBCT scanner is a nonmechanical sequential scanner (Fig. 20-1). After each acquisition, a 216-degree electron beam sweep that requires only 100 ms, the table is advanced 1.5 or 2.0 mm to the next slice position. By use of prospective ECG-triggering, single slices are acquired at every second heartbeat to allow for the table translations. A greater number of slices can be acquired at higher heart rates, which can be promoted by administration of a small dose of atropine prior to the test. Two angiographic protocols are being used: a consecutive 1.5 mm–slice protocol or an overlapping 3.0 mm–slice protocol, with a table increment of 2.0 mm. Generally, a Z-range of 7 to 10 cm can be covered during a breath hold lasting 35 to 45 seconds.

Multislice Spiral Computed Tomography

The MSCT scanner is a mechanical spiral scanner (Fig. 20-2). Contrary to sequential scanners, the table moves continuously while spiral CT data from up to four detector rows are acquired simultaneously. Most scanners use a 4 mm × 1 mm collimation protocol at a table increment of 1.5 mm per gantry rotation, which results in a Z-coverage of about 12 cm per breath hold. Retrospectively, the data are matched to the recorded ECG and an overlapping set of 1.25 mm slices can be reconstructed at any given cardiac phase. As a consequence of continuous data acquisition and retrospective image reconstruction, exposure to radiation is currently higher than with EBCT. At an x-ray tube rotation time of 500 ms, images can be created using advanced reconstruction algorithms requiring 250 ms of data or less. This relatively lower temporal resolution, compared with EBCT, can be compensated by use of β-blocking medication prior to the examination.

The calcium quantification scan can be performed in spiral mode with a collimation protocol of 4 mm × 2.5 mm. Because of concerns over x-ray exposure, however, a prospectively triggered sequential mode, with a 4 mm × 2.5 mm collimation, is mostly used.

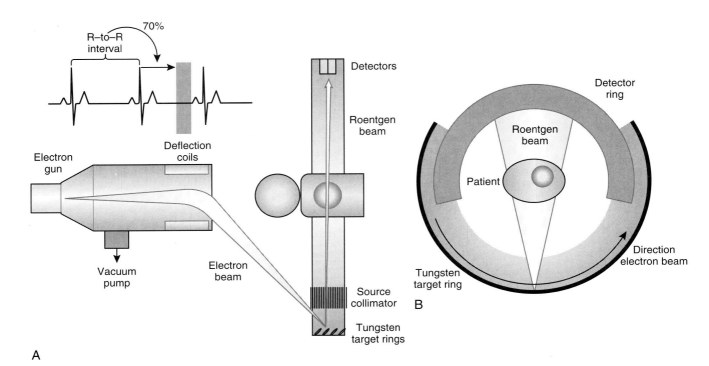

A

FIGURE 20–1. The EBCT scanner is a nonmechanical scanner without a rotating x-ray tube. Instead, an electron beam is directed by deflection coils along a 210-degree tungsten ring. *A,* A complete sweep can be performed within 100 ms or less. *B,* After collision with the target rings, roentgen rays are produced. The roentgen rays are collimated, and a narrow fan beam is directed through the patient. Attenuation projections are collected by a stationary 216-degree detector ring at the opposite side. The electron gun is triggered by the patient's electrocardiogram. According to a number of preceding heart beats, the moment of data acquisition is determined, at for instance 70% of the R-to-R interval, at which time the electron gun is activated and CT data are acquired. After the acquisition, the table is advanced to the next slice position.

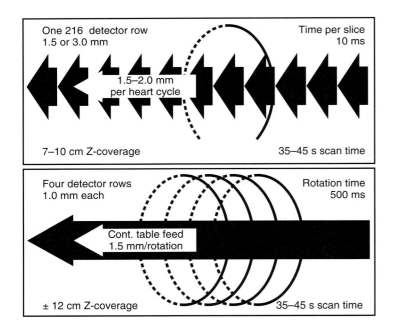

FIGURE 20–2. Sequential versus spiral imaging. The electron beam CT scanner acquires one slice at every second heart beat. Depending on the collimation protocol and the heart rate, a Z-range of 7 to 10 cm can be covered within the time of a breath hold. The multislice spiral CT scanner continuously acquires four channels of data while the table continuously advances through the gantry. For angiographic imaging, the table increment is set at 3 mm per gantry rotation, which, at a rotation time of 500 ms, results in a Z-coverage of about 12 cm in one breath hold. From 250 ms of spiral data per heart cycle, an overlapping number of 1.25 mm slices can be reconstructed at any phase within the cardiac cycle, after the acquisition has been completed.

QUANTIFICATION OF CORONARY CALCIFICATION

EBCT is a safe and sensitive tool to detect and quantify coronary artery calcification. The epicardial arteries can be readily identified because the density of the coronary artery (blood and wall) is higher than that of the surrounding peri-arterial fat. Coronary wall calcium is easily identified because the density of calcium is much higher than that of peri-arterial fat and coronary blood (Fig. 20–3).

Histologic studies have shown that a tissue density of 130 Hounsfield units (HU) is highly correlated with calcified coronary plaques.[1] A calcium scoring system has been devised based on the density of the calcific plaque and the area of calcium deposits: the *Agatston score*.[2] The threshold for a calcific lesion is set at a density of 130 HU for an area of 1 mm[2]. The Agatston score is calculated by multiplying the area of each calcific lesion by a density measure defined by the peak density number of the lesion. The density measure is 1 for a peak density of 130 to 199 HU, 2 for 200 to 299 HU, 3 for 300 to 399 HU, and 4 for 400 HU. The total calcium score is determined by adding up all lesion scores (see Fig. 20–3).

Coronary Calcium to Predict Obstructive Coronary Artery Disease in Patients Undergoing Diagnostic Coronary Angiography

The diagnostic accuracy of the presence of coronary calcium detected with EBCT to predict significant obstructive coronary artery disease was recently established by the Writing Group appointed by the American College of Cardiology and American Heart Association.[3] In a meta-analysis, a total of 3683 patients were enrolled in 16 studies. All patients underwent diagnostic coronary angiography. The prevalence of coronary artery disease averaged 60%. The weighted average sensitivity,

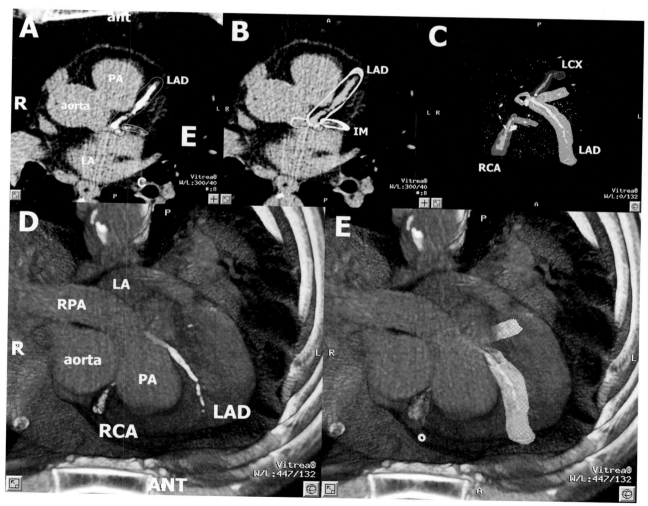

FIGURE 20–3. An example of detection and quantification of coronary calcium. *A,* To selectively quantify coronary calcified deposits, the coronary arteries are manually contoured in the axial slices. *B* and *C,* These contours are then connected and voxels within the boundaries of the segmented volume, which have density values beyond the threshold (130 HU) and are labeled *(red). D* and *E,* In the three-dimensional volume-rendered representations of the nonenhanced MSCT scans, the calcifications in the left anterior descending artery (LAD) and right coronary artery (RCA) are easily spotted. The respective Agatston and volume score of the main branches were: left main 0, 0; LAD 988, 629; left circumflex branch (LCX): 673, 445; RCA: 1629, 1061; posterior descending artery: 40, 35. The total score for this patient was 3330 or 2170, respectively, which can be considered high, regardless of his age. ANT, anterior; LA, left atrium; PA, Pulmonary artery; R, right; RPA, right pulmonary artery. (See color plates.)

specificity, and predictive accuracy was 80.4%, 40%, and 59%, respectively. The individual study sensitivity values ranged from 68% to 100%, whereas the specificity values ranged from 21% to 100%. The wide variation in outcomes reflects the differences in study patients, minimum area of calcified tissue required for a calcific lesion (areas ranged from 0.5 mm^2 to 2.0 mm^2), number of acquired tomograms, and slice thickness (3 to 6 mm).

Coronary Calcium to Predict Coronary Death or Nonfatal Myocardial Infarction in Asymptomatic High-Risk Persons

Coronary calcification is a specific component of coronary atherosclerosis. Individual patients exhibit a wide spectrum of coronary lesions, varying from early noncalcified lesions to far-advanced complicated calcific lesions. The presence of coronary calcium implies the presence of coronary atherosclerosis but cannot reliably distinguish between a stable or a vulnerable plaque. The presence and extent of coronary calcium appears closely related to the overall atherosclerotic plaque burden. Therefore, a large amount of calcium increases the likelihood of the presence of a vulnerable plaque but does not identify a specific vulnerable plaque. On the other hand, absence of calcium does not exclude atherosclerotic disease, including a vulnerable plaque, but its presence is very unlikely.[4]

The presence and extent of coronary calcium may have predictive value for subsequent coronary events in asymptomatic persons.[5-9] Data of three long-term follow-up studies have been published (Table 20–1).[5,7,9] All three studies investigated high risk asymptomatic populations. First, the predictive value of a calcium score is only relevant if it adds incremental predictive value to traditional risk factors. Second, because calcium deposition increases with age and is sex-related, these scores should be adjusted for age as well as for sex to provide optimal predictive value.

Detrano et al demonstrated that assessment of calcium score was not an accurate predictor of death or nonfatal myocardial infarction.[5] Furthermore, the calcium score did not add incremental information to traditional risk factors. However, a calcium score greater than 44 HU was associated with a 2.3 times higher likelihood of suffering a nonfatal myocardial infarction or death than study subjects with lower scores. When the population was divided into tertiles according to the height of the calcium score values, it appeared that the highest tertile was associated with the highest event rate.

Arad et al demonstrated that a coronary calcium score of 160 was associated with an odds ratio of 22.2 for risk of death or nonfatal myocardial infarction compared with persons with a lower score.[7] The calcium scores remained independently associated with outcome after adjustments for self-reported risk factors.

Finally, Raggi et al showed that, in high-risk persons, a calcium score of zero was associated with a 0.12% risk per year of death and nonfatal myocardial infarction; if calcium was present, the risk was 3% per year.[9] The calcium score, when adjusted for age and sex, provided incremental prognostic value to traditional risk factors for coronary artery disease.

In an earlier study, Raggi et al, reporting about 632 individuals followed for 32 ± 7 months, it appeared that both the height of the absolute calcium score and the calcium score divided into quartiles were closely related to the annualized event rate (Table 20–2).[8]

Thus, although the data conflict about the precise predictive value of coronary calcium scoring, it may be concluded that overall the presence of calcium is associated with a higher risk of adverse coronary events (Table 20–3).

Coronary Calcium to Predict Coronary Death and Nonfatal Myocardial Infarction in Symptomatic Patients after Coronary Angiography

Coronary lumen stenosis and coronary calcium are different manifestations of coronary atherosclerosis. Both coronary angiography and coronary calcium assessment provide an estimate of the total coronary plaque burden, but both techniques underestimate the extent and severity of the total plaque burden when compared to histologic studies.[4]

Extent and severity of coronary artery disease as assessed by coronary angiography has been shown to provide predictive value for coronary death and nonfatal myocardial infarction. Coronary calcium may have additional predictive value in patients who have undergone coronary angiography.

Two studies have addressed this issue (Table 20–4).[10,11] Detrano et al demonstrated that the risk of coronary death

■ ■ ■

TABLE 20–1　RISK STRATIFICATION IN ASYMPTOMATIC PERSONS

AUTHOR	NO. OF PATIENTS	RISK	FOLLOW-UP (MONTHS)	MEAN AGE	END POINTS			AGATSTON SCORE
					Male	Death	Nonfatal MI	
Detrano[5]	1196	High	41 ± 5	66 ± 8	89	17	29	>0
Arad[7]	1172	High*	43 (38–47)	53 ± 11	71	3	15	≥ 160
Raggi[9]	676	High†	32 ± 7	52 ± 12	51	9	21	≥0

*Self-referred.
†Referred by primary care physician.
MI, myocardial infarction.

■■■

TABLE 20–2 CALCIUM SCORE AND ANNUALIZED EVENT RATE

ABSOLUTE CA-SCORE CALCIUM SCORE	N	EVENT RATE ANNUALIZED %	QUARTILE	EVENT RATE ANNUALIZED %	ODDS RATIO
0	292	0.11	1	0.2	1.0
1–99	219	2.1	2	0.2	1.0 (0.1, 16.1)
100–400	74	4.1	3	1.4	6.2 (0.7, 52.1)
>400	28	4.8	4	4.5	21.5 (2.8, 162.4)

From Raggi P, et al: Identification of patients at increased risk of first unheralded acute myocardial infarction by electron-beam computed tomography. Circulation 101: 850–855, 2000.

■■■

TABLE 20–3 PREDICTIVE VALUE OF CALCIUM SCORE

	DETRANO[5]	ARAD[7]	RAGGI[9]	
Calcium score	≥44	≥ 160	0	>0
Relative risk of death, nonfatal MI compared with lower Ca scores	2.3	22.2	0.12%*	3.0%*

*Risk per year.

or nonfatal myocardial significantly increased with the calcium load.[10] Patients with a calcium score above median (i.e., > 75) had a six times higher event rate than those with lower scores. When patients were divided into quartiles according to ascending order of calcium amount, it was shown that 1 event occurred in the first quartile, 2 in the second quartile, 8 in the third quartile, and 10 in the fourth quartile. The calcium score predicted hard events just as well as the number of angiographically diseased coronary arteries; however, logistic regression showed that calcium amount independently contributed toward the probability of subsequent coronary events.

Keelan et al showed that patients with a calcium score of 100 had a relative risk of death or nonfatal myocardial infarction of 3.2 (95% CI, 1.2 to 8.7) compared with those who had a lower score.[11]

Multivariate analysis, including traditional risk factors, previous coronary event history, angiographic findings, and calcium score, showed that only age and extent of coronary artery calcification were independent predictors of hard events: relative risk ratios of 1.72 (95% CI, 1.02, 2.9) and 1.9 (95% CI, 1.0, 3.5), respectively, suggest that calcium extent adds significant prognostic information.

Coronary Calcification in Acute Coronary Syndromes

Histopathologic and intracoronary ultrasound studies have shown that early nonobstructive atherosclerotic lesions that contain a large lipid pool and carry a high risk of rupturing are not calcified and thus may not be detected by EBCT.[1] Although calcific lesions are thought to be stable, the extent of coronary calcium is an indicator of the total atherosclerotic plaque burden and thus is associated with a higher likelihood of vulnerable plaques. Coronary calcium is not a marker for stable or unstable plaques, and a negative result on calcium scanning does not rule out a vulnerable plaque.

Schmermund et al reported on the value of EBCT-detected coronary calcium in acute coronary syndromes.[12] They studied 118 patients, 57 ± 11 years of age, with previous myocardial infarction (n = 101) or unstable angina (n = 17). Calcium scan results were positive in 105 (95%) of 110 patients with significant obstructive disease and in 1 of the 8 patients (13%)

■■■

TABLE 20–4 CORONARY CALCIFICATION TO PREDICT CORONARY DEATH OR NONFATAL MYOCARDIAL INFARCTION AFTER CORONARY ANGIOGRAPHY

AUTHOR	NO. OF PATIENTS	AGE (YEARS)	MALES (%)	FOLLOW-UP	DEATH/NONFATAL MI (NO. OF PATIENTS)	CALCIUM SCORE	ADVERSE EVENT RISK*
Detrano[10]	422	55±12	57	30±13 months	13, 8	≥ 75	6 × higher
Keelan[11]	288	56±11	77	Mean 6.9 yrs	22	≥ 100	RR 3.2

*Compared with lower risk scores.
MI, myocardial infarction; RR, relative risk.

without significant obstructive disease. Calcium scan results were negative in five patients (5%) with and in seven (87%) patients without significant obstructive disease. These patients were younger and were active smokers. Raggi et al[8] confirmed these findings in 172 patients with an acute myocardial infarction. Ninety-six percent of these patients showed coronary calcium, and the extent of calcium was higher than expected with regard to age and sex. These studies confirm the idea that the vast majority of patients with an acute coronary syndrome have calcium and that absence of coronary calcium does not exclude the presence of an unstable plaque, although the likelihood of the presence of an unstable plaque is low.

COMPUTED TOMOGRAPHY IN THE EMERGENCY DEPARTMENT

Three studies have evaluated the merits of CT in screening patients admitted to an emergency department who have new chest pain of recent onset, nonspecific ECG findings, no enzyme rise, and no history of coronary artery disease.[13-15]

Laudon et al compared EBCT scan findings with cardiac evaluation findings including treadmill stress testing, radio nuclide testing, dobutamine echo-stress testing, and coronary angiography in 100 patients presenting at the emergency department.[13] Because the prevalence of coronary calcium greatly increases with age, the authors studied men (54%) between the ages of 30 and 55 years and women (46%) between 40 and 65 years. The scan was "positive" if the calcium score was greater than zero. The sensitivity of the positive calcium scan was 100% (95% CI, 77% to 100%) and the specificity was 63% (95% CI, 54% to 75%), resulting in a negative predictive value of 100% (95% CI, 94% to 100%).

McLaughlin et al studied 134 patients, 53 ± 2 years old, 63% of whom were women, who presented with chest pain at the emergency room.[14] A calcium score of greater than 1 was considered a positive result. The patients were followed for 30 days and the occurrence of sudden death, nonfatal myocardial infarction, percutaneous coronary angioplasty, or bypass surgery was recorded. Results were positive in 86 patients; in this group, seven coronary events (8%)—four nonfatal myocardial infarctions, two bypasses, and one angioplasty—occurred. Results were negative in 48 patients (36%); no events occurred in this group (Table 20–5).

Thus, the negative predictive value of 100% suggested that patients with a negative calcium scan result can be safely discharged.

Georgiou et al conducted a prospective observational study of 192 patients admitted to the emergency department for chest pain syndromes.[15] The mean age was 53 ± 9 years; 46% were women. The authors followed these patients for a mean of 50 ± 10 months. Hard events occurred in 30 patients: cardiac death (11) and nonfatal MI (19). Soft events occurred in another 28 patients: coronary artery bypass graft (9), percutaneous coronary angioplasty (4), hospitalization for angina (11), and ischemic stroke (4).

■ ▦ ■

TABLE 20–5   VALUE OF CALCIUM SCAN TO PREDICT CARDIAC DEATH AND NONFATAL MI IN PATIENTS PRESENTING AT EMERGENCY DEPARTMENT

CALCIUM SCAN	EVENT RATE* 30 DAYS (P)	EVENT RATE† 50±10 MONTHS (P)
Negative	0% (48)	0% (76)
Positive	4.4% (86)	15.6% (116)

*Data from McLaughlin et al.[14]
†Data from Georgiou et al.[15]

Patients with a negative result were event-free; among those with a positive result, the hard adverse event rate was 15.6% (see Table 20–5). It appeared that higher calcium scores were associated with a higher annualized event rate (Fig. 20–4). Adjustment for age and gender further stratified risk: Relative risks for total cardiovascular events were significantly higher in the third and fourth quartiles (Fig. 20–5). Multivariate analyses showed that calcium score and age- and gender-adjusted risk profiles were stronger independent predictors than the traditional risk factors and age.

It should be mentioned that all three studies investigated relatively small number of patients and that they studied relatively young patients because the higher prevalence of calcium in elderly patients would reduce the specificity of the calcium scan, making it less clinically useful.

It may be concluded that middle-aged patients with new chest pain, a nonspecific ECG result, and no enzyme rise, who are admitted to an emergency department and who have a negative calcium scan result, can be safely discharged without further provocative testing. However,

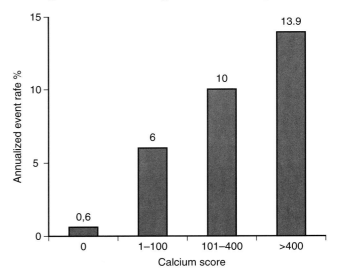

FIGURE 20–4. Annualized rates of cardiovascular events (death, MI, coronary artery bypass graft, percutaneous coronary angioplasty, hospitalization for angina, and ischemic stroke). (From Georgiou D, et al: Screening patients with chest pain in the emergency department using electron beam tomography: A follow-up study. J Am Coll Cardiol 38:105–110, 2001.)

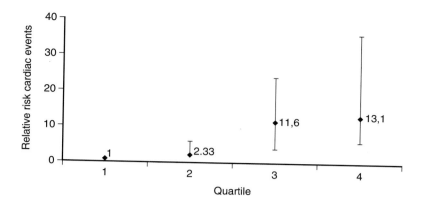

FIGURE 20–5. Relative risk for cardiac vascular events using age- and gender-adjusted quartiles. Confidence intervals (95%) are presented for each quartile. (From Georgiou D, Budoff MJ, Kaufer E, et al: Screening patients with chest pain in the emergency department using electron beam tomography: A follow-up study. J Am Coll Cardiol 38:105–110, 2001.)

a positive calcium scan test result is essentially useless and necessitates further testing.

COMPUTED TOMOGRAPHY OF THE CORONARY ARTERIES—THE FUTURE

EBCT and MSCT have emerged as two noninvasive diagnostic tools that can visualize the proximal and middle segments of the coronary tree and that may detect significant obstructive coronary artery disease (Fig. 20-6). The diagnostic value of both techniques is described in Tables 20-6[16-21] and 20-7.[22,23]

The diagnostic power of these techniques has been evaluated in elective symptomatic patients but has not specifically been evaluated in patients with acute coronary syndromes, but there is no reason to think that power would be different in patients with acute coronary syndromes. Obviously, the preliminary results are not sufficient to warrant replacement of conventional diagnostic angiography.

CT angiography has limited spatial and temporal resolution, whereas calcification of the coronary wall seriously hinders assessment of the coronary lumen so that underlying obstructive disease may remain unnoticed.

COMPUTED TOMOGRAPHY OF THE CORONARY PLAQUE—THE FUTURE

Rupture of a vulnerable plaque with superimposed coronary thrombosis is the most common cause of an acute coronary event. The risk of plaque disruption depends on plaque composition, and plaques containing a large lipid pool are more prone to disruption than fibrous or calcific plaques.

Noninvasive assessment of plaque components would be a desirable step forward in the risk stratification of patients with known or suspected coronary artery disease. MSCT does allow classification of plaque components into soft, intermediate, and calcific based on the x-ray attenuation characteristics of tissues, resulting in specific CT density values expressed in Hounsfield units. This method resembles the intracoronary ultrasound classification of plaques into soft, fibrous, and calcific based on the echogenicity of its components. Schroeder et al investigated 34 plaques in 15 patients.[24] Intracoronary ultrasonography classified these plaques into soft, intermediate, and calcific. MSCT showed that soft plaques had a density of 14 ± 26 HU, intermediate plaques 91 ± 21 HU, and calcific plaques 419 ± 194 HU. The identification of plaque components

■ ■ ■

TABLE 20–6   ELECTRON BEAM COMPUTED TOMOGRAPHY (EBCT) CORONARY ANGIOGRAPHY: ACCURACY TO DETECT SIGNIFICANT (>50% DIAMETER REDUCTION) STENOSES IN ASSESSABLE VESSEL SEGMENTS

AUTHORS	PATIENTS (N)	ASSESSABLE* (%)	SENSITIVITY (%)	SPECIFICITY (%)
Nakanishi et al[16]	37	NR	74	91
Reddy et al[17]	23	90	88	79
Schermund et al[18]	28	88	83	91
Rensing et al[19]	37	81	77	94
Achenbach et al[20]	125	75	92	94
Budoff et al[21]	52	90	78	91
Overall	302	81	84	92

NR, not reported.
*Image quality adequate for classification.

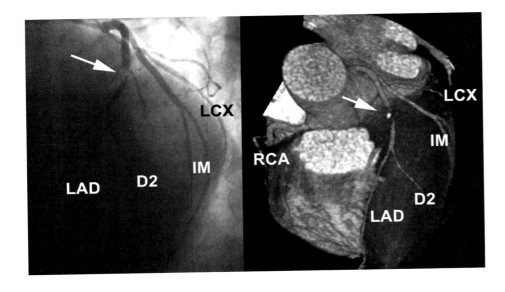

FIGURE 20–6. Conventional CT and MSCT coronary angiograms (three-dimensional volume-rendered) of a patient with a stenotic coronary lesion in the middle left anterior descending branch (LAD), just distal from the small first diagonal branch. The calcified contents of the plaque are visualized on the MSCT angiogram. The left circumflex coronary artery (LCX), right coronary artery (RCA), second diagonal branch (D2), and intermediate branch (IM) can also be appreciated. (*B*, see color plate.)

■ ▦ ■

TABLE 20–7   MULTISLICE SPIRAL COMPUTED TOMOGRAPHY (MSCT) CORONARY ANGIOGRAPHY: ACCURACY TO DETECT SIGNIFICANT (>50% DIAMETER REDUCTION) STENOSES IN ASSESSABLE VESSEL SEGMENTS

AUTHORS	PATIENTS (N)	ASSESSABLE* (%)	SENSITIVITY (%)	SPECIFICITY (%)
Nieman et al[22]	31	73	81	97
Achenbach et al[23]	64	68	91[†]	84[†]

*Image quality adequate for classification.
[†]High grade (>75% diameter reduction) stenoses.

is rather crude and should require histologic confirmation. However, these first results demonstrated the ability of MSCT to identify soft rupture-prone lesions. This technique may find future use as a tool for risk stratification.

REFERENCES

1. Rumberger JA, Simons DB, Fitzpatrick LA, et al: Coronary artery calcium area by electron-beam computed tomography and coronary atherosclerotic plaque area. A histopathologic correlative study. Circulation 1995;92:2157–2162.
2. Agatston AS, et al: Quantification of coronary artery calcium using ultrafast computed tomography. J Am Coll Cardiol 1990;15:827–832.
3. O'Rourke RA, Brundage BH, Froelicher VF, et al: American College of Cardiology/American Heart Association Expert Consensus Document on electron-beam computed tomography for the diagnosis and prognosis of coronary artery disease. J Am Coll Cardiol 2000;36:326–340.
4. Wexler L, Brundage B, Crouse J, et al: Coronary artery calcification: Pathophysiology, epidemiology, imaging methods, and clinical implications. A statement for health professionals from the American Heart Association Writing Group. Circulation 1996;94:1175–1192.
5. Detrano RC, Wong ND, Doherty TM, et al: Coronary calcium does not accurately predict near-term future coronary events in high-risk adults. Circulation 1999;99:2633–2638.
6. Arad Y, Spadaro LA, Goodman K, et al: Predictive value of electron beam computed tomography of the coronary arteries: 19-month follow-up of 1173 asymptomatic subjects. Circulation 1996;93:1951–1953.
7. Arad Y, Spadaro LA, Goodman K, et al: Prediction of coronary events with electron beam computed tomography. J Am Coll Cardiol 2000;36:1253–1260.
8. Raggi P, Callister TO, Cooil B, et al: Identification of patients at increased risk of first unheralded acute myocardial infarction by electron-beam computed tomography. Circulation 2000;101:850–855.
9. Raggi P, Cooil B, Callister TQ: Use of electron beam tomography data to develop models for prediction of hard coronary events. Am Heart J 2001;141:375–382.
10. Detrano R, Hsiai T, Wang S, et al: Prognostic value of coronary calcification and angiographic stenoses in patients undergoing coronary angiography. J Am Coll Cardiol 1996;27:285–290.
11. Keelan PC, Bielak LF, Ashai K, et al: Long-term prognostic value of coronary calcification detected by electron-beam computed tomography in patients undergoing coronary angiography. Circulation 2001;104:412–417.
12. Schmermund A, Baumgart D, Gorge G, et al: Coronary artery calcium in acute coronary syndromes: A comparative study of electron-beam computed tomography, coronary angiography, and intracoronary ultrasound in survivors of acute myocardial infarction and unstable angina. Circulation 1997;96:1461–1469.
13. Laudon DA, Vukov LF, Breen JF, et al: Use of electron-beam computed tomography in the evaluation of chest pain patients in the emergency department. Ann Emerg Med 1999;33:15–21.

14. McLaughlin VV, Balogh T, Rich S: Utility of electron beam computed tomography to stratify patients presenting to the emergency room with chest pain. Am J Cardiol 1999;84:327–328.

15. Georgiou D, Budoff MJ, Kaufer E, et al: Screening patients with chest pain in the emergency department using electron beam tomography: A follow-up study. J Am Coll Cardiol 2001;38:105–110.

16. Nakanishi T, Ito K, Imazu M, Yamakido M: Evaluation of coronary artery stenoses using electron-beam CT and multiplanar reformation. J Comput Assist Tomogr 1997;21:121–127.

17. Reddy GP, Chernoff DM, Adams JR, Higgins CB: Coronary artery stenoses: Assessment with contrast-enhanced electron-beam CT and axial reconstructions. Radiology 1998;208:167–172.

18. Schmermund A, Rensing BJ, Sheedy PF, et al: Intravenous electron-beam computed tomographic coronary angiography for segmental analysis of coronary artery stenoses. J Am Coll Cardiol 1998;31:1547–1554.

19. Rensing BJ, Bongaerts A, van Guens RJ, et al: Intravenous coronary angiography by electron beam computed tomography: A clinical evaluation. Circulation 1998;98:2509–2512.

20. Achenbach S, Moshage W, Ropers D, et al: Value of electron-beam computed tomography for the noninvasive detection of high-grade coronary-artery stenoses and occlusions. N Engl J Med 1998;339:1964–1971.

21. Budoff MJ, Oudiz RJ, Zalace CP, et al: Intravenous three-dimensional coronary angiography using contrast enhanced electron beam computed tomography. Am J Cardiol 1999;83:840–845.

22. Nieman K, Oudkerk M, Rensing BJ, et al: Coronary angiography with multi-slice computed tomography. Lancet 2001;357:599–603.

23. Achenbach S, Giesler T, Ropers D, et al: Detection of coronary artery stenoses by contrast-enhanced, retrospectively electrocardiographically-gated, multislice spiral computed tomography. Circulation 2001;103:2535–2538.

24. Schroeder S, Kopp AF, Baumbach A, et al: Noninvasive detection and evaluation of atherosclerotic coronary plaques with multislice computed tomography. J Am Coll Cardiol 2001;37:1430–1435.

Emerging Diagnostic Procedures for the Vulnerable Plaque

Richard Gallo
Cezar Staniloae

Atherosclerosis is a multifocal disease generally confined to the intima of coronary arteries. Confluent atherosclerotic plaques carpet the vessel wall,[1] but individual plaques vary greatly in composition and consistency even within the same coronary artery. In patients presenting with acute coronary syndromes, most culprit lesions have a significant atheromatous core.[2] No obvious relationship among plaque size, stenosis severity, and plaque composition has yet been elucidated. Atherogenesis and lesion progression may be expected to be linear with time. However, angiographic studies show that the progression of coronary artery disease in humans is neither linear nor predictable. New high-grade lesions often appear in segments of artery that appeared normal or near normal on previous angiographic examinations.[1,3] Two thirds or more of the culprit lesions responsible for unstable angina or myocardial infarction were only mildly to moderately stenotic on prior angiograms.[4] Giroud and colleagues[5] demonstrated that over three quarters of myocardial infarctions were in areas supplied by mildly stenosed (<50%) coronary arteries on a previous angiogram. Ambrose et al[4] and Little et al[6] further supported these observations by showing that the average degree of stenosis in lesions progressing to a later myocardial infarction was less than 50%.

Angiographic, angioscopic, and pathologic data have established an association between plaque rupture and the development of unstable angina, acute myocardial infarction, and sudden ischemic death. Additionally, there is ample evidence that plaque rupture, thrombosis, and fibrous organization of the thrombus may also account for the progression of atherosclerotic disease in asymptomatic patients and in those persons with stable coronary artery disease.[7] The cellular and biochemical structure and composition of atherosclerotic plaques, rather than the severity of the stenosis, are now considered to be the major determinants for acute coronary events. Fissuring or rupture of an atherosclerotic plaque in the coronary arteries is the principal event in the development of the acute coronary syndromes.[3] Disrupted atherosclerotic plaques are commonly associated with the formation of mural thrombi anchored to fissures in the disrupted plaque.

Detection of vulnerable plaques remains difficult and elusive with current imaging technologies. With the exception of relatively small, uncontrolled, and open-label studies using angioscopy or intravascular ultrasonography (IVUS), no prospective studies have clearly identified the characteristics of a coronary vulnerable plaque with long-term clinical outcomes. It is fair to say that almost all our understanding about the vulnerable plaque is based on retrospective data obtained from histologic ex vivo and in vitro experiments.[8]

The major limitation of current technologies lies in their inability of to characterize plaque content. Modalities capable of characterizing the atherosclerotic lesion may be helpful in understanding its natural history and detecting lesions that are at high risk for acute events. There is a visible need for newer imaging technologies with the ability to detect the most vulnerable of plaques. Other imaging modalities, including angiography, magnetic resonance imaging, IVUS, and nuclear medicine, are discussed in Chapters 18 and 19, respectively. This chapter explores four emerging technologies for the detection and characterization of atherosclerotic lesions. These newer technologies are in various stages of development, and many have very limited experience in humans. Nevertheless, impressive preclinical work has signaled their potential and warrants our attention. Other technologies that still remain at a proof-of-concept phase are not dealt with in this chapter.

OPTICAL COHERENCE TOMOGRAPHY

Optical coherence tomography (OCT) is a recently developed technique for noncontact imaging of microscopic tissue structures that can generate images with micrometer-scale resolution. This technique is analogous to ultrasound imaging but uses low-coherent infrared laser light back-reflected from tissue structures for image assembly. This technology has been successfully applied as a diagnostic imaging tool in ophthalmology.[9,10] OCT has unparalleled resolution in the imaging of the anterior ocular chamber and retina. It is now used to diagnose and monitor the progression of macular disease and glaucoma.[11-13] Additional applications for OCT technology include diagnostic imaging of dermatologic, respiratory, and urologic tracts.[14] Furthermore, OCT offers the possibility of becoming an optical biopsy with applications for diagnosing and assessing preneoplastic lesions such as Barrett esophagitis.[15,16] Cardiovascular applications have until recently been limited to in vitro experiments using postmortem aortic and coronary artery specimens.[17,18] Numerous in vivo animal experiments have shown the potential to identify vascular structures with remarkable resolution.[19,20]

Initial feasibility studies with OCT in humans are rather limited but encouraging. An initial series in 10 patients with coronary artery disease has been reported.[21] When OCT is compared with IVUS images, more detailed structural information of human coronary atherosclerotic plaques is obtained in vivo (Fig. 21-1).[22]

The greatest advantage of OCT as an intravascular imaging modality is its exceptionally high resolution. The unique capability of OCT to resolve micrometer-scale features of coronary plaques in patients suggests that this new technique holds promise for identifying features of coronary plaques at risk for rupture. OCT has demonstrated qualitatively superior delineation of plaque morphology when compared with IVUS in vitro and in vivo analysis of human atherosclerotic lesions.[18,21] Experimental studies have suggested that the high image contrast of OCT may qualitatively and quantitatively identify thrombus, intimal flaps and fissures, the thickness of intimal caps, internal and external elastic lamina, and the size of the lipid core, thus potentially identifying plaques vulnerable to rupture. Precise quantitative measurements of parameters such as plaque area and percentage of stenosis severity can be used to assess the benefits of therapies such as statins or future drugs on the progression or regression of atherosclerotic plaques. Additionally, the high resolution of OCT permits differentiation between lipid and water-based tissue, which with the exception of magnetic resonance imaging is a major limitation of conventional imaging technologies. When applied to humans, this ability may provide a precise modality for the characterization of tissue and subsequently the identification of vulnerable atherosclerotic plaques (Fig. 21-2).

Comparison with Current Imaging Technology

Although some complex atherosclerotic lesions can be identified by angiography, it is a rather poorly sensitive and specific imaging technology for identifying vulnerable atherosclerotic plaques. Angioscopy can directly visualize the surface of blood vessels. If its field of view is not obstructed by blood, angioscopy can clearly visualize thrombus and plaque fissures. However, it is poor for evaluating luminal dimensions and like angiography offers no insight into pathologic processes in the vessel wall. High-frequency (30 Mhz) IVUS is superior to angiography for the identification of coronary artery dissections, for quantitative assessment of stenosis, and as a

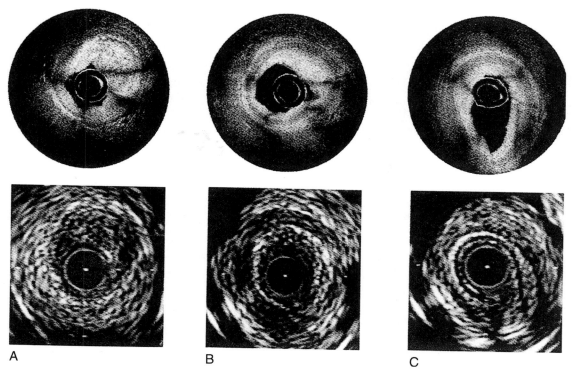

FIGURE 21-1. Comparison of optical coherence tomography with intravascular ultrasonography in a human postmortem coronary artery. *A,* Contains a subocclusive plaque. *B,* Demonstrates clearly defined layers of the vessel wall. *C,* Vessel lumen is well defined compared with intravascular ultrasonography. (From Patwari P, Weissman NJ, Boppart SA, et al: Assessment of coronary plaque with optical coherence tomography and high-frequency ultrasound. Am J Cardiol 2000;85:641-644.)

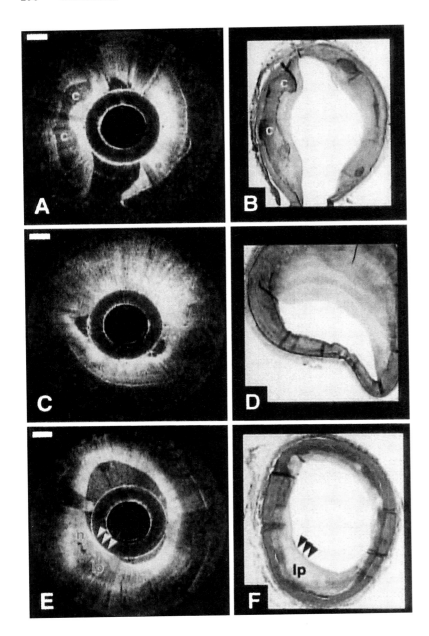

FIGURE 21–2. Correlation between optical coherence tomography images *(left)* and histologic findings *(right)* of human coronary artery plaques obtained at autopsy. *A,* Optical coherence tomography image of a calcium-rich *(C)* fibrous plaque as documented histologically *(B). C,* A predominantly fibrous plaque documented by optical coherence tomography imaging and histology *(D). E,* Lipid-rich plaque with a lipid pool (lp) and an overlying dense fibrous cap *(arrowheads)* documented histologically *(F).* Areas of neovascularization (n) are visible as open spaces within the lipid core. (From Jang IK, Bouma BE, Kang DH, et al: Visualization of coronary atherosclerotic plaques in patients using optical coherence tomography: Comparison with intravascular ultrasound. J Am Coll Cardiol 2002;39:604–609.)

guide to coronary interventions. However, its spatial resolution (essentially defined as the size of an object it can see) is only 110 µm compared with 5 to 20 µm for current OCT prototypes. This limits the ability of IVUS to delineate plaque morphology and tissue at a microscopic level as compared with OCT. The maximum resolution of the newer 50-MHz IVUS system is 70 µm, which remains a significant shortcoming compared with OCT. Moreover, unlike OCT, IVUS can not penetrate calcified tissue.[17,22] Additionally, IVUS is limited in its ability to appraise lipid content and evaluate the presence and amount of thrombus, and IVUS suffers from significant interobserver discrepancies.

As with all nascent technologies, OCT does present certain limitations. Currently, penetration depth is limited to 1 to 3 mm, depending on the light source used. This limits image acquisition to the atherosclerotic plaque and media. Full circumferential views of larger coronary arteries may not be possible. In normal coronary vessels, only the inner adventitia can be visualized. Further refinements in light sources should permit high-resolution imaging of the outer adventitia. Light waves can not propagate through metal, limiting the use of OCT in the evaluation of intracoronary stent-covered tissue. The greatest limitation of OCT is its reduced effectiveness when imaging through blood.[19,20] Red blood cells are a major source of light scattering and absorption, resulting in significant attenuation of the light signal. Certain in vivo experiments circumvented this problem by simultaneously injecting saline into the vessel, permitting unimpeded OCT imaging. Increasing the refractive index of serum with certain solutions such as contrast agents and dextran can also improve OCT imaging.[20] However, this concept remains to be evaluated in humans.

Technical Aspects

Ultrasound images represent a cross-sectional picture of the acoustic reflectance or echo properties of tissue. An image is produced by electronically measuring the delay time or echo for an acoustic pulse (ultrasound) to be reflected back from tissue to its source. In contrast with sound, light waves travel too fast for electronic equipment to capture and directly measure optical echoes. To overcome this physical barrier, OCT uses light interferometry.[23]

Light waves generated from a source are split evenly between a reference and sample arm in an interferometer (optical splitter). Light sent to the sample arm via a conventional intravascular catheter is then focused on the tissue. Simultaneously, light to the reference arm is focused on a mirror that constantly shifts to a precisely predetermined and controlled distance, inducing a known Doppler shift in the returned light. The reflections from both arms are then recombined by the interferometer (optical coupler). Interference between the light reflected from the tissue and light reflected from the reference mirror occurs when the distance their paths have traveled coincide and fall within the pulse duration of the source light (coherence length).[18,23] The use of interferometry permits the echo delay of the light reflected from the tissue to be measured as a function of depth with precise accuracy. The cross-sectional (tomographic) image finally produced is actually a two-dimensional map of the profile of all reflected light from the tissue that has been scanned. Images are displayed either in gray scale or in computer-generated colors to differentiate structures.

OCT catheters are small, ranging from 2.6 F (or 0.87 mm) to 2.9 F (or 0.97 mm) and have a central imaging core consisting of relatively simple and inexpensive fiberoptics. Unlike IVUS catheters, OCT catheters contain no electronic transducers within their sheath. The axial resolution of current cardiovascular systems range from 10 m to 20 μm, with acquisition rates of 4 to 10 frames per second. In addition, some OCT prototype models can be coupled to standard IVUS consoles, permitting combined IVUS and OCT imaging with the same console system.

Conclusions

OCT has emerged as a potential alternative imaging modality with superior imaging qualities and a potential for in vivo tissue characterization. Compared with IVUS, OCT provides sharper delineation among the intima, fibrous caps, and the lipid core of atherosclerotic plaques. In addition to furthering our knowledge of plaque vulnerability, the identification of vulnerable plaques may lead to therapies specifically designed for a given patient and may permit in situ monitoring of structural changes that occur in atherosclerotic plaques over time or, more precisely, with plaque progression after pharmacologic intervention.

CORONARY THERMOGRAPHY: RELATIONSHIP BETWEEN PLAQUE TEMPERATURE AND PLAQUE RUPTURE

Pathophysiology of Heat Production in Atherosclerotic Plaques

The rich cellular environment of atherosclerotic plaques contributes to the generation of heat. Cells of the immune system produce endogenous pyrogens known as cytokines. These structurally diverse proteins are mediators of inflammation angiogenesis and numerous internal cellular processes. In addition to contributing to the generation of heat, cytokines mediate the acute phase response by increased production of C-reactive protein; serum amyloid A; fibrinogen; complement proteins B, C3, and C4; interleukin-6; and a variety of proteinase inhibitors. Some of them, like tumor necrosis factor α and interleukin-1α, are able to increase endothelial cell adhesiveness and associated procoagulant effects.[24,25]

Macrophages and, to a lesser extent, T and B lymphocytes are the main cytokine producers in atherosclerotic plaques. Macrophages are abundant in atherosclerotic plaques within the plaque, often observed in the shoulder region where the fibrous cap meets normal intima.[3] Dense cellular regions in specimens of carotid plaques showed significantly higher temperatures when compared with the neighboring fatty core, which is often densely populated by lipid-laden macrophages.[26]

Another contributor to local heat production is plaque angiogenesis. Mediated by cytokines such as vascular endothelial growth factor, new capillaries that penetrate into the atherosclerotic plaque contribute to the elevation in the temperature profile.

There is a correlation between plaque angiogenesis and inflammation[27]; in addition, both are thought to be risk factors for plaque rupture. The release of matrix-digesting enzymes such as metalloproteinases secreted by macrophages soften the fibrous cap, enhancing the vulnerability of atherosclerotic plaques to rupture.[28,29]

Because inflamed plaques are at high risk for rupture with subsequent thrombosis, the development of a catheter-based or noninvasive imaging technique able to detect and distinguish vulnerable plaques could yield a valuable tool for assessing prognosis and developing treatment strategies. Oscillations in the temperature of an inflamed or hot-vulnerable plaque have led to a new technique that attempts to detect local temperature fluctuations of different plaques.

Applying Principles to Practice

It is now clear that before a plaque rupture, vulnerable plaques experience active inflammation and progressive matrix degeneration. Despite improvements in coronary imaging and identification of inflammatory markers, plaque rupture cannot be predicted by clinical means.[4,30,31] Casscells and colleagues were the first to postulate that plaques covering areas infiltrated by monocytes and inflammatory cells could be identified by the heat released by the activated inflammatory cells.[26] Further studies showed that ex vivo atherosclerotic plaques taken during carotid endarterectomy have thermal heterogeneity: Plaques with dense macrophage infiltration give off more heat than noninflamed plaques, and plaque temperature varies inversely with the thickness of the fibrous overlying cap. With the later development of a catheter-based technique to measure the temperature of human coronary arteries, thermal heterogeneity within human atherosclerotic coronary arteries was demonstrated.[32] Interestingly, this heterogeneity is markedly greater in patients presenting with unstable angina or acute myocardial infarction, implying that this heterogeneity may be related to the pathogenesis of these syndromes (Fig. 21–3). Furthermore, the presence of higher temperatures at the site of culprit lesions in patients with unstable angina or myocardial infarction is associated with higher levels of C-reactive protein and serum amyloid A.[33]

A recent experimental rabbit atherosclerotic model demonstrated a direct correlation between macrophage content in atherosclerotic plaques and temperature variations. In addition, lipid-lowering therapy not only reduced macrophage plaque content as determined by histology but subsequently resulted in reduced temperature heterogeneity within the plaque, suggesting that thermography may be a novel method of following the macrophage burden of atherosclerotic plaques.[34]

One of the few prospective studies to correlate plaque temperature and clinical outcomes involved 86 patients with stable coronary artery disease, unstable angina, and recent acute myocardial infarction.[35] The difference in temperature between the atherosclerotic plaque and healthy vessel wall is a strong predictor of event-free survival 1.5 years after a percutaneous coronary interven-

tion in patients with coronary artery disease. The mean change in temperature was greater in patients with adverse cardiac events within each subgroup, although there was a nonsignificant trend in patients with a recent acute myocardial infarction. The threshold value of temperature variation above which the rate of adverse cardiac events was significantly increased was 0.5°C. Interestingly, the majority of the cardiac events were related to restenosis of the treated lesion and not further acute coronary syndromes.

The results of these preliminary investigations should be interpreted with caution because there is a significant potential for interaction between known prognostic factors after percutaneous coronary intervention and change in plaque temperature.

Thermography Catheter

The technology of thermography catheters is rapidly progressing. There is no lack of interest from industry to develop an applicable catheter-based technology. Here we describe two advanced designs of thermography catheters presently under development: a contact-based temperature measurement catheter and an infrared side-viewing catheter. The last-generation prototype of an intravascular thermosensor basket catheter to be used in clinical studies was recently described.[36] This new thermosensor basket catheter system consists of the following:

- A 4 F catheter with an expandable and externally controllable basket with nine built-in thermosensors
- A computer board with digital transistors for high-speed sampling
- A personal computer
- A custom software package for real-time data acquisition, tracking, and thermographic imaging
- A circulating microbath for automatic thermal calibration.

The expandable basket at the end of catheter is made of four to eight highly flexible hollow wires (inside diameter, 0.003 inches; outside diameter, 0.05 inches) with 0.001-inch built-in thermocouples. Each wire has two sensors located at the maximum curve, 0.5 mm apart, allowing monitoring of temperature between and within plaques. The catheter also has a central wire with a thermal sensor to monitor the blood temperature simultaneously. Real-time data acquisition software supports digital transmitters for each channel with a thermal resolution of 0.0025°C and a sampling rate of 20 readings per second. The software can also display the circumferential and longitudinal thermal map of the vessel wall.[36]

An alternative side-viewing catheter is capable of imaging the temperature of the vessel wall with 180 degrees of freedom. The size of the coronary catheter is 4 F (1.33 mm). Nineteen chalcogenide fibers, each 100 μm in diameter, are bundled hexagonally with a total length of 1.5 m. At the tip of the catheter is a 1 mm wide wedge-shaped mirror assembly made of zinc selenide. It is transparent to infrared radiation and is placed in a way that reflects the temperature only from the side of the catheter. A guidewire lumen passes through the bundle.

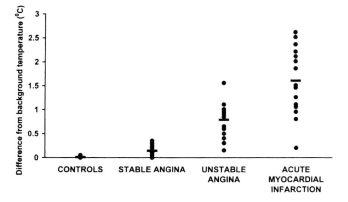

FIGURE 21–3. Progressive increase in the measured difference in maximum temperature from background temperature in patients with stable angina, unstable angina, and acute myocardial infarction. (From Stefanadis C, Diamantopoulos L, Vlachopoulos C, et al: Thermal heterogeneity within human atherosclerotic coronary arteries detected in vivo: A new method of detection by application of a special thermography catheter. Circulation 1999;99:1965–1971.)

The fiberoptic catheter is connected to a focal plane array–cooled infrared camera. The system has a thermal resolution of 0.01°C and spatial resolution of 100 μm. Real-time image reconstruction software continuously records the linear images obtained through the 1 mm window and processes them into two-dimensional and virtual longitudinal color-coded thermographic images of the lumen.[37]

This catheter was tested in a phantom model simulating blood vessels and hot plaques with continuous flow of normal saline in a silicon tube on which multiple hot spots were created. The catheter successfully detected temperature changes along the side of the tube. Some of the technical challenges that need to be overcome with both catheter-based systems are the need for temporary occlusion of the coronary vessel during temperature analysis; confounding temperature measurements from blood flow in the lumen and adjacent structures; and the inability to detect vulnerable eroded or thrombotic plaques with little inherent inflammation. This is an important consideration because 40% to 50% of thrombotic coronary events are due to plaque erosions, particularly in smokers.[38]

Conclusions

At present, strong pathophysiologic data support the role of heat production by vulnerable plaques. The technology to precisely measure the heat within the coronary plaques is available. However promising this technology is, larger clinical trials are required to determine its the sensitivity and specificity before it becomes widely available.

SPECTROSCOPY

Spectroscopy is the absorption, emission, or scattering of electromagnetic radiation by atoms or molecules to qualitatively or quantitatively study the atoms or molecules or to study physical processes. Spectroscopy is based on the fact that different chemical compounds absorb and scatter different amounts of energy at different wavelengths, leaving a unique chemical fingerprint.[8,39] Common medical applications use light or photonic energy as the radiation source. Currently, two forms of photonic spectroscopy show potential for clinical detection of atherosclerotic and particularly vulnerable plaques; Raman spectroscopy and near-infrared diffuse reflectance spectroscopy.

Raman Spectroscopy

Raman spectroscopy is a universal analytic technique for identification of molecules in gases, liquids, and solids by scattering of laser light. The Raman effect arises when incident light excites molecules in a sample, which subsequently scatters the light. Although most of this scattered light is at the same wavelength as the incident light, some is scattered at different wavelengths. Light that is scattered because of vibrations in molecules or optical photons in solids is called *Raman scattering*. It

results from the molecule changing its molecular motions. The energy difference between the incident light (Ei) and the Raman scattered light (Es) is equal to the energy involved in changing the molecule's vibrational state (i.e., getting the molecule to vibrate, Ev). This energy difference is called the *Raman shift*, defined by the formula Ev = Ei − Es.

A plot of the incident light intensity versus Raman shift is a Raman spectrum. Different Raman spectrums are often observed, each associated with the different vibrational or rotational motions of molecules in a sample. When Raman spectroscopy is applied to an atherosclerotic plaque, the resultant spectrums can be considered a molecular fingerprint of that plaque (Fig. 21-4).[40] This makes Raman spectroscopy potentially ideal for identifying the chemical makeup of different atherosclerotic plaques.[41]

Recent years have seen a remarkable increase in the application of Raman spectroscopy to the field of medicine. As disease leads to changes in the molecular composition of affected tissues, these changes should be reflected in the spectra.[39] Furthermore, if the spectral changes are specific enough for a particular disease state, they can, in principle, be used as a marker or more precisely a fingerprint of the disease. In vitro studies

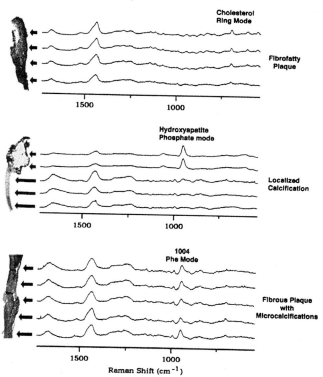

FIGURE 21–4. Cross-sections from three typical human atherosclerotic arterial lesions and their corresponding Raman spectra. Each individual plaque type reveals a unique spectra or "fingerprint." *Top,* Fibroatheromatous plaque with a lipid-rich core. *Center,* Heavily calcified plaque. *Bottom,* Fibrous plaque with scattered microcalcifications. (From Salenius J, Brennan J, Miller A, et al: Biochemical composition of human peripheral arteries examined with near-infrared Raman spectroscopy. J Vasc Surg 1998;27:710–719.)

have demonstrated that spectral analysis allows for the discrimination of coronary arterial tissue in three categories: nonatherosclerotic, calcified, and noncalcified plaque.[42,43] In addition, quantification of cholesterol content calculated by Raman spectroscopy correlates strongly with histologic findings.[44] Recent animal experiments have demonstrated the ability of Raman spectroscopy to follow the evolution of atherosclerotic plaques and to quantitatively determine the size and distribution of cholesterol and calcium depositions in plaques.[45]

Thus, the great appeal of Raman spectroscopy lies in its potential for in vivo discrimination of lipid-rich atheroma and calcified and fibrous plaques. However, Raman spectroscopy has yet to be evaluated in vivo and remains some years away from significant human validation studies. Penetration depth is limited to 1 to 1.5 mm, depending on the light source used.[42] This limits image acquisition to the fibrous cap and within the atheromatous core. To date, experiments have been limited to direct contact with tissue; full noncontact circumferential imaging has not been evaluated. In addition, strong background fluorescence and the blood's absorbance of emitted light are technical challenges. Raman spectroscopy does not in itself provide spatial orientation or plaque geometry, and it remains to be determined whether vulnerable plaques can be differentiated from more stable sclerotic plaques solely by chemical composition. Therefore, the future development of Raman spectroscopy as a catheter-based technology may involve a combination with another imaging modality such as IVUS or OCT.

Near-Infrared Diffuse Reflectance Spectroscopy

Similar to Raman spectroscopy, near-infrared diffuse reflectance spectroscopy uses light to detect and determine the composition of organic substances. However, unlike Raman spectroscopy, which uses high-energy laser light in the visible light spectrum, near-infrared diffuse reflectance spectroscopy is the process of understanding how infrared light (750 to 2500 nm) interacts with various molecules (e.g., water, fat, protein, and glucose). Near-infrared light occurs just beyond the location of red light in the visible spectrum.

Each type of molecule reacts and absorbs near-infrared light differently. The amount of light that is absorbed is proportional to the concentration of that particular molecule, revealing both qualitative and quantitative information about the pathologic process under investigation. Histologic correlation with reflectance patterns of different tissues can potentially detect and distinguish the lipid-rich atheromatous core and become a useful diagnostic tool for the detection of vulnerable plaque.

Spectroscopic systems using infrared light have demonstrated the ability to identify cholesterol, high-density lipoprotein, and low-density lipoprotein in arterial wall samples obtained at autopsy. Chemical analysis showed that correlation of the atheromatous core content using high-pressure liquid chromatography was high.[46] In another experiment, near-infrared diffuse reflectance spectroscopy correctly identified histologic features of plaque vulnerability, including the presence of lipid-rich atherosclerotic plaques, with a high degree of sensitivity (90%) and specificity (93%) in 199 human aortic specimens taken at autopsy.[47]

There have been few in vivo experiments with near-infrared diffuse reflectance spectroscopic systems. One study using a cholesterol fed rabbit model evaluated a catheter-based system and again demonstrated the superior sensitivity and specificity of infrared light spectroscopy (P. Moreno, 2001, personal communication). Despite limited experience, the technology does appear promising: Its potential advantages include the proven safety of the energy source and the fact that the fiberoptics required to deliver the energy source are readily available at reasonable cost. In addition, unlike the case with OCT, thermography, and potentially Raman spectroscopy, it does not appear that flowing blood interferes with the reflectance patterns of the longer wavelengths of infrared light. This should permit noncontact imaging of the circumference of the vessel without the need to occlude blood flow. However, this has yet to be proven in an in vivo model.[47,48]

INTRACORONARY DOPPLER AND PRESSURE MONITORING

Principles of Doppler Velocimetry

Christian Johann Doppler, an Austrian physicist, first described the phenomenon of increasing sound frequency as the sound source moves toward the observer, inversely decreasing as the source moves away.[49] Applying this principle to the circulatory system requires conceptualizing the red blood cell as the moving sound source. When an ultrasound beam with known frequency (fo) is transmitted to the blood stream, it is reflected by the moving erythrocyte. The frequency of the reflected ultrasound wave (fr) increases when the red blood cells are moving toward the source of ultrasound and decreases when they are moving away from it. The change in frequency between the transmitted sound and the reflected sound is called *Doppler shift* or *frequency shift* ($\Delta f = fo - fr$). The frequency of the reflected ultrasound wave (fr) and implicit Δf Doppler shift depends on (1) the transmitted frequency fo, (2) the velocity of the moving target (v), and (3) the angle θ (theta) between the ultrasound beam and the direction of the moving target. This relationship is expressed by the Doppler equation:

$$\Delta f = 2fo \times v \times \cos\theta/c$$

where c is the speed of sound in blood (1560 m/sec).

There are two types of Doppler forms. The pulsed-wave Doppler is a single piezoelectric crystal mounted at the tip of an intravascular catheter that both sends and receives sound beams. The crystal emits a short burst of ultrasound at a certain frequency called a *pulse repetition frequency*. The ultrasound is reflected by moving red blood cells and is received by the same crystal. Therefore, the pulsed-waved Doppler allows determination of the magnitude of the flow at a predetermined distance from the transducer. In contrast, in the continuous-wave mode, the transducer has two crystals: one to send and the other to receive the reflected ultrasound waves continuously. It measures all the velocities encountered by the exploring ultrasound beam. This mode is advantageous for measuring the highest flow velocity available.

The Doppler flow meters are easily introduced to epicardial vessels, and local flow velocities can be measured. Because there is a direct relation between the velocity and volumetric flow (i.e., blood flow = mean flow velocity × cross-sectional area), every change in measured velocity represents a similar change in blood flow, assuming that the cross-sectional area remains constant.

Doppler Guidewire Velocity Data

The Doppler guidewire is 0.014 inches in diameter, 175 cm long, flexible, and steerable with handling characteristics similar to the traditional angioplasty guidewire. An ultrasound transducer with a 12 MHz piezoelectric cell is mounted on the tip. The minimal cross-sectional area of a Doppler wire is only 0.1 mm^2, which does not create any significant stenosis when introduced into a human coronary artery. When a Doppler guidewire is substituted for a standard angioplasty guidewire, phasic coronary flow velocity characteristics are easily incorporated into an angioplasty procedure.[50,51] The Doppler wire is able to assess both the velocity and the direction of flow of the red blood cells. When blood flows away from the transducer, the Doppler spectrum appears above the baseline (Fig. 21–5).

Among the physical parameters measured are the maximum velocity of blood flow (peak velocity) and the average peak velocity, which is the average of peak velocity as a function of time. Calculations show that within an epicardial coronary artery, the average peak velocity represents twice the true mean flow velocity. By measuring maximal flow velocity and measuring the cross-sectional area of the epicardial vessel by quantitative coronary angiography, one can calculate the volumetric flow rate. Further calculations include the ratio of diastolic to systolic velocity and flow deceleration times. On a practical note, most interventional cardiologists use

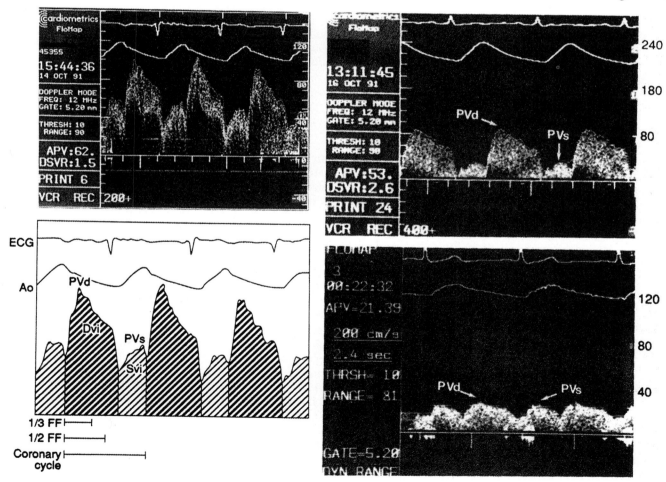

FIGURE 21–5. *Top left,* Normal coronary spectral flow pattern. Electrocardiogram and aortic pressure readings are shown above the spectral velocity signal. *Bottom left,* Measurements obtained from spectral signal. DV$_I$, diastolic velocity integral; FF, flow fraction; PV$_d$, peak diastolic velocity; Sv$_i$, systolic velocity integral; V$_i$, velocity integral. *Right,* Coronary flow velocity pattern in abnormal proximal *(top)* and distal coronary arteries *(bottom).* (From Ofili EO, Labovitz AJ, Kern MJ: Coronary flow velocity dynamics in normal and diseased arteries. Am J Cardiol 1993;71:3D–9D.

Doppler guidewires to measure the coronary flow reserve (CFR), which is calculated as the ratio between hyperemic and basal average peak velocities (see later).

Comparing values with those obtained by an electro-magnetic flowmeter validated the parameters measured by a Doppler guidewire.[52] The excellent correlation (r^2 = 0.94) found between these two techniques supports the use of the Doppler guidewire for accurate measurements of coronary flow velocities.

Coronary Blood Flow Velocity Patterns

Normal Blood Flow Velocity

Coronary flow velocity patterns were defined and validated in an initial study performed on 81 proximal coronary arteries without significant coronary stenosis.[50] Definitions of the systolic and diastolic flow measurements were based on simultaneous electrocardiogram and aortic pressure recordings. The flow velocity recordings show a predominant diastolic component in all coronary arteries. During systole, contraction of the myocardium impedes systolic inflow while enhancing systolic venous outflow. Comparisons of the phasic patterns of coronary arterial inflow and coronary venous outflow in the working human heart demonstrate that coronary inflow is higher in diastole and that coronary venous outflow is higher in systole. This phase shift between inflow and outflow indicates that a fraction of the intramural blood content is squeezed out of the myocardium with each systolic contraction.[53] Large differences between flow patterns also occur between left and right coronary arteries. The greater systolic compressive force of the left ventricle probably explains this difference.

Reproducibility of the analysis is excellent, with an interobserver and intraobserver variability of less than 5%. Although the peak diastolic/systolic flow velocity ratio is less in the right coronary artery compared with the left anterior descending or left circumflex artery, the coronary flow reserve determined after hyperemic response (see later) is similar in all three arteries. Thus, proximal and distal normal coronary arteries have similar relative flow velocity parameters and vasodilator reserve, with a diastolic predominant pattern.

Applications of Flow Velocity Patterns in Acute Coronary Syndromes

The primary therapeutic objective of patients with acute myocardial infarction is to restore infarct-related artery patency and re-establish adequate flow. However, the objective of reperfusion therapy is not merely restoration of blood flow in the coronary artery but also complete and sustained reperfusion of the myocardium at risk.[54] Studies performed with the help of intracoronary myocardial contrast echocardiography (MCE) have shown that up to 30% of patients undergoing primary angioplasty lack myocardial reperfusion despite recanalization of the infarct-related artery.[55-59] Furthermore, angiographically successful recanalization of the infarct-related artery does not necessarily guarantee adequate

myocardial salvage.[56,60] These regions of "no-reflow" may develop because of microvascular disruption, plugging by thromboembolic debris, or endothelial and myocardial edema.[61]

Angiography is currently the gold standard for assessing coronary artery patency and the efficacy of different reperfusion protocols. Although the latest refinements in quantifying the degrees of arterial patency such as Thrombolysis in Myocardial Infarction (TIMI) flow and frame count score have improved the prognostic value of this technique, they do not adequately define the level of microvascular perfusion or predict the recovery of myocardial function after successful reperfusion therapy. Newer techniques, such as MCE and physiologic testing with Doppler wire analysis, have been developed and are undergoing constant refinement in an attempt to better characterize the microvascular circulation. The assessment of perfusion by intracoronary MCE has been shown to provide information on perfusion territories, collateral flow, infarct size, myocardial viability, and success of reperfusion.[62] Recent advances in ultrasound technology and contrast agents have enabled the detection of myocardial perfusion after intravenous injection of transpulmonary contrast agents.[63-65] Physiologic assessment of the infarct-related artery and the underlying microcirculation, particularly by coronary flow reserve measurements, is also emerging as a complementary diagnostic tool to assess myocardial perfusion in patients undergoing percutaneous coronary interventions.

Coronary Blood Flow Velocity Pattern and Microvascular Dysfunction

Much of the information on coronary blood flow velocities has been gathered by coronary angiography and MCE. Microvascular dysfunction occurring during an acute myocardial infarction influences coronary flow dynamics. Slow radiopaque contrast runoff in the infarct-related artery (TIMI flow grade 2) after coronary intervention is considered a sign of the no-reflow phenomenon. Angiographic studies in patients with acute myocardial infarction have confirmed that TIMI flow grade 2 is caused by the microvascular dysfunction of the ischemic region[57,66] and may be regarded as failure to reperfuse the infarct-related artery.[67,68] The coronary blood flow velocity pattern observed in patients with no reflow phenomenon despite the absence of residual coronary stenosis is different from that observed in patients with lumen obstruction caused by coronary stenosis.[60] In patients with substantial no-reflow phenomenon, the coronary blood flow velocity pattern is characterized by a reduction in systolic antegrade flow, the appearance of abnormal retrograde flow in early systole, and rapid deceleration of the diastolic flow velocity. The diastolic/systolic velocity ratio or flow ratio is higher in patients with no reflow than in those with reflow. These distinct coronary flow patterns are associated with lack of reperfusion and correlate with angiographic TIMI flow grade 2.[60]

The precise mechanisms of slow contrast filling in the infarct-related artery and of the alterations in the coronary blood flow velocity pattern are not fully understood. A back-and-forth feature appears to exist in the epicardial coronary blood flow in patients with TIMI flow grade 1 or 2: a rapid decrease in the diastolic antegrade flow velocity and a subsequent rapid retrograde flow in early systole. It is hypothesized that the early systolic retrograde flow could be explained by an increase in microvascular impedance due to elevated pressures in the distal bed. Normally increased myocardial stress during systole, even in an infarcted region, would usually squeeze the intramyocardial blood pool into the coronary venous circulation. However, in patients with no reflow or diminished flow, pooled blood in the myocardium is not pressured into the venous circulation during systole because of the diffuse obstruction of microvasculature and, thus, would be pushed retrogradely back to the epicardial coronary artery to produce an early systolic retrograde flow.

If systolic retrograde movement is observed in patients with TIMI flow grade 2 after coronary interventions, it would indicate microvascular dysfunction rather than the presence of a flow-restricting lesion in the epicardial coronary artery. Among the characteristic flow patterns shown by MCE in which there was no reflow or reduced flow, the appearance of early systolic retrograde flow is the most remarkable sign to identify patients with severe microvascular dysfunction.[69]

Early systolic reverse flow detected in the peripheral coronary arteries, such as the septal branch, sometimes occurs in normal subjects. It is characterized by a slow or even sluggish reverse flow, often called "slosh."[70] This reverse flow is caused by the milking effect produced by the contracting myocardium. Systolic retrograde flow in normal subjects differs from that observed in patients with reduced coronary flow or no reflow due to microvascular dysfunction in that such flow is absent in large-conduit epicardial coronary arteries.[71,72]

In normal persons, it is during diastole that the coronary blood flow predominantly fills the intramyocardial blood pool and partially runs through the coronary microcirculation into the venous circulation. In patients with no reflow, the coronary microvasculature is profoundly damaged; subsequently, the intramyocardial blood pool is reduced considerably. The coronary blood flow should rapidly fill the residual intramyocardial blood pool, and the distal coronary pressure should increase in the very early phase of diastole. Therefore, the coronary flow rapidly decreases its velocity in mid to late diastole in patients with no reflow, resulting in a decrease in duration of the diastolic antegrade flow.[60] Additionally, the blood flow dynamics in a recanalized coronary artery may also depend on several other complex, inter-related factors, such as myocardial mass supplied by the infarct-related artery, vasodilator reserve, the extent of reperfusion injury, and hemodynamics.

Coronary Blood Flow Velocity and TIMI Perfusion Grade

TIMI flow grade is commonly used as a marker of successful reperfusion after myocardial infarction. Coronary blood flow as determined by angiography and graded using TIMI perfusion scores was compared with intracoronary Doppler flow velocity in a study involving 41 patients undergoing a percutaneous coronary intervention for acute myocardial infarction.[73] Coronary flow velocity correlated well in infarct-related vessels with a TIMI flow grade of 2. The lower the TIMI flow grade, the lower the flow velocity. However, there was significant heterogeneity in coronary flow velocities for infarct-related vessels with TIMI flow grade 3. This suggests that a TIMI grade of 3 does not necessarily guarantee successful myocardial reperfusion. The lower flow velocities observed possibly represent patients with different degrees of microvascular dysfunction, embolization, or significant residual stenosis. The wide range in coronary velocities observed with TIMI grade 3 flow after primary angioplasty may explain the disparity observed between expected and observed mortality rates among patients with acute myocardial infarctions. Additional studies are required to confirm these initial results.

Flow Velocity Patterns and Myocardial Recovery after Acute Myocardial Infarction

In patients with no reflow phenomenon, recovery of left-ventricular function is poor after myocardial infarction independent of the TIMI grade score.[74] The relationship between left-ventricular function and coronary blood flow velocity after successful reperfusion was studied in 23 consecutive patients with anterior acute myocardial infarctions. After successful angioplasty, a Doppler wire was placed distal to the culprit lesion and coronary blood flow to the area at risk was assessed. Follow-up echocardiography was performed at 1 month to examine the regional wall-motion recovery. Patients with viable myocardium at 1 month showed almost normal blood velocity patterns; the group with nonviable myocardium showed reduced anterograde systolic velocity caused by the combination of systolic retrograde flow and rapid diastolic deceleration time of diastolic flow velocity. The authors determined optimal cutoff values of 6.5 cm/sec for anterograde systolic velocities and 600 ms for diastolic deceleration time to predict myocardial viability. Higher antegrade systolic velocities and longer diastolic deceleration velocities of the coronary blood flow velocity after primary percutaneous coronary interventions were predictive of greater myocardial recovery within a region of acute ischemic injury. The sensitivity and specificity were between 80% and 90%.

Lower antegrade systolic velocities are probably due to backflow during systole in patients with microvasculature dysfunction, a common finding with the no-reflow phenomenon. Short diastolic deceleration times are in turn due to an increase in coronary vascular resistance caused by ischemic microvasculature damage and peripheral embolization.

Monitoring coronary blood flow velocity patterns with a Doppler guidewire is a promising method to detect different grades of no-reflow phenomenon in patients after reperfused acute myocardial infarction. This method an be applied easily to patients undergoing coronary interventions. In addition, it may provide useful prognostic information and help orient treatment strategies in this group of patients.

Coronary Flow Reserve and Fractional Flow Reserve in Acute Coronary Syndromes

Visual assessment of the coronary arteriogram as a means of predicting the functional significance of intermediate coronary stenosis is inaccurate. Coronary flow resistance varies according to the lesion length and morphology (entrance/exit angles, length, eccentricity, and luminal topography) as well as the status of the microvasculature. Because net coronary flow is the result of a complex system involving both conduit and microvascular bed resistances, qualitative anatomic variables such as angiography and intravascular imaging techniques are generally poor predictors of the functional response of flow through a given stenosis.[75]

The physiologic influence of a coronary stenosis on the distal arterial pressure/flow relationship can now be easily and safely determined with sensor-tipped angioplasty guidewires that measure the poststenotic absolute CFR, the relative coronary flow reserve (rCFR), and the pressure-derived fractional flow reserve of the myocardium (FFR). These measurements provide an understanding of the separate functions of the epicardial, microvascular, and collateral coronary circulation.

When an epicardial stenosis increases resistance to flow, the distant microvascular resistance vessels dilate to maintain regional basal flow at a level appropriate for concurrent myocardial oxygen demand. The increased dilation reduces the available potential maximal flow reserve. Because the distal microcirculation has compensated for the reduction in regional flow, the resting poststenotic epicardial conduit blood flow, depending on the severity of the stenosis, may be diminished (lower coronary flow reserve). Under normal resting conditions, epicardial flow is sufficient to satisfactorily maintain myocardial function and metabolism. However, any increase in myocardial oxygen demand or other hyperemic stimuli results in a smaller increment in poststenotic flow relative to the coronary flow increase that would be elicited in the same myocardial region without a stenosis (diminished relative coronary flow reserve).[76]

A significant stenosis also produces distal artery pressure loss (i.e., a translesional pressure gradient) because of a loss of kinetic (flow) energy due to viscous friction, turbulence, and flow separation. The reduction of the distal distending arterial pressure results in a pressure differential or gradient between the driving aortic pressure and the poststenotic coronary pressure. The degree of pressure loss is directly related to the flow rate as described by a curvilinear pressure/flow relationship of the particular lesion resistance.

CFR is affected by all factors that influence the basal blood flow, such as heart rate, blood pressure, contractility, and microvascular disease. Also, interposition of side branches between stenosis and the site of measurement may complicate the CFR determination. Collateral blood flow and the microcirculation also influence the results of CFR. To overcome the limitation of CFR, the concept of FFR was introduced by Piljs and colleagues.[77-79] FFR is defined as the ratio of maximal hyperemic flow in a stenotic artery compared with what maximum flow would be in the same artery in the absence of stenosis. It is calculated from intracoronary measurements obtained during basal and hyperemic states. Unlike the Doppler methods, FFR is unaffected by increased blood flow because measurements are performed in a pharmacologically induced state of maximum vasodilatation. Whereas CFR can not discriminate between epicardial disease and microcirculatory disease, FFR is a lesion-specific index for epicardial stenosis.

Translesional pressure gradients are measured using high-fidelity pressure guidewires. FFR is calculated from the ratio of poststenotic coronary pressure to aortic pressure at maximal hyperemia (usually after an intracoronary bolus injection of adenosine) corrected for the mean central venous pressure (assumed to be 5 mm Hg). Assuming that no epicardial stenosis is present, the mean aortic pressure should reflect the mean distal coronary pressure and the FFR should be equal to 1. In patients with normal left-ventricular function, a well-defined cut-off value of 0.75 has been shown to accurately distinguish stenosis capable of inducing myocardial ischemia (FFR < 0.75) from stenosis that is not (FFR $\geq$ 0.75).[79] There are several caveats to interpreting absolute CFR, rCFR, or FFR in the presence of impaired microcirculatory flow. If the presumed target vessel is abnormal, as in patients with an acute myocardial infarction, neither the absolute CFR nor the rCFR can identify the ischemic contribution of the lesion. Conditions such as myocardial hypertrophy, hypertension, and diabetes may blunt the CFR and may not permit accurate assessment of a stenosis. Furthermore, in patients with three-vessel coronary artery disease, no suitable reference vessel may be found, invalidating and precluding the use of rCFR. Coronary stenosis in these situations is best assessed by FFR.[75]

Because it is calculated only at peak hyperemia, as opposed to coronary flow reserve, FFR is independent of microvascular responses or hemodynamics such as basal blood flow, driving pressure, heart rate, and systemic blood pressure.[80] In the setting of microvascular disease, a normal FFR indicates that the conduit resistance is not a major contributing factor to perfusion impairment and that the enlargement of such a conduit obstruction would not restore normal perfusion. However, distal pressure is also a function of epicardial flow and epicardial resistance. A change in the latter affects the distal pressure as reflected by FFR and flow as reflected by CFR in opposite directions. Therefore, the results of these diagnostic techniques are often discordant in patients with intermediate coronary lesions. In such diagnostic dilemmas, FFR and Doppler velocimetry are complementary, describing the physiology of both the epicardial stenosis and the microvascular disease as potential contributors to myocardial ischemia.[75,81]

Coronary Flow Reserve and Myocardial Reperfusion in Acute Coronary Syndromes

Angiographic studies on coronary and myocardial perfusion were the initial studies that established the importance of coronary physiology after acute myocardial infarction and reperfusion strategies as a determinant of clinical outcomes.[82] FFR is a more accurate physiologic measure that can discriminate between coronary microcirculatory dysfunction and epicardial flow impairment.

CFR of an infarct-related artery is severely impaired immediately after myocardial reperfusion, recovering partially shortly thereafter.[83,84] After an initial depletion of vasoconstrictor reserves during ischemia, partial improvement of CFR after adequate reperfusion may be expected because of the greater availability of vasodilating mediator substances.[85]

Recent studies have demonstrated the prognostic capability of CFR after successful myocardial reperfusion. An increase of CFR within 24 hours after recanalization of the infarct-related artery was predictive of superior left-ventricular function at 4 weeks. In patients in whom the CFR remained depressed (CFR ratios < 1.6 are usually taken as a cutoff value), recovery of left-ventricular function at 4 weeks was significantly reduced or absent.[86,87]

Although the CFR is not the most highly sensitive indicator of microvascular integrity, in situations wherein hemodynamic parameters are stable, the value of CFR is principally a function of the resistance in the microcirculation and indirectly reflects microvascular function. After myocardial infarction, patients demonstrate a close correlation between the CFR of the infarct-related artery and the size of perfusion defects as determined by MCE.[86] Reduction of MCE perfusion defects was associated with improvement of CFR, whereas persistent MCE perfusion defects were associated with unchanged depression of CFR, indicating a relation between microvascular integrity assessed by CFR and myocardial perfusion as assessed by MCE.

Further insight in the ability of CFR measurements to predict the functional status of the microcirculation come from pharmacologic studies with abciximab. Abciximab is known to reduce microcirculatory embolization. Coronary flow and left-ventricular function at 2 weeks was greater in patients receiving abciximab during a percutaneous coronary intervention despite similar degrees of residual epicardial coronary artery stenosis. Coronary physiologic responses correlated with left-ventricular functional recovery. This suggests that physiologic testing in patients with acute coronary syndromes may have prognostic value and allow therapeutic strategies to be tailored to individual patients.

Fractional Flow Reserve in Acute Coronary Syndromes

Data on FFR are mostly derived from a selected stable patient population with single-vessel coronary disease and normal left-ventricular function. Information on FFR for patients with microvascular disease, acute or remote myocardial infarction, and unstable angina is limited. An important prerequisite of the principle of pressure-derived FFR is to achieve maximal arteriolar vasodilation in order to obtain the pressure measurements under conditions of minimal myocardial resistance. The presence of an acute myocardial infarction changes both the mass of viable myocardium and the maximal hyperemic response in the territory supplied by the infarct-related vessel. As a result, the usual cutoff value of 0.75 might not be valid for patients with recent myocardial infarction.

A relatively recent study by de Bruyne and colleagues[88] looked at the role of FFR in patients with a recent myocardial infarction. Fifty-seven patients with recent acute myocardial infarction (at least 6 days old) underwent FFR measurement before and after angioplasty of the infarct-related artery. The values obtained by FFR were compared with the occurrence of residual reversible flow maldistribution seen by adenosine-Tc^{99m} sestamibi nuclear scintigraphy. Consequently, the authors demonstrated that even for patients with recent myocardial infarction, a pressure-derived FFR value of 0.75 can accurately identify patients with residual reversible perfusion defects in partially infracted areas.

In conclusion, the practical application of physiologic concepts strongly complements coronary lumenology and has important clinical implications for the care of patients with coronary artery disease. Nevertheless, further pivotal clinical trials are required before physiological measurements can be fully incorporated into the management of acute coronary syndromes.

REFERENCES

1. Fuster V, Lewis A: Connor Memorial Lecture: Mechanisms leading to myocardial infarction: Insights from studies of vascular biology. Circulation 1994;90:2126–2146.
2. Ross R: The pathogenesis of atherosclerosis: A perspective for the 1990s. Nature 1993;362:801–809.
3. Fuster V, Badimon L, Badimon J, Chesebro J: The pathogenesis of coronary artery disease and the acute coronary syndromes, Parts 1 and 2. N Engl J Med 1992;326:242–250, 310–318.
4. Ambrose JA, Tannenbaum MA, Alexopoulos D, et al: Angiographic progression of coronary artery disease and the development of myocardial infarction. J Am Coll Cardiol 1988;12:56–62.
5. Giroud D, Li J, Urban P, Meier B, Rutishauser W: Relation of the site of acute myocardial infarction to the most severe coronary arterial stenosis at prior angiography. Am J Cardiol 1992;69:729–732.
6. Little W, Constantinescu M, Applegate R, et al: Can coronary angiography predict the site of a subsequent myocardial infarction in patients with mild-to-moderate coronary artery disease? Circulation 1988;78:1157–1166.
7. Libby P: Molecular bases of the acute coronary syndromes. Circulation 1995;91:2844–2850.
8. Naghavi M, Madjid M, Khan MR, et al: New developments in the detection of vulnerable plaque. Curr Atheroscler Rep 2001;3:125–135.
9. Ripandelli G, Coppe AM, Capaldo A, Stirpe M: Optical coherence tomography. Semin Ophthalmol 1998;13:199–202.
10. Fujimoto JG, Brezinski ME, Tearney GJ, et al: Optical biopsy and imaging using optical coherence tomography. Nat Med 1995;1:970–972.
11. Izatt JA, Hee MR, Swanson EA, et al: Micrometer-scale resolution imaging of the anterior eye in vivo with optical coherence tomography. Arch Opthalmol 1994;112:1584–1589.
12. Hee MR, Izatt JA, Swanson EA, et al: Optical coherence tomography of the human retina. Arch Opthalmol 1995;113:325–332.
13. Swanson EA, Izatt JA, Hee MR, et al: In vivo retinal imaging by optical coherence tomography. Optics Lett 1993;18:1864–1866.
14. Welzel J: Optical coherence tomography in dermatology: A review. Skin Res Technol 2001;7:1–9.
15. Brand S, Ponero JM, Bouma BE, et al: Optical coherence tomography in the gastrointestinal tract. Endoscopy 2000;32:796–803.
16. Li XD, Boppart SA, Van Dam J, et al: Optical coherence tomography: Advanced technology for the endoscopic imaging of Barrett's esophagus. Endoscopy 2000;32:921–930.

17. Brezinski ME, Tearney GJ, Bouma BE, et al: Optical coherence tomography for optical biopsy. Properties and demonstration of vascular pathology. Circulation 1996;93:1206-1213.

18. Brezinski ME, Tearney GJ, Weissman NJ, et al: Assessing atherosclerotic plaque morphology: comparison of optical coherence tomography and high frequency intravascular ultrasound. Heart 1997;77:397-403.

19. Fujimoto JG, Boppart SA, Tearney GJ, et al: High resolution in vivo intra-arterial imaging with optical coherence tomography. Heart 1999;82:128-133.

20. Brezinski M, Saunders K, Jesser C, et al: Index matching to improve optical coherence tomography imaging through blood. Circulation 2001;103:1999-2003.

21. Jang IK, Bouma BE, Kang DH, et al: Visualization of coronary atherosclerotic plaques in patients using optical coherence tomography: Comparison with intravascular ultrasound. J Am Coll Cardiol 2002;39:604-609.

22. Patwari P, Weissman NJ, Boppart SA, et al: Assessment of coronary plaque with optical coherence tomography and high-frequency ultrasound. Am J Cardiol 2000;85:641-644.

23. Huang D, Swanson EA, Lin CP, et al: Optical coherence tomography. Science 1991;254:1178-1181.

24. Libby P, Sukhova G, Lee RT, Galis ZS: Cytokines regulate vascular functions related to stability of the atherosclerotic plaque. J Cardiovasc Pharmacol 1995;25:S9-S12.

25. Libby P, Ridker PM, Maseri AM: Inflammation and atherosclerosis. Circulation 2002;105(9):1135-1143.

26. Casscells W, Hathorn B, David M, et al: Thermal detection of cellular infiltrates in living atherosclerotic plaques: Possible implications for plaque rupture and thrombosis. Lancet 1996;347:1447-1451.

27. Nikkari ST, O'Brien KD, Ferguson M, et al: Interstitial collagenase (MMP-1) expression in human carotid atherosclerosis. Circulation 1995;92:1393-1398.

28. Falk E: Morphologic features of unstable atherothrombotic plaques underlying acute coronary syndromes. Am J Cardiol 1989;63:114E-120E.

29. van der Wal AC, Becker AE, van der Loos CM, Das PK: Site of intimal rupture or erosion of thrombosed coronary atherosclerotic plaques is characterized by an inflammatory process irrespective of the dominant plaque morphology. Circulation 1994;89:36-44.

30. Little WC, Constantinescu M, Applegate RJ, et al: Can coronary angiography predict the site of a subsequent myocardial infarction in patients with mild-to-moderate coronary artery disease? Circulation 1988;78:1157-1166.

31. de Feyter PJ, Ozaki Y, Baptista J, et al: Ischemia-related lesion characteristics in patients with stable or unstable angina. A study with intracoronary angioscopy and ultrasound. Circulation 1995;92:1408-1413.

32. Stefanadis C, Diamantopoulos L, Vlachopoulos C, et al: Thermal heterogeneity within human atherosclerotic coronary arteries detected in vivo: A new method of detection by application of a special thermography catheter. Circulation 1999;99:1965-1971.

33. Stefanadis C, Diamantopoulos L, Dernellis J, et al: Heat production of atherosclerotic plaques and inflammation assessed by the acute phase proteins in acute coronary syndromes. J Mol Cell Cardiol 2000;32:43-52.

34. Verheye S, De Meyer G, Van Langenhove G, et al: In vivo temperature heterogeneity of atherosclerotic plaques is determined by plaque composition. Circulation 2002;105:1596-1601.

35. Stefanadis C, Toutouzas K, Tsiamis E, et al: Thermography of human arterial system by means of new thermography catheters. Catheter Cardiovasc Interv 2001;54:51-58.

36. Naghavi M, Gul K, O'Brien T, et al: Coronary thermosensor basket catheter with thermographic imaging software for thermal detection of vulnerable atherosclerotic plaques. Am J Cardiol 2001;88:80E.

37. Naghavi M, Melling P, Gul K, et al: First prototype of a 4-French, 180-degree, side-viewing infrared fiberoptic catheter for thermal imaging of atherosclerotic plaque. Am J Cardiol 2001;88:81E.

38. Falk E: Why do plaques rupture? Circulation 1992;86:III30-III42.

39. Choo-smith L, Edwards H, Hendtz H, et al: Medical applications of Raman spectroscopy: From proof of principle to clinical implementation. Biopolymers (Biospectroscopy) 2002;67:1-9.

40. Salenius J, Brennan J, Miller A, et al: Biochemical composition of human peripheral arteries examined with near-infrared Raman spectroscopy. J Vasc Surg 1998;27:710-719.

41. Pasterkamp G, Falk E, Woutman H, Borst C: Techniques characterizing the coronary atherosclerotic plaque: Influence on clinical decision making? J Am Coll Cardiol 2000;36:13-21.

42. Romer T, Brennan JI, Fitzmaurice M, et al: Histopathology of human atherosclerosis by quantifying its chemical composition by Raman spectroscopy. Circulation 1998;97:878-885.

43. Brennan JI, Romer T, Lees R, et al: Determination of human coronary artery composition by Raman Spectroscopy. Circulation 1997;96:99-105.

44. Romer T, Brennan JI, Baker-Schutt T, et al: Raman spectroscopy for quantifying cholesterol in intact coronary artery wall. Atherosclerosis 1998;141:117-124.

45. van De Poll S, Romer T, Volger O, et al: Raman spectroscopic evaluation of the effects of diet and lipid-lowering therapy on atherosclerotic plaque development in mice. Arterioscler Thromb Vasc Biol 2001;10:1630-1635.

46. Jarros W, Neumeister V, Lattke P, et al: Determination of cholesterol in atherosclerotic plaques using near infrared diffuse reflection spectroscopy. Atherosclerosis 1999;147:327-337.

47. Moreno P, Lodder R, Purushothaman R, et al: Detection of Lipid Pool, thin fibrous cap, and inflammatory cells in human aortic atherosclerotic plaques by near-infrared spectroscopy. Circulation 2002;105:923-927.

48. Cassis L, Lodder R: Near-IR imaging of atheromas in living arterial tissue. Annal Chem 1993;65:1247-1256.

49. Hatle L, Angelsen B: Doppler Ultrasound in Cardiology: Physical Principles and Clinical Applications. Philadelphia, Lea & Febiger, 1985.

50. Ofili EO, Labovitz AJ, Kern MJ: Coronary flow velocity dynamics in normal and diseased arteries. Am J Cardiol 1993;71:3D-9D.

51. Tadaoka S, Kagiyama M, Hiramatsu O, et al: Accuracy of 20-MHz Doppler catheter coronary artery velocimetry for measurement of coronary blood flow velocity. Cathet Cardiovasc Diagn 1990;19:205-213.

52. Doucette JW, Corl PD, Payne HM, et al: Validation of a Doppler guide wire for intravascular measurement of coronary artery flow velocity. Circulation 1992;85:1899-1911.

53. Spaan JA: Mechanical determinants of myocardial perfusion. Basic Res Cardiol 1995;90:89-102.

54. Anderson JL, Karagounis LA, Becker LC, et al: TIMI perfusion grade 3 but not grade 2 results in improved outcome after thrombolysis for myocardial infarction. Ventriculographic, enzymatic, and electrocardiographic evidence from the TEAM-3 Study. Circulation 1993;87:1829-1839.

55. Ito H, Tomooka T, Sakai N, et al: Lack of myocardial perfusion immediately after successful thrombolysis. A predictor of poor recovery of left ventricular function in anterior myocardial infarction. Circulation 1992;85:1699-1705.

56. Ito H, Okamura A, Iwakura K, et al: Myocardial perfusion patterns related to thrombolysis in myocardial infarction perfusion grades after coronary angioplasty in patients with acute anterior wall myocardial infarction. Circulation 1996;93:1993-1999.

57. Ito H, Maruyama A, Iwakura K, et al: Clinical implications of the "no reflow" phenomenon. A predictor of complications and left ventricular remodeling in reperfused anterior wall myocardial infarction. Circulation 1996;93:223-228.

58. Ragosta M, Camarano G, Kaul S, et al: Microvascular integrity indicates myocellular viability in patients with recent myocardial infarction. New insights using myocardial contrast echocardiography. Circulation 1994;89:2562-2569.

59. Kenner MD, Zajac EJ, Kondos GT, et al: Ability of the no-reflow phenomenon during an acute myocardial infarction to predict left ventricular dysfunction at one-month follow-up. Am J Cardiol 1995;76:861-868.

60. Iwakura K, Ito H, Takiuchi S, et al: Alternation in the coronary blood flow velocity pattern in patients with no reflow and reperfused acute myocardial infarction. Circulation 1996;94:1269-1275.

61. Kloner RA, Ganote CE, Jennings RB: The "no-reflow" phenomenon after temporary coronary occlusion in the dog. J Clin Invest 1974;54:1496-1508.

62. Sabia PJ, Powers ER, Ragosta M, et al: An association between collateral blood flow and myocardial viability in patients with recent myocardial infarction. N Engl J Med 1992;327:1825-1831.

63. Sheil ML, Kaul S, Spotnitz WD: Myocardial contrast echocardiography: Development, applications, and future directions. Acad Radiol 1996;3:260-275.

64. Porter TR, D'Sa A, Turner C, et al: Myocardial contrast echocardiography for the assessment of coronary blood flow reserve: Validation in humans. J Am Coll Cardiol 1993;21:349-355.

65. Kaul S, Senior R, Dittrich H, et al: Detection of coronary artery disease with myocardial contrast echocardiography: Comparison with 99mTc-sestamibi single-photon emission computed tomography. Circulation 1997;96:785-792.

66. Piana RN, Paik GY, Moscucci M, et al: Incidence and treatment of "no-reflow" after percutaneous coronary intervention. Circulation 1994;89:2514-2518.

67. Kleiman NS, White HD, Ohman EM, et al: Mortality within 24 hours of thrombolysis for myocardial infarction. The importance of early reperfusion. The GUSTO Investigators, Global Utilization of Streptokinase and Tissue Plasminogen Activator for Occluded Coronary Arteries. Circulation 1994;90:2658-2665.

68. Karagounis L, Sorensen SG, Menlove RL, et al: Does thrombolysis in myocardial infarction (TIMI) perfusion grade 2 represent a mostly patent artery or a mostly occluded artery? Enzymatic and electrocardiographic evidence from the TEAM-2 study. Second Multicenter Thrombolysis Trial of Eminase in Acute Myocardial Infarction. J Am Coll Cardiol 1992;19:1-10.

69. Akasaka T, Yoshida K, Kawamoto T, et al: Relation of phasic coronary flow velocity characteristics with TIMI perfusion grade and myocardial recovery after primary percutaneous transluminal coronary angioplasty and rescue stenting. Circulation 2000;101:2361-2367.

70. Goto M, Kimura A, Tsujioka K, Kajiya F: Characteristics of coronary artery inflow and its significance in coronary pathophysiology. Biorheology 1993;30:323-331.

71. Kern MJ, Donohue TJ, Bach RG, et al: Quantitating coronary collateral flow velocity in patients during coronary angioplasty using a Doppler guidewire. Am J Cardiol 1993;71:34D-40D.

72. Ofili E, Kern MJ, Tatineni S, et al: Detection of coronary collateral flow by a Doppler-tipped guide wire during coronary angioplasty. Am Heart J 1991;122:221-225.

73. Kern MJ, Moore JA, Aguirre FV, et al: Determination of angiographic (TIMI grade) blood flow by intracoronary Doppler flow velocity during acute myocardial infarction. Circulation 1996;94:1545-1552.

74. Kawamoto T, Yoshida K, Akasaka T, et al: Can coronary blood flow velocity pattern after primary percutaneous transluminal coronary angioplasty (correction of angiography) predict recovery of regional left ventricular function in patients with acute myocardial infarction? Circulation 1999;100:339-345.

75. Kern MJ, Meier B: Evaluation of the culprit plaque and the physiological significance of coronary atherosclerotic narrowings. Circulation 2001;103:3142-3149.

76. Kern MJ: Coronary physiology revisited: Practical insights from the cardiac catheterization laboratory. Circulation 2000;101:1344-1351.

77. Pijls NH, van Son JA, Kirkeeide RL, et al: Experimental basis of determining maximum coronary, myocardial, and collateral blood flow by pressure measurements for assessing functional stenosis severity before and after percutaneous transluminal coronary angioplasty. Circulation 1993;87:1354-1367.

78. Pijls NH, Van Gelder B, Van der Voort P, et al: Fractional flow reserve. A useful index to evaluate the influence of an epicardial coronary stenosis on myocardial blood flow. Circulation 1995;92:3183-3193.

79. Pijls NH, De Bruyne B, Peels K, et al: Measurement of fractional flow reserve to assess the functional severity of coronary-artery stenoses. N Engl J Med 1996;334:1703-1708.

80. de Bruyne B, Bartunek J, Sys SU, et al: Simultaneous coronary pressure and flow velocity measurements in humans. Feasibility, reproducibility, and hemodynamic dependence of coronary flow velocity reserve, hyperemic flow versus pressure slope index, and fractional flow reserve. Circulation 1996;94:1842-1849.

81. Meuwissen M, Chamuleau SA, Siebes M, et al: Role of variability in microvascular resistance on fractional flow reserve and coronary blood flow velocity reserve in intermediate coronary lesions. Circulation 2001;103:184-187.

82. Gibson CM, Murphy SA, Rizzo MJ, et al: Relationship between TIMI frame count and clinical outcomes after thrombolytic administration. Thrombolysis In Myocardial Infarction (TIMI) Study Group. Circulation 1999;99:1945-1950.

83. Ishihara M, Sato H, Tateishi H, et al: Impaired coronary flow reserve immediately after coronary angioplasty in patients with acute myocardial infarction. Br Heart J 1993;69:288-292.

84. Neumann FJ, Kosa I, Dickfeld T, et al: Recovery of myocardial perfusion in acute myocardial infarction after successful balloon angioplasty and stent placement in the infarct-related coronary artery. J Am Coll Cardiol 1997;30:1270-1276.

85. Vanhaecke J, Flameng W, Borgers M, et al: Evidence for decreased coronary flow reserve in viable postischemic myocardium. Circ Res 1990;67:1201-1210.

86. Lepper W, Hoffmann R, Kamp O, et al: Assessment of myocardial reperfusion by intravenous myocardial contrast echocardiography and coronary flow reserve after primary percutaneous transluminal coronary angioplasty (correction of angiography) in patients with acute myocardial infarction. Circulation 2000;101:2368-2374.

87. Mazur W, Bitar JN, Lechin M, et al: Coronary flow reserve may predict myocardial recovery after myocardial infarction in patients with TIMI grade 3 flow. Am Heart J 1998;136:335-344.

88. De Bruyne B, Pijls NH, Bartunek J, et al: Fractional flow reserve in patients with prior myocardial infarction. Circulation 2001;104:157-162.

Risk Stratification in Non–ST-Segment Elevation Acute Coronary Syndromes

Marc S. Sabatine
David A. Morrow
Elliott M. Antman

Unstable angina (UA) is classically defined as ischemic discomfort that occurs at rest (or with minimal exertion), occurs with a crescendo pattern, or is severe and of new onset.[1] If these symptoms are accompanied by release of cardiac biomarkers of necrosis (e.g., creatinine kinase MB [CK-MB] or cardiac troponin), then the diagnosis of non–ST-elevation myocardial infarction (NSTEMI) may be made.[2] Both entities typically share a common pathobiologic basis: development of a severe but nonocclusive coronary artery thrombus superimposed on a recently disrupted vulnerable plaque.[3-5] Thus, treatments for UA and NSTEMI are identical and consist of a combination of anti-ischemic and antithrombotic therapies (and, potentially, coronary revascularization).[6] Nonetheless, among patients presenting with UA/NSTEMI, the risk of death and major cardiac ischemic events over the ensuing several weeks shows substantial heterogeneity. In the Thrombolysis in Myocardial Infarction (TIMI) III registry, the rates of death or (re)infarction by 30 days were 2.5% and 2.9%, respectively. In clinical trials, which tend to enroll higher-risk patients who manifest objective evidence of ischemia on presentation, the rates are somewhat higher and range from 3.5% to 4.5% for death and 5% to 12% for (re)infarction by 30 days.[1]

Risk stratification, aimed at providing a more accurate estimate of a patient's prognosis, is pivotal in the clinical management of patients with UA/NSTEMI.[6] Such information is important to patients and their families and allows for more effective triage and allocation of clinical resources. Several trials have demonstrated the efficacy of new pharmacologic agents, such as low-molecular-weight heparins (LMWHs)[7,8] and glycoprotein (GP) IIb/IIIa inhibitors,[9,10] as well as an early invasive strategy of management.[11,12] However, these treatment options are often expensive and not without complications. Therefore, risk stratification is an integral part of clinical decision-making and may guide the use of more aggressive therapy in those who are likely to derive the greatest benefit.

Data from observational studies and clinical trials have documented the prognostic utility of individual factors for risk stratification. Demographic and historical features as well as data collected during the initial evaluation, including physical examination findings and electrocardiographic changes, have been used in simple risk-stratification schemes.[13] Elevations in various cardiac biomarkers have now been proven useful in identifying high-risk populations. All of these data may be used to help clinicians more completely and accurately assess a patient's risk for recurrent events.[14]

DEMOGRAPHIC AND HISTORICAL RISK FACTORS

Age

Increasing age has been shown to be a risk factor across the spectrum of acute coronary syndromes (ACS). For the sake of simplicity, age is often treated as a dichotomous variable (e.g., <64 vs. ≥65). However, in an analysis based on data from the TIMI III registry, age was treated as a continuous variable and each decade was found to confer a relative risk of 1.43 ($P < .001$) for the composite of death or MI.[15] Moreover, in the Platelet Glycoprotein IIb/IIIa in Unstable Angina: Receptor Suppression Using Integrilin Therapy (PURSUIT) trial, use of cubic spline functions[16,17] revealed that the univariate relationship between age as a continuous variable and mortality was, in fact, curvilinear.[18] Fortuitously, in both patients with UA and patients with NSTEMI, an inflection point is evident at approximately 65 years, thus supporting the use of 65 years as a cut point when a binary approach is desired. An alternative approach has been to treat age as a categorical variable, with the clinician assigning increasing weight for each decade above a certain threshold.[18,19] The increase in risk with age may be steeper in patients with NSTEMI than in patients with UA.[18] Thus, clinicians should bear in mind that advanced age likely conveys increased prognostic importance as one shifts from UA to NSTEMI to STEMI.[18-20]

Gender

The impact of gender on outcomes in ACS is complex. Because women with ACS tend to have more traditional risk factors, crude univariate associations showing either a harmful or a protective effect of female gender are likely significantly confounded. For example, Hochman and colleagues found that in TIMI IIIB (a clinical trial involving patients with UA/NSTEMI)[21] and in the GUSTO [Global Use of STrategies to Open occluded coronary arteries] IIb trial (a clinical trial that enrolled patients across the spectrum of ACSs),[22] women presenting with an acute coronary syndrome were older and were more likely to have hypertension, diabetes, and hyperlipidemia.[23,24] Studies have also revealed that women are also more likely to present with atypical features and thus may seek medical attention more slowly and may not receive appropriate care after presentation.[25,26] In angiographic studies, women presenting with ACSs tend to have less severe coronary artery disease than do their male counterparts.[23] In recent large clinical trials, the rates of death and cardiac ischemic events were similar between men and women.[9-11,27] In several multivariable analyses, female sex was not associated with outcome,[14,23] whereas in others it has been associated with a statistically significant protective effect,[18,24] although this effect may be restricted to patients with UA and not those with NSTEMI. Thus, after adjusting for other established predictors, it is not clear that female sex independently conveys either harm or protection.

Diabetes

In both patients at risk and patients with known coronary artery disease, diabetes has emerged as a potent risk indicator and is of increasing importance because of the rise in the incidence of diabetes. Approximately 6% of the population has diabetes.[28] Moreover, it is estimated that twice that number have prediabetic states, such as impaired fasting glucose and impaired glucose tolerance. In addition, there is the even more common metabolic syndrome, which is defined as the presence of at least three of the following[29]:

- Waist circumference greater than 102 cm in men and 88 cm in women
- Serum triglycerides level of at least 150 mg/dL
- High-density lipoprotein cholesterol level of less than 40 mg/dL in men and 50 mg/dL in women
- Blood pressure of at least 130/85 mm Hg
- Serum glucose level of at least 110 mg/dL

As is the case for type II diabetes, insulin resistance is thought to be the underlying cause.[30] A study from the Third National Health and Nutrition Examination Survey (1988 to 1994) revealed that approximately 20% to 25% of the population in the United States has the metabolic syndrome.[31] The high prevalence of the metabolic syndrome also illustrates how patients with glucose intolerance or overt diabetes tend to have other traditional cardiovascular risk factors. For example, half of diabetic patients have concomitant hypertension and a third have concomitant hyperlipidemia.

Pathophysiologically, diabetes results in increased oxidative stress[32] and the development of advanced gly-cation end products, which may be pro-atherogenic.[33] Hemostatic sequelae include heightened platelet aggregation,[34,35] increased levels of fibrinogen and plasminogen activator inhibitor type 1,[36,37] upregulated cell surface adhesion molecules,[38,39] and impaired endothelial function.[40]

In population-based studies, the risk of first or recurrent MI among diabetic patients without a prior MI was approximately equal to the risk among nondiabetic patients with a prior MI.[41] In two trials of patients with STEMI, Thrombolysis and Angioplasty in Myocardial Infarction (TAMI)[42] and GUSTO 1,[43] patients with diabetes were found to have nearly twice the risk of death as did their nondiabetic counterparts despite similar rates of infarct-related artery patency.[44,45] In multiple contemporary clinical trials in UA/NSTEMI, including GUSTO IIb,[46] Platelet Receptor Inhibition in Ischemic Syndrome Management in Patients Limited by Unstable Signs and Symptoms (PRISM-PLUS),[9] FRagmin and Fast Revascularisation during InStability in Coronary artery disease (FRISC) II,[12] Treat angina with Aggrastat and determine Cost of Therapy with an Invasive or Conservative Strategy (TACTICS)-TIMI 18,[11] and GUSTO IV-ACS,[27] diabetics were found to have 1.5 to 2.0 times the rates of death and cardiac ischemic events. The independent prognostic significance of diabetes was demonstrated using data from the Organization to Assess Strategies for Ischemic Syndrome (OASIS) registry, which showed that diabetes was an independent risk factor for mortality in non–ST-elevation ACS (relative risk, 1.57; 95% CI, 1.38 to 1.81).

Smoking

The smoker's paradox in ACSs has been well-described.[47] Current smokers tend to have lower rates of death and ischemic events than nonsmokers. This paradoxical benefit appears to be explained largely by the fact that smokers present at an earlier age than do nonsmokers and hence have less comorbidity and less extensive coronary artery disease. Thus, among patients with ACSs, *univariate* analyses show that current smokers have lower event rates than do nonsmokers[9,12,18] but *multivariable* analyses show that current smoking is not a significant independent prognostic factor.[18,48]

Peripheral Arterial Disease

Patients with peripheral arterial disease frequently have significant coronary artery disease; thus, it is not surprising that peripheral arterial disease is a risk factor for death and ischemic complications in patients with UA/NSETMI. However, what is striking is that in a multivariable analysis in the Orbofiban in Patients with Unstable coronary Syndromes (OPUS)-TIMI 16 trial that adjusted for other traditional risk factors, peripheral arterial disease remained an independent risk factor for death (odds ratio, 1.44; *P* = .0045) as well as for a composite of cardiac ischemic events (odds ratio, 1.21; *P* = .0035). Results were similar in the PURSUIT study.[18,49]

Prior Aspirin Use

Multiple studies have confirmed that patients with prior aspirin use are at increased risk.[14,50,51] Whether this is due to the presence of "aspirin-resistant" platelet-rich thrombi or to the greater likelihood of severe coronary artery disease in patients who present with UA/NSTEMI despite taking aspirin remains unclear.[52,53]

ACUTE PRESENTATION

The tempo of the acute presentation, specific physical findings, electrocardiographic changes, and biochemical evidence of myocardial necrosis have all been shown to convey important prognostic information.

Severity of Angina

In 1989, Braunwald differentiated among primary angina (due to plaque rupture and a reduction in myocardial blood supply), secondary angina (due to non–cardiac-induced mismatch), and postinfarction angina. He further differentiated between new-onset, crescendo, and rest angina. The importance of these distinctions have been supported in several studies, in which multiple episodes of angina in the preceding 24 hours, angina at rest, and postinfarction angina each has been shown to convey a worse prognosis.[14,54-57]

Physical Examination

Physical findings indicative of severe left-ventricular contractile dysfunction, such as the presence of an S_3 gallop, rales, a mitral regurgitation murmur, hypotension, and tachycardia, are more common in the setting of STEMI than of UA/NSTEMI. Such findings also confer a worse prognosis in UA/NSTEMI. In 1967, Killip and Kimball noted the significance of these physical findings in

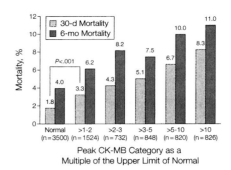

FIGURE 22–1. Mortality rates at 30 days and 6 months by peak creatinine kinase MB levels in the PURSUIT trial. (Reproduced with permission from Alexander JH, Sparapani RA, Mahaffey KW, et al: Association between minor elevations of creatine kinase-MB level and mortality in patients with acute coronary syndromes without ST-segment elevation. PURSUIT Steering Committee. Platelet Glycoprotein IIb/IIIa in Unstable Angina: Receptor Suppression Using Integrilin Therapy. JAMA 2000;283:347–353. ©2000, American Medical Association.

patients with STEMI.[58] Such findings remain important components of contemporary integrated risk scores.[19,20] Although these findings are rarer in UA/NSTEMI, their presence suggests significant underlying coronary artery disease and they are associated with mortality rates in excess of 60%.[59]

Electrocardiogram

The admission electrocardiogram (ECG) is one of the most useful and powerful predictors of adverse outcomes in ACSs. ST-segment depression on the presenting ECG indicates severe acute ischemia and is correlated with a worse in-hospital prognosis.[60,61] ST-segment depression is also associated with greater complexity of the culprit lesion[61] and hence a greater likelihood of requiring revascularization.[15] ST-segment depression is also indicative of more extensive coronary artery disease[15,61] and is associated with worse

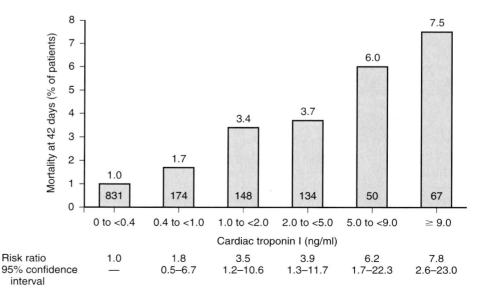

FIGURE 22–2. Mortality rate at 42 days by baseline cardiac troponin I levels in the TIMI IIIB Trial. (Reproduced with permission from Antman EM, Tanasijevic MJ, Thompson B, et al: Cardiac-specific troponin I levels to predict the risk of mortality in patients with acute coronary syndromes. N Engl J Med 1996;335:1342-1349. ©1996, Massachusetts Medical Society.)

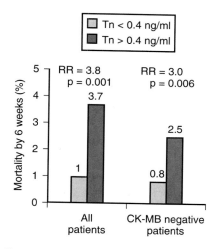

FIGURE 22–3. Mortality rate at 42 days by baseline cardiac troponin I status in the total group *(left)* and in patients with positive creatine kinase MB (CK-MB) results *(right)*. Tn, troponin. (Data from Antman EM, Tanasijevic MJ, Thompson B, et al: Cardiac-specific troponin I levels to predict the risk of mortality in patients with acute coronary syndromes. N Engl J Med 1996;335:1342–1349.)

outcomes at 6 months,[61] 1 year,[15] 4 years,[62] and 10 years.[63]

Importantly, ST-segment deviation of as little as 0.05 mV is associated with a higher rate of adverse events. In the TIMI III registry, patients with 0.05 mV ST-segment depression had an approximately twofold higher risk of death or MI at 30 days and at 1 year.[15,61] Moreover, there appears to be a gradient of increasing risk with increasing degree of ST depression. Among patients with non–ST-elevation ACSs, the 4-year survival rates for patients with 0.05 mV, 0.10 mV, or 0.20 mV (or greater) ST-segment depression were 82%, 77%, and 53%, respectively (P < .0001).[62]

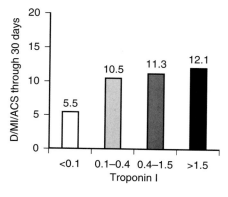

FIGURE 22–4. Death (D), myocardial infarction (MI), or rehospitalization through 30 days by baseline cardiac troponin I levels in the TACTICS-TIMI 18 trial. For the Bayer troponin I assay, the 97.5th percentile in healthy controls is 0.1 ng/mL, the level at which the assay has a 10% coefficient of variation is 0.4 ng/mL, and the level that corresponds to an MI defined by creatinine kinase MB elevation is 1.5 ng/mL. ACS, acute coronary syndrome; D, death. (Data from Morrow DA, Cannon CP, Rifai N, et al: Ability of minor elevations of troponins I and T to predict benefit from an early invasive strategy in patients with unstable angina and non-ST elevation myocardial infarction. JAMA 2001;286: 2405–2412.)

In contrast with ST depressions, T-wave inversions in general have not been shown to be associated with a worse prognosis.[15] However, deep (≥0.20 mV) precordial T-wave inversions are suggestive of left anterior descending artery disease and are associated with a worse prognosis.[64,65]

Detection of Necrosis

Another important predictor of outcome is the detection of myocyte necrosis. Patients with documented biochemical evidence of myocyte necrosis have higher mortality rates than do patients without elevations.[66] Moreover, there is a quantitative relationship between the magnitude of creatinine kinase MB (CK-MB) elevation and the risk of death (Fig. 22–1).[67]

Cardiac-specific troponins, with their superior sensitivity and specificity, have emerged as the biomarkers of choice for detecting myocyte necrosis.[2] As with CK-MB, there is a clear relationship between the magnitude of troponin elevation and mortality (Fig. 22–2).[68,69] With greater clinical sensitivity, troponins have enabled the detection of "microinfarctions" in approximately 30% of patients in whom the diagnosis would otherwise have been UA.[68] These patients, with an elevated troponin level but a negative CK-MB result, have been shown to be at three to four times the risk of dying compared with patients without an elevated troponin level and positive CK-MB results (Fig. 22–3).[6,68-70]

Debate has emerged about appropriate cut points for troponin assays. Some manufacturers have identified both a "diagnostic" cut point for MI that was selected from receiver-operating-curve analyses to correspond to CK-MB–defined MI and a "prognostic" cut point based on an upper limit of normal defined at the 97.5th percentile of a control population. With the emergence of troponins over CK-MB as the new gold standard for MI and questions of precision at the very low end of many assays, others have argued that a single cut point be adopted at the 99th percentile (assuming the coefficient of variation is < 10%).[2,71] However, work from trials of UA/NSTEMI have supported the prognostic importance of low-level troponin elevations even with more-sensitive current-generation assays (Fig. 22–4).[72]

Myoglobin is a small cytosolic protein found in both myocardial and skeletal muscle and is one of the earliest markers to be released in the circulation after an MI. Although not specific for myocardial injury, myoglobin is a sensitive marker, especially in the first 4 to 8 hours after the onset of necrosis.[73-75] In two separate UA/NSTEMI cohorts (TIMI IIB and TACTICS-TIMI 18), we have shown that an elevated baseline myoglobin is associated with increased 6-month mortality, independent of baseline characteristics, ECG changes, CK-MB, and troponin.[76] The pathobiologic underpinnings for this independent prognostic information are not yet defined.

INTEGRATED APPROACHES

Although the prognostic information associated with each of the discussed variables is useful, focusing on a single variable does not permit the clinician to use all of the information at their disposal. For example, a patient may have negative results for cardiac biomarkers; however, the patient may be elderly, have multiple cardiac risk factors, have had a prior MI, and be presenting with severe angina with ST depressions despite being on an aspirin. Clearly this patient is at high risk for death or cardiac ischemic events over the ensuing days and weeks despite a normal CK-MB level. Thus, relying on one predictor while ignoring others may lead to misclassification of risk.

In 1989, the need for an integrated approach was recognized with the Braunwald classification of UA.[13] Although typically used only to grade the severity of the acute presentation, the Braunwald system actually contains four axes: severity of acute symptoms, clinical circumstances, intensity of medical treatment, and electrocardiographic changes. The acute presentation was categorized as new-onset or crescendo angina without rest pain (class I); angina at rest but not within the preceding 48 hours (class II); and angina at rest within 48 hours (class III). The clinical circumstances (A, B, or C) were divided into secondary angina due to an extracardiac condition that intensified myocardial ischemia (A), primary angina presumably due to plaque rupture (B), and postinfarction angina (C). The intensity of medical treatment (denoted with subscripts 1, 2, or 3) ranged from angina occurring in the setting of no treatment, during treatment for chronic angina, and despite maximal anti-ischemic therapy. Finally, patients were divided into those with and without transient changes in ST-T wave during pain. Prospective validation of the Braunwald classification system confirmed the utility of such an approach.[77,78]

The completion of several recent clinical trials in which a wealth of baseline clinical, electrocardiographic, and serum marker data were gathered offered the opportunity to develop modern, integrated approaches to prognostication in UA/NSTEMI. These data have been used to develop several risk scores,[14,18,51] an example of which is the TIMI Risk Score for UA/NSTEMI, which was designed to provide clinicians with a prognostic tool with high discriminatory ability using baseline variables that are part of the routine medical evaluation.[14]

TIMI RISK SCORE FOR UNSTABLE ANGINA/NON–ST-SEGMENT ELEVATION MYOCARDIAL INFARCTION

Developing a Model

The TIMI Risk Score for UA/NSTEMI was developed in a derivation cohort consisting of 1957 patients who were randomized to the unfractionated heparin (UFH) arm of the TIMI IIB trial. TIMI IIB was a phase III, international, randomized, double-blind UA/NSTEMI trial comparing UFH with the LMWH enoxaparin.[7] The primary end point was the composite of all-cause mortality, new or recurrent MI, or severe recurrent ischemia prompting urgent revascularization by day 14.

Potential predictor variables were selected from baseline characteristics that could be readily identified at presentation and that had previously been reported to be important variables in predicting outcome (Table 22–1). Using multivariable logistic regression, seven independent, statistically significant predictors of the composite end point at 14 days were identified:

- Age ≥65 years
- Three or more risk factors for coronary artery disease
- Prior coronary artery stenosis ≥50%
- Severe anginal symptoms (two or more anginal events in the preceding 24 hours)
- Use of aspirin in the last 7 days

■ ■ ■

TABLE 22–1   BASELINE CHARACTERISTICS ANALYZED FOR DEVELOPMENT OF THE TIMI RISK SCORE FOR UA/NSTEMI

CHARACTERISTIC	UNIVARIATE ANALYSIS		MULTIVARIABLE ANALYSIS	
	OR (95% CI)	P Value	OR (95% CI)	P Value
Age ≥65 years	1.60 (1.25–2.04)	<.001	1.75 (1.35–2.25)	<.001
Three or more risk factors for CAD*	1.45 (1.10–1.91)	.009	1.54 (1.16–2.06)	.003
Prior coronary stenosis ≥50%	1.73 (1.34–2.23)	<.001	1.70 (1.30–2.21)	<.001
Prior MI	1.27 (0.99–1.63)	.06		
Prior CABG	1.35 (0.97–1.88)	.07		
Prior PTCA	1.62 (1.16–2.26)	.004		
ST deviation ≥0.05 mV	1.40 (1.06–1.85)	.02	1.51 (1.13–2.02)	.005
Severe anginal symptoms (≥two anginal events in prior 24 hours)	1.57 (1.24–2.00)	<.001	1.53 (1.20–1.96)	.001
Use of aspirin in last 7 days	1.86 (1.26–2.73)	.002	1.74 (1.17–2.59)	.006
Use of IV UFH within 24 hours of enrollment	1.18 (0.92–1.51)	.19		
Elevated serum cardiac markers (CK-MB or troponin)	1.42 (1.12–1.80)	.004	1.56 (1.21–1.99)	<.001
Prior history of CHF	0.90 (0.53–1.53)	.70		

*Risk factors included family history of CAD, hypertension, hypercholesterolemia, diabetes, or being a current smoker.
CABG, coronary artery bypass graft; CAD, coronary artery disease; CHF, congestive heart failure; CI, confidence interval; MI, myocardial infarction; NSTEMI, non–ST-elevation MI; OR, odds ratio; PTCA, percutaneous transluminal coronary angioplasty; UA, unstable angina; UFH, unfractionated heparin.
Adapted from Antman EM, Cohen M, Bernink PJ, et al: The TIMI risk score for unstable angina/non–ST elevation MI: A method for prognostication and therapeutic decision making. JAMA 2000; 284:835–842. ©2000, American Medical Association.

- ST deviation ≥0.05 mV
- Elevated serum cardiac marker (CK-MB or cardiac-specific troponin)

The final model demonstrated excellent calibration of the model predictions to the observed event rates (Hosmer-Lemeshow statistic[79] 3.56_{df8}; $P = .89$) as well as good overall predictive capacity of the model (C-statistic, 0.65).

Development of the Risk Score

Using a multivariable logistic regression model, one can calculate the probability of the outcome of interest for any given patient using a complex equation that weights each of the individual predictors. Such an approach, however, requires computational support and thus typically precludes rapid point-of-care bedside application. However, a simple integer-weighting scheme may be devised to enable application of such a risk model at the point of care.

Because the magnitudes of the prognostic significance (i.e., the odds ratios) for each independent predictor variable were similar, the TIMI Risk Score for UA/NSTEMI was constructed as the simple arithmetic sum of the number of predictors. Thus, the risk score is calculated by assigning 1 point for each variable that is present (Table 22-2).

Clinical Utility of the Model

Application of the TIMI Risk Score for UA/NSTEMI to patients in the UFH derivation cohort revealed that the score has several features desirable in risk stratification. First, the pattern of TIMI risk scores within that population followed a normal distribution (see bottom row of Fig. 22-5). Second, there was a progressive, significant pattern of increasing event rates for the composite endpoint of death, MI, and urgent revascularization ($P < .001$ by χ^2 for trend; see Fig. 22-5) with increasing TIMI Risk Score. Third, this pattern was also apparent for each component of the composite end point ($P < .001$ by χ^2 for trend for each component).[14] Fourth, the TIMI Risk Score categorized patients into a wide range of risk. The

■ ▪ ■

TABLE 22–2   TIMI RISK SCORE FOR UA/NSTEMI

CHARACTERSITIC	POINTS
Historical	
Age ≥65 years	1
Three or more risk factors for CAD	1
Known CAD (stenosis ≥50%)	1
Aspirin use in past 7 days	1
Presentation	
Recent (≤24 hr) severe angina	1
ST deviation ≥0.5 mm	1
↑ Cardiac markers	1
Risk Score = Total Points	(0–7)

CAD, coronary artery disease; NSTEMI, non–ST-elevation myocardial intervention; UA, unstable angina.

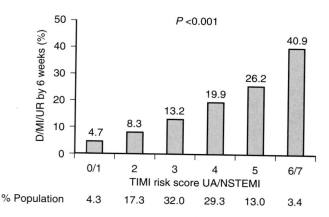

FIGURE 22–5. Death (D), myocardial infarction (MI), or need for urgent revascularization (UR) through 6 weeks by TIMI Risk Score in the unfractionated heparin arm of the TIMI IIB trial. NSTEMI, non-ST-segment elevation MI; UA, unstable angina. (Data from Antman EM, Cohen M, Bernink PJ, et al: The TIMI risk score for unstable angina/non-ST elevation MI: A method for prognostication and therapeutic decision making. JAMA 2000;284:835–842.)

rate of death, MI, or urgent revascularization was less than 5% in patients with a score of 0 or 1; the rate exceeded 40% in patients with a score of 6 or 7.

Validation of the Model

Although a well-constructed prediction model may perform adequately within its own derivation cohort, this is no guarantee that it will perform well in other cohorts. Therefore, prospective validation is required to ensure generalizability to other patient populations. The TIMI Risk Score for UA/NSTEMI was validated in three separate cohorts of patients: the enoxaparin group from TIMI IIB (n = 1953), the UFH group from the Efficacy and Safety of Subcutaneous Enoxaparin in Unstable Angina and Non–Q-Wave MI (ESSENCE) trial (n = 1564), and the enoxaparin group from the ESSENCE trial (n = 1564).[8] For all three validation cohorts, the rate of events increased significantly as the TIMI Risk Score increased ($P < .001$ by χ^2 for trend) and the C-statistics ranged from 0.59 to 0.65, confirming the generalizability of the risk score. Moreover, the slope of the increase in event rates was not statistically different between the UFH arms in TIMI IIB and ESSENCE ($P = .18$), demonstrating a homogeneous risk pattern among patients receiving similar treatments across different trials.[14]

The TIMI Risk Score has also been tested retrospectively in another UA/NSTEMI clinical trial population: PRISM-PLUS.[9] The pattern of TIMI risk scores within that population followed a normal distribution. As it did in TIMI IIB and ESSENCE, stratification by the TIMI Risk Score in PRISM-PLUS revealed an increasing gradient of risk for the prespecified composite end point of death, MI, and refractory ischemia by 14 days ($P < .001$ by χ^2 for trend).[80] The C-statistic (0.64) was similar to what was observed in the derivation cohort, and the Hosmer-Lemeshow goodness-of-fit test statistic was 3.85 with 3 degrees of freedom, yielding $P = .28$ and demonstrating good calibration.

The risk score was *prospectively* applied in the TACTICS-TIMI 18 UA/NSTEMI clinical trial,[11] using the prespecified composite end point of death, MI, or readmission for an ACS by 6 months. Once again, the pattern of TIMI risk scores within that population followed a normal distribution and there was a statistically significant increasing gradient of risk with an increasing risk score ($P < .001$ by χ^2 for trend).

The TIMI Risk Score was designed to facilitate risk stratification in patients with UA/NSTEMI. It was *not* designed to aid in the diagnosis of UA/NSTEMI, which remains a clinical diagnosis that may be supported by appropriate ECG changes and, in the case of NSTEMI, requires that myonecrosis biomarkers be elevated. Nonetheless, the TIMI Risk Score has been applied to unselected patients presenting to an emergency department with chest pain and has performed well in terms of predicting major cardiac adverse events, including death, MI, and severe ischemia requiring coronary revascularization: The event rates ranged from 0% among patients with a score of 0 to 70% among patients with a risk score of 6 or 7 ($P < .0001$).[81]

Thus, integrated risk scores such as the TIMI Risk Score for UA/NSTEMI serve as simple bedside tools for predicting death and cardiac ischemic events. Clinicians can use the prognostic information from risk scores to guide their decisions regarding triage and clinical resource allocation during the patient's index hospitalization. Moreover, such risk scores appear to predict not only which patients will suffer acute events but also which patients are at risk for dying or suffering cardiac ischemic events after discharge.[82]

NOVEL CARDIAC BIOMARKERS

Previously, cardiac biomarkers were limited to CK-MB, aspartate aminotransferase, and lactate dehydrogenase and were used to diagnose myocardial necrosis. Cardiac specific troponins offer a more sensitive and specific marker of myocyte necrosis and have proven to be an excellent prognostic indicator. More recently, however, several new biomarkers have been developed that provide insight into different aspects of the pathophysiology of ACSs.

C-Reactive Protein

C-reactive protein (CRP) has been used for decades as a marker of systemic inflammation. We now appreciate that inflammation plays a central role in atherosclerosis and that CRP itself may play a direct role in causing thrombosis.[83] Data from the Physician's Health Study revealed that among healthy persons with a supposedly normal CRP level (<1.5 mg/dL), there was a gradient of risk for MI with increasing CRP levels.[84] Studies in patients with ACSs revealed that patients with an elevated CRP level experienced worse short-term and long-term outcomes.[85,86] In several studies, CRP proved to be a potent predictor of short-term and long-term mortality, even after adjusting for troponin (Fig. 22–6).[86,87] Still, there is some discordance in the data with respect to

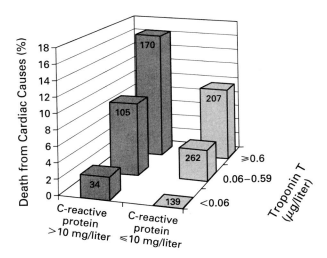

FIGURE 22–6. Cardiovascular mortality rate through 2 years by baseline C-reactive protein and cardiac troponin T status in the FRISC trial. (Reproduced with permission from Lindahl B, Toss H, Siegbahn A, Venge P, et al: FRagmin during Instability in Coronary Artery Disease. Markers of myocardial damage and inflammation in relation to long-term mortality in unstable coronary artery disease. N Engl J Med 2000;343: 1139-1147. ©2000, Massachusetts Medical Society.

predictive capacity of CRP for short-term outcomes. Moreover, the optimal timing of CRP measurements, precise clinical cut points, and methods of handling necrosis as a confounder remain to be firmly established.

B-Type Natriuretic Peptide

B-type natriuretic peptide (BNP) is synthesized and released by the ventricles in response to overload. Measuring BNP levels has proven useful in diagnosing and optimizing treatment for heart failure.[88,89] BNP levels have also been shown to be elevated in ACSs.[90] de Lemos et al demonstrated that the baseline level of BNP is correlated with the risk of death, MI, and congestive heart failure through 10 months (Fig. 22–7).[91] This relationship held true for STEMI, NSTEMI, and UA. It may be that ischemia-triggered transient left-ventricular systolic and diastolic dysfunction leads to the release of BNP; thus, BNP levels may reflect not only any underlying impairment in left-ventricular function but also the severity of the acute ischemic insult.[92]

Now that CRP and BNP assays are widely available, these biomarkers may improve our ability to stratify the risk of patients with UA/NSTEMI via a multimarker approach. Using data from two contemporary trials of ACS (OPUS-TIMI 16[93] and TACTICS-TIMI 18[11]), we categorized patients on the basis of the number of elevated biomarkers at presentation.[94] Each additional biomarker that was elevated led to a doubling of mortality risk (Fig. 22–8). Similar relationships existed for the end points of MI, congestive heart failure, and the composite end point. In a multivariable analysis that adjusted for clinical factors (including age, diabetes, prior MI, and ST depression), patients with one, two, and three elevated biomarkers experienced 2.1-fold, 3.1-fold, and 3.7-fold increases in the risk of death, MI, or congestive heart failure through 6 months ($P < .01$ for each hazard ratio). The

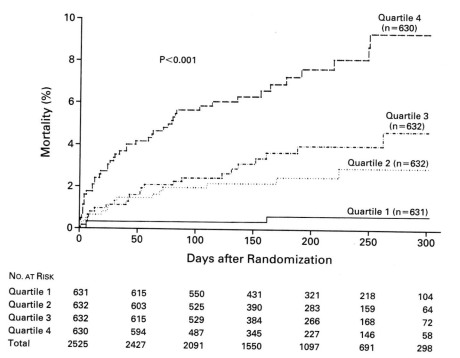

FIGURE 22–7. Mortality rate through 10 months by baseline B-type natriuretic peptide quartile in the TACTICS-TIMI 18 trial. (Reproduced with permission from de Lemos JA, Morrow DA, Bentley JH, et al: The prognostic value of B-type natriuretic peptide in patients with acute coronary syndromes. N Engl J Med 2001;345:1014–1021. ©2000, Massachusetts Medical Society.)

No. AT RISK						
Quartile 1	631	615	550	431	321	218	104
Quartile 2	632	603	525	390	283	159	64
Quartile 3	632	615	529	384	266	168	72
Quartile 4	630	594	487	345	227	146	58
Total	2525	2427	2091	1550	1097	691	298

incorporation of these new markers into existing integrated risk scores is the next logical step.

RISK STRATIFICATION AND CLINICAL DECISION MAKING

Not only is risk stratification useful for prognosis, it helps guide the use of specific therapies. In particular, LMWHs, GP IIb/IIIa inhibitors, and early invasive strategy are three treatment decisions about which clinicians continue to debate.[6] Each of the three treatments has been shown to be beneficial in large randomized trials. Nonetheless, the cost and potential complications associated with each of these treatments suggest the need for identifying patients who would derive particular benefit from these therapies.

In addition to their powerful prognostic role, troponin levels can also be used to guide therapy. In several of the trials of GP IIb/IIIa inhibitors in UA/NSTEMI, baseline blood samples were available for assessment of troponin levels. The message from the trials is remarkably consistent. In CAPTURE,[95] PRISM,[96] PRISM-PLUS,[97] and PARAGON-B,[98] among patients with elevated baseline troponin levels, the addition of a GP IIb/IIIa inhibitor was associated with relative risk reductions of 40% to 80% (see Fig. 22–7). In contrast, there was no demonstrable benefit among patients with normal troponin levels. Troponins have also proven useful in the setting of other potent medical therapies such as LMWH. Patients with elevated troponins have been shown to derive particular benefit from both short-term and extended therapy with LMWH.[99,100]

A similar interaction between troponin status and the benefits of an early invasive strategy was detected in the TACTICS-TIMI 18 trial. Patients with an elevated troponin (troponin I > 0.1 mg/L or troponin T > 0.01) showed a 39% relative risk reduction in the primary end point with the early invasive strategy versus the conservative strategy.[72] In contrast, the early invasive strategy showed no benefit in patients with normal troponin levels.

However, such binary categorization of troponin status—either positive or negative—may be too simplistic.[101] Although there is a steady monotonic rise in mortality risk with increasing troponin levels,[68] the risk of recurrent myocardial infarction appears to have a U-shaped relation with troponin levels.[102] Furthermore, although troponin-positive patients (as a whole) benefit from GP IIb/IIIa inhibitors and an early invasive strategy, the magnitude of benefit follows a U-shaped curve in relation to the degree of troponin elevation. In the PRISM study, the benefit of tirofiban in reducing death or MI was nonexistent in patients with undetectable or minimal levels of troponin, greatest among patients with intermediate elevations of troponin, and more modest in patients with higher levels of troponin.[96] A similar U-shaped interaction was seen in TACTICS-TIMI 18 in regard to troponin elevations and the benefit from an early invasive strategy.[72]

Moreover, despite the large amount of data supporting the prognostic utility of cardiac-specific troponins, they should not be viewed in isolation. For example, treatment with the GP IIb/IIIa inhibitor abciximab was not associated with a reduction in death or MI in the subset of patients in GUSTO IV-ACS in whom the baseline troponin level was elevated. Admittedly, abciximab was not effective in the overall GUSTO IV trial population. However, lamifiban was not efficacious in the overall cohort of patients in PARAGON-B, but the troponin-positive subset did show a robust benefit with GP

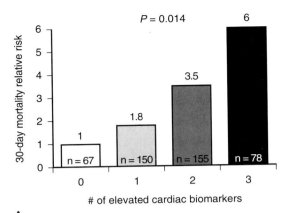

A

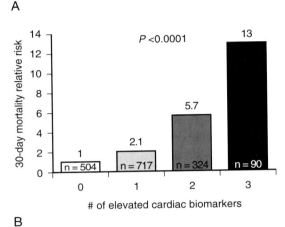

B

FIGURE 22–8. Relative 30-day mortality risks in patients stratified by number of elevated cardiac biomarkers (troponin I, C-reactive protein, and B-type natriuretic peptide) in OPUS-TIMI *(A)* and TACTICS-TIMI 18 *(B).* (Reproduced with permission from Sabatine MS, Morrow DA, de Lemos JA, et al: Multimarker approach to risk stratification in non-ST elevation acute coronary syndromes: Simultaneous assessment of troponin I, C-reactive protein, and B-type natriuretic peptide. Circulation 2002;105:1760-1763. ©2002, American Heart Association.

IIb/IIIa inhibition. There were also issues regarding the patient population and study drug dosing in GUSTO IV. Nonetheless, this example shows that a single positive

risk factor, even an elevated troponin, may be misleading when not viewed in the broader clinical context of integrated risk assessment. To that end, in their UA/NSTEMI guidelines, the American College of Cardiology/American Heart Association notes that "troponins should not be relied on as the sole markers for risk, because patients without troponin elevations may still exhibit a substantial risk of an adverse outcome. Neither [cardiac troponin I] nor [cardiac troponin T] is totally sensitive and specific in this regard."[6]

Diabetes is another prognostic factor with therapeutic implications. In a meta-analysis of the six major trials examining the use of GP IIb/IIIa inhibitors in UA/NSTEMI, treatment with a GP IIb/IIIa was associated with a statistically significant 26% reduction in mortality in diabetics (Fig. 22–9).[103] In contrast, there was no treatment effect in nondiabetics. It is pathobiologically plausible that inhibition of platelet aggregation is particularly important in diabetics. However, as noted earlier, many other comorbid states aggregate in diabetics; furthermore, because this was a univariate analysis, it would be premature to deny GP IIb/IIIa inhibitors to nondiabetics.[104]

The advantages of an integrated approach to risk stratification also hold true for therapeutic decision-making. Using the TIMI Risk Score for UA/NSTEMI, we have demonstrated a gradient of benefit for the use LMWH, GP IIb/IIIa inhibitors, and an early invasive strategy. In TIMI IIB and ESSENCE, treatment with the LMWH enoxaparin had a similar effect as treatment with UFH in patients with a risk score of 0 to 2, conferred a 17% relative risk reduction ($P = .016$) in patients with a risk score of 3 or 4, and conferred a 25% relative risk reduction ($P = .0025$) in patients with a risk score of 5 to 7 ($P_{interaction} = .02$) (Fig. 22–10).[14] As the TIMI Risk Score increases, the absolute and relative risk reductions in the composite end point with enoxaparin increase and, consequently, the number of patients needed to treat to prevent one event decreases.

Similarly, in PRISM-PLUS, treatment with the combination of the GP IIb/IIIa inhibitor tirofiban and UFH had an effect similar to that of treatment with UFH alone in

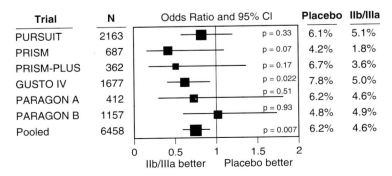

30-DAY MORTALITY DIABETIC PATIENTS

Trial	N	Odds Ratio and 95% CI		Placebo	IIb/IIIa
PURSUIT	2163		p = 0.33	6.1%	5.1%
PRISM	687		p = 0.07	4.2%	1.8%
PRISM-PLUS	362		p = 0.17	6.7%	3.6%
GUSTO IV	1677		p = 0.022	7.8%	5.0%
PARAGON A	412		p = 0.51	6.2%	4.6%
PARAGON B	1157		p = 0.93	4.8%	4.9%
Pooled	6458		p = 0.007	6.2%	4.6%

Breslow-Day: $P = 0.50$

FIGURE 22–9. Odds ratios and 95% confidence intervals (CI) for treatment effect of GP IIb/IIIa inhibitors on 30-day mortality in diabetic patients in six trials of GP IIb/IIIa inhibitors in unstable angina/non–ST-segment elevation myocardial infarction. (Reproduced with permission from Roffi M, Chew DP, Mukherjee D, et al: Platelet glycoprotein IIb/IIIa inhibitors reduce mortality in diabetic patients with non-ST-segment elevation acute coronary syndromes. Circulation 2001;104:2767. ©2001, American Heart Association.)

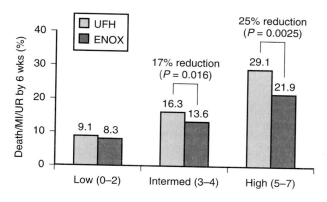

FIGURE 22–10. Death (D), myocardial infarction (MI), or need for urgent revascularization (UR) through 6 weeks by TIMI Risk Score and randomized treatment arm in the combined TIMI IIB and ESSENCE meta-analysis. ENOX, enoxaparin; UFH, unfractionated heparin. (Data from Antman EM, Cohen M, Bernink PJ, et al: The TIMI risk score for unstable angina/non-ST elevation MI: A method for prognostication and therapeutic decision making. JAMA 2000;284:835-842.)

patients with a risk score of less than 4, but the combination conferred a 34% relative risk reduction (P = .016) in patients with a risk score of 4 or higher ($P_{interaction}$ = .05) (Fig. 22-11).[80] Subgroup analyses from the GP IIb/IIIa inhibitor trials in UA/NSTEMI have suggested that the benefit of GP IIb/IIIa inhibition occurs primarily in patients who undergo percutaneous intervention. However, not only are these analyses potentially confounded by the fact that patients who undergo revascularization during their index hospitalization tend to be a sicker group, but the implications are less than practical as the decision to undergo revascularization may occur relatively late in the patient's hospital course. Instead,

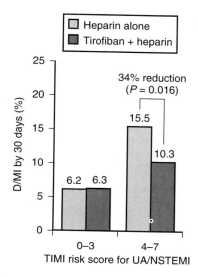

FIGURE 22–11. Death (D) or myocardial infarction (MI) through 30 days by TIMI Risk Score and randomized treatment arm in the PRISM-PLUS trial. NSTEMI, non–ST-segment elevation MI; UA, unstable angina. (Data from Morrow DA, Antman EM, Snapinn SM, et al: An integrated clinical approach to predicting the benefit of tirofiban in non-ST elevation acute coronary syndromes. Application of the TIMI Risk Score for UA/NSTEMI in PRISM-PLUS. Eur Heart J 2002;23:223-229.)

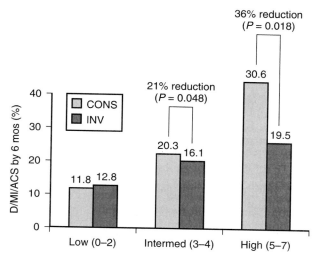

FIGURE 22–12. Death (D), myocardial infarction (MI), or rehospitalization for an acute coronary syndrome (ACS) through 6 months by TIMI Risk Score and randomized treatment arm in the TACTICS-TIMI 18 trial. NSTEMI, non–ST-segment elevation MI; UA, unstable angina. CONS, conservative strategy; INV, invasive strategy. (Data from Cannon CP, Weintraub WS, Demopoulos LA, et al: Comparison of early invasive and conservative strategies in patients with unstable coronary syndromes treated with the glycoprotein IIb/IIIa inhibitor tirofiban. N Engl J Med 2001;344:1879-1887.)

when patients were stratified by their baseline TIMI Risk Score, those with a risk score of 4 or higher who received tirofiban experienced relative risk reductions in death, MI, or refractory ischemia of 25% to 30%, regardless of whether they underwent percutaneous intervention.[105]

Finally, in TACTICS-TIMI 18, the TIMI Risk Score again defined a gradient of benefit: Treatment using an early invasive strategy had an effect similar to that of treatment with a conservative strategy in patients with a risk score of 0 to 2, conferred a 21% relative risk reduction (P = .048) in patients with a risk score of 3 or 4, and conferred a 36% relative risk reduction (P = .018) in patients with a risk score of 5 to 7 (Fig. 22-12).[11]

ALGORITHM

An algorithm for the approach to patients with suspected UA/NSTEMI is presented in Figure 22-13. This approach combines elements from the recent American College of Cardiology/American Heart Association 2002 Practice Update Guidelines for UA/NSTEMI with the pathways in place at Brigham and Women's Hospital.[106] A focused history and physical examination, 12-lead ECG, and cardiac biomarker determination provides all the elements necessary for appropriate risk stratification. The superior bioavailability, clinical efficacy, and ease of use of LMWHs suggest they should be the anticoagulant of choice. Recent data also suggest that LMWHs can safely be combined with a GP IIb/IIIa inhibitor.[107,108] However, depending on institutional

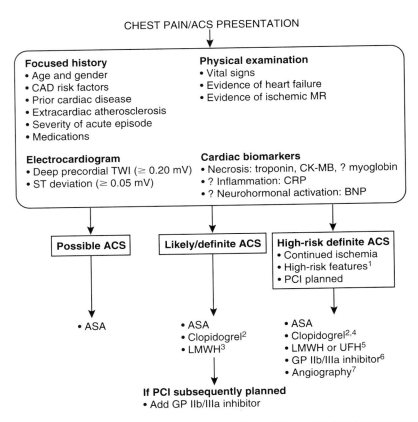

CHEST PAIN/ACS PRESENTATION

Focused history
- Age and gender
- CAD risk factors
- Prior cardiac disease
- Extracardiac atherosclerosis
- Severity of acute episode
- Medications

Physical examination
- Vital signs
- Evidence of heart failure
- Evidence of ischemic MR

Electrocardiogram
- Deep precordial TWI ($\geq$ 0.20 mV)
- ST deviation ($\geq$ 0.05 mV)

Cardiac biomarkers
- Necrosis: troponin, CK-MB, ? myoglobin
- ? Inflammation: CRP
- ? Neurohormonal activation: BNP

Possible ACS

Likely/definite ACS

High-risk definite ACS
- Continued ischemia
- High-risk features[1]
- PCI planned

- ASA

- ASA
- Clopidogrel[2]
- LMWH[3]

- ASA
- Clopidogrel[2,4]
- LMWH or UFH[5]
- GP IIb/IIIa inhibitor[6]
- Angiography[7]

If PCI subsequently planned
- Add GP IIb/IIIa inhibitor

FIGURE 22–13. Algorithm for risk stratification and treatment decision in patients with non–ST-elevation acute coronary syndromes. ACS, acute coronary syndrome; ASA, aspirin; BNP, B-type natriuretic peptide; CAD, coronary artery disease; CK-MB, creatinine kinase MB fraction; CRP, C-reactive protein; GP, glycoprotein; LMWH, low-molecular weight heparin; MR, mitral regurgitation; PCI, percutaneous intervention; TWI, T-wave inversion; UFH, unfractionated heparin.
[1]High-risk features include TIMI Risk Score $\geq$ 3, age > 75 years, diabetes, prior myocardial infarction, hemodynamic compromise, ST-segment depression, or an elevated cardiac biomarkers of necrosis.
[2]Clopidgrel should be given as a 300 mg loading dose followed by 75 mg PO four times daily.
[3]Tested LMWH regimens include enoxaparin 1 mg/kg[AU] SC twice a day ($\pm$30 mg IV bolus) and dalteparin 120 IU/kg SC twice a day. A greater benefit has been shown with enoxaparin than with other LMWHs, but few direct comparisons exist.
[4]In the setting of early angiography, clopidogrel may be withheld until it is clear that the patient will *not* be undergoing coronary artery bypass grafting.
[5]Enoxaparin has been shown to be superior to UFH, particularly in high-risk patients. Preliminary data also indicate that enoxaparin can safely be combined with a GP IIb/IIIa inhibitor. However, depending on institutional preferences, UFH can be considered if patient proceeding immediately to angiography. UFH should be administered using a weight-adjusted regimen: 60–70 U/kg IV bolus (maximum 5000 U) in an initial infusion of 12–15 U/kg/hr (maximum 1000 U/hr), titrated to an activated partial thromboplastin time of 60–80 sec.
[6]If PCI is planned, any of the GP IIb/IIIa inhibitors, including abciximab [0.25 mg/kg IV bolus followed by an infusion of 0.125 µg/kg/min [maximum, 10 µg/min)] can be given. If invasive management is *not* planned, either eptifibatide (180 µg/kg IVB followed by an infusion of 2.0 µg/kg/hr) or tirofiban (0.4 µg/kg/min × 30 min, followed by an infusion of 0.1 µg/kg/hr) should be given.
[7]Routine angiography should occur within 48 hr.

preferences, UFH can be considered in patients proceeding immediately to angiography. Based on the data presented earlier, GP IIb/IIIa inhibitors and early angiography are reserved for patients with definite ACS with continued ischemia, patients with high-risk features (including a TIMI Risk Score $\geq$3, troponin elevation, ST depression, and diabetes), or when percutaneous intervention is planned. As always, the appropriateness of guidelines must be viewed in the context of the specific patient.

REFERENCES

1. Cannon CP, Braunwald E: Unstable angina. In Braunwald E, Zipes DP, Libby P (eds): Heart Disease: A Textbook of Cardiovascular Medicine. Philadelphia, WB Saunders, 2001, pp 1232-1271.

2. Myocardial infarction redefined—a consensus document of The Joint European Society of Cardiology/American College of Cardiology Committee for the redefinition of myocardial infarction. Eur Heart J 2000;21:1502-1513.

3. Fuster V, Badimon L, Badimon JJ, Chesebro JH: The pathogenesis of coronary artery disease and the acute coronary syndromes (Part 1). N Engl J Med 1992;326:242-250.

4. Fuster V, Badimon L, Badimon JJ, Chesebro JH: The pathogenesis of coronary artery disease and the acute coronary syndromes (Part 2). N Engl J Med 1992;326:310-318.

5. Libby P: Molecular bases of the acute coronary syndromes. Circulation 1995;91:2844.

6. Braunwald E, Antman EM, Beasley JW, et al: ACC/AHA guidelines for the management of patients with unstable angina and non-ST-segment elevation myocardial infarction. A report of the American College of Cardiology/American Heart Association Task Force on Practice Guidelines (Committee on the Management of Patients With Unstable Angina). J Am Coll Cardiol 2000;36:970-1062.

7. Antman EM, McCabe CH, Gurfinkel EP, et al: Enoxaparin prevents death and cardiac ischemic events in unstable angina/non-Q-wave

myocardial infarction: Results of the thrombolysis in myocardial infarction (TIMI) IIB trial. Circulation 100:1593–1601, 1999.

8. Cohen M, Demers C, Gurfinkel EP, et al: A comparison of low-molecular-weight heparin with unfractionated heparin for unstable coronary artery disease. N Engl J Med 1997;337:447–452.

9. The Platelet Receptor Inhibition in Ischemic Syndrome Management in Patients Limited by Unstable Signs and Symptoms (PRISM-PLUS) Study Investigators: Inhibition of the platelet glycoprotein IIb/IIIa receptor with tirofiban in unstable angina and non-Q-wave myocardial infarction. N Engl J Med 338:1488–1497, 1998.

10. The PURSUIT Trial Investigators: Inhibition of platelet glycoprotein IIb/IIIa with eptifibatide in patients with acute coronary syndromes. N Engl J Med 1998;339:436–443.

11. Cannon CP, Weintraub WS, Demopoulos LA, et al: Comparison of early invasive and conservative strategies in patients with unstable coronary syndromes treated with the glycoprotein IIb/IIIa inhibitor tirofiban. N Engl J Med 2001;344:1879–1887.

12. FRagmin and Fast Revascularisation during InStability in Coronary artery disease (FRISC II) Investigators: Invasive compared with non-invasive treatment in unstable coronary-artery disease: FRISC II prospective randomised multicentre study. Lancet 1999;354:708–715.

13. Braunwald E: Unstable angina. A classification. Circulation 1989;80:410–414.

14. Antman EM, Cohen M, Bernink PJ, et al: The TIMI risk score for unstable angina/non-ST elevation MI: A method for prognostication and therapeutic decision making. JAMA 2000;284:835–842.

15. Cannon CP, McCabe CH, Stone PH, et al: The electrocardiogram predicts one-year outcome of patients with unstable angina and non-Q wave myocardial infarction: Results of the TIMI III Registry ECG Ancillary Study. J Am Coll Cardiol 1997;30:133–140.

16. Smith PL: Splines as a useful and convenient statistical tool. Am Statistician 1979;33:57–62.

17. Harrell FE, Lee KL, Pollack BG: Regression models in clinical studies: Determining relationships between predictors and response. J Nat Can Inst 1988;80:1198–1202.

18. Boersma E, Pieper KS, Steyerberg EW, et al: Predictors of outcome in patients with acute coronary syndromes without persistent ST-segment elevation. Results from an international trial of 9461 patients. The PURSUIT Investigators. Circulation 2000;101:2557–2567.

19. Morrow DA, Antman EM, Charlesworth A, et al: TIMI risk score for ST-elevation myocardial infarction: A convenient, bedside, clinical score for risk assessment at presentation: An intravenous nPA for treatment of infarcting myocardium early II trial substudy. Circulation 2000;102:2031–2037.

20. Morrow DA, Antman EM, Giugliano RP, et al: A simple risk index for rapid initial triage of patients with ST-elevation myocardial infarction: an InTIME II substudy. Lancet 2001;358:1571–1575.

21. The TIMI IIIB Investigators: Effects of tissue plasminogen activator and a comparison of early invasive and conservative strategies in unstable angina and non-Q-wave myocardial infarction: Results of the TIMI IIIB Trial. Circulation 1994;89:1545–1556.

22. The Global Use of Strategies to Open Occluded Coronary Arteries (GUSTO) IIb Investigators: A comparison of recombinant hirudin with heparin for the treatment of acute coronary syndromes. N Engl J Med 1996;335:775–782.

23. Hochman JS, McCabe CH, Stone PH, et al: Outcome and profile of women and men presenting with acute coronary syndromes: A report from TIMI IIIB. TIMI Investigators. Thrombolysis in Myocardial Infarction. J Am Coll Cardiol 1997;30:141–148.

24. Hochman JS, Tamis JE, Thompson TD, et al: Sex, clinical presentation, and outcome in patients with acute coronary syndromes. Global Use of Strategies to Open Occluded Coronary Arteries in Acute Coronary Syndromes IIb Investigators. N Engl J Med 1999;341:226–232.

25. Weaver WD, White HD, Wilcox RG, et al: Comparisons of characteristics and outcomes among women and men with acute myocardial infarction treated with thrombolytic therapy. GUSTO-I investigators. JAMA 1996;275:777–782.

26. Tunstall-Pedoe H, Morrison C, Woodward M, et al: Sex differences in myocardial infarction and coronary deaths in the Scottish MONICA population of Glasgow 1985 to 1991. Presentation, diagnosis, treatment, and 28-day case fatality of 3991 events in men and 1551 events in women. Circulation 1996;93:1981–1992.

27. The GUSTO IV-ACS Investigators: Effect of glycoprotein IIb/IIIa receptor blocker abciximab on outcome in patients with acute coronary syndromes without early coronary revascularisation: the GUSTO IV-ACS randomised trial. Lancet 2001;357:1915–1924.

28. Harris MI. Diabetes in America: Epidemiology and scope of the problem. Diabetes Care 1998;21(Suppl 3):C11–C14.

29. National Institutes of Health: Third Report of the National Cholesterol Education Program Expert Panel on Detection, Evaluation, and Treatment of High Blood Cholesterol in Adults (Adult Treatment Panel III). Bethesda, National Institutes of Health, 2001.

30. Grundy SM: Hypertriglyceridemia, insulin resistance, and the metabolic syndrome. Am J Cardiol 1999;83:25F–29F.

31. Ford ES, Giles WH, Dietz WH: Prevalence of the metabolic syndrome among US adults: findings from the third National Health and Nutrition Examination Survey. JAMA 2002;287:356–359.

32. Baynes JW, Thorpe SR: Role of oxidative stress in diabetic complications: A new perspective on an old paradigm. Diabetes 1999;48:1–9.

33. Stitt AW, Bucala R, Vlassara H: Atherogenesis and advanced glycation: promotion, progression, and prevention. Ann N Y Acad Sci 1997;811:115–127; discussion 127–129.

34. Sagel J, Colwell JA, Crook L, Laimins M: Increased platelet aggregation in early diabetes mellitus. Ann Intern Med 1975;82:733–738.

35. Knobler H, Savion N, Shenkman B, et al: Shear-induced platelet adhesion and aggregation on subendothelium are increased in diabetic patients. Thromb Res 1998;90:181–190.

36. Auwerx J, Bouillon R, Collen D, Geboers J: Tissue-type plasminogen activator antigen and plasminogen activator inhibitor in diabetes mellitus. Arteriosclerosis 1988;8:68–72.

37. Calles-Escandon J, Mirza SA, Sobel BE, Schneider DJ: Induction of hyperinsulinemia combined with hyperglycemia and hypertriglyceridemia increases plasminogen activator inhibitor 1 in blood in normal human subjects. Diabetes 1998;47:290–293.

38. Jilma B, Fasching P, Ruthner C, et al: Elevated circulating P-selectin in insulin dependent diabetes mellitus. Thromb Haemost 1996;76:328–332.

39. Tschoepe D, Roesen P, Kaufmann L, et al: Evidence for abnormal platelet glycoprotein expression in diabetes mellitus. Eur J Clin Invest 1990;20:166–170.

40. Williams SB, Cusco JA, Roddy MA, et al: Impaired nitric oxide-mediated vasodilation in patients with non-insulin-dependent diabetes mellitus. J Am Coll Cardiol 1996;27:567–574.

41. Haffner SM, Lehto S, Ronnemaa T, et al: Mortality from coronary heart disease in subjects with type 2 diabetes and in nondiabetic subjects with and without prior myocardial infarction. N Engl J Med 1998;339:229–234.

42. Topol EJ, Califf RM, George BS, et al: A randomized trial of immediate versus delayed elective angioplasty after intravenous tissue plasminogen activator in acute myocardial infarction. N Engl J Med 1987;317:581–588.

43. The GUSTO Investigators: An international randomized trial comparing four thrombolytic strategies for acute myocardial infarction. N Engl J Med 1993;329:673–682.

44. Granger CB, Califf RM, Young S, et al: Outcome of patients with diabetes mellitus and acute myocardial infarction treated with thrombolytic agents. The Thrombolysis and Angioplasty in Myocardial Infarction (TAMI) Study Group. J Am Coll Cardiol 1993;21:920–925.

45. Woodfield SL, Lundergan CF, Reiner JS, et al: Angiographic findings and outcome in diabetic patients treated with thrombolytic therapy for acute myocardial infarction: The GUSTO-I experience. J Am Coll Cardiol 1996;28:1661–1669.

46. McGuire DK, Emanuelsson H, Granger CB, et al: Influence of diabetes mellitus on clinical outcomes across the spectrum of acute coronary syndromes. Findings from the GUSTO-IIb study. GUSTO IIb Investigators. Eur Heart J 2000;21:1750–1758.

47. Barbash GI, White HD, Modan M, et al: Significance of smoking in patients receiving thrombolytic therapy for acute myocardial infarction. Experience gleaned from the International Tissue Plasminogen Activator/Streptokinase Mortality Trial. Circulation 1993;87:53–58.

48. Barbash GI, Reiner J, White HD, et al: Evaluation of paradoxic beneficial effects of smoking in patients receiving thrombolytic therapy for acute myocardial infarction: Mechanism of the "smoker's

paradox" from the GUSTO-I trial, with angiographic insights. Global Utilization of Streptokinase and Tissue-Plasminogen Activator for Occluded Coronary Arteries. J Am Coll Cardiol 1995;26: 1222-1229.

49. Cotter G, Cannon CP, McCabe CH, et al: Prior peripheral vascular disease and cerebrovascular disease are independent predictors of increased 1 year mortality in patients with acute coronary syndromes: Results from OPUS-TIMI 16. J Am Coll Cardiol 2000;35:410A.

50. Alexander JH, Harrington RA, Tuttle RH, et al: Prior aspirin use predicts worse outcomes in patients with non-ST-elevation acute coronary syndromes. Am J Cardiol 1999;83:1147-1151.

51. Sabatine MS, Januzzi JL, Snapinn S, et al: A risk score system for predicting adverse outcomes and magnitude of benefit with glycoprotein IIb/IIIa inhibitor therapy in patients with unstable angina pectoris. Am J Cardiol 2001;88:488-492.

52. Helgason CM, Bolin KM, Hoff JA, et al: Development of aspirin resistance in persons with previous ischemic stroke. Stroke 1994;25:2331-2336.

53. Weber AA, Zimmermann KC, Meyer-Kirchrath J, Schror K: Cyclooxygenase-2 in human platelets as a possible factor in aspirin resistance. Lancet 1999;353:900.

54. Califf RM, Phillips HR III, Hindman MC, et al: Prognostic value of a coronary artery jeopardy score. J Am Coll Cardiol 1985;5: 1055-1063.

55. Califf RM, Mark DB, Harrell FE Jr, et al: Importance of clinical measures of ischemia in the prognosis of patients with documented coronary artery disease. J Am Coll Cardiol 1988;11:20-26.

56. White LD, Lee TH, Cook EF, et al: Comparison of the natural history of new onset and exacerbated chronic ischemic heart disease. The Chest Pain Study Group. J Am Coll Cardiol 1990;16:304-310.

57. van Miltenburg-van Zijl AJ, Simoons ML, Veerhoek RJ, Bossuyt PM: Incidence and follow-up of Braunwald subgroups in unstable angina pectoris. J Am Coll Cardiol 1995;25:1286-1292.

58. Killip T, 3rd, Kimball JT: Treatment of myocardial infarction in a coronary care unit. A two year experience with 250 patients. Am J Cardiol 1967;20:457-464.

59. Holmes DR Jr, Berger PB, Hochman JS, et al: Cardiogenic shock in patients with acute ischemic syndromes with and without ST-segment elevation. Circulation 1999;100:2067-2073.

60. Cohen M, Hawkins L, Greenberg S, Fuster V: Usefulness of ST-segment changes in greater than or equal to 2 leads on the emergency room electrocardiogram in either unstable angina pectoris or non-Q-wave myocardial infarction in predicting outcome. Am J Cardiol 1991;67:1368-1373.

61. Savonitto S, Ardissino D, Granger CB, et al: Prognostic value of the admission electrocardiogram in acute coronary syndromes. JAMA 1999;281:707-713.

62. Hyde TA, French JK, Wong CK, et al: Four-year survival of patients with acute coronary syndromes without ST-segment elevation and prognostic significance of 0.5-mm ST-segment depression. Am J Cardiol 1999;84:379-385.

63. Gazes PC, Mobley EM Jr, Faris HM Jr, et al: Preinfarctional (unstable) angina—a prospective study—ten year follow-up. Prognostic significance of electrocardiographic changes. Circulation 1973;48: 331-337.

64. Haines DE, Raabe DS, Gundel WD, Wackers FJ: Anatomic and prognostic significance of new T-wave inversion in unstable angina. Am J Cardiol 1983;52:14-18.

65. de Zwaan C, Bar FW, Janssen JH, et al: Angiographic and clinical characteristics of patients with unstable angina showing an ECG pattern indicating critical narrowing of the proximal LAD coronary artery. Am Heart J 1989;117:657-665.

66. Anderson HV, Cannon CP, Stone PH, et al: One-year results of the Thrombolysis in Myocardial Infarction (TIMI) IIIB clinical trial. A randomized comparison of tissue-type plasminogen activator versus placebo and early invasive versus early conservative strategies in unstable angina and non-Q wave myocardial infarction. J Am Coll Cardiol 1995;26:1643-1650.

67. Alexander JH, Sparapani RA, Mahaffey KW, et al: Association between minor elevations of creatine kinase-MB level and mortality in patients with acute coronary syndromes without ST-segment elevation. PURSUIT Steering Committee. Platelet Glycoprotein IIb/IIIa in Unstable Angina: Receptor Suppression Using Integrilin Therapy. JAMA 2000;283:347-353.

68. Antman EM, Tanasijevic MJ, Thompson B, et al: Cardiac-specific troponin I levels to predict the risk of mortality in patients with acute coronary syndromes. N Engl J Med 1996;335:1342-1349.

69. Ohman EM, Armstrong PW, Christenson RH, et al: Cardiac troponin T levels for risk stratification in acute myocardial ischemia. GUSTO IIA Investigators. N Engl J Med 1996;335:1333-1341.

70. Hamm CW, Ravkilde J, Gerhardt W, et al: The prognostic value of serum troponin T in unstable angina. N Engl J Med 1992;327: 146-150.

71. Jaffe AS, Ravkilde J, Roberts R, et al: It's time for a change to a troponin standard [editorial]. Circulation 2000;102:1216-1220.

72. Morrow DA, Cannon CP, Rifai N, et al: Ability of minor elevations of troponins I and T to predict benefit from an early invasive strategy in patients with unstable angina and non-ST elevation myocardial infarction. JAMA 2001;286:2405-2412.

73. de Winter RJ, Koster RW, Sturk A, Sanders GT: Value of myoglobin, troponin T, and CK-MBmass in ruling out an acute myocardial infarction in the emergency room. Circulation 1995;92:3401-3407.

74. Zimmerman J, Fromm R, Meyer D, et al: Diagnostic marker cooperative study for the diagnosis of myocardial infarction. Circulation 1999;99:1671-1677.

75. Newby LK, Storrow AB, Gibler WB, et al: Bedside multimarker testing for risk stratification in chest pain units: The chest pain evaluation by creatine kinase-MB, myoglobin, and troponin I (CHECKMATE) study. Circulation 2001;103:1832-1837.

76. de Lemos JA, Morrow DA, Gibson CM, et al: The prognostic value of serum myoglobin in patients with non-ST segment elevation acute coronary syndromes: Results from the TIMI IIB and TACTICS-TIMI 18 studies. J Am Coll Cardiol 2002; 40:238-244.

77. Cannon CP, McCabe CH, Stone PH, et al: Prospective validation of the Braunwald classification of unstable angina: Results from the Thrombolysis in Myocardial Infarction (TIMI) III Registry. Circulation 1995;92:I-19.

78. Calvin JE, Klein LW, VandenBerg BJ, et al: Risk stratification in unstable angina. Prospective validation of the Braunwald classification. JAMA 1995;273:136-141.

79. Hosmer DW, Lemeshow S: Applied Logistic Regression. New York, John Wiley & Sons, 1989.

80. Morrow DA, Antman EM, Snapinn SM, et al: An integrated clinical approach to predicting the benefit of tirofiban in non-ST elevation acute coronary syndromes. Application of the TIMI Risk Score for UA/NSTEMI in PRISM-PLUS. Eur Heart J 2002;23:223-229.

81. Bartholomew BA, Sheps DS, Monroe S, et al: A prospective evaluation of the TIMI Risk Score for unstable angina and non-ST-elevation myocardial infarction. Circulation 2001;104 (Suppl II):728.

82. Sabatine MS, McCabe CH, Morrow DA, et al: Predicting risk of postdischarge events in unstable angina. Circulation 2000;102:II-589.

83. Lagrand WK, Visser CA, Hermens WT, et al: C-reactive protein as a cardiovascular risk factor: More than an epiphenomenon? Circulation 1999;100:96-102.

84. Ridker PM, Cushman M, Stampfer MJ, et al: Inflammation, aspirin, and the risk of cardiovascular disease in apparently healthy men. N Engl J Med 1997;336:973-979.

85. Liuzzo G, Biasucci LM, Gallimore JR, et al: The prognostic value of C-reactive protein and serum amyloid a protein in severe unstable angina. N Engl J Med 1994;331:417-424.

86. Lindahl B, Toss H, Siegbahn A, et al: Fragmin during Instability in Coronary Artery Disease. Markers of myocardial damage and inflammation in relation to long-term mortality in unstable coronary artery disease. N Engl J Med 2000;343:1139-1147.

87. Morrow DA, Rifai N, Antman EM, et al: C-reactive protein is a potent predictor of mortality independently and in combination with troponin T in acute coronary syndromes: A TIMI 11A substudy. J Am Coll Cardiol 1998;31:1460-1465.

88. Cowie MR, Struthers AD, Wood DA, et al: Value of natriuretic peptides in assessment of patients with possible new heart failure in primary care. Lancet 1997;350:1347-1351.

89. Troughton RW, Frampton CM, Yandle TG, et al: Treatment of heart failure guided by plasma aminoterminal brain natriuretic peptide (N-BNP) concentrations. Lancet 2000;355:1126-1130.

90. Omland T, Aakvaag A, Bonarjee VV, et al: Plasma brain natriuretic peptide as an indicator of left ventricular systolic function and long-term survival after acute myocardial infarction. Comparison with plasma atrial natriuretic peptide and N-terminal proatrial natriuretic peptide. 1996;Circulation 93:1963-1969.

91. de Lemos JA, Morrow DA, Bentley JH, et al: The prognostic value of B-type natriuretic peptide in patients with acute coronary syndromes. N Engl J Med 2001;345:1014–1021.

92. Sabatine MS, Morrow DA, de Lemos JA, et al: Elevation of B-type natriuretic peptide in the setting of myocardial ischemia. Circulation 2001;104(Suppl II):485.

93. Cannon CP, McCabe CH, Wilcox RG, et al: Oral glycoprotein IIb/IIIa inhibition with orbofiban in patients with unstable coronary syndromes (OPUS-TIMI 16) trial. Circulation 2000;102:149–156.

94. Sabatine MS, Morrow DA, de Lemos JA, et al: Multimarker approach to risk stratification in non-ST elevation acute coronary syndromes: Simultaneous assessment of troponin I, C-reactive protein, and B-type natriuretic peptide. Circulation 2002;105:1760–1763.

95. Hamm CW, Heeschen C, Goldmann B, et al: Benefit of abciximab in patients with refractory unstable angina in relation to serum troponin T levels. N Engl J Med 1999;340:1623–1629.

96. Heeschen C, Hamm CW, Goldmann B, et al: Troponin concentrations for stratification of patients with acute coronary syndromes in relation to therapeutic efficacy of tirofiban. Lancet 1999;354:1757–1762.

97. Januzzi JL, Chae CU, Sabatine MS, Jang IK: Elevation in serum troponin I predicts the benefit of tirofiban. J Thromb Thrombolys 2001;11:211–215.

98. Newby LK, Ohman EM, Christenson RH, et al: Benefit of glycoprotein IIb/IIIa inhibition in patients with acute coronary syndromes and troponin T-positive status: The Paragon-B troponin T substudy. Circulation 2001;103:2891–2896.

99. Lindahl B, Venge P, Wallentin L, et al: Troponin T identifies patients with unstable coronary artery disease who benefit from long-term antithrombotic protection. J Am Coll Cardiol 1997;29:43–48.

100. Morrow DA, Antman EM, Tanasijevic M, et al: Cardiac troponin I for stratification of early outcomes and the efficacy of enoxaparin in unstable angina: A TIMI-IIB substudy. J Am Coll Cardiol 2000;36:1812–1817.

101. Antman EM: Troponin measurements in ischemic heart disease: more than just a black and white picture. J Am Coll Cardiol 2001;38:987–990.

102. Lindahl B, Diderholm E, Lagerqvist B, et al: Mechanisms behind the prognostic value of troponin T in unstable coronary artery disease: A FRISC II substudy. J Am Coll Cardiol 2001;38:979–986.

103. Roffi M, Chew DP, Mukherjee D, et al: Platelet glycoprotein IIb/IIIa inhibitors reduce mortality in diabetic patients with non-ST-segment elevation acute coronary syndromes. Circulation 2001;104:2767.

104. Sabatine MS, Braunwald E: Will diabetes save the platelet blockers? Circulation 2001;104:2759–2761.

105. Morrow DA, Sabatine MS, Cannon CP, Theroux P: Benefit of tirofiban among patients treated without coronary intervention: Application of the TIMI Risk Score for Unstable Angina/Non-ST Elevation MI in PRISM-PLUS. Circulation 2001;104(Suppl II):782.

106. Cannon CP, O'Gara PT: Critical Pathways in Cardiology. Philadelphia, Lippincott Williams & Wilkins, 2001.

107. Cohen M, Théroux P, Borzak S, et al: Randomized double-blind safety study of enoxaparin versus unfractionated heparin in patients with non–ST-segment elevation acute coronary syndromes treated with tizofiban and aspirin: the ACUTE II Study. Am Heart J 2002;144:470–477.

108. Goodman S: INTERACT, 51st Scientific Sessions of the American College of Cardiology, Atlanta, March 17–20, 2002.

Continuous Risk Stratification in Acute Coronary Syndromes

Xavier Bosch
Pierre Théroux

In the 1980s and 1990s, the diagnosis and management of unstable angina underwent profound changes, and a new nomenclature has emerged fitted to pathophysiology and therapy to define acute coronary syndromes (ACS). The more accurate and more standardized diagnostic criteria have led to the identification of a population of patients whose risk may be greater than that of populations previously studied.

Data from various registries have shown an 8% to 12% risk of death or myocardial infarction (MI) at 6 months after the initial presentation.[1,2] In the ongoing International Global Registry of Acute Coronary Events (GRACE), the incidence of death or MI at 6 months after hospital discharge is 7.3% for non–ST-segment elevation MI, 5.9% for ST-segment elevation MI, and 4.9% for unstable angina.[3] Almost 25% of patients die or experience MI or acute refractory angina within 6 months of their initial presentation.[1,3,4] Despite these data, risk is not a linear function of time because half of the events occur within the first 7 days of presentation. Clinical trials that have excluded patients with normal electrocardiograms (ECGs) have shown that death and MI rates at 30 days are approximately 10%, even with optimal treatment.[5]

Risk assessment is an integral part of the management of ACS. Assessment is initiated when the diagnosis is first suspected and permits selective admission of higher risk patients to a coronary care unit. Because the patient's risk extends past the acute phase of the illness, risk assessment is not a one-time but a continuous process that is updated in-hospital and after discharge. Recognition of this dynamic approach coupled with a therapy that is usually effective and safe have rendered somewhat obsolete the previous concerns on the optimal timing for performing diagnostic procedures and coronary interventions. Early risk stratification in the emergency department and at hospital admission is discussed in Chapters 12 and 22. The present chapter concentrates on risk stratification once the patient has been admitted to an observation unit or hospital.

EARLY RISK STRATIFICATION

Risk stratification in ACS aims at prompt identification of the higher-risk patient who will profit from aggressive investigation and therapy and of the lower-risk patient who can advantageously be treated more conservatively. No clinical or laboratory marker is faultless. Coronary angiography identifies patients with no coronary artery disease but does not differentiate patients with unstable disease from patients with stable disease. ST-segment shifts and elevated levels of troponin T or I independently identify high-risk patients; their combination, and other markers such as C-reactive protein, enhance the diagnostic sensitivity. Early risk stratification is currently best achieved by combining clinical, ECG and troponin data. These parameters, incorporated into algorithms, have been validated for the orientation of patients into more or less aggressive management strategies. Yet, other markers may be useful and markers of disease processes other than ischemia and thrombosis are emerging that may add new dimensions to diagnosis and management: clinical and ECG data, and blood markers of necrosis.

The Electrocardiogram

The more severe the ischemia, the more extensive in general are the ST-T changes (see Chapter 13). Thus the prognosis of recurrent angina is worse when accompanied with ST-T changes. Persistent changes may indicate myocardial infarction. The changes are often transient and may show only during the ischemic episode, as is the case in Prinzmetal's variant angina. It is therefore important to obtain a 12-lead ECG during one or many episodes of chest pain.[6] New ST-T changes may appear or previously present abnormalities may intensify. Pseudonormalization of a previously abnormal ECG can also be seen, indicating severe ischemia. Such pseudonormalization can occur in vasoplastic angina, although transient ST-segment elevation is the hallmark of Prinzmetal's angina. Such transient ST-segment elevation can be associated with a critical coronary artery stenosis and is an indication for coronary angiography.

A frequently encountered ECG abnormality is the evolution from a nondiagnostic ECG at admission to an ECG in following hours that shows deep T-wave inversion in the anterior leads in the absence of recurrent chest pain.[7] This finding is usually diagnostic of a severe left anterior coronary artery stenosis, located proximally when the T-wave inversion involves the anterior and lateral leads, and in the midsection of the artery when the T-wave inversion is limited to the precordial leads.

The ECG can provide other useful information. The leads showing the ischemic changes usually permits identification of the location of the culprit lesion. Diffuse ST-T changes are often associated with multivessel disease or left main disease. ST-elevation in lead AVR may indicate left main disease, a poorly collateralized proximal left anterior descending coronary occlusion, or three-vessel disease.[8,9] The ECG may also be silent or show non-specific changes.

Markers of Cell Damage

The importance of blood markers for diagnosis and risk evaluation is stressed in many sections of this textbook (see Chapter 14). A single determination may not rule out the diagnosis of ACS, however, since the initial rise in troponin values in peripheral blood follows approximately that of CK-MB and is seen only 4-6 hours after the event, with peak values after 24 hours. Measurements should therefore be repeated 6 to 12 hours after admission to avoid false-negative results. In a study of 737 patients enrolled in the Global Use of Strategies to Open Occluded Coronary Arteries (GUSTO-2) trial, 260 patients had elevated troponin T levels at admission, 323 became positive later, and 151 remained negative. Mortality at 30 days was 10% in the baseline positive group, 5% in the late positive patients, and 0% in the negative patients. Both 8-hour and 16-hour results added to the strength of the baseline results ($P = 0.0007$ and 0.004 respectively).[10] Serial troponin determination is therefore required. A non–ST-segment elevation acute coronary syndrome is an admission working diagnosis. The final diagnosis can be a non-coronary syndrome, a Q-wave MI when new Q-waves have appeared, and a non–Q-wave MI when confirmed by the elevation of CK-MB or troponin levels. An isolated elevation of troponin T or T value is not diagnostic. The consensus of the Joint European Society of Cardiology/American College of Cardiology Committee for the redefinition of myocardial infarction proposed the following criteria:[11]

1) Typical rise and gradual fall (troponin) or more rapid rise and fall (CK-MB) of biochemical markers of myocardial necrosis with at least one of the following:
   a) ischemic symptoms;
   b) development of pathologic Q-wave on the ECG;
   c) ECG changes indicative of ischemia (ST-segment elevation or depression); or
   d) coronary artery intervention (e.g. coronary angioplasty);
2) Pathologic findings of an acute MI.[11]

Risk Scores

Risk scores were developed to facilitate early risk stratification. They incorporate important demographic, clinical, ECG and blood marker parameters shown to be independent predictors of prognosis in multiple or regression analyses of different databases.[12,14] The results of such analyses are influenced by the characteristics of the test populations and by the baseline data recorded. For the 9461 patients enrolled in the PURSUIT

(Platelet glycoprotein IIG/IIIa in Unstable angina: Receptor Suppression Using Integration Therapy) trial, more than 20 parameters were predictive of mortality alone and of the composite of death or nonfatal MI, the most important being age, heart rate, systolic blood pressure, ST-segment depression, signs of heart failure, and cardiac enzyme elevation.[12] The Thrombolysis in Myocardial Infarction (TIMI) score[13] has been validated in many datasets (see Chapter 22) and has gained popularity since it can be simply and readily applied by the simple mathematical addition of 7 parameters available at admission or shortly thereafter. The Predicting Risk of Death in Cardiac Disease Tool (PREDICT) score developed for risk assessment after myocardial infarction or unstable angina has shown enhanced performance by including comorbidities.[14] Including ejection traction also provides incremental information over that provided by the score and the comorbidity.[14] Risk scores are particularly useful to early risk stratification; they are used in the context of individual patients. Once a level of risk has been determined, the evaluation is updated to the clinical evolution and a more thorough evaluation of the patient. Table 23–1 summarizes some of the information that becomes available after admission and that requires consideration in patient evaluation, orientation, and management.

■ ■ ■

TABLE 23–1   IN-HOSPITAL RISK STRATIFICATION

Clinical Features

Ongoing chest pain
Recurrent angina
Recurrent ischemia
Refractory ischemia
Hemodynamic instability
Significant arrhythmias

Electrocardiogram Findings

ST-T changes during pain
Spontaneous evolution to T-wave inversion in anterior leads
Clinically silent ischemia
Total ischemic burden

Blood Markers

Late troponin T or I elevation
Typical changes in curve of troponin levels
Elevation in C-reactive protein
Elevation in brain natriuretic factor

Left Ventricular Function

Ejection fraction <45%
Ejection fraction <40%

Coronary Angiography

Intracoronary thrombus and complex plaques
Multiple complex plaques
Left main disease
Three-vessel disease
Proximal left anterior descending artery disease
Extent score

Provocative Testing

Positive treadmill test
Low tolerance to exercise
Inducible regional dysfunction
Significant perfusion deficit

GLOBAL RISK EVALUATION

Global risk is determined by prior risk and acute risk; the former magnifies the latter, and vice versa. Prior risk is affected by systemic factors such as age, diabetes, hypertension, cerebrovascular disease, peripheral vascular disease, impaired renal function, previous infarction, left ventricular dysfunction, and heart failure. All of these factors are related to the extent of the underlying coronary artery disease and left ventricular dysfunction and the general health status of the patient. Echocardiography, stress testing, perfusion scanning, and coronary angiography help evaluate the impact of these factors on the cardiovascular status of the patient. Acute ischemic risk is determined by the severity of impaired perfusion, the extent of myocardium involved, and the resulting changes in mechanical and electrical function of the heart. A patient with severe three-vessel disease may sustain a minor acute ischemic event; in contrast, a patient with limited disease may experience a fatal ischemic event. The most powerful discriminators of acute ischemic risk are ischemia associated with hemodynamic instability or arrhythmia, refractory angina with ECG evidence of ischemia, the release of troponin or other biomarkers of cell necrosis or inflammation, and the presence of high-risk coronary lesions. Management strategies must address prior and acute aspects of risk.

Faced with these numerous determinants of risk, clinicians should select the investigation they believe is most important to complement the early risk assessment. Results of these tests should be interpreted in light of the clinical, ECG, and biochemical data already available. In patients with an uncomplicated early in-hospital course, risk status is difficult to evaluate on clinical grounds alone, so further testing is required. This testing usually includes an evaluation of left ventricular function and of residual myocardial ischemia (see Table 23-1). Cardiac chest pain that fails to resolve or recurs early after admission indicates a high risk of further myocardial damage and provides a clear indication for angiography with a view to revascularization. Such is the case for post-infarction angina and ischemia.[15-17] Similarly, heart failure is a determinant of high risk and mandates additional investigation. Risk stratification is a dynamic process that demands continuous reevaluation in the hospital and after hospital discharge.

Recurrent Angina, Recurrent Ischemia, and Refractory Ischemia

The recurrence of ischemia once treatment has been instituted is an indicator of an uncontrolled disease process and a harbinger of a more serious ischemic event.[18-22] Reported incidences are influenced by definitions used, the characteristics of the studied populations, and the type and intensity of treatment. Incidences are higher in patients with ST-segment changes at admission and in patients with positive markers of necrosis. In one study of 125 patients referred to the Cleveland Clinic for refractory ischemia, a more aggressive medical regimen rendered 83% of patients pain-free. Of the truly refractory patients, coronary arteriography revealed an increased likelihood of left main or three-vessel disease. In-hospital treatment strategies for patients stabilized with medical therapy included continued medical therapy (n = 37), coronary angioplasty (n = 46), and coronary artery bypass graft (CABG) surgery (n = 31). The rate of MI or death in patients managed medically was 3%.[23]

A gradient in severity and prognosis is recognized from *recurrent angina to recurrent ischemia* (Fig. 23-1), and to *refractory ischemia* (Fig. 23-2), although the definitions are often partly subjective and influenced by the patient's and physician's tolerance to pain. Recurrent ischemia is diagnosed when objective signs of evolving ischemia are present in a patient receiving proper antianginal therapy. The ischemia is usually recognized promptly by the recording of a 12-lead ECG at the time of pain and occasionally by the physical examination with hemodynamic abnormalities, left heart heart failure, or mitral regurgitation.[16] When the ECG is silent and the pain suggestive, a two-dimensional echocardiogram or an injection of technetium-99m sestamibi at the time of pain can aid diagnosis. The myocardial perfusion study can be obtained later once the patient has stabilized.[24] Refractory ischemia is defined as recurrent angina or ischemia that persists despite an intensification in antianginal therapy comprising intravenous nitroglycerin, β-blockers, and calcium antagonists, or a prolonged episode of chest pain lasting more than 10 or 20 minutes that responds poorly to measures instituted for the immediate control of pain and that may require the administration of morphine.

Numerous studies have determined that a poor outcome is associated with recurrent spontaneous chest pain and ST-segment depression. In one study of post-MI patients,[15] in-hospital infarct extension occurred in 28% of patients with early post-MI ischemia, in 3.5% of patients with recurrent angina, and in 2% of patients

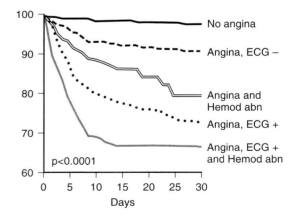

FIGURE 23-1. Cumulative survival without reinfarction, unstable angina, or need for revascularization in patients with early post-myocardial infarction angina. Long-term prognosis is impaired in patients with post-myocardial infarction angina (angina, no ST-T changes) and more so when the angina is associated with ST-T changes (angina plus ST-T changes). ECG, electrocardiogram; Hemod abn, hemodynamic abnormalities. (From Bosch X, Théroux P, Pelletier GB, et al: Clinical and angiographic features and prognostic significance of early post-infarction angina with and without electrocardiographic signs of transient ischemia. Am J Med 1991;91:493–501.)

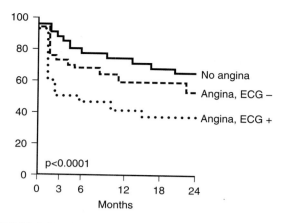

FIGURE 23–2. Data from the GUSTO-IIb trial show the negative impact on 1-year survival of recurrent ischemia. The prognosis was worse when the ischemia was refractory. Nonrefractory ischemia was defined in this study as symptoms of ischemia with ST-segment deviation or frank T-wave inversion. Refractory recurrent ischemia consisted of symptoms of ischemia with electrocardiogram (ECG) changes persisting for 10 minutes or longer despite the use of nitrates and either β-blockers or calcium channel blockers. (From Armstrong PW, Fu Y, Chang WC, Topol EJ, et al: Acute coronary syndromes in the GUSTO-IIb trial: Prognostic insights and impact of recurrent ischemia. The GUSTO-IIb Investigators. Circulation 1998;98:1860–1868.)

without post-MI angina ($P < 0.0001$). In this study, post-MI ischemia was a predictor of long-term mortality and of mortality and MI. In the overall population of patients with ACS, the appearance of recurrent ischemia during hospitalization increases the risk of adverse cardiac events by 5 to 10 times.[15-22]

In the Estudios Cardiologicos Latino America (ECLA)-3 study, recurrent angina occurred in 41% of patients; half of these patients were receiving full medical therapy.[19] In another study, half of patients with unstable angina had recurrent pain in the hospital, usually (80%) within the first 48 hours after admission.[20] Recurrent angina was more frequent in patients with acute angina at rest (64%) and less frequent in patients with subacute angina (45%) and accelerated effort angina (28%). The strongest predictor of recurrent ischemia was the time interval since the previous episode: the incidence was maximal shortly after admission; it was less than 20% after a pain-free interval of 48 hours and less than 10% after an interval of 72 hours.

In the Global Use of Strategies to Open Occluded Coronary Arteries (GUSTO)-IIb trial,[21] the incidence of recurrent ischemia was higher in patients with non–ST-segment elevation acute coronary syndrome (NSTEACS) than in patients with ST-segment elevation (35% versus 23%); in the former group, it was considerably less frequent among patients who had primary angioplasty compared with those who received thrombolysis (2.6% versus 11.2%). The most important predictor of recurrent ischemia in the study was a history of previous angina. Another study documented a high correlation between presence of a complex plaque at angiography and recurrent ischemia.[22] Transient ischemia observed on continuous ECG recordings also was more frequent in these patients. In the Platelet Receptor Inhibition in Ischemic Syndrome Management

in Patients Limited by Unstable Signs and Symptoms (PRISM-PLUS) trial, the persistence of an intracoronary thrombus on medical treatment correlated with occurrence of refractory ischemia.[25] In this trial, recurrent ischemia was associated with a twofold increase in the risk of death or MI at 30 days, from 8.5% to 15.5%. Treatment with tirofiban modified the impact of recurrent ischemia: it reduced by 50% the risk of death or MI at 30 days and by 25% the need for an urgent intervention for failure of medical treatment ($P = 0.01$).

Continuous ST-Segment Monitoring

Ischemia frequently occurs in the absence of chest pain, providing the rationale for continuous ST-segment monitoring. Incidences reported before the routine use of aspirin and heparin were in the range of 70%; since the routine use of aspirin and heparin, this incidence decreased to less than 30%.[18,21] The incidence is higher during the first 24 hours of hospitalization because of natural history of the disease, the effects of medical treatment, and the exclusion from analysis of high-risk patients who undergo early coronary angiography and revascularization.

Continuous ST-segment monitoring can be performed either with a Holter system or with a microprocessor-controlled and fully programmable system.[26] Demonstration of its presence and of its severity is valuable because it identifies patients who have an increased risk of recurrent ischemic events.[27,28] Silent ischemia during continuous monitoring correlates with high-risk coronary lesions,[29,30] decreased myocardial perfusion, and decreased ventricular function.[31,32] It permits detection of the total ischemic burden, most episodes of ST-segment depression being silent. Despite this higher sensitivity, its incremental value beyond other risk stratifiers remains poorly validated.

In the TIMI-IIIB substudy, patients randomized to the conservative strategy arm underwent noninvasive risk stratification with exercise ECG, exercise thallium scintigraphy, and 24-hour Holter monitoring before hospital discharge.[33] The thallium test identified 34% of the patients at risk, the exercise ECG test 33%, and the Holter monitoring only 3%. The most important value of continuous ST-segment monitoring is that it can be applied early after admission when the risk is highest, and during the observation period in chest pain units.[34] Routine continuous ST-segment monitoring is not part of the recommendations of the European (see Chapter 49) or the American College of Cardiology/American Heart Association (see Chapter 50) guidelines for the management of patients with a non–ST-segment elevation ACS.

Imaging for Ischemia

Imaging techniques are particularly useful in patients with atypical or typical symptoms in whom the ECG is silent or confounding. The 12-lead ECG lacks sensitivity to detect posterior and lateral ischemia; recording of right precordial leads (V_2R, V_3R) and dorsal leads (V_7, V_8, V_9) may increase sensitivity. Confounding ECGs are those with a left bundle branch block, a ventricular or paced rhythm, a Wolff-Parkinson-White or a Brugada pattern, and also those with significant left ventricular hypertrophy or a previous MI. Sestamibi single-proton emission computed tomography has proved useful in this setting for differentiating patients with coronary artery disease from patients without this disease (see Chapter 19), by showing the existence of perfusion defects. In one study, the sensitivity and specificity of the test for detecting significant coronary artery disease were 96% and 79% when sestamibi was injected during the episode of pain and 65% and 84% when it was injected during a pain-free state.[24] In another study of 532 consecutive patients consulting for chest pain and with a nondiagnostic ECG, the perfusion imaging was positive for 32% of patients and was a strong predictor of MI and of the need for revascularization with a sensitivity of 93% and of 81% respectively and negative predictive values of 99% and 97%.[35] Performance of a T_c^{99m} sestamibi scintigraphy in a setting of an emergency department in patients at a moderate risk reduced total admissions and altered resource utilization, allowing detection of a significant number of high-risk patients not otherwise identified.[36]

Two-D echocardiography is also useful in that regard, providing anatomic and functional data that are useful for diagnosis and prognosis (see Chapter 17).[37] The presence of a previous MI with wall motion abnormality is a confounder. Ischemia is associated with transient wall motion abnormalities. Echocardiography also is an invaluable tool to evaluate left ventricular ejection fraction, valvular and pericardial disease, acute pulmonary embolism, and suspected aortic dissection.

Provocative Testing

An exercise of pharmacologic provocative testing can be performed safely in patients with an ACS in the absense of evolving or recurrent ischemia and of hemodynamic instability.[38-40] In patients with no known coronary artery disease, atypical or more typical symptoms, normal troponin levels, and normal or nondiagnostic ECG, a diagnostic test is performed rapidly with the goal of identifying significant ischemia. Such provocative testing also is indicated in medium-risk patients with a normal or a nondiagnostic ECG at admission who remain asymptomatic during the first 24 to 48 hours.

As for patients with stable angina and patients recovering from MI, the sensitivity of a stress test for detecting ischemia is increased when imaging is obtained. This may be particularly true in women with a low pre-test likelihood of coronary artery disease.

Imaging further improves the capability of provocative testing to assess prognosis.[41-43] Since no large studies have reported the prognostic value of a positive test in patients with "stabilized" ACS, the interpretation of results are extrapolated from data obtained in other populations. This could be misleading, however, because of different underlying pathophysiological mechanisms. Thus, it is assumed that a positive test marks a significant flow restricting stenosis. The stenosis is usually fixed in stable angina. In unstable angina, a dynamic component is present. Thus, an occasional patient may experience an acute MI even with a negative treadmill test since a thrombus could have been nonflow restrictive at the time of the treadmill to subsequently progress to complete occlusion. Therefore the provocation testing may not exclude an unstable plaque. ECG features of a high-risk treadmill test are: magnitude of ST-segment shift and number of leads involved, and timing of appearance of the changes during the test and of normalization after the test.[44] A fall in blood pressure and multiple perfusion or contraction defects are markers of a severe disease.[45] Inability to perform a stress test and low exercise tolerance are independent predictors of recurrent adverse cardiac events. The negative predictive accuracy of predischarge stress testing is high: patients with a normal test result usually have a good prognosis without the need for additional investigation. Only small studies have directly compared the respective value of the various provocative tests after stabilization from ACS. The selection of a test is influenced by the patient's characteristics, the clinical presentation, the baseline ECG, the availability of various methods, and the local expertise. Treadmill exercise is usually a first choice since it is widely available, possesses a high negative prognostic value, and is low cost. Imaging is added when the baseline ECG is confounded. Pharmacologic testing is preferred when patients cannot perform adequately on the treadmill. The dipyridamole nuclear scan has become a standard. A false negative value can, however, occasionally be seen in patients with severe three-vessel disease and diffuse ischemia with no gradient in perfusion. Dobutamine stress echocardiography may be particularly useful in patients with good acoustical windows because both resting left ventricular function and the functional consequences of a coronary stenosis can be assessed.[41-45] The stress echo is as performing in selected patients and the dobutamine echo allows the study of reversibility of regional dysfunction at low dose of inducible ischemia at high dose (see Chapter 18).

Left Ventricular Function

Left ventricular function is a strong predictor of prognosis in patients with coronary artery disease and left ventricular ejection is the most important determinant of survival after an acute MI. Treatment with beta blockers and with angiotensin-converting enzyme inhibitors improves the prognosis of patients with left ventricular dysfunction. Reperfusion procedures can also improve left ventricular function and prolongs life especially when myocardium hibernation is present. Improved survival with bypass surgery compared with medical management in patients with three-vessel disease and left ventricular dysfunction has been documented in the first large trial that has compared surgery to medical therapy.[46]

Although routine evaluation of ejection fraction is not recommended as a routine procedure in various practice guidelines,[6-8] it should be obtained promptly in patients in whom a doubt exists regarding its integrity, such as patients with a previous MI, with a left bundle-branch block, or with any signs or symptoms suggestive of heart failure. The presence of ventricular dysfunction, especially when reversibility can be shown, is an incentive to perform a reperfusion procedure to improve prognosis.

Coronary Angiography

Coronary angiography is currently the only diagnostic procedure that can accurately characterize the presence and extent of significant coronary artery disease and define its anatomy for decisions to perform revascularization procedures. Among patients with ACS, 30% to 40% have single-vessel disease, and 15% to 20% have nonsignificant coronary artery disease. The incidence of left main coronary artery disease varies from 4% to 8%.[47] In risk stratification, coronary angiography allows rapid identification of patients with nonobstructed coronary arteries, who can be discharged promptly from the hospital, and of patients with severe disease, who would profit from intervention procedures.

A culprit lesion commonly is found, whereas many patients can show more than one complex plaque (see Chapter 17).[48] In one study in which angiography was performed after 48 hours of medical management, one third of patients still had a definite thrombus, and half had a possible or definite thrombus.[25] The angiographic persistence of thrombus predicted twofold increase in the risk of death, MI, and recurrent ischemia in the following weeks. A complicated course was observed in 20% of patients with a thrombus compared with 10% of patients with no thrombus. The independent predictors of a persisting thrombus in the study were previous CABG surgery, elevation of cardiac markers, and more extensive coronary artery disease.

Coronary angiography is usually performed to explore the option of reperfusion procedures with PCI or CABG[49]. Occasionally, it is performed for diagnostic purposes or for risk stratification. An invasive management strategy is a strong recommendation in patients with a non–ST-segment ACS at high risk by severe pain, troponin elevation, ST-segment changes, a high risk score, heart failure, recurrent ischemia, and by a depressed ejection traction, ischemia at a low threshold on the treadmill, or multiple perfusion defects on the perfusion scan (see Table 23–1). The guidelines also recommend coronary angiography in patients with prior PCI and prior CABG unless the coronary anatomy is already known not to be amenable to revascularization procedures. It could be useful to revise the angiogram in these patients and reevalute the reasons for the previous decision. An intra-aortic pump is inserted in patients with recurrent ischemia despite maximal medical management and in patients with hemodynamic instability until coronary angiography and revascularization can be completed. Patients with suspected Prinzmetal's variant angina also are candidates for coronary angiography.

The general indications for coronary angiography and revascularization are tempered by the characteristics and preferences of the individual patient. Patient and physician judgments regarding risks and benefits are particularly important for patients who may not be candidates for coronary revascularization, such as frail elderly patients and patients with serious comorbid conditions such as severe hepatic, pulmonary, or renal failure, or active or inoperable cancer.

BEYOND TRADITIONAL MANAGEMENT

Most cardiac events in patients with a non–ST-segment elevation occur within the first 3 months after the index hospitalization, half of them after hospital discharge. Management so far has focused on the major determinants of early prognosis: severity and extent of ischemia and left ventricular function. It has left untouched the fundamental causes of the disease that convert the stable plaque to an unstable plaque, resulting in an acute coronary syndrome. Time has now come to incorporate a new dimension in our management strategy that includes the control of atherosclerosis and of the factors that lead to instability. The terminology of plaque passivation has been introduced to describe these goals (see Chapter 30). Plaque activation can now, at least partly, be recognized and treated.

Markers of Inflammation

Among inflammatory markers and acute phase reactants that are elevated in a large proportion of patients with an ACS, the C-reactive protein (CRP) level holds a privileged role and is currently the marker recommended in clinical practice (see Chapter 16). In contrast to fibrinogen levels, which have been reported to correlate with short-term prognosis,[24] increased levels of C-reactive protein correlate better with long-term outcome.[50-52] In one study, the predictive value of C-reactive protein levels obtained at hospital admission was enhanced when another sample was assayed just before hospital discharge.[53] The prognostic value of C-reactive protein seems less related to the acute thrombotic process and more to the processes of inflammation associated with plaque destabilization and rupture. Accordingly, the prognostic value associated with elevated CRP is not profoundly altered by antithrombotic therapy, including GPIIb/IIa antagonists.[51] CRP levels also predict an impaired outcome after PCI and after CABG.[54-56] Statins reduce the CRP levels[57] and prevent refraction ischemia in the acute phase of ACS[58] and death, MI, and stroke in high-risk individuals and in patients with coronary artery disease.[59-60]

Neurohormonal Activation

Elevated blood levels of B-type natriuretic peptide have been associated with an impaired long-term prognosis in patients with ACS.[61-63] The association is better in patients with NSTEACS than in patients with ST-segment elevation ACS and is independent of clinical characteristics, troponin levels, and ECG changes at admission.[61] Based on these findings, it has been suggested that neurohormonal activation plays a role in ACS. The BNP levels could also be elevated in patients with left ventricular dysfunction associated with ischemia. The time course of the elevation remains to be determined.

ACS as a Systemic Inflammation and Auto-Immune Disease

Acute coronary syndromes are hallmarks of disease progression.[64] Antithrombotic therapy controls the immediate risk of occlusion, and revascularization the underlying flow obstruction, assuring optimal flow conditions and partly controlling the thrombotic process. Yet the pathophysiology may differ in intensity or in immediate triggers in some patients and many patients remain at risk. A low-grade systemic inflammation response syndrome (SIRS) can exist in many of these patients, likely caused by a combination of various triggers. Risk factors have a major role in these mechanisms. Continuous risk stratification is therefore indicated and an aggressive secondary prevention program individualized to patients is initiated early (see Chapter 43). Aspirin and a statin are indicated long term and an angiotensin-converting enzyme inhibitor is indicated in selected patients. Follow-up is required to assess clinical evaluation, tolerance of and response to therapy, and control of risk factors. Meanwhile, a variety of new agents are being developed, some being under clinical investigation, mostly anti-inflammatory agents which hold the promise of a more in-depth control of the disease.

REFERENCES

1. Yusuf S, Flather M, Pogue, et al, for the OASIS Registry Investigators: Variations between countries in invasive cardiac procedures and outcomes in patients with suspected unstable angina or myocardial infarction without initial ST elevation. Lancet 1998;352: 507–514.
2. Collinson J, Flather MD, Fox KAA, et al, for the PRAIS-UK Investigators: Clinical outcomes, risk stratification and practice patterns of unstable angina and myocardial infarction without ST elevation: Prospective Registry of Acute Ischaemic Syndromes in the UK (PRAIS-UK). Eur Heart J 2000;21:1450–1457.
3. Goldberg RJ, Spencer F, Gore JM, et al: Six month prognosis after hospital discharge in patients with acute coronary syndromes: The GRACE Project. J Am Coll Cardiol 2001;37(Suppl A):315A.
4. Sionis-Green A, Bosch X, Miranda-Guardiola F, et al: In-hospital evolution and current prognosis of unstable angina. Rev Esp Cardiol 2000;53:1573–1582.
5. Global Use of Strategies to Open Occluded Coronary Arteries (GUSTO IIb) Investigators: A comparison of recombinant hirudin with heparin for the treatment of acute coronary syndromes. N Engl J Med 1996;335:775–782.
6. López de Sá E, López-Sendón J, Bethencourt A, Bosch X: Prognostic value of ECG changes during chest pain in patients with unstable angina. Results of the Proyecto de Estudio del Pronóstico de la Angina (PEPA). J Am Coll Cardiol 1998;31(Suppl A):79.
7. de Zwaan C, Bar FW, Janssen JH, et al: Angiographic and clinical characteristics of patients with unstable angina showing an ECG pattern indicating critical narrowing of the proximal LAD coronary artery. Am Heart J 1989;117:657–665.
8. Yamaji H, Iwasaki K, Kusachi S, et al: Prediction of acute left main coronary artery obstruction by 12-lead electrocardiography. ST segment elevation in lead aVR with less ST segment election in lead V_1. J Am Coll Cardiol 2001; 38: 1348–1354.
9. Martinez-Dolz, Arnau MA, Almenar L, et al: Usefulness of the electrocardiogram in predicting the occlusion site in acute myocardial infarction with isolated disease of the left anterior descending coronary artery. Rev Esp Cardiol 2002; 55: 1036–10341.
10. Newby LK, Christenson RH, Ohman EM, et al: Value of serial troponin T measures for early and late risk stratification in patients with acute coronary syndromes. The GUSTO-IIa Investigators. Circulation 1998;98:1853–1859.
11. Myocardial infarction redefined: A consensus document of The Joint European Society of Cardiology/American College of Cardiology Committee for the redefinition of myocardial infarction. J Am Coll Cardiol 2000;36:959–969.
12. Boersma E, Pieper KS, Steyerberg EW, et al: Predictors of outcome in patients with acute coronary syndromes without persistent ST-segment elevation: Results from an international trial of 9461 patients. Circulation 2000;101:2557–2567.
13. Antman EM, Cohen M, Bernink PJL, et al: The TIMI risk score for unstable angina/non-ST elevation MI: A method for prognostication and therapeutic decision-making. JAMA 2000;284:835–842.
14. Singh M, Reeder GS, Jacobsen SJ, et al: Scores for post-myocardial infarction risk stratification in the community. Circulation 2002; 106: 2309–2314.
15. Bosch X, Théroux P, Waters DD, et al: Early postinfarction ischemia: Clinical, angiographic and prognostic significance. Circulation 1987;75:988–995.
16. Bosch X, Théroux P, Pelletier GB, et al: Clinical and angiographic features and prognostic significance of early post-infarction angina with and without electrocardiographic signs of transient ischemia. Am J Med 1991;91:493–501.
17. Betriu A, Califf RM, Bosch X, et al: Recurrent ischemia after thrombolysis: Importance of associated clinical findings. J Am Coll Cardiol 1998;31:94–102.
18. Akkerhuis KM, Klootwijk PAJ, Lindeboom W, et al: Recurrent ischemia during continuous multilead ST-segment monitoring identifies patients with acute coronary syndromes at high risk of adverse cardiac events: Meta-analysis of three studies involving 995 patients. Eur Heart J 2001;22:1997–2006.
19. Bazzino O, Díaz R, Tajer C, et al: Clinical predictors of in-hospital prognosis in unstable angina: ECLA 3. Am Heart J 1999;137:322–331.
20. Van Miltenburg-van Zijl AJ, Simoons ML, Veerhoek RJ, Bossuyt PM: Incidence and follow-up of Braunwald subgroups in unstable angina pectoris. J Am Coll Cardiol 1995;25:1286–1292.
21. Armstrong PW, Fu Y, Chang WC, et al: Acute coronary syndromes in the GUSTO-IIb trial: Prognostic insights and impact of recurrent ischemia. The GUSTO-IIb Investigators. Circulation 1998;98: 1860–1868.
22. Patel DJ, Gomma AH, Knight CJ, et al: Why is recurrent myocardial ischaemia a predictor of adverse outcome in unstable angina? An observational study of myocardial ischaemia and its relation to coronary anatomy. Eur Heart J 2001;22:1991–1996.
23. Grambow DW, Topol EJ: Effect of maximal medical therapy on refractoriness of unstable angina pectoris. Am J Cardiol 1992;70: 577–581.
24. Bilodeau L, Theroux P, Gregoire J, et al: Technetium-99m sestamibi tomography in patients with spontaneous chest pain: Correlations with clinical, electrocardiographic and angiographic findings. J Am Coll Cardiol 1991;18:1684–1691.
25. Zhao XQ, Theroux P, Snapinn SM, Sax FL: Intracoronary thrombus and platelet glycoprotein IIb/IIIa receptor blockade with tirofiban in unstable angina or non-Q-wave myocardial infarction: Angiographic results from the PRISM-PLUS trial (Platelet Receptor Inhibition for Ischemic Syndrome Management in Patients Limited by Unstable Signs and Symptoms). PRISM-PLUS Investigators. Circulation 1999;100:1609–1615.
26. Selker HP, Zalenski RJ, Antman EM, et al: An evaluation of technologies for identifying acute cardiac ischemia in the emergency department: A report from a national heart attack alert program working group. Ann Emerg Med 1997;29:13–87.
27. Patel DJ, Knight CJ, Holdright DR, et al: Long-term prognosis in unstable angina: The importance of early risk stratification using continuous ST segment monitoring. Eur Heart J 1998;19:240–249.
28. Wilcox I, Breedman S, Kelly D, et al: Clinical significance of silent ischemia in unstable angina pectoris. Am J Cardiol 1990;65: 1313–1316.
29. Bugairdini R, Borghi A, Pozzati A, et al: Relation of severity of symptoms to transient myocardial ischemia and prognosis in unstable angina. J Am Coll Cardiol 1995;25:597–604.
30. Chierchia S, Lazzari M, Freedman B, et al: Impairment of myocardial perfusion and function during painless myocardial ischemia. J Am Coll Cardiol 1983;1:924–930.
31. Klootwijk P, Meij S, Melkert R, et al: Reduction of recurrent ischemia with abciximab during continuous ECG-ischemia monitoring in patients with unstable angina refractory to standard treatment (CAPTURE). Circulation 1998;98:1358–1364.

32. Gottlieb SO, Weisfeldt ML, Ouyang P, et al: Silent ischemia as a marker for early unfavorable outcomes in patients with unstable angina. N Engl J Med 1986;314:1214-1219.

33. Stone PH, Thopson B, Zaret BL, et al: Factors associated with failure of medical therapy in patients with unstable angina and non-Q wave myocardial infarction: A TIMI-IIIB database study. Eur Heart J 1999;20:1084-1093.

34. Fesmire FM, Percy RF, Bardoner JB, et al: Usefulness of automated serial 12-lead ECG monitoring during the initial emergency department evaluation of patients with chest pain. Ann Emerg Med 1998;31:3-11.

35. Kontos MC, Jesse RL, Schmidt KL, et al: Value of acute rest sestamibi perfusion imaging for evaluation of patients admitted to the emergency department with chest pain. J Am Coll Cardiol 1997; 30: 976-982.

36. Knott JC, Baldey AC, Grigg LE, et al: Impact of acute chest pain T_c^{99m} sestamibi myocardial perfusion imaging on clinical management. J Nucl Cardiol 2002; 9: 257-262.

37. Gomez MA, Anderson JL, Karagounis LA, et al, for the ROMIO Study Group: An emergency department–based protocol for rapid ruling out myocardial ischemia reduces hospital time and expense: Results of a randomized study (ROMIO). J Am Coll Cardiol 1994;23:1390-1396.

38. Amsterdam EA, Kirk JD, Diercks DB, et al: Immediate exercise testing to evaluate low-risk patients presenting to the emergency department with chest pain. J Am Coll Cardiol 2002;40:251-256.

39. Bosch X, Magriñá J, March R, et al: Prediction of in-hospital cardiac events using dipyridamole-thallium scintigraphy performed very early after acute myocardial infarction. Clin Cardiol 1996;19: 189-196.

40. Sitges M, Paré C, Azqueta M, et al: Feasibility and prognostic value of dobutamine-atropine stress echocardiography early in unstable angina. Eur Heart J 2000;21:1063-1071.

41. Amanullah AM, Lindvall K, Bevegard S: Prognostic significance of exercise thallium-201 myocardial perfusion imaging compared to stress echocardiography and clinical variables in patients with unstable angina who respond to medical treatment. Int J Cardiol 1993;39:71-78.

42. Brown KA: Prognostic value of thallium-201 myocardial perfusion imaging in patients with unstable angina who respond to medical treatment. J Am Coll Cardiol 1991;17:1053-1057.

43. Santoro GM, Sciagra R, Buonamici P, et al: Head-to-head comparison of exercise stress testing, pharmacologic stress echocardiography, and perfusion tomography as first-line examination for chest pain in patients without history of coronary artery disease. J Nucl Cardiol 1998;5:19-27.

44. Nyman I, Larsson H, Areskog M, et al: The predictive value of silent ischemia at an exercise test before discharge after an episode of unstable coronary artery disease. Am Heart J 1992;123: 324-331.

45. Cheitlin MD, Alpert JS, Armstrong WF, et al: ACC/AHA guidelines for the clinical application of echocardiography: A report of the American College of Cardiology/American Heart Association Task Force on Practice Guidelines (Committee on Clinical Application of Echocardiography). Developed in collaboration with the American Society of Echocardiography. Circulation 1997;95: 1686-1744.

46. Parisi AF, Khuri S, Deupree RH, et al: Medical compared with surgical management of unstable angina: 5-year mortality and morbidity in the Veterans Administration Study. Circulation 1989;80: 1176-1189.

47. TIMI IIIB Investigators: Effects of tissue plasminogen activator and a comparison of early invasive and conservative strategies in unstable angina and non-Q-wave myocardial infarction: Results of TIMI IIIB trial. Circulation 1994;89:1545-1556.

48. Goldstein JA, Demetriou D, Grines CL, et al: Multiple complex coronary plaques in patients with acute myocardial infarction. N Engl J Med 2000;343:915-922.

49. Scanlon PJ, Faxon DP, Audet A, et al: ACC/AHA guidelines for coronary angiography: A report of the American College of Cardiology/American Heart Association Task Force on Practice Guidelines (Committee on Coronary Angiography). J Am Coll Cardiol 1999;33:1756-1824.

50. Toss H, Lindahl B, Siegbahn A, Wallentin L: Prognostic influence of increased fibrinogen and C-reactive protein levels in unstable coronary artery disease. FRISC Study Group. Fragmin During Instability in Coronary Artery Disease. Circulation 1997;96: 4204-4210.

51. Heeschen C, Hamm CW, Bruemmer J, Simoons ML: Predictive value of C-reactive protein and troponin T in patients with unstable angina: A comparative analysis. CAPTURE Investigators. Chimeric c7E3 Antiplatelet Therapy in Unstable Angina REfractory to Standard Treatment trial. J Am Coll Cardiol 2000;35:1535-1542.

52. Liuzzo G, Biasucci LM, Gallimore JR, et al: The prognostic value of C-reactive protein and serum amyloid A protein in severe unstable angina. N Engl J Med 1994;331:417-424.

53. Ferreirós ER, Boissonnet CP, Pizarro R, et al: Independent prognostic value of elevated c-reactive protein in unstable angina. Circulation 1999;100:1958-1963.

54. Blake GJ, Ridker PM: C-reactive protein and prognosis after percutaneous coronary intervention. Eur Heart J 2000; 23: 923-925.

55. Chew DP, Bhatt DL, Robbins MA, et al: Incremental prognostic value of elevated baseline C-reactive protein among established markers of risk in percutaneous coronary intervention. Circulation 2001; 104: 992-997.

56. de Winter RJ, Heyde GS, Koch KT, et al: The prognostic value of elevated baseline C-reactive protein in patients undergoing elective coronary angioplasty. Eur Heart J 2002; 23: 960-966.

57. Jialal I, Stein D, Balis D, et al: Effect of hydroxymethyl glutaryl coenzyme A reductase inhibitor therapy on high sensitive C-reactive protein levels. Circulation 2002; 103: 1933-1935.

58. Pitt B, Waters D, Brown WV, et al: Aggressive lipid-lowering therapy compared with angioplasty in stable coronary artery disease. Atorvastatin versus Revascularization Treatment Investigators. N Engl J Med 1999; 341: 70-76.

59. Heart Protection Study Collaborative Group: MRC/BHF Heart Protection Study of cholesterol lowering with simvastatin in 20,536 high-risk individuals: A randomised placebo-controlled trial. Lancet 2002;360:7-22.

60. Ridker PM, Hennekens CH, Buring JE, et al: C-reactive protein and other markers of inflammation in the prediction of cardiovascular disease in women. N Engl J Med 2000; 342: 836-843.

61. De Lemos JA, Morrow DA, Bentley JH, et al: The prognostic value of B-type natriuretic peptide in patients with acute coronary syndromes. N Engl J Med 2001;345:1014-1021.

62. Jernberg T, Stridsberg M, Lindahl, B: N-terminal pro brain natriuretic peptide on admission for early risk stratification of patients with chest pain and no ST-segment elevation. J Am Coll Cardiol 2000; 40: 437-445.

63. Omland T, deLemos JA, Morrow DA, et al: Prognostic value of N-terminal pro-atrial and pro-brain natriuretic peptide in patients with acute coronary syndromes. Am J Cardiol 2002; 89: 463-465.

64. Moise A, Theroux P, Taeymans Y, et al: Unstable angina and progression of coronary atherosclerosis. N Engl J Med 1983; 309: 685-689.

■ ■ ■ c h a p t e r 2 4

Nitrates and Nitric Oxide Donors

Balkrishna K. Singh
Jacob Joseph
Jawahar L. Mehta

HISTORICAL BACKGROUND

The organic nitrates are one of the most commonly used drugs in the management of coronary artery disease (CAD) in a variety of clinical situations such as stable angina, unstable angina, myocardial infarction (MI), and congestive heart failure (CHF). In 1867, Brunton first described the clinical effectiveness of amyl nitrite in angina pectoris; in 1879, Murrell reported that a 1% solution of nitroglycerin administered orally relieved angina and prevented subsequent attacks.[1] Organic nitrates were among the first drugs to be used in the treatment of CAD and have, for more than a century, continued to be used in the treatment of this condition. It is now evident that most of the observed effects of nitrates are mediated through the generation of nitric oxide (NO), leading to relaxation of peripheral and coronary vascular smooth muscle. Improvements in our understanding of vascular biology and the mechanisms of action and efficacy of nitrates has led to intense research in this area and hence to the prospect of novel therapies.

PHARMACOLOGY OF ORGANIC NITRATES

The most commonly used organic nitrates are nitroglycerin (glyceryl trinitrate), isosorbide dinitrate, and isosorbide mononitrate. These drugs are available in a variety of formulations with different routes of administration. The nitrates are rapidly absorbed from the gastrointestinal tract, skin, and mucous membranes.[2] Isosorbide dinitrate and nitroglycerin undergo extensive first-pass hepatic metabolism when given orally.[3] Nitroglycerin has a plasma half-life of approximately 1 to 4 minutes. Nitroglycerin undergoes hepatic and intravascular metabolism, yielding biologically active dinitrate metabolites that have a half-life of approximately 40 minutes.[2,4]

Despite early studies that suggested that isosorbide was completely metabolized during its first pass through the liver and lacked any hemodynamic effect,[5] subsequent studies have consistently demonstrated substantial hemodynamic and anti-ischemic effects of isosorbide dinitrate.[6-8] Isosorbide dinitrate is rapidly metabolized

and has a half-life of approximately 40 minutes. Its major metabolites, isosorbide-2-mononitrate and isosorbide-5-mononitrate, are both biologically active and have half-lives of approximately 2 and 4 hours, respectively. Isosorbide mononitrate (isosorbide-5-mononitrate) does not undergo first-pass hepatic metabolism and has 100% bioavailability.[9]

MECHANISMS OF ACTION OF THE ORGANIC NITRATES

Various mechanisms of action of organic nitrates are summarized in Table 24-1.

Cellular Effects

Organic nitrates are prodrugs and must be biodegraded to exert therapeutic effects. This biotransformation involves denitration of the nitrate, with subsequent liberation of NO. Hence, nitrates can cause vasodilation whether or not the endothelium is intact.[10] These agents are accordingly often called *endothelium-independent vasodilators*. After entering vascular smooth muscle cells, nitrates are converted to reactive NO or S-nitrosothiols, which activate intracellular guanylate cyclase to produce cyclic guanosine monophosphate (cGMP), which in turn triggers smooth muscle relaxation.[11,12] The exact mechanism by which organic nitrates undergo denitration-liberating NO remains controversial.[13,14] Although it was originally proposed that reduced sulfhydryl (SH) groups were an essential substrate for bioconversion,[15,16] they are probably required only as cofactors.[13,14] In accordance with this hypothesis, nitroglycerin-induced vasodilation can be enhanced by prior administration of N-acetylcysteine, an agent that increases the availability of SH groups,[17] as well as by SH-containing angiotensin-converting enzyme (ACE) inhibitors such as captopril.[18] This action of N-acetylcysteine potentiates the peripheral and coronary vasodilator effect of nitroglycerin and reverses the partial tolerance to the effect of nitrates.

In addition to exerting vasodilating effects, nitroglycerin has modest platelet aggregation inhibitory effect,

■ ■ ■

TABLE 24–1 MECHANISM OF ACTION OF THE ORGANIC NITRATES

Cellular Effects

Denitration of the organic nitrate with liberation of nitric oxide
Intracellular conversion to reactive nitric oxide or S-nitrosothiols
Activation of intracellular guanylate cyclase to produce cGMP
cGMP triggers smooth muscle cell relaxation and platelet inhibition
Inhibition of vascular growth and decrease in myocardial contractility

Vascular Effects of Nitrates

Dilation of capacitance venous bed (reduction in preload)
Modest dilator effect on medium-sized arteries (reduction in
    afterload)
Reduction in ventricular volume
Reduction in myocardial-wall tension and oxygen requirement
Dilation of epicardial coronary arteries and collateral channels,
    particularly in the subendocardial region

cGMP, cyclic guanosine monophosphate.

particularly at high doses.[19,20] NO is also involved in the control of endothelial function and vascular growth[21] as well as myocardial contractility.[22] The expression of NO synthase, and hence the availability of endogenous NO, is decreased in a variety of conditions associated with endothelial dysfunction, such as diabetes mellitus, hypertension, and smoking. In blood vessels with dysfunctional endothelium, exogenous NO donors cause intense vasodilation, perhaps because of lack of competition with endogenous NO. Accordingly, organic nitrates and other NO donors are particularly beneficial in conditions associated with endothelial dysfunction.

Hemodynamic Effects

Our understanding of the vascular effects of nitrates has progressed considerably. Currently, the hemodynamic and antianginal actions of the organic nitrates are thought to be mediated primarily through dilation of capacitance venous beds, although these agents also have a modest vasodilatory effect on medium-sized arterioles. Dilation of capacitance vessels reduces ventricular volume and preload,[23] which in turn reduces myocardial wall tension and oxygen requirements, resulting in improved subendocardial blood flow. Coupled with modest decrease in afterload, nitrates are useful in the treatment of CHF as well as myocardial ischemia.

Nitrates dilate epicardial coronary arteries, including stenotic segments.[24] Nitrates also dilate collateral channels with enhanced blood flow to the ischemic areas.[25] In doses used in clinical practice, however, these agents do not affect coronary resistance vessels or result in "coronary steal," a phenomenon that often occurs with drugs such as dipyridamole and short-acting dihydropyridines, which cause dramatic arteriolar dilation and result in ischemia.[26,27] This unique combination of the vascular effects of nitrates can favorably affect the mismatch between myocardial oxygen supply and demand in patients with CAD and CHF. The preload- and afterload-reducing effects of nitrates may also be of clinical benefit in aortic or mitral valvular regurgitation.

Antithrombotic Effects

Platelet accumulation of soluble cGMP upon administration of nitrates results in modest inhibitory actions on platelets in addition to vasodilation, particularly in high doses. Although the antithrombotic effects of intravenous nitroglycerin have been demonstrated in both patients with unstable angina and those with chronic stable angina,[28-30] the clinical significance of these actions is not clear.

USE OF NITRATES IN CLINICAL SETTING

Stable Angina Pectoris

Nitrates are the cornerstone of therapy of stable angina pectoris. These agents are available as sublingual or oral tablets, sprays, and transdermal ointments and patches. Each has its own benefits and limitations.

Treatment of Acute Episodes

Nitroglycerin is the most frequently used drug for treating acute episodes of angina pectoris. It is usually given as a sublingual tablet or as a sublingual spray. The disadvantage of the sublingual tablet is its rapid and unpredictable deterioration once exposed to air, and thus the supply needs to be replaced every 3 months. The spray, however, remains stable for at least 3 years. Isosorbide dinitrate is also available as a sublingual tablet, but its onset of action is slower than that of the nitroglycerin preparations.

Prevention of Angina with Nitroglycerin

Many patients can predict which activity will induce angina and are thus able to prevent it by using sublingual nitroglycerin 2 to 5 minutes before undertaking such activity. In some patients, this practice obviates the need for further anti-anginal therapy.[31,32] Oral preparation of nitroglycerin is usually not preferred for the prevention of angina because of the limited data on efficacy with sustained therapy and the absence of data on efficacy throughout the dosing interval.[33] Nitroglycerin ointment also has a clinically important anti-anginal effect and is efficacious during sustained therapy[34] when an intermittent regimen with a 12-hour dose-free interval is followed. Nitroglycerin transdermal patches have the theoretical advantage of stable therapeutic plasma concentrations throughout a 24-hour period, but the results of studies with transdermal nitroglycerin therapy demonstrate some loss of effects during continuous therapy.[35,36] Nitrate tolerance can be prevented or at least reduced by implementing a patch-free period that involves a regimen of 12 hours on and 12 hours off.[37-41] Such a regimen may improve exercise performance in patients with chronic stable angina pectoris.

Prevention of Angina with Isosorbide Dinitrate

Sublingual isosorbide dinitrate is useful in the prevention of angina. Because of its long half-life, this agent provides effective prophylaxis against episodes of angina for up to 1 hour.[42] Oral isosorbide dinitrate is also an effective antianginal drug when given over the short term.[7] Partial tolerance to the hemodynamic and antianginal effects develops with long-term therapy when given without interruption.[8] Sustained-release isosorbide dinitrate has a slower rate of absorption and results in therapeutic concentrations lasting 12 hours, but when given in doses of 80 mg every 12 hours, tolerance develops.[43] This preparation continues to have the anti-ischemic effect when given once daily.

Prevention of Angina with Isosorbide Mononitrate

When the drug is given in an eccentric fashion (i.e., twice daily with 7 hours between doses), its antianginal efficacy lasts for about 12 hours.[44,45] Sustained-release isosorbide mononitrate does not have an advantage over the standard formulation because of the need for a nitrate-free interval. The standard formulation of isosorbide mononitrate in doses of 20 to 40 mg induces tolerance when given every 12 hours for 1 week.[46,47]

Combination Therapy

Nitrates are commonly prescribed in combination with other anti-anginal agents, such as β-blockers and calcium channel blockers. When given with these agents, nitrates increase time to angina and exercise time in patients with stable CAD. In one study, nitrates alone were found to be as potent as dihydropyridine calcium channel blockers.[48] Generally, combination therapy results in less frequent side effects. The results of the Gruppo Italiano per lo Studio della Sopravvivenza nell'infarto Miocardico (GISSI) 3 trial[49] suggest that nitrates can produce some additive beneficial effect when used along with an ACE inhibitor, but this effect was not apparent in the fourth International Study of Infarct Survival (ISIS 4) (discussed later).

Unstable Angina

Nitroglycerin has been incorporated in the treatment of unstable angina because of clinical observations and perceived hemodynamic benefit, but studies showing such benefit in rigorous comparison with placebo are lacking. Studies on the use of intravenous nitroglycerin in patients with unstable angina have been relatively small in sample size, and dose regimens have varied considerably.[50] Further, the trials have been of brief duration. The phenomena of nitrate tolerance and recurrent ischemic events imply that nitrates are not definitive therapy for unstable angina beyond the acute phase. Regarding long-term outcome with nitrates in unstable angina, only one trial has compared transdermal nitroglycerin with placebo therapy over 4 months, each arm receiving conventional medical treatment in addition. Outcome events such as death, MI, or refractory angina were similar in the nitrate- and placebo-treated patients.[51]

In a limited study of the comparison of diltiazem and nitrates, diltiazem was found to be more effective in relieving angina, but the study does not reflect clinical

approach, which usually involves combination of nitrates with a β-blocker or rate-limiting calcium antagonist.[52] The widespread use of oral, topical, and intravenous nitrates in unstable angina is based on reasonable extrapolation from pathophysiologic observations, clinical experience, case series, and evidence of a modest reduction of mortality in acute MI.[49,53,54] Once a patient's condition has stabilized for about 48 hours in hospital, intravenous nitrate therapy is generally tapered with the substitution of oral or topical nitrates.

Acute Myocardial Infarction

Nitrates can reduce oxygen demand and myocardial wall stress during acute MI by reducing preload and afterload.[55] Furthermore, nitrates can increase coronary blood flow to the ischemic region by relieving coronary vasospasm.[56] The antiplatelet effects of nitrates may also be beneficial. In both animals and humans, nitrates have been shown to reduce infarct size and improve left-ventricular function.[53,57] However, controlled clinical trials and overviews provide conflicting results.

In a meta-analysis of seven small trials of intravenous nitroglycerin and three trials of intravenous nitroprusside in a total of 2041 patients, Yusuf et al[60] showed that nitrate treatment reduced mortality by about 35%.[58] The effect of different nitrate treatments in patients with acute MI has been tested in two recent large-scale mortality trials enrolling more than 77,000 patients. The patients were receiving currently recommended concomitant therapies (90% received aspirin and about 70% received thrombolysis).[49,54] Both trials showed that routine nitrate use does not improve survival, either in the total population of patients with acute MI or in the subgroups at different risks for death. However, a large number of patients in the control group received out-of-protocol nitrate treatment because of a specific indication such as angina, CHF, or hypertension, thus obscuring a true benefit in terms of mortality reduction. In the ISIS 4 study, investigators analyzed the effects of nitrates in the subgroup of patients not receiving out-of-protocol nitrate treatment; the results of this subanalysis also showed no decrease in mortality with nitrates.[54] A further overview of all existing trials, including 10 small trials plus the two recent large-scale trials, confirms the lack of mortality reduction.[54] The use of the NO donor molsidomine in the European Study of Prevention of Infarction with Molsidomine (ESPRIM) trial also failed to show any mortality benefit in acute MI.[59]

A concern with any treatment for CHF in the acute phase of MI is how it might influence infarct size. Nitroglycerin may increase collateral blood flow to the infarct zone and thus limit infarct size, particularly if the heart rate is controlled.[60] Others have shown a detrimental effect of nitrates in the setting of acute MI.[61] The hypotensive effect of nitrates combined with bradycardia can increase the current of injury on the electrocardiogram, which is partly reversed by atropine.

One must be cautious about the concomitant use of nitrates with tissue-type plasminogen activator (t-PA). There are two provocative studies on the combination of thrombolytic drug given with intravenous nitroglycerin.

In both studies, nitroglycerin (vs. placebo) given with t-PA resulted in a somewhat bigger infarct size, perhaps because nitroglycerin administration resulted in enhanced hepatic catabolism of t-PA. In an earlier animal model of coronary artery thrombosis, we showed that the use of nitrates along with t-PA may diminish the efficacy of t-PA and thus lead to inadequate thrombolysis.[62] Part of the explanation for the attenuation of the effect of t-PA may be improved hepatic blood flow with nitrates, leading to rapid catabolism of t-PA. These observations should be kept in mind as one routinely prescribes nitrates along with thrombolytics.

The available data show that nitrates are not recommended routinely for all patients with acute MI. However, nitrates are well tolerated along with other treatments such as β-blockers, aspirin, thrombolytics, and ACE inhibitors, suggesting that nitrates used in patients with specific indications in the setting of acute MI (such as angina, CHF, mitral regurgitation, and hypertension) is safe and likely beneficial. We lack definitive data on the short-term mortality benefit of intravenous nitroglycerin started in the first 24 hours after acute MI.

Specific situations such as right-ventricular MI may be a contraindication to the use of nitrates. In these situations, right-ventricular output depends on the preload; reduction of preload may cause marked hypotension. However, excessive preload leads to right-ventricular dilation and compression of the left ventricle. Left-ventricular filling thus may be impaired because of ventricular interdependence and the restraining effect of pericardium. Under these circumstances, despite the diagnosis of right-ventricular MI, nitrates may have a theoretical advantage in reducing right-ventricular preload and thus reducing left-ventricular compression and improving filling.

Post Myocardial Infarction

Oral or transdermal nitrates did not improve prognosis in the first few weeks after MI in the ISIS 4[54] and GISSI 3[49] trials. In a small study from Japan, long-term nitrate treatment increased cardiac events in patients with healed MI.[63] The trial was not blinded and raises doubts about the randomization technique.

Percutaneous Coronary Intervention

Sublingual or intracoronary nitroglycerin is routinely used during coronary angiography to relieve coronary spasm and to define the severity of fixed obstructive disease. This technique also helps in defining the vessel diameter for optimal selection of balloon and stent size. Though nitroglycerin does not improve the "no-reflow phenomenon" that occurs in the setting of percutaneous coronary intervention, nitroglycerin is frequently used to relieve coronary spasm during atherectomy.

Congestive Heart Failure

Vasodilators reduce left-ventricular afterload and preload, and these beneficial effects were first observed in 1956,[64,65] but it was not until the 1970s that the concept was widely accepted.[66,67] The first drugs used for this purpose were pure vasodilators, such as nitroprusside, nitroglycerin, and phentolamine. Subsequently, the use of ACE inhibitors and inodilators became common.

Reduction of afterload and preload in CHF improves left-ventricular performance in keeping with the classic Frank-Starling relationship, with reduced myocardial oxygen demand leading to increased cardiac output.[68,69] Vasodilation, particularly afterload reduction, may also reduce valvular regurgitation and may improve organ function by acting directly on selected vascular beds, such as the coronary and the renal vasculature.

When used as acute vasodilator therapy in CHF, nitrates cause reduction in left-ventricular filling pressures within 3 to 5 minutes, mainly by venodilation and to some extent by lowering of preload.[70,71] Reduction in systemic vascular resistance may also lead to improvement in cardiac output. Although the effect of nitroglycerin on coronary blood flow has not been studied in CHF, it is conceivable that nitrate therapy favorably affects myocardial perfusion and the oxygen supply/demand ratio.[72,73] Acute administration of nitrates appears to be especially useful in patients with elevated filling pressures and concurrent myocardial ischemia. When used in the setting of CHF after acute MI, nitroglycerin causes a marked reduction in left-ventricular filling pressure more than arterial pressure and causes a small decrease in cardiac output and a reflex increase in heart failure. Nitrates and hydralazine have been used as long-term vasodilator therapy in CHF.

The effects on left-ventricular function and hemodynamics are similar to the acute effects of combination of afterload and preload reduction described earlier.[74,75] The addition of a nitrate to hydralazine causes a greater effect on the reduction in filling pressures than can be achieved by hydralazine alone.[76] In view of the beneficial hemodynamic effects of nitrates on coronary circulation, nitrates should be added to hydralazine therapy in patients with significant CAD.[77] Although hydralazine-nitrate therapy is marginally superior to ACE inhibitors in improving exercise capacity, this combination may not be as well tolerated.[78]

The first Vasodilator Heart Failure Trial (V-HeFT I) was the first placebo-controlled trial to study the effect of vasodilator on survival in patients with chronic CHF. The study recruited 642 patients with mild to moderate CHF, who were randomized to receive placebo, prazosin, or the combination of hydralazine and isosorbide dinitrate. Two years after randomization, survival in the hydralazine-nitrate treated group was significantly better than in the placebo group. For the entire follow-up period, the difference was not significant, however. The mortality in the prazosin arm was no different from that in the placebo group.[79] The second V-HeFT study examined the efficacy of hydralazine and isosorbide dinitrate with that of the ACE inhibitor enalapril. There were 804 patients, randomized to the two treatment strategies. Two years after randomization, the all-cause mortality rate was 18% in the enalapril group compared with 25% in the hydralazine-nitrate group ($P = .016$). Over the entire follow-up period, however, the difference was not significant ($P = .08$).

ADVERSE REACTIONS FROM NITRATES

Common minor side effects with use of nitrates include headache, flushing, and hypotension. Hypotension is sometimes severe in patients with volume depletion and unstable ischemic syndromes and can be aggravated by upright posture and meals. Nitroglycerin-induced severe hypotension is sometimes associated with bradycardia, consistent with a vasovagal or vasodepressor response. The partial pressure of oxygen in arterial blood may fall after large doses of nitroglycerin because of a ventilation-perfusion imbalance due to inability of pulmonary vascular bed to constrict in areas of alveolar hypoxia, thereby leading to perfusion of less hypoxic tissues.[80] The commonly used doses of nitrates cause small elevations of methemoglobin as NO combines with oxyhemoglobin, but these elevations are not clinically significant. Rarely, methemoglobinemia is a significant complication after ingestion of very large doses of nitrates.

NITRATE TOLERANCE

Mechanisms

The use of nitrates in treatment of angina is limited by the development of tolerance. Nitrate tolerance has been defined as "the loss of hemodynamic and antianginal effect during sustained therapy."[81] Although a subject of intense study, the precise cause of nitrate tolerance remains elusive. Many mechanisms have been postulated that are based on interference in pathways thought to be necessary for mediating the effects of nitrates on coronary and systemic vasculature. Various mechanisms of nitrate tolerance are summarized in Table 24-2.

Defects in Biotransformation

Animal studies have shown a defect in the biotransformation of nitroglycerin to its effector molecule NO.[82] Sage et al studied the phenomenon of nitrate tolerance in internal mammary and saphenous vein graft segments from patients undergoing elective coronary artery bypass surgery.[83] Preoperative exposure to nitroglycerin was associated with a decreased response of vessel walls to nitroglycerin but a preserved response to nitroprusside, which acts as a direct NO donor. Furthermore, bio-

■ ■ ■

TABLE 24–2   NITRATE TOLERANCE: MECHANISMS

Defective biotransformation of nitroglycerin to its effector molecule nitric oxide

Depletion of sulfhydryl groups, possibly reducing conversion of nitrate to its effector molecule nitric oxide

Expansion of plasma volume can counter the effects of nitrates on ventricular preload

Neurohormonal activation

Oxidative stress with increased production of superoxide anion

conversion of nitroglycerin to 1,2 glyceryl dinitrate was reduced in the group exposed to nitrates, NO oxide synthase after administration of nitroglycerin, and reversal with folate administration.[84]

Depletion of Sulfhydryl Groups

The hypothesis of depleted sulfhydryl groups is based on the knowledge that thiol groups play a role in action of nitrates, with their depletion causing nitrate tolerance, possibly by reducing conversion of nitrate to NO.[85] However, the exact nature of this interaction remains controversial because supplementation of SH groups has produced conflicting results in preventing nitrate tolerance. Some ACE inhibitors that contain an SH group have been studied in terms of preventing nitrate tolerance; for example, one study showed that captopril prevented nitrate tolerance, whereas the non–SH-containing ACE inhibitor enalapril was devoid of this effect.[86] However, in another study, the ACE inhibitor benazepril, which does not possess an SH group, preserved the effect of nitrates on exercise tolerance.[87] Further complicating this issue is the fact that acetylcysteine, an SH-containing agent, can augment the vascular effect of nitrates,[17,88] indicating that the benefit of SH supplementation may be independent of nitrate tolerance.[89]

Expansion of Plasma Volume

Therapy with nitrates leads to expansion of plasma volume.[90] It has been suggested that plasma volume expansion can counteract the effects of nitrates on ventricular preload and contribute to tolerance. Sodium retention does not appear to play a major role in this process.[91] Studies with diuretics to reduce plasma volume have yielded conflicting results, with some studies showing prevention of tolerance by diuretic treatment.[92] However, a study using hydrochlorothiazide showed no benefit in preventing nitrate tolerance.[93]

Neurohumoral Activation

Vasodilatation from nitrate therapy can lead to activation of compensatory vasoconstrictor neurohumoral systems and possibly to a reversal of nitrate effects. Studies have shown that plasma concentrations of angiotensin II, renin, catecholamines, and endothelin are elevated during nitrate therapy.[94] Autocrine production of endothelin has been proposed to contribute to nitrate tolerance by enhancing the vasoconstrictor response of angiotensin II and serotonin.[95] Another postulated mechanism of nitrate tolerance relates to a neurohumorally mediated increase in oxidative stress, as described later. However, neurohormonal activation is not a consistent finding in nitrate tolerance. Furthermore, use of neurohumoral antagonists such as ACE inhibitors has yielded conflicting results, as discussed earlier.

Oxidative Stress

Animal studies have shown an association of nitrate tolerance with increased production of superoxide anion and its reversal by antioxidants.[96] Kurz et al showed increased NADH/NADPH oxidase activity and vascular superoxide production as a result of activation of the renin-angiotensin system and endothelin in nitrate tolerance. One study showed that the antioxidant vitamin E prevents nitrate tolerance.[97] A preliminary study showed that vitamin C prevents nitrate tolerance, presumably by preventing superoxide-induced deactivation of NO.[98] Hydralazine, a drug that inhibits the membrane-bound oxidases responsible for superoxide anion production, has also been shown to prevent nitrate tolerance in animal studies.[99] Gogia et al[100] showed that hydralazine prevents nitrate tolerance. However, this benefit was not seen in another study.[101] The effect of hydralazine is interesting, considering the substantial benefit of the combination of hydralazine and isosorbide dinitrate in heart failure in spite of a nitrate-dosing schedule known to induce tolerance.[79]

Therapy

Although a number of interventions have been tested, including ACE inhibitors, hydralazine, and diuretics, results have been inconsistent. The most effective strategy is to reduce exposure to nitrates by employing a nitrate-free or low-nitrate interval.[102] Because nitrate tolerance prevents anti-ischemic protection round the clock, it is important to use regimens that prevent nitrate tolerance and maximize the anti-ischemic effect. The beneficial effect can be maintained during the day by regimens such as isosorbide/5-mononitrate, 120 to 240 mg once daily, or transdermal nitroglycerine for 10 to 12 hours per day. Dosing intervals have to be appropriately adjusted in patients experiencing predominant nocturnal angina.

NITRIC OXIDE DONORS

The identification of NO as the endothelium-derived relaxing factor has allowed a thorough investigation of the effects of organic nitrate esters as well as other nitrogen-containing vasodilators such as nitrites, nitrosothiols, sydnonomines, and nitroprusside. These substances can release NO or mediators derived from it and are thus known as *NO donors*. For organic nitrates, clinical tolerance arises because mechanisms involved in their bioactivation become exhausted. In contrast, both the molsidomine metabolite SIN-1 and nitroprusside are considered to act as direct NO donors because their biologic activity is not limited by the mode of their bioactivation. Newly acquired knowledge therefore justifies consideration of NO donors as therapeutic substitutes for the protective autacoid NO, which is the basis for further pharmacologic and clinical development of these compounds. Of the different NO donors, molsidomine and its active metabolite SIN-1 has been used extensively in both experimental and clinical situations. The need for intravenous administration, its pharmacokinetic action, and potent vascular effects make nitroprusside a poor agent in the treatment of ischemic coronary syndromes. Hence, most of the discussion pertaining to NO donors

is limited to the class of compounds called *sydnonomines* and of which molsidomine and its metabolite SIN-1 are important members.

Comparison of Nitrates and Sydnonomines

Organic nitrates and the sydnonomine-derivative molsidomine exhibit similar pharmacodynamic actions. Both drugs cause relaxation of smooth muscle cells and thus lead to preload reduction and some afterload reduction with some direct coronary vasodilator actions. The net effect is a reduction in myocardial oxygen consumption and increased delivery, which is beneficial in the treatment of CAD and various ischemic syndromes. In contrast with nitrate-induced tolerance, long-term use of molsidomine is not associated with clinically relevant tolerance. With regard to maximal anti-ischemic and hemodynamic effects, organic nitrates and molsidomine are similar.[103] Thus, molsidomine may be an alternative to nitrate interval treatment or can be used as an adjunct to interval treatment should it become necessary to bridge the therapeutic gap. Despite the theoretic advantage of NO donors, clinical experience with the use of these compounds is rather limited. In clinical studies such as the ESPRIM trial, the use of NO donor molsidomine failed to show any mortality benefit in acute MI.[63]

Mechanism of Action of Molsidomine

Molsidomine is enzymatically metabolized in the liver to SIN-1 and readily converted into the active metabolite SIN-1A, which carries a free nitroso group. Molsidomine and its active metabolite SIN-1 and SIN-1A have pharmacologically active NO, which rapidly increases levels of soluble cGMP, decreases levels of intracellular calcium ions in smooth muscle cells, and induces vasodilation. These compounds increase cGMP levels in close association with, but before, their relaxing action. Relaxation and rises in cGMP by SIN-1 are potentiated by an inhibitor of cGMP phosphodiesterase and attenuated by methylene blue, a dye that inhibits activation of guanylate cyclase by SIN-1 and various nitrosovasodilators.[104] A single significant correlation between rise in cGMP and relaxation was obtained for both SIN compounds and various nitrovasodilators. Relaxation by SIN-1A was independent of the presence of endothelium and was not affected by various inhibitors of arachidonic acid metabolism. In contrast with nitroglycerin, SIN-1 did not induce substantial tolerance, nor were its actions reduced in arterial strips that were tolerant to nitroglycerin. The results indicate that SIN-1A relaxes coronary smooth muscle by a direct stimulant effect on soluble guanylate cyclase in vascular smooth muscle cell. Nitroprusside and SIN-1 show little to negligible tolerance. These drugs stimulate soluble guanylate cyclase in vitro in the absence of cysteine, whereas organic nitrates require the presence of thiol. Thus, it appears that nitroglycerin must be converted into a cyclase stimulator by a cysteine-dependent reaction.

However, Rinaldi et al[105] have used in vitro experiments on precontracted canine coronary arteries to show that both molsidomine and SIN-1 cause a delayed and greater relaxation than nitroglycerin. This was accompanied by less increase in cGMP levels; the peak cGMP level did not precede the onset of relaxation. The authors questioned the relationship between elevated cGMP levels and the relaxation effect after molsidomine or SIN-1 administration.

The pharmacokinetics of molsidomine suggest rapid absorption and hydrolysis. The time to peak plasma drug concentration is 1 to 2 hours. The bioavailability of the parent compound is 44% to 59%.[106] Further metabolism to form polar metabolites such as SIN-1 is rapid, and the half-life of SIN-1 is 1 to 2 hours. Most of the administered molsidomine undergoes biodegradation to the active metabolite, and urinary excretion accounts for 90% of the part of the administered dose of molsidomine. Protein binding of the parent compound is very low. The pharmacokinetics of molsidomine are not markedly altered by impaired renal function. The duration of action of molsidomine is longer than would be expected on the basis of the elimination half-life and is partly due to the metabolic delay in the formation of NO from SIN-1.

Other beneficial effects of molsidomine include its inhibitor effect on platelet aggregation and antiproliferative action. Kukovetz et al showed that the active metabolite SIN-1 of the prodrug molsidomine exerts its inhibitory effect on platelet aggregation by its direct stimulatory effect on soluble guanylate cyclase in the cytosol of platelets.[107] Other investigators have shown similar antiplatelet actions.[108] Nitz et al showed that this effect is also related to the stimulation of prostacyclin synthesis and inhibition of thromboxane release.[109] They suggested that molsidomine exerts its beneficial effect by activation of fibrinolytic system and drug-induced release of a plasminogen activator favoring the antiplatelet aggregatory effect. The drugs that inhibit lipooxygenase enzyme in the arachidonate cascade may theoretically shift prostaglandin catabolism to cyclo-oxygenase products, such as prostacyclin, that may protect against the expansion of ischemia and the induction of coronary spasm. Experimental studies showed a reduction of myocardial infarct size when molsidomine was administered before or after a cardiac insult.[109] However, Kober et al showed that SIN-1 has no direct myocardial anti-ischemic action.[110]

The combination of molsidomine and sodium nitroprusside inhibits monocyte chemotaxis along with an increase in cGMP levels, supporting earlier observations that NO inhibits monocyte function in vitro via a cGMP-mediated mechanism. The differential effects of the spontaneous and thiol-dependent NO donating nitrovasodilators on monocyte function suggest that monocytes, like platelets, are not able to directly metabolize organic nitrates. If in vivo observations prove similar, certain nitrovasodilators might be used therapeutically to inhibit monocyte function (e.g., during atherogenesis).[111]

Le Quan et al showed the influence of SIN-1 on platelet calcium handling. SIN-1 generates both NO and superoxide anion.[112] SIN-1 elicits dose-dependent vasodilatation in vivo in spite of the opposite effects of its breakdown products on vascular tone and platelet aggregation. SIN-1 administration reduced cytosolic calcium in unstimulated platelets by decreasing calcium influx. It attenuated calcium mobilization from internal stores evoked by thrombin or thapsigargin. Superoxide dismutase, the superoxide scavenger, enhanced the capacity of SIN-1 to inhibit calcium mobilization, but catalase had no effect. This suggests that the effects of SIN-1 on platelet calcium handling resemble those of NO but are modulated by simultaneous superoxide anion release, independently of hydrogen peroxide formation.

In recent interesting studies, Jaworski et al demonstrated that S-nitrosothiols, unlike other NO donors such as nitroprusside and SIN-1, do not induce oxidative stress.[113] These authors studied the oxidation of low-density lipoproteins in cultures of vascular endothelial or smooth muscle cells. Thus, some NO donors, despite their advantages, might also induce oxidative stress. Hempelmann et al showed that the vascular relaxation induced by the NO donors DEA/NO and SIN-1 are partly mediated via activation of potassium channels.[114]

CONCLUSIONS

Organic nitrates are powerful drugs that are effective in the therapy of myocardial ischemia and CHF. It is interesting that after nearly a century of use, we do not know the precise mechanisms of their action or the basis of nitrate tolerance. The fact that NO is a molecule that exerts many effects similar to those of organic nitrates will lead to development of compounds that are clinically more effective than organic nitrates and yet have few associated problems.

REFERENCES

1. Murrell W: Nitroglycerin as a remedy for angina pectoris. Lancet 1879;80–81:113–116.
2. Murad F: Drugs used for the treatment of angina: Organic nitrates calcium-channel blockers and adrenergic antagonists. In Gilman AG, Rall TW, Nies AS, Taylor P (eds): Goodman and Gilman's the Pharmacological Basis of Therapeutics, 8th ed. New York, Pergamon Press, 1990, pp 764–783.
3. Bogaert MG: Pharmacokinetics of organic nitrates in man: An overview. Eur Heart J 1988;9(Suppl A):33–37.
4. Armstrong PW, Moffat JA, Marks GS: Arterial-venous nitroglycerin gradient during intravenous infusion in man. Circulation 1982;66:1273–1276.
5. Needleman P, Lang S, Johnson EM Jr: Organic nitrates: Relationship between biotransformation and rational angina pectoris therapy. J Pharmacol Exp Ther 1972;181:489–497.
6. Glancy DL, Richter MA, Ellis EV, Johnson W: Effect of swallowed isosorbide dinitrate on blood pressure, heart rate and exercise capacity in patients with coronary artery disease. Am J Med 1977;62:39–46.
7. Thadani U, Fung H-L, Darke AC, Parker JO: Oral isosorbide dinitrate in the treatment of angina pectoris: Dose-response relationship and duration of action during acute therapy. Circulation 1980;62:491–502.
8. Thadani U, Fung H-L, Darke AC, Parker JO: Oral isosorbide dinitrate in the treatment of angina pectoris: Comparison of duration of action and dose-response relation during acute and sustained therapy. Am J Cardiol 1982;49:411–419.
9. de Belder MA, Schneeweiss A, Camm AJ: Evaluation of the efficacy and duration of action of isosorbide mononitrate in angina pectoris. Am J Cardiol 1990;65:6.
10. Murad F: Cyclic guanosine monophosphate as a mediator of vasodilation. J Clin Invest 1986;78:1–5.

11. Katskuki S, Murad F: Regulation of adenosine cyclic 3′, 5′-monophosphate and guanosine cyclic 3′, 5′-monophosphate levels and contractility in bovine tracheal smooth muscle. Mol Pharmacol 1977;13:330-341.

12. Axelsson KL, Wikberg JES, Andersson RGG: Relationship between nitroglycerin, cyclic GMP and relaxation of vascular smooth muscle. Life Sci 1979;24:1779-1786.

13. Fung HL, Chung SJ, Bauer JA, et al: Biochemical mechanism of organic nitrate action. Am J Cardiol 1992;70:4B-10B.

14. Harrison DG, Bates JN: The nitrovasodilators: New ideas about old drugs. Circulation 1993;87:1461-1467.

15. Needleman P, Jakshik B, Johnson EM Jr: Sulfhydryl requirement of relaxation of vascular smooth muscle. J Pharmacol Exp Ther 1973;187:324-331.

16. Ignarro LJ, Lippton H, Edwards JC, et al: Mechanism of vascular smooth muscle relaxation by organic nitrates, nitroprusside and nitrous oxide: Evidence for the involvement of S-nitrosothiols as active intermediates. J Pharmacol Exp Ther 1981;218:739-749.

17. Horowitz JD, Antman EM, Lorell BH, et al: Potentiation of the cardiovascular effects of nitroglycerine by N-acetyl cysteine. Circulation 1983;68:1247-1253.

18. Lawson DL, Nichols WW, Mehta P, Mehta JL: Captopril-induced reversal of nitroglycerin tolerance: Role of sulfhydryl group vs. ACE-inhibitory activity. J Cardiovasc Pharmacol 1991;17:805-811.

19. Mehta JL, Mehta P: Comparative effects of nitroprusside and nitroglycerin on platelet aggregation in patients with heart failure. J Cardiovasc Pharmacol 1980;2:25-33.

20. Diodati J, Théroux P, Latour JG, et al: Effects of nitroglycerine at therapeutic doses on platelet aggregation in unstable angina pectoris and acute myocardial infarction. Am J Cardiol 1990;66:683-688.

21. Mocada S, Higgs A: The l-arginine-nitric oxide pathway. N Engl J Med 1993;329:2002-2012.

22. Kelly RA, Balligand JL, Smith TW: Nitric oxide and cardiac function. Circ Res 1996;79:363-380.

23. Williams JF Jr, Glick G, Braunwald E: Studies on cardiac dimensions in intact unanesthetized man. V: Effects of nitroglycerin. Circulation 1965;32:767-771.

24. Brown BG, Bolson E, Petersen RB, et al: The mechanisms of nitroglycerin action: Stenosis vasodilatation as a major component of drug response. Circulation 1981;64:1089-1097.

25. Goldstein RE, Stinson EB, Scherer JL, et al: Intraoperative coronary collateral function in patients with coronary occlusive disease: Nitroglycerin responsiveness and angiographic correlations. Circulation 1974;49:298-308.

26. Fam WM, McGregor M: Effect of nitroglycerin and dipyridamole on regional coronary resistance. Circ Res 1968;22:649-659.

27. Early treatment of unstable angina in the coronary care unit: A randomized, double blind, placebo controlled comparison of recurrent ischaemia in patients treated with nifedipine or metoprolol or both: report of the Holland Interuniversity Nifedipine/Metoprolol Trial (HINT) Research Group. Br Heart J 1986;56:400-413.

28. Chirkov YY, Naukalis JI, Sage E, Horowitz JD: Antiplatelet effects of nitroglycerin in healthy subjects and in patients with stable angina pectoris. J Cardiovasc Pharmacol 1993;21:384-389.

29. Lacoste LL, Theroux P, Lidon RM, et al: Antithrombotic properties of transdermal nitroglycerin in stable angina pectoris. Am J Cardiol 1994;73:1058-1062.

30. Andrews R, May JA, Vickers J, Heptinstall S: Inhibition of platelet aggregation by transdermal glyceryl trinitrate. Br Heart J 1994;72:575-579.

31. Reichek N, Priest C, Chandler T, et al: Comparison of time of onset of hemodynamic effects of sustained-release buccal nitroglycerin and sublingual nitroglycerin. In Goldberg AAJ, Parkson DG (eds): Modern Concepts of Nitrate Delivery Systems. London, Royal Society of Medicine, 1983, pp 143-149.

32. Parker JO, Vankoughnett KA, Farrell B: Nitroglycerin lingual spray: clinical efficacy and dose-response relation. Am J Cardiol 1986;57: 1-5.

33. Winsor R, Berger HJ: Oral nitroglycerin as a prophylactic antianginal drug: Clinical, physiologic, and statistical evidence of efficacy based on a three-phase experimental design. Am Heart J 1975;90:611-626.

34. Reichek N, Goldstein RE, Redwood DR, Epstein SE: Sustained effects of nitroglycerin ointment in patients with angina pectoris. Circulation 1974;50:348-352.

35. Reichek N, Priset C, Simrin D, et al: Antianginal effects of nitroglycerin patches. Am J Cardiol 1984;54:1-7.

36. Parker JO, Fung H-L: Transdermal nitroglycerin in angina pectoris. Am J Cardiol 1984;54:471-476.

37. Steering Committee, Transdermal Nitroglycerin Cooperative Study: Acute and chronic antianginal efficacy of continuous twenty-four-hour application of transdermal nitroglycerin. Am J Cardiol 1991;68:1263-1273.

38. Cowan JC, Bourke JP, Reid DS, Julian DG: Prevention of tolerance to nitroglycerin patches by overnight removal. Am J Cardiol 1987;60:271-275.

39. DeMots H, Glasser SP: Intermittent transdermal nitroglycerin therapy in the treatment of chronic stable angina. J Am Coll Cardiol 1989;13:786-795.

40. Ferratini M, Pirelli S, Merlini P, et al: Intermittent transdermal nitroglycerin monotherapy in stable exercise-induced angina: A comparison with a continuous schedule. Eur Heart J 1989;10: 998-1002.

41. Parker JO, Amies MH, Hawkinson RW, et al: Intermittent transdermal nitroglycerine therapy in angina pectoris: Clinically effective without tolerance or rebound: Minitran Efficacy Study Group. Circulation 1995;91:1368-1374.

42. Goldstein RE, Rosing DR, Redwood DR, et al: Clinical and circulatory effects of isosorbide dinitrate: Comparison with nitroglycerin. Circulation 1971;43:629-640.

43. Silber S, Vogler AC, Krause KH, et al: Induction and circumvention of nitrate tolerance applying different dosage intervals. Am J Med 1987;83:860-870.

44. Parker JO: Eccentric dosing with isosorbide-5-mononitrate in angina pectoris. Am J Cardiol 1993;72:871-876.

45. Thadani U, Maranda CR, Amsterdam E, et al: Lack of pharmacologic tolerance and rebound angina pectoris during twice-daily therapy with isosorbide-5-mononitrate. Ann Intern Med 1994;120:353-359.

46. Kohli RS, Rodrigues EA, Kardash MM, et al: Acute and sustained effects of isosorbide 5-mononitrate in stable angina pectoris. Am J Cardiol 1987;58:727-731.

47. Thadani U, Prasad R, Hamilton SF, et al: Usefulness of twice-daily isosorbide-5-mononitrate in preventing development of tolerance in angina pectoris. Am J Cardiol 1987;60:477-482.

48. Hill JA, Feldman RL, Pepine CJ, Conti CR: Randomized double-blind comparison of nifedipine and isosorbide dinitrate in patients with coronary arterial spasm. Am J Cardiol 1982;49:431-438.

49. Gruppo Italiano per lo Studio della Sopravvivenza nell'infarto Miocardico (GISSI-3): Effects of lisinopril and transdermal nitrate singly and together on 6-week mortality and ventricular function after acute myocardial infarction. Lancet 1994;343:1115-1122.

50. Orlander R: Use of nitrates in the treatment of unstable and variant angina. Drugs 1987;33:131-139.

51. Ardissino D, Merlini PA, Savonito S, et al: Effect of transdermal nitroglycerin on N-acetylcysteine, or both, in the long-term treatment of unstable angina pectoris. J Am Coll Cardiol 1997;29:941-947.

52. Gobel EJAM, Hautvast RWH, van Gilst WH, et al: Randomized, double-blind trial of intravenous diltiazem versus glyceryl trinitrate for unstable angina pectoris. Lancet 1995;346:1653-1657.

53. Jugdutt BI, Warnica JW: Intravenous nitroglycerin therapy to limit myocardial infarction size, expansions and complications. Effective timing, dosage and infarct location. Circulation 1988;78:906-920.

54. ISIS-4 Collaborative Group: ISIS-4: A randomized factorial trial assessing early oral captopril, oral mononitrate, and intravenous magnesium sulphate in 58,050 patients with suspected acute myocardial infarction. Lancet 1995;345:669-685.

55. Jugdutt BI, Becker LC, Hutchins GM, et al: Effect of intravenous nitroglycerin on collateral blood flow and infarct size in the conscious dog. Circulation 1981;63:17-28.

56. Hackett D, Davies G, Chierchia S, Maseri A: Intermittent coronary occlusion in acute myocardial infarction: Value of combined thrombolytic and vasodilator therapy. N Engl J Med 1987;317:1055-1059.

57. Jugdutt BI, Sussex BA, Tymchak WJ, Warnice JW: Intravenous nitroglycerin in the early management of acute myocardial infarction. Cardiovasc Rev Rep 1989;10:29-35.

58. Yusuf S, Collins R, MacMahon S, Peto R: Effect of intravenous nitrates on mortality in acute myocardial infarction: An overview of the randomized trials. Lancet 1988;1:1088-1092.

59. The European Study of Prevention of Infarction with molsidomine (ESPRIM) Group: The ESPRIM trial: Short-term treatment of acute myocardial infarction with molsidomine. Lancet 1994;344:91-97.

60. Yusuf S, Sleight P, Rossi PRF, et al: Reduction in infarct size, arrhythmias, chest pain and morbidity by early intravenous beta-blockade

in suspected acute myocardial infarction. Circulation 1983;67: 32–41.

61. Miller RR, Awan NA, DeMaria AN, et al: Importance of maintaining systemic blood pressure during nitroglycerin administration for reducing ischemic injury in patients with coronary disease. Effects on coronary blood flow, myocardial energetics and left ventricular function. Am J Cardiol 1977;40:504–508.

62. Mehta JL, Nicolini FA, Nichols WW, Saldeen TGP: Concurrent nitroglycerin administration decreases thrombolytic potential of tissue-type plasminogen activator. J Am Coll Cardiol 1991;17:805–811.

63. Ishikawa K, Kanmasa K, Ogawa I, et al: Long-term nitrate treatment increases cardiac events in patients with healed myocardial infarction. Jpn Circ J 1996;60:779–788.

64. Eichna LW, Sobel BJ, Kessler RH: Hemodynamic and renal effects produced in congestive heart failure by the intravenous administration of a ganglionic blocking agent. Trans Assoc Am Phys 1956;69:207–213.

65. Burch GE: Evidence for increased venous tone in chronic heart failure. Arch Intern Med 1956;98:750–766.

66. Zells R, Mason DT, Braunwald E: A comparison of the effects of vasodilator stimuli on peripheral resistance vessels in normal subjects and in patients with congestive heart failure. J Clin Invest 1968;47:960–970.

67. Id PA, Sharma B, Taylor SH: Phentolamine for vasodilator treatment of severe heart failure. Lancet 1971;2:719–724.

68. Franciosa JA, Guiha NH, Limas CJ, et al: Improved left ventricular function during nitroprusside infusion in acute myocardial infarction. Lancet 1972;1:650–654.

69. Cohn JN, Franciosa JA: Vasodilator therapy of cardiac failure. N Engl J Med 1977;297:27–31.

70. Lavine SJ, Campbell CA, Held AC, Johnson V: Effect of nitroglycerin-induced reduction of left ventricular filling pressure on diastolic filling in acute dilated heart failure. J Am Coll Cardiol 1989;14:233–241.

71. Mason DT, Braunwald E: The effects of nitroglycerin and amyl nitrate on arteriolar and venous tone in the human forearm. Circulation 1965;32:755–765.

72. DeMarco T, Chatterjee K, Rouleau JL, Parmley WW: Abnormal coronary hemodynamics and myocardial energetics in patients with chronic heart failure caused by ischemic heart disease and dilated cardiomyopathy. Am Heart J 1988;115:809–815.

73. Unverferth DV, Magorien RD, Lewis RP, Leier CV: The role of subendocardial ischemia in perpetuating myocardial failure in patients with non-ischemic congestive cardiomyopathy. Am Heart J 1983;105:176–179.

74. Chattejee K, Ports TA, Brundage BH, et al: Oral hydralazine in chronic heart failure: sustained beneficial hemodynamic effects. Ann Intern Med 1980;92:600–604.

75. Franciosa JA, Jordan RA, Wilen MM, Leddy CL: Minoxidil in patients with chronic left heart failure: Contrasting hemodynamic and clinical effects in a controlled trial. Circulation 1984;70:63–68.

76. Massie B, Chatterjee K, Werner J, et al: Hemodynamic advantage of combined administration of hydralazine orally and nitrates non-parenterally in the vasodilator therapy of chronic heart failure. Am J Cardiol 1977;40:794–801.

77. Packer M, Meller J, Medina N, et al: Provocation of myocardial ischemia events during initiation of vasodilator therapy for severe chronic heart failure. Clinical and hemodynamic evaluation of 52 consecutive patients with ischemic cardiomyopathy. Am J Cardiol 1981;48:939–946.

78. Cohn JN, Johnson G, Ziesche S, et al: A comparison of enalapril with hydralazine-isosorbide dinitrate in the treatment of chronic congestive heart failure. N Engl J Med 1991;325:303–310.

79. Cohn JN, Archibald DG, Ziesche S, et al: Effect of vasodilator therapy on mortality in chronic congestive heart failure. N Engl J Med 1986;314:1547–1552.

80. Hales CA, Westphal D: Hypoxemia following the administration of sublingual nitroglycerin. Am J Med 1978;65:911–918.

81. Parker JD, Parker JO: Drug therapy: Nitrate therapy for stable angina pectoris. N Engl J Med 1998;338:520–531.

82. Omura T, Matsumoto T, Nakae I, et al: Two possible mechanisms underlying nitrate tolerance in monkey coronary arteries. Clin Exp Pharmac Physiol 2001;28:256–265.

83. Sage PR, de la Lande IS, Stafford I, et al: Nitroglycerine tolerance in human vessels: Evidence for impaired nitroglycerine bioconversion. Circulation 2000;102:2810–2815.

84. Gori T, Burstein JM, Ahmed S, et al: Folic acid prevents nitroglycerine-induced nitric oxide synthase dysfunction and nitrate tolerance: A human in vivo study. Circulation 2001;104:1119–1123.

85. Needleman P, Johnson EM Jr: Mechanism of tolerance development to organic nitrates. J Pharmacol Exp Ther 1973;184: 709–715.

86. Katz RJ, Levy WS, Buff L, Wasserman AG: Prevention of nitrate tolerance with angiotensin-converting enzyme inhibitors. Circulation 1991;83:1271–1277.

87. Muiesan ML, Boni E, Castellano M, et al: Effects of transdermal nitroglycerine combination with an ACE-inhibitor in patients with chronic stable angina pectoris. Eur Heart J 1993;14:1701–1708.

88. Winniford MD, Kennedy PL, Wells PJ, Hillis DL: Potentiation of nitroglycerine induced coronary dilatation by N-acetyl cysteine. Circulation 1986;73:138–142.

89. Fung HL, Chong S, Kowaluk E, et al: Mechanisms for the pharmacologic interaction of organic nitrates with thiols: existence of an extracellular pathway for the reversal of nitrate vascular tolerance by N-acetyl cysteine. J Pharmacol Exp Ther 1988;245:524–530.

90. Dupis J, Lalonde G, Lemieux R, Rouleau JL: Tolerance to intravenous nitroglycerine in patients with congestive heart failure: Role of increased intravascular volume, neurohumoral activation and lack of prevention with N-acetyl cysteine. J Am Coll Cardiol 1990;16:923–931.

91. Parker JD, Parker JO: Effect of therapy with an angiotensin-converting enzyme inhibitor on hemodynamic and counter-regulatory responses during continuous therapy with nitroglycerine. J Am Coll Cardiol 1993;21:1445–1453.

92. Sussex BA, Campbell NRC, Raju MK, McKay DW: The antianginal efficacy of isosorbide dinitrate therapy is maintained during diuretic treatment. Clin Pharmacol Ther 1994;56:229–234.

93. Parker JD, Parker AB, Farrell B, Parker JO: The effects of diuretic therapy on the development of tolerance to nitroglycerine and exercise capacity in patients with chronic stable angina. Circulation 1996;93:691–696.

94. Kurz S, Hink U, Nickenig G, et al: Evidence for a causal role of the renin-angiotensin system in nitrate tolerance. Circulation 1999;99:3181–3187.

95. Parker JD, Farrell B, Fenton T, et al: Counter-regulatory responses to continuous and intermittent therapy with nitroglycerin. Circulation 1991;84:2336–2345.

96. Munzel T, Sayegh H, Freman BA, et al: Evidence for enhanced vascular superoxide anion production in nitrate tolerance: A novel mechanism underlying tolerance and cross-tolerance. J Clin Invest 1995;95:187–194.

97. Watanabe H, Kakihana M, Ohtsuka S, Sugishita Y: Randomized, double blind, placebo-controlled study of supplemental vitamin E on attenuation of the development of nitrate tolerance. Circulation 1997;96:2545–2550.

98. Daniel TA, Nawarskas JJ: Vitamin C in the prevention of nitrate tolerance. Ann Pharmacother 2000;34:1193–1197.

99. Bauer JA, Fung HL: Concurrent hydralazine administration prevents nitroglycerine-induced hemodynamic tolerance in experimental heart failure. Circulation 1991;84:35–39.

100. Gogia H, Mehra A, Parikh S, et al: Prevention of tolerance to hemodynamic effects of nitrates with concomitant use of hydralazine in patients with chronic heart failure. J Am Coll Cardiol 1995;26:1575–1580.

101. Parker JD, Parker AB, Farrell B, Parker JO: The effect of hydralazine on the development of tolerance to continuous nitroglycerine. J Phamacol Exp Ther 1997;280:866–875.

102. Thadani U: Nitrate tolerance, rebound, and their clinical relevance in stable angina pectoris, unstable angina and heart failure. Cardiovasc Drugs Ther 1997;10:735–742.

103. Rudolph W, Dirschinger J: Clinical comparison of nitrates and sydnonimines. Eur Heart J 1991;12(Suppl E):33–41.

104. Kukovetz WR, Holzman S: Cyclic GMP as the mediator of molsidomine-induced vasodilation. Eur J Pharmacol 1986;122: 103–109.

105. Rinaldi G, Cingolani H: The efficacy of substituted sydnonimines on coronary smooth muscle relaxation and cyclic guanosine monophosphate levels. Circulation 1983;68:1315–1320.

106. Rosenkranz B, Winkelmann BR, Parnham MJ: Clinical pharamacokinetics of molsidomine. Clin Pharmacokinet 1996;950:3 72–384.

107. Kukovetz WR, Holzman S: Mechanism of the vasodilating effect and blood platelet antiaggregating activity of molsidomine and SIN-1. Pathol Biol (Paris) 1987;35:260–265.

108. Wautie JL, Weill D, Kadeva H, et al: Modulation of platelet function by SIN-1A, a metabolite of molsidomine. J Cardiovasc Pharmacol 1989;14(Suppl 11):S111–S114.

109. Nitz RE, Fielder VB: Molsidomine: Alternative approaches to treat myocardial ischemia. Pharmacotherapy 1987;7:28–37.

110. Kober G, Bender M, Vallbracht C, et al: SIN-1 has no direct myocardial anti-ischemic action. Clin Cardiol 1993;16:717–722.

111. Bath PM: The effect of nitric oxide–donating vasodilators on monocyte chemotaxis and intracellular cGMP concentration in vitro. Eur J Clin Pharmacol 1993;45:53–58.

112. Le Quan Sang KH, Le Feuvre C, Brunet A, et al: Influence of SIN-1 on platelet Ca2+ handling in patients with suspected coronary artery disease: Ex vivo and in vitro studies. Thromb Haemost 2000;83:752–758.

113. Jaworski K, Kinard F, Goldstein D, et al: S-nitrosothiols do not induce oxidative stress, contrary to other nitric oxide donors, in cultures of vascular endothelial or smooth muscle cells. Eur J Pharmacol 2001;425:11–19.

114. Hemplemann RG, Seebeck J, Kruse ML, et al: Role of potassium channels in the relaxation induced by the nitric oxide (NO) donor DEA/NO in the isolated rat basilar artery. Neurosci Lett 2001;313:21–24.

β-Blockers and Calcium Channel Blockers: Use in Acute Coronary Syndromes

Lionel H. Opie
Patrick J. Commerford

The medical management of acute coronary syndromes (ACS) is focused increasingly on antithrombotic and antiplatelet agents, with a strong trend toward early revascularization. ACS is by definition a syndrome, with an underlying disease that needs to be diagnosed. The patient needs to be carefully assessed clinically with specific attention to associated diabetes mellitus, hypertension, heart failure, anemia, thyroid dysfunction, and renal failure, besides risk stratification of the ACS. The use of β-blockers and calcium channel blockers (CCBs) as antiischemic agents is only part of the picture (Fig. 25–1). Ideally, there should be large decisive outcome trials defining whether β-blockers, CCBs, neither, or both are effective add-on therapy in ACS. That these drugs relieve ischemia and pain is beyond doubt. If we take the modern view that the range of ACS extends to include acute myocardial infarction (MI), it could be argued that this is the one situation in which β blockade has evidence favoring its use. Studies favoring β blockade were done in an era when acute MI was diagnosed differently, however; thrombolytic therapy was not common. Taking into account the paucity of good data, much of the frequent use of β-blockers in ACS is based on extrapolation from other situations. The choice is not evidence based but based on the recommendation of expert committees, essentially B or C in category, which makes it a reasonable, but not an essential, choice. In the case of CCBs, there are data warning against their use (particularly short-acting nifedipine)[1] and data favoring their use (particularly diltiazem).[2,3]

PATHOPHYSIOLOGY

Coronary Spasm or Inappropriate Coronary Vasoconstriction?

Unstable angina, only one component of ACS, is itself "a veritable mosaic, with considerable overlap, of diverse clinical clusters."[4] Previously, localized coronary spasm, as in Prinzmetal's vasospastic angina, was thought to be a major factor in precipitating unstable angina, but the spastic theory has been downgraded, at least in part through the failure of the vasodilatory CCBs to give results clearly better than β-blockers, which tend to cause coronary vasoconstriction. Only in some specific situations is there good evidence that true coronary spasm is a dominant factor, such as in Japanese patients

with unstable angina (this may reflect local dietary customs) and in cocaine users. Nonetheless, the defects in the coronary arteries in unstable angina extend beyond anatomic occlusive vascular disease. *Inappropriate coronary vasoconstriction* accompanies coronary stenosis, and the activity of endothelin-1 may account for much of the increased resting tone found in atherosclerotic coronary arteries.[5] Other factors, such as temporary increases in sympathetic activity or in inflammatory markers such as C-reactive protein, are probably also important.

Closely related entities are impaired coronary vascular reserve and *endothelial dysfunction*. The latter currently is regarded as an important mechanism contributing to vascular dysfunction in diseased coronary arteries. Almost all coronary risk factors can be related to endothelial dysfunction. The current treatment for endothelial dysfunction is not clearly defined, however, and there is no evidence that acute manipulation of endothelial function by any agent would provide clinical benefit. These are ideas for the future. For example, folate may protect the endothelium from the dysfunction associated with hyperlipidemia[6] and from the changes found in nitrate tolerance.[7] A host of other agents also have been reported to improve endothelial function, including vitamin C, angiotensin-converting enzyme (ACE) inhibitors, angiotensin receptor blockers, and β-blockers. With the use of a statin, improvement in endothelial dysfunction is possible within 3 days.[8] With CCBs, cholesterol-induced abnormal vasomotion and coronary constriction can be opposed.[9] In no case, however, has endothelial function been studied in ACS, at least not in the acute phase.

Microvascular Dysfunction

Microvascular dysfunction is another functional abnormality of the coronary vascular system.[10] In this case, myocardial ischemic episodes cannot be ascribed to fixed or dynamic epicardial coronary stenosis or to inappropriate vasoconstriction of the larger arteries, but rather to constriction of small coronary arterioles or prearterioles. Such functional disease could predispose to and sometimes precipitate obstructive lesions.[10]

It is likely that most patients with ACS would have some additional functional coronary disease beyond obstructive atheroma. The one way to treat this vascular dysfunction at present is by risk factor manipulation, a long-term process.

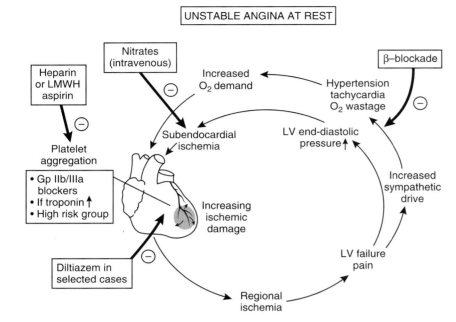

UNSTABLE ANGINA AT REST

FIGURE 25–1. Hypothetical mechanisms for unstable angina at rest and proposed therapy. Increasing emphasis is being placed on the role of antithrombotics and antiplatelet agents, such as glycoprotein (Gp) IIb/IIIa blockers and clopidogrel. β blockade may be particularly effective in the presence of sympathetic activation with increased heart rate and blood pressure. Calcium channel blockers need to be differentiated. Diltiazem, a heart rate–lowering calcium channel blocker, may be used intravenously or orally. Dihydropyridines, such as nifedipine and amlodipine, should be used with care and only in combination with β blockade. LMWH, low-molecular-weight heparin; LV, left ventricular. (Copyright, L.H. Opie, 2001.)

Coronary Steal

Coronary steal occurs when vasodilation by drugs or by an increased oxygen demand siphons blood to normally perfused myocardial areas away from a flow-limiting stenosis, potentially aggravating ischemia in the poststenotic ischemic zone.[11] Classic agents that evoke steal are adenosine and dipyridamole, thought to act by vigorous dilation of small coronary vessels. It sometimes is feared that CCBs can cause steal and assumed that β-blockers do not. Measurements of coronary blood flow by xenon clearance show, however, that nifedipine maintains coronary flow in poststenotic areas during pacing, whereas nitroglycerin vasodilates in such a way that poststenotic flow falls.[12] Perhaps unexpectedly, propranolol also may decrease poststenotic flow, perhaps by the combination of reduction of the coronary perfusion driving pressure and coronary vasoconstriction near the stenotic site. It would be useful to have such studies repeated with more modern techniques for measuring regional coronary blood flow.

PHARMACOLOGIC PROPERTIES

β-Blockers and CCBs act through improving the myocardial oxygen supply/demand balance, albeit by different mechanisms. β-Blockers act primarily to reduce myocardial oxygen demand, with well-known negative chronotropic and inotropic effects that reduce heart rate, stroke volume, and arterial blood pressure, and have a lesser known metabolic effect by reducing blood free fatty acid levels and in this way improving ischemic metabolism. β-Blockers also have major antiarrhythmic

effects, whereby serious ventricular arrhythmias can be lessened.

Properties of β-Blockers

β-Blockers are sometimes divided into arbitrary *generations.* First-generation agents, such as propranolol, nonselectively block all the β-receptors (β_1 and β_2). Second-generation agents, such as atenolol, metoprolol, acebutolol, bisoprolol, and others, have relative selectivity when given in low doses for the β_1 (largely cardiac) receptors. Third-generation agents have added vasodilatory properties, acting chiefly through two mechanisms: (1) agents with intrinsic sympathomimetic β-adrenergic activity, also sometimes called *partial agonist activity,* which stimulates formation of vascular cyclic AMP to relax blood vessels, and (2) agents with added α-adrenergic blockade, as in the case of labetalol and carvedilol. Other nonvasodilatory β-blockers tend to promote vascular and coronary vasoconstriction by unopposed α-adrenergic activity.

Other marked differences between β-blockers are in the pharmacokinetic properties, with half-lives varying from about 9 minutes to more than 30 hours and in differing lipid or water solubility. Nonetheless, there is no evidence that any of these ancillary properties has any compelling therapeutic advantage in the therapy of chronic effort angina or hypertension. When considering ACS, the short half-life and intravenous availability of esmolol is of particular advantage.

Esmolol (Brevibloc) is an ultrashort-acting β_1-blocker with a half-life of 9 minutes, rapidly converting to inactive metabolites by blood esterases. Full recovery from β blockade occurs within 30 minutes in patients with a normal cardiovascular system. Esmolol is ideally suited when on-off control of β blockade is desired, as in unstable angina,[13] especially if there is associated severe hypertension or supraventricular tachycardia. *Cautions* include extravasation of the acid solution with risk of skin necrosis.

Properties of Calcium Channel Blockers

CCBs are divided into (1) the more vascular-active dihydropyridines (DHPs), such as nifedipine, amlodipine, and others, and (2) the more cardiac-active non-DHPs, which are also called the *heart rate–slowing agents.* Both types of CCBs, but especially the DHPs, inhibit the vascular long-lasting calcium channels to diminish calcium ion entry and to cause coronary vasodilation, with improvement in the myocardial blood supply. Another vascular action, well studied experimentally, is increased production of nitric oxide by the vascular endothelium, a process that can be expected to be protective by the vasodilatory and antiplatelet aggregation properties of nitric oxide. Consonant with these observations, in humans, CCBs oppose the vasoconstrictory effects of high levels of oxidized low-density lipoprotein.[14] The chief non-DHPs are verapamil and diltiazem, which both have some β-blocking–like properties in reducing heart rate and myocardial contractility. Added to peripheral vasodilation, there is substantial oxygen conservation with these agents. With the DHPs, especially with short-acting nifedipine, the more marked peripheral vasodilation stimulates adrenergic reflexes and tachycardia, which could account for the adverse effects of nifedipine capsules in unstable angina.

β-BLOCKERS IN ACUTE CORONARY SYNDROMES

It is appropriate briefly to consider the diagnosis of ACS. As pointed out elsewhere in this book, ACS are acute chest pain conditions that include the previous diagnoses of unstable angina, non–ST-segment elevation MI, and ST-segment elevation MI. According to the current view, any detectable release of any cardiac-specific enzyme, such as one of the troponins, provides proof of myocardial necrosis and qualifies for the laboratory diagnosis of MI. I take the view that the outcome evidence and proof of the benefit of β-blockers are restricted to what used to be called acute MI, as defined by the World Health Organization guidelines, that is, two of the following: prolonged chest pain (often ≥30 minutes), a typical large rise in serum enzymes, and sequential electrocardiogram changes often involving early ST-segment elevation and later formation of Q waves. In this situation, β-blockers are well established, especially their postinfarct protective effect. It is in very early stage acute and clinically obvious MI in the prethrombolytic era that intravenous followed by oral β blockade has been best tested (Table 25–1).

Unstable Angina Pectoris

Regarding what used to be called unstable angina pectoris, with the relative demise of the coronary spasm theory, β-blockers are conventionally and preferentially used to CCBs. It is equally true that there is no reliable outcome study beyond one placebo-controlled trial,[1] in which patients who were not on prior β-blockers were

■ ■ ■

TABLE 25–1 TRIAL OUTCOME DATA ON USE OF β BLOCKADE IN ACUTE CORONARY SYNDROMES*

TRIAL	ENTRY CRITERIA	DRUG AND DOSE	OUTCOME
Kirshenbaum[45]	16 patients with acute MI or unstable angina with wedge pressure 15–25 mm Hg	Esmolol up to 300 μg/kg/min IV up to 48 h	Rate-pressure product fell, wedge pressure the same, drug effect over by 30 min. In 4 of 16, drug stopped, oliguria or hypotension
MIAMI[46]	5778 patients with definite or suspected acute MI	Metoprolol 15 mg IV (3 × 5 mg), then 100 mg every 12 h until day 16	No overall difference, but in high-risk group (retrospective) 29% fall in deaths
Ryden[47]	1395 patients with suspected or later proven MI	As above but oral metoprolol for 3 mo	Less ventricular fibrillation (*P* < .05)
Norris[20]	735 patients with suspected MI within 4 h of onset	Propranolol 7 mg over 5 min (weight adjusted); oral 40 mg 1, 3, 7, 11, 15, 19, 23, 27 h after start	Less ventricular fibrillation (*P* = .006)
HINT[1]	338 patients with unstable angina	Metoprolol, 100 mg twice a day	MI at 48 h odds ratio, 1.07 (95% CI, 0.54–2.09)
Roberts,[18] TIMI II-B	All tPA; early vs late β blockade	Early metoprolol 1 mg as above, then 100 mg in first 12 h, then 200 mg/day in split doses	Mortality and ejection fraction at discharge unchanged; less early reinfarction and recurrent pain in early group; trend toward fewer intracranial bleeds
ISIS-1[17]	16,027 patients within 12 h of onset of suspected MI	Atenolol 5–10 mg at once, then 100 g/day orally for 7 days	Vascular mortality on first day reduced, *P* < .003; days 1–365, *P* < .01

*All except HINT are suspected or proved early-phase clinical acute myocardial infarction. CI, confidence interval; IV, intravenously; MI, myocardial infarction.

randomized to metoprolol, to short-acting nifedipine, or to the combination. The relative risk (RR) in favor of β blockade for recurrent ischemia was 0.76 (confidence interval [CI], 0.49 to 1.16), but for recurrent infarction only, RR was 1.07 (CI, 0.54 to 2.09). Maybe if the trial had not been stopped because of the increase in MI with nifedipine only (RR, 2.0; CI, 1.1 to 3.6), the β-blocker–alone group would have fared better. Taking relief of chest pain as the only parameter, β blockade is better than short-acting nifedipine, the latter generally increasing the heart rate.[15]

That chest pain is often relieved by β blockade is beyond clinical doubt, and that myocardial oxygen consumption is conserved is beyond physiologic doubt. Logically the lower the heart rate, within limits, the less the risk of recurrent ischemia. Despite the missing outcome data, two factors swing toward β blockade. First, the clinician may be under the impression that, with outcome studies in diverse conditions such as hypertension and heart failure, there should already be outcome evidence in ACS even though that is not the case. Second, ACS encompass a gradation of events. Unstable angina can develop into a situation in which there is clinical deterioration with large-scale enzyme release and typical electrocardiogram changes of clinical acute MI. In that case, most clinicians would be happy to have β blockade "on board" as a protective measure. One pilot study suggested that threatened MI may be prevented from becoming overt.[16]

Very Early Acute Myocardial Infarction

There are not many definitive studies on very early acute MI. In the International Study of Infarct Survival (ISIS-1) trial on acute MI (not defined), intravenous followed by short-term oral atenolol for 7 days, starting within 12 hours of the onset of symptoms, gave an advantage to β blockade at a time when thrombolysis was not used.[17] In the thrombolytic era, there is only one study with very early administration of a β-blocker, Thrombolysis in Myocardial Infarction (TIMI II), in which acute MI was defined as typical chest pain for 30 minutes or more plus ST-segment elevation.[18] Early metoprolol started intravenously within 2 hours reduced recurrent MI compared with later β blockade started after 6 days. The primary end point, global ejection fraction at discharge, was the same in early and in late β-blocker groups. In the Global Use of Strategies to Open Occluded Coronary Arteries (GUSTO-I) study, use of atenolol overall was associated with better outcomes, but in patients given intravenous atenolol, there was more heart failure, shock, recurrent ischemia, and need for pacemakers.[19] In patients with ischemic chest pain for more than 30 minutes but less than 4 hours, propranolol started intravenously lessened ventricular fibrillation but did not change mortality.[20] Of specific interest is a retrospective analysis from the National Registry of Myocardial Infarction in the United States, in which immediate intravenous β-blocker therapy was associated with a 31% reduction in intracra-

nial hemorrhage, a dreaded complication of thrombolysis with tissue plasminogen activator.[21]

Theoretically, intravenous β blockade is of most use in the early hours after the onset of acute MI when the adrenergic reflex response is most evident and when ventricular fibrillation might be most prevalent. In the United States, only two selective agents, metoprolol and atenolol, are licensed for intravenous use in acute MI. If the hemodynamic status is uncertain, ultrashort-acting esmolol is the logical drug of choice,[13] although it is not licensed for this purpose in the United States. Logically, β blockade should be of most use in the presence of ongoing pain, tachycardia, hypertension, or ventricular rhythm instability.

Taking all the evidence into account, *early intravenous β blockade* is recommended for patients without contraindications by the task force of the American College of Cardiology/American Heart Association on acute MI, using the prior definitions of MI.[22] There are no data on ACS with non–ST-segment elevation acute MI, now regarded as a relatively common condition, which might not have satisfied the definitions of acute MI used at the time of the studies.

Summary

There is little direct evidence that β blockade given for ACS (whether non-MI or MI by modern definitions) has more than an antianginal effect. The appropriate trial data for ACS without clinical MI are lacking. Common-sense says that β blockade should benefit by reducing heart rate contractility, improving myocardial metabolism, and lessening early ventricular fibrillation. By contrast, if there is a full-scale classical MI, overall evidence favors the early use of β blockade and continuation into the postinfarct follow-up period. The expectancy would be that intravenous β blockade would be most effective in patients with clinical adrenergic activation, but the trial data to support this proposal are lacking.

CALCIUM CHANNEL BLOCKERS IN ACUTE CORONARY SYNDROMES

In the heyday of the coronary spasm hypothesis for unstable angina, the use of CCBs was almost routine. With the near-demise of this theory and the negative results of the HINT (Holland Inter-university Nifedipine Trial) study,[1] far greater circumspection is required before the use of CCBs in ACS. Of all the potential anti-ischemic drugs, including β-blockers, only diltiazem has a study showing that it is more powerfully antianginal than a nitrate, and this benefit extends to the follow-up period (Table 25–2). In *Prinzmetal's variant angina*, a cause of ACS now thought to be relatively rare except in Japan, the CCBs are used in preference to β-blockers as a result of short-term trial data and because theoretically only the CCBs lessen the severe coronary spasm that underlies this condition.

■ ■ ■

TABLE 25–2 TRIAL OUTCOME DATA ON USE OF CALCIUM CHANNEL BLOCKERS IN ACUTE CORONARY SYNDROMES INCLUDING UNSTABLE ANGINA

TRIAL	ENTRY CRITERIA	DRUG AND DOSE	OUTCOME
HINT[1]	515 patients with unstable angina	Nifedipine 10 mg every 4 h; with metoprolol 200 mg daily or placebo	Nifedipine-only group: double clinical MI at 48 h; for nifedipine added to prior metoprolol, MI 48 h reduced OR 0.56 (CI, 0.30–0.99)
Göbel[2,3]	129 patients with unstable angina	Diltiazem 25 mg IV over 5 min, then 5–15 mg/h to maximum 25 mg/h vs nitroglycerin infusion over 48 h	Reduced refractory angina in diltiazem group; fewer events over 1 year of follow-up
DATA[48]	59 patients with early phase acute MI and ST-segment elevation treated with tPA	Diltiazem IV 10 mg bolus, then 10 mg/h for 48 h, then oral up to 4 wk	Composite end point of death and reinfarction in recurrent ischemia reduced by 78% at 35 days ($P = .027$)
DAVIT 1[28]	3498 patients with clinical acute MI admitted to CCU	Verapamil 0.1 mg/kg IV and 120 mg orally followed by 120 mg thrice daily for 6 mo	No effect on mortality or reinfarction at 6 mo

CCU, coronary care unit; CI, confidence interval; IV, intravenously; MI, myocardial infarction; OR, odds ratio; tPA, tissue plasminogen activator.

Dihydropyridines for Acute Coronary Syndromes

The DHPs all bind to the same sites on the α_1-subunit (the DHP or N sites), establishing their common property of calcium channel antagonism. Vascular selectivity refers to the greater inhibitory effect on vascular smooth muscle than on the myocardium or nodal tissue. For practical purposes, effects on the sinoatrial and atrioventricular nodes can be ignored. Nifedipine is the prototype of the DHPs. In the originally available, short-acting capsule form, it rapidly vasodilates to relieve severe hypertension and to terminate attacks of coronary spasm. The peripheral vasodilation may lead to rapid reflex adrenergic activation with tachycardia, stimulation of the renin-angiotensin system, and increased myocardial ischemia. Such intermittent adrenergic activation may explain why the short-acting DHPs in high doses have adverse outcome effects.[23] The inappropriate use of short-acting nifedipine in situations similar to ACS can explain much of the adverse publicity that previously surrounded the CCBs as a group, so that the focus has now changed to the long-acting DHPs.

On the basis of the HINT study, DHPs as a group including amlodipine are contraindicated in unstable angina in the absence of β blockade.[1] The use of nifedipine capsules now is totally contraindicated in ACS, in stark contrast to the situation in the early 1980s, when capsular nifedipine was often given to patients with unstable angina to stop the supposed coronary spasm. What is often neglected in an evaluation of the HINT study, however, is that the addition of nifedipine to prior β blockade was the only group with improved results. In my view, in the patient with ACS already given maximum doses of β blockade, also receiving nitrates, and still in significant pain, and without the facilities for rapid percutaneous intervention, the cautious addition of low doses of DHPs is acceptable. The capsules give large swings in blood levels, however, and long-acting DHPs

are undesirable in the context of ACS, in which treatment is often evolving.

There are no studies with long-acting DHPs in ACS. Because DHPs as a group tend to increase variable adrenergic stimulation, their use without concomitant β blockade must be avoided. By contrast, there are several smaller medium-size studies suggesting use of the non-DHPs in ACS (see next sections). The practical choice is often the addition of a non-DHP, with the added advantage that it also can be given intravenously.

Nondihydropyridines for Acute Coronary Syndromes

Verapamil and diltiazem bind to two different sites on the α_1-subunit of the calcium channel, but they have many properties in common. They both act on nodal tissue, being effective in supraventricular tachycardias. Both tend to decrease the sinus rate. Both inhibit myocardial contraction more than the DHPs or, put differently, are less vascular selective. These properties, added to peripheral vasodilation, lead to substantial reduction in myocardial oxygen demand. Such oxygen conservation makes the non-DHPs much closer than the DHPs to the β-blockers, with which they share a similar spectrum of therapeutic activity. Two important exceptions are (1) the almost total lack of beneficial effect of verapamil and diltiazem on standard types of ventricular tachycardia, which is a strong contraindication to their use, and (2) the benefits of β blockade in heart failure, in which the non-DHPs are also contraindicated.

In *unstable angina*, verapamil has not been tested against placebo, although it is licensed for this condition in the United States. Vasospastic angina is an approved indication for diltiazem in the United States, but not unstable angina. Data for diltiazem are better. One good, albeit relatively small study shows that intravenous diltiazem (not licensed for this purpose in the United States) gives better pain relief than does intravenous nitrate.[2] At

1-year follow-up, there were fewer events of note in the group initially treated by diltiazem despite lesser use of β-blockers.[3] It seems as if diltiazem conferred long-term advantages compared with nitrates, but that is no proof of superiority over β blockade. Compared with β blockade (propranolol), diltiazem is about as good using relief of ischemia as the end point.[24] Long-term, there was no survival benefit of diltiazem over β blockade for unstable angina according to one observational post-ACS follow-up study.[25]

In a pilot study on *early-phase acute MI,* defined as chest pain within the previous 6 hours with ST-segment elevation, intravenous diltiazem added to tissue plasminogen activator reduced postinfarct ischemia and reinfarction with decrease in the combined end point of death, reinfarction, or recurrent ischemia at 35 days.[26] In the INTERCEPT (Incomplete Infarction Trial of European Research Collaborators Evaluating Prognosis Post-Thrombolysis) study on post-thrombolysis patients with acute MI, long-acting oral diltiazem plus aspirin started within 36 to 96 hours of the onset of MI was compared with aspirin alone and given for 6 months.[27] Although there was a 24% reduction in the combined primary end point of death, recurrent MI, or refractory ischemia, the CIs just overlapped unity (0.59 to 1.02). Regarding verapamil, one early-phase trial[28] disappointingly gave no benefit, but 40% of the patients were admitted more than 6 hours after the onset of symptoms.

Summary

The DHP CCBs may not be used in ACS without concurrent β blockade. The non-DHPs, verapamil and diltiazem, previously were used often for unstable angina, although now β blockade seems to be preferred. There are, however, no direct comparative trials with adequate outcome events. There are small trials favoring the use of intravenous diltiazem over intravenous nitrates in unstable angina and the protective effect of intravenous diltiazem in patients given tissue plasminogen activator for thrombolysis.

COMBINATIONS OF CALCIUM CHANNEL BLOCKERS AND β-BLOCKERS IN UNSTABLE ANGINA

Because β-blockers and CCBs have different and potentially complementary properties, logically they should act synergistically in unstable angina. Four studies support this point of view. In the largest, the HINT study,[1] "of all the treatments studied, only the addition of nifedipine to previous maintenance with a β-blocker was clearly beneficial" at 48 hours.[1] Only nifedipine added to prior β blockade reduced recurrent ischemia (RR, 0.68; CI, 0.47 to 0.97) and recurrent MI (RR, 0.56; CI, 0.30 to 0.99). Similar arguments for combination therapy arise from the Gerstenblith study,[29] in which capsule nifedipine was added to prior β blockade with reduction of the combined end points of sudden death, myocardial infarction, or coronary artery bypass graft surgery within

4 months. Similarly, in the third study, the addition of nifedipine to prior β blockade gave better pain relief than did increasing the dose of propranolol or nitrates or both.[15] In the fourth study, the addition of propranolol to prior nifedipine reduced symptomatic and silent ischemic episodes.[30] There is good evidence for the benefits of the DHP/β-blocker combination in unstable angina. In every case, the DHP was short-acting nifedipine, however, and there is no good evidence favoring the combination of non-DHPs and β-blockers. In the study by Göbel and colleagues[2] that showed the superiority of intravenous diltiazem over nitroglycerin for pain relief in unstable angina, 37% of the diltiazem patients (22 of 60) received β blockade on admission and at a minimum started off with diltiazem/β blockade, but this subgroup was not reported separately. The diltiazem/β blockade combination is attractive, possibly allowing the additive benefits of calcium channel blockade with those of β blockade. These advantages may be especially important when planning long-term treatment for patients with no option for revascularization. If this combination were started in hospital, any problems, such as excess bradycardia or atrioventricular conduction defects or negative inotropy, could readily be detected.

COMORBID CONDITIONS

Comorbid conditions may complicate the clinical picture. I could not find any evidence-based outcome studies to guide the therapy of choice, and the following are my personal opinions.

Severe Hypertension

With severe hypertension, intravenous therapy is indicated to achieve smooth blood pressure reduction without any sudden hypotension or tachycardia. Sodium nitroprusside, although often regarded as the gold standard for emergency hypertension, has no outcome data in its favor and has no anti-ischemic properties. The antihypertensive anti-ischemics are β blockade, non-DHP CCBs, or nitrates. Nitrates generally produce tachycardia and so are not the agents of choice unless added to preexisting β blockade. Theoretically, nitrates would be especially suitable when there is evidence of an increased preload, such as pulmonary congestion. Among β-blockers, ideal when there is coexisting tachycardia, the β_1-selective agent esmolol is attractive because of its short half-life and ready reversibility. In the presence of left ventricular failure, although gradually increasing β blockade over many days is now used for this purpose, sudden ablation of sympathetic support remains risky. Cautious β blockade, reducing dose if needed, is one option. Labetalol, an α/β-blocker with a half-life of 6 to 8 hours, has vasodilating properties and may be considered if heart rate reduction is not the top priority. Intravenous diltiazem, with a half-life of 4 to 5 hours, is likely to produce blood pressure and heart rate reduction similar to esmolol and is a good alternative if chronic pulmonary disease is present but is contraindicated if clinical heart failure is present.[2]

Atrial Arrhythmias

Esmolol is licensed in the United States for supraventricular tachycardia and intravenous diltiazem for treatment of paroxysmal supraventricular tachycardia and for reduction of the ventricular response rate in atrial flutter or fibrillation. Verapamil, although not licensed for this purpose, is the approximate equivalent of diltiazem.

Asthma or Other Clear Contraindications to β Blockade

In a patient with overt asthma, β blockade is contraindicated. Acute anti-ischemic treatment should be based on intravenous or oral diltiazem, followed by long-term therapy with either diltiazem or verapamil. After MI, verapamil is better documented:[31] 120 mg three times daily, started 7 to 15 days after MI and continued for 12 to 18 months. In the United States, this is an off-label use of verapamil. Heart failure is a contraindication to the use of verapamil and diltiazem. A meta-analysis[32] showed that verapamil decreased the combined outcome of death or reinfarction (RR, 0.82; CI, 0.70 to 0.97).

Strongly Suspected Coronary Artery Spasm

No β-blockers are licensed in the United States for strongly suspected coronary artery spasm because they tend to promote coronary spasm by unopposed α-adrenergic activity. CCBs are used preferentially. For intravenous therapy, diltiazem and verapamil are best tested, but neither diltiazem nor verapamil is licensed for this purpose in the United States. Oral verapamil and amlodipine are approved for use in the United States. In resistant cases, amlodipine can be combined with either diltiazem or verapamil; it must be in mind that verapamil as a non-DHP has prominent heart rate–lowering effects and that amlodipine as a DHP has strong vascular effects.

Left Ventricular Dysfunction and Clinical Heart Failure

In left ventricular dysfunction and clinical heart failure, it is essential to give a diuretic to treat fluid retention and to give an ACE inhibitor. During pacing-induced myocardial ischemia, adrenergic and renin-angiotensin activation occurs in the heart.[33] It would be logical, although unsubstantiated by trials, to give an ACE inhibitor for its antiadrenergic and anti–renin-angiotensin system effects, which are desirable in heart failure and in unstable angina. During cotherapy with diuretics and an ACE inhibitor, carefully started and up-titrated oral β-blockers have reduced mortality in large clinical trials of heart failure patients with no unstable angina. The slow dose increase over several weeks as used in heart failure trials is impractical in unstable angina, in which rapid β blockade must be achieved. Intravenous β blockade by esmolol may be started cautiously with the hemody-

namic status carefully watched. When β blockade has been achieved successfully in the patient, a switch to an oral agent, such as metoprolol, is logical. Among the oral agents, metoprolol is attractive because it has the shortest half-life of the three β-blockers that have convincing trial data favoring their use in heart failure; the other two are carvedilol and bisoprolol. Also, metoprolol is cardioselective, which carvedilol is not.

CCBs generally are thought to be contraindicated unless the left ventricular failure is due to severe hypertension, which may present as acute pulmonary edema with an ejection fraction greater than 50%.[34] Two small trials show the benefits of short-acting nifedipine in severe hypertension.[35,36] In one of these trials, nifedipine was superior to verapamil. This finding is not surprising given the capacity of short-acting nifedipine to activate the sympathetic nervous system with a more modest negative inotropic effect than with verapamil. The modern equivalent of capsular nifedipine is intravenous nicardipine (1 to 3 µg/kg/min), which has not been tested in ACS. Intravenous diltiazem is another option, although it is untested in ACS from the hemodynamic point of view. Relatively high doses (0.4 mg/kg over 5 minutes followed by 0.4 mg/kg over 10 minutes) were as well tolerated during atrial pacing in coronary disease patients with low ejection fractions less than 45% as in patients with higher mean ejection fractions of 58%.[37] Although indices of contractility held well during the diltiazem infusion, left ventricular end-diastolic pressure rose toward the end of the study.

Before Planned Coronary Artery Bypass Graft Surgery

It is already known that β blockade can protect from some of the adverse effects of peripheral vascular surgery.[38] The situation is not the same as ACS, but it does represent a temporary strain to the cardiovascular system in high-risk patients that has some analogy to the development of ACS. Perioperative deaths from cardiac causes and MI could be reduced by bisoprolol in high-risk patients. Logically, one could extrapolate that coronary artery bypass graft surgery, another form of stress reaction, also calls for prior β blockade. A further benefit, not yet fully reported, is reduction of postoperative atrial fibrillation. A further extrapolation would be to give β blockade to patients undergoing intra-aortic counterpulsation.

OTHER MANAGEMENT PROBLEMS

The most important management problem is that the therapy must be geared to the patient's symptoms and signs. Practical issues include when to use intravenous and when to use oral agents, whether to titrate the β-blockers and CCBs or to start with high doses, and whether the drugs should be continued after hospital discharge. No trial data offer guidance on these issues. Some clinical and pathophysiologic considerations might lead to educated guesses, however.

Clinical Picture

Good clinical judgment remains as important as ever. Judgment on the requirement for β blockade could be simplified as follows. First, the more the clinical picture veers toward clinical acute MI, the more likely is a vigorous adrenergic response with an adverse tachycardia and elevation of blood free fatty acids. The latter changes reflect catecholamine activation, as when comparing larger with smaller infarcts.[39] In a patient with ACS, a brisk adrenergic reaction with severe pain is reflected by a rise in heart rate and blood pressure. The greater the adrenergic response, the greater is the logic for β blockade; a second choice could be a non-dihydropyridine calcium channel blocker. Second, a low blood pressure does not exclude adrenergic activation if there is clinical MI. Of interest is the simple risk index for triage of patients with acute ST-segment elevation MI.[40] Three adverse factors are age, high heart rate, and low blood pressure. Here it seems likely that the low blood pressure results from a large infarct with a compensatory tachycardia. Although such a patient is at high risk, with clear adrenergic activation, there would be definite hemodyamic problems with acute β blockade unless carefully administered esmolol is used to reduce the tachycardia. Prime attention must be on rapid revascularization, whether by thrombolytics or mechanical means. Third, the more the evidence favors vasospastic angina, the stronger the argument for beginning with a non-DHP CCB, such as diltiazem. Although a DPH would relieve coronary spasm, it might be difficult to ensure that the ST-segment elevation was purely due to vasospastic angina, which could be relieved by coronary vasodilation, or whether true MI with ST-segment elevation was developing, as in some of the original cases described by Prinzmetal. In the latter case, the DHP would be undesirable.

Diabetics

Diabetics generally have a worse prognosis, with greater benefit from glycoprotein IIb/IIIa antagonists,[41] and are more likely to present with more serious ACS and be stronger candidates for therapy by β blockade. A nonselective agent, such as propranolol, can be expected to have extra benefit by inhibiting the release of free fatty acids from adipose tissue with decreased blood levels and decreased myocardial uptake of fatty acids. Additionally (not supported by trial data), with greater myocardial metabolic abnormalities, diabetics with ACS should be candidates for intravenous insulin therapy, as in clinical MI.[42]

Intravenous or Oral Route for Anti-Ischemic Agents

Whether to give the β-blocker or non-DHP intravenously or orally is a clinical judgment. In clinical acute MI, intravenous β blockade relieves pain[43] and probably helps to prevent ventricular fibrillation.[20] Factors influencing the decision are adrenergic markers, such as the severity of the pain, tachycardia, and hypertension and evidence of high-risk, including the diabetic state.

Truly Low-Risk Patients

In patients with a persistently normal electrocardiogram, no history of coronary artery disease, and normal blood troponin levels, there is no argument for the use of either β-blockers or CCBs.

Post–Acute Coronary Syndrome Policy

First, there is now growing evidence that statins should be started early and continued in post-ACS patients. The Heart Protection Study (HPS) has shown that statins are of benefit even in patients with vascular disease and normal blood cholesterol levels.[44] Second, even an ACS that is not an ST-segment elevation MI has a clear risk of future clinical MI. It makes empirical sense to continue to use β blockade or a non-DHP[3,31] on a long-term basis. A β-blocker is the first choice because it is likely better to protect against development of heart failure. It is only after clinical MI, however, that good appropriate trial data for such protection exist. Third, because patients with ACS are by definition high-risk patients, an ACE inhibitor should be given long-term.

SUMMARY

There are no adequate outcome trials concerning the use of β-blockers or of currently used CCBs in ACS, here taken to mean predominantly unstable angina. β blockade is often used because heart rate reduction is seen as logical and because of its protective effects in full-blown acute MI, especially in the follow-up phase. Of the CCBs, only the non-DHPs may be used in the absence of concurrent β blockade. Verapamil and diltiazem have been used widely in unstable angina, but the trial data focusing on outcome measures are limited to one study with diltiazem showing benefit over nitrates that extended to a 1-year follow-up. There are no comparative studies of non-DHPs with β blockade with adequate outcome measures. Based on the inadequate data presently available, these agents may be used in unstable angina, especially when β blockade is contraindicated or when vasospastic angina is suspected. One of the few trials with a positive outcome in unstable angina added nifedipine to prior β blockade, which lends support to the primary use of β blockade with an added DHP. Short-acting capsular nifedipine is no longer favored, however, and long-acting DHPs have no data in ACS and may be a disadvantage in a situation in which clinical management may change rapidly according to the clinical status of the patient.

Diltiazem also may be used as a first-line agent for unstable angina and has a trial with 1-year follow-up in its favor. Data for verapamil in unstable angina are weak. In practice, many physicians first use a β-blocker with nitrates, because of the stronger data for β blockade in acute-phase MI and post-MI follow-up.

REFERENCES

1. HINT Study: Early treatment of unstable angina in the coronary care unit, a randomised, double-blind placebo controlled comparison of recurrent ischemia in patients treated with nifedipine or metoprolol or both. Holland Inter-university Nifedipine Trial. Br Heart J 1986;56:400-413.

2. Göbel EJ, Hautvast RW, van Gilst WH, et al: Randomised, double-blind trial of intravenous diltiazem versus glyceryl trinitrate for unstable angina pectoris. Lancet 1995;346:1653-1657.

3. Göbel EJAM, van Gilst WH, de Kam PJ, et al: Long-term follow-up after early intervention with intravenous diltiazem or intravenous nitroglycerin for unstable angina pectoris. Eur Heart J 1998;19: 1208-1213.

4. Bentivoglio LG, Detre K, Yeh W, et al: Outcome of percutaneous transluminal coronary angioplasty in subsets of unstable angina pectoris: A report of the 1985-1986 National Heart, Lung and Blood Institute Percutaneous Transluminal Coronary Angioplasty Registry. J Am Coll Cardiol 1994;24:1195-1206.

5. Kinlay S, Behrendt D, Wainstein M, et al: Role of endothelin-1 in the active constriction of human atherosclerotic coronary arteries. Circulation 2001;104:1114-1118.

6. Verhaar MC, Wever RMF, Kastelein JJP, et al: Effects of oral folic acid supplementation on endothelial function in familial hypercholestolemia: A randomized placebo-controlled trial. Circulation 1999;100:335-338.

7. Gori T, Burstein JM, Ahmed S, et al: Folic acid prevents nitroglycerin-induced nitric oxide synthase dysfunction and nitrate tolerance. Circulation 2001;104:1119-1123.

8. Tsunekawa T, Hayashi T, Kano H, et al: Cerivastatin, a hydroxy-methylglutaryl coenzyme A reductase inhibitor, improves endothelial function in elderly diabetic patients within 3 days. Circulation 2001;104:376-379.

9. Kaufmann PA, Frielingsdorf J, Mandinov L, et al: Reversal of abnormal coronary vasomotion by calcium antagonists in patients with hypercholesterolemia. Circulation 1998;97:1348-1354.

10. Maseri A, Lanza GA, Sanna T, Rigattieri S: Coronary blood flow and myocardial ischemia. In Fuster V, Alexander RW, O'Rourke RA (eds): Hurst's The Heart, 10th ed. New York, McGraw-Hill, 2001, pp 1109-1129.

11. Holmvang G, Fry S, Skopicki HA, et al: Relation between coronary "steal" and contractile function at rest in collateral-dependent myocardium of humans with ischemic heart disease. Circulation 1999;99:2510-2516.

12. Lichtlen PR, Engel H-J, Rafflenbeul W: Calcium entry blockers especially nifedipine, in angina of effort: Possible mechanisms and clinical implications. In Opie LH (ed): Calcium Antagonists and Cardiovascular Disease. New York, Raven Press, 1984, pp 221-236.

13. Hohnloser SH, Meinertz T, Klingenheben T, et al: For the European Esmolol Study Group. Usefulness of esmolol in unstable angina pectoris. Am J Cardiol 1991;67:1319-1323.

14. Cooper RS, Rotimi CN, Kaufman JS, et al: Hypertension treatment and control in sub-Saharan Africa: The epidemiological basis for policy. BMJ 1998;316:614-617.

15. Muller J, Turi Z, Pearl D, et al: Nifedipine and conventional therapy for unstable angina pectoris: A randomized, double-blind comparison. Circulation 1984;69:728-733.

16. Yusuf S, Sleight P, Rossi R, et al: Reduction in infarct size, arrhythmias and chest pain by early intravenous beta blockade in suspected acute myocardial infarction. Circulation 1983;67 (Suppl I): I-32-I-41.

17. ISIS-1 Study: Randomised trial of intravenous atenolol among 16 027 cases of suspected acute myocardial infarction: ISIS-1. Lancet 1986;1:921-923.

18. Roberts R, Rogers WJ, Mueller HS, et al, for the TIMI Investigators: Immediate versus deferred β-blockade following thrombolytic therapy in patients with acute myocardial infaction: Results of the Thrombolysis in Myocardial Infarction (TIMI) II-B study. Circulation 1991;83:422-437.

19. Pfisterer M, Cox JL, Granger CB, et al: Atenolol use and clinical outcomes after thrombolysis for acute myocardial infarction: The GUSTO-I Experience. Global Utilization of Streptokinase and TPA (Alteplase) for Occluded Coronary Arteries. J Am Coll Cardiol 1998;32:634-640.

20. Norris RM, Brown MA, Clarke ED, et al: Prevention of ventricular fibrillation during acute myocardial infarction by intravenous propranolol. Lancet 1984;2:883-886.

21. Barron HV, Rundle AC, Gore JM, et al: Intracranial hemorrhage rates and effect of immediate beta-blocker use in patients with acute myocardial infarction treated with tissue plasminogen activator. Am J Cardiol 2000;85:294-298.

22. Ryan TJ, Antman EM, Brooks NH, et al: 1999 Update of the ACC/AHA Guidelines for the Management of Patients with Acute Myocardial Infarction: A report of the American College of Cardiology/American Heart Association Task Force on Practice Guidelines (Committee and Management of Acute Myocardial Infarction). J Am Coll Cardiol 1999;34:890-911.

23. Furberg CD, Psaty BM, Meyer JV: Nifedipine dose-related increase in mortality in patients with coronary heart disease. Circulation 1995;92:1326-1331.

24. Théroux P, Taeymans Y, Morissette D, et al: A randomized study comparing propranolol and diltiazem in the treatment of unstable angina. J Am Coll Cardiol 1985;5:717-722.

25. Smith NL, Reiber GE, Psaty BM, et al: Health outcomes associated with beta-blocker and diltiazem treatment of unstable angina. J Am Coll Cardiol 1998;32:1305-1311.

26. Théroux P, Gregoire J, Chin C, Pelletier G, de Guise P, Juneau M. Intravenous diltiazem in acute myocardial infarction. Diltiazem as Adjunctive Therapy to Activase (DATA) trial. J Am Coll Cardiol 1998; 32:620-628.

27. Boden WE, Fox K, Whitehead A, et al: Incomplete Infarction Trial of European Research Collaborators Evaluating Prognosis Post-Thrombolysis (INTERCEPT trial): Diltiazem in acute myocardial infarction treated by thrombolytic agents. Lancet 2000;355: 1751-1756.

28. DAVIT 1 Study: Danish Study Group of Verapamil in Myocardial Infaction: Verapamil in acute myocardial infarction. Eur Heart J 1984;5:516-528.

29. Gerstenblith G, Ouyang P, Achuff SC, et al: Nifedipine in unstable angina: A double-blind, randomized trial. N Engl J Med 1982;306: 885-889.

30. Gottlieb SO, Weisfeldt ML, Ouyang P, et al: Effect of the addition of propranolol to therapy with nifedipine for unstable angina pectoris: A randomized, double-blind, placebo-controlled trial. Circulation 1986;73:331-337.

31. The Danish Study Group on verapamil in myocardial infarction. Secondary prevention with verapamil after myocardial infarction. Am J Cardiol 1990;66:331-40I.

32. Pepine CJ, Faich GF, Makuch R: Verapamil use in patients with cardiovascular disease: An overview of randomized trials. Clin Cardiol 1998;21:633-641.

33. Remme WJ, Kruyssen DA, Look MP, et al: Systemic and cardiac neuroendocrine activation and severity of myocardial ischemia in humans. J Am Coll Cardiol 1994;23:82-91.

34. Little WC: Hypertensive pulmonary oedema is due to diastolic dysfunction [editorial]. Eur Heart J 2001;22:1961-1964.

35. Guazzi MD, Cipolla E, Bella PD, et al: Disparate unloading efficacy of the calcium channel blockers, verapamil and nifedipine on the failing hypertensive left ventricle. Am Heart J 1984;108:116-123.

36. Ellrodt AG, Ault MJ, Riedinger MS, Murati GH: Efficacy and safety of sublingual nifedipine in hypertensive emergencies. Am J Med 1985;79 (Suppl 4A): 19-25.

37. Remme WJ, Drauss XH, van Hoogenhuyze DCA, Kruyssen DACM: Hemodynamic tolerability and anti-ischemic efficacy of high dose intravenous diltiazem in patients with normal versus impaired ventricular function. J Am Coll Cardiol 1993;21:709-720.

38. Poldermans D, Boersma E, Bax JJ, et al: The effect of bisoprolol on perioperative mortality and myocardial infarction in high-risk patients undergoing vascular surgery. N Engl J Med 1999;341: 1789-1794.

39. Opie LH, Tansey MJ, Kenelly BM: Proposed metabolic vicious circle in patients with large myocardial infarcts and high plasma free fatty acid concentrations. Lancet 1977;2:890-892.

40. Morrow DA, Antman EM, Giuliano RP, et al: A simple risk index for rapid initial triage of patients with ST-elevation myocardial infarction: An InTIME II substudy. Lancet 2001;358:1571-1575.

41. Sabatine MS, Braunwald E: Will diabetes save the platelet blockers? Circulation 2001;104:2759-2761.

42. Malmberg K, Ryden L, Hamsten A, et al: Effects of insulin treatment on cause-specific one-year mortality and morbidity in diabetic patients with acute myocardial infarction. DIGAMI study group. Diabetes Insulin-Glucose in Acute Myocardial Infarction. Eur Heart J 1996;17:1337–1344.

43. Herlitz J, Hjalmarson A, Holmberg S, et al: Effect of metoprolol on chest pain in acute myocardial infarction. Br Heart J 1984;51: 438–444.

44. Heart Protection Study Collaborative Group: MRC/PHF Heart Protection Study of cholesterol lowering with simvastatin in 20,536 high-risk individuals: a randomized placebo-controlled trial. Lancet 2002;630:7–22.

45. Kirshenbaum JM, Kloner RF, McGowan N, Antman EM: Use of an ultrashort-acting beta-receptor (esmolol) in patients with acute myocardial ischemia and relative contraindications to beta-blockade therapy. J Am Coll Cardiol 1988;12:773–780.

46. MIAMI Trial Research Group: Metoprolol in Acute Myocardial Infarction (MIAMI): A randomized placebo-controlled international trial. Eur Heart J 1985;6:199–226.

47. Ryden L, Ariniego R, Arnman K, et al: A double-blind trial of metoprolol in acute myocardial infarction. N Engl J Med 1983;308:614–618.

48. Stewart JT, French JK, Théroux P, et al: Early noninvasive identification of failed reperfusion after intravenous thrombolytic therapy in acute myocardial infarction. J Am Coll Cardiol 1998;31:1499–1505.

ATP-Sensitive Potassium Channels, Adenosine, and Preconditioning

Fabrizio Tomai

EXPERIMENTAL ISCHEMIC PRECONDITIONING

Ischemic preconditioning refers to the ability of short periods of ischemia to make the myocardium more resistant to a subsequent ischemic insult. This term was introduced by Murry and colleagues,[1] who found in a canine model that four consecutive periods of coronary occlusion of 5 minutes reduced the infarct size caused by a subsequent period of occlusion of 40 minutes by 75%. This classic form of ischemic preconditioning has been observed in several animal species.[2]

Although ischemic preconditioning initially referred to the ability of short periods of ischemia to limit infarct size,[1] some investigators extended this definition to include a beneficial effect on ischemia and reperfusion–induced arrhythmias[3] and on myocardial stunning.[4] It is controversial, however, whether the reduction in the incidence of arrhythmias by ischemic preconditioning is due to a direct antiarrhythmic effect or whether it is a consequence of the delay of ischemic cell death.[1,3] Regarding the beneficial effects of ischemic preconditioning on postischemic contractile dysfunction, Cohen and associates[4] showed that in rabbits, preconditioning can lead to enhanced recovery of contractile function of the myocardial region at risk. In this case also, the beneficial effects of preconditioning on acute recovery of contractile function might be a consequence of the delay of ischemic cell death; parameters of necrosis extent (i.e., infarct size and enzyme leakage) correlate with the enhancement of functional recovery.[4]

The chain of events that confers resistance to ischemia is only partially understood. Cohen and coworkers[5] developed the hypothesis that binding of surface receptors by agonists (including adenosine, bradykinin, opioids, acetylcholine, catecholamines, and oxygen radicals) results in the activation of protein kinase C (PKC). This seems to be the first element of a complex kinase cascade that ultimately causes opening of mitochondrial adenosine triphosphate (ATP)-sensitive potassium (K_{ATP}) channel, which may be the final mediator of protection for ischemic preconditioning.[5] How the opening of mitochondrial K_{ATP} channel may be protective is still uncertain, however. Three hypotheses have been proposed: (1) mitochondrial swelling and optimization of respiration, (2) decrease in the extent of mitochondrial calcium overload, and (3) stimulation of mitochondrial reactive oxygen species production.[6] Figure 26-1

shows the proposed mechanism of preconditioning at the cellular level.

It is now well established that the protective effects of preconditioning are transient and last for less than 2 hours.[2,5] A so-called second window of protection or delayed ischemic preconditioning has been shown in different species, however, occurring 24 hours after the preconditioning stimulus and lasting for about 48 hours.[7,8] This time course is consistent with the concept that the second window of protection is mediated by the activation of genes encoding for cytoprotective proteins.[7,8] Similar to the early phase of preconditioning, aside from a delayed anti-infarct effect, a delayed antiarrhythmic effect after preconditioning has been reported.[9] Sun and colleagues[10] described a delayed preconditioning against myocardial stunning, independent of ischemic necrosis, since the ischemic challenge used was insufficient to induce myocardial infarction (MI).

EVIDENCE FOR PRECONDITIONING IN HUMAN MYOCARDIUM

Ischemic preconditioning represents the most powerful form of protection against experimental MI described to date.[2,5] This endogenous form of myocardial protection has been shown in all animal species investigated.[2,5] It seems reasonable to assume that such a form of endogenous cardioprotection also might occur in the clinical setting. If this were the case, the possibility of exploiting this endogenous form of protection by pharmacologic means would be important in the attempt to reduce myocardial infarct size. Experimental findings on ischemic preconditioning cannot be directly extrapolated to humans, however. For logistic and ethical reasons, no clinical study can meet the strict conditions of experimental studies on preconditioning in which infarct size is the end point. Surrogate end points have been used, including contractile function, electrocardiogram (ECG) ischemic changes, and biochemical evidence of cell damage. This fact has to be taken into account in the evaluation of clinical studies on preconditioning because the mechanisms of such nonclassic forms of ischemic preconditioning may differ from those involved in the reduction of infarct size in the experimental models. Another important limitation of several published clinical studies is the extent of coronary collateral flow, which in humans is a major determinant of the severity

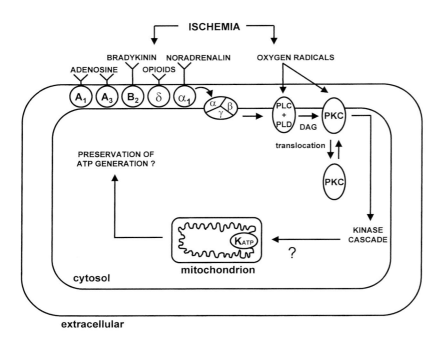

FIGURE 26–1. Proposed mechanism of preconditioning at the cellular level. Ischemia leads to release of adenosine, bradykinin, opioids, noradrenalin, and free radicals that together produce stimulation of phospholipase C (PLC) or D (PLD) that, in turn, activate protein kinase C (PKC). This seems to be the first element of a complex kinase cascade that ultimately causes opening of mitochondrial ATP-sensitive potassium (K_{ATP}) channel, which may be the final mediator of protection for ischemic preconditioning. ATP, adenosine triphosphate; DAG, diacylglycerol.

of myocardial ischemia during coronary occlusion; it cannot always be accurately quantified.

In vitro human studies, in which confounding effects secondary to coronary collateral flow can be overcome, showed that human cardiomyocytes can be preconditioned.[11-14] Carr and coworkers[11] showed that isolated superfused isometrically contracting human atrial trabeculae can be preconditioned against a combined hypoxic and substrate depletion challenge by simulated ischemia and by A_1 and A_3 adenosine receptor activation. The same group also showed that protection against contractile dysfunction caused by a combined hypoxic and substrate depletion challenge can be induced by activation of PKC and by the opening of K_{ATP} channels and that the protection induced by PKC activation and preconditioning can be blocked by blockade of K_{ATP} channels.[12] Cleveland and associates[13] showed that no such protection was evident when the myocardium was obtained from diabetic patients exposed to long-term oral hypoglycemic agents, suggesting important clinical implications. Morris and Yellon[14] showed in human atrial trabeculae that angiotensin-converting enzyme inhibitors can potentiate the protective effects of a subthreshold preconditioning stimulus, possibly secondary to bradykinin degradation inhibition resulting in enhanced B_2-bradykinin receptor activation. Such a demonstration may help explain the mechanisms involved in the reduction of fatal ischemic events in patients treated with angiotensin-converting enzyme inhibitors.[15-18]

The limitations of the model of isolated superfused isometrically contracting human atrial trabeculae are the use of hypoxia rather than ischemia to initiate protection, of recovery of contractile function as surrogate end

point, and of atrial rather than ventricular tissue. In vitro human studies do not provide answers about the clinical situations in which preconditioning does occur, and they do not clarify which mechanisms are involved in mediating ischemic preconditioning in different clinical settings. Ischemic preconditioning in humans has been studied in the following clinical settings: (1) preinfarction angina, (2) exercise-induced ischemia (warm-up phenomenon), (3) coronary angioplasty, and (4) cardiac surgery.[19-22]

Preinfarction Angina

Studies showed that patients with MI preceded by angina have smaller infarcts and a better in-hospital outcome after thrombolytic therapy than patients without preinfarction angina.[23-25] At least three mechanisms may explain this difference between MIs that are preceded by angina and MIs that are not: (1) coronary collaterals, (2) reperfusion rate, and (3) ischemic preconditioning. Kloner and associates[23] found that patients with angina within 48 hours of MI had a lower in-hospital death rate and a smaller infarct size than patients without angina, despite similar development of coronary collateral vessels assessed at angiography 90 minutes after MI, suggesting that preconditioning by preinfarction angina might render the myocardium more resistant to infarction from the subsequent prolonged ischemic episode. Another attractive hypothesis about the protective role of preinfarction angina was suggested by Andreotti and colleagues.[24] They compared the infarct size of patients with or without unstable angina during the week before MI, taking into account the speed of recanalization. In patients with preinfarction angina, compared with patients without, thrombolytic therapy resulted in more rapid reperfusion and smaller infarcts, suggesting that the benefit of preinfarction angina on infarct size might depend on a speedier coronary thrombolysis in addition to or perhaps instead of preconditioning. Also in this study, there was no significant difference in collateral development between patients with and without preinfarction angina, implying that collaterals are unlikely to play a major role in explaining the beneficial effects of preinfarction angina. Ishihara and associates[25] confirmed that reperfusion was achieved more frequently in patients with than in patients without prodromal angina in the 24 hours before infarction, suggesting a more efficient response of the infarct-related artery to thrombolytic therapy in the former. These investigators also showed that prodromal angina in the 24 hours before infarction, but not angina occurring at an earlier time, was independently associated with a better 5-year outcome, suggesting a role for ischemic preconditioning.

Warm-Up Phenomenon

The warm-up phenomenon (i.e., the improved performance exhibited by more than half of patients with coronary artery disease after a first exercise test)[26,27] may be another clinical correlate of ischemic preconditioning. Okazaki and colleagues[26] showed that in patients with a single lesion of the left anterior descending coronary artery, great cardiac vein flow is similar during the first and second exercise stress test, suggesting that the warm-up phenomenon is not accompanied by an increase in total myocardial blood flow. Myocardial oxygen consumption was reduced during the second test, suggesting increased metabolic efficiency, a feature of preconditioning. A role for preconditioning is also supported by the demonstration that the time course of the warm-up phenomenon is consistent with that of classic ischemic preconditioning (lasting 60 to 90 minutes).[27] We found that in patients with stable angina undergoing three consecutive exercise tests, the warm-up phenomenon observed within minutes of a first exercise test is a result of adaptation to ischemia, whereas warm-up phenomenon observed 2 hours after the second exercise test is a result of a training effect caused by peripheral mechanisms.[27] Studies that have examined the cellular mechanisms of the warm-up phenomenon do not fully support this hypothesis, however. The involvement of K_{ATP} channels in the warm-up phenomenon is uncertain. K_{ATP} channel blockade by glibenclamide, given in an attempt to prevent the warm-up phenomenon at a dose previously shown to block adaptation to ischemia during coronary angioplasty,[28] yielded conflicting results.[29-32] Adenosine receptors, which have been identified as key mediators in experimental ischemic preconditioning, do not seem to play a major role in the setting of the warm-up phenomenon. Aminophylline, a nonselective antagonist of adenosine receptors, and bamifylline, a selective antagonist of A_1 adenosine receptors, fail to prevent the warm-up phenomenon.[33,34] Future work is warranted to understand better the

mechanisms of the warm-up phenomenon, including studies on transmural distribution of myocardial perfusion and on triggers of ischemic preconditioning different from adenosine.

Coronary Angioplasty

Since its introduction in 1976, coronary angioplasty has provided a useful model for studying the effects of transmural myocardial ischemia because of controlled coronary occlusions in patients with coronary artery disease. Studies during coronary angioplasty have contributed greatly to the understanding of several pathophysiologic aspects of myocardial ischemia in humans, including the role of collateral circulation, stenosis severity, and small vessel function.[35-38] More recently, the experimental demonstration of preconditioning with the common clinical observations of fewer ECG ischemic changes and less anginal pain during sequential coronary balloon occlusion led to the use of coronary angioplasty as a model for the study of ischemic preconditioning in humans. The procedure usually involves repeated intracoronary balloon inflations with intervening periods of reperfusion; the first period of ischemia may enhance the myocardial tolerance to subsequent balloon inflations via classic ischemic preconditioning. The first formal study aimed at assessing adaptation to ischemia during coronary angioplasty was published by Deutsch and coworkers[39] and involved 12 patients with an isolated obstructive stenosis in the left anterior descending coronary artery undergoing two sequential 90-second balloon inflations. Compared with the initial balloon occlusion, the second occlusion was characterized by less subjective anginal pain, less ST-segment shift, and lower mean pulmonary artery pressure, despite a reduction in cardiac vein flow and unchanged coronary wedge pressure. These findings have been observed in several other angioplasty studies,[28,40-43] confirming an adaptive response of the myocardium to repeated ischemic episodes, akin to ischemic preconditioning. Some angioplasty studies failed to show adaptation to ischemia during repeated coronary occlusions, probably because they neglected some crucial methodologic aspects (i.e., short balloon inflations of <90 seconds, preinflation ischemia, or inadequate end points).[19,44]

A limitation of the angioplasty model of ischemic preconditioning is that the myocardial adaptation to ischemia observed after repeated coronary balloon occlusions is related at least partially to collateral recruitment.[45-47] Although collateral recruitment during a first coronary balloon inflation does occur, however, further recruitment during subsequent inflations is infrequent (in about 30% of patients) and occurs only after multiple inflations.[19,44] It is still controversial whether ST-segment changes are a reliable indicator of a protected state[48-50]; several studies in patients undergoing coronary angioplasty have shown that the ST-segment shift correlates with metabolic (i.e., lactate production), mechanical (i.e., regional wall motion abnormalities), and clinical (i.e., anginal pain) parameters of myocardial ischemia.[19,44]

The most convincing evidence that the adaptation to ischemia during repeated balloon inflations is mediated by ischemic preconditioning comes from the observation that in this setting the adaptation to ischemia can be prevented or mimicked by agents that specifically prevent or mimic preconditioning in experimental models. Adaptation to ischemia during repeated coronary occlusions is prevented by glibenclamide,[28] adenosine antagonists,[40,41] phentolamine,[43] and naloxone,[51] whereas it is mimicked by adenosine,[42] morphine sulfate,[52] and bradykinin.[53] Finally, in the setting of coronary angioplasty, Leesar and colleagues[54] reported a delayed preconditioning-mimetic effect of nitroglycerin.

Cardiac Surgery

Intermittent ischemia achieved by aortic cross-clamping in a fibrillating heart during coronary artery bypass graft surgery has been used as a clinical model of ischemic preconditioning. In this model, the confounding effects resulting from collateral flow are overcome by using global rather than regional ischemia. Yellon and associates[55] examined the effect of two ischemic episodes of 3 minutes, each followed by 2-minute reperfusion, on high-energy phosphate metabolism during 10-minute cross-clamping, while the first distal coronary anastomosis was performed. Myocardial biopsy specimens taken after the 10-minute ischemic insult exhibited a significantly higher ATP content than that found in controls not previously exposed to brief ischemic episodes, proving that the human myocardium shows the typical biochemical features of preconditioning observed by Murry and colleagues[1] in their classic canine model of ischemic preconditioning. Perrault and coworkers[56] reported, however, that 3-minute aortic cross-clamping followed by 2-minute reperfusion before warm-blood cardioplegic arrest during coronary artery bypass graft surgery fails to provide any beneficial effect. Nevertheless, evidence that preconditioning may offer patients protection against irreversible myocyte injury comes from another study by Jenkins and coworkers,[57] who showed a reduction of troponin T release in patients exposed to two periods of myocardial ischemia of 3 minutes each at the beginning of the revascularization operation. It has been shown that, in the setting of coronary artery bypass graft surgery, adenosine[58] and acadesine[59] are effective in improving postoperative left ventricular function. Studies have shown that volatile anesthetics, including enflurane and isoflurane, are able to optimize myocardial protection during cardiac surgery, probably through activation of K_{ATP} channels.[60-63]

ATP-SENSITIVE POTASSIUM CHANNEL OPENERS AND ADENOSINE IN ACUTE CORONARY SYNDROMES

A tantalizing clinical application of pharmacologic preconditioning is in patients with acute coronary syndromes, in the attempt to slow down the progression of myocardial necrosis, increasing the time available for

effective reperfusion. The exploitation of preconditioning depends, however, on the possibility of administering preconditioning drugs before ischemia, making this approach difficult in patients at low risk of MI, such as patients with chronic stable angina. Conversely, it is well known that patients with unstable angina or with a recent MI have a higher risk of MI in the few months following the initial ischemic episode.[64] In this group of patients, the administration of drugs mimicking ischemic preconditioning in the time period at increased risk might slow necrosis rate in patients who eventually would develop an acute MI, increasing the time available for reperfusion therapy. The myocardium of patients with unstable angina already might be preconditioned, however, by prior ischemic episodes, limiting the potential advantages of preconditioning drugs. Another theoretical problem may be the development of tachyphylaxis to preconditioning agents. Tsuchida and colleagues[65] showed in a rabbit model that continuous infusion of a selective A_1 adenosine receptor agonist led to downregulation of the signaling mechanism and loss of protection. More encouraging data have been obtained, however, using a different dosing schedule, in which the same drug was administered to rabbits by intermittent dosing over 10 days with persistence of myocardial protection assessed 48 hours after the last dose.[66]

Few studies have evaluated the protective role of pharmacologic preconditioning strategies in patients with acute coronary syndromes (Table 26–1). In particular, the preconditioning-mimetic drugs investigated so far are adenosine and the only clinically available K_{ATP} channel opener licensed for cardiovascular use, nicorandil. Adenosine was the first endogenous ligand to be identified as a trigger of the cardioprotective action of experimental ischemic preconditioning, and the mitochondrial K_{ATP} channel is thought to be the distal target or effector of protection.

Nicorandil

The first clinical trial aimed at assessing the cardioprotective role of nicorandil in patients with unstable angina was published by Patel and associates [Clinical European Studies in Angina and Revascularization (CESAR 2) investigation].[67] This study suggested that opening of K_{ATP} channel with nicorandil, in addition to standard maximal antianginal therapy, results in a significant reduction in the incidence of myocardial ischemic episodes and tachyarrhythmias.[67] Because most patients were already receiving treatment with either oral or intravenous nitrates, it is unlikely that the beneficial effects of oral nicorandil were due to its vasodilatory properties. It is possible that the protection observed in the nicorandil group was due to pharmacologic preconditioning resulting in a significant reduction in the number of ischemic events.[67] Further large-scale randomized trials are warranted to assess the effects of nicorandil on prognosis and adverse outcome in this setting.

As pointed out previously, the exploitation of ischemic preconditioning depends on the possibility of administering preconditioning drugs before the prolonged, potentially lethal ischemic insult (e.g., patients with

■ ■ ■

TABLE 26–1   STUDIES ON NICORANDIL AND ADENOSINE IN ACUTE CORONARY SYNDROMES

CLINICAL SETTING	REPERFUSION TREATMENT	AGENT	POTENTIAL MECHANISM	RESULTS	REFERENCE
Unstable angina	—	IV nicorandil	Preconditioning	↓ Ischemic episodes and arrhythmias	Patel et al[67]
AMI	Thrombolysis or PTCA	IC nicorandil	↓ Reperfusion injury	↑ LV function	Sakata et al[69]
AMI	Thrombolysis	Oral nicorandil	↓ Reperfusion injury	↓ Arrhythmias	Sen et al[70]
AMI	PTCA	IV nicorandil	↓ Reperfusion injury	↑ LV function and in-hospital outcome	Ito et al[71]
AMI	PTCA	IV adenosine	↓ Reperfusion injury	↓ Infarct size	Garratt et al[73]
AMI	Thrombolysis	IV adenosine	↓ Reperfusion injury	↓ Infarct size (anterior infarction)	Mahaffey et al[74]
AMI	PTCA	IC adenosine	↓ Reperfusion injury	↑ LV function and in-hospital outcome	Marzilli et al[76]
AMI	PTCA	AMP579*	↓ Reperfusion injury	↓ Infarct size (anterior infarction)	Kopecky et al[77]

*AMP579 is an adenosine receptor agonist.
AMI, acute myocardial infarction; IC, intracoronary; IV, intravenous; LV, left ventricular; PTCA, percutaneous transluminal coronary angioplasty.

unstable angina). Some authors have proposed, however, that the cardioprotective effects of preconditioning also might be operative during the reperfusion phase of ischemia-reperfusion injury, resulting in a reduction in cytosolic calcium oscillations and free radical formation.[68] These observations prompted investigation into the potential cardioprotective properties of nicorandil after acute MI. Sakata and colleagues[69] investigated the effects of an intracoronary bolus of nicorandil after successful coronary thrombolysis or primary angioplasty. They found that compared with controls, nicorandil-treated patients exhibited improved restoration of myocardial blood flow to the infarcted myocardium, as assessed by contrast echocardiography and improved regional wall motion at 1 month. Similar findings were obtained by Sen and coworkers,[70] who evaluated the safety and efficacy of oral nicorandil as an adjunct to routine therapeutic management in patients with acute MI. They showed that nicorandil was safe and well tolerated in the setting of acute MI with no increase in adverse events compared with controls. They also showed a trend toward a reduction in development of Q waves in patients presenting with subendocardial infarction and a reduced incidence of arrhythmias in the nicorandil-treated group. Finally, Ito and associates[71] investigated the effects of intravenous infusion of nicorandil in patients with acute MI undergoing primary coronary angioplasty. They found that intravenous nicorandil in conjunction with coronary angioplasty is associated with better functional and in-hospital clinical outcomes compared with angioplasty alone. In the setting of acute MI, the cardioprotective effects of nicorandil probably are related to an improvement in microvascular perfusion rather than to myocardial preconditioning, as suggested by the lesser frequency of no-reflow phenomenon in nicorandil-treated patients than in controls.[69,71]

All these studies provide evidence for safety and tolerability of nicorandil in the setting of acute MI; they suggest that either intravenous or oral administration of this drug as an adjunct to standard reperfusion strategies improves microvascular perfusion of the ischemic myocardium and possibly improves left ventricular function. Further large-scale randomized studies are warranted to assess the effects of nicorandil on prognosis and adverse outcome in this setting.

Adenosine

Adenosine and acadesine, an adenosine-regulating agent, have been shown to confer cardioprotection in the settings of coronary angioplasty and cardiac surgery,[19] but no clinical trial in patients with unstable angina has been reported yet. A potential therapeutic exploitation of preconditioning with adenosine or its analogues in the setting of unstable angina remains to be investigated.

Adenosine, in addition to its role in myocardial ischemic preconditioning, has been shown to attenuate ischemia-reperfusion injury in animals, through inhibition of neutrophil activation, inhibition of oxygen free radical formation, and improvement of microvascular function, resulting in a reduction of infarct size and an improvement of left ventricular function and coronary blood flow.[72] These data prompted investigation into the potential cardioprotective properties of adenosine in patients with acute MI. Garratt and associates[73] investigated the effects of intravenous adenosine and lidocaine in patients with acute MI undergoing primary angioplasty. They found that moderate doses of adenosine may be given intravenously in this setting without unacceptable risk of complication and that compared with historical controls, adenosine-treated patients had smaller infarcts at 6-week follow-up. These findings were confirmed by a relatively larger multicenter, randomized trial (AMISTAD [Acute Myocardial Infarction Study of Adenosine]) designed to test the hypothesis that intravenous adenosine as an adjunct to thrombolysis would reduce myocardial infarct size.[74] Patients with anterior acute MI assigned to adenosine had a 67% relative reduction in final infarct size as assessed by single-photon emission computed tomography 6 days after the infarct; however, there was no reduction in the final infarct size observed in patients with nonanterior infarction or evidence of morbidity and mortality in-hospital benefit.[74] Experimental studies showed, however, that the beneficial effect of adenosine on infarct size is remarkable and consistent when this agent is given before coronary occlusion and that it is still present, although weaker, when adenosine is given before reperfusion and negligible and inconsistent when adenosine is given during reperfusion.[72,75] The lack of an obvious beneficial impact of adenosine on clinical outcome observed in the AMISTAD trial[74] may be at least partially due to delayed adenosine administration (after thrombolytic administration) in about 50% of the patients. This drawback was overcome in a small randomized trial in patients with acute MI undergoing primary angioplasty, in whom intracoronary adenosine was given right before balloon dilation.[76] In this study, intracoronary adenosine administration prevented the no-reflow phenomenon, improved ventricular function, and was associated with a more favorable clinical course.[76]

Finally, in the randomized, placebo-controlled ADMIRE (AMP579 Delivery for Myocardial Infarction Reduction) trial, the administration of a novel adenosine agonist with high affinity for A_1 and A_2 receptors, AMP579, intravenously before primary angioplasty was associated with a trend toward smaller infarct size and greater myocardial salvage in patients with anterior MI.[77] Given the small sample size and the methodologic limitations of the studies reported to date, larger and better designed clinical trials are needed to confirm the cardioprotective effects of adenosine (or its agonists) in the setting of acute coronary syndromes.

CONCLUSIONS

Several lines of evidence indicate that adaptation of the myocardium to ischemia observed during in vitro studies on human atrial trabeculae and in different clinical settings is mainly due to ischemic preconditioning and is mediated at least partially by the stimulation of adenosine receptors and by the opening of K_{ATP} channels. These findings suggest that in patients at high risk of MI (i.e., patients with unstable angina or recent MI), drugs known to elicit this endogenous form of protection might have a relevant therapeutic role. In this regard, a first clinical trial conducted in patients with unstable angina shows that nicorandil, in addition to standard maximal antianginal therapy, results in a significant reduction in the incidence of myocardial ischemic episodes and tachyarrhythmias.[67] No other clinical trials aimed at assessing the cardioprotective role of preconditioning-mimetic agents in patients with unstable angina are available to date. In addition to preconditioning-mimetic agents such as adenosine and nicorandil, another promising therapeutic approach to cardioprotection in patients with unstable angina may be the use of sodium/hydrogen exchange inhibitors (e.g., cari-

poride), proved to be cardioprotective in experimental studies[78-80] and in the clinical setting of cardiac surgery.[81]

In patients with acute myocardial infarction, pharmacologic agents given after the onset of coronary ischemia may be useful adjuncts to reperfusion treatment if they reduce reperfusion injury. In this regard, both K_{ATP} channel openers and adenosine have been shown to be cardioprotective (probably independently of their preconditioning-mimetic effects) particularly when given right before reperfusion, thus making this approach mainly feasible in the setting of primary coronary angioplasty.[71,76]

REFERENCES

1. Murry CE, Jennings RB, Reimer KA: Preconditioning with ischemia: A delay of lethal cell injury in ischemic myocardium. Circulation 1986;74:1124-1136.
2. Yellon DM, Baxter GF, Garcia-Dorado D, et al: Ischaemic preconditioning: Present positions and future directions. Cardiovasc Res 1998;37:21-33.
3. Shiki K, Hearse DJ: Preconditioning of ischemic myocardium: Reperfusion-induced arrhythmias. Am J Physiol 1987;253: H1470-1476.
4. Cohen MV, Liu GS, Downey JM: Preconditioning causes improved wall motion as well as smaller infarcts after transient coronary occlusion in rabbits. Circulation 1991;84:341-349.
5. Cohen MV, Baines CP, Downey JM: Ischemic preconditioning: From adenosine receptor to K_{ATP} channel. Annu Rev Physiol 2000;62: 79-109.
6. O'Rourke B: Myocardial K_{ATP} channels in preconditioning. Circ Res 2000;87:845-855.
7. Yellon DM, Baxter GF: A "second window of protection" or delayed preconditioning phenomenon: Future horizons for myocardial protection? J Mol Cell Cardiol 1995;27:1023-1034.
8. Bolli R: The late phase of preconditioning. Circ Res 2000;87: 972-983.
9. Vegh A, Papp JG, Parrat JR: Prevention by dexamethasone of the marked antiarrhythmic effects of preconditioning induced 20 h after rapid cardiac pacing. Br J Pharmacol 1994;113:1081-1082.
10. Sun JZ, Tang XL, Knowlton AA, et al: Late preconditioning against myocardial stunning: An endogenous protective mechanism that confers resistance to postischemic dysfunction 24 hours after brief ischemia in conscious pigs. J Clin Invest 1995;95:388-403.
11. Carr CS, Hill RJ, Masamune H, et al: Evidence for a role for both A_1 and A_3 receptors in protection of isolated human atrial muscle against simulated ischemia. Cardiovasc Res 1997;36:52-59.
12. Speechly-Dick ME, Grover GJ, Yellon DM: Does ischemic preconditioning in the human involve protein kinase C and the ATP-dependent K^+ channel? Studies of contractile function after simulated ischemia in an atrial in vitro model. Circ Res 1995;77: 1030-1035.
13. Cleveland JC, Meldrum DR, Cain BS, et al: Oral sulfonylurea hypoglycemic agents prevent ischemic preconditioning in human myocardium: Two paradoxes revisited. Circulation 1997;96:29-32.
14. Morris SD, Yellon DM: Angiotensin-converting enzyme inhibitors potentiate preconditioning through bradykinin B_2 receptor activation in human heart. J Am Coll Cardiol 1997;29:1599-1606.
15. SOLVD (Study of Left Ventricular Dysfunction): Effect of enalapril on mortality and development of heart failure in asymptomatic patients with reduced left ventricular ejection fractions. N Engl J Med 1992;327:685-691.
16. SAVE (Survival and Ventricular Enlargement): Effects of captopril on ischemic events after myocardial infarction. Circulation 1994;90:1731-1738.
17. GISSI-3 (Gruppo Italiano per lo Studio della Sopravvivenza nell'Infarto Miocardico III): Effects of lisinopril and transdermal glycerin trinitrate singly and together on 6 week mortality and ventricular function after acute myocardial infarction. Lancet 1994;343:1115-1122.

18. ISIS-4 (Fourth International Study of Infarct Survival): A randomized factorial trial assessing early oral captopril, oral mononitrate, and intravenous magnesium sulphate in 58,050 patients with suspected acute myocardial infarction. Lancet 1995;345:669-685.

19. Tomai F, Crea F, Chiariello L, et al: Ischemic preconditioning in humans. Circulation 1999;100:559-563.

20. Yellon DM, Dana A: The preconditioning phenomenon: A tool for the scientist or a clinical reality? Circ Res 2000;87:543-550.

21. Yellon DM, Baxter GF: Protecting the ischaemic and reperfused myocardium in acute myocardial infarction: Distant dream or near reality? Heart 2000;83:381-387.

22. Nakano A, Cohen MV, Downey JM: Ischemic preconditioning: From basic mechanisms to clinical applications. Pharmacol Ther 2000;86:263-275.

23. Kloner RA, Shook T, Przyklenk K, et al, for the TIMI 4 investigators: Previous angina alters in hospital outcome in TIMI 4: A clinical correlate to preconditioning? Circulation 1995;91:37-47.

24. Andreotti F, Pasceri V, Hackett DR, et al: Preinfarction angina as a predictor of more rapid coronary thrombolysis in patients with acute myocardial infarction. N Engl J Med 1996;334:7-12.

25. Ishihara M, Sato H, Tateishi H, et al: Implications of prodromal angina pectoris in anterior wall acute myocardial infarction: Acute angiographic findings and long-term prognosis. J Am Coll Cardiol 1997;30:970-975.

26. Okazaki Y, Kodama K, Sato H, et al: Attenuation of increased regional myocardial oxygen consumption during exercise as a major cause of warm-up phenomenon. J Am Coll Cardiol 1993;21:1597-1604.

27. Tomai F, Crea F, Danesi A, et al: Mechanisms of the warm-up phenomenon. Eur Heart J 1996;17:1022-1027.

28. Tomai F, Crea F, Gaspardone A, et al: Ischemic preconditioning during coronary angioplasty is prevented by glibenclamide, a selective ATP-sensitive K^+ channel blocker. Circulation 1994;90:700-705.

29. Tomai F, Danesi A, Ghini AS, et al: Blockade of ATP-sensitive K^+ channels prevents the warm-up phenomenon. Eur Heart J 1999;20:196-202.

30. Ovunc K: Effects of glibenclamide, a K_{ATP} channel blocker, on warm-up phenomenon in type II diabetic patients with chronic stable angina pectoris. Clin Cardiol 2000;23:535-539.

31. Correa SD, Schaefer S: Blockade of K_{ATP} channels with glibenclamide does not abolish preconditioning during demand ischemia. Am J Cardiol 1997;79:75-78.

32. Bogaty P, Kingma JG, Robitaille M, et al: Attenuation of myocardial ischemia with repeated exercise in subjects with chronic stable angina: Relation to myocardial contractility, intensity of exercise and the adenosine triphosphate-sensitive potassium channel. J Am Coll Cardiol 1998;32:1665-1671.

33. Bogaty P, Kingma JG, Guimon J, et al: Myocardial perfusion imaging findings and the role of adenosine in the warm-up angina phenomenon. J Am Coll Cardiol 2001;37:463-469.

34. Tomai F, Crea F, Danesi A, et al: Effects of A_1 adenosine receptor blockade on the warm-up phenomenon. Cardiologia 1997;42:385-392.

35. Rentrop KP, Cohen M, Blanke H, et al: Changes in collateral filling immediately following controlled coronary artery occlusion by an angioplasty balloon in man. J Am Coll Cardiol 1985;5:587-592.

36. Cohen M, Rentrop KP: Limitation of myocardial ischemia by collateral circulation during sudden controlled coronary artery occlusion in human subjects: A prospective study. Circulation 1996;74:469-476.

37. Tomai F, Crea F, Gaspardone A, et al: Determinants of myocardial ischemia during percutaneous transluminal coronary angioplasty in patients with significant narrowing of a single coronary artery and stable or unstable angina pectoris. Am J Cardiol 1994;74:1089-1094.

38. El-Tamini H, Davies GT, Sritara P, et al: Inappropriate constriction of small coronary vessels as a possible cause of a positive exercise test early after successful coronary angioplasty. Circulation 1991;84:2307-2312.

39. Deutsch E, Berger M, Kussmaul WG, et al: Adaptation to ischemia during percutaneous transluminal coronary angioplasty: Clinical, hemodynamic, and metabolic features. Circulation 1990;82:2044-2051.

40. Claeys MJ, Vrints CJ, Bosmans JM, et al: Aminophylline inhibits adaptation to ischemia during angioplasty: Role of adenosine in ischemic preconditioning. Eur Heart J 1996;17:539-544.

41. Tomai F, Crea F, Gaspardone A, et al: Effects of A_1 adenosine receptor blockade by bamiphylline on ischemic preconditioning during coronary angioplasty. Eur Heart J 1996;17:846-853.

42. Leesar MA, Stoddard M, Ahmed M, et al: Preconditioning of human myocardium with adenosine during coronary angioplasty. Circulation 1997;95:2500-2507.

43. Tomai F, Crea F, Gaspardone A, et al: Phentolamine prevents adaptation to ischemia during coronary angioplasty: Role of α-adrenergic receptors in ischemic preconditioning. Circulation 1997;96:2171-2177.

44. Tomai F: Ischemic preconditioning during coronary angioplasty. In Marber MS, Yellon DM (eds): Ischemia: Preconditioning and Adaptation. Oxford, UCL Molecular Pathology Series, BIOS Scientific Publishers, 1996, pp 163-185.

45. Kyriakidis MK, Petropoulakis PN, Tentolouris CA, et al: Relation between changes in blood flow of the contralateral coronary artery and the angiographic extent and function of recruitable collateral vessels arising from this artery during balloon coronary occlusion. J Am Coll Cardiol 1994;23:869-878.

46. Billinger M, Fleisch M, Eberli FR, et al: Is the development of myocardial tolerance to repeated ischemia in humans due to preconditioning or to collateral recruitment? J Am Coll Cardiol 1999;33:1027-1035.

47. Tomai F, Crea F, Gioffrè PA: Preconditioning, collateral recruitment and adenosine [letter]. J Am Coll Cardiol 2000;35:259-260.

48. Shattock MJ, Lawson CS, Hearse DJ, et al: Electrophysiological characteristics of repetitive ischemic preconditioning in the pig heart. J Mol Cell Cardiol 1996;28:1339-1347.

49. Cohen MV, Yang X, Downey JM: Attenuation of S-T segment elevation during repetitive coronary occlusions truly reflects the protection of ischemic preconditioning and is not an epiphenomenon. Basic Res Cardiol 1997;92:426-434.

50. Birincioglu M, Yang XM, Critz SD, et al: S-T segment voltage during sequential coronary occlusion is an unreliable marker of preconditioning. Am J Physiol 1999;277:H2435-H2441.

51. Tomai F, Crea F, Gaspardone A, et al: Effects of naloxone on myocardial ischemic preconditioning in humans. J Am Coll Cardiol 1999;33:1863-1869.

52. Xenopoulos NP, Leesar M, Bolli R: Morphine mimics ischemic preconditioning in human myocardium during PTCA. J Am Coll Cardiol 1998;31(Suppl A):65A.

53. Leesar MA, Stoddard MF, Manchikalapudi S, et al: Bradykinin-induced preconditioning in patients undergoing coronary angioplasty. J Am Coll Cardiol 1999;34:639-650.

54. Leesar MA, Stoddard MF, Dawn B, et al: Delayed preconditioning-mimetic action of nitroglycerin in patients undergoing coronary angioplasty. Circulation 2001;103:2935-2941.

55. Yellon DM, Alkhulaifi AM, Pugsley WB: Preconditioning the human myocardium. Lancet 1993;342:276-277.

56. Perrault LP, Menasché P, Bel A, et al: Ischemic preconditioning in cardiac surgery: A word of caution. J Thorac Cardiovasc Surg 1996;112:1378-1386.

57. Jenkins DP, Pugsley WB, Alkhulaifi AM, et al: Ischemic preconditioning reduces troponin T release in patients undergoing coronary artery bypass surgery. Heart 1997;77:314-318.

58. Mentzer RM, Rahko PS, Molina-Viamonte V, et al: Safety, tolerance, and efficacy of adenosine as an additive to blood cardioplegia in humans during coronary artery bypass surgery. Am J Cardiol 1997;79:38-43.

59. Menasché P, Jamieson WRE, Flameng W, et al: Acadesine: A new drug that may improve myocardial protection in coronary artery bypass grafting (CABG). J Thorac Cardiovasc Surg 1995;110:1096-1106.

60. Tomai F, De Paulis R, Penta de Peppo A, et al: Beneficial impact of isoflurane during coronary artery bypass surgery on troponin I release. G Ital Cardiol 1999;29:1007-1014.

61. Penta de Peppo A, Polisca P, Tomai F, et al: Recovery of LV contractility in man is enhanced by preischemic administration of enflurane. Ann Thorac Surg 1999;68:112-118.

62. Belhomme D, Peynet J, Louzy M, et al: Evidence for preconditioning by isoflurane in coronary artery bypass graft surgery. Circulation 1999;100(Suppl II):II340-II344.

63. Haroun-Bizri S, Khoury SS, Chehab IR, et al: Does isoflurane optimize myocardial protection during cardiopulmonary bypass? J Cardiothorac Vasc Anesth 2001;15:418-421.

64. Mulcahy R, Al Awadhi AH, de Buitleor M, et al: Natural history and prognosis of unstable angina. Am Heart J 1985;109:753–758.

65. Tsuchida A, Thompson R, Olsson RA, et al: The anti-infarct effect of an adenosine A₁-selective agonist is diminished after prolonged infusion as is the cardioprotective effect of ischaemic preconditioning in rabbit heart. J Mol Cell Cardiol 1994;26:303–311.

66. Dana A, Baxter GF, Walker JM, et al: Prolonging the delayed phase of myocardial protection: Repetitive adenosine A₁ receptor activation maintains rabbit myocardium in a preconditioned state. J Am Coll Cardiol 1998;31:1142–1149.

67. Patel DJ, Purcell HJ, Fox KM: Cardioprotection by opening of the K$_{ATP}$ channel in unstable angina: Is this a clinical manifestation of myocardial preconditioning? Results of a randomized study with nicorandil. Eur Heart J 1999;20:51–57.

68. Opie LH: Preconditioning: We do not need more experiments, because our current knowledge already permits us to develop pharmacological agents. Basic Res Cardiol 1997;92(Suppl 2): 46–47.

69. Sakata Y, Kodama K, Komamura K, et al: Salutary effect of adjunctive intracoronary nicorandil administration on restoration of myocardial blood flow and functional improvement in patients with acute myocardial infarction. Am Heart J 1997;133:616–621.

70. Sen S, Neuss H, Berg G, et al: Beneficial effects of nicorandil in acute myocardial infarction: A placebo-controlled, double blind pilot safety study. Br J Cardiol 1998;5:208–220.

71. Ito H, Taniyama Y, Iwakura K, et al: Intravenous nicorandil can preserve microvascular integrity and myocardial viability in patients with reperfused anterior wall myocardial infarction. J Am Coll Cardiol 1999;33:654–660.

72. Sommerschild HT, Kirkebøen KA: Adenosine and cardioprotection during ischaemia and reperfusion—an overview. Acta Anaesthesiol Scand 2000;44:1038–1055.

73. Garratt KN, Holmes DR, Molina-Viamonte V, et al: Intravenous adenosine and lidocaine in patients with acute myocardial infarction. Am Heart J 1998;136:196–204.

74. Mahaffey KH, Puma JA, Barbagelata NA, et al: Adenosine as an adjunct to thrombolytic therapy for acute myocardial infarction: Results of a multicenter, randomized, placebo-controlled trial: The Acute Myocardial Infarction Study of Adenosine (AMISTAD) trial. J Am Coll Cardiol 1999;34:1711–1720.

75. Miura T, Tsuchida A: Adenosine and preconditioning revisited. Clin Exp Pharmacol Physiol 1999;26:92–99.

76. Marzilli M, Orsini E, Marraccini P, et al: Beneficial effects of intracoronary adenosine as an adjunct to primary angioplasty in acute myocardial infarction. Circulation 2000;101:2154–2159.

77. Kopecky S, Midei MG, Kellett MA, et al: Report of AMP579 Delivery for Myocardial Infarction Reduction (ADMIRE) [abstract]. Circulation 1999;100(Suppl):I-651.

78. Bugge E, Munch-Ellingsen J, Ytrehus K: Reduced infarct size in the rabbit heart in vivo by ethylisopropyl-amiloride: A role for Na⁺/H⁺ exchange. Basic Res Cardiol 1996;91:203–209.

79. Gumina RJ, Mizumura T, Beier N, et al: A new sodium/hydrogen exchange inhibitor, EMD 85131, limits infarct size in dogs when administrated before or after coronary artery occlusion. J Pharmacol Exp Ther 1998;286:175–183.

80. Linz W, Albus U, Crause P, et al: Dose-dependent reduction of myocardial infarct mass in rabbits by the NHE-1 inhibitor cariporide (HOE 642). Clin Exp Hypertens 1998;20:733–749.

81. Théroux P, Chaitman BR, Danchin N, et al: Inhibition of the sodium-hydrogen exchanger with cariporide to prevent myocardial infarction in high-risk ischemic situations: Main results of the GUARDIAN trial. Circulation 2000;102:3032–3038.

chapter 27

Metabolic Interventions

Gary D. Lopaschuk

The therapeutic management of ischemic heart disease and its complications has undergone dramatic changes since the 1980s. Introduction of thrombolytic therapy, antiplatelet therapy, anticoagulation, angiotensin-converting enzyme inhibition, β blockade, and other therapies has resulted in greatly reduced mortality and morbidity in patients who have had a myocardial infarction (see the other chapters in this section for detailed discussion). Despite these advances, cardiovascular disease continues to be a major clinical problem, and it is imperative to explore new avenues to treat ischemic heart disease. One promising new approach to treating ischemic heart disease is by *metabolic modulation*. Pharmacologic agents that target metabolism act either by increasing energy production or by increasing the efficiency of energy production and use in the heart.[1-5] The interruption of oxygen supply that occurs during myocardial ischemia results in a dramatic decrease in energy production by heart muscle. Although traditional approaches to treating ischemic heart disease involve interventions aimed at either increasing oxygen supply to the heart muscle or decreasing the oxygen demand, metabolic modulation is aimed at improving the efficiency of oxygen use by the tissue. In particular, switching energy metabolism from fatty acid to glucose oxidation is one approach to improving cardiac efficiency. This chapter discusses some of the emerging metabolic agents that can be used to treat myocardial ischemia.

Another potential application of metabolic modulation is in the treatment of heart failure. Heart failure, characterized by progressive deterioration of heart pump function, is a highly lethal disease with an annual mortality of 5% to 10% in patients with mild symptoms and 30% to 40% in patients with severe symptoms.[6] The morbidity associated with heart failure is also substantial, resulting in a huge socioeconomic impact on society. The need to prevent and, when necessary, effectively treat heart failure is crucial. Presently, angiotensin-converting enzyme inhibitors, β-adrenergic receptor antagonists, and diuretics, with or without aldosterone antagonists and digoxin, are mainstays of long-term pharmacologic treatment of heart failure.[4] Inotropic therapy to increase contractility in heart failure is not used routinely because currently used inotropic agents simultaneously increase myocardial oxygen demand, a clinically undesirable effect.[7] One potential approach to this problem is to optimize energy metabolism in the failing heart in the absence or presence of inotropic therapy. Metabolic modulation as an approach to treating heart failure also is discussed in this chapter.

ENERGY METABOLISM IN THE AEROBIC HEART

The heart has a high energy demand because of the constant and large amount of ATP necessary to maintain muscle contraction. The heart is an omnivore and can produce this energy by metabolizing a variety of carbon substrates, including carbohydrates, lipids, and ketone bodies.[1-5] Of these substrates, fatty acids and glucose normally provide most of the substrate for ATP production (Fig. 27-1). The predominance of either source varies according to the physiologic state of myocardial workload and relative oxygen supply.

Energy production from the metabolism of glucose by the heart can be separated into two main components, glycolysis and glucose oxidation (see Fig. 27-1). Most of the glucose is derived from the blood, although glucose can be mobilized rapidly from endogenous glycogen stores if necessary. Glycolysis is the initial sequence of reactions involved in the breakdown of glucose to pyruvate and contributes small yields of ATP (normally <10% of total ATP produced by the aerobic heart).[1] Although ATP yield from glycolysis is small, this supply of ATP is thought to be essential to maintain ionic stability and cell integrity.[2,8]

Glucose oxidation is the second part of the glucose metabolic pathway, where the pyruvate generated from glycolysis and, to a lesser extent, from lactate is metabolized further within the mitochondria to produce most carbohydrate-derived ATP. The conversion of pyruvate in the mitochondria to acetyl coenzyme A (CoA) is catalyzed by the enzymes contained within the pyruvate dehydrogenase (PDH) complex. This complex comprises the rate-limiting step in glucose oxidation and is tightly regulated by a kinase/phosphatase (inactivation/activation) process, which is itself subject to allosteric regulation.[1] Acetyl CoA or reducing equivalents generated by fatty acid oxidation can reduce dramatically the activity of PDH via this mechanism.

Within the TCA cycle, acetyl CoA undergoes further metabolism, with the resultant production of reducing equivalents for the electron transport chain. The electron transport chain transfers electrons through a series of reduction and reoxidation reactions culminating in the pumping of protons out of the mitochondria and the synthesis of ATP by the process of oxidative phosphorylation. Molecular oxygen is the eventual final proton recipient and is essential for most ATP produced by the heart.

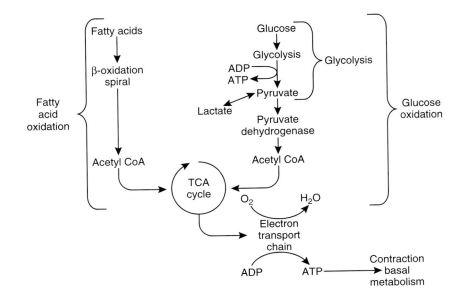

FIGURE 27–1. Catabolic pathway for glucose and fatty acids in the myocardium. Fatty acids and glucose share a common oxidative pathway after the formation of acetyl CoA, although glucose is able to continue with glycolysis without further oxidation under anaerobic conditions. Acetyl CoA, acetyl coenzyme A; ADP, adenosine diphosphate; ATP, adenosine triphosphate; TCA, tricarboxylic acid.

Fatty acids are the other major source of acetyl CoA for the TCA cycle and the oxidative production of myocardial ATP. Under normal aerobic conditions, fatty acids are the predominant substrate of the myocardium, contributing approximately 60% to 80% of ATP of the myocardial acetyl CoA when supplied at physiologic levels.[1,5] Fatty acids are not as efficient as glucose as a source of myocardial energy (with respect to oxygen consumption) and require approximately 10% more oxygen to produce the equivalent amount of ATP.

Long-chain fatty acids enter the mitochondria via a process of active transport involving a carnitine-dependent shuttle. Fatty acid oxidation is tightly controlled, with the translocation of fatty acids into the mitochondria being a key step in the regulation of fatty acid oxidation. The "gatekeeper" in this process is carnitine palmitoyl transferase (CPT) 1, which is regulated by myocardial levels of malonyl CoA, a potent endogenous inhibitor of fatty acid oxidation. During and after ischemia, malonyl CoA control of fatty acid oxidation decreases,[9] resulting in an increase in the contribution of fatty acid oxidation to overall energy production (see next section).[10-12] When fatty acids are transported into the mitochondria, fatty acyl CoA undergoes β-oxidation in the mitochondrial matrix, producing several acetyl CoAs, which then enter the TCA cycle.

ENERGY METABOLISM DURING AND AFTER ISCHEMIA

The interruption of oxygen supply that occurs during myocardial ischemia results in a dramatic decrease in energy production by heart muscle. Mitochondrial oxidative metabolism decreases during ischemia; the extent of this decrease depends on the degree of oxygen deprivation to the heart, which in turn depends on the severity of ischemia.[1,8] During a mild ischemic episode, such as

occurs during an angina attack, fatty acid oxidation and glucose oxidation decrease, with glycolysis becoming a more prominent source of ATP production.[1] Glycogen stores also are mobilized to support glycolysis. If the ischemic insult is more severe, sources of ATP production other than glycolysis effectively cease. Since coronary blood flow and the glucose it provides is now greatly reduced or halted, a marked depletion of intracellular glycogen stores occurs.

Whether ischemia is mild or severe, the acceleration of glycolysis and the decrease in glucose oxidation result in an uncoupling of glycolysis from glucose oxidation. The consequences are an increased production of lactate by the heart and the production of cytosolic protons.[2,3,5,13,14] Because uncoupling of glycolysis from glucose oxidation increases the production of protons in the ischemic heart and because coronary flow is diminished at this time, protons accumulate, resulting in an increase in intracellular acidosis. These protons exchange for other cations and can lead to increases in intracellular Na^+ and Ca^{2+}.[3,5] The need to use ATP to reestablish H^+, Na^+, and Ca^{2+} homeostasis leads to a decrease in cardiac efficiency, as ATP is used to reestablish ion homeostasis instead of supporting contractile function. Intracellular proton accumulation directly decreases the efficiency of the contractile proteins, which also contributes to a decrease in contractile efficiency.[12] This decrease in cardiac efficiency occurs at a time when the heart is starved of energy. As a result of these two actions, proton accumulation can be an important contributor to contractile failure and myocardial injury during ischemia.

If reversibly injured ischemic myocardium is reperfused (e.g., during thrombolysis after an acute myocardial infarction), contractile function recovers when energy production has been restored and cytosolic calcium levels normalize. During this period, myocardial oxygen consumption (MVO_2) and TCA cycle activity rapidly recover.[13-15] During reperfusion, fatty acid oxidation is the predominant source of ATP production and can provide greater than 90% of the heart's energy requirements.[10] These high rates of fatty acid oxidation are due to an increase in circulating fatty acid levels that occurs during and after ischemia[16-18] and subcellular alterations in the control of fatty acid oxidation[9] that result in increased mitochondrial uptake and oxidation of fatty acids.[10,11,15,19] The consequence of these high rates of fatty acids is that glucose oxidation rates are low because fatty acids are potent inhibitors of glucose oxidation. The increase in glycolysis that occurs during ischemia persists into reperfusion, resulting in a continued uncoupling of glycolysis from glucose oxidation and a continued production of protons and lactate by the heart.[13,14] Similar to what happens during ischemia, an increased need for ATP to clear these protons results in a decrease in contractile efficiency during reperfusion.[13,14] As discussed subsequently, inhibiting fatty acid oxidation and stimulating glucose oxidation is a therapeutic approach that can be used to improve cardiac efficiency significantly.

ENERGY METABOLISM IN THE FAILING HEART

Many abnormalities in energy metabolism and contractile function have been identified in failing cardiac muscle. Metabolic changes include decreases in high-energy phosphorylation potential, decreases in mitochondrial oxidative metabolism, reduced ATP content, and dysfunctional mitochondria.[20-28] Also, the proportion of fatty acid oxidation oxidized relative to glucose increases in patients with heart failure compared with normal age-matched healthy volunteers.[22,23,25,27] This low-carbohydrate oxidation in the failing heart, in the presence of high glycolytic rates, probably contributes to the development of contractile dysfunction in heart failure. This possibility is supported by studies showing that the contractile performance of the heart at a given rate of oxygen consumption is greater when the heart is oxidizing glucose and lactate rather than fatty acids.[29-31]

In addition to alterations in energy metabolism, heart failure is characterized by alterations in contractile protein function, including changes in myosin isoform profile and alterations in calcium cycling during diastole and systole.[32] Failing and hypertrophied hearts are known to have abnormalities in calcium homeostasis that likely contribute to the poor contractile function of these hearts[32]; this probably contributes to a decrease in contractile efficiency of an already energetically compromised heart.

MODULATING MYOCARDIAL METABOLISM DURING ISCHEMIA

The classic approach to treating ischemic heart disease involves interventions aimed at either increasing oxygen supply to the heart muscle or decreasing oxygen demand of the muscle. A novel approach to treating ischemia involves improving the efficiency of oxygen use by the tissue. Because myocardial energy metabolism during ischemia and during reperfusion is linked closely to cardiac function, metabolic modulation presents the clinician an arena for possible intervention. Current approaches that are used to manipulate myocardial energy metabolism involve either inhibiting fatty acid oxidation or stimulating glucose metabolism. These approaches are discussed individually.

Inhibitors of Myocardial Fatty Acid Oxidation

Since high fatty acid oxidation rates markedly decrease glucose oxidation, one approach to increasing glucose oxidation is to inhibit fatty acid oxidation. This approach has proved effective during and after ischemia, and this pharmacologic approach increasingly is being used clinically. Three pharmacologic agents that act by inhibiting fatty acid oxidation include trimetazidine, ranolazine, and etomoxir.

Trimetazidine

Trimetazidine is the first antianginal agent widely used that has a mechanism of action that can be attributed to an optimization of energy metabolism. Trimetazidine acts by inhibiting fatty acid oxidation, stimulating glucose oxidation in the heart (Fig. 27–2).[33-35] Earlier studies showed that trimetazidine inhibits mitochondrial palmitoylcarnitine oxidation, while only slightly altering pyruvate oxidation and preserving mitochondrial oxidative functions.[33] In isolated working rat hearts, it was shown that trimetazidine directly inhibits fatty acid oxidation, resulting in an increase in glucose oxidation and PDH, the rate-limiting enzyme of glucose oxidation.[34,35] Trimetazidine inhibits fatty acid oxidation by inhibiting long-chain 3-ketoacyl CoA thiolase (3-KAT), an enzyme of the fatty acid β-oxidation pathway.[35] Based on this mechanism of action, trimetazidine is now classified as a 3-KAT inhibitor. Inhibition of fatty acid oxidation by trimetazidine and the resultant stimulation of glucose oxidation improves the coupling of glycolysis to glucose oxidation, resulting in a decrease in proton production and a decrease in intracellular acidosis during ischemia.[36]

Experimental studies in vivo showed that trimetazidine decreases ST-segment elevation in regionally ischemic rabbit hearts and reduces infarct size in rabbit and dog models of cardiac ischemia.[37] This agent also has been shown to be cardioprotective in in vitro models of ischemia and reduces intracellular acidosis during low-flow simulated ischemia.[36,38-40]

Several clinical studies have confirmed the beneficial effects of trimetazidine seen in experimental studies. Trimetazidine has been shown to improve ergometric exercise duration and total work output of patients with effort angina, increasing the time to 1-mm ST-segment depression compared with placebo.[41-44] Patients with chronic stable angina reported a greater than 50%

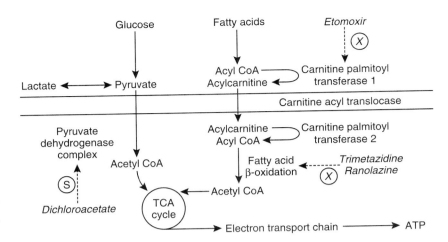

FIGURE 27–2. Potential sites for pharmacologic intervention that can protect the ischemic heart in the pathways involved in glucose and fatty acid metabolism. Acetyl CoA, acetyl coenzyme A; ATP, adenosine triphosphate; S, stimulation; TCA, tricarboxylic acid; X, inhibition.

decline in attack frequency and a reduction in nitroglycerin requirement while taking trimetazidine[45] and displayed improved effort tolerance on ergometric testing.[46] Multicenter trials of trimetazidine have been undertaken by a European collaborative working group, which have confirmed the antianginal efficacy of trimetazidine.[47] The antianginal efficacy of trimetazidine was found to be equivalent to that of propranolol[47] and nifedipine[48] but without any reduction in cardiac rate-pressure product or coronary blood flow. In combination with diltiazem, additive antianginal effects were observed.[49] In a study by Szwed and colleagues,[50] trimetazidine combined with metoprolol resulted in a significant improvement in exercise stress tests and the symptoms of angina relative to patients treated with metoprolol alone. Trimetazidine has been considered unique among antianginal agents for its lack of vasodilator activity and has been found to have beneficial effects on the acute ischemic changes associated with coronary angioplasty.[51] It has been approved for clinical use throughout Europe and in more than 80 countries worldwide.

Ranolazine

Similar to trimetazidine, ranolazine is another inhibitor of fatty acid β-oxidation that seems to achieve its anti-ischemic effect through direct inhibition of β-oxidation.[52-55] Because of this mode of action, it has been termed a *pFOX inhibitor* (partial fatty acid oxidation inhibitor). In isolated rat hearts[53] and skeletal muscle,[54] ranolazine partially inhibits fatty acid oxidation and reciprocally increases glucose oxidation at concentrations that correspond to clinically efficacious plasma levels. This increase in glucose oxidation is accompanied by an increase in PDH activity.[52] The beneficial effect on energy metabolism is accompanied by beneficial effects in experimental models of ischemia. Studies in isolated rat, rabbit, and guinea pig hearts showed that ranolazine improves contractile function during or after ischemia or at both times.[53,55,56]

Clinical trials show that ranolazine is an effective antianginal agent in patients with chronic stable angina. Similar to trimetazidine, ranolazine exerts its beneficial effects without any direct hemodynamic effects.[57] In double-blind, placebo-controlled trials, high doses of ranolazine increased treadmill exercise times in patients with chronic stable angina without decreasing rest or exercise heart rate or blood pressures,[55,59,60] whereas lower doses proved ineffective.[61] Ranolazine is not yet clinically approved for the treatment of angina, but two pivotal phase III trials have been completed with promising results. In the first trial, MARISA (Monotherapy Assessment of Ranolazine In Stable Angina), patients with reproducible angina-limited exercise durations and 1 mm or more ST-segment depression during graded exercise tests were withdrawn from all other antianginal drugs and randomized to receive a sustained-release ranolazine preparation.[62] Exercise duration, time to the onset of angina, and time to 1-mm ST-segment depression were increased significantly compared with placebo. Although ranolazine had no clinically meaningful effects on blood pressure or heart rate either at rest or during exercise, there was a small dose-dependent lengthening of the QT segment on the electrocardiogram that was not associated with any adverse events.[62] The second pivotal trial with ranolazine was reported at the 2001 Sessions of the American Heart Association. In this study, ranolazine was used in combination with standard therapy in a double-blind, randomized, placebo-controlled trial, CARISA (Combination Assessment of Ranolazine In Stable Angina).[63] Chronic stable angina patients were randomized to either placebo or ranolazine according to background therapy (atenolol, diltiazem, or amlodipine). Twelve weeks of ranolazine treatment significantly increased total exercise duration and exercise time to onset of angina compared with placebo and decreased the frequency of angina attacks. The type of background therapy did not affect the efficacy of ranolazine. Similar to trimetazidine, ranolazine is an effective antianginal drug when administered either alone or in combination with β-adrenergic antagonists or calcium antagonists.

Etomoxir

Another potential target for inhibiting fatty acid oxidation is CPT 1. Several CPT 1 inhibitors have been developed (etomoxir, oxfenicine, and methylpalmoxirate), although etomoxir is the only agent presently undergoing clinical trials.[64,65] In fatty acid–perfused isolated working hearts, etomoxir increases glucose oxidation, which is associated with an improved functional recovery of the ischemic heart during reperfusion.[66] In rodents, etomoxir induces cardiac hypertrophy, possibly by accumulating long-chain acyl residues, as this is circumvented by feeding a medium-chain fatty acid (non–CPT 1-dependent) diet.[67] Despite this effect, etomoxir seems to improve heart function and contractile protein function in pressure-overload hypertrophy.[68-70] The hypertrophy observed in rodents does not seem to be a problem in studies involving humans.[64,65]

Direct Stimulation of Glucose Oxidation

Numerous experimental studies have shown that directly stimulating glucose oxidation during and after ischemia can benefit the ischemic heart.[3,5] Dichloroacetate, the prototype of this class, acts by stimulating pyruvate dehydrogenase (PDH).[71] By improving the coupling of glycolysis to glucose oxidation,[72] dichloroacetate decreases proton production in the heart, resulting in a decrease in tissue acidosis and an improvement in cardiac efficiency.[13,14] In isolated working rat hearts reperfused after ischemia, dichloroacetate results in a marked improvement in mechanical recovery.[13,14,72,73] The anti-ischemic effects of dichloroacetate also have been shown in vivo. In dogs subjected to coronary artery occlusion, dichloroacetate reduced the degree of epicardial ST-segment elevation under basal conditions and in the presence of isoproterenol.[74] This reduction was accompanied by increased glucose extraction and decreased lactate release from the ischemic zone.

Clinical use of dichloroacetate is complicated by the fact that dichloroacetate has a short half-life and must be administered intravenously at high doses. A small study showed, however, that acute intravenous administration of dichloroacetate could stimulate myocardial lactate usage, augment stroke volume, and enhance myocardial efficiency in nine patients with coronary artery disease.[75]

Another approach to stimulating glucose oxidation is to lower the intramitochondrial acetyl CoA-to-Coa ratio, resulting in an increase in PDH activity.[1-6] In addition to its role in regulating mitochondrial fatty acid uptake, L-carnitine is a carrier molecule for the principal shuttle removing acetyl CoA from the mitochondria and increasing PDH activity and glucose oxidation.[76] L-carnitine and its analogue propionyl L-carnitine have been shown to increase glucose oxidation and benefit myocardial function.[76,77]

Although most commonly employed therapeutically in the setting of hypertrophied and failing ventricles,[78] ani-mal studies also revealed a cardioprotective effect of L-carnitine in models of experimental ischemia.[79] An increase in tissue carnitine content is associated with a lessening of ischemic injury and improved contractile function during reperfusion.[76]

Clinically, L-carnitine has been shown to be beneficial in many angina studies.[80-82] In a multicenter trial, L-carnitine was shown to reduce ventricular end-diastolic pressure and attenuate the progression of left ventricular dilation in patients after myocardial infarction (Table 27-1).[83]

Altering Energy Supply to the Heart

Since high levels of fatty acids dramatically inhibit glucose oxidation, one potential metabolic approach to treating ischemic heart disease is to decrease circulating fatty acid levels. During most clinically relevant conditions of myocardial ischemia, fatty acid levels in the blood increase dramatically.[16-18] One pharmacologic approach to lowering fatty acids involves the use of nicotinic acid, which acts by decreasing free fatty acid release from adipocytes and by inhibiting hepatic very-low-density lipoprotein secretion.[84] Effective in the setting of long-term reduction of blood lipid levels, nicotinic acid can increase glucose uptake acutely, with a twofold to threefold rise in myocardial glucose oxidation rates.[84] Data from the in situ pig ischemia-reperfusion model[85] show reduced fatty acid oxidation and a myocardial protective effect with nicotinic acid. No clinical trial data addressing this specific effect of nicotinic acid are available at present. The many side effects of this agent are a drawback to its use in myocardial ischemia–reperfusion.

β-Blockers are effective in blunting the catecholamine-mediated release of free fatty acids from adipocytes during acute ischemia; this may convey a theoretic benefit to the ischemic myocardium. β blockade has been shown to be of benefit in the long-term survival of patients with ischemic heart disease.[86] More recently, acute intravenous therapy in small-scale studies also proved beneficial. Although the beneficial effects of β blockade have been attributed primarily to its effects on decreasing oxygen demand, a component of this beneficial effect may be related to a lowering of fatty acid levels in the blood.

Glucose-Insulin-Potassium Therapy

The use of glucose-insulin-potassium (GIK) solutions to protect the ischemic myocardium dates back to the 1960s.[87] Early clinical trials in the prethrombolytic era were encouraging,[87] and newer data from the ECLA (Estudios Cardiologicos Latinoamerica) collaborative group report a dramatic reduction in acute myocardial infarction in-hospital mortality relative risk with GIK.[88] Ongoing studies continue to evaluate the effects of GIK in various models of ischemia.

Several metabolic mechanisms may be invoked to explain the beneficial effect of a GIK infusion for the

■ ■ ■

TABLE 27-1   METABOLIC MODULATORS USED TO TREAT HEART DISEASE

AGENT	METABOLIC ACTION	LIMITATIONS	CURRENT USAGE
Trimetazidine	Inhibits fatty acid oxidation by inhibiting long-chain 3-ketoacyl CoA thiolase (3-KAT) Increases glucose oxidation	Not available for clinical use in North America	Approved for clinical use as antianginal agent in >80 countries in Europe, Asia, and South America
Ranolazine	Partial fatty acid oxidation inhibitor Increases glucose oxidation	Not available for clinical use in North America	Approval for clinical use pending Potential application as an antianginal agent
Dichloroacetate	Activates pyruvate dehydrogenase Increases glucose oxidation, lactate oxidation Reduces MVO_2	Parenteral infusion at high concentration required Limited clinical data in acute ischemia-reperfusion	Experimental Limited clinical trials in progress Nonproprietary
L-carnitine	Decreases mitochondrial acetyl CoA / CoASH ratio	Not available for clinical use in North America	Congestive heart failure
Propionyl-L-carnitine	Activates pyruvate dehydrogenase Increases glucose oxidation		Cardiomyopathy Some antianginal applications
CPT 1 antagonists (etomoxir)	Specific antagonism of carnitine palmitoyl transferase 1 Inhibits oxidation of long-chain fatty acids and increases glucose oxidation	Accumulation of cytoplasmic long-chain acyl-CoA residues Long-term use causes hypertrophy in rat hearts	Not currently in clinical use Ongoing clinical studies for treatment of chronic heart failure

ischemic heart. Although the benefits of GIK usually are ascribed to an increase in glucose supply for the heart, one possible benefit of GIK may be related to a decrease in circulating fatty acid levels, since insulin inhibits the mobilization of free fatty acids from adipocytes, an early and potentially adverse systemic event in myocardial ischemic syndromes. It has yet to be determined clinically, however, what effect GIK has on circulating fatty acid levels in the clinical setting of ischemia (Table 27–2).

METABOLIC MODULATION OF THE FAILING HEART

Beneficial effects of pharmacologic agents that influence myocardial energy substrate metabolism, including pyruvate, have been shown in experimental and clinical studies of cardiac hypertrophy[89] and heart failure.[90] Although the mechanisms by which metabolic agents influence myocardial metabolism differ, all generally alter it by shifting energy metabolism away from fatty acids toward carbohydrates (see Fig. 27–2). Specifically the agents improve coupling of glycolysis and glucose oxidation by stimulating glucose oxidation via activation of the pyruvate dehydrogenase complex.

At present, there are no routine therapies aimed at increasing the mechanical efficiency of the failing myocardium through optimization of myocardial energy metabolism. Current medical therapies are directed at the relief of symptoms, as is the case with diuretics and acute administration of β-adrenergic agonists and phosphodiesterase inhibitors and at attenuation of progressive left ventricular remodeling with a goal toward improved survival, as is the case with long-term therapy

■ ■ ■

TABLE 27-2   INDIRECT APPROACHES TO MODULATING CARDIAC ENERGY METABOLISM

AGENT	METABOLIC ACTION	LIMITATIONS	CURRENT USAGE
Glucose-insulin-potassium solutions	Increases glucose uptake and oxidation Reduces circulating fatty acids	May increase glycolytic H^+ production	Reduced post-reperfusion mortality risk in multicenter pilot studies
Nicotinic acid	Antilipolytic that decreases circulating fatty acids Stimulates myocardial glucose transport May increase glucose oxidation during reperfusion	Limited experimental data showing some protective effects in acute ischemia and reperfusion Numerous side effects	Decreased mortality in hyperlipidemic patients No definitive data regarding clinical use in reperfusion
β-Blocking agents	Blunts catecholamine release Reduces circulating fatty acids Decreases myocardial oxygen consumption	Unclear if the benefits are directly attributable to metabolic effects	Established benefit in acute ischemic syndromes Improves short-term and long-term survival

with angiotensin-converting enzyme inhibitors, β-adrenergic receptor blockers, and possibly aldosterone antagonists. Of the many drugs currently used in the treatment of heart failure, only β-blockers may act, in part, by modulating myocardial energy metabolism. Drugs designed specifically to improve myocardial efficiency by optimizing myocardial energy metabolism, such that greater cardiac work can be achieved for a given amount of oxygen consumed, would be a welcome addition to the existing arsenal of therapies aimed at the treatment of chronic heart failure. Experimental and clinical evidence has suggested that this approach may be feasible. Studies have been done with trimetazidine, ranolazine, etomoxir, and dichloroacetate.

Trimetazidine

Although originally developed to treat angina, evidence is accumulating to suggest that trimetazidine may be beneficial in heart failure. Experimentally, trimetazidine has been shown to decrease mortality in Syrian cardiomyopathic hamsters, an animal model of congenital heart failure that also manifests impaired cardiac PDH activity.[91] Clinically, trimetazidine has been shown to improve cardiac function in heart failure patients (New York Heart Association class II or III) with prior myocardial infarction and multivessel coronary artery disease.[92] In patients randomized to trimetazidine for 2 months, a significant increase in left ventricular ejection fraction was observed under resting conditions compared with patients treated with placebo. A similar trimetazidine-induced increase in ejection fraction was observed during high-dose dobutamine infusion, which was accompanied by a significant improvement in regional contractile function in formerly dyskinetic segments.[92]

Ranolazine

Experimental studies have shown that ranolazine is effective in treating heart failure.[93,94] In dogs with chronic microembolism-induced heart failure, acute administration of ranolazine resulted in an increase in left ventricular ejection fraction, stroke volume, and cardiac output without an increase in myocardial oxygen consumption, heart rate, or blood pressure. Ranolazine resulted in an increase in the power of the left ventricle without an increase in energy expenditure (i.e., greater left ventricular efficiency).[94]

Clinically the effects of ranolazine in heart failure have not been assessed. In a subgroup of patients from the phase III MARISA trial, angina patients with New York Heart Association class I or II heart failure had greater improvement in total exercise duration with ranolazine than chronic stable angina patients without heart failure.[63]

Etomoxir

Although etomoxir results in hypertrophy in rodent hearts, evidence suggests that etomoxir may be beneficial in the treatment of heart failure. Chronic treatment with the CPT 1 inhibitor etomoxir in rats with left ven-tricular hypertrophy produced by aortic banding also prevented the deterioration in left ventricular function and sarcoplasmic reticulum Ca^{2+} handling compared with placebo.[68-70] Clinically a pilot study in 15 New York Heart Association class II to III heart failure patients showed that after treatment for 3 months with etomoxir there was a significant improvement in maximal cardiac output, ejection fraction, and stroke volume during exercise; however, the study was not blinded or controlled.[96]

Stimulation of Pyruvate Dehydrogenase

The clinical utility of directly stimulating pyruvate dehydrogenase as an approach to treating heart failure has not been extensively examined. Acute administration of dichloroacetate to patients with coronary artery disease undergoing catheterization showed that left ventricular stroke volume is increased, which was accompanied by an increase in myocardial efficiency.[75] In association with improved performance of failing myocardium, an experimental study in human heart samples found that pyruvate caused decreases in proton concentration and in improved homeostasis of and responsiveness to Ca^{2+}.[90] Specifically, pyruvate decreased proton concentration and increased Ca^{2+} transients, presumably related to greater accumulation and release of Ca^{2+} from the sarcoplasmic reticulum, and myofilament sensitivity to Ca^{2+}, with the latter change likely caused by the reduced proton concentration. Modification of proton and Ca^{2+} and Na^+ homeostasis is considered a crucial factor underlying the beneficial functional effects of the previously described metabolic modulators.

SUMMARY

Optimizing energy metabolism in the heart is a novel approach for management of ischemic heart disease and heart failure. In particular, promoting myocardial glucose metabolism can enhance heart function or lessen tissue injury or both. Many pharmacologic agents are now available that directly stimulate myocardial glucose oxidation or indirectly stimulate glucose oxidation secondary to an inhibition of fatty acid oxidation. This includes the use of metabolic modulators, such as trimetazidine, ranolazine, and etomoxir. These agents increase glucose metabolism in the heart secondary to a direct inhibition of fatty acid metabolism. With emerging experimental and clinical studies on other agents, it is clear that metabolic modulation may provide a new approach to treating cardiovascular disease that should complement and improve existing therapies.

REFERENCES

1. Neely JR, Morgan HE: Relationship between carbohydrate metabolism and energy balance of heart muscle. Ann Rev Physiol 1974; 36:413-459.
2. Opie LH, King LM: Glucose and glycogen utilization in myocardial ischemia—changes in metabolism and consequences for the myocyte. Mol Cell Biochem 1998;180:3-26.

3. Stanley WC, Lopaschuk GD, Hall JL, McCormack JG: Regulation of myocardial carbohydrate metabolism under normal and ischaemic conditions. Cardiovasc Res 1997;33:243–257.

4. Taegtmeyer H: Energy substrate metabolism as target for pharmacotherapy in ischaemic and reperfused heart muscle. Heart Metab 1998;1:5–9.

5. Lopaschuk GD, Belke DD, Gamble J, et al: Regulation of fatty acid oxidation in the mammalian heart in health and disease. Biochem Biophys Acta 1994;1213:263–276.

6. Gomberg-Maitland M, Baran DA, Fuster V: Treatment of congestive heart failure: Guidelines for the primary care physician and the heart failure specialist. Arch Intern Med 2001;161:342–352.

7. Felker GM, O'Conor CM: Rational use of inotropic therapy in heart failure. Curr Cardiol Rep 2001;3:108–113.

8. Opie L: The Heart: Physiology, from Cell to Circulation. Philadelphia, Lippincott-Raven, 1998.

9. Kudo N, Kung L, Witters LA, et al: Heart contains an active 5'AMP-activated protein kinase that is involved in the regulation of fatty acid oxidation. Circulation 1996;92:I-771(abstract).

10. Saddik M, Lopaschuk GD: Myocardial triglyceride turnover during reperfusion of isolated rat hearts subjected to a transient period of global ischemia. J Biol Chem 1991;267:3825–3831.

11. Liedtke AJ: Alterations in carbohydrate and lipid metabolism in the acutely ischaemic heart. Prog Cardiovasc Dis 1981;23:321–326.

12. Orchard CH, Kentish JC: Effects of changes of pH on the contractile function of cardiac muscle. Am J Physiol 1990;258:C967–C981.

13. Liu B, Clanachan AS, Schulz R, Lopaschuk GD: Cardiac efficiency is improved after ischemia by altering both the source and fate of protons. Circ Res 1996;79:940–948.

14. Liu B, El Alaoui-Talibi Z, Clanachan AS, et al: Uncoupling of contractile function from mitochondrial TCA cycle activity and MVO$_2$ during reperfusion of ischemic hearts. Am J Physiol 1996;270: H72–H80.

15. Lopaschuk GD, Spafford M, Davies NJ, Wall SR: Glucose and palmitate oxidation in isolated working rat hearts reperfused following a period of transient global ischemia. Circ Res 1989;66:546–553.

16. Oliver MF, Opie LH: Effects of glucose and fatty acids on myocardial ischemia and arrhythmias. Lancet 1994;343:155–158.

17. Mueller HS, Ayres ST: Metabolic responses of the heart in acute myocardial infarction in man. Am J Cardiol 1978;42:363–371.

18. Lopaschuk GD, Collins-Nakai R, Olley PM, et al: Plasma fatty acid levels in infants and adults following myocardial ischemia. Am Heart J 1995;128:61–67.

19. Benzi RH, Lerch R: Dissociation between contractile function and oxidative metabolism in postischemic myocardium. Circ Res 1991;71:567–576.

20. Lopaschuk GD, Rebeyka IM, Allard MF: Metabolic modulation: A means to mend a broken heart. Circulation 2002;105:140–142.

21. Barger PM, Kelly DP: Fatty acid utilization in the hypertrophied and failing heart: Molecular regulatory mechanisms. Am J Med Sci 1999;318:36–42.

22. Sabbah HN, Stanley WC: Partial fatty acid oxidation inhibitors: A potentially new class of drugs for heart failure. Eur J Heart Fail 2002;4:3–6.

23. Allard MF, Schonekess BO, Henning SL, Lopaschuk GD: Contribution of oxidative metabolism and glycolysis to ATP production in hypertrophied hearts. Am J Physiol 1994;267:H742–H750.

24. Hoppel CL, Tandler B, Parland W, et al: Hamster cardiomyopathy: A defect in oxidative phosphorylation in the cardiac interfibrillar mitochondria. J Biol Chem 1982;257:1540–1548.

25. Sabbah HN, Sharov VG, Riddle JM, et al: Mitochondrial abnormalities in myocardium of dogs with chronic heart failure. J Mol Cell Cardiol 1992;24:1333–1347.

26. Sharov VG, Sabbah HN, Cook JM, et al: Abnormal mitochondrial respiration in failed human and dog myocardium. J Mol Cell Cardiol 1998;30:1757–1762.

27. Stanley WC, Hoppel CL: Mitochondrial dysfunction in heart failure: Potential for therapeutic interventions? Cardiovasc Res 2000; 45:805–806.

28. Paolisso G, Gambardella A, Galzerano D, et al: Total body and myocardial substrate oxidation in congestive heart failure. Metabolism 1994;43:174–178.

29. Mjøs OD: Effect of free fatty acids on myocardial function and oxygen consumption in intact dogs. J Clin Invest 1971;50:1386–1389.

30. Simonsen S, Kjekshus JK: The effect of free fatty acids on myocardial oxygen consumption during atrial pacing and catecholamine infusion in man. Circulation 1978;58:484–491.

31. Korvald C, Elvenes OP, Myrmel T: Myocardial substrate metabolism influences left ventricular energetics in vivo. Am J Physiol 2000; 278:H1345–H1351.

32. Houser SR, Placentino V III, Weisser J: Abnormalities of calcium cycling in the hypertrophied and failing heart. J Mol Cell Cardiol 2000;32:1595–1607.

33. Fantini E, Demaison L, Sentex E, et al: Some biochemical aspects of the protective effect of trimetazidine on rat cardiomyocytes during hypoxia and reoxygenation. J Mol Cell Cardiol 1994;26:949–958.

34. Lopaschuk GD, Kozak R: Trimetazidine inhibits fatty acid oxidation in the heart. J Mol Cell Cardiol 1998;30:A112.

35. Kantor PF, Lucien A, Kozak R, Lopaschuk GD: The antianginal drug trimetazidine shifts cardiac energy metabolism from fatty acid oxidation to glucose oxidation by inhibiting mitochondrial long-chain 3-ketoacyl coenzyme a thiolase. Circ Res 2000;86:580–588.

36. El Banani H, Bernard M, Baertz D, et al: Changes in intracellular sodium and pH during ischemia-reperfusion are attenuated by trimetazidine: comparison between low- and zero-flow ischaemia. Cardiovasc Res 2000;47:688–696.

37. d'Alache P, Clauser P, Morel M, Guathier V: Assessment with potential mapping of the cardiac protective effect of a drug: Example of trimetazidine. J Pharmacol Methods 1991;26:43–51.

38. Libersa C, Honore E, Adamantidis M, et al: Anti-ischemic effect of trimetazidine—enzymatic and electrical response in a model of in vitro myocardial ischemia. Cardiovasc Drugs Ther 1990;4:808–809.

39. Boucher FR, Hearse DJ, Opie LH: Effects of trimetazidine on ischemic contracture in isolated perfused rat heart. J Cardiovasc Pharmacol 1994;24:45–49.

40. El Banani H, Bernard M, Cozzone P, et al: Ionic and metabolic imbalance as potential factors of ischemia reperfusion injury. Am J Cardiol 1998;82:25K–29K.

41. Mehrotra TN, Bassadone ET: Trimetazidine in the treatment of angina pectoris. Br J Clin Pract 1967;21:553–554.

42. Brodbin P, O'Conner CA: Trimetazidine in the treatment of angina pectoris. Br J Clin Pract 1967;22:395–396.

43. Sellier P: The effects of trimetazidine on ergometric parameters in exercise-induced angina: Controlled multicenter double blind versus placebo study. Arch Mal Coeur Vaiss 1986;79:1331–1336.

44. Sellier P, Audouin P, Payen B, et al: Ergometric effects of a single administration of trimetazidine. Presse Med 1986;15:1771–1774.

45. Passerson J: Effectiveness of trimetazidine in stable effort angina due to chronic coronary insufficiency: A double-blind versus placebo study. Presse Med 1986;15:1775–1778.

46. Gallet M: Clinical effectiveness of trimetazidine in stable effort angina: A double blind versus placebo controlled study. Presse Med 1986;15:1779–1782.

47. Detry JM, Sellier P, Pennaforte S, et al: Trimetazidine: A new concept in the treatment of angina: Comparison with propranolol in patients with stable angina. Br J Clin Pharmacol 1994;37:279–288.

48. Dalla-Volta S, Maraglino G, Della-Valentina P, et al: Comparison of trimetazidine with nifedipene in effort angina: A double-blind, crossover study. Cardiovasc Drugs Ther 1990;4(Suppl 4):853–859.

49. Levy S: Combination therapy of trimetazidine with diltiazem in patients with coronary artery disease. Group of South of France Investigators. Am J Cardiol 1995;76:12B–16B.

50. Szwed H, Sadowski Z, Elikowski W, et al: Combination treatment in stable effort angina using trimetazidine and metroprolol: Results of a randomized, double-blind, multicentre study (TRIMPOL II). Eur Heart J 2001;22:2267–2274.

51. Kober G, Buck T, Sievert H, Vallbracht C: Myocardial protection during percutaneous transluminal coronary angioplasty: Effects of trimetazidine. Eur Heart J 1992;13:1109–1115.

52. Clarke B, Wyatt KM, McCormack JG: Ranolazine increases active pyruvate dehydrogenase in perfused normoxic rat hearts: Evidence for an indirect mechanism. J Mol Cell Cardiol 1996;28:341–350.

53. McCormack JG, Barr RL, Wolff AA, Lopaschuk GD: Ranolazine stimulates glucose oxidation in normoxic, ischaemic, and reperfused ischaemic rat hearts. Circulation 1996;93:135–145.

54. McCormack JG, Baracos VE, Barr R, Lopaschuk GD: Effects of ranolazine on oxidative substrate preference in epitrochlearis muscle. J Appl Physiol 1996;81:905–910.

55. McCormack JG, Stanley WC, Wolff AA: Pharmacology of ranolazine: A novel metabolic modulator for the treatment of angina. Gen Pharmacol 1998;30:639–645.

56. Gralinski MR, Black SC, Kilgore KS, et al: Cardioprotective effects of ranolazine (RS-43285) in the isolated perfused rabbit heart. Cardiovasc Res 1994;28:1231–1237.

57. Schofield RS, Hill JA: The use of ranolazine in cardiovascular disease. Expert Opin Invest Drugs 2002;11:117-123.
58. Cocco G, Rousseau MF, Bouvy T, et al: Effects of a new metabolic modulator, ranolazine, on exercise tolerance in angina pectoris patients treated with beta-blocker or diltiazem. J Cardiovasc Pharmacol 1992;20:131-138.
59. Pepine CJ, Wolff AA, for the Ranolazine Study Group: A controlled trial with a novel anti-ischaemic agent, ranolazine, in chronic stable angina pectoris that is responsive to conventional antianginal agents. Am J Cardiol 1999;84:46-50.
60. Cocco G, Rousseau MF, Bouvy T, et al: Effects of a new metabolic modulator, ranolazine, on exercise tolerance in angina pectoris treated with beta blocker or diltiazem. J Cardiovasc Pharmacol 1992;20:131-138.
61. Thadani U, Ezekowitz M, Fenney L, Chiang YK: Double-blind efficacy and safety study of a novel anti-ischaemic agent, ranolazine, versus placebo in patients with chronic stable angina pectoris. Ranolazine Study Group. Circulation 1994;90:726-734.
62. Wolff AA, for the MARISA Investigators: MARISA: Monotherapy Assessment of Ranolazine In Stable Angina. J Am Coll Cardiol 2000;35(Suppl A):408A.
63. Chaitman BR, for the CARISA Investigators: Improved exercise capacity using a novel pFOX inhibitor as antianginal therapy: Results of the Combination Assessment of Ranolazine In Stable Angina (CARISA). Circulation 2001;104:2B.
64. Schmidt-Schweda S, Holubarsch C: First clinical trial with etomoxir in patients with chronic congestive heart failure. Clin Sci 2000;99:27-35.
65. Bristow M: Etomoxir: A new approach to treatment of chronic heart failure. Lancet 2000;356:1621-1622.
66. Lopaschuk GD, Wall SR, Olley PM, Davies NJ: Etomoxir, a carnitine palmitoyltransferase I inhibitor, protects hearts from fatty acid-induced ischaemia injury independent of changes in long chain acylcarnitine. Circ Res 1988;63:1036-1043.
67. Rupp H, Schulze W, Vetter R: Dietary medium chain triglycerides can prevent changes in myosine and SR due to CPT 1 inhibition by etomoxir. Am J Physiol 1995;269:R630-R640.
68. Zarain-Herzberg A, Rupp H, Elimban V, Dhalla NS: Modification of sarcoplasmic reticulum gene expression in pressure overload cardiac hypertrophy by etomoxir. FASEB J 1996;10:1303-1309.
69. Rupp H, Elimban V, Dhalla NS: Modification of subcellular organelles in pressure-overloaded heart by etomoxir, a carnitine palmitoyltransferase I inhibitor. FASEB J 1992;6:2349-2353.
70. Turcani M, Rupp H: Etomoxir improves left ventricular performance of pressure-overloaded rat heart. Circulation 1997;96:3681-3686.
71. Stacpoole PW: The pharmacology of dichloroacetate. Metabolism 1989;38:1124-1144.
72. Lopaschuk GD, Wambolt RB, Barr RL: An imbalance between glycolysis and glucose oxidation is a possible explanation for the detrimental effects of high levels of fatty acids during aerobic reperfusion of ischemic hearts. J Pharm Exp Ther 1993;264:135-144.
73. McVeigh JJ, Lopaschuk GD: Dichloroacetate stimulation of glucose oxidation improves recovery of ischemic rat hearts. Am J Physiol 1990;29:H1079-H1085.
74. Mjos OD, Miller NE, Riemersma RA, Oliver MF: Effects of dichloroacetate on myocardial substrate extraction, epicardial ST-segment elevation, and ventricular blood flow following coronary occlusion in dogs. Cardiovasc Res 1976;19:427-436.
75. Wargovich TJ, Macdonald RG, Hill JA, et al: Myocardial metabolic and hemodynamic effects of dichloroacetate in coronary artery disease. Am J Cardiol 1988;61:65-70.
76. Broderick TL, Quinney HA, Barker CC, Lopaschuk GD: The beneficial effect of carnitine on mechanical recovery of rat hearts reperfused after a transient period of global ischemia is accompanied by a stimulation of glucose oxidation. Circulation 1993;87:972-981.
77. Schonekess BO, Allard MF, Lopaschuk GD: Propionyl-L-carnitine improvement of hypertrophied heart is accompanied by an increase in carbohydrate oxidation. Circ Res 1995;77:726-734.
78. Ferrari R, Anard I: Utilization of propionyl-L-carnitine for the treatment of heart failure. In De Jong JW, Ferrari R (eds): The Carnitine System: A New Therapeutical Approach to Cardiovascular Diseases. Dordrecht, Kluwer Academic Publishers, 1995, pp 323-336.
79. Paulson DJ, Shug AL: Experimental evidence for the anti-ischemic effects of L-carnitine. In De Jong JW, Ferrari R (eds): The Carnitine System: A New Therapeutical Approach to Cardiovascular Diseases. Dordrecht, Kluwer Academic Publishers, 1995, pp 183-198.
80. Cherchi A, Lai C, Angelino F, et al: Effects of L-carnitine in exercise tolerance in chronic stable angina: A multi-center, double-blinded, randomized, placebo controlled crossover study. J Clin Pharmacol Therap Toxicol 1985;23:569-572.
81. Ferrari R, Cucchina F, Visioli O: The metabolic effects of L-carnitine in angina pectoris. Int J Cardiol 1984;5:213-216.
82. Kawikawa T, Suzuki Y, Kobayashi A, et al: Effects of L-carnitine on exercise tolerance in patients with stable angina pectoris. Jpn Heart J 1984;25:587-597.
83. Iliceto S, Scrutinio D, Bruzzi P, et al (on behalf of the CEDIM investigators): Effects of L-carnitine administration on left ventricular remodeling after acute anterior myocardial infarction: The L-carnitine ecocardiografia digitalizzata infarto miocardico (CEDIM). J Am Coll Cardiol 1995;26:380-387.
84. Datta S, Das DK, Engelman RM, et al: Enhanced myocardial protection by nicotinic acid, an antilipolytic compound: Mechanism of action. Basic Res Cardiol 1989;84:63-76.
85. Vik-Mo H, Mjos O, Neely JR, et al: Limitation of myocardial infarct size by metabolic interventions that reduce accumulation of fatty acid metabolites in ischaemic myocardium. Am Heart J 1986;111:1048.
86. Hjalmarson A: Effects of beta blockade on sudden cardiac death during acute myocardial infarction and the post infarction period. Am J Cardiol 1997;80:35J-39J.
87. Fath Ordoubadi F, Beatt KJ: Glucose-insulin-potassium therapy for the treatment of acute myocardial infarction: An overview of randomized placebo-controlled trials. Circulation 1997;96:1132-1136.
88. Diaz R, Paolasso EC, Piegas LS, et al, on behalf of the ECLA (Estudios Cardiologicos Latinoamerica) collaborative group: Metabolic modulation of acute myocardial infarction: The ECLA Glucose-Insulin-Potassium Pilot trial. Circulation 1998;98:2227-2234.
89. Schonekess BO, Allard MF, Lopaschuk GD, Propionyl L-carnitine improvement of hypertrophied heart function is associated with an improvement in cardiac efficiency. Eur J Pharmacol 1995;286:155-166.
90. Hasenfuss G, Maier LS, Hermann H-P, et al: Influence of pyruvate on contractile performance and Ca^{2+} cycling in isolated failing human myocardium. Circulation 2002;105:194-199.
91. D'hahan N, Taouil K, Dassouli A, Morel JE: Long-term therapy with trimetazidine in cardiomyopathic Syrian hamster BIO 14:6. Euro J Pharmacol 1997;328:163-174.
92. Bellardinelli R, Purcario A: Effects of trimetazidine on the contractile response of chronically dysfunctional myocardium to low-dose dobutamine in ischaemic cardiomyopathy. Eur Heart J 2001;23:2164-2170.
93. Stanley WC, Mishima T, Biesiadecki BJ, et al: Ranolazine, a partial fatty acid oxidation inhibitor, improves left ventricular performance in dogs with chronic heart failure. Eur J Heart Fail 2000;2(Suppl 2):97.
94. Stanley WC, Chandler MP, Mishima T, et al: Ranolazine, a partial fatty acid oxidation (pFOX) inhibitor, improves left ventricular efficiency in dogs with heart failure. Cardiovasc Drug Ther 2001;15(Suppl 1):107.
95. Schmidt-Schweda S, Holubarsch C: First clinical trial with etomoxir in patients with chronic heart failure NYHA II-III. J Mol Cell Cardiol 1997;29:A55.
96. Bersin RM, Wolfe C, Kwasman M, et al: Improved hemodynamic function and mechanical efficiency in congestive heart failure with sodium dichloroacetate. J Am Coll Cardiol 1994;23:1617-1624.

Antiplatelet Therapy

Richard C. Becker
Annemarie Armani

The development of pharmacologic agents designed to attenuate platelet-mediated physiologic responses is a "bench-to-bedside" metamorphosis, which bases therapeutic strategies on an understanding of adaptive and maladaptive cellular biology in atherothrombotic vascular disease. This chapter summarizes knowledge of antiplatelet therapy for acute coronary syndromes (ACS) with emphasis on pathology, pharmacology, and use in clinical practice.

PLATELET BIOLOGY

Platelets are small, anucleated cells in peripheral blood at an average concentration of 150 to 400×10^9/L. They are derived from cytoplasmic fragmentation of megakaryocytes found in relatively small numbers (0.02% to 0.05% of the nucleated cell population) within bone marrow. When required, however, mature megakaryocytes exhibit unique physical characteristics, which allow them to produce several thousand platelets per cell. Thrombopoietin and a variety of cytokines are the major regulators of megakaryocyte development, maturation, and activity.

Platelet Structure

The complex structure-function relationship of platelets is appreciated best by dividing them into four anatomically distinct zones: (1) the peripheral zone, containing an exterior coat, platelet unit membrane, and submembrane region; (2) the sol-gel zone (microtubules allowing cell contraction and microfilaments allowing pseudopodia production); (3) the organelle zone (alpha and dense granules); and (4) the membrane zone. Platelet ultrastructure can be simplified further by subdividing into three topographic components (from outside to inside) that define its functional characteristics: (1) platelet membranes (responsible for intracellular and extracellular interactions), (2) cytoskeleton (containing motor proteins that participate in contraction and shape change), and (3) granules/intracytoplasmic organelles (required for platelet secretion).

Platelet membranes are similar to other biologic membranes, containing proteins and lipids that are vital for the maintenance of vascular integrity and complete hemostatic potential. The platelet surface plays a pivotal role in adhesion and aggregation; the latter provides a stable platform for coagulation protease assembly and fibrin formation (Table 28–1). The activated platelet membrane undergoes a variety of structural changes, presenting a catalytic surface for plasma proteins and facilitating cell-cell interactions. The glycoprotein (GP) Ib receptor is cleared rapidly from the cell surface, whereas the GP IIb/IIIa receptor is expressed in greater numbers as a result of surface conformational changes (exposing additional receptors) and mobilization from internal storage pools.

The platelet cytoskeleton contains three specific types of filaments: microtubules, microfilaments, and intermediate filaments. The cytoskeleton provides structural integrity (static function) and the means to change shape on activation (dynamic function).

Platelets contain four specific types of secretory granules: α-granules, dense granules, lysosomes, and peroxisomes. The α-granules contain an impressive array of adhesive proteins, biochemicals, coagulation factors, growth factors, protease inhibitors, and immunoglobulins. Dense granules, found in relatively small numbers (two to seven per platelet), are the major storage site for serotonin, catecholamines, divalent cations (calcium and magnesium), adenosine diphosphate (ADP), and adenosine triphosphate (ATP). Lysosomes, found in small numbers (two to three per platelet), are involved with platelet–vessel wall interactions, which are facilitated by the secretion of several glycoproteins. A similar functional role has been suggested for peroxisomes.

The final structural component of platelets that deserves mention is the microparticle. In electron microscopy preparations of activated platelets, microparticles can be observed adjacent to pseudopods, providing an expanded and highly efficient procoagulant surface. P-Selectin expression on microparticles facilitates platelet-monocyte interactions and tissue factor expression.

Platelet Function

General Principles

Under normal circumstances, platelets circulate freely, undergoing limited interactions with other cells and the blood vessel wall. In contrast, on exposure to areas of vessel damage, a rapid chain of events is triggered, leading to platelet-rich clot formation. The specific "trigger" determines whether the response ultimately is considered physiologic (hemostasis) or pathologic (coronary arterial thrombosis). The platelet's programmed response includes five well-defined and integrated steps: adhesion, activation, secretion, aggregation, and support of coagulation.[1]

TABLE 28-1 CELLULAR ADHESION MOLECULES ON PLATELETS AND THEIR LIGANDS

LIGANDS

Integrin Superfamily

$\alpha_2 \beta_1$	Collagen, laminin
$\alpha_5 \beta_1$	Fibronectin
$\alpha_6 \beta_1$	Fibronectin, laminin
$\alpha_{IIb} \beta_3$	Fibrinogen, vitronectin, vWF
$\alpha_V \beta_3$	Vitronectin

Ig Gene Superfamily

PECAM 1 (?)

Selectins

p-Selectin   Sialyl Lewis X

Leucine-Rich Motif Family

GP Ib	vWF
GP IX	
GP V	

Other

GP IV
vWF (von Willebrand factor)
GP (glycoprotein)
Thrombospondin

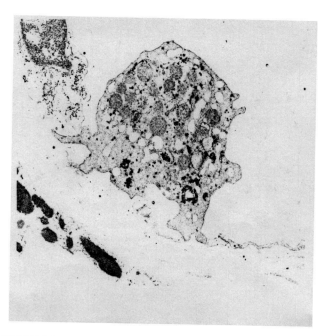

FIGURE 28–1. The initial step in physiologic hemostasis and pathologic thrombosis is platelet adhesion to a disrupted vascular surface.

Platelet Adhesion

Platelets adhere avidly to damaged, disrupted, or topographically distorted blood vessel walls. The initial event, referred to as *platelet contact,* is a process mediated by a specific surface membrane glycoprotein complex (Ib/IX/V) and von Willebrand factor—a large protein synthesized by endothelial cells.[2-4] von Willebrand factor has functional domains that facilitate its binding to platelets and exposed vessel wall constituents, serving as a "bridge" for adhesion (Fig. 28-1).

Platelet Activation

A wide variety of biochemical and mechanical stimuli initiate platelet activation—a pivotal step in protective hemostasis and pathologic thrombosis. Platelet agonists typically are classified as either weak or strong, based on their ability to (1) provoke a full range of responses and (2) cause activation despite inhibition of one or more intracellular pathways. Thrombin is considered a strong platelet agonist, whereas collagen is characterized best as a weak agonist (Table 28-2).[5,6]

Platelet Secretion

Platelet secretion quickly follows activation and is considered an energy-dependent contractile process that causes extrusion of granule contents. Fusion of α-granules with one another and with deep invaginations of plasma membrane (open canalicular system) followed by emptying of their contents has been shown.[7,8] The responsible mechanisms for dense granule and lysosome secretion are less well characterized (Tables 28-3 and 28-4).

Platelet Aggregation

The goal of platelet activation is aggregation, representing the final step toward thrombus growth and development. For platelets to link with one another requires a specific surface receptor and protein ligand. In the context of aggregation, the surface receptor and protein ligand are the GP IIb/IIIa integrin and fibrinogen.

The GP IIb/IIIa (αIIb/β3) receptor, found solely on platelets and their precursors, is a heterodimer composed of two distinct subunits. There are five calcium ion binding sites contained within the complex. Fibrinogen, a dimeric glycoprotein found in high concentrations within plasma and platelet α-granules, contains six potential binding sites that allow platelet cross-linking via GP IIb/IIIa receptor interactions (Figs. 28–2 and 28–3).

Other Platelet Functions

Platelets Support of Coagulation

The phospholipid membrane of activated platelets, platelet-derived microparticles, and particularly platelet aggregates forms the preferred template for coagulation protein assembly and thrombus development (Table 28–5; Fig. 28–4).[8]

Platelets and Inflammation

It could be stated that platelets are to thrombosis as leukocytes are to inflammation; however, it now is recognized that cellular elements and inflammatory processes are linked closely. Platelets and leukocytes adhere to one another and to regions of vessel wall damage. A variety of inflammatory modulators are produced by platelets (Table 28–6; Fig. 28–5).[9-11]

Text continues on page 372.

TABLE 28-2 AGONIST AND ANTAGONIST RECEPTORS ON PLATELETS

LIGAND	RECEPTOR(S)	RESPONSE TO STIMULATION	NO. PLATELETS
Thrombin*	PAR-1	PLC; P13K; AC(−)	2000
	PAR-3	—	?
	PAR-4	—	?
TxA_2	TxA_2R	PLC	1000
Epinephrine	α_{2A}-AR	AC(−)	300
PAF	PAF R	PLC	200–2000
Vasopressin	V_1R	PLC	100
ADP	P_{2Y1}	PLC	?
	$P2Y_{AC}$†	AC(−)	?
	$P2X_1$	Ca^{2+} influx	?
Collagen	$\alpha_2\beta_1$	?	?
	GPV1	Syk, PLC_γ	
	GPIb/IX (via v WF)	?	25,000
	$\alpha_{IIb}\beta_3$ (via v WF)	?	40,000–80,000
PGI_2‡	PGI_2R	AC(+)	?

* Thrombin is also known to bind to GP Ib. It has not been shown that this leads to intracellular signaling.
† $P2Y_{AC}$ receptors have been defined pharmacologically but not yet cloned.
‡ PGI_2 receptors stimulate adenylyl cyclase and cause an increase in cyclic adenosine monophosphate formation, antagonizing platelet activation.
α_{2A}-AR, α_2-adrenergic receptors; AC(+), stimulates adenylyl cyclase; AC(−), inhibits adenylyl cyclase; ADP, adenosine diphosphate; GP, glycoprotein; GPCR, G protein–coupled receptor; PAF, platelet-activating factor; PAR, protease-activated receptor; PGI_2, prostacyclin; P13K, phosphatidylinositol 3-kinase; PLC, phospholipase C; TXA_2, thromboxane A_2; vWF, von Willebrand factor.
Modified from Brass LF: The molecular basis for platelet activation. In Benz E, Cohen H, Furie B, et al (eds): Hematology: Basic Principles and Practice, 3rd ed. New York, Churchill Livingstone, 1999, p 1757.

TABLE 28-3 BIOCHEMICAL AGONISTS FOR PLATELET GRANULE SECRETION

AGONIST	α-GRANULES	DENSE GRANULES	LYSOSOMES
Weak*			
Thromboxane A_2	+	+	−
Serotonin	+	+	−
Vasopressin	+	+	−
ADP	+	+	−
Platelet-activating factor	+	+	−
Epinephrine	+	+	−
Strong†			
Thrombin	+	+	+
Collagen	+	+	+

*Affect arachidonate metabolism (dependent on thromboxane A_2 formation).
†Affect phosphoinositide hydrolysis and arachidonate metabolism.

TABLE 28-4 CONSTITUENTS OF PLATELET α-GRANULES, DENSE GRANULES, AND LYSOSOMES

RELATIVE AMOUNT PER PLATELET (VERSUS PLASMA)

α-Granules

Protein
Platelet factor 4	++
α-Thromboglobulin	++
Thrombospondin	++
Platelet-derived growth factor	+
von Willebrand factor	+
Fibrinogen	+
Factor V	+
Fibronectin	+
Plasminogen	+

Dense Granules

Substance
Adenosine diphosphate	++
Serotonin	+
Calcium	++

Lysomes

Glycosidases	
α-Galactosidase	++
β-Galactosidase	++
α-Glucosidase	++
β-Glucosidase	++
Heparinase	++
α-Fucosidase	++
α-Mannosidase	++
Proteinase	
Cathepsin D	++
Cathepsin E	++
Other	
Phospholipase A_2	++
Acid Phosphatase	++

+, low concentration; ++, high concentration.

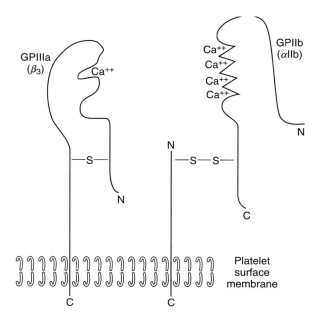

FIGURE 28–2. The αIIb/β3 receptor belongs to the integrin family of adhesion receptors and is the most abundant protein on the platelet surface (approximately 50,000 copies). It is a noncovalently linked heterodimeric with five cation (principally calcium) binding sites (four on the αIIb subunit and one on the β3 subunit) that stabilize the complex by decreasing dissociation rates for ligands (principally fibrinogen).

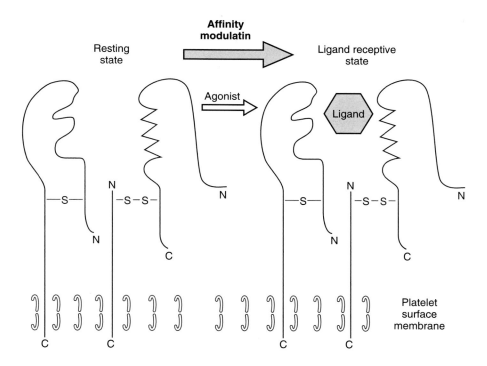

FIGURE 28–3. The process of platelet aggregation requires activation of the αIIb/β3 receptor. Affinity modulation (achieved predominantly through conformational change) converts the receptor from its resting state (low affinity for ligand binding) to its active state (high affinity for ligand binding).

TABLE 28-5   AGONIST AND ANTAGONIST RECEPTORS ON PLATELETS

PROTEIN	AMOUNT PRESENT	LOCALIZATION	MECHANISM OF RELEASE OR EXPOSURE	BIOLOGIC FUNCTION
Fibrinogen	5–25 mg/10^{11} platelets			
Surface-associated	0.3–10 mg/10^{11} platelets	Adsorbed to plasma membrane	Not released	Platelet aggregation following stimulation by ADP
Intracellular	3–7 mg/10^{11} platelets	α-Granules	Secretion	Platelet aggregation by thrombin
Factor V	0.25–0.77 mg/10^{11} platelets	α-Granules	Secretion	Receptor for factor X_a
von Willebrand factor	10–64 mg/10^{11} platelets	α-Granules	Secretion	Platelet adherence
High-molecular weight kininogen	0.06 mg/10^{11} platelets	α-Granules	Secretion	Contact-phase activation
Factor XI	1.2–6.1 U/10^{11} platelets	Plasma membrane	Unknown	Substitute for plasma factor XI in contact activation α
Factor XIII	50% of the total in blood	Cytoplasm	Not released	Source of plasma factor XIII

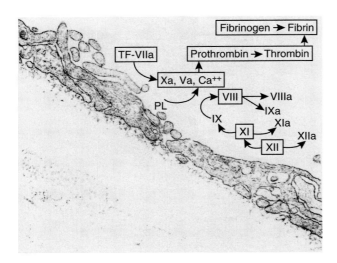

FIGURE 28–4. Platelet aggregates provide the phospholipid (PL) substrate required for coagulation processes occurring at sites of vessel wall injury. Tissue factor (TF) complexes with factor VIIa to accelerate the conversion of factor X to its active state (Xa). In the presence of factor Va, calcium (Ca^{2+}), and PL (prothrombinase complex), prothrombin is converted to thrombin, which converts fibrinogen to fibrin. The contribution of factors XIIa, XIa, IXa, and VIIIa to hemostatic processes is recognized and suggests biologic crossover between the coagulation cascades (intrinsic and extrinsic) in vivo.

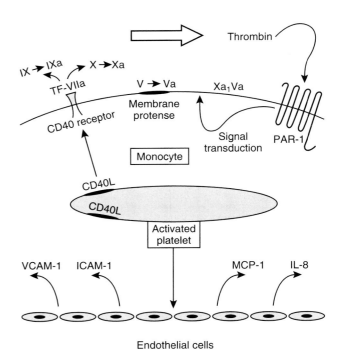

Endothelial cells

FIGURE 28–5. The link between thrombotic and inflammatory events is evident in coronary atherothrombosis. Coagulation protease assembly and activation occurring on monocytes, through CD40L causes platelet activation, which provides a stimulus for adhesion molecule expression, monocyte recruitment, and release of inflammatory mediators.

Platelet Immunology

A variety of alloantigens, expressed typically on surface integrins, have been identified on platelets. Although their role in specific immune disorders, such as idiopathic thrombocytopenic purpura, thrombotic thrombocytopenic purpura, and transfusion reactions, is recognized, it is conceivable that genetic alterations in one or more alleles also may contribute a predisposition toward arterial thrombosis and determine the degree of inhibitory response to platelet antagonist.

ARTERIAL THROMBOSIS

Hemostasis and pathologic arterial thrombosis are distinct for several reasons. First, vascular thromboresistance, a vital regulatory defense mechanism, is impaired and

poorly regulated in coronary atherosclerosis. Second, platelet-rich thrombi develop on several cell surfaces, including dysfunctional endothelial cells and monocytes. Third, the underlying substrate for thrombosis remains active for an abnormal length of time. Fourth, there is a greater tendency toward distal thromboembolism (reflecting impaired thromboregulatory mechanisms). Last, in the setting of arterial thrombosis, platelet-predominant thromboembolism and platelet-leukocyte aggregates contribute directly to microvascular dysfunction and compromised myocardial perfusion, setting the stage for ventricular arrhythmias and sudden cardiac death. This process has been referred to as the *activation-relocation phenomenon*.

CELL-BASED MODEL OF HEMOSTASIS AND THROMBOSIS

The traditional view of clot formation is based on coagulation proteases assembling on cell surfaces solely because of their requirement for phosphatidyl serine (found within cell membranes). An emerging cell-based model considers three overlapping stages: (1) *initiation*, occurring on a tissue factor–bearing cell; (2) *amplification*, characterized by activation of platelets and cofactors; and (3) *propagation*, during which thrombin is generated on platelet surfaces (Fig. 28–6).[12] The individual processes take place on specific cells that are best suited for particular events. The cell-based model of

■ ▦ ■

TABLE 28-6   PLATELET-RELATED INFLAMMATORY MODULATORS

Nitric oxide
Thrombospondin
Transforming growth factor-β
CD 154 (CD40 ligand)
Platelet factor 4
Platelet-derived growth factor
RANTES
Thromboxane A_2
Serotonin
Adenosine

RANTES, regulated on activation, normal T cell expressed and secreted.

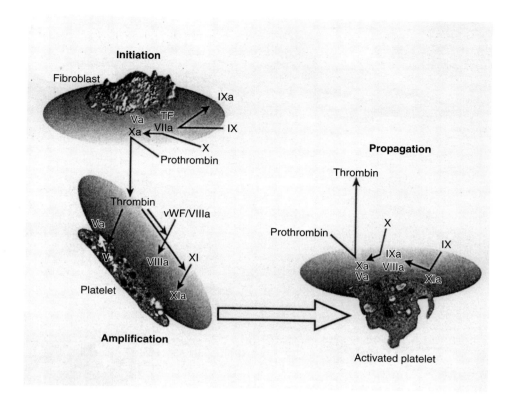

FIGURE 28–6. The cell-based model of coagulation suggests that three phases of coagulation occur on different cell surfaces: *initiation* on a tissue factor–bearing cell; *amplification* on the platelet surface as it becomes activated; and *propagation* on the activated platelet surface. (From Hoffman M, Monroe III DM: A cell-based model of hemostasis. Thromb Haemost 2001;85:958–965.)

thrombosis and hemostasis fosters a unique view of coagulopathies and thrombophilias, raising the possibility that mechanistic differences between physiologic and pathologic events would permit targeted therapies that are safer and more effective.

LINKING PLATELET BIOLOGY AND PHARMACOLOGIC THERAPY IN ACUTE CORONARY SYNDROMES

The fundamental role of platelets in arterial thrombosis provides a variety of attractive targets for pharmacologic therapy in ACS.

Pharmacologic Agents

The primary objective for platelet-directed therapy in ACS is to decrease platelet contribution to arterial thrombosis and thromboembolism by (1) preventing platelet adherence, activation, aggregation, and support of coagulation; (2) attenuating platelet-leukocyte interactions; and (3) reducing the participation of platelet-derived growth factors in the atherothrombotic process.

Aspirin

Aspirin, the prototypic salicylate, is a nonsteroidal anti-inflammatory drug (NSAID). In vivo, the drug is hydrolyzed rapidly to salicylate and acetate. Each gram of

aspirin contains approximately 760 mg of salicylate (Table 28–7).

Mechanism of Action

Aspirin irreversibly acetylates cyclooxygenase (COX), impairing prostaglandin metabolism and thromboxane A_2 (TXA_2) synthesis in platelets. Other potential mechanisms include (1) facilitation of neutrophil-mediated platelet inhibition, (2) increased endothelial cell nitric oxide synthesis, and (3) reduced low-density lipoprotein cholesterol oxidation.

Pharmacokinetics

Approximately 80% to 100% of an oral dose of aspirin is absorbed. Although hydrolysis is an important step in the production of salicylate (the compound responsible for most of the observed pharmacologic effects), unhydrolyzed aspirin is pharmacologically active, as are several acetylated proteins (particularly those found on platelet surfaces). Food does not decrease the bioavailability of either unhydrolyzed aspirin or salicylate. After rectal administration as a suppository, aspirin is slowly and variably absorbed. In general, 20% to 60% of the dose is absorbed if the suppository is retained for 2 to 4 hours, and 70% to 100% is absorbed if the suppository is retained for at least 10 hours. The overall rate-limiting step in absorption is dissolution.

TABLE 28-7   ASPIRIN PREPARATIONS*

FORMULATION	DOSAGE	TRADE NAMES
Tablets	325 mg	Empirin aspirin
	500 mg	Norwich aspirin maximum strength
	650 mg	
Chewable tablets	81 mg	Bayer Children's Chewable Aspirin
		St. Joseph adult chewable aspirin caplets
Delayed-release tablets	81 mg	Acuprin adult low-dose aspirin
		Bayer enteric aspirin adult low strength
		Ecotrin adult low strength
		Halfprin
	162 mg	Halfprin
	325 mg	Bayer enteric aspirin regular strength caplets
		Ecotrin
		Genacote
		Norwich aspirin enteric safety coated
	500 mg	Bayer aspirin arthritis pain regimen extra-strength caplets
		Ecotrin maximum strength
		Genacote maximum
		Norwich aspirin strength enteric safety coated
	650 mg	Aspirin delayed-release tablets
		Easprin
Extended-release tablets	650 mg	8-hour Bayer timed-release aspirin caplets
	800 mg	Aspirin SR tablets
		Sloprin
		ZORprin
Film-coated tablets	325 mg	Bayer aspirin caplets
		Bayer aspirin tablets
	500 mg	Bayer aspirin extra-strength caplets
		Bayer aspirin extra-strength tablets
Rectal suppositories	60 mg	Aspirin suppositories
	120 mg	
	200 mg	
	300 mg	
	325 mg	
	600 mg	
	650 mg	
Aspirin with buffer tablets	81 mg	Bayer aspirin regimen
	325 mg	Magnaprin improved
	500 mg	Bayer plus aspirin extra strength
Film-coated tablets	325 mg	Adprin B tribuffered caplets
		Ascriptin regular strength
		Ascriptin arthritis pain caplets
		Bufferin tablets
	500 mg	Ascriptin maximum extra-strength caplets
		Bufferin arthritis-strength caplets
		Bufferin extra strength
Enteric-coated tablets	81 mg	Ascriptin enteric adult low strength
		Bufferin enteric low dose
Tablets, for solution	325 mg	Alka-Seltzer effervescent pain reliever and antacid
		Alka-Seltzer flavored effervescent pain reliever and antacid
	500 mg	Alka-Seltzer extra-strength effervescent pain reliever and antacid

*This list is not exhaustive, is evolving, and varies between countries.

After oral ingestion of non–enteric-coated aspirin, salicylate is detected in serum within 5 to 30 minutes, and peak concentrations are attained within 0.25 to 2 hours. Enteric coating delays absorption (peak 4 hours), whereas buffering does not. Extended-release aspirin preparations yield peak salicylate levels at 4 to 8 hours.[13,14]

Aspirin is weakly bound to plasma proteins and distributed widely into most body tissues and fluids. The elimination half-life in plasma is 15 to 20 minutes. Unhydrolyzed aspirin is metabolized rapidly and almost completely by esterases within the liver, plasma, erythrocytes, and synovial fluid. The rate of hydrolysis may be decreased in women. Salicylate and its metabolites are excreted in urine. The most effective means for removal of salicylate are hemodialysis and plasmapheresis with exchange transfusion.

Pharmacodynamics

Aspirin inhibits COX-1 activity (found predominantly within platelets) to a greater extent than COX-2 activity (expressed in tissues after an inflammatory stimulus). Platelet aggregation in response to collagen, ADP, thrombin (in low concentrations), and TXA_2 is inhibited.[15,16] TXA_2, produced from arachidonate, diffuses across plasma membranes and is responsible for platelet "recruitment." The short half-life of TXA_2 (30 seconds) confines platelet activation to the original area of injury.

Adverse Effects

Adverse reactions to aspirin mainly involve the gastrointestinal tract and include dyspepsia, erosive gastritis, and peptic ulcers. Symptomatic gastrointestinal disturbances occur in 5% to 10% of patients and correlate strongly with aspirin dose. Sensitivity reactions, manifested principally as bronchospasm, occur in 0.3% of the general population, 20% of patients with chronic urticaria, 4% of patients with asthma (particularly with coexisting nasal polyps), and 1.5% of individuals with chronic rhinitis. Hepatic and renal toxicity are observed with high salicylate levels (>250 mg/mL). The adverse-effect profile of aspirin in general and its associated risk for major hemorrhage in particular are determined largely by the following:

- Dose
- Duration of administration
- Associated structural (peptic ulcer disease, *Helicobacter pylori* infection) and hemostatic (inherited, acquired) abnormalities
- Concomitant use of other antithrombotic agents

Aspirin is usually well tolerated when given in low doses (80 to 325 mg daily) for brief periods (6 to 8 weeks) to patients at low risk for bleeding complications. Most conditions for which aspirin is considered the standard of care persist over time (e.g., atherosclerotic vascular disease), necessitating prolonged periods of exposure. For this reason, aspirin, similar to all antithrombotic drugs that compromise hemostatic capacity, should be given only after a comprehensive evaluation of the patient's thrombotic and hemorrhagic risk has been established.

Enteric coating of aspirin has *not* been shown to reduce the likelihood of adverse effects involving the gastrointestinal tract. Patients with gastric erosions or peptic ulcer disease who require treatment with aspirin should receive concomitantly a proton-pump inhibitor to minimize the risk of hemorrhage.[17]

The impact of aspirin use on the hemodynamic properties of angiotensin-converting enzyme inhibitors is a subject of considerable clinical relevance. Because COX-1 participates in prostaglandin production, which influences vascular tone, drugs with preferential COX-1 activity would be expected to interact with angiotensin-converting enzyme inhibitors to a greater extent than COX-2 antagonists. The available evidence, derived from retrospective analyses, suggests that the antihypertensive and hemodynamic benefits are attenuated when doses of aspirin greater than 100 mg are administered daily. This effect may be particularly important in patients with poor ventricular performance and clinical heart failure. In these settings, alternative vascular/hemodynamic (e.g., angiotensin II receptor antagonists) and antithrombotic therapies (e.g., clopidogrel) should be considered.

The interaction of aspirin and angiotensin-converting enzyme inhibitors does not influence short-term outcome after acute myocardial infarction (MI),[18] but must be considered with prolonged coadministration, particularly in patients with poor left ventricular function and moderate-to-severe congestive heart failure. In this setting, the aspirin dose should be limited to 100 mg or less.

Administration in Older Patients

Dose adjustments in older patients have not been recommended.

Dose Adjustment with Renal Impairment

Patients with renal insufficiency may experience a decrease in creatinine clearance after initiation of aspirin therapy; this is particularly common in the setting of concomitant congestive heart failure (and other conditions associated with sodium and fluid retention). Although dose adjustments have not been recommended on the basis of renal function, maintenance doses of 80 to 100 mg/day may be adequate in most patients.

Clinical Trials

Aspirin's beneficial effects are determined largely by the absolute risk for vascular events. Patients at low risk (healthy individuals without predisposing risk factors for atherosclerotic vascular disease or prior events) derive minimal benefit, whereas patients at high risk (ACS) derive considerable benefit (Fig. 28–7).

Several clinical trials conducted in the 1980s[19] coupled with observations made by the Antiplatelet Trialists group[20] provide strong support for aspirin's ability to prevent vascular events, including nonfatal MI, nonfatal stroke, and vascular death in a wide range of high-risk patients with ACS (Figs. 28–8, 28–9, and 28–10).[21-25] The benefit occurs regardless of age, sex, blood pressure, and diabetes. Considering high-risk patients as a whole, antiplatelet therapy (predominantly with aspirin) reduces nonfatal MI by approximately one third and vascular death by nearly one quarter.

Prior Aspirin Use

Patients with prior aspirin use who experience ACS are at risk for MI and death over the ensuing weeks to months, suggesting a thrombotic stimuli that overcomes the relatively modest platelet-inhibiting potential of aspirin.[26] Combination pharmacotherapy should be considered strongly in these patients.

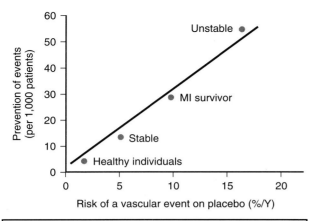

The risk-benefit ratio of aspirin administration is determined by a patient's overall likelihood of experiencing a vascular event. Patients at greatest risk derive the greatest benefits from daily treatment.

FIGURE 28–7. The benefit derived from aspirin therapy is a function of inherent risk for vascular events. (From Patrono C, Coller B, Dalen JE, et al: Chest 2001;119:39S–63S.)

Aspirin Resistance

Despite its proven benefit, aspirin does have inherent limitations. A review of the existing literature reveals a sizable proportion of serious vascular events in patients treated with aspirin (Table 28–8). Several explanations must be considered. First, aspirin is a relatively weak platelet antagonist. Second, relatively strong thrombotic stimuli can overcome aspirin's inhibitory effects. Third, some patients do not respond to aspirin (i.e., have little or no platelet inhibition). Fourth, some patients develop a tolerance to aspirin (i.e., an initial platelet inhibitory response that wanes over time). Last, the contribution of platelets to clinical events varies among patients.[27-29] Aspirin's ability to inhibit platelet aggregation is discordant, and 30% of individuals either are nonresponders or exhibit a paradoxical increase in platelet aggregation and activation.

Duke[30] reported that patients with anemia and thrombocytopenia experience a shortening of their bleeding time after transfusion, raising the possibility that platelet behavior is influenced directly by erythrocytes.[30] In vitro, erythrocytes augment platelet activation through several mechanisms, including:

- Physical interactions
- ADP-mediated activation
- Facilitated TXA_2 production

The interplay between erythrocytes and platelets has important clinical implications with regard to aspirin dosing. Low-dose aspirin (80 mg) inhibits TXA_2 production; however, the relationship between TXA_2 concentration and platelet activation is nonlinear, suggesting one or more alternative pathways of platelet activation that include thrombin, serotonin, and platelet-activating factor. Erythrocytes can activate platelets in the presence of low-dose aspirin (Fig. 28–11).[31]

TXA_2, a potent platelet agonist, must be suppressed by 90% or more for complete inhibition. Aspirin's ability to reduce COX activity varies considerably among individuals, and atherosclerosis is associated with increased tissue level expression resulting from cytokine-mediated induction. Genetic polymorphisms and resulting gene expression of COX and thromboxane synthase could limit aspirin's overall effectiveness (Fig. 28–12).[32]

Aspirin Dosing

Aspirin dosing has varied widely in clinical trials of patients with vascular disease including ACS (range, 75 to 1500 mg/day). Although indirect comparisons (Table 28–9) conducted by the Antiplatelet Trialist group[20] failed to identify outcome differences that favor higher over lower doses, the recognized variability in aspirin pharmacodynamics and cumulative event rates over time in aspirin-treated patients supports future studies that directly compare doses and administration strategies (e.g., daily treatment with monthly "pulse" therapy).[33] Research efforts also should include the development of readily available measurement tools to determine specific aspirin-mediated thresholds for platelet inhibition that can be applied specifically to individual subsets of patients (coronary artery disease, cerebrovascular disease, peripheral vascular disease) rather than extrapolating across groups.

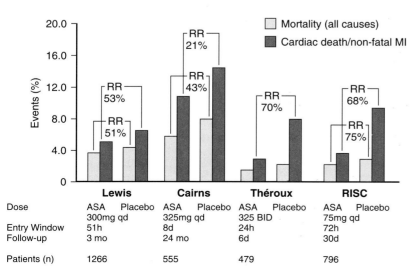

FIGURE 28–8. Impact of aspirin (ASA) therapy on mortality (all-cause) and the composite of death and nonfatal myocardial infarction (MI).

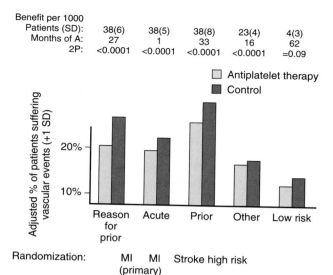

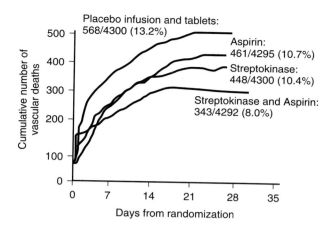

FIGURE 28–10. The benefit of aspirin therapy in acute myocardial infarction: ISIS-2 (Second International Study of Infarct Survival Collaborative Group) study. (From ISIS-2 study. Lancet 1988;2: 349-360.)

FIGURE 28–9. Absolute benefit of antiplatelet therapy (145 trials) on vascular events (myocardial infarction [MI], stroke, and vascular death) in high-risk (including acute coronary syndromes) and low-risk patients. (From Antiplatelet Trialists' Collaboration: Collaborative overview of randomized trials of antiplatelet therapy: I. Prevention of death, myocardial infarction, and stroke by prolonged antiplatelet therapy in various categories of patients. BMJ 1994;308:81-106.)

Aspirin Use According to Published Guidelines

Myocardial Infarction All patients with MI should receive non–enteric-coated aspirin to chew and swallow immediately on consideration of the diagnosis. The initial dose should be at least 162 mg. Long-term treatment with aspirin (75 to 162 mg/day) also is recommended.[34,35]

Unstable Angina All patients with unstable angina should receive non–enteric-coated aspirin to chew and swallow immediately on consideration of the diagnosis. The initial dose should be at least 162 mg. Long-term treatment with aspirin (75 to 162 mg/day) also is recommended.[34,35]

Other Nonsteroidal Anti-Inflammatory Agents

A wide variety of nonaspirin, reversible, competitive inhibitors of COX are available.

Mechanisms of Action

The anti-inflammatory, analgesic, and antipyretic effects of NSAIDs are mediated principally by inhibition of prostaglandin synthesis mediated by COX-2. The concomitant inhibition of COX-1 is responsible for decreased platelet aggregation and prolongation of the bleeding time.[36]

Pharmacokinetics

Similar to aspirin, other NSAIDs are well absorbed from the gastrointestinal tract, with peak concentrations being reached in 2 hours. Elimination is predominantly through renal mechanisms.

Pharmacodynamics

Competitive, reversible inhibition of platelet COX-1 activity (by 70% to 90%) reduces TXA_2-mediated platelet aggregation to a variable degree. The degree of platelet inhibition is modest, with the exception of indobufen and naproxen, which exert similar biochemical properties to aspirin at doses used clinically.[37]

Clinical Trials

The reversible COX inhibitors that have been studied for their potential antithrombotic potential include

■ ■ ■

TABLE 28-8   STRENGTHS AND WEAKNESSES OF ASPIRIN THERAPY

PATIENT GROUP	RELATIVE RISK REDUCTION (%)*	ABSOLUTE RISK REDUCTION (%)†	MOST PATIENTS REMAIN AT RISK
Chronic stable angina	33	45	Yes
Unstable angina	39	50	Yes
Acute myocardial infarction	29	38	**Yes**
Post–myocardial infarction	25	36	Yes

*Effect on major vascular events.
†Per 1000 patients

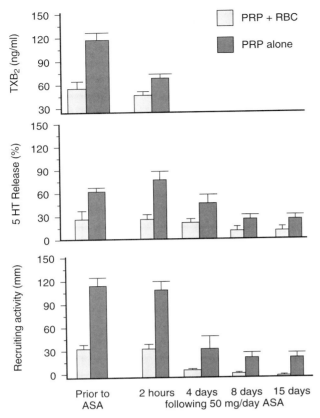

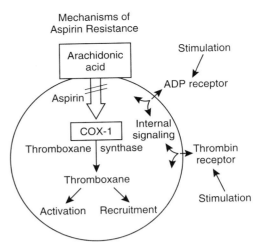

FIGURE 28–12. Aspirin reduces platelet activation (and recruitment) by limiting the synthesis of thromboxane A_2, a potent agonist. The platelet can be activated (in the presence of aspirin) by other mediators. Local concentrations of cyclooxygenase (COX-1) are elevated in atherosclerotic vascular disease (increasing thromboxane A_2-generating potential).

FIGURE 28–11. Erythrocyte enhancement of platelet reactivity in the presence of aspirin (ASA, 50 mg/d). Platelet reactivity was measured in normal donors before aspirin; 2 hours after aspirin; and 4, 8, and 15 days later. *A*, Within 4 days of aspirin treatment, thromboxane B_2 (TXB_2) was blocked in platelet and platelet-erythrocyte mixtures. *B* and *C*, Erythrocytes continue to promote platelet activation (serotonin-5 HT) release *(B)* and recruitment even after 15 days of treatment *(C)*. A "pulse" dose of aspirin (500 mg) abolished erythrocyte enhancement of platelet reactivity. PRP, platelet-rich plasma; RBC, red blood cells. (From Santos MT, Valles J, Aznar J, et al: Prothrombotic effects of erythrocytes on platelet activity: Reduction by aspirin. Circulation 1997;95:63–68.)

sulfinpyrazone, flurbiprofen, triflusal, and indobufen. Although most clinical trials had small sample sizes and yielded negative results, two studies of indobufen suggested that it may reduce saphenous vein bypass graft occlusion,[38,39] and a single placebo-controlled trial of flurbiprofen revealed lower 6-month reinfarction rates.[40]

■ ■   ■

TABLE 28-9   INDIRECT COMPARISON OF ASPIRIN DOSE AND REDUCTION IN VASCULAR EVENTS

ASPIRIN DOSE (mg/d)	CLINICAL TRIALS (n)	PATIENTS (n)	EVENT REDUCTION (%)
500–1500	30	18,471	21.4
160–325	12	23,670	28.3
75	4	5012	**29.7**

At present, none of the reversible COX inhibitors are approved for their platelet-inhibiting effects. Until further information is available, they should not be used either in place of or concomitantly with aspirin in patients with atherosclerotic vascular disease.

Coxibs

Celecoxib and rofecoxib are structurally and functionally related compounds with anti-inflammatory properties.

Mechanism of Action

Celecoxib and rofecoxib belong to a unique drug class known as *COX-1-sparing NSAIDs*. The selective inhibition of COX-2 by those drugs is based on its large binding site, providing access to a side pocket that is readily bound by both compounds.[41]

Pharmacokinetics

Coxibs are well absorbed from the gastrointestinal tract, with peak plasma concentrations attained within 3 hours of oral ingestion. Peak plasma levels are increased by 40% to 50% in patients greater than 65 years old. Metabolism takes place in the liver (cytochrome P-450), and elimination is through the urine and feces.

Pharmacodynamics

In contrast to prototypical NSAIDs, coxibs do not inhibit platelet aggregation or prolong the binding time. Prolongation of the international normalized ratio has been observed in patients concomitantly receiving warfarin, principally in older patients.[41]

Clinical Trials

Concern has emerged for the potential prothrombotic effects of selective COX-2 inhibitors because of their absence of platelet-inhibiting potential and selective inhibition of COX-2-derived endothelial prostacyclin.[42] The VIGOR (Vioxx Gastrointestinal Outcomes Research) study[43] reported a higher incidence of thrombotic cardiovascular events in patients receiving rofecoxib compared with patients randomized to naproxen. A safety analysis including more than 28,000 patients who had participated in a total of 23 studies (>14,000 patient-years of treatment)[44] failed to show that rofecoxib was associated with an excess of cardiovascular events (fatal MI, fatal stroke, sudden death, nonfatal cardiac events, nonfatal cerebrovascular events). Event rates were higher in studies comparing rofecoxib with naproxen (relative risk 1.69 [95% confidence interval, 1.07 to 2.69]), supporting a protective antiplatelet effect derived from the latter agent.

Ticlopidine

Ticlopidine (Ticlid) is a thienopyridine derivative that is structurally and functionally distinct from most platelet antagonists.

Mechanism of Action

Ticlopidine selectively inhibits ADP-mediated platelet activation, reducing intracellular calcium stores, inositol triphosphate formation (a strong stimulator of calcium mobilization), and phospholipase A_2 activation (with subsequent release of arachidonate from membrane phospholipids).

Pharmacokinetics

Ticlopidine is well absorbed after oral administration, with peak plasma concentrations occurring within 1 to 3 hours. It is metabolized rapidly and extensively in the liver to one or more metabolites that are responsible for the drug's platelet-inhibiting properties.

Pharmacodynamics

In Vitro Effects In vitro, ticlopidine is a weak inhibitor of platelet aggregation. Against low concentrations of collagen, arachidonic acid, or ADP, ticlopidine exhibits much less antiaggregative activity than aspirin.[45] In addition to its modest in vitro platelet-inhibiting properties, ticlopidine (1) attenuates endothelial cell growth and (2) increases endothelial cell–associated von Willebrand factor concentrations.[46]

Ex Vivo Effect on Platelet Function After oral administration, ticlopidine becomes a concentration-dependent inhibitor of ADP-mediated platelet aggregation.[47,48] With standard dosing, platelet inhibition is evident within 24 hours; however, peak effects are not observed for 3 to 6 days. The platelet-inhibiting effects of ticlopidine persist for 72 hours after discontinuation of the drug and progressively decline over the next 4 to 8 days. A synergistic effect on platelet inhibition has been reported with the combined administration of aspirin and ticlopidine.[49]

Although ticlopidine has lipophilic properties that can affect the fluidity of platelet membrane lipids, there is no evidence that it directly inhibits ADP binding. Ticlopidine does inhibit fibrinogen binding but does so without inducing a quantitative change in the surface GP IIb/IIIa receptor.[51,52]

Nonplatelet Effects Ticlopidine binds to erythrocyte membranes and improves cellular deformability in response to shear stress. In vitro, ticlopidine inhibits platelet-mediated neutrophil activation in a dose-dependent fashion, and in patients undergoing hemodialysis, ticlopidine reduces complement-mediated leukocyte trapping within the pulmonary circulation.[52]

Administration in Older Patients

Total plasma clearance of ticlopidine is lower and plasma concentrations are higher among older patients. In clinical trials, 45% of patients were older than age 65 years and 12% were older than age 75 years. There were no age-related differences in safety or efficacy.

Dose Adjustment with Renal Impairment

The experience to date suggests that ticlopidine can be administered safely to patients with mild renal impairment. There are no data regarding its use in moderate-to-severe renal insufficiency.

Adverse Effects

Approximately 10% to 15% of patients receiving ticlopidine at the recommended dosage of 250 mg twice daily (taken with food) experience side effects, the most common of which are gastrointestinal complaints and skin rash. Bleeding is relatively uncommon but can occur. Cholestatic jaundice and hepatitis also have been reported.

Ticlopidine's hematologic side effects, including agranulocytosis, neutropenia, erythroleukemia, thrombocytopenia, and thrombotic thrombocytopenic purpura, are the most concerning and potentially life-threatening. In an overview of 60 cases of thrombotic thrombocytopenic purpura associated with ticlopidine administration, the drug had been taken for less than 1 month by 80% of patients, and a normal platelet count was documented within 2 weeks of onset of the disorder.[53] A retrospective analysis of 43,322 patients undergoing coronary stenting at study sites participating in the EPISTENT (Evaluation of Platelet GPIIb/IIIa Inhibitor for Stenting) study revealed an incidence of 1 case per 4814 patients treated.[54] Although an infrequent occurrence, the 0.02% incidence is noteworthy (and clinically relevant) when the estimated 0.0004% incidence in the general population is considered. Close monitoring of platelet counts is recommended, particularly if therapy is continued beyond 2 weeks.

Clinical Trials

The ability of ticlopidine to inhibit platelet aggregation in a dose-dependent manner, coupled with the synergistic effects observed when it is combined with aspirin, has led to a relatively large clinical experience that spans a variety of cardiovascular settings, including ACS.

Unstable Angina   In a multicenter trial of 652 patients admitted to the hospital with a diagnosis of unstable angina, conventional therapy (β-blocker, nitrates, calcium channel antagonists) plus ticlopidine (250 mg twice a day) reduced the likelihood of vascular death or nonfatal MI by nearly 50% compared with conventional therapy alone. The composite end point of fatal MI and nonfatal MI was reduced by greater than 50% (Fig. 28-13).[55]

Myocardial Infarction   The administration of ticlopidine in the early hours after acute MI has received limited attention, perhaps because of the delayed onset (48 to 72 hours) of its antiplatelet effect. A study of patients treated with ticlopidine within 12 hours of symptom onset reported a lower peak creatine kinase concentration (suggesting reduced infarct size) compared with patients not treated.

Coronary Arterial Stenting   Since its introduction by Sigwart and colleagues in 1987,[56] coronary stent implantation has been hampered by two major complications: subacute stent thrombosis and hemorrhage (related to vascular access and antithrombotic therapy regimens). An initial report generated by the French Multicenter Registry suggested that the combination of aspirin and ticlopidine was superior to strategies that included conventional anticoagulant therapy.[57] The rates of stent thrombosis, major cardiac events, and hemorrhage were reduced with antiplatelet therapy. In a randomized study

of 257 patients, the combination of ticlopidine and aspirin reduced the incidence of cardiac death, MI, repeated angioplasty, and bypass surgery (composite end point) by 75% compared with unfractionated heparin followed by warfarin (plus aspirin).[58] Subacute stent thrombosis occurred in less than 1% of patients treated with the combination antiplatelet regimen (Fig. 28-14). Hemorrhagic complications occurred only in the anticoagulant therapy group. The results of several multicenter trials confirmed these observations. Evidence provided by the FANTASTIC (Full Anticoagulation Versus Aspirin and Ticlopidine) and MATTIS (Multicenter Aspirin and Ticlopidine Trial After Coronary Stenting) trials suggests that antiplatelet strategies are superior to anticoagulant (or combined anticoagulant plus aspirin) strategies in terms of efficacy and safety for low-risk and high-risk patients.[59,60]

Although improved techniques of stent deployment, operator experience, and the development of less thrombogenic materials and design have contributed substantially to improved outcomes, the available evidence suggests that antithrombotic therapy is required for the initial 2 to 4 weeks. Whenever possible, treatment should be initiated 2 to 3 days before the procedure. In the EPISTENT trial,[61] ticlopidine pretreatment was associated with a significant decrease in the composite end point of death, MI, or target vessel revascularization at 1 year. The benefit was most robust in patients who did not receive abciximab. Some low-risk patients may require only aspirin therapy; however, combination antiplatelet therapy represents the standard of care.[62]

Ticlopidine Use According to Published Guidelines

Unstable Angina   Patients with unstable angina who have aspirin allergy or intolerance can be treated with ticlopidine (250 mg twice a day) for several months. The more favorable experience with clopidogrel supports its preferential use.[34,35]

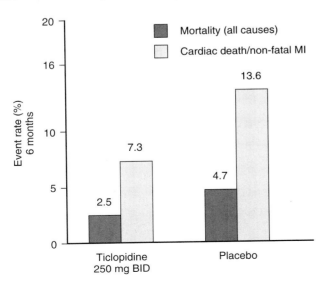

FIGURE 28-13. The benefit of platelet inhibition with ticlopidine (250 mg twice a day) compared with placebo in patients with unstable angina. MI, myocardial infarction.

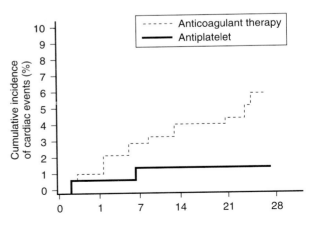

FIGURE 28-14. The combination of ticlopidine and aspirin (antiplatelet therapy) reduced cardiac event rates (predominantly through the prevention of subacute thrombosis) by 75% compared with anticoagulation therapy after coronary arterial stenting. (From Schomig A, Neumann FJ, Kastrati A, et al: N Engl J Med 1996;334:1084-1089.)

Myocardial Infarction   The lack of data in the setting of MI precludes recommendations for ticlopidine administration.[34,35]

Coronary Arterial Stents   Patients undergoing balloon angioplasty or atherectomy who cannot tolerate aspirin should receive ticlopidine, 500 mg, as a loading dose followed by 250 mg twice daily before the procedure. Ticlopidine also can be used as an adjunct to aspirin in coronary arterial stenting. Treatment should be continued for 10 to 14 days. The side effect profile of ticlopidine is clinically important.[34,35]

Clopidogrel

Clopidogrel is a novel platelet antagonist that is several times more potent than ticlopidine, a related thienopyridine.

Mechanism of Action

Clopidogrel selectively inhibits the binding of ADP to its platelet receptor (P2Y12) and the subsequent G protein–linked mobilization of intracellular calcium and activation of the GP IIb/IIIa complex.[63,64] The specific receptor has been cloned and is present in large amounts on the platelet surface.[65,66] Clopidogrel has no direct effect on COX-1, phosphodiesterase, or adenosine uptake.

Pharmacokinetics

After repeated 75-mg daily doses of clopidogrel administered orally, plasma concentrations of the parent compound, which lacks platelet-inhibiting properties, are low. Clopidogrel is metabolized extensively in the liver. Its main circulating metabolite (with platelet antagonist effects) is a carboxylic acid derivative with a plasma half-life of 7.7 ± 2.3 hours. Approximately 50% of an oral dose is excreted in the urine, and the remaining 50% is excreted in feces over the following 5 days.

Pharmacodynamics

Dose-dependent inhibition of platelet aggregation in response to ADP is observed 2 hours after a single oral dose of clopidogrel, with marked inhibition ($\geq 80\%$) being achieved after loading doses of 300 mg or more. Repeated doses of 75 mg/day achieve steady-state inhibition (40% to 60%) between day 3 and day 7. Based on ex vivo studies, clopidogrel is 100-fold more potent than ticlopidine. There are no cumulative antiplatelet effects with prolonged oral administration.[67,68]

Administration in Older Patients

There are no dose adjustments recommended for patients greater than 65 years old.

Dose Adjustment with Renal Impairment

There are no dose adjustments recommended for patients with renal impairment. There are limited data, however, regarding its use in moderate-to-severe renal insufficiency.

Adverse Effects

Bone marrow suppression and hematologic abnormalities observed with ticlopidine are encountered rarely with clopidogrel. Although thrombotic thrombocytopenic purpura has been reported,[69] it too is rare (11 cases reported in 3 million patients treated).

Clinical Trials

The well-documented benefit derived from platelet inhibition among patients with vascular disease, coupled with existing concerns regarding aspirin resistance and the attractive nature of "multitargeted" or combined antithrombotic therapy, has fostered clopidogrel's development.

Acute Coronary Syndromes   The benefit of continued therapy with aspirin and clopidogrel was confirmed in the CURE (Clopidogrel in Unstable Angina to Prevent Recurrent Events) trial.[70] A total of 12,562 patients experiencing ACS without ST-segment elevation received clopidogrel (300 mg immediately, 75 mg daily) plus aspirin (75 to 325 mg daily) or aspirin alone for 3 to 12 months. The composite end point of death, MI, or stroke occurred in 9.3% and 11.4% of patients (relative risk reduction 20%). In hospital-refractory ischemia, congestive heart failure and revascularization procedures also were less likely in clopidogrel-treated patients (Figs. 28–15 and 28–16). Although there was a greater risk of major hemorrhage with combination therapy, life-threatening bleeding and hemorrhagic stroke occurred with similar frequency.

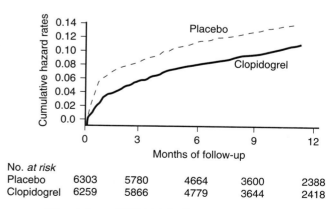

No. *at risk*				
Placebo	6303	5780	4664	3600	2388
Clopidogrel	6259	5866	4779	3644	2418

Abbreviations: CURE (trial), Clopidogrel in unstable angina to prevent recurrent events.

FIGURE 28–15.   Cumulative hazard rates for the first primary outcome of death from cardiovascular causes, nonfatal myocardial infarction, or stroke during 12-month follow-up—CURE (Clopidogrel in Unstable Angina to Prevent Recurrent Events) trial. (From Yusuf S, Zhao F, Mehta SR, et al: Effects of Clopidogrel in addition to aspirin in patients with acute coronary syndromes without ST-segment elevation. N Engl J Med 2001;358:527–533.)

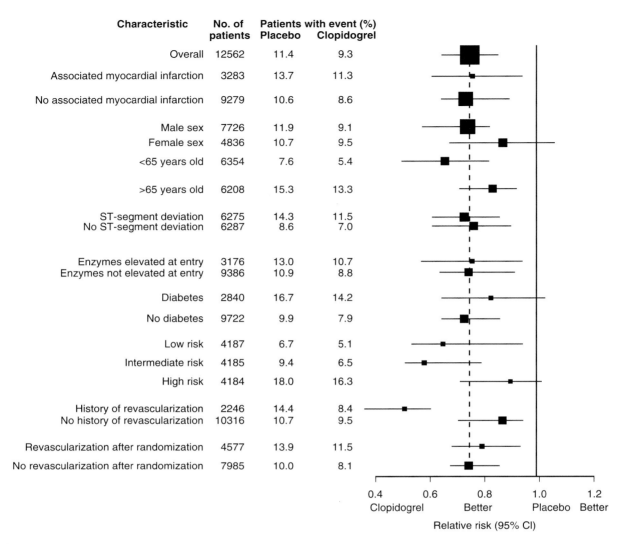

FIGURE 28–16. Rates and relative risks of the first primary outcome of death from cardiovascular causes, nonfatal myocardial infarction, or stroke in various subgroups—CURE trial. (From Yusuf S, Zhao F, Mehta SR, et al: Effects of clopidogrel in addition to aspirin in patients with acute coronary syndromes without ST-segment elevation. N Engl J Med 2001;358:527–533.)

Coronary Stenting A multicenter, randomized, controlled trial, CLASSICS (Clopidogrel Plus ASA vs Ticlopidine Plus ASA in Stent Patients Study),[71] included 1020 patients undergoing coronary stent placement who received aspirin (325 mg/day) plus ticlopidine (250 mg twice a day), aspirin plus clopidogrel (75 mg/day), or aspirin plus front-loaded clopidogrel (300 mg as an initial dose followed by 75 mg/day). Treatment was continued for 28 days after stent placement. Intravenous GP IIb/IIIa antagonists were not administered to patients enrolled in the trial. The primary safety end point was a composite of neutropenia, thrombocytopenia, bleeding, and drug discontinuation for adverse events (noncardiac). The secondary efficacy end point was a composite of MI, target vessel revascularization, and cardiovascular death.

The primary end point was experienced by 9.1% of ticlopidine-treated patients, 6.3% of clopidogrel-treated patients (75 mg), and 2.9% of front-loaded clopidogrel–treated patients. Early drug discontinuation occurred in

8.2%, 5.1%, and 2% of patients. The most commonly reported adverse effects prompting drug discontinuation were allergic reactions, gastrointestinal distress, and skin rashes. The secondary cardiovascular end points were reached by 0.9%, 1.5%, and 1.3% of patients.

In patients undergoing coronary arterial stent placement, clopidogrel (plus aspirin) compares favorably with ticlopidine in preventing thrombotic closure. It is associated with fewer noncardiac adverse events that cause discontinuation of treatment.[72]

The importance of adequate platelet inhibition before and after percutaneous coronary intervention (PCI) (with stenting) was confirmed in the PCI-CURE study.[73] A total of 2658 patients undergoing PCI were randomized to double-blind treatment with clopidogrel or placebo (aspirin alone) for a median of 6 days before the procedure followed by 4 weeks of open-label thienopyridine (after which study drug was resumed for 8 months). The primary end point (cardiovascular death,

MI, or urgent target vessel revascularization within 30 days) was reached in 4.5% of clopidogrel-treated patients and 6.4% of placebo-treated patients (30% relative reduction) (Fig. 28–17). Long-term administration of clopidogrel was associated with a lower rate of death, MI, or any revascularization (Fig. 28–18) with no increased bleeding complications.

The TARGET trial[74] investigated the safety and efficacy of two GP IIb/IIIa receptor antagonists in patients undergoing PCI (with the intent to perform stenting). All patients received aspirin and, when possible, clopidogrel (300 mg) 3 to 6 hours before the procedure. Both antiplatelet agents were continued throughout the study period. Urgent revascularization (<1.0%) and MI (creatine kinase value five times normal) were low in both groups, as was major hemorrhage.

Intracoronary radiation therapy is an available means to treat in-stent restenosis; however, late total occlusion and thrombosis are serious complications, with rates approaching 10% to 15%. Accumulating evidence suggests that prolonged treatment with clopidogrel and aspirin (≥6 months) is a more effective means to prevent last thrombosis than an abbreviated course (1 month).[75]

Clopidogrel Use According to Published Guidelines

Unstable Angina   Patients with unstable angina who have aspirin allergy or intolerance can be treated with clopidogrel (75 mg daily).[34,35] The combined administration of aspirin and clopidogrel is promising.

Myocardial Infarction   Patients with myocardial infarction who have contraindications to aspirin should receive clopidogrel (75 mg/day) indefinitely. The combined administration of aspirin and clopidogrel is promising.[34,35]

Coronary Arterial Stents   Patients undergoing balloon angioplasty or atherectomy who cannot tolerate aspirin should be pretreated with clopidogrel (300-mg oral loading dose, followed by 75 mg/day). As an adjunct to aspirin therapy in patients undergoing coronary arterial stenting, clopidogrel (300-mg oral loading dose, followed by 75 mg/day) for 14 to 30 days is recommended.[34,35]

Platelet Glycoprotein IIb (αIIb)/IIIa (β3) Receptor Antagonists

The GP IIb/IIIa receptor antagonists are a major advance in clinical practice and represent the end result of scientific insight and clinical trials involving more than 100,000 patients with ischemic heart disease.

Mechanism of Action

The αIIb/β3 receptor belongs to the integrin family of adhesion receptors that are found predominantly on the surface of platelets and megakaryocytes. This receptor is found in large numbers (80,000 copies per platelet) and consists structurally of a non–covalently linked heterodimer. GP IIb/IIIa receptor antagonists occupy the αIIb/β3 receptor, inhibiting fibrinogen-mediated platelet aggregation.[76] There are currently three intravenous platelet GP IIb/IIIa receptor antagonists approved in the United States: abciximab, tirofiban, and eptifibatide.

Abciximab (ReoPro)

Abciximab is the Fab fragment of the chimeric human-murine monoclonal antibody c7E3.

Pharmacokinetics

After an intravenous bolus, free plasma concentrations of abciximab decrease rapidly with an initial half-life of less than 10 minutes and a second-phase half-life of 30 minutes, representing rapid binding to the platelet GP IIb/IIIa receptor. Abciximab remains in the circulation for 10 or more days in the platelet-bound state.

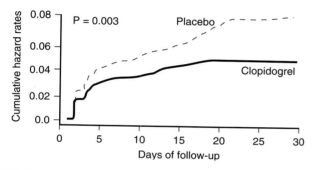

FIGURE 28–17. Kaplan-Meier cumulative hazard rates for primary outcome of cardiovascular death, nonfatal myocardial infarction, or urgent target vessel revascularization at 30 days after percutaneous coronary intervention (PCI) in the PCI-CURE Trial. (From Mehta SR, Yusuf S, Peters RJ, for the CURE investigators: Effects of pretreatment with clopidogrel and aspirin following by long-term therapy in patients undergoing percutaneous coronary intervention: The PCI-CURE study. Lancet 2001;358:527–533.)

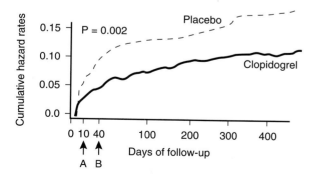

FIGURE 28–18. Kaplan-Meier cumulative hazard rates for cardiovascular death or myocardial infarction from randomization to long-term follow-up in the PCI-CURE Trial. (From Mehta SR, Yusuf S, Peters RJ, for the CURE investigators: Effects of pretreatment with clopidogrel and aspirin following by long-term therapy in patients undergoing percutaneous coronary intervention: The PCI-CURE study. Lancet 2001;358:527–533.)

Pharmacodynamics

Intravenous administration of abciximab in doses ranging from 0.15 mg/kg to 0.3 mg/kg produces a rapid dose-dependent inhibition of platelet aggregation in response to ADP. At the highest dose, 80% of platelet GP IIb/IIIa receptors are occupied within 2 hours, and platelet aggregation, even with 20 mM of ADP, is completely inhibited. Sustained inhibition is achieved with prolonged infusions (12 to 24 hours), and low-level receptor blockade is present for 10 days after cessation of the infusion; however, platelet inhibition during infusions beyond 24 hours has not been well characterized. Platelet aggregation in response to 5 mM of ADP returns to greater than or equal to 50% of baseline within 24 hours in most cases (Fig. 28–19).[77]

Administration in Older Patients

In large Phase III clinical trials,[78-80] 37% of the patients were 65 years old or older, whereas 8% were 75 years old or older. The experience to date shows no difference in safety or efficacy for patients 65 to 75 years old (compared with younger patients). The data for patients older than 75 years are inadequate to determine whether they respond differently to abciximab than patients younger than age 75.

Dose Adjustment with Renal Impairment

There are no specific recommendations for dose adjustment in patients with renal insufficiency.

Hematologic Effects

Thrombocytopenia Platelet counts should be monitored beginning 2 to 4 hours after the bolus dose of abciximab and again at 24 hours. The incidence of thrombocytopenia ($<100,000/mm^3$) in the EPIC (Evaluation of Platelet IIb/IIIa Inhibition For Prevention Of Ischemic Complications),[78] CAPTURE (c7E3 Fab Antiplatelet Therapy in Unstable Refractory Angina),[79] and EPILOG (Evaluation in PTCA to Improve Long-term Outcome with Abciximab GPII/IIIa Blockage)[80] trials was 5.2%, 5.6%, and 2.6%; platelet counts less than $50,000/mm^3$ occurred in 1% to 1.5% of patients treated. Profound thrombocytopenia ($<20,000/mm^3$) has been observed rarely with abciximab administration.

Other Adverse Effects Administration of abciximab may cause human antichimeric antibody formation that potentially could cause allergic/hypersensitivity reactions (including anaphylaxis), thrombocytopenia, or diminished benefit on readministration.

Clinical Trials

In nearly 2100 patients undergoing either balloon coronary angioplasty or atherectomy who were judged to be at high risk for ischemic (thrombotic) complications, a bolus of abciximab (0.25 mg/kg) followed by a 12-hour continuous infusion (10 μg/min) reduced the occurrence of death, MI, or the need for an urgent intervention (repeat angioplasty, stent placement, balloon pump insertion, or bypass grafting) by 35%.[81] At 6 months,[79] the absolute difference in patients with a major ischemic event or elective revascularization was 8.1% comparing patients who received abciximab (bolus plus infusion) with patients given placebo (35.1% versus 27%; 23% reduction). All patients received aspirin and unfractionated heparin during the procedure. At 3 years,[82] the composite end point occurred in:

- 41.1% of patients receiving an abciximab bolus plus infusion
- 47.4% of patients receiving an abciximab bolus only
- 47.2% of patients receiving placebo

The greatest benefit was observed in patients with refractory angina or evolving MI.

The EPILOG study[80] included 2792 patients undergoing elective or urgent percutaneous coronary revascularization who received either abciximab with standard, weight-adjusted unfractionated heparin (initial bolus,

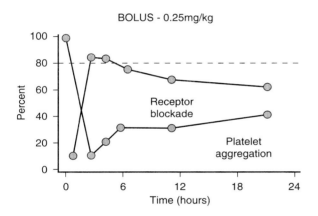

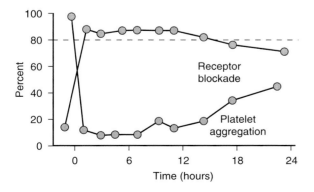

FIGURE 28–19. Duration of receptor blockade and inhibition of platelet aggregation (5 μm ADP) *(top)* in five patients receiving a 0.25 mg/kg bolus dose (intravenous) of abciximab and *(bottom)* in five patients receiving a bolus followed by an infusion (10 μg/min). Data are presented as mean ± SEM. (From Uprichard A: Handbook of Experimental Pharmacology. Berlin, Springer Verlag, 1995, pp 175-208.)

100 U/kg; target activated clotting time, ≥300 seconds) or placebo with standard-dose, weight-adjusted heparin. At 30 days, the composite event rate was 5.4%, 5.2%, and 11.7%. The benefit was observed in high-risk and low-risk patients.

The CAPTURE study[79] was uniquely designed to assess whether abciximab, given 18 to 24 hours before coronary angioplasty, could improve clinical outcome in patients with refractory (myocardial ischemia despite nitrates, heparin, and aspirin) unstable angina. A total of 1265 patients (of 1400 scheduled) were randomly assigned to abciximab or placebo. By 30 days, the primary end point (death, MI, urgent revascularization) occurred in 11.3% of abciximab-treated patients and in 15.9% of placebo-treated patients ($P = .012$). The rate of MI was lower *before* and *during* coronary interventions in patients given abciximab.

Patients participating in the GUSTO (Global Use of Strategies to Open Occluded Arteries) IV-ACS trial[83] (n = 7800) had chest pain and either ST-segment depression or elevated troponin (T or I) levels. They were randomized to receive placebo or abciximab for 24 hours or abciximab for 48 hours. All patients received aspirin and heparin (unfractionated or low molecular weight). Neither abciximab group fared better than the placebo group with respect to death or MI at 30 days. At 48 hours, a higher mortality rate was observed in patients receiving abciximab than in patients given placebo that was more marked in the 48-hour infusion group. No patient subgroup experienced a significant treatment benefit with abciximab.

Tirofiban (Aggrastat)

Tirofiban, a synthetic 495-kd nonpeptide tyrosine derivative, is a selective competitive antagonist of the platelet GP IIb/IIIa receptor.

Pharmacokinetics

The pharmacokinetics of tirofiban are linear, and plasma concentrations are proportional to dose after intravenous infusions of 0.05 to 0.4 μg/kg/min for 1 hour or 0.1 to 0.2 μg/kg/min for 4 hours in healthy individuals. Concomitant administration of aspirin or clopidogrel does not affect pharmacokinetics.

Tirofiban is approximately 65% bound to plasma proteins, and binding is independent of drug concentrations over a wide range. The steady-state volume of distribution ranges from 22 to 42 L.

After intravenous administration, plasma concentrations of tirofiban decline in a biphasic manner. The half-life averages 1.5 to 2 hours. Clearance is predominantly (65% to 70%) through renal excretion, and metabolism of the drug is limited. Plasma clearance of tirofiban is 20% to 25% lower in older patients (≥65 years old) and can be reduced by 50% or more in patients with marked renal insufficiency (creatinine clearance <30 mL/min). Drug clearance is not influenced by gender, race, or mild-to-moderate hepatic insufficiency. Tirofiban is removed to a variable degree by hemodialysis.

Pharmacodynamics

Tirofiban mimics the geometric stereotactic and conformational characteristics of the αIIb/β3 receptor arginine-glycine-aspartic acid (RGD) sequence, interfering with fibrinogen surface binding and platelet aggregation.

Three doses of tirofiban were studied in phase I clinical trials: bolus dose of 5, 10, or 15 μg/kg followed by a continuous intravenous infusion of 0.05, 0.10, or 0.15 μg/kg/min. A dose-dependent inhibition of ex vivo platelet aggregation was observed within several minutes of bolus administration with sustained inhibition during the maintenance infusion.[84] Further studies to investigate dosing strategies that achieve maximal platelet inhibition are under way.

Hematologic Effect

Thrombocytopenia In controlled clinical trials of tirofiban,[85-87] the incidence of thrombocytopenia (<90,000/mm^3) was 1.5% for the combination of tirofiban and unfractionated heparin compared with 0.6% for heparin monotherapy; reductions to less than 50,000/mm^3 were observed in 0.3% and 0.1% of patients. Microscopic hematuria and occult blood in the stool were reported in 10.7% and 18.3% of patients receiving combination therapy and 7.8% and 12.2% of patients given monotherapy.

Other Adverse Effects Anaphylaxis or urticaria requiring discontinuation of therapy has not been reported in clinical trials.

Administration in Older Patients

Clinical trials of tirofiban[85-87] have included patients older than age 65 (43% of patients) and older than age 75 (11.7% of patients). The experience to date has not revealed age-related differences in response to treatment. Although the overall incidence of bleeding has been higher, the incremental risk is similar for combination therapy and monotherapy. Dose adjustment of tirofiban is not recommended for older patients.

Dose Adjustment with Renal Impairment

Plasma clearance of tirofiban is decreased substantially in patients with severe renal impairment (creatinine clearance <30 mL/min), including patients requiring hemodialysis. These patients should receive half the usual infusion rate.

Clinical Trials

The RESTORE (Randomized Efficacy of Tirofiban Outcomes and Restenosis) trial[85] was a randomized, double-blind, placebo-controlled trial of tirofiban in patients undergoing coronary intervention within 72 hours of hospital presentation with ACS.

Patients (n = 2139) received tirofiban as a 10-μg/kg intravenous bolus over a 3-minute period and a continuous infusion of 0.15 μg/kg/min over 36 hours. All patients received unfractionated heparin and aspirin. The primary composite end point (death, MI, angioplasty) at 30 days was reduced from 12.2% in the placebo group to 10.3% in the tirofiban group (16% relative reduction).

The PRISM (Platelet Receptor Inhibition in Ischemic Syndrome Management) trial[86] included 3231 patients with unstable angina/non–ST-segment elevation MI. All patients received aspirin and were randomized to treatment with either unfractionated heparin or tirofiban, given as a loading dose of 0.6 µg/kg/min over 30 minutes followed by a maintenance infusion of 0.15 µg/kg/min for 48 hours (angiography/revascularization was discouraged during the infusion period). The primary composite end point (death, MI, refractory ischemia) at 48 hours was 5.6% in tirofiban-treated patients and 3.8% in placebo (aspirin/heparin)-treated patients (risk reduction 33%). Benefit was maintained but overall was less impressive at 7 and 30 days.

The PRISM PLUS (Patients Limited by Unstable Signs and Symptoms) trial[87] included 1915 patients with unstable angina and non–ST-segment elevation MI who were treated with aspirin and unfractionated heparin and randomized to either tirofiban (0.4 µg/kg/min × 30 min, then 0.1 µg/kg/min for a minimum of 48 hours and a maximum of 108 hours) or placebo (unfractionated heparin). Angiography and revascularization were encouraged in that trial. Tirofiban-treated patients had a lower composite event rate of 7 days than the placebo group (12.9% versus 17.9%, risk reduction 34%). The benefit was due mainly to a reduced incidence of MI (47% risk reduction) and refractory ischemia (30% risk reduction). The benefit was maintained at 30 days (22% risk reduction in composite event rate) and at 6 months (Table 28-10). The trial originally included a tirofiban-alone arm (no unfractionated heparin), which was dropped because of excess mortality at 7 days.

The importance of early intervention among patients with non–ST-segment elevation ACS was emphasized in the TACTICS TIMI-18 (Treat Angina With Aggrastat and Determine Cost of Therapy With an Invasive or Conservative Strategy—Thrombolysis in Myocardial Infarction) trial,[88] as was the benefit of aggressive pharmacologic therapy (GP IIb/IIIa receptor antagonists) combined with PCI for patients at greatest risk for adverse ischemic outcomes (prior MI, ST-segment changes, elevated cardiac enzymes).

Eptifibatide (Integrilin)

Eptifibatide, a synthetic cyclic heptapeptide, is a selective competitive antagonist of the platelet GP IIb/IIIa receptor.

■ ▓ ■

TABLE 28-10 CLINICAL TRIALS OF TIROFIBAN: PRISM AND PRISM-PLUS STUDIES

EVENTS (%)	PRISM			PRISM-PLUS		
	Tirofiban	Heparin	Risk Ratio	Tirofiban + Heparin	Heparin	Risk Ratio
48 Hours						
Composite	3.8	5.6	0.67*	7.8	5.7	0.71
Refractory ischemia	3.5	5.3	0.65*	4.8	5.9	0.78
MI or death	1.2	1.6	0.76	0.9	2.6	0.34*
MI	0.9	1.4	0.64	0.8	2.4	0.32*
Death	0.4	0.2	1.48	0.3	0.1	0.51
7 Days						
Composite	10.3	11.2	0.90	12.9	17.9	0.68*
Refractory ischemia	9.1	9.9	0.91	9.3	12.7	0.70*
MI or death	3.3	4.2	0.77	4.9	8.3	0.57*
MI	3.6	3.1	0.84	3.9	7.0	0.53*
Death	1.0	1.6	0.63	1.9	1.9	1.01
30 Days						
Composite	15.9	17.1	0.92	18.5	22.3	0.78*
Refractory ischemia	10.6	10.8	0.98	10.6	13.4	0.76
MI or death	5.8	7.1	0.80	8.7	11.9	0.70*
MI	4.1	4.3	0.95	6.6	9.2	0.70
Death	2.3	2.6	0.62*	3.6	4.5	0.79
6 Months						
Composite	—	—	—	27.7	32.1	0.81*
Refractory ischemia	—	—	—	10.6	13.4	0.76
MI or death	—	—	—	12.3	15.3	0.78
MI	—	—	—	8.3	10.5	0.76
Death	—	—	—	6.9	7.0	0.97
Readmission for unstable angina	—	—	—	6.9	10.7	1.00

*$P < .05$.
PRISM, Platelet Receptor Inhibition in Ischemic Syndrome Management; PRISM-Plus, Platelet Receptor Inhibition in Ischemic Syndrome Management—Patients Limited by Unstable signs and Symptoms; MI, myocardial infarction

Pharmacokinetics

The pharmacokinetics of eptifibatide are linear, and plasma concentrations are proportional to dose after intravenous administration of 90 to 250 µg/kg and infusions of 0.5 to 3 µg/kg/min. Concomitant administration of aspirin or heparin does not influence the pharmacokinetics of eptifibatide.[89]

Eptifibatide is approximately 25% bound to plasma proteins, principally albumin. The volume of distribution ranges from 185 to 260 mL/kg.

Plasma concentrations of eptifibatide decline in a biexponential manner after intravenous administration. The half-life ranges from 2.5 to 2.8 hours. Eptifibatide is eliminated by renal and nonrenal mechanisms. The drug undergoes deamination within plasma to a metabolite that is responsible for approximately 40% of the platelet inhibitory effects. Clearance of eptifibatide is proportional to body weight and creatinine clearance and inversely proportional to age. Renal clearance is responsible for 40% to 50% of total body clearance. Eptifibatide is removed to a variable degree by hemodialysis.

Pharmacodynamics

Early studies of patients undergoing PCI determined that bolus doses of 135 µg/kg or higher yielded greater than 80% inhibition of ADP-mediated platelet aggregation in most (75%) patients. A double bolus strategy (180 µg/kg × 2 administered 10 minutes apart) achieved maximal inhibition in a greater proportion of patients.[90] Platelet aggregation returns to 50% of baseline 4 hours after infusion termination.

Hematologic Effects

Thrombocytopenia   The incidence of thrombocytopenia (<100,000/mm³ or a decrease of 50% from baseline) in clinical trials of eptifibatide has been low and similar to patients receiving placebo. Profound thrombocytopenia (<20,000/mm³) occurs rarely (0.2% of patients).[91-93]

Other Adverse Effects   Anaphylaxis was reported in seven patients (0.16%) receiving eptifibatide in the Platelet Glycoprotein IIb/IIIa in Unstable Angina Receptor Suppression Using Integrilin Therapy (PURSUIT) trial (0.15% in placebo group).

Administration in Older Patients

Clinical trials of eptifibatide[91-93] have included patients older than age 65 (65% of patients) and older than age 75 (12% of patients). There are no clear age-related differences in efficacy; however, bleeding complications were higher among older individuals. Although dose adjustments based on age have not been recommended, patients greater than 75 years of age were required to be at least 50 kg in weight to enter the PURSUIT trial.[92]

Dose Adjustments with Renal Impairment

Dose adjustments have not been recommended with mild renal impairment (serum creatinine <2 mg/dL); however, patients with serum creatinine levels between 2 and 4 mg/dL should receive a reduced initiating bolus dose (135 µg/kg) and infusion rate (0.5 µg/kg/min). Eptifibatide is not recommended in patients with marked renal insufficiency, including patients requiring hemodialysis.

Clinical Trials

The Integrilin to Minimize Platelet Aggregation and Coronary Thrombosis (IMPACT-II) trial[91] enrolled 4010 patients undergoing elective, urgent, or emergency coronary interventions. Patients were assigned to placebo, a bolus of 135 µg/kg of eptifibatide followed by an infusion of 0.5 µg/kg/min for 20 to 24 hours, or a bolus of 135 µg/kg followed by an infusion of 0.75 µg/kg/min. By 30 days, the composite end point (death, MI, unplanned revascularization, stent placement for abrupt closure) occurred in 11.4%, 9.2%, and 9.9% of patients. Although the benefit of treatment was maintained at 6 months, the differences between groups were not statistically significant.

The PURSUIT trial[92] included patients with unstable angina or non–ST-segment elevation MI with symptoms within 24 hours and electrocardiogram changes within 12 hours (of ischemia). A total of 10,948 patients were randomized to eptifibatide, 180 µg/kg bolus plus 1.3 µg/kg/min infusion or 180 µg/kg bolus plus 2 µg/kg/min infusion, or placebo for 3 days (in addition to unfractionated heparin [in most patients] and aspirin). The group receiving the lower dose was discontinued when the higher dose was shown safe. The 30-day event rate of death or nonfatal MI was 14.2% with eptifibatide and 15.7% with placebo (1.5% absolute reduction) (Fig. 28-20). A reduction in MI or death (composite) with eptifibatide was observed at 96 hours, 7 days, and 30 days in medically or interventionally treated patients; however, the benefit was less impressive at later time points.

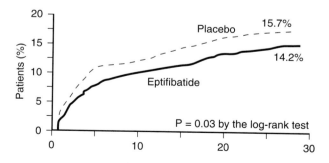

FIGURE 28–20. Incidence of death or nonfatal myocardial infarction illustrated by Kaplan-Meier curves in the PURSUIT (Platelet Glycoprotein IIb/IIIa in Unstable Angina Receptor Suppression Using Integrilin Therapy) trial. (From Platelet Glycoprotein IIb/IIIa in Unstable Angina Receptor Suppression Using Integrilin Therapy [PURSUIT] trial investigators: Inhibition of platelet glycoprotein IIb/IIIa with eptifibatide in patients with acute coronary syndromes. N Engl J Med 1998;339:436–443.)

The ESPRIT (Enhanced Suppression of the Platelet GPIIb/IIIa Receptor with Integrilin) trial was designed to test the hypothesis that a minimum threshold of 80% GP IIb/IIIa receptor blockade was required for benefit.[93] A total of 2064 patients received either eptifibatide (two 180-μg/kg boluses 10 minutes apart, continuous infusion of 2 μg/kg/min for 18 to 24 hours) or placebo before PCI. The trial was terminated early for efficacy because patients receiving eptifibatide had a 4% absolute reduction in death, MI, urgent target vessel revascularization, or "bail out" GP IIb/IIIa antagonist use within 48 hours compared with placebo. Major events were significantly lower at 30 days as well.

Similarities and Differences Between Intravenous Glycoprotein IIb/IIIa Antagonists

Although considered collectively as GP IIb/IIIa receptor antagonists, abciximab, tirofiban, and eptifibatide differ at several levels, including their:

- Molecular size
- Binding characteristics
- Clearance
- Plasma concentrations
- Platelet-bound and biologic half-life
- Potential reversibility (Table 28-11)
- Non–platelet-related effects

The duration of platelet inhibition after drug discontinuation and the potential for reversing the pharmacologic effect are particularly important properties in cases of emergent surgery and major hemorrhagic complications. In general, a return of platelet function toward a physiologic state (≤50% inhibition) occurs within 4 hours after the cessation of tirofiban and eptifibatide. In contrast, 12 hours are required for abciximab (Fig. 28-21). Some of the delayed return of physiologic platelet function after abciximab termination may be counterbalanced by its low free plasma concentration and drug-to-receptor ratio. These properties are responsible for the rapid return of hemostatic potential after platelet transfusions. In contrast, the high plasma concentrations observed with the small-molecule inhibitors limit the effectiveness of platelet transfusions. Fibrinogen supplementation (fresh frozen plasma, cryoprecipitate) is the more logical first choice for restoration of hemostatic potential, given the competitive nature of binding and relative availability of platelet GP IIb/IIIa receptors (Fig. 28-22).[94]

The non–platelet-related effects of GP IIb/IIIa receptor antagonists may have important implications. In contrast to tirofiban and eptifibatide, which selectively bind the $\alpha IIb/\beta 3$ receptor, abciximab binds the vitronectin receptor ($\alpha V/\beta 3$) with similar affinity. The vitronectin receptor mediates procoagulant properties of platelets and proliferative properties of endothelial and smooth muscle cells. Abciximab also reduces platelet-leukocyte interactions through inhibition of MAC-1 binding[95] and exhibits anticoagulant properties that exceed those of tirofiban and eptifibatide.[96]

Several studies have suggested that RGD peptides and RGD-mimetic GP IIb/IIIa receptor antagonists promote cellular apoptosis through CASPASE-1 and CASPASE-3 activation.[97-99] CASPASES promote nuclear enzyme activity involved in DNA degeneration. Long-term administration of compounds that passively diffuse into the

■ ▪ ■

TABLE 28-11 INDIVIDUAL CHARACTERISTICS AND DOSING OF GLYCOPROTEIN IIb/IIIa RECEPTOR ANTAGONISTS

CHARACTERISTICS	ABCIXIMAB	EPTIFIBATIDE	TIROFIBAN
Type	Antibody	Peptide	Nonpeptide
Molecular weight (d)	~50,000	~800	~500
Platelet-bound half-life	Long (hr)	Short (sec)	**Short (s)**
Plasma half-life	Short (min)	Extended (2 hr)	Extended (2 h)
Drug-to-GP IIb/IIIa receptor ratio	1.5–2.0	250–2500	>250
50% return of platelet function (without transfusion)	12 hr	~4 hr	~4 h
Antagonist Dosing			
PCI			
Bolus	0.25 mg/kg	Double bolus 180 μg/kg/min (10 min apart)	10 μg/kg
Infusion	0.125 μg/kg/min × 12 hr	2 μg/kg/min × 20–24 hr	0.5 μg/kg/min × 18–24 hours*
ACS			
Bolus	Not recommended†	180 μg/kg over 30 min	0.4 μg/kg over 30 min
Infusion		2 μg/kg/min up to 72 hr	0.1 μg/kg/min for 48–108 hrs
Renal dysfunction			
Creatinine ≥2 mg/dL	No adjustment required	135 μg/kg over 30 min; 0.5 μg/kg/min infusion	0.2 μg/kg over 30 min
Creatinine ≥4 mg/dL	No adjustment required	Contraindicated	0.5 μg/kg/min infusion‡

*Not approved, but PCI trials have used this dosing regimen.
†Use of abciximab for ACS in absence of planned PCI not recommended.
‡Dose of tirofiban for patients with creatinine clearance < 30 mL/min. Experience limited.
ACS, acute coronary syndrome; GP, glycoprotein; PCI, percutaneous coronary intervention.

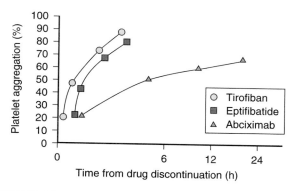

FIGURE 28–21. The time course for restoration of platelet aggregability after cessation of glycoprotein IIb/IIIa receptor antagonists.

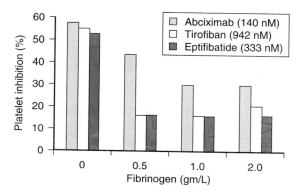

FIGURE 28–22. Fibrinogen supplementation restores platelet aggregability in the presence of competitive glycoprotein IIb/IIIa receptor antagonists. [From Li YF, Spencer FA, Becker RC: Comparative efficacy of fibrinogen and platelet supplementation on the in vitro reversibility of fibrinogen and platelet supplementation on the in vitro reversibility of competitive glycoprotein IIb/IIIa (alphaIIb/beta3) receptor–directed platelet inhibition. Am Heart J 2001;142:204–210.]

cell cytoplasm (e.g., oral GP IIb/IIIa receptor antagonists) could promote myocyte death.

Major Clinical End Points

The intravenous GP IIb/IIIa receptor antagonists have been shown to reduce cardiac event rates in patients with ACS who are treated by pharmacologic means alone or undergo PCI. The available data suggest that the greatest overall benefit occurs in high-risk patients, many of whom require mechanical revascularization.

Methodologic differences between the major clinical trials make it difficult to compare the GP IIb/IIIa receptor antagonists; however, there is clear consistency among the agents with regard to efficacy and safety.[100] Meticulous attention to femoral arterial access, sheath care, and periprocedural heparin dosing has reduced vascular and major hemorrhagic complications substantially.

The Do Tirofiban And ReoPro Give Similar Efficacy Trial (TARGET) randomized 5308 patients to either tirofiban (RESTORE trial dosing strategy) or abciximab before PCI (with the intent to perform stenting). The primary end point, a composite of death, nonfatal MI, or urgent revascularization at 30 days, was reached in 7.6% and 6% of tirofiban-treated patients (hazard ratio 1.26).[101] There were no differences in the rates of major bleeding complications or transfusions, but tirofiban was associated with a lower rate of minor bleeding and thrombocytopenia (Fig. 28–23).

Oral Gycoprotein IIb/IIIa Receptor Antagonists

The success enjoyed by intravenous GP IIb/IIIa receptor antagonists, coupled with the recognized risk for recurrent cardiac events incurred by patients with atherosclerotic coronary artery disease, stimulated interest in the development of oral agents that would provide continued, low-level GP IIb/IIIa receptor inhibition. To date, more than 30,000 patients have been enrolled in four large-scale, double-blind, placebo-controlled clinical

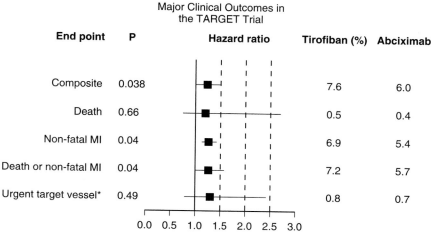

Major Clinical Outcomes in the TARGET Trial

End point	P	Hazard ratio	Tirofiban (%)	Abciximab
Composite	0.038		7.6	6.0
Death	0.66		0.5	0.4
Non-fatal MI	0.04		6.9	5.4
Death or non-fatal MI	0.04		7.2	5.7
Urgent target vessel*	0.49		0.8	0.7

Abbreviations: MI, myocardial infaction; * Revascularization

FIGURE 28–23. Hazard ratios for the end point of death, nonfatal myocardial infarction, urgent target vessel revascularization, and their combination in the TARGET (Do Tirofiban and ReoPro Give Similar Efficacy?) trial. (From Topol EJ, Moliterno DJ, Herrman HC, et al: Comparison of two platelet glycoprotein IIb/IIIa inhibitors, tirofiban and abciximab, for the prevention of ischemic events with percutaneous coronary revascularization. N Engl J Med 2001;334: 1888–1894.)

trials. Individually, each trial failed to identify a reduction in ischemic outcomes. Collectively a significant excess in mortality with three different oral GP IIb/IIIa receptor antagonists was observed (Fig. 28–24).[102]

Intravenous Glycoprotein IIb/IIIa Receptor Antagonists Use According to Published Guidelines

Unstable Angina/Non–ST-Segment Elevation Myocardial Infarction   A platelet GP IIb/IIIa receptor antagonist should be administered, in addition to aspirin and heparin, to patients with continuing ischemia or with other high-risk features (see Chapters 49 and 50) and to patients in whom PCI is planned. Eptifibatide and tirofiban are approved for this use. Abciximab can be used for 12 to 24 hours in patients scheduled to undergo PCI within the next 24 hours.[34,35]

Miscellaneous Platelet Antagonists

A wide variety of pharmacologic agents with platelet-inhibiting properties have undergone testing in patients with atherosclerotic vascular disease. Although not approved specifically for use in patients with ACS, several compounds are discussed briefly.

Aggrenox

Aggrenox is a combination platelet antagonist that includes aspirin (25 mg twice daily) and dipyridamole (200 mg extended-release preparation).

Mechanisms of Action   Aspirin's mechanism of action has been discussed previously. Dipyridamole inhibits cyclic adenosine monophosphate (cAMP)-phosphodiesterase (PDE) and cyclic-3′,5′-GMP-PDE.[103,104]

Pharmacokinetics   The pharmacokinetic profile of aspirin has been summarized previously. Peak dipyridamole levels in plasma are achieved within several hours of oral administration (400-mg dose of Aggrenox). Extensive metabolism via conjugation with glucuronic acid occurs in the liver. There are no significant pharmacokinetic interactions between aspirin and dipyridamole coadministered as Aggrenox.

Pharmacodynamics   Dipyridamole inhibits platelet aggregation by two distinct mechanisms. First, it attenuates adenosine uptake into platelets, endothelial cells, and erythrocytes. The resulting increase elicits a rise in cellular adenylate cyclase concentrations, resulting in elevated cAMP levels, which inhibit platelet activation to several stimuli, including ADP, collagen, and platelet-activating factor. Dipyridamole also inhibits PDE.[105] The subsequent increase in cAMP elevates nitric oxide concentration, facilitating platelet inhibitory potential.[106]

Adverse Effects   ESPS 2 (European Stroke Prevention Study) reported that 79.9% of patients experienced at least one on-treatment adverse event. The most common side effects were gastrointestinal complaints and headache.

Dipyridamole has vasodilatory effects and should be used with caution in patients with severe coronary artery disease in whom episodes of angina pectoris may increase. Dipyridamole administration has not been

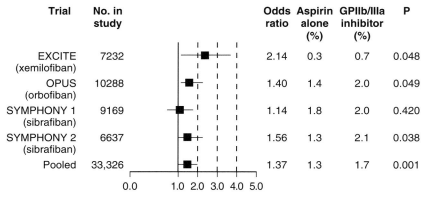

Major Outcomes in Trials of
Oral GPIIb/IIIA Receptor Antagonists

Trial	No. in study		Odds ratio	Aspirin alone (%)	GPIIb/IIIa inhibitor (%)	P
EXCITE (xemilofiban)	7232		2.14	0.3	0.7	0.048
OPUS (orbofiban)	10288		1.40	1.4	2.0	0.049
SYMPHONY 1 (sibrafiban)	9169		1.14	1.8	2.0	0.420
SYMPHONY 2 (sibrafiban)	6637		1.56	1.3	2.1	0.038
Pooled	33,326		1.37	1.3	1.7	0.001

Abbreviations:
 EXCITE, Evaluation of Oral Xemilofiban in Controlling Thrombotic Events;
 OPUS, Orbofiban in Patients with Unstable Coronary Syndromes;
 SYMPHONY, Sibrafiban vs Aspirin to Yield Maximum Protection from
 Ischemic Heart Events Post-acute Coronary Syndromes.

Odds ratio and 95% confidence intervals for death beyond 30 days in trials of oral GPIIb/IIIa receptor antagonists.

FIGURE 28–24. Pooled analysis of the oral glycoprotein IIb/IIIa antagonist trials. An increased mortality rate was observed at 30 days. (From Chew DP, Bhatt DL, Sapp S, Topol EJ: Increased mortality with oral platelet glycoprotein IIb/IIIa antagonists. Circulation 2001;103: 201–206.)

associated with hepatic enzyme elevation. Patients receiving Aggrenox should not receive adenosine for myocardial perfusion studies.[107]

Administration in Older Patients Plasma concentrations of dipyridamole are approximately 40% higher in patients greater than 65 years of age compared with patients less than age 55 years.

Administration in Patients with Renal Insufficiency Urinary excretion of the parent compound is negligible; however, to date, studies of Aggrenox have not been done in patients with renal insufficiency.

Clinical Trials There have been no clinical trials studying the use of Aggrenox in ACS. ESPS 2[108] was a randomized, double-blind, placebo-controlled, 24-month study that included 6602 patients with a history of either ischemic stroke (76%) or transient ischemic attack (24%). Patients were randomized to receive Aggrenox b.i.d., dipyridamole alone, aspirin alone, or placebo. Aggrenox reduced the risk of stroke by 22.1% ($P = .008$) compared with aspirin ($P = .008$) and by 24.4% compared with dipyridamole ($P = .002$).[109]

Aggrenox Use According to Published Guidelines Aggrenox is not interchangeable with the individual components of aspirin and dipyridamole tablets. Dipyridamole has vasodilatory effects and should be used cautiously in patients with advanced coronary artery disease, particularly patients with ACS. Patients with cerebrovascular disease (transient ischemic attack or prior stroke) and concomitant coronary artery disease may require higher aspirin doses than contained in Aggrenox. An alternative platelet antagonist is recommended in this setting.[109]

Cilostazol

Cilostazol is a quinolinone derivative that inhibits cellular phosphodiesterase.

Mechanism of Action Cilostazol inhibits PDE III, which suppresses cAMP degradation. The resulting increase of cAMP in platelets and endothelial cells leads to inhibition of platelet aggregation and vasodilation.[110-112] Cilostazol also increases lipoprotein lipase activity, lowering serum triglyceride levels and raising high-density lipoprotein concentrations.[113]

Cardiovascular Effects The vasodilatory effects of cilostazol affect peripheral vascular and cardiovascular beds.

Pharmacokinetics Cilostazol is well absorbed after oral administration. Although absolute bioavailability has not been determined, high-fat meals have been shown to significantly increase (by 90%) absorption. Metabolism occurs via the hepatic cytochrome P-450 enzymes, and most of the metabolites are excreted in the urine (75% of overall clearance). One of the two active metabolites is responsible for more than 50% of PDE III inhibition. The elimination half-life of cilostazol (and its metabolites) is approximately 12 hours.

Pharmacodynamics Increasing cAMP concentrations within endothelial cells causes vasodilation, whereas elevated levels in platelets impair aggregation.

Adverse Effects The most common adverse effect associated with cilostazol administration is headache. Other relatively frequent causes of drug discontinuation include palpitations and diarrhea.

Several PDE III inhibitors have been associated with decreased survival in patients with class III/IV congestive heart failure. Cilostazol should *not* be administered to patients with congestive heart failure (of any severity).

Use in Older Patients The clearance of cilostazol (and its metabolites) has not been determined in patients older than age 65.

Use in Patients with Renal Insufficiency Moderate-to-severe renal impairment increases cilostazol metabolite levels and alters protein binding of the parent compound. Patients with advance renal insufficiency have not been studied.

Clinical Studies Cilostazol is approved for the treatment of intermittent claudication. Across eight clinical trials, the improvement in walking distance (compared with placebo) was approximately 40% to 50%.[114,115] Although there is experience with cilostazol after coronary arterial stenting,[116-118] its long-term administration to patients with coronary artery disease has not been studied. Short-term coadministration with aspirin reduced ADP-mediated platelet aggregation by 30% to 40% (compared with aspirin alone). There are no randomized clinical trials of cilostazol in ACS.

Use According to Published Guidelines Cilostazol is recommended for patients with disabling claudication, particularly when revascularization cannot be offered.[34] Although it has platelet-inhibiting properties, cilostazol should not be considered a substitute for aspirin or clopidogrel in patients with ACS who have concomitant peripheral vascular disease.

OTHER AGENTS

Prostaglandin E and Prostacyclin Several natural prostanoids (PGE_1 and PGI_2) inhibit platelet activation and aggregation by elevating cAMP levels. The primary mechanism of inhibition is through the activation of adenylate cyclase (with a subsequent rise in cAMP concentrations), which prevents calcium mobilization. The clinical application of PGE$_1$ and PGI$_2$ has been limited by their effect on vascular tone, producing substantial systemic hypotension,[119] and by extensive first-pass metabolism in the lungs (70% of the active compound is rapidly cleared).[120] The prostanoid analogues (e.g., iloprost, beraprost, cicaprost, ciprostene) are more stable compounds than PGE$_1$ and PGI$_2$.

Thromboxane/Endoperoxide Receptor Antagonists

This class of compounds is designed to prevent platelet activation in response to TXA$_2$ and other endoperoxides. There is a limited experience with the thromboxane receptor antagonists ridogrel, sulotraban, and SQ 30741 in patients with MI treated with fibrinolytics.[121,122]

Agents that Inhibit Platelet Aggregation

Serotonin Receptor Antagonists

Ketanserin, a serotonin receptor antagonist, has been studied in animal models of coronary thrombosis and thrombolysis, in which it has been shown, when administered concomitantly with a TXA$_2$ receptor antagonist, to improve reperfusion and decrease reocclusion after tissue plasminogen activator administration.[123]

Thromboxane Synthetase Inhibitors

Thromboxane synthetase antagonists, including dazoxiben and pirmagrel, suppress platelet thromboxane synthesis and platelet aggregation.[124,125] Clinical development has been hampered by the aggregating potential of endoperoxide intermediates and by the incomplete inhibition of thromboxane synthesis by currently available compounds.

Dextran

Dextran is a polysaccharide preparation that ranges in molecular weight from 65 to 80 kd. It prolongs the bleeding time, probably by interfering with surface membrane receptor function and fibrinogen binding.[126] Dextran also reduces plasma viscosity.

Nitric Oxide

Nitric oxide (NO) is a naturally occurring molecule derived from the amino acid L-arginine. It is a product of normal vascular endothelial cells and plays a crucial role in maintaining vasoreactivity and thromboresistance.

NO prevents platelet adhesion and inhibits agonist-dependent G protein–mediated phospholipase C activation with subsequent calcium release. Accordingly, NO prevents P-selectin expression and calcium-dependent conformation change in platelet surface GP IIb/IIIa. It also has been shown to potentiate platelet disaggregation by preventing the stabilization of fibrinogen–GP IIb/IIIa interactions.[127] Beyond having potent platelet-inhibitory effects, NO also inhibits neutrophil aggregation in vitro and prevents leukocyte adhesion to vascular endothelium.[128,129] Inhaled NO is undergoing clinical evaluation in the setting of acute MI. In patients with ACS, S-nitrosoglutathione reduced platelet activation and GP IIb/IIIa expression.

NONOates

Complexes of NO with nucleophiles, known as NONOates, are capable of spontaneously generating NO and, as a result, may offer therapeutic benefit in the treatment of NO deficiency states. The biologic potency and duration of action can be modified by altering the carrier nucleophile. DEA (diethylamine)/NO possesses a shorter half-life that SPER (spermine)/NO (2.1 minutes versus 39 minutes) resulting in an earlier peak activity (5 minutes versus 15 minutes) and a shorter duration of action. In contrast to the acid stability of 5-nitrosothiols (RSNOs), NONOates are alkali stable and decompose rapidly at low pH.[130]

DEA/NO and SPER/NO have been shown to have potent antiplatelet properties. Platelet aggregation measured in whole blood or platelet-rich plasma after the addition of collagen was reduced by DEA/NO in a dose-dependent manner. The effect was similar to aspirin in whole blood. In vivo, both agents showed antiplatelet activity that correlated with the rate of release of NO in solution.[131]

A rapid NO donor, PROLI/NO, formed by the reaction of nitric acid with L-proline in methanolic sodium methoxide, dissociates to proline (1 mole) and NO (2 moles) with a half-life of 1.8 seconds at a pH of 7.4 (37°C) and possesses antiplatelet and vasodilatory properties. When infused into an unheparinized polyester vascular graft (baboon model), platelet deposition was reduced significantly.[132]

Molsidomine and SIN-1

A novel class of nitrosovasodilators, the sydnonimines, that include molsidomine and its active metabolite SIN-1, has been evaluated clinically as effective NO donors. SIN-1 reacts with molecular oxygen resulting in the spontaneous release of NO through a process that involves a 1-electron abstraction.[133]

It has been suggested that administration of molsidomine and SIN-1 may decrease mortality associated with acute MI by 35%. To confirm this observation, the ESPRIM (European Study of Prevention of Infarct with Molsidomine) trial randomized 4017 patients with acute MI to receive either SIN-1 (1 mg/hr intravenously for 48 hours) followed by molsidomine (16 mg orally for 12 days) or placebo. Although there was no difference in all-cause mortality between groups at either 35 days or 13 months, the study was considered inconclusive, based on the inclusion of predominantly low-risk patients.[134]

Pirsidomine

Pirsidomine, N-p-anisoyl-3 (cis-2,6-dimethylpiperidino) sydnonimine, possesses hemodynamic properties similar to molsidomine, but has a longer duration of action.[135]

Nitric Oxide Donors

Several novel NO donors are currently under development. The compound FK 409, (±)(E)-4-ethyl-3 [(Z)-hydroxyimino]-5-nitro-3-hexene-1-yl]-3-pyridinecarboxamide, similarly releases NO but at a slower rate. When compared with FR 14420 in an isolated rat aortic preparation, FK 409 showed greater vasorelaxant potency and hemodynamic effects, although its duration of action was shorter than that seen with FR 144420.[136]

IFT 296

The nitrate ester IFT 296, [3-2-nitro-oxyethyl)-3-4dihydro-2H-1,3-benzoxazin-4-one] has shown anti-ischemic effects in an isolated rabbit heart model subjected to global ischemia.[137]

SPM-5185

The compound SPM-5185, (N-nitratopivaloyl]-S-(N'-acetylalanyl)-cysteine ethylester, is an effective NO donor.[138]

Compounds with Platelet-Inhibiting Properties

The management of patients with atherosclerotic coronary artery disease includes a variety of compounds with secondary platelet-inhibiting properties. Several with potentially important clinical effects are discussed.

3-Hydroxy-3-Methylglutaryl Coenzyme A Inhibitors

The 3-hydroxy-3-methylglutaryl coenzyme A (HMG-CoA) reductase inhibitors (or statins) are potent antagonists of cholesterol biosynthesis; however, the clinical benefits may exceed what is expected from changes in lipids alone, suggesting other mechanisms. The pleiotropic effects attributable to statins, in addition to those on endothelial cells, smooth muscle cells, monocytes/macrophages, and inflammatory cells, include platelets. Statins have been shown to reduce platelet reactivity,[139,140] TXA_2 biosynthesis,[141] cytosolic calcium concentrations,[142] and deposition on damaged vessels.[143,144]

Omega-3 Fatty Acids

Polyunsaturated fatty acids are obtained from coldwater fish and plants. A major omega-3 fatty acid in fish oil is eicosapentaenoic acid (EPA). EPA enters the phospholipid of cell membranes and competes with arachidonic acid for COX. The resulting thromboxane produced (TXA_3) cannot activate platelets. The prostaglandin produced by EPA, PGI_3, has the same vasodilatory effects as the arachidonic-derived PGI_2 and platelet-inhibiting effects.[145] Favoring EPA-derived prostaglandin synthesis produces the desirable state of vasodilation and reduced platelet aggregation.[146] Anti-inflammatory properties also have been described.[147] Although potential benefits in patients at risk for coronary events have been

reported,[148,149] the impact on more acute processes has not been investigated.

MONITORING OF PLATELET ACTIVITY

Despite the well-recognized benefits of platelet inhibition for the prevention and treatment of ACS, studies using traditional monitoring tools have not successfully achieved "proof of concept" in determining the degrees of inhibition that are capable of assessing underlying atherosclerotic disease activity, prothrombotic potential, and response to treatment. The advent of near-patient assays and point-of-care technology may change management substantially, facilitating a more targeted and comprehensive approach.

Platelet Aggregometry

The current laboratory evaluation of platelet function is based predominantly on *turbidometric platelet aggregometry* (also known as *light transmission aggregometry*). This test is performed by preparing platelet-rich plasma (with platelet-poor plasma as a control) and eliciting an aggregation response with ADP, epinephrine, collagen, arachidonic acid, and ristocetin.[150]

Impedance platelet aggregometry[151] has been introduced as an alternative to turbidometric methods, with the potential physiologic advantage of using whole-blood samples. The reproducibility of platelet aggregometry is influenced by a variety of factors that include:

- Concentration of sodium citrate in the collecting tubes
- Adjustment of the platelet count
- Storage time
- Stirring rate
- Temperature
- pH of the blood sample

Bedside Assays and Instruments

Bedside assays, near-patient testing, and point-of-care monitoring instruments are attractive for several reasons. First, they provide a rapid, reliable, and reproducible means to assess hemostatic potential and treatment response. Second, the techniques involved require minimal training, reagent handling, calibration, and physical space. Third, emerging technology will offer a full complement of coagulation and platelet tests that can be used for management in the home, ambulatory clinic, emergency department, angioplasty suite, coronary care unit, and operating room.[152]

Platelet Function Analyzer-100

The platelet function analyzer (PFA)-100 simulated primary hemostasis under high shear stress conditions. Citrated whole blood is drawn by capillary action through a membrane coated with either collagen and epinephrine or collagen and ADP.[153] An aperture in the membrane occludes after platelet adhesion and aggregation, and the test results are recorded as closure time. The

PFA-100 is most useful in detecting primary hemostatic abnormalities (primary platelet function disorders and von Willebrand disease) and determining response to replacement therapy.[154]

Clot Retraction Assay

The strength of clot retraction can serve as a measure of platelet function,[155] and a hemostasis analyzer has been developed for this purpose. Citrated whole blood or platelet-rich plasma is placed in a sample chamber, where calcium and thrombin are added to stimulate clot formation. As platelets bind, undergo cellular contraction, and polymerize with fibrin strands, the force developed by the platelets is measured by a probe transducer that produces an electrical output (a voltage signal converted to force reported in dynes) proportional to the amount of force generated.

The clot retraction assay provides information, and can use whole blood or plasma obtained from standard citrated blood collection tubes. Potential uses include the evaluation of hemostatic defects in uremia and after bypass surgery.[156]

Rapid Platelet Function Assay

The rapid platelet function assay is a semiautomated turbidometric system that is based on the ability of activated platelets to interact with fibrinogen, yielding macroscopically visible agglutination. Fibrinogen-coated polystyrene beads, buffers, and a modified thrombin receptor activating peptide (iso-TRAP) are incorporated into a disposable cartridge and exposed to samples of citrated whole blood. The instrument detects agglutination between the fibrinogen-coated beads and activated platelets, providing a quantitative digital display. Because agglutination is proportional to the proportion of unblocked GP IIb/IIIa receptors, this device is well suited for determining platelet inhibitory response to currently available GP IIb/IIIa receptor antagonists.[157] The time required to obtain results is 2 minutes.

The semiautomated system is easy to use and correlates closely with traditional measurements of platelet function, turbidometric platelet aggregation ($r^2 = 0.95$), and the percentage of free GP IIb/IIIa molecules ($r^2 = 0.96$).[158] The use of whole blood and duplicate analysis eliminated variables in sample preparation and minimizes random errors. Results can be reported as an absolute rate of aggregation or as a percentage of the baseline aggregation.

A rapid bedside assay that provides a reliable measurement of GP IIb/IIIa receptor blockade offers a broad range of medical, interventional, and surgical applications. Dose titration with intravenous agents could be performed, achieving a safe and effective degree of platelet inhibition.[159]

The intensity or level of platelet inhibition (achieved with GP IIb/IIIa antagonist therapy) required to prevent thrombotic complications after PCI was determined in 485 patients participating in the GOLD study.[160] One quarter of all patients did not achieve greater than or equal to 95% inhibition (rapid platelet function assay)

10 minutes after the initiation of treatment and experienced a significantly higher incidence of death, MI, or urgent target vessel revascularization (14.4% versus 6.4%). Those with less than 70% inhibition at 8 hours were also at increased risk (25% versus 8.1%). A reliable and readily available means to assess inhibitory response to GP IIb/IIIa receptor antagonists also may provide guidance for dose titration in patients at risk for bleeding complications, including patients with thrombocytopenia, prior hemorrhagic events, and known coagulopathies (Table 28-12).[161]

PLATELET POLYMORPHISMS

Genetic factors play an important role in the development and expression of atherosclerotic coronary artery disease. Although the hereditary link traditionally has been considered in the context of atherosclerotic risk factors, it has become increasingly clear that an inherited predisposition to arterial thrombosis (more often in the context of concomitant abnormalities in the vascular endothelium that impair thromboresistance) plays a pivotal role in disease expression and, in all probability, response to antithrombotic therapy.[162-172]

Several polymorphisms specific to platelets and their potential ligands have been described (Table 28-13). Because overall risk (or protection) may be determined by the coexistence of several variant alleles, ongoing efforts must consider a broader genetic pool.

FUTURE DIRECTIONS

The participation of platelets to vascular atherothrombosis is well established and serves fundamentally as the basis for pharmacologic management of ACS. Further strides will be made through genomics, proteomics, and pharmacogenomics that will foster targeted therapy that maximizes efficacy and safety. Pending developments on

■ ▨ ■

TABLE 28-12 CLINICAL SETTINGS IN WHICH PLATELET MONITORING MIGHT BE USEFUL

Patient-Related (Confirmed Target Inhibition)

Before percutaneous coronary intervention
Patients with refractory ischemia or recurrent symptoms despite receiving glycoprotein IIb/IIIa receptor antagonist therapy
Interruption of infusion
Thrombocytopenia
Qualitative platelet abnormality
Renal insufficiency
Low or high body weight

Clinically Related

Bleeding
    Confirm intensity of inhibition
    Confirm reversal of inhibition after replacement therapy
Emergent surgery
    Guidance to reverse platelet inhibition (if clinically necessary)
Transition from one glycoprotein IIb/IIIa receptor antagonist to another

■ ■ ■

TABLE 28-13 PLATELET POLYMORPHISMS AND THEIR IMPACT ON CARDIOVASCULAR EVENTS AND TREATMENT RESPONSE

POLYMORPHISM	CLINICAL RELEVANCE
Pl^{A2} (GP IIIa)	Increased risk for myocardial infarction
	Reduced response to aspirin
GP Ibα	Increased risk for coronary heart disease and acute coronary syndromes
GP Ia	Increased cardiovascular events
vWF promoter variant	Increased risk for acute coronary syndromes
Fibrinogen promoter variant	Increased cardiovascular events
P-Selectin (715 pro)	Reduced cardiovascular events

GP, glycoprotein; vWF, von Willebrand factor.

the genomolecular level, further clinical investigation is needed to define optimal dosing strategies for existing therapies, including those that are most widely available to clinicians and their patients worldwide.

REFERENCES

1. Marcus AJ: Platelet function. N Engl J Med 1969;280:1213–1220.
2. Roth GJ: Platelets and blood vessels: The adhesion event. Immunol Today 1992;13:100.
3. Fauvel F, Grant ME, Legrand YJ, et al: Interaction of blood platelets with a microfibrillar extract from adult bovine aorta: Requirement for von Willebrand factor. Proc Natl Acad Sci U S A 1983;80:551.
4. Birembaur P, Legrand YJ, Bariety J, et al: Histochemical and ultrastructural characterization of subendothelial glycoprotein microfibrils interacting with platelets. J Histochem Cytochem 1982;30:75.
5. Packham MA: Platelet reactions in thrombosis. In Gottllieb AI, Langille BL, Federoff S (eds): Atherosclerosis: Cellular and Molecular Interactions in the Artery Wall. New York, Plenum Press, 1991, p 209.
6. Kinlough-Rathborn RI, Packham MA, Reimers HJ, et al: Mechanisms of platelet shape change, aggregation and release induced by collagen, thrombin, or A23, 187. J Lab Clin Med 1977;90:707.
7. Stenberg PE, Shuman MA, Levine SP, Bainton DF: Redistribution of alpha-granules and their contents in thrombin-stimulated platelets. J Cell Biol 1984;98:748.
8. Ginsberg MH, Taylor L, Painter RG: The mechanism of thrombin-induced platelet factor 4 secretion. Blood 1980;55:661.
9. Redl H, Hammerschmidt DE, Schlag G: Augmentation by platelets of granulocyte aggregation in response to chemotaxins: Studies utilizing an improved cell preparation technique. Blood 1983;61:125.
10. Deuel TF, Huang JS: Platelet derived growth factor: Structure, function and roles in normal and transformed cells. J Clin Invest 1984;74:669.
11. De Gaetano G, Evangelista V, Ratjar G, et al: Activated polymorphonuclear leukocytes stimulate platelet function. Thromb Res 1990;11:25.
12. Hoffman M, Monroe III DM: A cell-based model of hemostasis. Thromb Haemost 2001;85:958–965.
13. Patrono C: Aspirin as an antiplatelet drug. N Engl J Med 1994;330:1287–1294.
14. O'Brien JR: Effects of salicylates on human platelets. Lancet 1968;1:779–783.
15. Roth GJ, Majerus PW: The mechanism of the effect of aspirin on human platelets: I. Acetylation of a particulate fraction protein. J Clin Invest 1975;56:624–632.
16. Burch JW, Stanford N, Majerus PW: Inhibition of platelet prostaglandin synthetase by oral aspirin. J Clin Invest 1978;61:314–319.
17. Hawkey CJ, Karrasch JA, Szczepanski L, et al: Omeprazole compared with misoprostol for ulcers associated with nonsteroidal antiinflammatory drugs. Omeprazole versus Misoprostol for NSAID-induced Ulcer Management (OMNIUM) study group. N Engl J Med 1998;338:727–734.
18. Latini R, Tognoni G, Maggioni AP, et al: Clinical effects of early angiotension-converting enzyme inhibitor treatment of acute myocardial infarction are similar in the presence and absence of aspirin: Systemic overview of individual data from 96,712 randomized patients. Angiotension-Converting Enzyme Inhibitor Myocardial Infarction Collaborative Group. J Am Coll Cardiol 2000;35:1801–1807.
19. Awtry EH, Loscalzo J: Aspirin. Circulation 2000;101:1206–1207.
20. Antiplatelet Trialists' Collaboration: Collaborative overview of randomized trials of antiplatelet therapy: I. Prevention of death, myocardial infarction, and stroke by prolonged antiplatelet therapy in various categories of patients. BMJ 1994;308:81–106.
21. Lewis HD, Davis JW, Archibald DG, et al: Protective effects of aspirin against acute myocardial infarction and death in men with unstable angina: Results of Veterans Administration Cooperative Study. N Engl J Med 1985;313:1369–1375.
22. Cairns JA, Gent M, Singer J, et al: Aspirin, sulfinpyrazone, or both, in unstable angina: Results of a Canadian multicentre clinical trial. N Engl J Med 1985;313:1369–1375.
23. Theroux P, Ouimet H, McCans J, et al: Aspirin, heparin, or both to treat acute unstable angina. N Engl J Med 1988;319:1105–1111.
24. Theroux P, Waters D, Qui S, et al: Aspirin versus heparin to prevent myocardial infarction during the acute phase of unstable angina. Circulation 1993;88:2045–2048.
25. RISC Group: Risk of myocardial infarction and death during treatment with low-dose and intravenous heparin in men with unstable coronary artery disease. Lancet 1990;336:827–830.
26. Alexander JH, Harrington RA, Tuttle RH, et al: Prior aspirin use predicts worse outcomes in patients with non-ST elevation acute coronary syndromes: PURSUIT investigators. Platelet IIb/IIIa in Unstable Angina: Receptor Suppression Using Integrilin Therapy. Am J Cardiol 1999;83:1147–1151.
27. Becker RC, Tracy RP, Bovill EG, et al: The clinical use of flow cytometry for assessing platelet activation in acute coronary syndromes. Coron Artery Dis 1994;5:339–345.
28. Becker RC, Bovill EG, Corrao JM, et al: Platelet activation determined by flow cytometry persist despite antithrombotic therapy in patients with unstable angina and non-Q-wave myocardial infarction: For the TIMI III Thrombosis and Coagulation Study Group. J Thromb Thrombol 1994;1:95–100.
29. Becker RC, Bovill EG, Corrao JM, et al: Dynamic nature of thrombin generation, fibrin formation, and platelet activation in unstable angina and non-Q-wave myocardial infarction. J Thromb Thrombol 1995;2:57–64.
30. Duke WW: The relation of blood platelets to hemorrhagic disease. JAMA 1983;250:1201–1209.
31. Santos MT, Valles J, Aznar J, et al: Prothrombotic effects of erythrocytes on platelet activity: Reduction by aspirin. Circulation 1997;95:63–68.
32. Nair GV, Davis CJ, McKenzie ME, et al: Aspirin in patients with coronary artery disease: Is it simply irresistible? J Thromb Thrombol 2001;11:117–126.
33. Rocca B, FitzGerald GA: Simple read: Erythrocytes modulate platelet function: Should we rethink the way we give aspirin? Circulation 1997;95:11–13.
34. Sixth ACCP Consensus Conference on Antithrombotic Therapy. Chest 2001;119(Suppl):1–370S.
35. ACC/AHA Guidelines for the management of patients with unstable angina and non-ST segment elevation myocardial infarction. J Am Coll Cardiol 2001;36:970–1062.
36. Patrono C, Coller B, Dalen JE, et al: Platelet-active drugs: The relationship among dose, effectiveness, and side-effects. Chest 1998;114(Suppl):470S–488S.
37. Cipollone F, Patrignani P, Greco A, et al: Differential suppression of thromboxane biosynthesis by indobufen and aspirin in patients with unstable angina. Circulation 1997;96:1109–1116.

38. Rajah SM, Rees M, Walker D, et al: Effects of antiplatelet therapy with indobufen or aspirin-dipyridamole on graft patency 1 year after coronary artery bypass grafting. J Thorac Cardiovasc Surg 1994;107:1146-1153.

39. SINBA group: Indobufen versus aspirin plus dipyridamole after coronary artery surgery. Coron Artery Dis 1991;2:897-906.

40. Brochier ML: Evaluation of flurbiprofen for prevention of reinfarction and reocclusion after successful thrombolysis or angioplasty in acute myocardial infarction: The Flurbiprofen French Trial. Eur Heart J 1993;14:951-957.

41. Brooks P, Emery P, Evans JF, et al: Interpreting the clinical significance of the differential inhibition of cycloxygenase-1 and oxygenase-2. Rheumatology 1999;39:779-788.

42. McAdam BF, Catella-Lawson F, Mardino IA, et al: Systemic biosynthesis of prostacyclin by cyclooxygenase (COX)-2: The human pharmacology of selective inhibitors of COX-2 [erratum appears in Proc Natl Acad Sci U S A 1999;96:5890]. Proc Natl Acad Sci U S A 1999;96:272-277.

43. Bombardier C, Laine L, Rercin A, et al: Comparison of upper gastrointestinal toxicity of rofecoxib and naproxen in patients with rheumatoid arthritis. N Engl J Med 2000;343:1520-1528.

44. Konstam MA, Matthew R, Weir MD, et al: Cardiovascular thrombotic events in controlled, clinical trials of rofecoxib. Circulation 2001;104:2280-2288.

45. Bruno JJ: The mechanism of action of ticlopidine. Thromb Res 1983;4(Suppl):59-67.

46. Piovella F, Ricetti MM, Almasioni P, et al: The effect of ticlopidine on human endothelial cells in culture. Thromb Res 1984;33:323-332.

47. O'Brien JR, Etherington MD, Shuttleworth RD: Ticlopidine—an antiplatelet drug: Effects in human volunteers. Thromb Res 1978;13:245-254.

48. Ellis DJ, Roe RI, Bruno JJ, et al: The effects of ticlopidine hydrochloride on bleeding and platelet function in man [abstract]. Thromb Haemost 1981;46:176.

49. De Caterina R, Sicari R, Bernini W, et al: Benefit/risk profile of combined antiplatelet therapy with ticlopidine and aspirin. Thromb Haemost 1991;65:504-510.

50. De Minno G, Cerbone AM, Mattioli PL, et al: Functionally thromboasthenic state in normal platelets following the administration of ticlopidine. J Clin Invest 1985;75:328-338.

51. Berglund U, von Scheneck H, Wallentin L: Effect of ticlopidine on platelet function in men with stable angina pectoris. Thromb Haemost 1985;54:808-812.

52. Panak E, Blanchard J, Roe RI: Evaluation of the antithrombotic efficacy of ticlopidine in man. Agents Action 1984;15(Suppl):148-166.

53. Bennett CL, Weinberg PD, Rozenberg-Ben-Dror K, et al: Thrombotic thrombocytopenic purpura associated with ticlopidine: A review of 60 cases. Ann Intern Med 1998;128:541-544.

54. Steinhubl SR, Tan WA, Foody JM, for the EPISTENT investigators: Incidence and clinical course of thrombotic thrombocytopenic purpura due to ticlopidine following coronary stenting. JAMA 1999;281:806-810.

55. Balsano F, Rizzon P, Violi F, et al: Antiplatelet treatment with ticlopidine unstable angina: A controlled multicenter clinical trial. Studio della Ticlopidina nell'Angina Instablie group. Circulation 1990;82:17-26.

56. Sigwart U, Puel J, Mirkovitch V, et al: Intravascular stents to prevent occlusion and restenosis after transluminal angioplasty. N Engl J Med 1987;316:701-706.

57. Morice MC, Zemour G, Benveniste E, et al: Intracoronary stenting without coumadin: One month results of a French multicenter study. Cathet Cardiolvasc Diagn 1995;35:1-7.

58. Schömig A, Neumann FJ, Kastrati A, et al: A randomized comparison of antiplatelet and anticoagulant therapy after the placement of coronary-artery stents. N Engl J Med 1996;334:1084-1089.

59. Bertrand ME, Legrand V, Boland J, et al: Randomized multicenter comparison of conventional anticoagulation versus antiplatelet therapy in unplanned and elective coronary stenting. Full Anticoagulation Versus Aspirin and Ticlopidine (FANTASTIC) study. Circulation 1998;98:1597-1603.

60. Urban P, Macaya C, Rupprecht HJ, et al, for the MATTIS investigators: Randomized evaluation of anticoagulation versus antiplatelet therapy after coronary stent implantation in high risk patients. Multicenter Aspirin and Ticlopidine Trial After Intracoronary Stenting (MATTIS). Circulation 1998;98:2126-2132.

61. Steinhubl SR, Ellis SG, Wolski K, et al, for the EPISTENT investigators: Ticlopidine pretreatment before coronary stenting is associated with sustained decrease in adverse cardiac events. Circulation 2001;103:1403-1409.

62. Leon MB, Baim DS, Gordon P, et al: Clinical and angiographic results from the Stent Anticoagulation Regimen Study (STARS). Circulation 1996;94(Suppl I):I685.

63. Gachet C, Stierlé A, Cazenave JP, et al: The thienopyridine PCR 4099 selectively inhibits ADP-induced platelet aggregation and fibrinogen binding without modifying the membrane glycoprotein IIb-IIIa complex in rat and in man. Biochem Pharmacol 1990;40:229-238.

64. Gachet C, Savi P, Ohlmann P, et al: ADP receptor induced activation of guanine nucleotide binding proteins in rat platelet membranes—an effect selectively blocked by the thienopyridine clopidogrel. Thromb Haemost 1992;68:79-83.

65. Mills DC, Puri R, Hu CJ, et al: Clopidogrel inhibits the binding of ADP analogues to the receptor mediating inhibition of platelet adenylate cyclase. Arterioscler Thromb 1992;12:430-436.

66. Hollopter G, Jantzen HM, Vincent D, et al: Identification of the platelet ADP receptor targeted by antithrombotic drugs. Nature 2001;409:202-207.

67. Cadroy Y, Bossavy JP, Thalamas C, et al: Early potent antithrombotic effect with combined aspirin and a loading dose of clopidogrel on experimental arterial thrombogenesis in humans. Circulation 2000;101:2823-2828.

68. Helft G, Osende JI, Worhtley SG, et al: Acute antithrombotic effect of a front-loaded regimen of clopidogrel in patients with arthrosclerosis on aspirin. Arterioscler Thromb Vasc Biol 2000;20:2316-2321.

69. Bennett CL, Connors JM, Carwile JM, et al: Thrombotic thrombocytopenia purpura associated with clopidogrel. N Engl J Med 2000;342:1773-1777.

70. Clopidogrel in Unstable Angina to Prevent Recurrent Events Trial investigators: Effects of clopidogrel in addition to aspirin in patients with acute coronary syndromes without ST-segment elevation. N Engl J Med 2001;345:494-502.

71. Bertrand ME: Double-blind study of the safety of clopidogrel with and without a loading dose in combination with aspirin after coronary stenting: The Clopidogrel Aspirin Stent Internation Cooperative Study (CLASSICS). Circulation 2000;102:624-629.

72. Muller C, Buttner HJ, Peterson J, et al: A randomized comparison of clopidogrel and aspirin versus ticlopidine and aspirin after the placement of coronary-artery stents. Circulation 2000;101:590-593.

73. Mehta SR, Yusuf S, Peters RJ, for the CURE investigators: Effects of pretreatment with clopidogrel and aspirin following by long-term therapy in patients undergoing percutaneous coronary intervention: The PCI-CURE study. Lancet 2001;358:527-533.

74. Topol EJ, Moliterno DJ, Herrman HC, et al: Comparison of two platelet glycoprotein IIb/IIIa inhibitors, tirofiban and abciximab, for the prevention of ischemic events with percutaneous coronary revascularization. N Engl J Med 2001;334:1888-1894.

75. Waksman R, Ajani AE, White RI, et al: Prolonged antiplatelet therapy to prevent late thrombosis after intracoronary γ-radiation in patients with restenosis: Washington Radiation for In-Stent Restenosis Trial Plus 6 Months of Clopidogrel (WRIST PLUS). Circulation 2001;103:2332-2335.

76. Lefkovits J, Plow EF, Topol EJ: Platelet glycoprotein IIb/IIIa receptors in cardiovascular medicine. N Engl J Med 1995;332:1553-1559.

77. Frederickson BJ, Turner NA, Kleiman NS, et al: Effects of abciximab, ticlopidine, and combined abciximab/ticlopidine therapy on platelet and leukocyte function in patients undergoing coronary angioplasty. Circulation 2000;101:1122-1129.

78. Evaluation of Platelet IIb/IIIa Inhibition For Prevention Of Ischemic Complications (EPIC) investigators: Use of a monoclonal antibody directed against the platelet glycoprotein IIb/IIIa receptor in high-risk coronary angioplasty. N Engl J Med 1994;330:956-961.

79. CAPTURE investigators: Randomized placebo-controlled trial of abciximab before and during coronary intervention in refractory unstable angina: The CAPTURE study. Lancet 1997;349: 1429-1435.

80. EPILOG investigators: Platelet glycoprotein IIb/IIIa receptor blockade and low-dose heparin during percutaneous coronary revascularization. N Engl J Med 1997;336:1689-1696.

81. Topol EJ, Califf RM, Weisman HF, et al, for the EPIC investigators: Randomized trial of coronary intervention with antibody against platelet IIb/IIIa integrin for reduction of clinical restenosis: Results at six months. Lancet 1994;343:881-886.

82. Topol EJ, Ferguson JJ, Weisman HF, et al, for the EPIC investigator group: Long-term protection from myocardial ischemic events in a randomized trial of brief integrin B, blockade with percutaneous coronary intervention. JAMA 1997;278:479-484.

83. GUSTO IV investigators: Randomized placebo controlled trial of abciximab before early coronary revascularization: The GUSTO IV-ACS randomized trial. Lancet 2001;357:1915-1924.

84. Kereiakes DJ, Kleiman NS, Ambrose J, et al: Randomized, double-blind, placebo-controlled dose-ranging study of tirofiban (MK-383) platelet IIb/IIIa blockade in high risk patients undergoing coronary angioplasty. J Am Coll Cardiol 1996;27:536-542.

85. Randomized Efficacy Study of Tirofiban for Outcomes and Restenosis (RESTORE) investigators: Effects of platelet glycoprotein IIb/IIIa blockade with tirofiban on adverse cardiac events in patients with unstable angina or acute myocardial infarction undergoing coronary angioplasty. Circulation 1997;96:1445-1453.

86. Platelet Receptor Inhibition in Ischemic Syndrome Management (PRISM) study investigators: A comparison of aspirin plus tirofiban with aspirin plus heparin for unstable angina. N Engl J Med 1998;338:1498-1505.

87. Platelet Receptor Inhibition in Ischemic Syndrome Management in Patients Limited by Unstable Signs and Symptoms (PRISM PLUS) study investigators: Inhibition of the platelet glycoprotein IIb/IIIa receptor with tirofiban in unstable angina and non-Q wave myocardial infarction. N Engl J Med 1998;338:1488-1497.

88. Cannon CP, Weintraub WS, Demopoulos LA, et al, for the TACTICS-TIMI 18 investigators: Comparison of early invasive and conservative strategies for patients with unstable coronary syndromes treated with the glycoprotein IIb/IIIa inhibitor tirofiban. N Engl J Med 2001;334:1879-1887.

89. Phillips DR, Scarborough RM: Clinical pharmacology of eptifibatide. Am J Cardiol 1997;80:11B-20B.

90. Harrington RA, Kleiman NS, Kottke-Marchant K, et al: Immediate and reversible platelet inhibition after intravenous administration of a peptide glycoprotein IIb/IIIa inhibitor during percutaneous coronary intervention. Am J Cardiol 1995;76:1222-1227.

91. Integrilin to Minimize Platelet Aggregation and Coronary Thrombosis (IMPACT)-II investigators: Randomized placebo-controlled trial of effect of eptifibatide on complications of percutaneous coronary intervention: IMPACT-II. Lancet 1997;349: 1422-1428.

92. Platelet Glycoprotein IIb/IIIa in Unstable Angina Receptor Suppression Using Integrilin Therapy (PURSUIT) trial investigators: Inhibition of platelet glycoprotein IIb/IIIa with eptifibatide in patients with acute coronary syndromes. N Engl J Med 1998;339:436-443.

93. ESPIRIT investigators: Novel dosing regimen of eptifibatide in planned coronary stent implantation (ESPRIT): A randomized, placebo-controlled trial. Lancet 2000;356:2037-2044.

94. Becker RC, Spencer FA, Liu T: Fibrinogen exerts varying effects on GPIIb/IIIa receptor-directed platelet inhibition in vitro. Am Heart J 2001;142:204-210.

95. Weber C, Springer TA: Neutrophil accumulation on activated, surface-adherent platelets in flow is mediated by interaction of Mac-1 with fibrinogen bound to alphaIIbbeta3 and stimulated by platelet-activating factor. J Clin Invest 1997;100:2085-2093.

96. Li YF, Spencer FA, Ball S, Becker RC: Inhibition of platelet-dependent prothrombinase activity and thrombin generation by glycoprotein IIb/IIIa receptor-directed antagonists: Potential contributing mechanism of benefit in acute coronary syndromes. J Thromb Thrombol 2000;10:69-76.

97. Adderley SR, Fitzgerald DJ: Glycoprotein IIb/IIIa antagonists induce apoptosis in rat cardiomyocytes by caspase-3 activation. J Biol Chem 2000;275:5760-5766.

98. Buckley CD, Pilling D, Henriquez NV, et al: RGD peptides induce apoptosis by direct caspase-3 activation. Nature 1999;397: 534-539.

99. Mannick JB, Hausladen A, Liu L, et al: Fas-induced caspase denitrosylation. Science 1999;284:651-654.

100. Kong DF, Califf RM, Miller DP, et al: Clinical outcomes of therapeutic agents that block the platelet glycoprotein IIb/IIIa integrin in ischemic heart disease. Circulation 1998;98:2829-2835.

101. Topol EJ, Moliterno DJ, Herrmann HC, et al, for the TARGET investigators: Comparison of two platelet glycoprotein IIb/IIIa inhibitors, tirofiban and abciximab, for the prevention of ischemic events with percutaneous coronary revascularization. N Engl J Med 2001;344:1888-1894.

102. Chew DP, Bhatt DL, Sapp S, Topol EJ: Increased mortality with oral platelet glycoprotein IIb/IIIa antagonists. Circulation 2001;103: 201-206.

103. Bunag RD, Douglas CR, Imai S, Berne RM: Influence of pyrimidopyrimidine derivative on deamination of adenosine by blood. Circ Res 1964;15:83-88.

104. Born GVR, Cross MJ: Inhibition of the aggregation of blood platelets by substances related to adenosine diphosphate. J Physiol 1963;166:29P-30P.

105. FitzGerald GA: Dipyridamole. N Engl J Med 1987;316:1247-1257.

106. Eisert WG: Near-field amplification of antithrombotic effects of dipyridamole through vessel wall cells. Neurology 2001;57(5 Suppl 2):S20-23.

107. Bokhari S, Bergmann S: Warning to physicians performing pharmacologic stress tests. J Nucl Cardiol 2000;7:546.

108. Diener HC, Cunha L, Forbes C, et al: European Stroke Prevention Study-2: Dipyridamole and acetylsalicylic acid in the secondary prevention of stroke. J Neurol Sci 1996;143:1-13.

109. Hervey PS, Goa KL: Extended-release dipyridamole/aspirin. Drugs 1999;58:469-475.

110. Umekawa H, Tanaka T, Kimura Y, et al: Purification of cyclic adenosine monophosphate phosphodiesterase from human platelets using new-inhibitor sepharose chromatography. Biochem Pharmacol 1984;33:3339-3344.

111. Kimura Y, Tani T, Kanbe T, et al: Effect of cilostazol on platelet aggregation and experimental thrombosis. Arzneimittelforschung 1985;35:1144-1149.

112. Okuda Y, Kimura Y, Yamashita K: Effect of cilostazol on walking distances in patients with intermittent claudication caused by peripheral vascular disease. Drug Rev 1993;11:451-465.

113. Timi T: Cilostazol, a selective type III phosphodiesterase inhibitor, decreases triglyceride and increases HDL cholesterol levels by increasing lipoprotein lipase activity in rats. Atherosclerosis 2000;152:299-305.

114. Dawson DL, Cutler BS, Meissner MH, et al: Cilostazol has beneficial effects in treatment of intermittent claudication: Results from a multicenter, randomized, prospective, double-blind trial. Circulation 1998;98:678-686.

115. Beebe HG, Dawson DL, Cutler BS, et al: A new pharmacologic treatment for intermittent claudication: Results of a randomized, multicenter trial. Arch Intern Med 1999;159: 2041-2050.

116. Ochiai M, Isshiki T, Takeshita S, et al: Use of cilostazol, a novel antiplatelet agent, in a post-Palmaz-Schatz stenting regimen. Am J Cardiol 1997;79:1471-1474.

117. Park SW, Lee CW, Kim HS, et al: Comparison of cilostazol versus ticlopidine therapy after stent implantation. Am J Cardiol 1999;84:511-514.

118. Kozuma K: Effects of cilostazol on late lumen loss and repeat revascularization after Palmaz-Schatz coronary stent implantation. Am Heart J 2001;141:124-130.

119. Weksler BB: Prostaglandins and vascular-function. Circulation 1984;70(Suppl III):63-71.

120. Sharma B, Wheth RP, Gimenez HJ, et al: Intracoronary prostaglandin E1, plus streptokinase in acute myocardial infarction. Am J Cardiol 1986;58:1161.

121. Kopia GA, Kopaciwicz LJ, Ohlstein EH, et al: Combinations of the thromboxane receptor antagonists, sulotroban, with streptokinase: Demonstration of thrombolytic synergy. J Pharmacol Exp Ther 1989;250:887.

122. Grover GJ, Parham CS, Shumacher WA: The combined anti-ischemic effects of the thromboxane receptor antagonist SQ

30741 and tissue type plasminogen activator. Am Heart J 1991;121:426.

123. Golino P, Ashton JH, Glas-Greenwalt P, et al: Mediation of reocclusion by thromboxane A2 and serotonin after thrombolysis with tissue-type plasminogen activator in a canine preparation of coronary thrombosis. Circulation 1988;77:678.

124. Fitzgerald GA, Reilly LA, Pederson AK: The biochemical pharmacology of thromboxane synthase inhibition in man. Circulation 1985;72:1194–1201.

125. Mullane KM, Foinabaio D: Thromboxane synthetase inhibitors reduce infarct size by a platelet dependent, aspirin-sensitive mechanism. Circ Res 1988;62:668–678.

126. Evans RJ, Gordon JD: Mechanisms of the antithrombotic actions of dextran. N Engl J Med 1974;290:748–756.

127. Gries A, Bode C, Peter K, et al: Inhaled nitric oxide inhibits human platelet aggregation, P-selectin expression, and fibrinogen binding in vitro and in vivo. Circulation 1998;97:1481–1487.

128. Adams MR, Jessup W, Hailstones D, et al: L-Arginine reduces human monocyte adhesion to vascular endothelium and endothelial expression of cell adhesion molecules. Circulation 1997;95:662–668.

129. Loscalzo J: Antiplatelet and antithrombotic effects of organic nitrates. Am J Cardiol 1992;70(Suppl):18B–22B.

130. Morley D, Maragos CM, Zhang X-Y, et al: Mechanism of vascular relaxation induced by the nitric oxide (NO/nucleophile complexes), a new class of NO-based vasodilators. J Cardiovasc Pharmacol 1993;21:670–676.

131. Diodati JG, Quyyumi AA, Hussain N, et al: Complexes of nitric oxide with nucleophiles as agents for the controlled biological release of nitric oxide: Antiplatelet effect. Thromb Haemost 1993;70:654–658.

132. Saavedra JE, Southan GJ, Davies KM, et al: Localizing antithrombotic and vasodilatory activity with a novel, ultrafast nitric oxide donor. J Med Chem 1996;39:4361–4365.

133. Reden J: Molsidomine. Blood Vessels 1990;27:282–294.

134. ESPRIM trial: Short-term treatment of acute myocardial infarction with molsidomine. European Study of Prevention of Infarct with Molsidomine. Lancet 1994;334:91–97.

135. Wainwright CL, Martorona PA: Pirsidomine, a novel nitric oxide donor suppresses ischemic arrhythmias in anesthetized pigs. J Cardiovasc Pharmacol 1993;22:S44–S50.

136. Kita Y, Ohkubo K, Hiraswa Y, et al: FR 144420, a novel, slow, nitric oxide-releasing agent. Eur J Pharmacol 1995;275:125–130.

137. Rossoni G, Bert F, Bermareggi M, et al: Protective effects of ITF 296 in the isolated rabbit heart subjected to global ischemia. J Cardiovasc Pharmacol 1995;26:S44–S52.

138. Lefer DJ, Nakanishi K, Johnston WE, Vinter-Johansen J: Antineutrophil and myocardial protecting actions of a novel nitric oxide donor after acute myocardial ischemia and reperfusion of dogs. Circulation 1993;88:2337–2350.

139. Huhle G, Abletshauser C, Mayer N, et al: Reduction of platelet activity markers in type II hypercholesterolemic patients by a HMG-CoA-reductase inhibitor. Thromb Res 1999;95:229–234.

140. Hale LP, Craver KT, Berrier AM, et al: Combination of fosinopril and pravastatin decreases platelet response to thrombin receptor agonist in monkeys. Arterioscler Thromb Vasc Biol 1998;18:1643–1646.

141. Notarbartolo A, Davi G, Averna M, et al: Inhibition of thromboxane biosynthesis and platelet function by simvastatin in type IIa hypercholesterolemia. Arterioscler Thromb Vasc Biol 1995;15:247–251.

142. Le Quan Sang KH, Levenson J, Megnien JL, et al: Platelet cytosolic Ca^{2+} and membrane dynamics in patients with primary hypercholesterolemia: Effects of pravastatin. Arterioscler Thromb Vasc Biol 1995;15:759–764.

143. Alfon J, Royo T, Garcia-Mill X, Badimon L: Platelet deposition on eroded vessel walls at a stenotic shear rate is inhibited by lipid-lowering treatment with atorvastatin. Arterioscler Thromb Vasc Biol 1999;19:1812–1817.

144. Alfon J, Fernandez de Arriba A, Gomez-Casajus LA, et al: Alternative binding assay of GPIIb/IIIa antagonists with a nonradioactive labeling method of platelets. Thromb Res 2001;102:247–253.

145. Neuhof H: Eicosanoides in trauma and traumatic shock. In Schlag G, Redl H (eds): Pathophysiology of Shock, Sepsis, and Organ Failure. Berlin, Springer Verlag, 1993, pp 79–91.

146. Kramer HJ, Stevens J, Grimminger F, et al: Fish oil acids and human platelets: Dose dependent decrease in dienoic and increase in trienoic thromboxane generation. Biochem Pharmacol 1996;52:1211–1217.

147. Meydani SN, Dinarello CA: Influence of dietary fatty acids on cytokine production and its clinical implications. Nutr Clin Pract 1993;8:65–72.

148. Cerbone AM: Persistent impairment of platelet aggregation following cessation of a short-course dietary supplementation of moderate amounts of N-3 fatty acid ethyl esters. Thromb Haemost 1999;82:128–133.

149. Knapp HR, Reilly IAG, Alessandrini P, et al: In vivo indexes of platelet and vascular function during fish-oil administration in patients with atherosclerosis. N Engl J Med 1986;314:937–942.

150. Born GVR: Qualitative investigations into the aggregation of blood platelets. J Physiol (Lond) 1962;67:162.

151. Cardinal DC, Flower RJ: The electronic aggregometer: A novel device for assessing platelet behavior in blood. J Pharmacol Methods 1980;3:135–158.

152. Becker RC: Exploring the medical need for alternate site testing: A clinician's perspective. Arch Pathol Lab Med 1995;119:894–897.

153. Mammen EF, Comp PC, Cosselin R, et al: PFA-100 system: A new method for assessment of platelet dysfunction. Semin Thromb Hemost 1998;24:195–202.

154. Jennings LK, White MM: Expression of ligand induced binding sites on glycoprotein IIb/IIIa complexes and the effect of various inhibitors. Am Heart J 1998;135:S179–S183.

155. Greilich PE, Carr ME, Carr SL, Chang AS: Reduction in platelet force development by cardiopulmonary bypass are associated with hemorrhage. Anesth Analg 1995;80:459–465.

156. Carr ME, Zekert SL, Hantgan RR, Braaten J: Glycoprotein IIb/IIIa blockade inhibits platelet-mediated force development and reduces gel elastic modulus. Thromb Haemost 1995;73:499–505.

157. Coller BS, Scudder LE, Beer J, et al: Monoclonal antibodies to platelet glycoprotein IIb/IIIa as antithrombotic agents. Ann N Y Acad Sci 1991;614:193–213.

158. Smith JW, Steinhubl SR, Lincoff AM, et al: Rapid platelet-function assay: An automated and quantitative cartridge-based method. Circulation 1999;99:620–625.

159. Kereiakes DJ, Mueller M, Howard W, et al: Efficacy of abciximab induced platelet blockade using a rapid point of care assay. J Thromb Thrombol 1999;7:265–276.

160. Steinhubl SR, Talley JD, Braden GA, et al: Point-of-care measured platelet inhibition correlates with a reduced risk of an adverse cardiac event after percutaneous coronary intervention: Results of the GOLD (AU—Assessing Ultegra) multicenter study. Circulation 2001;103:2572–2578.

161. Mukherjee D, Chew DP, Robbins M, et al: Clinical application of procedural platelet monitoring during percutaneous coronary intervention among patients at increased bleeding risk. J Thromb Thrombol 2001;11:151–154.

162. Carter AM, Gerning-Ossei N, Wilson IJ, et al: Association of platelet P1A polymorphism of glycoprotein IIb/IIIa and the fibrinogen β-beta 448 polymorphism with myocardial infarction and extent of coronary artery disease. Circulation 1997;96:1424–1431.

163. Phillips DR, Charo IF, Scarborough RM: GPIIb/IIIa: The responsive integrin. Cell 1991;65:359–362.

164. Goodall AH, Curzen N, Panesar M, et al: Increased binding of fibrinogen to glycoprotein IIIa-proline33 (HPA-1b, Pla2, Zwb) positive platelets in patients with cardiovascular disease. Eur Heart J 1999;20:742–747.

165. Feng DL, Lindpainter K, Larson MG, et al: Increased platelet aggregability associated with platelet GPIIb/IIIa Pla2 polymorphism-the Framingham Offspring Study. Arterioscler Thromb Vasc Biol 1999;19:1142–1147.

166. Weiss EJ, Bray PF, Tayback M, et al: A polymorphism of a platelet glycoprotein receptor as in inherited risk for coronary thrombosis. N Engl J Med 1996;334:1090–1094.

167. Ardissino D, Mannucci PM, Merlini PA, et al: Prothrombotic genetic risk factors in young survivors of myocardial infarction. Blood 1999;94:46–51.

168. Ridker PM, Hennekens CH, Schmitz C, et al: P1$^{A1/A2}$ polymorphism of platelet glycoprotein IIIa and risk of myocardial infarction, stroke and venous thrombosis. Lancet 1997;349:385–358.

169. Michelson AD, Furman MI, Goldschmidt-Clermont P, et al: Platelet GPIIIa PI (A) polymorphism display different sensitivities to agonists. Circulation 2000;101:1013–1018.

170. Walter DH, Schachinger V, Elsner M, et al: Statin therapy is associated with reduced restenosis rates after coronary stent implantation in carriers of the P1^{A2} allele of the platelet glycoprotein IIIa gene. Eur Heart J 2001;22:587–595.

171. Kenny D, Muckian C, Fitzgerald DJ, et al: Platelet glycoprotein Iba receptor polymorphisms and recurrent ischaemic events in acute coronary syndrome patients. J Thromb Thrombolysis, 2000;13:13–19.

172. Undas A, Brummel K, Musial J, et al: P1A2 polymorphism of β3 integrins is associated with enhanced thrombin generation and impaired antithrombotic action of aspirin at the site of microvascular injury. Circulation 2001;104:2666–2672.

Anticoagulant Therapy

Jeffrey I. Weitz
Shannon M. Bates

ROLE OF THROMBOSIS IN ISCHEMIC HEART DISEASE

Although acute coronary syndromes (ACS) are divided for the purpose of treatment assignment into unstable angina, non–ST-segment elevation myocardial infarction (MI), and ST-segment elevation MI, the clinical manifestations in all three instances usually are triggered by thrombosis superimposed on disrupted atherosclerotic plaque.[1-3] After plaque disruption, platelets adhere to newly exposed subendothelial matrix components, particularly collagen and von Willebrand factor, via constitutively expressed receptors. Adherent platelets become activated and recruit additional platelets by synthesizing thromboxane A_2 and releasing ADP.[4] Platelet activation induces conformational changes in glycoprotein (GP) IIb/IIIa, the most abundant receptors on the platelet surface. By binding fibrinogen or, under high shear conditions, von Willebrand factor, conformationally activated GP IIb/IIIa cross-links adjacent platelets,[4] resulting in platelet aggregation.

Damage to the vascular wall also exposes tissue factor–expressing cells to blood.[4] Lipid-laden macrophages in the core of atherosclerotic plaques are particularly rich in tissue factor,[3] explaining the propensity for thrombus formation at sites of plaque disruption. Exposed tissue factor binds activated factor VII (factor VIIa), which is found in small amounts in plasma, and factor VII. When bound to tissue factor, factor VII can undergo autoactivation, augmenting the local concentration of factor VIIa.[5]

The factor VIIa/tissue factor complex, also known as extrinsic tenase, activates factors IX and X, leading to the generation of factors IXa and Xa.[4] Factor IXa binds to factor VIIIa on the surface of activated platelets to form intrinsic tenase, a complex that also activates factor X. Factor Xa, generated through the extrinsic and intrinsic tenase complexes, assembles on the surface of activated platelets as part of the prothrombinase complex (factor Xa, factor Va, and calcium) that converts prothrombin to thrombin.[4] Thrombin converts fibrinogen to fibrin and activates factor XIII, which, by cross-linking the fibrin network, stabilizes the platelet/fibrin thrombus. In addition, thrombin triggers thrombus growth via several mechanisms. It amplifies its own generation by feedback activation of factors V and VIII; it activates factor XI on the platelet surface, augmenting factor Xa generation[5]; and it serves as a potent platelet agonist.[4]

The resultant intraluminal thrombus impairs blood flow, increasing shear and promoting further platelet deposition.

Because arterial thrombosis involves activation of coagulation in addition to platelet aggregation, most current strategies for its prevention and treatment focus on attenuating thrombin generation and inhibiting platelet aggregation. Antithrombotic drugs inhibit thrombus formation by either of these two mechanisms. *Anticoagulant* is a more specific term, referring to an agent that interferes with the activity of coagulation enzymes. Traditionally, unfractionated heparin has been the anticoagulant of choice in ACS. The limitations of unfractionated heparin have prompted the development of new anticoagulant agents. This chapter focuses on anticoagulants used in the management of ACS. The mechanisms of action and clinical trial data for these agents are reviewed. Particular attention is given to more recently developed anticoagulants and the opportunities presented by these therapies.

TARGETS FOR NEW ANTICOAGULANTS

Initiation of coagulation can be inhibited by agents that target the factor VIIa/tissue factor complex, whereas propagation of coagulation can be blocked by drugs that target factors IXa or Xa or inactivate factors Va or VIIIa, key cofactors in coagulation. Thrombin inhibitors prevent fibrin formation; block thrombin-mediated feedback activation of factors V, VIII, and XI; and attenuate thrombin-induced platelet aggregation (Fig. 29-1).

THROMBIN INHIBITORS

The procoagulant effects of thrombin can be blocked either by inactivating the enzyme itself or by preventing its generation from precursor coagulation proteins. Indirect thrombin inhibitors, such as unfractionated heparin and low-molecular-weight heparin (LMWH), activate the naturally occurring thrombin inhibitor, antithrombin. Direct thrombin inhibitors act in an antithrombin-independent manner by binding directly to thrombin and blocking its interaction with its substrates. The most extensively studied direct thrombin inhibitors are hirudin and bivalirudin.

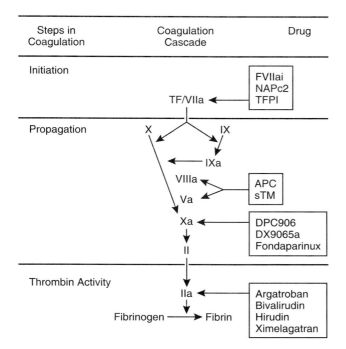

Steps in Coagulation	Coagulation Cascade	Drug

FIGURE 29–1. Sites of action of anticoagulant agents. The formation of the tissue factor/factor VIIa complex (TF/VIIa) triggers coagulation. This complex activates factors IX and X. The activated form of factor IX (factor IXa), along with the activated cofactor, factor VIIIa, propagates coagulation by activating factor X. Activated factor X (factor Xa), with its cofactor, activated factor V (factor Va), converts prothrombin to thrombin (IIa). Thrombin then converts fibrinogen to fibrin. Tissue factor pathway inhibitor (TFPI) and nematode anticoagulant protein (NAPc2) target TF/VIIa. Fondaparinux, DX9065a, and DPC 906 inactivate factor Xa. Activated protein C (APC) degrades and inactivates factors V and VIIIa, whereas soluble thrombomodulin (STM) binds thrombin and renders it a potent activator of protein C. Unfractionated heparin and low-molecular-weight heparin enhance antithrombin-mediated inactivation of thrombin and factor Xa, whereas the direct thrombin inhibitors (hirudin, bivalirudin, argatroban, and ximelagatran) inactivate thrombin directly.

Indirect Thrombin Inhibitors

Unfractionated Heparin

Mechanism of Action Unfractionated heparin acts as an anticoagulant by activating antithrombin.[6] A pentasaccharide sequence, randomly distributed along one third of the heparin chains, mediates the interaction between heparin and antithrombin (Fig. 29–2). On binding, heparin induces conformational change in the reactive site loop of antithrombin that changes it from a slow thrombin and factor Xa inhibitor to a rapid inhibitor of these coagulation enzymes. To enhance thrombin inhibition by antithrombin, heparin must bind simultaneously to the enzyme and the inhibitor, promoting formation of a ternary thrombin/antithrombin/heparin complex.[7,8] Only pentasaccharide-containing chains that contain at least 13 additional saccharide units and have a molecular mass of greater than or equal to 5400 are of sufficient length to perform this bridging reaction. In contrast, because bridging is unnecessary to enhance the inactivation of factor Xa by antithrombin, pentasaccharide-containing chains of any length catalyze this reaction.

Indications

Acute Myocardial Infarction with Thrombolysis The role of subcutaneous unfractionated heparin after thrombolysis in aspirin-treated patients has been examined in three large multicenter randomized trials.[9-11] Together, these studies indicate that high-dose subcutaneous unfractionated heparin (12,500 U twice daily, beginning 4 to 12 hours after initiation of thrombolytic therapy) produces no statistically significant reduction in mortality or other clinical benefit. Unfractionated heparin produces a small, but statistically significant, increase in major bleeds. The substitution of intravenous heparin for subcutaneous heparin provides little advantage in terms of reducing mortality and nonfatal stroke in patients receiving streptokinase.[11] Patients given streptokinase or anisoylated plasminogen streptokinase activator complex (APSAC) should receive intravenous heparin only if they are at high risk of systemic or venous thromboembolism (i.e., patients with acute anterior MI, congestive heart failure, previous embolic event, or atrial fibrillation).[12]

The results of small patency trials[13-15] and the first Global Utilization of Strategies to Open Occluded Coronary Arteries (GUSTO) trial[16] have been invoked to support the routine early administration of intravenous unfractionated heparin in patients given tissue plasminogen activator (t-PA) or reteplase. It is recommended that such patients be treated with heparin for 48 hours. Continuation beyond this time should be considered only in patients at high risk of systemic or venous thromboembolism.[12] Meta-analyses have shown no net mortality benefit associated with intravenous unfractionated heparin when used in conjunction with thrombolytics and full-dose aspirin.[17,18] The early termination of the Thrombolysis in Myocardial Infarction (TIMI)-9A[19] and GUSTO IIa[20] trials because of excessive major bleeding in patients receiving intravenous unfractionated heparin (despite the fact that the heparin dose used was only 20% higher than that used in previous trials) emphasizes the potential hazards of high-dose unfractionated heparin in this setting. This concern is reflected in recommendations to reduce the intensity of unfractionated heparin treatment in patients receiving thrombolytic therapy.[12,20] Unless a specific contraindication exists, patients undergoing coronary thrombolysis who do not receive high-dose unfractionated heparin should be given thromboprophylaxis with low-dose heparin therapy until ambulatory.[12]

Unstable Angina and Non–ST-Segment Elevation Myocardial Infarction Considerable confusion and controversy exist regarding recommendations for the use of unfractionated heparin in patients with unstable angina or non–ST-segment elevation MI. Interpretation of data is difficult because of variations in treatment regimens, patient population heterogeneity, and small trial size. Many small trials have shown limited benefit when heparin is added to aspirin in these patients.[22-24] A meta-analysis of these trials showed a 33% reduction in the relative risk of MI or death with the addition of intravenous

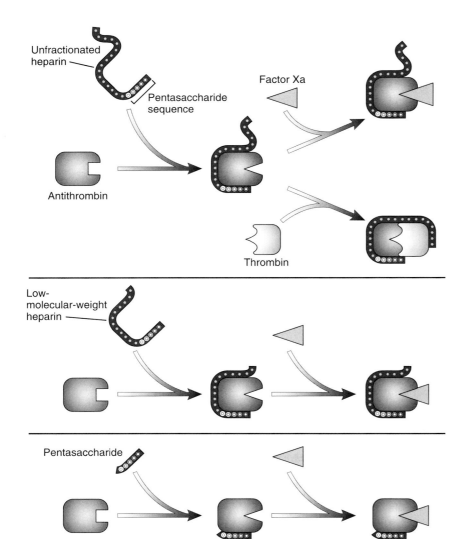

FIGURE 29–2. Mechanism of action of unfractionated heparin, low-molecular-weight heparin (LMWH), and synthetic pentasaccharide. The interaction of unfractionated heparin and LMWH with antithrombin is mediated by the pentasaccharide sequence of the drugs. Binding of these drugs or synthetic pentasaccharide to antithrombin causes a conformational change at the reactive center of antithrombin that accelerates its interaction with factor Xa. Consequently, unfractionated heparin, LMWH, and synthetic pentasaccharide (fondaparinux) catalyze the inactivation of factor Xa by antithrombin. In contrast, catalysis of antithrombin-mediated inactivation of thrombin requires the formation of a ternary heparin-antithrombin-thrombin complex. This complex can be formed only by chains at least 18 saccharide units long. Consequently, fondaparinux has no inhibitory activity against thrombin, whereas LMWH has less inhibitory activity against thrombin than does unfractionated heparin because most LMWH chains are not long enough to bridge antithrombin to thrombin.

unfractionated heparin to aspirin in patients with unstable angina.[25] Although this difference was not statistically significant, it suggests there may be a benefit. Current practice guidelines support the use of intravenous unfractionated heparin in addition to aspirin for treatment of unstable angina.[12]

Percutaneous Coronary Interventions   Intravenous unfractionated heparin has been used since the advent of percutaneous coronary interventions to prevent arterial thrombus formation at the site of arterial injury and to reduce the thrombogenicity of catheter equipment and guidewires used during the procedure.[26,27] There is no clinical trial evidence to support the routine use of postprocedural heparin in patients undergoing uncomplicated coronary angioplasty.[28,29]

Limitations of Unfractionated Heparin   The discontinuation of unfractionated heparin treatment in patients

with unstable angina or non–ST-segment elevation MI is associated with a clustering of recurrent ischemic events,[30,31] and abrupt vessel closure after successful coronary angioplasty occurs in 10% of patients despite the use of high-dose heparin in addition to aspirin.[26] This reactivation of the thrombotic process after heparin discontinuation has been attributed in part to the inability of the heparin/antithrombin complex to inactivate thrombin bound to fibrin,[32,33] fibrin degradation products,[32] and factor Xa bound to activated platelets trapped within the thrombus.[34,35] By activating prothrombin, bound factor Xa increases the amount of thrombin available to bind to fibrin.[34] Because thrombin bound to fibrin remains enzymatically active and protected from inactivation,[32] it can trigger thrombus growth by locally activating platelets[36] and amplifying coagulation.[37]

Nonspecific binding of unfractionated heparin to endothelial cells, plasma proteins or proteins released from activated platelets at the site of plaque rupture[38-40] results in reduced bioavailability, a dose-dependent half-life, and an unpredictable anticoagulant response.[41] Because the anticoagulant response to heparin is variable, careful laboratory monitoring is necessary when unfractionated heparin is given in therapeutic doses.

Dosages When unfractionated heparin is given in therapeutic doses, laboratory monitoring is essential to ensure that adequate anticoagulation is achieved.[42] Unfractionated heparin usually is monitored using the activated partial thromboplastin time (aPTT).[42] The therapeutic aPTT range, which targets a minimum and a maximum anticoagulant effect, differs depending on the aPTT reagent and coagulometer used to perform the test.[43] Several studies have shown that the use of a nomogram to adjust heparin doses improves the likelihood of obtaining a therapeutic effect.[42,44]

A lower therapeutic range is recommended for patients with acute myocardial ischemia receiving unfractionated heparin with thrombolytic agents or GP IIb/IIIa receptor antagonists than for patients receiving unfractionated heparin for other indications. Patients treated with t-PA or reteplase should receive a bolus of unfractionated heparin of 60 U/kg to a maximum dose of 4000 U at the initiation of thrombolysis, followed by an initial maintenance infusion of 12 U/kg/hr, to a maximum dose of 1000 U, adjusted to maintain the aPTT 1.5 to 2 times control. If intravenous unfractionated heparin is used in patients treated with streptokinase or APSAC, the unfractionated heparin infusion should be commenced once the aPTT is less than twice the control value. In patients not treated with thrombolytic therapy, intravenous unfractionated heparin should be initiated with a bolus of 75 U/kg, followed by an initial maintenance dose of 1250 U/hour adjusted to maintain the aPTT 1.5 to 2.0 times control. When heparin is given for prophylaxis, the dose ranges from 5000 to 7500 U subcutaneously twice daily,[12] and no anticoagulation monitoring is needed.

Percutaneous Coronary Interventions Monitoring of heparin anticoagulation in patients undergoing percutaneous coronary interventions is performed using the activated clotting time (ACT) rather than the aPTT because of the need for point-of-care results and because the large doses of heparin used in these settings produce unmeasurably high aPTT results. Patients undergoing percutaneous transluminal coronary angioplasty or stent placement without concomitant use of GP IIb/IIIa antagonists should receive a heparin bolus of 100 to 175 U/kg before the procedure. Incremental boluses should be given to maintain the ACT at 300 to 350 seconds during the procedure. The sheath should be removed 4 to 6 hours after an uncomplicated intervention. Continuation of heparin therapy depends on whether a thrombus or large vessel wall dissection is detected at the end of the procedure.[26] In patients receiving concomitant GP IIb/IIIa antagonists, the heparin bolus should be reduced to 70 U/kg and incremental boluses given to maintain the ACT at greater than 200 seconds.[26]

Side Effects The major complication of unfractionated heparin is hemorrhage.[45] The absolute risk of hemorrhage depends on the total dose of heparin; the patient's age; the tendency for bleeding; and the concomitant use of thrombolytic drugs, antiplatelet agents, and oral anticoagulants.[45] The risk of major hemorrhage ranges from 1% to 5% when heparin is added to aspirin in low-risk patients and is 19% in heparin-treated patients receiving concomitant thrombolytic therapy.[46]

Another complication is heparin-induced thrombocytopenia (HIT), which usually develops 5 to 15 days after heparin therapy is initiated, although it can occur within hours in patients previously exposed to heparin.[47] Although the incidence of arterial or venous thrombosis in patients with HIT has not been well defined, it has been estimated to occur in at least 20% of patients with this syndrome. HIT is initiated when heparin binds to platelets, causing platelet activation[48] and release of platelet factor 4. Heparin binds to platelet factor 4, alters its conformation, and stimulates the formation of antibodies against the heparin/platelet factor 4 complex.[49,50] Antibodies, usually of the IgG type, not only bind to these complexes, but also bind to platelet Fc receptors. Thrombosis is thought to be triggered by immune complex–mediated platelet activation, which causes platelet microparticle formation. By serving as a surface on which clotting factors assemble, these microparticles can promote thrombin generation,[51] triggering thrombosis.

When given for longer than 1 month, heparin may cause osteoporosis.[42,52] Allergic reactions,[53] alopecia, skin necrosis,[54] and hypoaldosteronism[55] are rare complications of unfractionated heparin therapy.

Contraindications and Drug Interactions Therapeutic doses of unfractionated heparin should not be given to patients who are actively bleeding or who are at high risk of life-threatening bleeding diatheses (Table 29–1). Unfractionated heparin should not be given to patients with a history of HIT. Concomitant use of oral anticoagulants, antiplatelet agents, thrombolytic drugs, and GP IIb/IIIa receptor antagonists increases the risk of hemorrhage.[12,45]

Low-Molecular-Weight Heparin

Mechanism of Action LMWHs are fragments of unfractionated heparin produced by chemical or enzymatic depolymerization processes that yield glycosaminoglycan chains with a mean molecular mass of approximately 5000 D.[56] Similar to unfractionated heparin, LMWHs act as anticoagulants by activating antithrombin via a pentasaccharide sequence found on about 20% of these smaller heparin chains (see Fig. 29–2).[6] LMWH exhibits less activity against thrombin than against factor Xa because less than half of the heparin chains are long enough to bridge antithrombin to thrombin.[7,57] Because heparin catalysis of factor Xa inhibition by antithrombin does not require bridging between factor Xa and antithrombin, the smaller

■ ■ ■

TABLE 29–1 CONTRAINDICATIONS TO ANTICOAGULANT THERAPY

Absolute

Active bleeding
Severe bleeding diathesis
Severe thrombocytopenia
Recent neurosurgery, ocular surgery, or intracranial bleed

Relative

Moderate thrombocytopenia
Bleeding diathesis
Brain metastases
Recent major trauma
Recent major abdominal surgery (<1 or 2 days)
Gastrointestinal or genitourinary bleeding within the past 14 days
Endocarditis
Severe hypertension
    Systolic blood pressure >200 mm Hg and/or diastolic blood
        pressure >120 mm Hg at presentation

pentasaccharide-containing chains in LMWH retain their ability to catalyze factor Xa inhibition. Consequently, LMWHs have greater inhibitory activity against factor Xa than against thrombin.

Because binding to endothelial cells and to plasma proteins is chain-length dependent, with longer heparin chains having greater affinity than shorter chains, LMWHs bind less avidly to plasma proteins[58,59] and endothelium[60] than unfractionated heparin. Consequently, LMWHs produce a more predictable dose response[61,62] than unfractionated heparin and have a longer half-life. With these pharmacokinetic advantages, routine laboratory monitoring of LMWHs is unnecessary. The advantages of LMWH over unfractionated heparin are summarized in Table 29–2. Because LMWHs are cleared principally by the kidneys and their biologic half-life is prolonged in patients with renal failure,[63] monitoring is necessary when therapeutic doses are given to patients with renal insufficiency.[63] In these patients, the dose of LMWH should be adjusted to achieve a peak anti–factor Xa level of 0.5 to 1.2 U/mL.

Indications

Myocardial Infarction with Thrombolysis There is limited experience with LMWH in ST-segment elevation acute MI. Although adjunctive therapy with LMWH seems to be as effective as unfractionated heparin in achieving infarct-related artery patency after thrombolysis,[64-67] the use of protocols with lower doses of LMWH seems necessary to reduce the risk of bleeding.[64,65,67,68] Because of the small size of these trials, however, confirmatory investigations are necessary.

Unstable Angina and Non–ST-Segment Elevation Myocardial Infarction Many randomized trials have examined the role of LMWH in aspirin-treated patients with unstable angina.[69-74] When added to aspirin in the acute setting, dalteparin is superior to placebo[69] but similar to unfractionated heparin for prevention of death and MI in patients with unstable angina and non–ST-segment elevation MI.[70] In contrast, a course of therapy with enoxaparin results in reduced risk of death, MI, and recurrent angina compared with unfractionated heparin that is sustained for at least 1 year.[71,72,75] Another LMWH, nadroparin (Fraxiparine), has not been shown to be more effective than unfractionated heparin in patients with unstable angina or non–ST-segment elevation MI.[73]

The reason for the difference between the results of studies using dalteparin[70] and nadroparin[73] and studies using enoxaparin[71,72] is uncertain. Dalteparin and nadroparin are depolymerized by different chemical methods than enoxaparin, and all three LMWHs have different molecular weight distributions. These differences are unlikely, however, to explain the more favorable results seen with enoxaparin because a more aggressive LMWH regimen (in terms of anti–factor Xa and anti–factor IIa units) was used in the study comparing dalteparin with unfractionated heparin[70] than in the enoxaparin-containing studies.[71,72] Although the unfractionated heparin dosage regimens were similar in all the studies, the average duration of unfractionated heparin therapy was shorter than that of LMWH therapy in one of the studies evaluating enoxaparin.[72] The event rates in patients assigned unfractionated heparin were higher in the stud-

■ ■ ■

TABLE 29–2 ADVANTAGES OF LOW-MOLECULAR-WEIGHT HEPARINS OVER UNFRACTIONATED HEPARIN

ADVANTAGE	EFFECT	CLINICAL CONSEQUENCE
Reduced binding to proteins	More predictable anticoagulant response	Routine monitoring of anticoagulant therapy unnecessary
Reduced binding to and clearance by endothelial cells and macrophages	Clearance predominantly by renal mechanisms	Longer plasma half-life; once-daily dosing effective
Reduced binding to osteoblasts	Reduced activation of osteoclasts	Lower incidence of osteopenia and reduced risk of heparin-associated osteoporosis and fracture with prolonged treatment
Reduced affinity for platelets and platelet factor 4	Less platelet activation with reduced release of platelet factor 4; reduced formation of complexes of heparin/platelet factor 4	Reduced incidence of heparin-induced thrombocytopenia

ies evaluating enoxaparin[71,72] than in the trial assessing dalteparin.[70] Although the favorable results with enoxaparin might have been the result of chance, this explanation is less likely given that there are two positive studies with this drug.[71,72] Whether one LMWH preparation is more effective than the others in the acute treatment of unstable angina is an open question that can be answered only by direct comparison of different LMWHs in randomized trials. Overall, LMWH is associated with at least as favorable outcomes as unfractionated heparin in this setting. Given these results, the practical convenience of use, and the lower incidence of heparin-induced thrombocytopenia (HIT), LMWHs seem to be a better choice in this setting than unfractionated heparin.[12]

The prolonged use of LMWH in patients with unstable angina has been examined in four trials.[69,70,72,74] In the first two, prolonged use of a reduced once-daily dose of dalteparin after day 6 did not provide any additional benefit over aspirin.[69,70] In the FRISC (Fast Revascularization during Instability in Coronary Artery Disease) II study, 3 months of treatment with a higher dose of twice-daily dalteparin significantly reduced the risk of death and MI compared with placebo at 30 days. These benefits were not sustained during longer term follow-up, however.[74] No additional benefit, beyond that seen with in-hospital administration, has been derived from continuing once-daily subcutaneous enoxaparin on an outpatient basis.[72] Given these results and the risk of increased bleeding complications with long-term anticoagulation, the role of outpatient LMWH remains controversial.

Studies evaluating combinations of LMWH and GP IIb/IIIa antagonists are under way. In a report of 525 patients with unstable angina and non–ST-segment elevation MI randomized to receive either tirofiban and enoxaparin or tirofiban and unfractionated heparin, major and minor bleeding were equally low in each group.[76]

Percutaneous Coronary Angioplasty To date, four trials have failed to show that LMWH therapy reduces the risk of late restenosis in patients undergoing coronary angioplasty,[77-80] and the use of LMWH cannot be recommended for this purpose. Increasing experience with short-term LMWH in place of unfractionated heparin in patients undergoing percutaneous coronary interventions[81-84] suggests, however, that safety and efficacy of these procedures is not diminished by this substitution.

Dosages When given in treatment doses, LMWH can be given once or twice daily subcutaneously in weight-adjusted doses without laboratory monitoring.[154] Only twice-daily dosing regimens have been evaluated in patients with unstable angina. For dalteparin, the recommended dose is 120 anti–factor Xa U/kg twice daily[69,70]; for enoxaparin, the recommended dose is 100 anti–factor Xa U/kg (1 mg/kg) twice daily,[71,72] with or without an initial intravenous bolus of 30 mg.

Side Effects and Drug Interactions Based on results of trials comparing LMWH with unfractionated heparin in patients with unstable angina, LMWH does not increase the risk of major bleeding.[69-72] In the TIMI 11A trial, however, patients receiving more than 1 mg/kg (100 U/kg) of enoxaparin subcutaneously twice daily were more likely to develop major hemorrhage.[86] These findings suggest that 1 mg of enoxaparin subcutaneously twice daily represents the maximum dose that can be given safely in this setting, but that the dosing should be reconsidered in high-risk subgroups, such as patients with decreased renal function.

Protamine sulfate, widely used as an antidote to neutralize the high doses of unfractionated heparin administered to patients undergoing cardiopulmonary bypass surgery and to antagonize its hemorrhagic side effects, completely blocks the inhibitory effects of LMWH on thrombin. Because only longer LMWH chains bind protamine sulfate, the anti–factor Xa activity of LMWH is incompletely reversed.[87] Although studies in laboratory animal models suggest that bleeding produced by high concentrations of LMWH is only incompletely controlled with protamine sulfate,[88] similar studies in humans are lacking.

There is evidence from a randomized trial that the incidences of heparin-induced IgG formation and of HIT are lower in patients treated with prophylactic doses of LMWH than in patients treated with low-dose unfractionated heparin,[89] possibly because LMWHs cause less platelet activation[48] and release of platelet factor 4 and because the lower affinity of LMWH for platelet factor 4 results in reduced formation of heparin/platelet factor 4 complexes.

Heparin binding to osteoblasts[90] and osteoclast activation are chain-length dependent, and bone loss in laboratory animals is less marked with LMWH than with unfractionated heparin.[91,92] These laboratory findings are consistent with the results of a small randomized study that showed a lower incidence of bone fracture in patients assigned to LMWH than in patients randomized to unfractionated heparin.[93] The risk of osteoporosis with long-term LMWH has not been established in large studies.

Contraindications LMWH should not be used in patients who have absolute contraindications to anticoagulant therapy (see Table 29–1). The risk of hemorrhage is increased with concomitant use of oral anticoagulants, antiplatelet agents, or thrombolytic drugs.[45]

Although the incidence of HIT is lower in patients treated with LMWH than in patients given unfractionated heparin,[89] there is a high degree of in vitro cross-reactivity between LMWHs and the antibody that causes HIT.[94] In addition, the administration of LMWH can be associated with the development of thrombocytopenia in previously unexposed individuals and in individuals with a history of HIT.[95-97] LMWH should not be given to patients with established HIT. It is probably best to avoid LMWHs in patients with significant renal dysfunction (creatinine clearance <30 mL/min) because these drugs are cleared via the kidneys.[63,85]

Oral Heparins

Delivery systems have been developed that make it possible to give heparin or LMWH orally. These systems use synthetic amino acids such as sodium N-(8[2-hydroxybenzoyl]amino) caprylate (SNAC) or disodium-(10-[2-hydroxybenzoyl]amino) decanoate (SNAD) that can form noncovalent bonds with heparin to facilitate heparin absorption by the gut.[98] Although absorption is limited and variable, sufficient amounts of heparin can be delivered orally to prolong the aPTT.[98] Phase II/III studies comparing SNAC/heparin with LMWH for venous thromboembolism prophylaxis in patients undergoing elective hip or knee arthroplasty have been completed, but the data have not been released.

Direct Thrombin Inhibitors

Direct thrombin inhibitors bind thrombin and block its interaction with substrates, preventing fibrin formation; thrombin-mediated activation of clotting factors V, VII, XI, or XIII; and thrombin-induced platelet aggregation. As a class, these agents have potential biologic and pharmacokinetic advantages over heparin. In contrast to unfractionated heparin and LMWH, direct thrombin inhibitors inactivate fibrin-bound thrombin,[32] in addition to fluid-phase thrombin. Consequently, direct thrombin inhibitors may attenuate thrombus accretion more effectively. Direct thrombin inhibitors also produce a more predictable anticoagulant effect than unfractionated heparin because they do not bind to plasma proteins and are not neutralized by platelet factor 4.[99,100]

In vitro and in vivo studies have suggested that direct thrombin inhibitors are more potent antithrombotic agents than unfractionated heparin.[101] Despite extensive evaluation in clinical trials, however, there has been uncertainty about their role in the management of patients with ACS. A meta-analysis based on individual data from 35,970 patients in 11 randomized trials comparing direct thrombin inhibitors (hirudin, bivalirudin, argatroban, inogatran, or efegatran) with heparin for management of ACS showed a lower risk of death or MI at the end of treatment and at 30 days with direct thrombin inhibitors than with heparin. This reduction primarily reflected a lower risk of MI.[102] Subgroup analyses indicated a benefit of direct thrombin inhibitors in ACS trials and percutaneous coronary intervention trials.[102] A reduction in death or MI was seen with hirudin and bivalirudin but not with univalent direct thrombin inhibitors.[102] Based on this analysis, additional studies are warranted to identify the role of direct thrombin inhibitors in the management of patients with ACS. The characteristics of the approved direct thrombin inhibitors are highlighted in Table 29–3.

Hirudin

Mechanism of Action Hirudin is a 65-amino acid polypeptide originally isolated from the saliva of the medicinal leech. A potent and specific inhibitor of thrombin, it binds to thrombin's active site by its globular amino-terminal domain and to thrombin's substrate recognition site (exosite 1) via its carboxy-terminal domain.[103,104] In contrast to natural hirudin, recombinant hirudin lacks a sulfate group on the tyrosine residue at position 63. Although this lack results in a 10-fold reduction in its affinity for thrombin, recombinant hirudin still binds tightly to the enzyme, forming a slowly reversible complex.[105] The almost irreversible nature of this complex may be considered a relative weakness because there is no available antidote should bleeding occur. Hirudin is not absorbed via the gastrointestinal tract and must be administered intravenously or by subcutaneous injection.[100] Hirudin is cleared predominantly by the kidneys and undergoes little hepatic metabolism.[100,106] It has a plasma half-life of 40 minutes after intravenous administration and approximately 120 minutes after subcutaneous injection.[100]

Indications Hirudin has been tested as an adjunct to thrombolytic therapy in patients with acute MI and as a replacement for heparin in patients with unstable angina or non–ST-elevation MI and patients undergoing percutaneous coronary interventions.

Acute Myocardial Infarction with Thrombolysis Three trials of hirudin as an adjunct to coronary thrombolysis were stopped prematurely because hirudin produced an unacceptable risk of intracranial hemorrhage.[19,20,107] Lower doses of hirudin were assessed in three studies.[108-110] Overall, hirudin was no more effective than heparin at 30 days,[110,111] although short-term benefits at 24 hours and 48 hours were observed in one study,[109] and a 35% reduction in the rate of death and reinfarction at 30 days was seen in a retrospective analysis of the subgroup of patients who received streptokinase.[112] No such favorable interaction was seen in patients receiving hirudin as an adjunct to t-PA. Although critics of these studies suggested that the hirudin dose was too low, treatment initiation too delayed, and treatment duration too short to obtain evidence of clinical efficacy, in the population of patients mentioned, therapy with hirudin was no better than unfractionated heparin in preventing adverse clinical outcomes.

■ ▪ ■

TABLE 29–3 PROPERTIES OF HIRUDIN, BIVALIRUDIN, AND ARGATROBAN

PROPERTY	HIRUDIN	BIVALIRUDIN	ARGATROBAN
Molecular mass	7000	1980	527
Site(s) of interaction with thrombin	Active site and exosite 1	Active site and exosite 1	Active site
Predominant mechanism of clearance	Renal	Proteolysis at sites other than kidneys and liver	Hepatic
Plasma half-life after intravenous administration (minutes)	40	24	45

Unstable Angina and Non–ST-Segment Elevation Myocardial Infarction Hirudin was compared with heparin in two large trials involving patients with unstable angina or non–ST-segment elevation MI. Among patients enrolled in the GUSTO-IIb trial who presented without ST-segment elevation and did not receive thrombolytic therapy, there was no significant difference in the rate of death or MI between patients who received intravenous unfractionated heparin and patients treated with hirudin,[109] although there was a trend for an early, but transient, benefit with hirudin. In the OASIS-2 (Organization to Assess Strategies for Ischemic Syndromes) study, hirudin was more effective than unfractionated heparin during the 3 days of treatment. There was no additional gain or loss of benefit after treatment stopped, and a nonstatistically significant advantage in favor of hirudin with respect to cardiovascular death or new MI was still present at days 7 and 35.[113] Combined data from the trials using this agent in patients with unstable angina or non–ST-segment elevation MI show,[108,109,113] however, that hirudin provides a statistically significant reduction in cardiovascular death and MI rates at 72 hours and 7 days. Although the effect persists beyond 7 days, its impact is attenuated statistically over time.[114]

Percutaneous Coronary Interventions Hirudin produced only transient advantages over heparin with respect to death; nonfatal MI; or need for coronary bypass surgery, stenting, or second angioplasty when used after coronary angioplasty.[115] Consequently the sole use of hirudin in this setting cannot be recommended until additional studies are performed.

Dosages Hirudin's narrow therapeutic window makes monitoring of anticoagulant effect necessary, particularly when the drug is given in conjunction with thrombolytic agents.[19,20,107] Generally, treatment is monitored with the aPTT, which should be determined before treatment, 4 hours after the start of intravenous hirudin therapy, 4 hours after every dosage change, and at least once daily.[116] If the aPTT is subtherapeutic, the infusion rate should be increased by 20%. If the aPTT is supratherapeutic, the aPTT should be stopped for 2 hours and if the aPTT is within the therapeutic range, the infusion should be restarted at 50% of the previous dose.[117] There are problems when the aPTT is used to monitor hirudin therapy, including variability in responsiveness between patients[118] and the lack of a linear correlation of the aPTT with plasma hirudin levels. At higher doses, use of the ecarin clotting time may be more appropriate because its correlation with plasma hirudin levels is more linear.[119,120] In patients with unstable angina or non–ST-segment elevation MI, hirudin has been given as a 0.4 mg/kg bolus, followed by a 0.15 mg/kg/hr infusion for 72 hours, adjusted to maintain the aPTT between 60 and 100 seconds.[113]

Side Effects Although major bleeding has been observed to occur more frequently in patients treated

with hirudin than in patients receiving adjusted-dose unfractionated heparin,[102,114] no excess of strokes or life-threatening bleeds has been shown.[115] The absolute risk of major bleeding with hirudin therapy is similar to that seen in other trials with the use of enoxaparin,[71,72] dalteparin,[70] and combined GP IIb/IIIa antagonist and unfractionated heparin therapy.[121,122] No specific antidote is available to neutralize hirudin. Hirudin-induced bleeding diathesis has been reversed by prothrombin complex concentrates,[123] hemodialysis, or hemofiltration.[124]

Contraindications and Drug Interactions Hirudin should not be given to patients with contraindications to anticoagulants (see Table 29–1). The drug is cleared by the kidneys, and dose adjustments and careful monitoring are required if this agent is used in patients with renal dysfunction.[116] The risk of hemorrhage is increased when hirudin is combined with antiplatelet agents and thrombolytic drugs; the interaction when hirudin is used in combination with GP IIb/IIIa receptor antagonists, unfractionated heparin, and LMWH has not been well studied.[116]

Bivalirudin

Mechanism of Action Similar to hirudin, bivalirudin also acts as a bivalent inhibitor of thrombin.[125] This synthetic 20-amino acid polypeptide comprises an active site-directed moiety, D-Phe-Pro-Arg-Pro, linked via a tetraglycine spacer to a dodecapeptide analogue of the carboxy-terminal of hirudin[125] that interacts with exosite 1 on thrombin.[126] In contrast to hirudin, bivalirudin produces only transient inhibition of the active site of thrombin because, when bound, thrombin cleaves the Arg-Pro bond within the amino-terminal of bivalirudin.[127,128] Without its amino-terminal segment, the carboxy-terminal portion of bivalirudin bound to thrombin's substrate recognition site is a much weaker thrombin inhibitor.[127]

Bivalirudin's plasma half-life after intravenous infusion is 24 minutes.[129] This shorter half-life may confer bivalirudin with a better safety profile than hirudin. Only a fraction of bivalirudin is renally excreted, suggesting that hepatic metabolism and proteolysis at other sites contribute to its clearance.[129] This agent must be administered parenterally.

Indications
Acute Myocardial Infarction with Thrombolysis As a result of bivalirudin's early promise in patency trials using streptokinase,[130-132] the HERO-2 (Hirulog Early Reperfusion/Occlusion) trial, an open-label randomized study of 17,073 patients, was performed comparing this agent with unfractionated heparin in patients receiving streptokinase for acute MI.[133] Although there was no difference between the two regimens with respect to the primary end point of 30-day mortality in this study, bivalirudin was associated with a reduction in the rate of reinfarction at 96 hours, a prespecified secondary end point. The composite net clinical benefit outcome of

death, MI, and nonfatal disabling stroke favored bivalirudin (P = .049). A reduction in MI in the absence of an effect on mortality is consistent with the results with other direct thrombin inhibitors.[102] There was a small but statistically significant increase in the rate of moderate bleeding in patients receiving bivalirudin (1.4% versus 1.1%). A similar trend was seen for excess severe bleeding (0.7% versus 0.5%, P = 0.07). This was an unexpected finding given the reduced risk of bleeding seen in earlier studies with bivalirudin. Post-hoc subgroup analysis indicated that the excess bleeding with bivalirudin could be accounted for by the fact that, in contrast to heparin, the dose of bivalirudin was not titrated to the aPTT. The rates of major bleeding and intracranial hemorrhage in this trial were substantially lower than those in trials evaluating heparin or other antithrombotic agents as adjuncts to thrombolysis in ACS.[134] Bivalirudin has not been evaluated in patients receiving t-PA or third-generation bolus thrombolytic therapy.

Unstable Angina   Early dose-ranging studies of bivalirudin in patients with unstable angina suggest that this drug is effective and well tolerated in this clinical situation.[135-137] These results require confirmation in large clinical studies.

Percutaneous Coronary Interventions   Bivalirudin has been studied as an alternative to heparin in patients with unstable angina undergoing percutaneous coronary angioplasty. Initial results of the bivalirudin (Hirulog) Angioplasty Study showed that bivalirudin is no more effective than heparin for patients undergoing percutaneous coronary angioplasty, although it produces less bleeding than high-dose heparin and is superior to heparin in high-risk patients undergoing intervention for postinfarction angina.[138] In a reanalysis of the study results, however, bivalirudin was more effective than heparin at reducing the risk of death, MI, and revascularization at 6 months.[139] Based on this reanalysis and meta-analyses,[102,140] bivalirudin seems to be an effective alternative to heparin in patients undergoing coronary angioplasty. Licensed for use as an alternative to heparin in patients undergoing percutaneous coronary interventions, studies are under way to determine whether bivalirudin obviates the need for GP IIb/IIIa antagonists in all but the highest risk patients.

Dosages   In contrast to hirudin, there is no evidence that bivalirudin requires laboratory monitoring in patients undergoing coronary angioplasty because the drug is safe when given in weight-adjusted doses (bolus of 1 mg/kg, followed by a 4-hour infusion at a rate of 2.6 mg/kg/hr, then a 14- to 20-hour infusion at a rate of 0.2 mg/kg/hr) to patients undergoing this procedure.[138,141] In contrast, the results of the HERO-2 trial suggest that the dose of bivalirudin should be titrated to achieve an aPTT 1.5 to 2.5 times control if bivalirudin is used as an adjunct to streptokinase and aspirin for treatment of acute MI.[130]

Side Effects   It has been suggested that the principal benefit of bivalirudin seems to be a reduction in the risk of major hemorrhage. In the Bivalirudin Angioplasty Study Investigators, major bleeding occurred less frequently in patients randomized to bivalirudin than in patients receiving unfractionated heparin (3.8% and 9.8%, P < .001).[148] There was no difference in the rate of intracranial hemorrhage between patients given unfractionated heparin and patients given bivalirudin. Although there was no statistically significant difference in the rates of major bleeding in patients receiving bivalirudin or heparin as an adjunct to streptokinase therapy for acute MI in the HERO-2 study,[133] the Direct Thrombin Inhibitor Trialists' Collaborative Group did find a reduced risk of major bleeding with bivalirudin treatment.[102]

Contraindications and Drug Interactions   Bivalirudin is contraindicated in patients with the conditions listed in Table 29-1. The concomitant use of antiplatelet agents, other anticoagulants, or thrombolytic agents with bivalirudin increases the risk of hemorrhage.

Active Site–Directed Direct Thrombin Inhibitors

Argatroban

A carboxylic acid derivative, argatroban binds noncovalently to the active site of thrombin.[142] This agent has a half-life of 20 to 60 minutes and prolongs the aPTT in a dose-dependent manner. Argatroban is extensively metabolized in the liver, and its plasma levels are not influenced by renal function.[142] This drug is an effective alternative to heparin in patients with HIT and is approved for this indication. Studies are under way to evaluate argatroban for the treatment of arterial thrombosis.[143,144]

Inogatran

In an animal model, inogatran, a noncovalent thrombin inhibitor, improved thrombolysis when given together with, but not after, t-PA.[145] When used in unstable angina, however, inogatran was associated with a statistically significant higher incidence of death, MI, and refractory or recurrent angina compared with unfractionated heparin.[146]

Efegatran

A phase II dose-finding study in patients with unstable angina suggested that intravenous efegatran, a covalent inhibitor that forms a slowly reversible complex with thrombin, had promising antithrombotic efficacy. Of patients receiving this direct thrombin inhibitor, 20% developed superficial thrombophlebitis, however.[147]

Ximelagatran

Ximelagatran, an uncharged lipophilic drug with little intrinsic activity against thrombin, is a prodrug of melagatran, an active site–directed thrombin inhibitor. Ximelagatran is well absorbed from the gastrointestinal tract and undergoes rapid biotransformation to melagatran.[148,149] The drug produces a predictable anticoagulant response after oral administration, and little or no laboratory monitoring seems to be necessary. In phase II studies, ximelagatran was shown to be safe and to have antithrombotic efficacy when used as prophylaxis against venous thromboembolism after elective hip or knee arthroplasty.[150,151] Phase III clinical trials comparing ximelagatran with warfarin for prevention and treatment of venous thromboembolism are under way. Ximelagatran also is being compared with warfarin for prevention of cardioembolic events in patients with nonvalvular atrial fibrillation based on promising phase II data. Ximelagatran also is undergoing phase II evaluation in patients with ACS.

INHIBITORS OF INITIATION OF COAGULATION

Because tissue factor in disrupted atherosclerotic plaques initiates thrombosis, alternative therapeutic approaches have focused on the development of agents that target the factor VIIa/tissue factor complex and block the initiation of coagulation.[4] The drugs in the most advanced stage of development are recombinant tissue factor pathway inhibitor (TFPI) and nematode anticoagulant peptide (NAPc2) (Fig. 29–3). Active site–blocked factor VIIa (factor VIIai) also has been evaluated in humans.

Tissue Factor Pathway Inhibitor

TFPI forms a complex with factor Xa that binds to factor VIIa/tissue factor and inhibits thrombin generation.[152] Only small amounts of TFPI circulate in the blood in the free state. Most of the circulating TFPI is associated with lipoproteins or is bound to the endothelium. Additional TFPI is stored in platelets.[153] Full-length TFPI is released from the endothelium when heparin or LWMH is given, presumably because these agents displace TFPI bound to endothelial glycosaminoglycans. When administered intravenously, TFPI has a short half-life because it is cleaved rapidly into nonfunctional truncated forms by an unknown protease. In pigs, TFPI attenuates injury-induced neointimal hyperplasia, and it inhibits smooth muscle cell migration in vitro.[154] TFPI attenuates the coagulopathy and improves survival in sepsis models in animal models.[155-157] Based on promising phase II results,[158] TFPI was compared with placebo in a large phase III clinical trial in patients with severe sepsis. Although the results have yet to be published, a preliminary report suggests that TFPI failed to reduce mortality in these high-risk patients.

Nematode Anticoagulant Protein c2

NAPc2, an anticoagulant protein isolated from the nematode *Ancylostoma caninum*, binds to a noncatalytic site

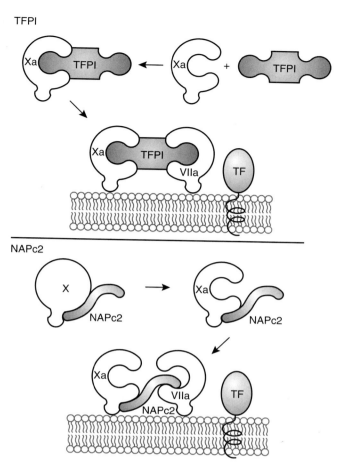

FIGURE 29–3. Inhibition of the initiation of coagulation. Tissue factor pathway inhibitor (TFPI) and nematode anticoagulant protein (NAPc2) inhibit factor VIIa bound to tissue factor in a factor Xa-dependent fashion. TFPI first binds and inactivates factor Xa, then factor Xa–bound TFPI inactivates factor VIIa. In contrast, NAPc2 binds to a noncatalytic site on factor X or factor Xa, then factor Xa–bound NAPc2 inhibits factor VIIa. Because NAPc2 binds to factor X and factor Xa, NAPc2 has a long half-life.

on factor X and factor Xa and inhibits factor VIIa within the factor VIIa/tissue factor complex.[159] Functionally, NAPc2 behaves similar to TFPI. Because NAPc2 binds to factor X and factor Xa, it has a half-life of almost 50 hours after subcutaneous injection. In a phase II study, NAPc2 showed promise in preventing venous thromboembolism after elective knee replacement surgery.[160] Studies are under way to evaluate the utility of NAPc2 in patients with unstable angina.

Active Site–Blocked Factor VIIa

FVIIai, an inactivated factor VIIa, is a competitive inhibitor of tissue factor-dependent factor IX or X activation. In in vitro studies and animal studies, infusions of FVIIai prevented thrombus formation on artificial surfaces or injured vasculature.[161-166] This agent is undergoing phase II evaluation in patients having percutaneous coronary interventions.

INHIBITORS OF PROPAGATION OF COAGULATION

The propagation of coagulation can be inhibited by drugs that block factors IXa or Xa or by agents that inactivate their respective cofactors, factor VIIIa or factor Va.

Factor IXa Inhibitors

Factor IXa is essential for amplification of coagulation.[167] Strategies to block factor IXa activity are in the early stages of development. Active site–blocked factor IX (factor IXai) competes with factor IXa for incorporation into the intrinsic tenase complex that assembles on the surface of activated platelets. Factor IXai inhibits clot formation in vitro and has been shown to block coronary artery thrombosis in a dog model.[168] Monoclonal antibodies against factor IX/IXa have been described.[169-171] One, a chimeric humanized derivative of an antibody that inhibits factor XI–mediated activation of factor IX and blocks factor IXa activity, has shown antithrombotic activity in a rat arterial thrombosis model.[170,171]

Factor Xa Inhibitors

Direct and indirect factor Xa inhibitors have been investigated. Direct factor Xa inhibitors, agents that bind directly to factor Xa and block its activity, include recombinant analogues of natural inhibitors and synthetic drugs that target the active site of factor Xa. Synthetic pentasaccharide, an analogue of the pentasaccharide sequence of heparin that mediates its interaction with antithrombin,[172] is a new indirect factor Xa inhibitor that blocks factor Xa in an antithrombin-dependent fashion. The ability of the direct factor Xa inhibitors to access and inhibit platelet-bound factor Xa,[173] in addition to free factor Xa, is a potential advantage of these agents over indirect inhibitors.

Direct Factor Xa Inhibitors

Natural inhibitors of factor Xa include tick anticoagulant peptide (TAP) and antistasin. TAP[174] and antistasin[175] originally were isolated from the soft tick and the Mexican leech. Both are available in recombinant forms. TAP is a 60-amino acid polypeptide that forms a stoichiometric complex with factor Xa.[174] TAP seems to bind to factor Xa in a two-step fashion[174] in which an initial low-affinity interaction involving a site distinct from the catalytic site of the enzyme is followed by a high-affinity interaction with the active site, resulting in the formation of a stable enzyme inhibitor complex. Antistasin, a 119-amino acid polypeptide, is also a tight-binding, slowly reversible inhibitor of factor Xa.[176] TAP and antistasin have been shown to reduce arterial thrombosis[177,178] and restenosis[179] in animal models. Because they are antigenic, neither TAP nor antistasin has been tested in humans.

DX-9065a[180] and DPC 906 are synthetic nonpeptidic, low-molecular-weight, reversible inhibitors of factor Xa. Although DX-9065 exhibits oral bioavailability,[181] high doses must be given to produce an antithrombotic effect. In a phase I study in patients with atherosclerotic disease, intravenous DX-9065 seemed safe and did not cause excess bleeding. DX-9065a is currently undergoing phase II evaluation in patients with ACS or patients having percutaneous coronary interventions. DPC906, an aminobenzisoxazole that binds factor Xa with high affinity, has good oral bioavailability and a half-life of approximately 12 hours. The antithrombotic potential of this agent is currently being investigated in a phase II trial of thromboprophylaxis in knee arthroplasty patients.

Indirect Factor Xa Inhibitors

Fondaparinux, a synthetic pentasaccharide analogue, has high affinity for antithrombin. Because it is too short to bridge antithrombin to thrombin, fondaparinux enhances the rate of factor Xa inactivation by antithrombin but has no effect on the rate of thrombin inhibition. This agent has almost complete bioavailability after subcutaneous injection and a dose-independent elimination half-life of approximately 15 hours.[182] Fondaparinux is not metabolized, and clearance is almost exclusively by the kidneys.[183] The antithrombotic efficacy of fondaparinux was shown in four phase III trials comparing this agent with LMWH for thromboprophylaxis after surgery for hip fracture or for elective hip or knee arthroplasty.[184-186] In a randomized, open-label, dose-finding trial, coadministration of fondaparinux and alteplase in ST-segment elevation acute MI produced similar angiographic patency rates at 90 minutes, as did treatment with unfractionated heparin and alteplase.[187] Fondaparinux also compared favorably with enoxparin in a large phase II trial of patients with ACS without ST-segment elevation; a pivotal phase III trial is now in the planning stages.

Inhibitors of Factors VIIIa and Va

Factors VIIIa and Va, key cofactors for intrinsic tenase and prothrombinase, are crucial for propagation of coagulation. Both cofactors are inactivated by activated protein C, a naturally occurring anticoagulant that is generated when thrombin binds to thrombomodulin, producing a complex that activates protein C. Strategies aimed at enhancing the protein C anticoagulant pathway include administration of protein C or activated protein C concentrates or soluble thrombomodulin.

Plasma-derived and recombinant forms of protein C and activated protein C are available. In a phase III trial, intravenous recombinant activated protein C, known as Drotrecogin Alpha (activated), reduced mortality in patients with severe sepsis compared with placebo.[188] These findings prompted licensing of recombinant activated protein C for this indication.

Similar to membrane-bound thrombomodulin, soluble thrombomodulin complexes thrombin and induces a conformational change in the active site of the enzyme that abolishes its procoagulant activity and converts it into a potent activator of protein C. Recombinant soluble thrombomodulin[189] has been shown to be an effective antithrombotic agent in a variety of animal models.[190,191]

A phase II trial examining the utility of soluble thrombomodulin for thromboprophylaxis after elective hip arthroplasty is forthcoming.

VITAMIN K ANTAGONISTS

Mechanism of Action

Coumarin derivatives are vitamin K antagonists that interfere with the cyclic interconversion of vitamin K and its 2,3 epoxide (vitamin K epoxide).[192] Vitamin K acts as a cofactor for post-translational carboxylation of glutamic acid residues found on the amino-terminal of vitamin K–dependent coagulation factors (factors II, VII, IX, and X) and anticoagulant proteins (protein C and protein S).[192] Gamma carboxylation is a prerequisite for calcium-dependent interaction of these coagulation proteins with activated phospholipid surfaces. Carboxylation of vitamin K–dependent cofactors is catalyzed by a carboxylase that requires the reduced form of vitamin K. During this reaction, reduced vitamin K is oxidized to vitamin K epoxide, which is recycled back to vitamin K by vitamin K epoxide reductase. Vitamin K then is converted to reduced vitamin K by vitamin K reductase. The vitamin K antagonists inhibit vitamin K epoxide reductase and, possibly, vitamin K reductase (Fig. 29–4). With depletion of reduced vitamin K, carboxylation of the vitamin K–dependent proteins is inhibited. The antithrombotic effect of coumarin derivatives, which probably reflects lowered factor II (prothrombin) and factor X levels, is delayed for 72 to 96 hours.

Indications

Although oral anticoagulants have been used in patients with ischemic heart disease for 50 years, their role in this patient population remains controversial.

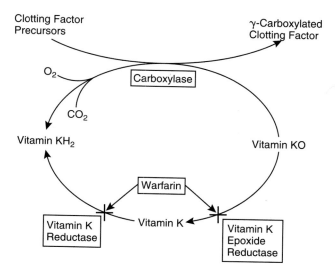

FIGURE 29–4. Mechanism of action of warfarin. Warfarin inhibits the carboxylation of glutamic acid residues on the precursors of the vitamin K–dependent clotting factors by blocking vitamin K epoxide reductase and vitamin K reductase, preventing the formation of reduced vitamin K in the liver.

Acute Myocardial Infarction

High-intensity oral anticoagulant treatment (target international normalized ratio [INR] of 2.8 to 4.8) after MI produces a reduction in mortality and clinically important vascular outcomes.[193-196] Although the efficacy of long-term high-intensity oral anticoagulant treatment has been compared directly with that of aspirin, interpretation of these results is limited by small sample size.[197] Moderate-intensity oral anticoagulation (INR of 2.0 to 3.0) is more effective than placebo at reducing recurrent ischemic events[198,199] but does not seem superior to aspirin.[200,201] These trials were too small, however, to claim equivalency with aspirin confidently.

The addition of low, fixed-dose warfarin (1 or 3 mg)[202] or low-intensity warfarin (target INR of 1.5)[203] to aspirin in patients with a recent MI does not seem to provide clinical benefit beyond that achieved with aspirin alone. Although the combination of aspirin with long-term moderate-intensity warfarin (target INR of 2.0 to 2.5) seems to result in lower rates of death, new MI, and stroke than aspirin alone, this benefit occurs at the expense of an appreciable increase in bleeding and therapeutic complexity.[203]

Although aspirin and oral anticoagulants are more effective than placebo after MI, the increased rate of major hemorrhage and the greater cost and complexity of oral anticoagulant therapy make aspirin a better choice in most patients. Oral anticoagulation is an alternative for patients at increased risk of thromboembolism (i.e., during the first 3 months after anterior MI; patients with MI complicated by severe left ventricular dysfunction; and patients with congestive heart failure, previous emboli, evidence of mural thrombi, or atrial fibrillation) and for patients who cannot tolerate aspirin.[12]

Primary Prevention of Ischemic Heart Disease

Low-intensity warfarin (target INR of 1.5) confers protection against fatal and nonfatal manifestations of ischemic heart disease in high-risk men, as does the combination of low-intensity warfarin and 75 mg of aspirin daily.[204] Combined treatment seems to be more effective than either warfarin or aspirin alone. The adverse effects associated with warfarin therapy are greater than those of aspirin, however, and monitoring of warfarin treatment is laborious. Consequently, low-intensity warfarin, with or without aspirin, cannot be recommended for the primary prevention of MI. In individuals who cannot tolerate aspirin, however, warfarin may be a useful alternative, and combination therapy can be considered in patients at high risk for ischemic events.

Dosages

The prothrombin time (PT) is sensitive to reductions in three of the four vitamin K–dependent clotting factors, prothrombin, factor VII, and factor IX. Because commercially available thromboplastin reagents vary in their sensitivity to reductions in these three clotting factors, the adequacy of warfarin dosing is measured using a standardized method of PT reporting. The INR is based on the use of an international sensitivity index (ISI) assigned to each thromboplastin reagent that standardizes sensitivity to reductions in vitamin K–dependent clotting factors against an international reference preparation provided by the World Health Organization. The PT is converted to an INR by using the formula INR = (observed PT/mean normal PT)^{ISI}.[192]

Oral anticoagulants have a narrow therapeutic window and a highly variable dose-response relation.[205] Consequently the use of these agents can be complicated by serious bleeding, and their anticoagulant effect must be monitored closely by laboratory tests. The total dose of warfarin required to reach a therapeutic INR varies from patient to patient. This interindividual variation in warfarin dosing may reflect differences in age, weight, liver function, diet, alcohol intake, concomitant medications, and comorbid illnesses.[192] More frequent monitoring is indicated if there are changes in the diet or drug regimen. A randomized trial suggests that an initial daily dose of warfarin of 5 mg is less likely to cause excessive anticoagulation or to produce a transient hypercoagulable state through the reduction of protein C levels than an initial daily dose of 10 mg.[206]

In the trials in which oral anticoagulant therapy after MI reduced mortality or clinically important vascular outcomes, oral anticoagulants were given in doses that achieved an INR of at least 2.8 to 4.8. Moderate-intensity oral anticoagulation (INR of 2.0 to 3.0) also seems effective in reducing recurrent MI and stroke. In contrast, fixed low-dose warfarin and low-intensity warfarin regimens (INR of <1.5) have not been effective in this patient population.

Side Effects

Bleeding is the most frequent complication of warfarin therapy. The risk of bleeding is influenced by the intensity of anticoagulation; the concomitant use of aspirin, nonsteroidal anti-inflammatory agents, or other drugs that influence hemostasis; a history of bleeding; advanced age; a history of stroke; or the presence of serious comorbid conditions.[45] With an INR of 2.0 to 3.0, the annual risk of a major bleed is 2%, and that of a fatal bleed is approximately 0.8%.[45] Warfarin-induced skin necrosis is a rare complication that usually develops soon after oral anticoagulant therapy is initiated in patients with congenital or acquired protein C or protein S deficiency.[207] It likely results from the rapid decrease in levels of these anticoagulant proteins that precedes reduction in prothrombin levels. To circumvent this complication, patients with known protein C or protein S deficiency should be started on maintenance, rather than loading, doses of warfarin after therapeutic doses of heparin have been given.

Contraindications and Drug Interactions

Patients who have contraindications to anticoagulation therapy should not be given warfarin (see Table 29–1). Because warfarin is teratogenic, its use should be avoided, if possible, by pregnant women.[207]

Combined therapy with warfarin and aspirin can benefit patients who have a high risk of thrombosis, who have failed single-agent therapy, and who have a relatively low risk of bleeding.[12,208] The risk of major hemorrhage, especially bleeding from the gastrointestinal tract, is greater when the drugs are used together. Because the dose of aspirin used in conjunction with warfarin seems to be a predictor of bleeding,[209-213] the dose of aspirin should be kept low (e.g., 80 to 100 mg/day), and warfarin should be given in doses that achieve an INR of 2.0 to 3.5.[208]

Numerous medications may influence patient response to warfarin.[214] Any change in medication profile should prompt more frequent anticoagulant monitoring.

CONCLUSIONS

Many new anticoagulants have been evaluated in patients with ACS. Of these, only LMWH and bivalirudin have shown consistent benefit: LMWH for acute treatment of patients with unstable angina or non–ST-segment MI and bivalirudin for patients undergoing percutaneous coronary interventions. Despite promising data, the role of the other agents in this patient population has not been clearly delineated. Orally active agents that target thrombin or factor Xa are particularly exciting. If these drugs can be given safely without the need for anticoagulation monitoring, they have the potential to replace warfarin, simplifying oral anticoagulant therapy. The challenge for the future will be to determine which of the numerous agents currently under development will provide the greatest efficacy with the greatest degree of safety.

REFERENCES

1. Fuster V: Elucidation of the role of plaque instability and rupture in acute coronary events. Curr Opin Cardiol 1996;11:351-360.
2. Falk E, Shah PK, Fuster V: Coronary plaque disruption. Circulation 1995;92:657-671.
3. Fuster V, Badimon L, Badimon JJ, et al: The pathogenesis of coronary artery disease and the acute coronary syndromes. N Engl J Med 1992;326:242-250.
4. Davie EW: Biochemical and molecular aspects of the coagulation cascade. Thromb Haemost 1995;75:1-6.
5. Yamamoto M, Nakagaki T, Kisiel W: Tissue factor-dependent autoactivation of human blood coagulation factor. J Biol Chem 1992;267:19089-19094.
6. Rosenberg RD, Bauer KA: The heparin-antithrombin system: A natural anticoagulant mechanism. In Colman RW, Hirsh J, Marder VJ, Salzman EW (eds): Hemostasis and Thrombosis: Basic Principles and Clinical Practice, 3rd ed. Philadelphia, JB Lippincott, 1994, pp 837-860.
7. Danielsson A, Raub E, Lindahl U, et al: Role of ternary complexes in which heparin binds both antithrombin and proteinase, in the acceleration of the reactions between antithrombin and thrombin or factor Xa. J Biol Chem 1986;261:15467-15473.
8. Jordan RE, Oostra GM, Gardner WT, et al: The kinetics of hemostatic enzyme antithrombin interactions in the presence of low molecular weight heparin. J Biol Chem 1980;255:100081-100090.
9. Gruppo Italiano per lo Studio della Sopravivenza ne'Infarto Miocardio: GISSI-2: A factorial randomised trial of alteplase versus streptokinase and heparin versus no heparin among 12,490 patients with acute myocardial infarction. Lancet 1990;336:65-71.

10. International Study Group: In-hospital mortality and clinical course of 20,891 patients with suspected acute myocardial infarction randomised between alteplase and streptokinase with or without heparin. Lancet 1990;336:71–75.

11. ISIS-3 Collaborative Group: ISIS-3: A randomized comparison of streptokinase vs. tissue plasminogen activator vs. anistreplase and of aspirin plus heparin vs. aspirin alone among 41,299 cases of suspected acute myocardial infarction. Lancet 1992;339:753–770.

12. Cairns JA, Theroux P, Lewis HD, et al: Antithrombotic agents in coronary artery disease. Chest 2001;119(Suppl):229S–252S.

13. Hsia J, Hamilton WP, Kleiman N, et al: A comparison between heparin and low-dose aspirin as adjunctive therapy with tissue-plasminogen activator for acute myocardial infarction. N Engl J Med 1990;323:1433–1437.

14. Bleich SD, Nichols TC, Schumacher RR, et al: Effect of heparin on coronary artery patency after thrombolysis with tissue plasminogen activator in acute myocardial infarction. Am J Cardiol 1990;66:1412–1417.

15. de Bono DP, Simoons ML, Tijssen J, et al, for the European Cooperative Study Group (ECSG): Effect of early intravenous heparin on coronary artery patency, infarct size, and bleeding complications after alteplase thrombolysis: Results of a randomized double-blind European Cooperative Study Group Trial. Br Heart J 1992;62:122–128.

16. GUSTO Investigators: An international randomised trial comparing four thrombolytic strategies for AMI. N Engl J Med 1993;329:673–682.

17. Mahaffey KW, Granger CB, Collins R, et al: Overview of randomized trials of intravenous heparin in patients with acute myocardial infarction treated with thrombolytic therapy. Am J Cardiol 1996;77:550–556.

18. Collins R, MacMahon S, Flather M, et al: Clinical effects of anticoagulant therapy in suspected acute myocardial infarction: Systematic overview of randomised trials. BMJ 1996;313:652–659.

19. Antman EM, for the TIMI-9A Investigators: Hirudin in acute myocardial infarction: Safety report from the thrombolysis and thrombin inhibition in myocardial infarction (TIMI) 9A trial. Circulation 1994;90:1624–1630.

20. Global Use of Strategies to Open Occluded Coronary Arteries (GUSTO) IIa Investigators: Randomized trial of intravenous heparin versus recombinant hirudin for acute coronary syndromes. Circulation 1994;90:1631–1637.

21. Ryan TJ, Antman EM, Brooks NH, et al: ACC/AHA guidelines for the management of patients with acute myocardial infarction: A report of the ACC/AHA taskforce on practice guidelines. J Am Coll Cardiol 1999;34:890–891.

22. RISC Group: Risk of myocardial infarction and death during treatment with low dose aspirin and intravenous heparin in men with unstable artery disease. Lancet 1990;336:827–830.

23. Holdright D, Patel D, Cunningham D, et al: Comparison of the effect of heparin and aspirin vs. aspirin alone on transient myocardial ischemia and in-hospital prognosis in patients with unstable angina. J Am Coll Cardiol 1994;24:39–45.

24. Gurfinkel EP, Manos EK, Mejail RI, et al: Low-molecular-weight heparin versus regular heparin or aspirin in the treatment of unstable angina and silent ischemia. J Am Coll Cardiol 1994;24:39–45.

25. Oler A, Whooley MA, Oler J, et al: Adding heparin to aspirin reduces the incidence of myocardial infarction and death in patients with unstable angina: A meta-analysis. JAMA 1996;26:313–318.

26. Popma JJ, Weitz J, Bittle JA, et al: Antithrombotic therapy in patients undergoing coronary angioplasty. Chest 1998;114(Suppl):728S–741S.

27. Grayburn PA, Willard JE, Brickner ME, et al: In vivo thrombus formation on a guidewire during intravascular ultrasound imaging: Evidence for inadequate heparinization. Cathet Cardiovasc Diagn 1991;23:141–143.

28. Ellis SB, Roubin GS, Wilentz J, et al: Effect of 18- to 24-hour heparin administration for prevention of restenosis after uncomplicated coronary angioplasty. Am Heart J 1989;117:777–782.

29. Friedman HZ, Cragg DR, Glazier SM, et al: Randomized prospective evaluation of prolonged versus abbreviated intravenous heparin therapy after coronary angioplasty. J Am Coll Cardiol 1994;24:1214–1219.

30. Theroux P, Waters D, Lam J, et al: Reactivation of unstable angina after the discontinuation of heparin. N Engl J Med 1992;327:141–145.

31. Oldgren J, Grip L, Wallentin L: Reactivation after cessation of thrombin inhibition in unstable coronary artery disease, regardless of aspirin dose [abstract 2515]. Circulation 1996;94:I-431.

32. Weitz JI, Hudoba M, Massel D, et al: Clot-bound thrombin is protected from inhibition by heparin-antithrombin III but is susceptible to inactivation by antithrombin III-independent inhibitors. J Clin Invest 1990;86:385–391.

33. Hogg PJ, Jackson CM: Fibrin monomer protects thrombin from inactivation by heparin-antithrombin III: Implications for heparin efficacy. Proc Natl Acad Sci U S A 1989;86:3619–3623.

34. Eisenberg PR, Siegel JE, Abendschein DR, et al: Importance of factor Xa in determining the procoagulant activity of whole-blood clots. J Clin Invest 1993;91:1877–1883.

35. Marciniak E: Factor Xa inactivation by antithrombin III: Evidence for biological stabilization of factor Xa by factor V-phospholipid complex. Br J Haematol 1973;24:391–400.

36. Kumar R, Beguin S, Hemker HC: The effect of fibrin clots and clot-bound thrombin on the development of platelet procoagulant activity. Thromb Haemost 1995;74:962–968.

37. Kumar R, Beguin S, Hemker HC: The influence of fibrinogen and fibrin on thrombin generation B evidence for feedback activation of the clotting system by clot-bound thrombin. Thromb Haemost 1994;72:713–721.

38. Lane DA: Heparin binding and neutralizing proteins. In Lane DA, Lindahl U (eds): Heparin: Chemical and Biological Properties and Clinical Applications. Boca Raton, FL, CRC, 1989, pp 1787–1793.

39. Lane DA, Pejler J, Flynn AM, et al: Neutralization of heparin related saccharides by histidine-rich glycoprotein and platelet factor 4. J Biol Chem 1984;261:3980–3986.

40. Young E, Prins M, Levine MN, et al: Heparin binding to plasma proteins, an important mechanism for heparin resistance. Thromb Haemost 1992;67:639–643.

41. Hirsh J: Heparin. N Engl J Med 1991;324:1565–1574.

42. Hirsh J, Fuster V: Guide to anticoagulant therapy: I. Heparin. Circulation 1994;89:1449–1468.

43. D'Angelo A, Seveso MP, D'Angelo SV, et al: Effect of clot-detection methods and reagents on activated partial thromboplastin time (aPTT): Implications in heparin monitoring by aPTT. Am J Clin Pathol 1990;94:297–306.

44. Raschke RA, Reilly BM, Guidry JR, et al: The weight-based heparin dosing nomogram compared with standard care: A randomized controlled trial. Ann Intern Med 1993;119:874–881.

45. Levine M, Raskob GE, Landefeld CS, et al: Hemorrhagic complications of anticoagulant treatment. Chest 1998;118(Suppl):511S–523S.

46. Bovill EG, Tracy RP, Knatterud GL, et al: Hemorrhagic events during therapy with recombinant tissue plasminogen activator, heparin and aspirin for unstable angina (Thrombolysis in Myocardial Ischemia-IIIB trial). Am J Cardiol 1997;79:391–396.

47. Hirsh J, Warkentin TE, Raschke R, et al: Heparin and low-molecular weight heparin: Mechanism of action, pharmacokinetics, dosing considerations, monitoring, efficacy, and safety. Chest 1998;114:489S–510S.

48. Salzman EW, Rosenberg RD, Smith MN, et al: Effect of heparin and heparin fractions on platelet aggregation. J Clin Invest 1980;65:64–73.

49. Amiral J, Bridey F, Wolf M, et al: Antibodies to macromolecular platelet factor 4-heparin complexes in heparin induced thrombocytopenia: A study of 44 cases. Thromb Haemost 1995;73:21–28.

50. Kelton JG, Smith JW, Warkentin TE, et al: Immunoglobulin G from patients with heparin-induced thrombocytopenia binds to a complex of heparin and platelet factor 4. Blood 1994;83:3232–3239.

51. Warkentin TE, Hayward CPM, Boshkov LK, et al: Sera from patients with heparin-induced thrombocytopenia generate platelet-derived microparticles with procoagulant activity: An explanation for the thrombotic complications of heparin-induced thrombocytopenia. Blood 1994;84:3691–3699.

52. Ginsberg JS, Kowalchuk G, Hirsh J, et al: Heparin effect on bone density. Thromb Haemost 1990;64:286–289.

53. Curry N, Bandana EJ, Pirofsky B: Heparin sensitivity: Report of a case. Arch Intern Med 1973;132:744–745.

54. White RW, Sadd JR, Nensel RE: Thrombotic complications of heparin therapy, including six cases of heparin-induced skin necrosis. Ann Surg 1979;190:595–608.

55. O'Kelly R, Magee F, McKenna J: Routine heparin therapy inhibits adrenal aldosterone production. J Clin Endocrinol Metab 1983;56:108–112.

56. Ofosu FA, Barrowcliffe TW: Mechanisms of action of low-molecular-weight heparins and heparinoids. Baillieres Clin Hematol 1990; 3:505–529.

57. Andersson L-O, Barrowcliffe TW, Holmer E, et al: Molecular weight dependence of the heparin potentiated inhibition of thrombin and activated factor X: Effect of heparin neutralization in plasma. Thromb Res 1979;15:531–541.

58. Young E, Wells PS, Holloway S, et al: Ex-vivo and in-vitro evidence that low-molecular-weight heparins exhibit less binding to plasma proteins than unfractionated heparin. Thromb Haemost 1994; 71:300–304.

59. Young E, Cosmi B, Weitz J, Hirsh J: Comparison of the non-specific binding of unfractionated heparin and low-molecular-weight heparin (enoxaparin) to plasma proteins. Thromb Haemost 1993;70:625–630.

60. Barzu T, Molho P, Tobelem G, et al: Binding and endocytosis of heparin by human endothelial cells in culture. Biochem Biophys Acta 1985;845:196–203.

61. Bara L, Billaud E, Gramond G, et al: Comparative pharmcokinetics of a low-molecular-weight heparin (PK 10169) and unfractionated heparin after intravenous and subcutaneous administration. Thromb Res 1985;30:630–636.

62. Handeland GF, Abilgaard U, Holm HA, et al: Dose-adjusted heparin treatment of deep venous thrombosis: A comparison of unfractionated and low-molecular-weight heparin. Eur J Clin Pharmacol 1990;30:107–112.

63. Cadroy Y, Pourrat J, Baladre MF, et al: Delayed elimination of enoxaparin in patients with chronic renal insufficiency. Thromb Res 1991;63:385–390.

64. Frostfeldt G, Ahlberg G, Gustafsson G, et al: Low molecular weight heparin (dalteparin) as adjuvant treatment of thrombolysis in acute myocardial infarction—a pilot study: Biochemical markers in acute coronary syndromes (BIOMACS II). J Am Coll Cardiol 1999;33:627–633.

65. Glick A, Kornowski R, Michowich Y, et al: Reduction of reinfarction and angina with use of low-molecular weight heparin therapy after streptokinase (and heparin) in acute myocardial infarction. Am J Cardiol 1996;77:1145–1148.

66. Chamuleau SA, de Winter RJ, Levi M, for the Fraxiparin Anticoagulant Therapy in Myocardial Infarction Study Amsterdam (FATIMA) study group: Low molecular weight heparin as an adjunct to thrombolysis for acute myocardial infarction: The FATIMA study. Heart 1998;80:35–39.

67. Ross AM, Molhoek P, Lundergan C, et al: Randomized comparison of enoxaparin, a low-molecular-weight heparin, with unfractionated heparin adjunctive to recombinant tissue plasminogen activator thrombolysis and aspirin. Second trial of Heparin and Aspirin Reperfusion Therapy (HART II). Circulation 2001;104:648–652.

68. Kontny F, Dale J, Abildgaard U, Pedersen TR, on behalf of the FRAMI Study Group: Randomized trial of low molecular weight heparin (Dalteparin) in prevention of left ventricular thrombus formation and arterial embolism after acute myocardial infarction: The Fragmin in Acute Myocardial Infarction (FRAMI) Study. J Am Coll Cardiol 1997;30:962–969.

69. Fragmin During Instability in Coronary Artery Disease (FRISC) study group: Low-molecular-weight heparin during instability in coronary artery disease. Lancet 1996;347:561–568.

70. Klein W, Buchwald A, Hillis SE, et al, for the FRIC investigators: Comparison of low-molecular-weight heparin with unfractionated heparin acutely and with placebo for 6 weeks in the management of unstable coronary artery disease: Fragmin in Unstable Coronary Artery Disease study (FRIC). Circulation 1997;96:61–68.

71. Cohen M, Demers C, Gurfinkel EP, et al, for the Efficacy and Safety of Subcutaneous Enoxaparin in Non-Q-Wave Coronary Events study group: A comparison of low-molecular-weight heparin with unfractionated heparin for unstable coronary artery disease. N Engl J Med 1997;337:447–452.

72. Antman E, McCabe CH, Gurfinkel EP, et al, for the TIMI 11B investigators: Enoxaparin prevents death and cardiac ischemic events in unstable angina/non-Q-wave myocardial infarction. Circulation 1999;100:1593–1601.

73. FRAX.I.S. study group: Comparison to two treatment durations (6 days and 14 days) of a low molecular weight heparin with a 6-day treatment of unfractionated heparin in the initial management of unstable angina or non-Q wave myocardial infarction: FRAX.I.S. Eur Heart J 1999;20:1553–1562.

74. Fragmin and Fast Revascularisation During Instability in Coronary Artery Disease (FRISC II) investigators: Long-term low-molecular-mass heparin in unstable coronary artery disease: FRISC II prospective randomised multicentre study. Lancet 1999;354:701–707.

75. Goodman S, Bigonzi F, Radley D, et al, for the ESSENCE group: One-year follow-up of the ESSENCE trial (enoxaparin versus heparin in unstable angina and non-Q-wave myocardial infarction) [abstract P477]. Eur Heart J 1998;50.

76. Cohen M, Theroux P, Borzak S, et al: Randomized double-blind safety study of enoxaparin versus unfractionated heparin in patients with non-ST-segment elevation acute coronary syndromes treated with tirofiban and aspirin: the ACUTE II Study. Am Heart J 2002;144:470–477.

77. Faxon DP, Spiro TE, Minor S, et al: Low molecular weight heparin in prevention of restenosis after angioplasty: Results of enoxaparin restenosis (ERA) trial. Circulation 1994;90:908–914.

78. Cairns JA, Gill J, Morton B, et al: Fish oils and low-molecular-weight heparin for the reduction of restenosis after percutaneous transluminal coronary angioplasty: The EMPAR study. Circulation 1996;94:1553–1560.

79. Lablanche JM, McFadden E, Meneveau N, et al: Effect of nadroparin, a low-molecular-weight heparin, on clinical and angiographic restenosis after coronary balloon angioplasty: The FACT study. Circulation 1997;96:3396–3402.

80. Karsch KR, Preisack MB, Baildow R, et al: LMWH in prevention of restenosis after PTCA: The REDUCE trial. J Am Coll Cardiol 1996; 28:1437–1443.

81. Montalescot G, Cohen M: Low molecular-weight heparins in the cardiac catheterization laboratory. J Thromb Thrombol 1999;7: 319–323.

82. Collet JP, Montalescot G, Drobinski G, et al: PTCA without heparin and without coagulation monitoring in unstable angina patients pre-treated with subcutaneous enoxaparin [abstract]. Circulation 1999;100(Suppl I):I-188.

83. Kereiakes D, Grines C, Fry E, et al: Abciximab-enoxaparin interaction during percutaneous coronary intervention: Results of the NICE 1 and 4 trials. J Am Coll Cardiol 2000;35(Suppl A):92A.

84. Kereiakes DJ, Fry E, Matthai W, et al: Combination enoxaparin and abciximab therapy during percutaneous coronary intervention: "NICE guys finish first." J Invas Cardiol 2000;12(Suppl A): 1A–5A.

85. Weitz JI: Low-molecular-weight heparins. N Engl J Med 1997;337: 688–698.

86. Thrombolysis in Myocardial Infarction (TIMI) 11A trial investigators: Dose ranging trial of enoxaparin for unstable angina: Results of the TIMI 11A. J Am Coll Cardiol 1997;29:1474–1482.

87. Woltzt M, Weltermann A, Nieszpaur-Los M, et al: Studies on the neutralizing effects of protamine on unfractionated and low-molecular weight heparin (Fragmin) at the site of activation of the coagulation system in man. Thromb Haemost 1995;73:439–443.

88. Van Ryn-McKenna J, Cai L, Ofosu FA, et al: Neutralization of enoxaparin-induced bleeding by protamine sulfate. Thromb Haemost 1990;63:271–274.

89. Warkentin TE, Levine MN, Hirsh J, et al: Heparin-induced thrombocytopenia in patients treated with low-molecular-weight heparin or unfractionated heparin. N Engl J Med 1995;332:1330–1335.

90. Bhandari M, Hirsh J, Weitz JI, et al: The effects of standard and low molecular weight heparin on bone nodule formation in vitro. Thromb Haemost 1998;80:413–417.

91. Shaughnessy SG, Young E, Deschamps P, et al: The effects of low-molecular-weight and standard heparin on calcium loss from fetal rat calvaria. Blood 1995;86:1368–1373.

92. Muir JM, Andrew M, Hirsh J, et al: Histomorphometric analysis of the effects of standard heparin on trabecular bone in vivo. Blood 1996;88:1314–1320.

93. Monreal M, Lafoz E, Olive A, et al: Comparison of subcutaneous unfractionated heparin with low-molecular-weight heparin (Fragmin) in patients with venous thromboembolism and contraindications to Coumadin. Thromb Haemost 1994;71:7–11.

94. Chong BH, Ismail F, Cade J, et al: Heparin-induced thrombocytopenia: Studies with a new low-molecular-weight heparinoid, Org 10172. Blood 1989;73:1592–1596.

95. Leroy J, Leclerc MN, Delahousse B, et al: Treatment of heparin-associated thrombocytopenia and thrombosis with low-molecular-weight heparin (CY 216). Semin Thromb Haemost 1985;11: 327–329.

96. Vitoux JF, Mathier JF, Roncata M, et al: Heparin-associated thrombocytopenia treatment with low-molecular-weight heparin. Thromb Haemost 1986;55:37-39.

97. Horellou MH, Conrad J, Lecrubier C, et al: Persistent heparin-induced thrombocytopenia despite therapy with low-molecular-weight heparin. Thromb Haemost 1986;55:37-39.

98. Rivera TM, Leone-Bay A, Paton DR, et al: Oral delivery of heparin in combination with sodium N-[8-2-(hydroxybenzoyl)amino] caprylate: Pharmacological considerations. Pharm Res 1997;14: 1830-1834.

99. Fox I, Dawson A, Loynds P, et al: Anticoagulant activity of Hirulog, a direct thrombin inhibitor, in humans. Thromb Haemost 1993;69:157-163.

100. Stringer KA, Lindenfeld J: Hirudins: Antithrombin anticoagulants. Ann Pharmacother 1992;26:1535-1540.

101. Heras M, Chesebro JH, Webster MWI, et al: Hirudin, heparin and placebo during deep arterial injury in the pig: The in vivo role of thrombin in platelet-mediated thrombosis. Circulation 1990;82: 1476-1484.

102. Direct Thrombin Inhibitor Trialists' Collaborative Group: Direct thrombin inhibitors in acute coronary syndromes: Principal results of a meta-analysis based on individual patients' data. Lancet 2002;359:294-302.

103. Stone SR, Maraganore JM: Hirudin interactions with thrombin. In Berliner LJ (ed): Thrombin: Structure and Function. New York, Plenum Press, 1992, pp 219-228.

104. Rydel TJ, Ravichandran KG, Tulinsky A, et al: The structure of a complex of recombinant hirudin and human alpha-thrombin. Science 1990;249:277-280.

105. Hosteenge J, Stone JR, Donella-Deane A, et al: The effect of substituting phosphotyrosine for sulphotyrosine on the activity of hirudin. Eur J Biochem 1990;188:55-59.

106. Walenga JM, Pifarre R, Fareed J: Recombinant hirudin as an antithrombotic agent. Drugs Future 1990;14:267-280.

107. Neuhaus KL, von Essen R, Tebbe U, et al: Safety observations from the pilot phase of the randomized r-Hirudin for Improvement of Thrombolysis (HIT-III) Study: A study of the Arbeitsgemeinschaft Leitender Kardiologischer Krankenausarzte (ALKK). Circulation 1994;90:1638-1642.

108. Antman EM, for the TIMI 9B investigators: Hirudin in acute myocardial infarction: Thrombolysis and Thrombin Inhibition in Myocardial Infarction (TIMI) 9B trial. Circulation 1996;94: 911-921.

109. Global Use of Strategies to Open Occluded Coronary Arteries (GUSTO) IIb investigators: A comparison of recombinant hirudin with heparin for the treatment of acute coronary syndromes. N Engl J Med 1996;335:775-782.

110. Neuhaus KL, Molhoek GP, Zeymer U, et al: Recombinant hirudin (lepirudin) for the improvement of thrombolysis with streptokinase in patients with acute myocardial infarction: Results of the HIT-4 trial. J Am Coll Cardiol 1999;34:966-973.

111. Simes R, Granger C, Antman E, et al: Impact of hirudin versus heparin on mortality and (re)infarction in patients with acute coronary syndromes: A prospective meta-analysis of the GUSTO IIb and TIMI 9B trials [abstract]. Circulation 1996;94(suppl 1): 1-430.

112. Metz BK, White HD, Granger CB, et al, for the Global Use of Strategies to Open Occluded Coronary Arteries in Acute Coronary Syndromes (GUSTO)-IIb investigators: Randomized comparison of direct thrombin inhibition versus heparin in conjunction with fibrinolytic therapy for acute myocardial infarction: Results from the GUSTO-IIb trial. J Am Coll Cardiol 1998;31:1493-1498.

113. OASIS-2 investigators: Effects of recombinant hirudin (lepirudin) compared with heparin on death, myocardial infarction, refractory angina, and revascularisation procedures in patients with acute myocardial ischaemia without ST elevation: A randomised trial. Lancet 1999;353:429-438.

114. Fox KAA: Implications of the organization to assess strategies for ischemic syndromes-2 (OASIS-2) study and the results in the context of other trials. Am J Cardiol 1999;84(Suppl 5):26M-31M.

115. Serruys PW, Herrman J-PR, Simon R, for the HELVETICA investigators: A comparison of hirudin with heparin in the prevention of restenosis after coronary angioplasty. N Engl J Med 1995;333: 757-763.

116. Greinacher A, Lubenow N: Recombinant hirudin in clinical practice: Focus on lepirudin. Circulation 2001;103:1479-1484.

117. Greinacher A, Volpel H, Janssens U, et al: Recombinant hirudin (lepirudin) provides safe and effective anticoagulation in patients with the immunologic type of heparin-induced thrombocytopenia: A prospective study. Circulation 1999;99:73-80.

118. Hafner G, Rupprecht HJ, Luz M, et al: Recombinant hirudin as a periprocedural antithrombotic in coronary angioplasty for unstable angina pectoris. Eur Heart J 1996;17:1207-1215.

119. Nurmohamed MT, Berckmans RJ, Morrien-Salomons WN, et al: Monitoring anticoagulant therapy by activated partial thromboplastin time: Hirudin assessment. Thromb Haemost 1994;72: 685-692.

120. Potzsch B, Madlener K, Seelig C, et al: Monitoring of r-hirudin anticoagulation during cardiopulmonary bypass: Assessment of the whole blood ecarin clotting time. Thromb Haemost 1997;77: 920-925.

121. CAPTURE investigators: Randomised placebo-controlled trial of abciximab before and during coronary intervention in refractory unstable angina: The CAPTURE study. Lancet 1997;349: 1429-1435.

122. PURSUIT trial investigators: Inhibition of platelet glycoprotein IIb/IIIa with eptifibatide in patients with acute coronary artery syndromes. N Engl J Med 1998;388:436-442.

123. Irami MS, Harvey JW, Sexon RG: Reversal of hirudin-induced bleeding diathesis by prothrombin complex concentrate. Am J Cardiol 1995;75:422-423.

124. Vanholder R, Dhondt A: Recombinant hirudin: Clinical pharmacology and potential applications in nephrology. Biol Drugs 1999;11:417-429.

125. Maraganore JM, Bourdon P, Jablonski J, et al: Design and characterization of hirulogs: A novel class of bivalent peptide inhibitors of thrombin. Biochemistry 1990;29:7095-7101.

126. Skrzpczak-Jankun E, Carperos VE, Ravichandran KG, et al: Structure of the hirugen and hirulog 1 complexes of A-thrombin. J Mol Biol 1991;221:1379-1393.

127. Witting JI, Bourdon P, Brezniak DV, et al: Thrombin-specific inhibition by slow cleavage of hirulog-1. Biochem J 1992;282:737-743.

128. Lyle TA: Small molecular inhibitors of thrombin. Perspect Drug Discov Design 1993;1:453-460.

129. Fox I, Dawson A, Loyonds P, et al: Anticoagulant activity of Hirulog, a direct thrombin inhibitor, in humans. Thromb Haemost 1993;69:157-163.

130. White HD, Aylward PE, Frey MJ, et al, for the Hirulog Early Reperfusion/Occlusion (HERO) trial investigators: Randomized, double-blind comparison of hirulog versus heparin in patients receiving streptokinase and aspirin for acute myocardial infarction (HERO). Circulation 1997;96:2155-2161.

131. Lindon RM, Theroux P, Bonana R, et al: A pilot early angiographic patency study using a direct thrombin inhibitor as adjunctive therapy to streptokinase in acute myocardial infarction. Circulation 1994;89:1567-1572.

132. Theroux P, Perez-Villa F, Waters D, et al: A randomized double-blind comparison of two doses of hirulog or heparin as adjunctive therapy to streptokinase to promote early patency of the infarct-related artery in acute myocardial infarction. Circulation 1994;91:2132-2139.

133. White H, for the Hirulog and Early Reperfusion or Occlusion (HERO)-2 trial investigators: Thrombin-specific anticoagulation with bivalirudin versus heparin in patients receiving fibrinolytic therapy for acute myocardial infarction: The HERO-2 randomised trial. Lancet 2001;358:1855-1863.

134. Mehta S, Eikelboom JW, Yusuf S: Risk of intracranial haemorrhage with bolus versus infusion thrombolytic therapy: A meta-analysis of over 100,000 patients. Lancet 2000;346:449-454.

135. Sharma GVRK, Lapsley DE, Vita JA, et al: Usefulness and tolerability of hirulog, a direct thrombin inhibitor in unstable angina pectoris. Am J Cardiol 1993;72:1357-1360.

136. Lindon RM, Theroux P, Juneau M, et al: Initial experience with a direct antithrombin, hirulog, in unstable angina: Anticoagulant, antithrombotic and clinical effects. Circulation 1993;88(Part 1): 1495-1501.

137. Fuchs J, Cannon CP, and the TIMI 7 investigators: Hirulog in the treatment of unstable angina: Results of the Thrombin Inhibition in Myocardial Ischemia (TIMI) 7 trial. Circulation 1995;92: 727-733.

138. Bittl JA, Strony J, Brinker J, et al, for the Hirulog Angioplasty Study investigators: Treatment with bivalirudin (hirulog) as compared

with heparin during coronary angioplasty for unstable or post-infarction angina. N Engl J Med 1995;333:764-769.

139. Bittl JA, Chairman BR, Feit F, et al: Bivalirudin versus heparin during coronary angioplasty for unstable or post-infarction angina: Final report reanalysis of the Bivalirudin Angioplasty Study. Am Heart J 2001;142:952-959.

140. Kong DF, Topol EJ, Bittl JA, et al: Clinical outcomes of bivalirudin for ischemic heart disease. Circulation 1999;100:2049-2053.

141. Bittle JA: Comparative safety profiles of hirulog and heparin in patients undergoing coronary angioplasty. The Hirulog Angioplasty Study investigators. Am Heart J 1995;130:658-665.

142. Fitzgerald D, Murphy N: Argatroban: A synthetic thrombin inhibitor of low relative molecular mass. Coron Artery Dis 1996;7:455-458.

143. Vermeer F, Vahanian A, Fels PW, et al, for the ARGAMI Study Group: Argatroban and alteplase in patients with acute myocardial infarction: The ARGAMI Study. J Thromb Thrombol 2000;10:233-240.

144. Kaplinsky E: Direct antithrombin-argatroban in acute myocardial infarction (ARGAMI-2). J Am Coll Cardiol 1998;32:1-7.

145. Chen L, Nichols WW, Mattsson C: Inogatran, a novel low-molecular-weight thrombin inhibitor, given with, but not after, tissue-plasminogen activator improves thrombolysis. J Pharmacol Exp Ther 1996;277:12276-12283.

146. Andersen K, Delbourg M: Heparin is more effective than inogatran, a low-molecular-weight thrombin inhibitor in suppressing ischemia and recurrent angina in unstable coronary disease: Thrombin Inhibition in Myocardial Ischemia (TRIM) Study Group. Am J Cardiol 1998;81:939-944.

147. Klootwijk P, Lenderink T, Meji S, et al: Anticoagulant properties, clinical efficacy and safety of efegatran, a direct thrombin inhibitor, in patients with unstable angina. Eur Heart J 1999;20:1101-1111.

148. Eriksson UG, Johansson L, Frison L, et al: Single and repeated oral dosing of H376/95, a prodrug of the direct thrombin inhibitor melagatran, to young healthy male subjects [abstract #101]. Blood 1999;94:26a.

149. Gustafsson D, Nystrom J-E, Carlsson S, et al: Pharmacodynamic properties of H376/95, a prodrug of the direct thrombin inhibitor melagatran, intended for oral use [abstract #102]. Blood 1999;94:26a.

150. Eriksson BI, Lindbratt S, Kalebo P, et al: METHRO II: Dose-response study of the novel oral, direct thrombin inhibitor, H376/95 and its subcutaneous formulation, melagatran, compared with dalteparin as thromboembolic prophylaxis after total hip or total knee replacement. Haemostasis 2000;30(Suppl 1):20-21.

151. Heit JA, Colwell DW, Francis CW, et al, for the AstraZeneca Arthroplasty Study Group: Comparison of the oral direct thrombin inhibitor ximelagatran with enoxparin as prophylaxis against venous thromboembolism after total knee replacement. Arch Intern Med 2001;161:2215-2221.

152. Girard TJ, MacPhail LA, Likert KM, et al: Inhibition of factor VIIa-tissue factor coagulation activity by a hybrid protein. Science 1990;248:1421-1424.

153. Broze GJ Jr: Tissue factor pathway inhibitor. Thromb Haemost 1995;74:90-93.

154. Oltrona L, Speidel CM, Recchia D, et al: Inhibition of tissue factor-mediated coagulation markedly attenuates stenosis after balloon-induced arterial injury in minipigs. Circulation 1997;96:646-652.

155. Creasey AA, Chang AC, Feigen L, et al: Tissue factor pathway inhibitor reduces mortality from *Escherichia coli* septic shock. J Clin Invest 1993;91:2850-2856.

156. Elsayed YA, Nakagawa K, Kamikubo YI, et al: Effects of recombinant human tissue factor pathway inhibitor on thrombus formation and its in vivo distribution in a rat DIC model. Am J Clin Pathol 1996;106:574-583.

157. Bajaj MS, Bajaj SP: Tissue factor pathway inhibitor: Potential therapeutic applications. Thromb Haemost 1997;78:471-477.

158. Creasey AA, Reihart K: Tissue factor pathway inhibitor activity in severe sepsis. Crit Care Med 2001;29(Suppl 7):S126-S129.

159. Stassens P, Bergum PW, Gansemans Y, et al: Anticoagulant repertoire of the hookworm *Ancylostoma caninim*. Proc Natl Acad Sci U S A 1996;93:2149-2154.

160. Lee A, Agnelli G, Buller H, et al: Dose-response study of recombinant factor VIIa/tissue factor inhibitor recombinant nematode anticoagulant protein c2 in prevention of postoperative venous thromboembolism in patients undergoing total knee replacement. Circulation 2001;104:74-78.

161. Banner DW, D'Arcy A, Chene C, et al: The crystal structure of the complex of blood coagulation factor VIIa with soluble tissue factor. Nature 1996;380:41-46.

162. Harker LA, Hanson SR, Kelly AB: Antithrombotic strategies targeting thrombin activities, thrombin receptors and thrombin generation. Thromb Haemost 1997;78:736-741.

163. Arnljots B, Ezban M, Hedner U: Prevention of experimental arterial thrombosis by topical administration of active site-inactivated factor VIIa. J Vasc Surg 1997;25:341-346.

164. Golino P, Ragni M, Cirillo P, et al: Antithrombotic effects of recombinant human, active site-blocked factor VIIa in a rabbit model of recurrent and arterial thrombosis. Circ Res 1998;82:39-46.

165. Jang Y, Guzman LA, Lincoff AM, et al: Influence of blockade at specific levels of the coagulation cascade on restenosis in a rabbit atherosclerotic femoral artery injury model. Circulation 1995;92:3041-3050.

166. Giesen PL, Rauch U, Bohrmann B, et al: Blood-borne tissue factor: Another view of thrombosis. Proc Natl Acad Sci U S A 1999;96:2311-2315.

167. Hoffman M, Monroe DM, Oliver JA, et al: Factors IXa and Xa play distinct roles in tissue-dependent initiation of coagulation. Blood 1995;86:1794-1801.

168. Benedict CR, Ryan J, Wolitzky B, et al: Active site-blocked factor IXa prevents intravascular thrombus formation in the coronary vasculature without inhibiting extravascular coagulation in a canine thrombosis model. J Clin Invest 1991;88:1760-1765.

169. Bajaj SP, Rapaprt SI, Maki SL: A monoclonal antibody to factor IX that inhibits the factor VII:Ca potentiation of factor X activation. J Biol Chem 1985;260:11574-11580.

170. Feuerstein GZ, Toomey JR, Valock R, et al: An inhibitory anti-factor IX antibody effectively reduces thrombus formation in a rat model of venous thrombosis. Thromb Haemost 1999;92:1443-1450.

171. Feuerstin GZ, Patel A, Toomey JR, et al: Antithrombotic efficacy of a novel murine antihuman factor IX antibody in rats. Arterioscler Thromb Vasc Biol 1999;19:2554-2562.

172. Herbert JM, Heralult JP, Bernat A, et al: Biochemical and pharmacological properties of SANORB 340006, a potent and long-acting synthetic pentasaccharide. Blood 1998;91:4197-4205.

173. Eisenberg PR, Siegel JE, Abendschein DR, et al: Importance of factor Xa in determining the procoagulant activity of whole-blood clots. J Clin Invest 1993;91:1877-1883.

174. Vlasuk GP: Structural and functional characterization of tick anticoagulant peptide (TAP): A potent and selective inhibitor of blood coagulation factor Xa. Thromb Haemost 1993;70:212-216.

175. Tuszyuski G, Gasic TB, Gasic GJ: Isolation and characterization of antistasin. J Biol Chem 1987;262:9718-9723.

176. Dunwidddie C, Thornberry NA, Bull HG, et al: Antistasin: A leech-derived inhibitor of factor Xa: Kinetic analysis of enzyme inhibition and identification of the reactive site. J Biol Chem 1989;264:16694-16699.

177. Beimond BJ, Friederich PW, Levi M, et al: Comparison of sustained antithrombotic effects of inhibitors of thrombin and factor Xa in experimental thrombosis. Circulation 1996;93:153-160.

178. Orvim U, Barstad RM, Vlasuk GP, et al: Effect of selective factor Xa inhibition on arterial thrombus formation triggered by tissue factor/factor VIIa or collagen in an ex vivo model of shear-dependent human thrombogenesis. Arterioscler Thromb Vasc Biol 1995;15:2188-2194.

179. Ragosta M, Gimple LW, Gertz SD, et al: Specific factor Xa inhibition reduces restenosis after balloon angioplasty of atherosclerotic femoral arteries in rabbits. Circulation 1994;89:1262-1271.

180. Herbert JM, Bernat A, Dol F, et al: CX-9065a, a novel synthetic, selective and orally active inhibitor of factor Xa: In vitro and in vivo studies. J Pharmacol Exp Ther 1996;276:1030-1038.

181. Murayama N, Tanaka M, Kunitada S, et al: Tolerability, pharmacokinetics and pharmacodynamics of DX-9065a, a new synthetic potent anticoagulant and specific factor Xa inhibitor, in healthy male volunteers. Clin Pharmacol Ther 1999;66:258-264.

182. Boneu B, Necciari J, Cariou R, et al: Pharmacokinetics and tolerance of the natural pentasaccharide (SR90107A/ORG31540) with high affinity to antithrombin III in man. Thromb Haemost 1995;74:1468-1473.

183. Walenga J, Jeske W, Bara L, et al: Biochemical and pharmacological rationale for the development of a synthetic heparin pentasaccharide. Thromb Res 1997;86:1–36.

184. Eriksson BI, Bauer KA, Lassen MR, et al, for the Steering Committee of the Pentasaccharide in Hip Fracture Surgery Study: Fondaparinux compared with enoxaparin for the prevention of venous thromboembolism after hip-fracture surgery. N Engl J Med 2001;345:1340–1342.

185. Turpie G: The PENTHATHLON 2000 Study: Comparison of the first synthetic factor Xa inhibitor with low molecular weight heparin in the prevention of venous thromboembolism (VTE) after elective hip replacement [abstract]. Blood 2000;96:491a.

186. Bauer KA, Eriksson MD, Lassen MR, et al, for the Steering Committee of the Pentasaccharide in Major Knee Surgery Study: Fondaparinux compared with enoxaparin for the prevention of venous thromboembolism after major elective knee surgery. N Engl J Med 2001;345:1305–1310.

187. Coussement PK, Bassand JP, Convens C, et al, for the PENTALYSE investigators: A synthetic factor Xa inhibitor (ORG31540/SR9017A) as an adjunct to fibrinolysis in acute myocardial infarction. Eur Heart J 2001;22:1716–1724.

188. Bernard GR, Vincent JL, Laterre PF, et al: Efficacy and safety of recombinant activated protein C for severe sepsis. N Engl J Med 2001;344:699–709.

189. Parkinson JF, Grinnell BW, Moore RE, et al: Stable expression of a secretable deletion mutation of recombinant human thrombomodulin in mammalian cells. J Biol Chem 1990;265:12602–12610.

190. Gomi L, Zushi M, Honda G, et al: Antithrombotic effect of recombinant human thrombomodulin on thrombin-induced thromboembolism in mice. Blood 1990;75:1369–1399.

191. Aoki Y, Ohishi R, Takei R, et al: Effects of recombinant human soluble thrombomodulin (rhs-TM) on a rat model of disseminated intravascular coagulation with decreased levels of plasma antithrombin III. Thromb Haemost 1994;71:452–455.

192. Hirsh J, Fuster V: Guide to anticoagulant therapy: II. Oral anticoagulants. Circulation 1994;89:1469–1480.

193. Sixty-Plus Reinfarction Study Research Group: A double-blind trial to assess long-term anticoagulant therapy in elderly patients after myocardial infarction. Lancet 1980;2:989–994.

194. Smith P, Arnesen H, Holme I: The effect of warfarin on mortality and reinfarction after myocardial infarction. N Engl J Med 1998;323:147–152.

195. Anticoagulants in the Secondary Prevention of Events in Coronary Thrombosis (ASPECT) Research Group: The effect of long-term oral anticoagulant treatment on mortality and cardiovascular morbidity after myocardial infarction. Lancet 1994;343:499–503.

196. Breddin K, Loew D, Ledner K, et al: Secondary prevention of myocardial infarction: A comparison of acetylsalicylic acid, placebo, and phenprocoumon. Haemostasis 1980;9:325–344.

197. Anand SS, Yusuf S: Oral anticoagulant therapy in patients with coronary artery disease: A meta-analysis. JAMA 1999;282:2058–2067.

198. Ebert RV: Long-term anticoagulant therapy after myocardial infarction. JAMA 1969;207:2263–2267.

199. Medical Research Council Working party: An assessment of long-term anticoagulant administration after myocardial infarction. BMJ 1964;2:837–843.

200. EPSIM Research Group: A controlled comparison of aspirin and oral anticoagulants in prevention of death after myocardial infarction. N Engl J Med 1982;307:701–708.

201. Julian DG, Chamberlain DA, Popcock SJ, for the AFTER study group: A comparison of aspirin and anticoagulation following thrombolysis for myocardial infarction (the AFTER study). BMJ 1996;313:1429–1431.

202. Coumadin Aspirin Reinfarction Study (CARS) investigators: Randomized double-blind trial of fixed low-dose warfarin with aspirin after myocardial infarction. Lancet 1997;350:389–396.

203. Anand SS, Yusuf S, Pogue J, et al: Long-term oral anticoagulant therapy in patients with unstable angina or suspected non-Q-wave myocardial infarction: Organisation to Assess Strategies for Ischemic Syndrome (OASIS) pilot study results. Circulation 1998;98:1064–1070.

204. Medical Research Council's General Practice Research Framework: Thrombosis prevention trial: Randomised trial of low-intensity oral anticoagulation with warfarin and low-dose aspirin in the primary prevention of ischaemic heart disease in men at increased risk. Lancet 1998;351:233–241.

205. Hirsh J: Oral anticoagulant drugs. N Engl J Med 1991;324:1865–1875.

206. Harrison L, Johnston M, Massicotte MP, et al: Comparison of 5-mg and 10-mg loading doses in initiation of warfarin therapy. Ann Intern Med 1997;126:133–136.

207. Broekmans AW, Bertina RM, Loeliger EA, et al: Protein C and the development of skin necrosis during anticoagulant therapy [letter]. Thromb Haemost 1983;49:251.

208. Goodnight SH: Antiplatelet therapy with aspirin: From clinical trials to practice. Thromb Haemost 1995;74:401–405.

209. Dale J, Myhre E, Storstein O, et al: Prevention of arterial thromboembolism with acetylsalicylic acid: Controlled clinical study in patients with aortic ball valves. Am Heart J 1977;94:101–111.

210. Chesebro JH, Fuster V, Elveback LR, et al: Trial of combined warfarin plus dipyridamole or aspirin therapy in prosthetic heart valve replacement: Danger of aspirin compared with dipyridamole. Am J Cardiol 1983;51:1537–1541.

211. Turpie AGG, Gent M, Laupacis A, et al: A comparison of aspirin with placebo in patients treated with warfarin after heart-valve replacement. N Engl J Med 1993;329:524–529.

212. Meade TW, Roderick PJ, Brennan PJ, et al: Extra-cranial bleeding and other symptoms due to low dose aspirin and low intensity oral anticoagulation. Thromb Haemost 1992;68:1–6.

213. Prichard PJ, Kitchingman GK, Walt RP, et al: Human gastric mucosal bleeding induced by low dose aspirin, but not warfarin. BMJ 1989;298:493–496.

214. Wells PS, Holbrook AM, Crowther M, et al: Interactions of warfarin with drugs and food. Ann Intern Med 1994;121:676–683.

■ ■ ■ chapter 3 0

Acute Plaque Passivation and Endothelial Therapy

Peter L. Thompson

The central role of the unstable plaque and disturbed endothelial function in acute coronary syndromes is described in Chapters 5 and 6. This chapter briefly reviews these mechanisms in and the potential for reversing them in patients with acute coronary syndromes. Several therapies that improve outcomes in acute coronary syndromes may act by acute plaque passivation and stabilization of endothelial dysfunction; these are reviewed, and future therapeutic possibilities are discussed.

CONCEPT OF PLAQUE PASSIVATION

The pathophysiologic processes that contribute to instability of the coronary atherosclerotic plaque are now well described,[1,2] and our understanding of the underlying processes that cause the inflammation and its consequences is growing.[3] A vulnerable plaque is characterized by increases in the lipid pool, macrophages, foam cells, and T lymphocytes and by a reduced collagen and smooth muscle cell population.[4,5] This leads to rupture or erosion at the margins or shoulder region of the plaque, where the overlying fibrous cap is thinnest and infiltrated by macrophages[6] and exposed to the greatest sheer stress.[7,8] The resultant platelet adhesion, aggregation, and consequent coronary thrombosis are the targets of the current aggressive antithrombotic strategies used to stabilize the patient with an acute coronary syndrome.

In contrast with the relatively advanced state of antithrombotic therapy and understanding of the underlying process of plaque instability, there are few diagnostic tools to identify the unstable plaque and only a few clearly identified therapeutic targets for preventing plaque rupture and enhancing plaque stabilization. Nevertheless, there is a huge potential to improve clinical outcomes in acute coronary syndromes if the balance of the complex processes within the unstable plaque can be tipped toward stabilization and passivation.

Multiple factors determine the balance between instability and stability of the atherosclerotic plaque and define the potential therapeutic targets. The options for enhancing passivation of the plaque are summarized in Table 30-1.

Enhancing the Thickness of the Overlying Fibrous Cap

Histopathologic observations confirm that a thin overlying cap is a typical feature of the unstable plaque, leading to rupture and erosion.[6] Both rupture and erosion are important, and shear stresses may mechanically damage the endothelium without causing rupture.[9] Therefore, plaque is strengthened by deposition of collagen in the fibrous cap. The challenge is to control this process in the unstable plaque without encouraging adverse vascular remodeling and without affecting matrix synthesis in other tissues and organs.

Enhancing the Synthetic Role of Vascular Smooth Muscle Cells

Smooth muscle cells can modulate their phenotype from normal contractile cells to a synthetic phenotype capable of proliferation and enhanced matrix synthesis.[10] Transition to the synthetic phenotype of smooth muscle cells is associated with an increase in collagen secretion, a key process in enhancing plaque stabilization.[11] In contrast, the unstable atherosclerotic plaque is typically characterized by reduced numbers of vascular smooth muscle cells and reduced collagen content and by an increase in the rate of smooth muscle cell apoptosis. The rate of apoptosis is a major determinant of the numbers of vascular smooth muscle cells in the atherosclerotic plaque and is governed by complex interactions of cells, cell matrix, and cell cytokine.[12] There is evidence of increased apoptosis of vascular smooth muscles in the atherosclerotic plaque of patients with unstable angina compared with patients with stable angina,[13] and apoptosis has been detected in the shoulder region of plaques at the sites that appear most likely to rupture.[14] A key determinant of the rate of smooth muscle cell apoptosis

■ ▪ ■

TABLE 30–1 POTENTIAL TARGETS FOR PLAQUE STABILIZATION AND PASSIVATION

Enhancing the thickness of the overlying fibrous cap
Enhancing the synthetic role of vascular smooth muscle cells
Reducing the extent of the inflammatory process
Reducing the size of the lipid pool
Preventing matrix degeneration by metalloproteinases

is the expression of nitric oxide, which is enhanced by pro-inflammatory cytokines such as interleukin-I β, interferon-γ, and tumor necrosis factor[15] and which acts via the production of peroxynitrite in combination with superoxide radicals.

Reducing the Extent of the Inflammatory Process

Atherosclerosis has been recognized as an inflammatory process,[3] and unstable plaques in particular are characterized by a dense inflammatory cell infiltrate.[6] Comparisons of atherectomy specimens taken from patients with acute versus chronic coronary syndromes show an increased frequency of macrophages and T lymphocytes in the specimens of patients with refractory unstable angina.[16] A potential approach to stabilizing the plaque is to control the inflammatory cell infiltrate into an unstable atherosclerotic plaque via modulation of cell adhesion molecules and migration factors.

Reducing the Size of the Lipid Pool

In addition to the thickness of the overlying cap and the degree of cellular infiltration, the degree of stability of the plaque is determined by the size of the lipid pool. Davies et al established that the critical threshold of vulnerability to rupture was a 50% volume of extracellular lipids.[17] Computer modeling of plaques has identified the circumferential tensile strength on the fibrous cap as the most important mechanical stress factor involved in plaque rupture.[18,19] Therefore, any intervention that can reduce the size of the lipid pool is likely to stabilize the plaque.

Preventing Matrix Degeneration by Metalloproteinases

Matrix degradation leading to plaque rupture appears to be primarily due to the action of matrix metalloproteinases (MMPs).[20] The expression of MMP by vascular smooth muscle cells and macrophages is increased in human atherosclerotic plaques.[21] The activity of MMPs is inhibited by naturally occurring tissue inhibitors of metalloproteinases. Exogenously administered tissue inhibitors of metalloproteinases are readily metabolized and denatured.[22] The CD40 pathway is a key signaling mechanism through which macrophages and vascular smooth muscle cells in atheroma can express matrix-degrading proteinases, leading to plaque

rupture.[23] This CD40–CD40 ligand interaction raises the intriguing therapeutic possibility that using a CD40 ligand antibody to interrupt CD40 signaling could result in plaque stabilization.[24]

ROLE OF THE ENDOTHELIUM AND ENDOTHELIAL DYSFUNCTION

The vascular endothelium is the most widely distributed but largest "organ" in the body, equivalent in area to a football field and in mass to five normal-sized hearts. Endothelial cells line the cardiovascular system and provide an interface between blood and tissues, allowing intercellular communication and exchange of solutes and ions. In addition, the endothelium has complex functions that modulate smooth muscle tone and mediate hemostasis, cellular proliferation, and inflammatory and immune mechanisms in the vessel wall.[25] The seminal observations of Furchgott and Zawadzki established that normal vasoregulation requires the presence of the endothelium.[26] The modulation of vascular tone depends on relaxing and contracting factors derived from the endothelium. These are summarized in Table 30–2.

Endothelium-Dependent Vasodilation

Endothelium-dependent vasodilation depends on at least three endothelium-derived vasodilators, each of which represents a potential therapeutic target. The first potent endothelium-derived vasoactive substance to be discovered was prostacyclin in the late 1970s.[27] A more labile, diffusible, nonprotanopic substance that mediated endothelium-dependent vasorelaxation was discovered in the 1980s[28] and was initially called *endothelium-derived relaxation factor*, although it is now well established as nitric oxide.[29,30] Nitric oxide is synthesized from its precursor, L-arginine, with the enzyme nitric oxide synthase (NOS). There are three isoforms of NOS: neuronal (n-NOS), inducible (i-NOS), and endothelial (e-NOS),[31] of which e-NOS is expressed ubiquitously in endothelial cells. Differing genotypes offer some potential for gene therapy.[32] The activity of nitric oxide depends on an intracellular rise in calcium that is signaled through stimulation with neurotransmitters such as acetylcholine or substance P, circulating hormones such as bradykinin, or shear stress. A third vasodilating

■ ▪ ■

TABLE 30–2 ENDOTHELIUM-DEPENDENT VASOACTIVE SUBSTANCES

Endothelium-Dependent Vasodilation
  Prostacyclin (PGI2)
  Endothelium-derived relaxation factor (EDRF), nitric oxide (NO)
  Endothelium-derived hyperpolarising factor (EDHF)
Endothelium-Dependent Vasoconstriction
  Ecosanoid family (especially thromboxane A$_2$)
  Endothelin-1

factor, called *endothelium-derived hyperpolarizing factor*, leads to hyperpolarization of smooth muscle cells via activation of potassium channels.[33]

Endothelium-Dependent Vasoconstriction

Endothelium-dependent vasoconstriction is mediated by two directly acting endothelium-derived contracting factors, the *eicosanoid family*, predominantly thromboxane A_2, and the *endothelins*.[34] The endothelin most active in the vasculature is endothelin-1, stimulated by numerous endogenous agents including interleukin-1, transforming growth factor β, shear stress, and hypoxia. Vasoconstriction is also enhanced by the final stage of production of angiotensin II by the angiotensin-converting enzyme (ACE) at the luminal surface of endothelial cells.[35]

In addition to its role in vasoregulation, the endothelium secretes a range of prothrombotic and antithrombotic factors, including tissue plasminogen activator and plasminogen activator inhibitor. The endothelium helps prevent spontaneous platelet aggregation adhesion by production of prostacyclin and nitric oxide.

The endothelium contains important mechanoreceptors that sense changes in shear stress and hydrostatic pressure. Flow-induced vessel dilatation requires an intact functional endothelium[36] and is the basis of the widely used flow-mediated dilatation test of endothelial function.[37] The concept of endothelial dysfunction has been intensively studied.[38] Endothelial cells are activated by the inflammatory cytokines interleukin-1, tumor necrosis factor α, and interferon-γ. Activated endothelial cells express leukocyte adhesion molecules and produce tissue factor, creating a procoagulant environment. Endothelial cell injury results in a dysfunctional endothelium that can no longer maintain a thromboresistant state and promotes vasoconstriction by diminished production of nitric oxide and synthesis of endothelin-1.[38] The production of reactive oxygen species as a consequence of endothelial injury potentiates endothelial dysfunction by depleting available nitric oxide and reacting to form peroxynitrite, which causes further oxidative injury to the endothelium. The production of lipid peroxides further depletes nitric oxide.[39] Oxidized low-density lipoprotein (LDL) acts as chemoattractant for macrophages, which in turn promote the expression of adhesion molecules on the endothelial surface.[40] Reversal of endothelial dysfunction is an important future target of therapy for acute coronary syndromes; some of the interventions currently used for acute coronary syndromes work by reversing endothelial dysfunction. These are discussed in the following.

THERAPIES DIRECTED AT PLAQUE PASSIVATION AND CORRECTION OF ENDOTHELIAL DYSFUNCTION

Hydroxy-Methylglutaryl Coenzyme A Reductase Inhibitors (Statins)

Statins influence a number of other mechanisms independent of their lipid-lowering effects, which are thought to be potentially important in the treatment of acute coronary syndromes. Animal studies have revealed potential roles for statins in plaque stabilization by increasing the collagen content of the unstable plaque,[41] reducing macrophage activation, expressing MMPs,[42] and modulating immune function. Reductions in plasma fibrinogen[43] and thrombogenic factors have been demonstrated in hypercholesterolemic patients.[44,45] A tendency for enhanced platelet thrombus formation in subjects with hypercholesterolemia can be reversed with only 2.4 months of treatment with pravastatin.[46] Early improvements in endothelial-dependent vasodilation have been demonstrated in hypercholesterolemic patients,[47-50] and these benefits occur within 6 weeks of the commencement of statin therapy in patients who are recovering from an acute coronary syndrome.[51]

Clinical trials in patients in stable condition after a coronary event have demonstrated beyond doubt that treatment with statins reduces the risk of future cardiovascular events and reduces mortality in patients with cardiovascular disease. These beneficial effects have been demonstrated not only when the initial plasma cholesterol level is elevated, as in the Scandinavian Simvastatin Survival Study,[52] but also when it is in the average range, as in the Cholesterol and Recurrent Events[53] and Long-term Intervention with Pravastatin in Ischemic Disease studies.[54] These major postcoronary studies have demonstrated clear-cut effects in patients who experience stabilization *after* a coronary event; the curves for coronary events diverge after a delay of at least a year. It would seem logical to initiate secondary preventive treatment as soon as possible after the acute event,[55] but there is a significant "evidence gap" to judge whether there is truly an early effect of statins in acute coronary syndromes.

Small-scale clinical trials have shown that statins started 2 to 10 days after acute myocardial infarction (AMI) or unstable angina pectoris are well tolerated and are associated with reductions in total and LDL cholesterol and improvements in endothelial function.[56,57] These studies did not assess long-term outcomes, but the Randomized Lipid-Coronary Artery Disease study, which commenced treatment with pravastatin at 6 ± 5 days, showed an improvement in the angiographic appearance and a significant reduction in the incidence of major cardiovascular events in patients followed up for 2 years ($P < .03$).[58]

Retrospective analyses of databases suggest that statin therapy confers a short-term benefit before or immediately following admission to the hospital for AMI. In one small hospital-based study, patients with AMI who received statins in the hospital were matched with those who did not; the results showed a possible benefit on hospital mortality and re-infarction.[59] In an observational study of patients with acute coronary syndromes who participated in two clinical trials of glycoprotein IIb/IIIa inhibitors (the Global Strategies to Open Occluded Arteries [GUSTO] IIb and Platelet Glycoprotein IIb/IIIa in Unstable Angina Receptor Suppression Using Integrilin Therapy [PURSUIT] trials), those who underwent lipid-lowering therapy were compared with those who did not.[60] The all-cause mortality of the 3653 patients who were discharged on lipid-lowering agents was compared with the 17,156 who were not. Lipid-lowering therapy at hospital discharge was associated with a halving of mortality at 30 days (hazard ratio, 0.44; 95% CI, 0.27 to 0.73; P = .001) and at 6 months (P < .0001). The reduction in mortality in those prescribed a lipid-lowering drug in the hospital was still significant at 6 months (hazard ratio, 0.67; 95% CI, 0.48 to 0.95; P = .023) after adjustment for the propensity to be prescribed lipid-lowering agents and other potential confounders.

In a 58-hospital registry study in Sweden between 1995 and 1998, the 5528 patients with AMI who received statins at or before hospital discharge were compared with the 14,071 who did not.[61] At 1 year, the unadjusted mortality rate was 9.3% in the no-statin group and 4.0% in the statin group. After adjustment for confounding factors and propensity score for statin use, early statin treatment was associated with a reduction in 1-year mortality (relative risk, 0.75; 95% CI, 0.63 to 0.89; P =. 001) in hospital survivors of AMI. In a preliminary report from the Orbofiban in Patients with Unstable coronary Syndromes/Thrombolysis In Myocardial Infarction (OPUS-TIMI) study, patients who were treated with lipid-lowering drugs experienced a similar reduction in mortality at 1 month after an acute coronary syndrome.[62] Despite the sophisticated matching techniques for assessing the propensity for being prescribed lipid-lowering therapy, the possibility of bias in the decision to treat cannot be excluded, and the effect of statins cannot be separated from the effect of other lipid-lowering therapies. Randomized trial data are still needed to fully assess the impact of early statin therapy.

The randomized clinical trials of early commencement of statins after a coronary event are summarized in Table 30-3.

The Myocardial Ischemia Reduction with Aggressive Cholesterol Lowering (MIRACL) study was the first complete large-scale clinical trial to investigate whether early treatment with a statin in patients with unstable angina pectoris or non–Q-wave AMI is beneficial.[63] MIRACL was a 16-week, randomized, double-blind, placebo-controlled trial that enrolled 3086 patients with unstable angina pectoris or non–Q-wave acute MI. Patients were randomized within 24 to 96 hours of hospital admission to atorvastatin (80 mg per day) or placebo. The primary effi-

cacy parameter was time at the first occurrence of death, resuscitated cardiac arrest, nonfatal MI, or angina pectoris with evidence of myocardial ischemia requiring rehospitalization. The relative risk of the primary efficacy measure was 0.84 (P = .048; 95% CI, 0.701 to 0.999). The relative risk for rehospitalization for unstable angina (a component of the primary efficacy measure) was 0.74 (P = .02; 95% CI, 0.57 to 0.95. There was no effect on death, nonfatal myocardial infarction, or resuscitated cardiac arrest. The stroke rate was unexpectedly halved from 1.6 to 0.8 (P = .05; 95% CI, 0.026 to 0.99). The primary efficacy measure in the MIRACL trial only just achieved its statistical significance, P = .048, and the 95% confidence intervals of the relative risk of the primary efficacy measure were wide and at the lower end of the confidence level. A relatively large number of patients were lost to follow-up. Patients undergoing planned coronary revascularization were excluded from the MIRACL trial. Although the MIRACL trial provides some support for the early initiation of statin therapy, the results are not definitive evidence of an early benefit for statins in the modern treatment of acute coronary syndromes. The investigators of the FLuvastatin On RIsk Diminishing After acute myocardial infarction (FLORIDA) trial commenced a statin within 24 hours of onset. A preliminary report from this study showed an apparent reduction in coronary events in those treated with fluvastatin compared with placebo.[64] Ongoing trials may provide further evidence of the extent and timing of the benefit. The timing of commencement of therapy in the published trials of statins after acute coronary syndromes is summarized in Figure 30-1.

The Pravastatin in Acute Coronary syndromes Trial (PACT) initiates statin therapy within 24 hours after the onset of the acute coronary syndrome, and its primary end point is the frequency of events within the first month. These design features make it likely that the investigators will gain further information on the capacity of statin therapy to stabilize the atherothrombotic plaque in acute coronary syndromes. The PRavastatin Or atorVastatin Evaluation and Infection Therapy (PROVE-IT) trial will compare the effect of pravastatin, 40 mg, with atorvastatin, 80 mg, as well as the effect of an antibiotic on clinical outcomes in acute coronary syndromes. The assumption for the statin arm of the study is that 80 mg of atorvastatin will be equivalent to 40 mg of pravastatin, and the statistical considerations are based on the effect of the antibiotic rather than the two alternative statin strategies. The A to Z study is a targeted study to evaluate the effect of statin therapy (simvastatin) in stabilizing the postcoronary course in patients who have received a glycoprotein IIb/IIIa inhibitor (tirofiban) in the early treatment of their acute coronary syndrome.

In summary, there are valid reasons, including convenience and no evidence of an adverse effect, for initiating lipid-lowering therapy with a statin in hospital after an acute coronary syndrome. At this stage, however, there is still no convincing evidence of benefit. Evidence from large-scale clinical trials is still required to assess whether early statin initiation is more effective in reducing clinical events than later commencement after an acute coronary syndrome.

■ ■ ■

TABLE 30–3 TRIALS OF EARLY INITIATION OF STATINS IN ACUTE CORONARY SYNDROMES

TRIAL	DRUGS	PATIENTS
MIRACL	Atorvastatin 80 mg, placebo	Non-STEMI
PACT	Pravastatin 20–40 mg, placebo	STEMI and Non-STEMI
A to Z	Tirofiban then simvastatin 40 mg vs. placebo	Non-STEMI
PRINCESS	Cerivastatin 400 μg vs. placebo	Non-STEMI
PROVE-IT	Pravastatin 40 mg vs. atorvastatin 80 mg/gatifloxacin vs. placebo	Non-STEMI

STEMI, ST-elevation myocardial infarction.

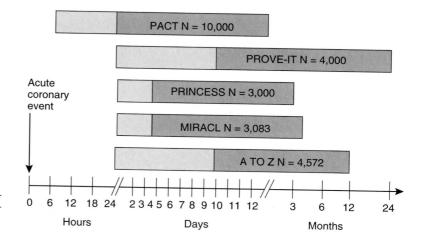

FIGURE 30–1. Timing of initiation and duration of therapy in the trials of early initiation of statins in acute coronary syndromes.

Angiotensin-Converting Enzyme Inhibitors

The presence of an important tissue renin-angiotensin system is now well recognized, and it is estimated that less than 10% of ACE is found circulating in the plasma.[65] The central role of the system in the vascular wall is summarized in Figure 30–2.

Angiotensin II can have a wide range of deleterious effects in the vascular wall, including vasoconstriction, by stimulating the production of norepinephrine and enhancing the production of endothelin-1, which further facilitates the conversion of angiotensin I to angiotensin II. It also promotes the release of inflammatory cytokines, metalloproteinases, and thrombotic factors.[65] Angiotensin II increases superoxide production via membrane-bound NADH/NADPH oxidase production in smooth muscle cells, leading to the degrading of nitric oxide.[66] The endothelium-based receptor that binds oxidized LDL (lectin-like oxidized low-density lipoprotein receptor type 1, or LOX) interacts with angiotensin II. Angiotensin II upregulates the receptor effects, which can be blocked with angiotensin receptor blockers and ACE inhibitors.[67] ACE inhibitors can block these effects, shifting the balance in favor of

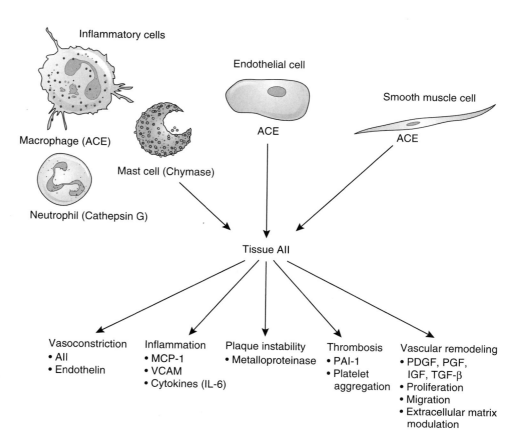

FIGURE 30–2. Effects of the tissue angiotensin system on the vessel wall.

vasodilatating, anti-inflammatory, and antiproliferative effects.

These effects have been demonstrated to be clinically significant.[68,69] Several clinical trials of ACE inhibitors have shown improvements in coronary endothelial dysfunction in patients with coronary artery disease. Quinapril, 20 mg per day, partly reversed the vasoconstricting effects of intracoronary acetylcholine in patients with coronary artery disease in the QUinapril Ischemic Event Trial (QUIET).[70] However, the effects on atherosclerotic progression were less impressive.[71] The benefits of quinapril on endothelial dysfunction were enhanced among smokers compared with nonsmokers.[72] Studies of an alternative ACE inhibitor, enalapril, showed that the benefits were restricted to those with depressed endothelial function and those with the ACE DD or ID genotypes and not in those homozygous for the I allele.[73] The benefits of ACE inhibitors in reversing endothelial dysfunction were confirmed in a study that compared quinapril (20 mg) with losartan (50 mg), amlodipine (5 mg), or enalapril (10 mg) [the Brachial Artery Normalization of Forearm Function (BANFF) study].[74] In this study, only quinapril was effective. The improvement did not occur in those with the DD ACE genotype but did occur in those with the ID and II genotypes.

It is not yet clear whether angiotensin II receptor antagonists will mimic these benefits of ACE inhibitors on endothelial function. A preliminary study with irbesartan suggests that it has effects on cytokines and adhesion molecules in patients with premature atherosclerosis, which may be of potential benefit in plaque passivation and restoration of endothelial dysfunction.[75]

The benefits of ACE inhibitors on improving ischemic outcomes have been the subject of detailed study in patients with stable coronary artery disease and those at high risk, but these inhibitors have not been tested directly in the setting of acute coronary syndromes. A benefit on ischemic events in chronically treated patients suggests a mechanism of benefit on coronary atherosclerosis independent of the well-established benefits in hypertension, cardiac failure, and left-ventricular dysfunction. This was initially suspected in retrospective analyses of the cardiac failure and post-infarction trials, which showed effects consistent with a benefit on myocardial ischemia in addition to the hypothesized effect on left-ventricular dysfunction.[76] The Survival and Ventricular Enlargement (SAVE) trial with captopril[77] and the Study On Left-Ventricular Dysfunction (SOLVD) with enalapril[78] both showed that the patients in the ACE inhibitor arms of the trials had an apparent reduction in ischemic events. In a meta-analysis of all the post-infarction ACE inhibitor trials (N = 5966), mortality was lower with ACE inhibitors than with placebo (odds ratio, 0.74; 95% CI, 0.66 to 0.83), as were the rates of reinfarction (odds ratio, 0.80; 95% CI, 0.69 to 0.94).[79]

These suspected benefits of ACE inhibitors on myocardial ischemia gleaned from meta-analysis were strikingly confirmed in a prospective randomized trial in high-risk patients using ramipril.[80] In the Health, Osteoporosis, Progestin, Estrogen (HOPE) study, 9297 high-risk patients (55 years old or older) with atherosclerotic disease and at high risk for an ischemic event by having diabetes or another risk factor were given ramipril (10 mg, once per day orally) or matching placebo for a mean of 5 years. There was a clear-cut benefit on mortality in terms of death from any cause (relative risk, 0.78; 95% CI, 0.70 to 0.86; P < .001) and death from cardiovascular causes (relative risk, 0.74; P < .001). The effects in this group without known left-ventricular dysfunction are consistent with a benefit on the atherosclerotic process, with a reduction in myocardial infarction (relative risk, 0.80; P < .001), stroke (relative risk, 0.68; P < .001), and the need for revascularization (relative risk, 0.85; P < .001). Whether the benefits are also seen with angiotensin receptor antagonists is being tested in a trial of telmisartan against ramipril [Ongoing Telmisartan Alone and in Combination with Ramipril Global Endpoint Trial (ONTARGET)].

Although the early administration of ACE inhibitors during AMI is well supported by randomized clinical trials, this effect is consistent with the known benefits on left-ventricular dysfunction and was less dramatic in those without left-ventricular dysfunction. The benefits on mortality in the acute phase are equivalent to a 7% (standard deviation, 2%) proportional reduction (95% CI, 2% to 11%; P < .004), representing approximately five deaths (standard deviation, 2%) per 1000 patients, with most of the benefit observed within the first week. These benefits occur at the expense of an excess of persistent hypotension (17.6% vs. 9.3%; P < .01) and renal dysfunction (1.3% vs. 0.6%, P < .01).[81] These data on early administration of ACE inhibitors in patients with AMI, many of whom have left-ventricular dysfunction, do not necessarily support the routine use of ACE inhibitors in patients with acute coronary syndromes. More data are needed before a clear recommendation can be made in patients without high-risk features or left-ventricular dysfunction.[82]

Aspirin–ACE Inhibitor Interaction?

In discussing the potential use of ACE inhibitors in acute coronary syndromes, it is important to address the controversy on the interaction between aspirin and ACE inhibitors. Several studies have suggested that in patients taking aspirin concomitantly with ACE inhibitors, the ACE inhibitor benefit is reduced because of the inhibition of prostaglandins by the aspirin.[83,84] However, there was no evidence of a clinically significant interaction in an observational study of ACE inhibitor use in a lipid-lowering trial[85] or in an overview of all the large postinfarction trials.[86] In view of this evidence in large-scale trials, it seems unlikely that this interaction would be significant in the setting of combined aspirin and ACE inhibitor use in acute coronary syndromes. However, an analysis of the combination in patients in acute coronary reperfusion studies and trials of antiplatelet therapy in patients undergoing percutaneous coronary intervention have suggested an interaction.[87] After adjusting for confounders, combined use of aspirin and ACE inhibitors was associated with increased mortality compared with aspirin alone. Despite the reassuring findings from the large trials in stable patients, the possibility of an interaction during the intensive therapy phase of an acute coronary syndrome cannot be discounted.

Other Drugs and Modifiers Used in Acute Coronary Syndromes

β-Adrenergic Blockers
β-Adrenergic blockers are widely used in acute coronary syndromes.[82] There is no evidence that the standard β-blockers exert their benefit on acute coronary syndromes through an effect on the unstable plaque or on endothelial function, but a reduction in shear stress and flexion stress has been thought to be important.[88] A third generation β-blocker, nebivolol, was shown to have some effects on in vitro markers of endothelial function,[89] but there are no firm data that this finding is relevant to the management of an acute coronary syndrome. Of the more widely used β-adrenergic blockers, it has been shown that atenolol has no effect on endothelium-dependent forearm blood flow in hypertensive patients when compared with an ACE inhibitor,[90] nor was any effect on endothelium-dependent coronary vasomotion shown in patients with coronary disease.[91]

It remains uncertain whether calcium channel blockers are effective in acute coronary syndromes,[92,93] and these agents are recommended only for symptom relief rather than for improving prognosis. There is no convincing evidence that any of the effects observed in clinical trials are due to an effect on plaque passivation or on endothelial dysfunction, although the results with third-generation calcium channel blockers suggest a possible role.[94]

Organic Nitrates
Organic nitrates are commonly used in acute coronary syndromes. Their action is similar to that of nitric oxide, causing vasodilatation via an increase in intracellular concentrations of cyclic guanosine monophosphate, resulting in smooth muscle cell relaxation and antiplatelet effects.[95] Exogenously administered nitrates can act in the presence of a damaged endothelium. The effects of nitrates have been studied in AMI, but no convincing effect benefits have been shown in patients with unstable angina or non–ST-segment elevation.[82]

Antioxidants
The production of reactive oxygen species in the vascular wall has several deleterious effects. The production of superoxide anion depletes bioavailable nitric oxide very rapidly by reacting with nitric oxide to produce peroxynitrite, which can damage the endothelium directly.[96] In addition, reactive oxygen species can cause oxidation of LDL to form oxidized LDL.[97] Oxidized LDL can further deplete nitric oxide levels by attenuating nitric oxide release.[98] Oxidized LDL is taken up by macrophages in the vascular wall, leading to formation of foam cells. Once localized within the vascular wall, oxidized LDL serves as a chemoattractant for circulating monocytes, encouraging their adhesion and migration into the subendothelial space and their differentiation into lipid-filled macrophages.[99,100]

Antioxidant vitamins can protect from oxidant damage by inhibiting lipid peroxidation.[101] A large number of epidemiologic observational studies has shown an association between atherosclerotic disease and low levels of antioxidant vitamins. Some clinical trials have demonstrated a benefit, but most of the well-conducted studies have failed to show a clear benefit.[102]

There are benefits of vitamin C[103] and vitamin E[104] on endothelial dysfunction, but there is no clear relationship to the extent of carotid intima medial thickness.[105]

The Cambridge Heart Antioxidant Study showed a benefit of α-tocopherol in patients with proven coronary artery disease.[106] In contrast, the HOPE study failed to show any effect of vitamin E supplementation in high-risk patients with coronary heart disease,[107] and there was no benefit in administration of vitamin E in a large randomized study of post-infarction patients.[108]

To date, there are no studies of the effect of antioxidant therapy administered in the early phases of acute coronary syndromes.

Estrogens
The effects of estrogen on the vascular wall are mediated by nongenomic and genomic mechanisms.[109,110] Estrogen causes rapid activation of NOS in a manner that does not require new gene transcription, resulting in nitric oxide–induced vasodilatation.[111] This occurs via the estrogen receptor A, and estrogen has been shown to cause coronary vasodilation in women[112] and in men.[113] These short-term coronary vasodilatory effects in humans have been shown to be due to the increased production of nitric oxide.[114] The genomic effects of estrogen refer to mechanisms in which gene expression is upregulated. These effects have been shown to affect the expression of I-NOS[115] and may be responsible for some of the observed effects on longer-term actions of restoration of disturbed coronary endothelial function.[116] Estrogens have been shown to have beneficial effects on restoration of endothelial integrity after vascular injury by local expression of endothelial growth factor.[117] Estrogen may inhibit apoptosis of endothelial cells via effects on the estrogen receptor.[118] Effects on inhibiting migration of vascular smooth muscles may have long-term benefits but, in the short term, these effects delay the stabilization of the unstable plaque.[119]

The effects of estrogen on clinical outcomes are unclear at present. There is abundant evidence of a benefit from long-term observational studies,[120,121] but the effect of selection bias cannot be quantitated in these studies. In the Heart and Estrogen/Progestin Replacement Study (HERS), the first randomized trial to examine the effect of hormone replacement therapy in postmenopausal women with coronary disease, treatment with conjugated equine estrogens plus medroxyprogesterone for an average of 4.1 years[122] failed to show a beneficial effect on congestive heart disease events after an average of 4.1 years of treatment. There was a statistically significant trend for more congestive heart disease events in the hormone group than in the placebo group in the first year (71 deaths from congestive heart disease in the hormone group compared with 58 such deaths in the placebo group). Dropout rates were greater and follow-up less than planned, limiting the power of the HERS study to reliably address the use of hormone replacement therapy. The reasons for the failure of combined estrogen progesterone therapy in the HERS study to confirm the expectations from the cohort and case-control studies has not been clarified but clearly demonstrates the hazard in drawing final conclusions on the benefits of hormone replacement therapy from cohort and case-control studies.[123,124]

The early hazard in treatment with hormone replacement with estrogen-progesterone therapy seen in the HERS study was not observed in a trial of the selective estrogen receptor modulator, raloxifene.[125] This trial also demonstrated a significant reduction in the risk of cardiovascular events in the subset of women at increased cardiovascular risk. At present, the use of estrogen in the stabilization of the plaque and restoration of endothelial function cannot be recommended in acute coronary syndromes. Obviously, further research is required to know whether alternative methods of utilizing the effects of estrogen on the vascular wall will deliver better clinical outcomes in the acute coronary syndromes.

Blood Sugar Control Disturbed endothelial function is well documented in diabetes.[126] The mechanism by which diabetes affects endothelial function is not well understood, but advanced glycation end products, glycated and oxidized LDLs, and reactive oxygen species linked to hyperglycemia have all been implicated.[127] Intensive blood glucose control with sulphonylureas of insulin is associated with a reduction in microvascular, though not macrovascular, complications in type 2 diabetes,[128] and intensive control with metformin in overweight patients with type 2 diabetes is associated with reduced vascular end points.[129] The mechanism of this improvement over a 20-year follow-up period is not clear, but improved metabolic control in diabetic patients, whatever the treatment used, is associated with reversal of endothelial dysfunction.[130] The thiazolidinediones may exert specific effects on endothelial function by their ability to bind to peroxisome proliferator-activated receptors, which have been shown to be present in the vessel wall.[131]

Exercise has been shown to improve endothelial dysfunction in subjects with type 2 diabetes.[132] Evidence shows that strict glycemic control is beneficial in critically ill patients. In the Diabetes and Insulin-Glucose Infusion in Acute Myocardial Infarction (DIGAMI) trial, strict control of blood sugar in the acute phase of myocardial infarction improved long-term mortality.[133] In a randomized but not blinded trial of critically ill patients treated in an intensive care unit, intensive insulin therapy resulted in a mortality one third lower than the mortality in those treated with conventional therapy.[134] The mechanism for the benefit of glycemic control in these clinical scenarios has not been adequately explained. A benefit on endothelial function is only speculative but consistent with the observation that hyperglycemia has an adverse effect on collateral blood flow by a mechanism related to nitric oxide.[135]

Smoking Cessation There is some evidence that the deleterious effects of smoking are mediated by an effect on endothelial dysfunction.[136] This may also occur with passive smoking.[137] The effects in acute coronary syndromes have not been documented for obvious reasons, but the available data support the universal clinical recommendation that a patient with an acute coronary syndrome should immediately and permanently desist from smoking.

Dietary Intervention There is evidence that dyslipidemia is associated with disturbed endothelial function.[138] A high-fat meal accompanied by a postprandial rise in serum triglycerides can impact endothelial dysfunction within hours.[139] These effects were minimized when the high-fat meal contained antioxidant-rich foods.[140] Animal experiments have shown that hypercholesterolemic rabbits fed a low-fat diet show a reduction in cellular infiltrate and MMP activity and an increase in collagen accumulation in the fibrous cap compared with animals fed a high-fat diet.[141] This demonstrates a likely mechanism by which a low-fat diet can contribute to plaque stabilization in acute coronary syndromes. It has been hypothesized that the postprandial state can precipitate unstable coronary syndromes because of effects on the vascular wall, leading to plaque instability.[142] Dietary interventions are discussed in more detail in Chapter 49.

ROLE OF PERCUTANEOUS CORONARY INTERVENTION IN PLAQUE PASSIVATION

The use of percutaneous coronary intervention in acute coronary syndromes is widespread, and the convincing results of recent trials of acute coronary intervention in acute coronary syndromes[143,144] confirm the validity of this approach. Until now, the target lesion for percutaneous coronary intervention in acute coronary syndrome patients has been the critical lesion, which is assumed to be the cause of the acute reduction in coronary blood flow. It is not clear whether the benefits of coronary stenting in acute coronary syndromes are achieved by plaque stabilization or by other mechanisms. The use of percutaneous coronary intervention with drug-eluting stents to treat plaques that are unstable but not critically obstructing the vessel is a potential future strategy for management of an acute coronary syndrome.

SHOULD COX-2 INHIBITORS BE AVOIDED IN ACUTE CORONARY SYNDROMES?

There have been some reports that patients on COX-2 inhibitors may be at higher risk for acute vascular thrombotic events than patients on nonsteroidal anti-inflammatory drugs.[145] There is some evidence that this may be due to an effect on endothelial function and thrombosis,[146] inhibition of prostacyclin production, or leucocyte adherence,[147] but the relevance of these post hoc analyses and in vitro observations to the management of an acute coronary syndrome is not clear. Until more observations become available, limited use of COX-2 inhibitors in acute coronary syndromes may be a sensible precaution.[148] A trial is now designed to compare aspirin alone with a combination of aspirin and rofecoxib in the secondary prevention of acute coronary syndromes; this will permit the evaluation of (1) the risk of the COX-2 inhibition in the presence of aspirin and (2) a potential benefit of combined COX-1 and COX-2 inhibition.

REFERENCES

1. Davies MJ, Thomas A: Thrombosis and acute coronary-artery lesions in sudden cardiac ischemic death. N Engl J Med 1984;310: 1137–1140.
2. Gorlin R, Fuster V, Ambrose IA: Anatomic-physiologic links between acute coronary syndromes. Circulation 1986;74:6–9.
3. Ross R: Atherosclerosis: An inflammatory disease. N Engl J Med 1999;340:115–125.
4. Davies MJ, Richardson PD, Woolf N, et al: Risk of thrombosis in human atherosclerotic plaques: Role of extracellular lipid, macrophage, and smooth muscle cell content. Br Heart J 1993;69:377–381.
5. van der Wal AC, Becker AE, van der Loos CM, Das PK: Site of intimal rupture or erosion of thrombosed coronary atherosclerotic plaques is characterized by an inflammatory process irrespective of the dominant plaque morphology. Circulation 1994;89:36–44.
6. Davies MJ: Stability and instability: Two faces of coronary atherosclerosis. Circulation 1996;94:2013–2020.
7. Burleigh MC, Briggs AD, Lendon CL, et al: Collagen types I and rn, collagen content, GAGs and mechanical strength of human atherosclerotic plaque caps: Span-wise variations. Atherosclerosis 1992;96:71–81.
8. Cheng GC, Loree HM, Kamm RD, Fishbein MC, Lee RT: Distribution of circumferential stress in ruptured and stable atherosclerotic lesions. A structural analysis with histopathological correlation. Circulation 1993;87:1179–1187.
9. Virman R, Kolodgie FD, Burke AP, et al: Lessons from sudden coronary death. Atheroscler Thromb Vasc Biol 2000;20:1262–1275.
10. Chamley-Campbell J, Campbell G: What controls smooth muscle phenotype? Atherosclerosis 1981;40:347–357.
11. Ang AH, Tachas G, Campbell JH, et al: Collagen synthesis by cultured rabbit smooth muscle cell. Alteration with phenotype. Biochem J 1999;265:461–469.
12. Bennett MR: Apoptosis of vascular smooth muscle cells in vascular remodeling and atherosclerotic plaque rupture. Cardiovasc Res 1999;41:361–368.
13. Bauriedel G, Schmucking I, Hutter R, et al: Increased apoptosis and necrosis of coronary plaques in unstable angina. Z Kardiol 1997; 86:902–910.
14. Geng Y, Libby P. Evidence for apoptosis in advanced human atheroma: Co-localization with interleukin 1b converting enzyme. Am J Pathol 1995;147:251–266.
15. Geng Y, Wu Q, Muszynzki M, Hansson G, et al: Apoptosis of vascular smooth-muscle cells induced by in vitro stimulation with interferon gamma, tumor necrosis factor-alpha, and interleukin 1 beta. Atheroscler Thromb Vasc Biol 1996;16:19–27.
16. Van der Wal AC, Becker AE, et al: Clinically stable angina is not necessarily associated with histologically stable atherosclerotic plaques. Heart 1996;76:112–117.
17. Davies MJ, Richardson P, Woolf N, et al: Risk of thrombosis in human atherosclerotic plaque: Role of extracellular lipid, macrophages and smooth muscle cell content. Br Heart J 1993;69: 377–381.
18. Falk E: Why do plaques rupture? Circulation 1992;86(Suppl III): II30–III42.
19. Cheng GC, Loree HM, Kamm RD, et al: Distribution of circumferential stress in ruptured and stable atherosclerotic lesions: A structural analysis with histopathologic correlation. Circulation 1993;87:1179–1187.
20. Dollery CM, McEwan JR, Henney AM: Matrix metalloproteinases and cardiovascular disease. Circ Res 1995;77:863–868.
21. Galis ZS, Sukhova GK, Lark MW, Libby P: Increased expression of matrix metalloproteinases and matrix degrading activity in vulnerable regions of human atherosclerotic plaques. J Clin Invest 1994;94:2493–2503.
22. Rabbini R, Topol EJ: Strategies to achieve coronary arterial plaque stabilization. Cardiovasc Res 1999;41:402–412.
23. Mach F, Schonbeck U, Bonnefoy JY, et al: Activation of monocyte/macrophage functions related to acute atheroma complications by ligation of CD40: Induction of collagenase, stromelysin, and tissue factor. Circulation 1997;96:396–399.
24. Schonbeck U, Mach F, Sukhova GK, et al: Regulation of matrix metalloproteinase expression in human vascular smooth muscle cells by T lymphocytes: A role for CD40 signalling in plaque rupture? Circ Res 1997;81:448–454.
25. Rubanyi GM: The role of endothelium in cardiovascular homeostasis and diseases. J Cardiovasc Pharmacol 1993;22:(Suppl 4): S1–S4.
26. Furchgott RF, Zawadzki JV: The obligatory role of endothelial cells in the relaxation of arterial smooth muscle by acetylcholine. Nature 1980;288:373–376.
27. Moncada S, Vane VR: Pharmacology and endogenous roles of prostaglandin endoperoxides, thromboxane A2 and prostacyclin. Pharmacol Rev 1979;30:293–331.
28. Vanhoutte PM, Rubanyi GM, et al: Modulation of vascular smooth muscle contraction by the endothelium. Annu Rev Physiol 1986;48:307–320.
29. Kinlay S, Libby P, Ganz P: Endothelial function and coronary artery disease. Curr Opin Lipidol 2001;12:383–389.
30. Moncada S, Higgs A: The l-arginine-nitric oxide pathway. N Engl J Med 1993;329:2002–2012.
31. Wever RM, Luscher TF, Cosentino F, Rabelink TJ: Atherosclerosis and the two faces of endothelial nitric oxide synthase. Circulation 1998;97:108–112.
32. von der Leyen HE, Dzau VJ: Therapeutic potential of nitric oxide synthase gene manipulation. Circulation 2001;103:2760–2765.
33. Feletou M, Vanhoutte PM: The third pathway: Endothelium-dependent hyperpolarization. J Physiol Pharmacol 1999;50: 525–534.
34. d'Uscio LV, Barton M, Shaw S, Luscher TF: Endothelin in atherosclerosis: Importance of risk factors and therapeutic implications. J Cardiovasc Pharmacol 2000;35(Suppl 2):S55–S59.
35. Luscher TF, Wenzel RR, Moreau P, Takase H: Vascular protective effects of ACE inhibitors and calcium antagonists: Theoretical basis for a combination therapy in hypertension and other cardiovascular diseases. Cardiovasc Drugs Ther Suppl 1995;3:509–523.
36. Holtz J, Forstermann U, et al: Flow-dependent, endothelium-mediated dilation of epicardial coronary arteries in conscious dogs: effect of cyclo-oxygenase inhibition. J Cardiovasc Pharmacol 1984;6:1161–1169.
37. Raitakari OT, Celermajer DS: Testing for endothelial dysfunction. Ann Med 2000;32:293–304.
38. Kinlay S, Libby P, Ganz P: Endothelial function and coronary artery disease. Curr Opin Lipidol 2001;12:383–389.
39. Forgione MA, Leopold JA, Loscalzo J: Roles of endothelial dysfunction in coronary artery disease. Curr Opin Cardiol 2000;15:409–415.
40. Henriksen T, Mahoney EM, Steinberg D: Interactions of plasma lipoproteins with endothelial cells. Ann N Y Acad Sci 1982;401: 102–116.
41. Weissberg P, Clesham GJ, Bennett MR: Is vascular smooth muscle cell proliferation beneficial? Lancet 1996;347:305–307.
42. Aikawa M, Rabkin E, Sugiyama S, et al: An HMG-CoA reductase inhibitor, cerivastatin, suppresses growth of macrophages expressing matrix metalloproteinases and tissue factor in vivo and in vitro. Circulation 2001;103:276–283.
43. Tsuda Y, Satoh K, Kitadai M, et al: Effects of pravastatin sodium and simvastatin on plasma fibrinogen level and blood rheology in type II hyperlipoproteinemia. Atherosclerosis 1996;122:225–233.

44. Wada H, Mori Y, Kaneko T, et al: Hypercoagulable state in patients with hypercholesterolemia: Effects of pravastatin. Clin Ther 1992;14:829–834.

45. Vaughan CJ, Murphy MB, Buckley BM: Statins do more than just lower cholesterol. Lancet 1996;348:1079–1082.

46. Lacoste J, Lam JYT, Hung J, et al: Hyperlipidemia and coronary disease: Correction of the increased thrombogenic potential with cholesterol reduction. Circulation 1995;92:3172–3177.

47. Egashira K, Hirooka Y, Kai H, et al: Reduction in serum cholesterol with pravastatin improves endothelium-dependent coronary vasomotion in patients with hypercholesterolemia. Circulation 1994;89:2519–2524.

48. O'Driscoll G, Green D, Taylor RR: Simvastatin, an HMG-coenzyme A reductase inhibitor, improves endothelial function within 1 month. Circulation 1997;95:1126–1131.

49. Perticone F, Ceravolo R, Maio R, et al: Effects of atorvastatin and vitamin C on endothelial function of hypercholesterolemic patients. Atherosclerosis 2000;152:511–518.

50. Vita JA, Yeung AC, Winniford M, et al: Effect of cholesterol-lowering therapy on coronary endothelial vasomotor function in patients with coronary artery disease. Circulation 2000;102:846–851.

51. Dupuis J, Tardif JC, Cernacek P, Theroux P: Cholesterol reduction rapidly improves endothelial function after acute coronary syndromes. The RECIFE (reduction of cholesterol in ischemia and function of the endothelium) trial. Circulation 1999;99:3227–3233.

52. Scandinavian Simvastatin Survival Study Group: Randomised trial of cholesterol lowering in 4444 patients with coronary heart disease: The Scandinavian Simvastatin Survival Study (4S). Lancet 1994;344:1383–1389.

53. Sacks FM, Pfeffer MA, Moye LA, et al: The effect of pravastatin on coronary events after myocardial infarction in patients with average cholesterol levels. Cholesterol and Recurrent Events Trial investigators. N Engl J Med 1996;335:1001–1009.

54. The Long-Term Intervention with Pravastatin in Ischemic Disease (LIPID) Study Group: Prevention of cardiovascular events and death with pravastatin in patients with coronary heart disease and a broad range of initial cholesterol levels. N Engl J Med 1996;339:1349–1357.

55. Arntz HR: Evidence for the benefit of early intervention with pravastatin for secondary prevention of cardiovascular events. Atherosclerosis 1999;147(Suppl 1):S17–S21.

56. den Hartog F, Verheugt F: Early HMG-COA reductase inhibition in acute coronary syndromes: Preliminary data of the pravastatin in acute ischemic syndromes study (PAIS) [abstract]. Eur Heart J 1998;19:2802.

57. Kesteloot H, Claeys G, Blanckaert N, Lesaffre E: Time course of serum lipids and apolipoproteins after acute myocardial infarction: Modification by pravastatin. Acta Cardiol 1997;52:107–116.

58. Arntz HR, Wunderlich W, Schnitzer L: The decisive importance of cholesterol lowering therapy for coronary lesions and clinical course immediately after an acute coronary event: Short and long-term results of a controlled study. Circulation 1998;98(Suppl 1):222.

59. Bybee KA, Wright RS, Williams BA, et al: Effect of concomitant or very early statin administration on in-hospital mortality and reinfarction in patients with acute myocardial infarction. Am J Cardiol 2001;87:771–774.

60. Aronow HD, Topol EJ, Roe MT, et al: Effect of lipid-lowering therapy on early mortality after acute coronary syndromes: An observational study. Lancet 2001;357:1063–1068.

61. Stenestrand U, Wallentin L: Early statin treatment following acute myocardial infarction and 1-year survival. JAMA 2001;285:430–436.

62. Cannon CP, McCabe CH, Bentley J, Braunwald E: Early statin therapy is asscociated with markedly lower mortality in patients with acute coronary syndromes. Observations from OPUS-TIMI 16 [Abstract]. J Am Coll Cardiol 2001;37 (Suppl A):334.

63. Schwartz GG, Olsson AG, Ezekowitz MD, et al: Myocardial Ischemia Reduction with Aggressive Cholesterol Lowering (MIRACL) Study Investigators. Effects of atorvastatin on early recurrent ischemic events in acute coronary syndromes: The MIRACL study—a randomized controlled trial. JAMA 2001;285:1711–1718.

64. Liem A, van Boven AJ, Withagen AP, et al: Fluvastatin in acute myocardial infarction: Effects on early aand late ischemia and events: the FLORIDA trial [Abstract]. Circulation 2000;102:2672.

65. Dzau VJ, Bernstein K, Celermajer D, et al: The relevance of tissue angiotensin-converting enzyme: Manifestations in mechanistic and endpoint data. Am J Cardiol 2001;88 (Suppl 1):1–20.

66. Rajagopalan S, Kurz S, et al: Angiotensin II–mediated hypertension in the rat increases vascular superoxide production via membrane NADH/NADPH oxidase activation. Contribution to alterations of vascular tone. J Clin Invest 1996;97:1916–1923.

67. Morawietz H, Rueckschloss U, Niemann B, et al: Angiotensin II induces LOX-1, the human endothelial receptor for oxidized low density lipoprotein. Circulation 1999;100:899–902.

68. Lonn EM, Yusuf S, Jha P, et al: Emerging role of angiotensin-converting enzyme inhibitors in cardiac and vascular protection. Circulation 1994;90:2056–2069.

69. Enseleit F, Hurlimann D, Luscher TF: Vascular protective effects of angiotensin converting enzyme inhibitors and their relation to clinical events. J Cardiovasc Pharmacol 2001;37 (Suppl 1):S21–S30.

70. Mancini GB, Henry GC, Macaya C, et al: Angiotensin-converting enzyme inhibition with quinapril improves endothelial vasomotor dysfunction in patients with coronary artery disease. The TREND (Trial on Reversing ENdothelial Dysfunction) Study. Circulation 1996;94:258–265.

71. Cashin-Hemphill L, Holmvang G, Chan RC, et al: Angiotensin-converting enzyme inhibition as antiatherosclerotic therapy: No answer yet. QUIET Investigators. QUinapril Ischemic Event Trial. Am J Cardiol 1999;83:43–47.

72. Schlaifer JD, Mancini GB, O'Neill BJ, et al: Influence of smoking status on angiotensin-converting enzyme inhibition-related improvement in coronary endothelial function. TREND Investigators. Trial on Reversing Endothelial Dysfunction. Cardiovasc Drugs Ther 1999;13:201–209.

73. Prasad A, Narayanan S, Husain S, et al: Insertion-deletion polymorphism of the ACE gene modulates reversibility of endothelial dysfunction with ACE inhibition. Circulation 2000;102:35–41.

74. Anderson TJ, Elstein E, Haber H, Charbonneau F: Comparative study of ACE-inhibition, angiotensin II antagonism, and calcium channel blockade on flow-mediated vasodilation in patients with coronary disease (BANFF study). J Am Coll Cardiol 2000;35:60–66.

75. Navalkar S, Parthasarathy S, Santanam N, Khan BV: Irbesartan, an angiotensin type 1 receptor inhibitor, regulates markers of inflammation in patients with premature atherosclerosis. J Am Coll Cardiol 2001;37:440–444.

76. Lonn EM, Yusuf S, Jha P, et al: Emerging role of angiotensin converting enzyme inhibitors in cardiac and vascular protection. Circulation 1994;90:2056–2069.

77. Rutherford JD, Pfeffer MA, Moye LA, et al: Effects of captopril on ischemic events after MI: Results of the Survival And Ventricular Enlargement trial (SAVE investigators). Circulation 1994;90:1731–1738.

78. Yusuf S, Pepine CJ, Garces C, et al: Effect of enalapril on MI and unstable angina in patients with low ejection fractions. Lancet 1992;340:1173–1178.

79. Flather MD, Yusuf S, Kober L, et al: Long-term ACE-inhibitor therapy in patients with heart failure or left-ventricular dysfunction: A systematic overview of data from individual patients. ACE-Inhibitor Myocardial Infarction Collaborative Group. Lancet 2000;355:1575–1581.

80. Yusuf S, Sleight P, Pogue J, et al: Effects of an angiotensin-converting enzyme inhibitor, ramipril, on cardiovascular events in high-risk patients: The Heart Outcomes Prevention Evaluation study investigators. N Engl J Med 2000;342:145–153.

81. ACE Inhibitor MI Collaborative Group: Indications for ACE inhibitors in the early treatment of acute MI: Systematic overview of individual data from 100,000 patients in randomized trials. Circulation 1998;97:2202–2012.

82. Braunwald E, Antman EM, Beasley JW, et al: ACC/AHA guidelines for the management of patients with unstable angina and non-ST-segment elevation myocardial infarction: Executive summary and recommendations. A report of the American College of Cardiology/American Heart Association task force on practice guidelines (committee on the management of patients with unstable angina). Circulation 2000;102:1193–1209.

83. Hall D, Zeider H, Rudolph W: Counteraction of the vasodilator effect of enalapril by aspirin in severe heart failure. J Am Coll Cardiol 1992;20:1549–1555.

84. Hour LMH, Schipperheyn JJ, van der Laarse A, et al: Combining salicylate and enalapril in patients with coronary artery disease and heart failure. Br Heart J 1995;73:227–236.

85. Leor J, Reicher-Reiss H, Goldbourt U, et al: Aspirin and mortality in patients treated with angiotensin-converting enzyme inhibitors: A cohort study of 11,575 patients with coronary artery disease. J Am Coll Cardiol 1999;33:1920–1925.

86. Latini R, Tognoni G, Maggioni AP, et al: Clinical effects of early angiotensin-converting enzyme inhibitor treatment for acute myocardial infarction are similar in the presence and absence of aspirin: systematic overview of individual data from 96,712 randomized patients. Angiotensin-converting Enzyme Inhibitor Myocardial Infarction Collaborative Group. J Am Coll Cardiol 2000;35:1801–1807.

87. Peterson JG, Topol EJ, Sapp SK, et al: Evaluation of the effects of aspirin combined with angiotensin-converting enzyme inhibitors in patients with coronary artery disease. Am J Med 2000;109:371–377.

88. Frishman WH, Lazar EJ: Reduction of mortality, sudden death and non-fatal re-infarction with beta-adrenergic blockers in survivors of acute myocardial infarction: A new hypothesis regarding the cardioprotective action of beta-adrenergic blockade. Am J Cardiol 1990;66:66G–70G.

89. Brehm BR, Bertsch D, von Fallois J, Wolf SC: Beta-blockers of the third generation inhibit endothelin-1 liberation, mRNA production and proliferation of human coronary smooth muscle and endothelial cells. J Cardiovasc Pharmacol 2000;36:S401–S403.

90. Higashi Y, Sasaki S, Nakagawa K, et al: A comparison of angiotensin-converting enzyme inhibitors, calcium antagonists, beta-blockers and diuretic agents on reactive hyperemia in patients with essential hypertension: A multicenter study. J Am Coll Cardiol 2000;35:284–291.

91. Burger W, Hampel C, Kaltenbach M, et al: Effect of atenolol and celiprolol on acetylcholine-induced coronary vasomotion in coronary artery disease. Am J Cardiol 2000;85:172–177.

92. Held PH, Yusuf S, Furberg CD: Calcium channel blockers in acute myocardial infarction and unstable angina: An overview. BMJ 1989;299:1187–1192.

93. Kizer JR, Kimmel SE: Epidemiologic review of the calcium channel blocker drugs. An up-to-date perspective on the proposed hazards. Arch Intern Med 2001;161:1145–1158.

94. Mason RP: Mechanisms of atherosclerotic plaque stabilization for a lipophilic calcium antagonist amlodipine. Am J Cardiol 2001;88 (Suppl 1):2–6.

95. Anderson TJ, Meredith IT, Ganz P, et al: Nitric oxide and nitrovasodilators: Similarities, differences and potential interactions. J Am Coll Cardiol 1994;24:555–566.

96. Beckman JS, Beckman TW, Chen J, et al: Apparent hydroxyl radical production by peroxynitrite: Implications for endothelial injury from nitric oxide and superoxide. Proc Natl Acad Sci U S A 1990;87:1620–1624.

97. Rubbo H, Radi R, Trujillo M, et al: Nitric oxide regulation of superoxide and peroxynitrite-dependent lipid peroxidation. Formation of novel nitrogen-containing oxidized lipid derivatives. J Biol Chem 1994;269:26066–26075.

98. Chin JH, Azhar S, Hoffman BB: Inactivation of endothelial derived relaxing factor by oxidized lipoproteins. J Clin Invest 1992;89:10–18.

99. Henriksen T, Mahoney EM, Steinberg D: Interactions of plasma lipoproteins with endothelial cells. Ann N Y Acad Sci 1982;401:102–116.

100. Chisolm GM, Steinberg D: The oxidative modification hypothesis of atherogenesis: An overview. Free Radic Biol Med 2000;28:1815–1826.

101. Esterbauer H, Striegl G, Puhl H, et al: The role of vitamin E and carotenoids in preventing oxidation of low density lipoproteins. Ann N Y Acad Sci 1989;570:254–267.

102. Jha P, Flather M, Lonn E, et al: The antioxidant vitamins and cardiovascular disease. A critical review of epidemiologic and clinical trial data. Ann Intern Med 1995;123:860–872.

103. Taddei S, Virdis A, Ghiadoni L, et al: Vitamin C improves endothelium-dependent vasodilation by restoring nitric oxide activity in essential hypertension. Circulation 1998;97:2222–2229.

104. Skyrme-Jones RA, O'Brien RC, Meredith IT, et al: Vitamin E supplementation improves endothelial function in type I diabetes mellitus: A randomized, placebo-controlled study. J Am Coll Cardiol 2000;36:94–102.

105. McQuillan BM, Hung J, Beilby JP, et al: Antioxidant vitamins and the risk of carotid atherosclerosis: the Perth Carotid Ultrasound Disease Assessment Study (CUDAS). J Am Coll Cardiol 2001;38:1788–1794.

106. Stephens NG, Parsons A, Schofield PM, et al: Randomised controlled trial of vitamin E in patients with coronary disease: Cambridge Heart Antioxidant Study (CHAOS). Lancet 1996;347:781–786.

107. Yusuf S, Dagenais G, Pogue J, et al: Vitamin E supplementation and cardiovascular events in high-risk patients. The Heart Outcomes Prevention Evaluation Study Investigators. N Engl J Med 2000;342:154–160.

108. GISSI-Prevenzione Investigators: Dietary supplementation with n-3 polyunsaturated fatty acids and vitamin E after myocardial infarction: Results of the GISSI-Prevenzione trial. Lancet 1999;354:447–455.

109. Mendelsohn ME, Karas RH: Estrogen and the blood vessel wall. Curr Opin Cardiol 1994;9:619–626.

110. Farhat MY, Lavigne MC, Ramwell PW: The vascular protective effects of estrogen. FASEB J 1996;10:615–624.

111. Chen Z, Yuhanna IS, Galcheva-Gargova ZI, et al: Estrogen receptor alpha mediates the nongenomic activation of endothelial nitric oxide synthase by estrogen. J Clin Invest 1999;103:401–406.

112. Collins P, Rosano GMC, Sarrel PM, et al: 17β-Estradiol attenuates acetylcholine-induced coronary arterial constriction in women but not men with coronary heart disease. Circulation 1995;92:24–30.

113. Blumenthal RS, Heldman AW, Brinker JA, et al: Acute effects of conjugated estrogens on coronary blood flow response to acetylcholine in men. Am J Cardiol 1997;80:1021–1024.

114. Guetta V, Quyyumi AA, Prasad A, et al: The role of nitric oxide in coronary vascular effects of estrogen in postmenopausal women. Circulation 1997;96:2795–2801.

115. Weiner CP, Lizasoain I, Baylis SA, et al: Induction of calcium-dependent nitric oxide synthases by sex hormones. Proc Natl Acad Sci U S A 1994;91:5212–5216.

116. Roqué M, Heras M, Roig E, et al: Short-term effects of transdermal estrogen replacement therapy on coronary vascular reactivity in postmenopausal women with angina pectoris and normal results on coronary angiograms. J Am Coll Cardiol 1998;31:139–143.

117. Krasinski K, Spyridopoulos I, Asahara T, van der Zee R, et al: Estradiol accelerates functional endothelial recovery after arterial injury. Circulation 1997;95:1768–1772.

118. Spyridopoulos I, Sullivan AB, Kearney M, et al: Estrogen-receptor-mediated inhibition of human endothelial cell apoptosis: Estradiol as a survival factor. Circulation 1997;95:1505–1514.

119. Kolodgie FD, Jacob A, Wilson PS, et al: Estradiol attenuates directed migration of vascular smooth muscle cells in vitro. Am J Pathol 1996;148:969–976.

120. Grodstein F, Stampfer MJ, Colditz GA, et al: Postmenopausal hormone therapy and mortality. N Engl J Med 1997;336:1769–1775.

121. Belchetz PE: Hormonal treatment of postmenopausal women. N Engl J Med 1994;330:1062–1071.

122. Hulley S, Grady D, Bush T, et al: Randomized trial of estrogen plus progestin for secondary prevention of coronary heart disease in postmenopausal women. JAMA 1998;280:605–613.

123. Furberg CD, Vittinghoff E, Davidson M, et al: Subgroup interactions in the Heart and Estrogen/Progestin Replacement Study: Lessons learned. Circulation 2002;105:917–922.

124. Barrett-Connor E: Looking for the pony in the HERS data. Heart and Estrogen/progestin Replacement Study. Circulation 2002;105:902–903.

125. Barrett-Connor E, Grady D, Sashegyi A, et al: Raloxifene and cardiovascular events in osteoporotic postmenopausal women: Four-year results from the MORE (Multiple Outcomes of Raloxifene Evaluation) randomized trial. JAMA 2002;287:847–857.

126. Guerci B, Kearney-Schwartz A, Bohme P, et al: Endothelial dysfunction and type 2 diabetes. Part 1: Physiology and methods for exploring the endothelial function. Diabetes Metab 2001;27:425–434.

127. Cooper ME, Bonnet F, Oldfield M, Jandeleit-Dahm K: Mechanisms of diabetic vasculopathy: An overview. Am J Hypertens 2001;14:475–486.

128. UK Prospective Diabetes Study (UKPDS) Group: Intensive blood-glucose control with sulphonylureas or insulin compared with conventional treatment and risk of complications in patients with type 2 diabetes (UKPDS 33). Lancet 1998;352:837–853.

129. Hermann LS, Kalen J, Katzman P, et al: Longterm glycaemic improvement after addition of metformin to insulin in insulin-treated obese type-2 diabetes patients. Diabetes Obes Metab 2001;3:428–434.

130. Guerci B, Bohme P, Kearney-Schwartz A, et al: Endothelial dysfunction and type 2 diabetes. Part 2: Altered endothelial function and the effects of treatments in type 2 diabetes mellitus. Diabetes Metab 2001;27:436–447.

131. Parulkar AA, Pendergrass ML, Granda-Ayala R, et al: Non-hypoglycemic effects of thiazolidinediones. Ann Intern Med 2001;134:61–71.

132. Maiorana A, O'Driscoll G, Cheetham C, et al: The effect of combined aerobic and resistance exercise training on vascular function in type 2 diabetes. J Am Coll Cardiol 2001;38:860–866.

133. Malmberg K, Norhammar A, Wedel H, Ryden L: Glycometabolic state at admission: Important risk marker of mortality in conventionally treated patients with diabetes mellitus and acute myocardial infarction: Long-term results from the Diabetes and Insulin-Glucose Infusion in Acute Myocardial Infarction (DIGAMI) study. Circulation 1999;99:2626–2632.

134. van den Berghe G, Wouters P, Weekers F, et al: Intensive insulin therapy in the surgical intensive care unit. N Engl J Med 2001;345:1359–1367.

135. Kersten JR, Toller WG, Tessmer JP, et al: Hyperglycemia reduces coronary collateral blood flow through a nitric oxide-mediated mechanism. Am J Physiol 2001;281:2097–2104.

136. Raij L, DeMaster EG, Jaimes EA: Cigarette smoke–induced endothelium dysfunction: Role of superoxide anion. J Hypertens 2001;19:891–897.

137. Raitakari OT, Adams MR, McCredie RJ, et al: Arterial endothelial dysfunction related to passive smoking is potentially reversible in healthy young adults. Ann Intern Med 1999;130:578–581.

138. Vogel RA, Corretti MC, Gellman J: Cholesterol, cholesterol lowering, and endothelial function. Prog Cardiovasc Dis 1998;41:117–136.

139. Vogel RA, Corretti MC, Plotnick GD: Effect of a single high-fat meal on endothelial function in healthy subjects. Am J Cardiol 1997;79:350–354.

140. Vogel RA, Corretti MC, Plotnick GD: The postprandial effect of components of the Mediterranean diet on endothelial function. J Am Coll Cardiol 2000;36:1455–1460.

141. Aikawa M, Rabkin E, Okada Y, et al: Lipid lowering by diet reduces matrix metalloproteinase activity and increases collagen content of rabbit atheroma: A potential mechanism of lesion stabilization. Circulation 1998;97:2433–2444.

142. Anderson RA, Jones CJ, Goodfellow J: Is the fatty meal a trigger for acute coronary syndromes? Atherosclerosis 2001;159:9–15.

143. Invasive compared with non-invasive treatment in unstable coronary-artery disease: FRISC II prospective randomised multicentre study. FRagmin and Fast Revascularisation during InStability in Coronary artery disease Investigators. Lancet 1999;354:708–715.

144. Cannon CP, Weintraub WS, Demopoulos LA, et al: Comparison of early invasive and conservative strategies in patients with unstable coronary syndromes treated with the glycoprotein IIb/IIIa inhibitor tirofiban. N Engl J Med 2001;344:1879–1887.

145. Mukherjee D, Nissen SE, Topol EJ: Risk of cardiovascular events associated with selective COX-2 inhibitors. JAMA 2001;286:954–959.

146. Hennan JK, Huang J, Barrett TD, et al: Effects of selective cyclooxygenase-2 inhibition on vascular responses and thrombosis in canine coronary arteries. Circulation 2001;104:820–825.

147. Muscara MN, Vergnolle N, Lovren F, et al: Selective cyclooxygenase-2 inhibition with celecoxib elevates blood pressure and promotes leukocyte adherence. Br J Pharmacol 2000;129:1423–1430.

148. Cleland LG, James MJ, Stamp LK, Penglis PS: COX-2 inhibition and thrombotic tendency: A need for surveillance. Med J Aust 2001;175:214–217.

chapter 31

Antithrombotic Therapy

Pierre Théroux

Antithrombotic therapy, in conjunction with intervention procedures, has become an essential component of management of patients with an acute coronary syndrome (ACS). The benefit is in line with the abundant evidence implicating intravascular thrombus formation as the direct trigger of these syndromes. The most convincing evidence, however, has emerged from numerous clinical trials that have demonstrated a striking reduction in the rates of death, myocardial infarction (MI), and recurrent ischemia. Figure 31–1 summarizes the progress made in treatment in recent decades, first with the introduction of aspirin, second with the addition of unfractionated heparin to aspirin, and more recently with enoxaparin, intravenous glycoprotein (GP) IIb/IIIa antagonists, and clopidogrel. Clinical research continues to flourish with the development of a host of different compounds and various combinations acting on platelets, the coagulation cascade, and the fibrinolytic system. This chapter focuses on the practical aspects of antithrombotic therapy in patients with a non–ST-segment ACS and affords a perspective on pathophysiology, mechanisms, and emerging new therapies. Antiplatelet drugs are reviewed in Chapter 28, and anticoagulants are reviewed in Chapter 29.

PLATELETS AND THE COAGULATION FACTORS IN ACUTE CORONARY SYNDROMES

Platelets and the coagulation system are the two major regulators of blood hemostasis in health and disease. The two components are activated in ACSs. Markers of an inflammatory state are also elevated in these patients, signaling the close interactions that exist between thrombosis, atherosclerosis, and inflammation (see Chapters 5 and 16).

The contemporary view of intracoronary thrombus formation involves a multicompartment model in which tissue factor expressed by the diseased plaque triggers intravascular coagulation on the surface of activated platelets. Tissue factor is expressed by endothelial cells and derived microparticles,[1] as well as by monocytes and macrophages within the plaque. It forms a complex with circulating factor VIIa, resulting in activation of the coagulation cascade and formation of factor Xa within the tenase complex. Factor Xa is pivotal to thrombin generation. Thrombin cleaves fibrinogen to fibrin and has multiple effects on cells and mediators of thrombus formation and inflammation. Amplifying loops and counteracting natural anticoagulants modulate this coagulation cascade. Thus, thrombin amplifies its own generation by feedback activation of factors V, VIII, and XI. On the other hand, thrombin binds thrombomodulin on the endothelium to activate protein C, which acts as an anticoagulant (by inactivating factor VIIIa and factor Va) and as a profibrinolytic (by inactivating the thrombin activable fibrinolysis inhibitor).

In parallel with the activation of the coagulation cascade, circulating platelets promptly adhere to the damaged endothelium through interactions between receptors and ligands. GPIb/IX present on circulating platelets promptly binds von Willebrand factor exposed to the circulation from endothelium storage sites. Platelet adhesion and other local agonists initiate intracellular signaling that increases cytosolic Ca^{2+} concentration, resulting in platelet activation and shape change, external translocation of the anionic phospholipid membrane layer, release of intracellular active compounds, and activation of the GPIIb/IIIa receptor. The activated GPIIb/IIIa receptors recognize and bind fibrinogen resulting in cross-bridging of platelets into aggregates.

Interactions: Platelets and Coagulation Factors

Whereas thrombin is the most potent platelet agonist in vivo, activated platelets secrete numerous coagulation proteins as fibrinogen and factors V, XI, and XIII and provide a well-suited template for rapid assembly of the coagulation complexes. These close interactions set the pathophysiologic basis for the efficacy of anticoagulant therapy and antiplatelet therapy and of their combination in the management of ACSs.

Interactions: Platelets, Coagulation Factors, and Inflammation

Platelets and the coagulation factors are linked to inflammation through numerous interactive pathways, many of which being promoted by platelet secretion products.[2] Adenosine diphosphate and thromboxane A_2 secreted by activated platelets upregulate CD11b/CD18 (also known as Mac-1) expression on neutrophils and monocytes. Other pro-inflammatory molecules released by platelets include P-selectin, CD40L, RANTES (regulated on activation, normal, T-cell expressed, and secreted), and platelet factor 4.

P-selectin binds the P-selectin glycoprotein ligand present on the endothelial cell and on myeloid cells, mediating heterotypic cell interactions. Early myocardial

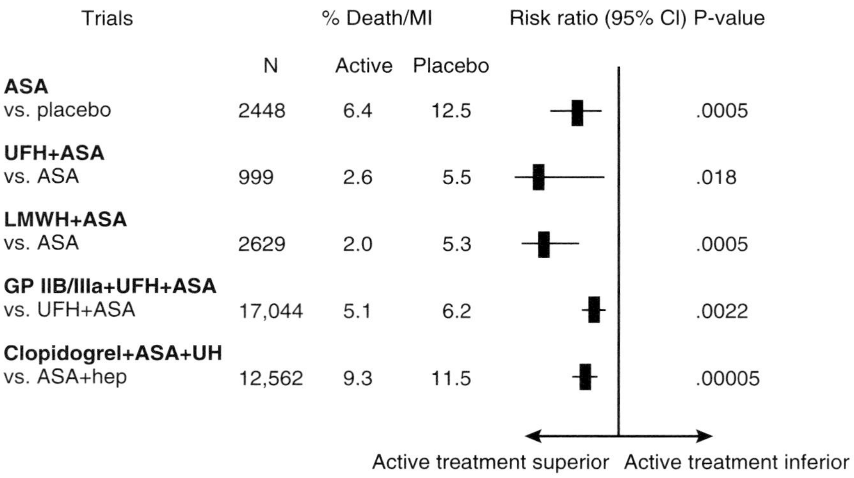

Trials		% Death/MI		Risk ratio (95% CI)	P-value
	N	Active	Placebo		
ASA vs. placebo	2448	6.4	12.5		.0005
UFH+ASA vs. ASA	999	2.6	5.5		.018
LMWH+ASA vs. ASA	2629	2.0	5.3		.0005
GP IIB/IIIa+UFH+ASA vs. UFH+ASA	17,044	5.1	6.2		.0022
Clopidogrel+ASA+UH vs. ASA+hep	12,562	9.3	11.5		.00005

Active treatment superior   Active treatment inferior

FIGURE 31–1. Progress in antithrombotic therapy for acute coronary syndromes. ASA, aspirin; CI, confidence interval; GP, glycoprotein; LMWH, low-molecular weight heparin; MI, myocardial infarction; UFH, unfractionated heparin.

cell injury is associated with the presence of platelet-neutrophil and platelet-monocyte aggregates in the circulation.[3] CD40L, a transmembrane protein member of the tumor necrosis factor family mainly secreted by platelets, interacts with the CD40 receptors present on endothelial cells, smooth muscle cells, and monocytes to promote tissue factor expression, activation of leukocytes, production of cytokines, and synthesis of adhesion molecules and of matrix metalloproteinases.[4] The pro-inflammatory cytokines prevent the anticoagulant and profibrinolytic effects of activated protein C by reducing the concentration of thrombomodulin.[5] They also promote production of C-reactive protein within the liver. C-reactive protein, beyond being a marker of risk, activates the complement, sensitizes T cells to kill endothelial cells, induces cell adhesion molecule expression, mediates macrophage low-density lipoprotein cholesterol uptake, recruits monocytes into the arterial wall, and promotes the expression of tissue factor and monocyte-chemoattractant protein-1.[6,7] Thrombin-stimulated platelets deposit the cytokine RANTES when in contact with endothelial cells to provide another link between platelets, autoimmunity, and inflammation.[8]

Coagulation factors can be pro-inflammatory, and cytokines can be thrombogenic. The tissue factor/factor VIIa complex induces leukocyte activation and production of reactive oxygen species by macrophages, and factor Xa and thrombin signal activation of nuclear factor-kappa-beta ($NF_{k\beta}$) and production of cytokines.[9] The pro-inflammatory effects of thrombin on endothelial cells and macrophages are mediated through binding to protease-activated receptors.[10]

As the mechanisms for these various interactions between thrombosis and inflammation become better understood, the management of ACSs improves. Thus, antithrombotic drugs inhibiting the interactions of thrombosis and inflammation can be envisioned and also anti-inflammation drugs that favorably influence thrombogenesis.

ANTITHROMBOTIC THERAPY

Anticoagulants

Currently available anticoagulants target inhibition of thrombin and of factor Xa (see Chapter 29). Unfractionated heparin (UFH), low-molecular-weight heparins (LMWHs), and fondaparinux are indirect inhibitors that accelerate the inhibitory effects of antithrombin by many 100 times. The length of saccharide chains modifies the pharmacokinetic and pharmacodynamic properties of the various heparins. Unfractionated heparins are heterogeneous mixtures of long and short polysaccharide chains and inhibit factor Xa and thrombin in a 1:1 ratio; LMWHs are enriched in short chains and more specifically inhibit factor Xa than thrombin to a ratio of 2:1 to 3:1. LMWHs present distinct advantages over UFH. They can be administered subcutaneously once or twice a day. They bind plasma proteins and endothelial cells less avidly than UFH, providing more predictable anticoagulation that usually does not require monitoring. LMWHs possess fewer platelet agonist effects and are less often associated with heparin-induced thrombocytopenia. They also have favorable effects on von Willebrand factor.[11] Fondaparinux is a synthetic pentasaccharide that modifies antithrombin to highly specifically bind to factor Xa. It is currently approved for the prevention of deep vein thrombosis in orthopedic surgery.

Direct thrombin inhibitors do not need a cofactor to highly specifically inhibit thrombin. Hirudin is the prototype of this class of agents. It binds the anion-binding and catalytic sites of thrombin almost irreversibly. Bivalirudin is a peptide that has been modeled on hirudin to inhibit the two active sites; the link between the two active sites is shorter and weaker than that of hirudin and can be cleaved by thrombin.[12] Other direct thrombin inhibitors that act selectively on the catalytic site do not appear to be very effective in coronary artery disease.

Antiplatelets

Antiplatelet drugs can act at different levels of platelet function from adhesion, to activation, to aggregation (see Chapter 28). The numerous pathways to platelet activation converge into a unique pathway to aggregation. Drugs acting more proximally are therefore more specific for a given mechanism of activation, and drugs acting distally have a more general effect in inhibiting platelet aggregation to any agonist. The combination of different drugs is therefore expected to produce complementary effects. Such is the case with the combination of aspirin and clopidogrel, the combination of aspirin and dipyridamole, and the combination of aspirin, clopidogrel, and a GPIIb/IIIa antagonist. On the other hand, GPIIb/IIIa antagonists block all aggregation but do not affect activation or secretion. Indeed, they are platelet agonists through outside-to-inside signaling.[13]

CLINICAL USE OF ANTITHROMBOTIC DRUGS

Aspirin

Aspirin remains the first choice antithrombotic therapy in ST-segment and non–ST-segment ACSs and in primary and secondary prevention. Aspirin is prescribed to all patients with an ACS whether another antiplatelet drug is used or not, unless a contraindication is present. Aspirin effects are dose-related, cumulative, and irreversible. A minimum loading dose of 160 is required to fully inhibit the platelet pool, followed by a daily dose of 80 to 160 mg to inhibit the 10% of the pool regenerated daily. Higher doses possess anti-inflammatory effects but have not been documented superior to the low doses for the control of the thrombotic process.[14] The Antiplatelet Trialists' Collaboration definitively documented the efficacy of aspirin in a meta-analysis that included 135,000 patients given antiplatelet therapy versus controls and 77,000 patients randomized to different antiplatelet regimens in 287 controlled trials.[15] The absolute benefit of aspirin increases with the risk inherent to the condition for which it is prescribed. The impact is considerable in patients with a non–ST-elevation ACS: a reduction of 25% in serious vascular events, 33% in nonfatal MIs, 25% in nonfatal strokes, and 16% in vascular mortality.

In addition to preventing vascular ischemic events, aspirin reduces their severity when they occur.[16] Events that occur on aspirin therapy, however, carry a worse long-term prognosis.[17] The apparent paradox may be linked to the emerging concept of aspirin resistance. It suggests that the failure is only partial, but that the patients with failure need supplemental antithrombotic therapy. Aspirin resistance is suspected on clinical grounds in patients who experience recurrent ischemic events despite aspirin therapy and, in a broader sense, in patients who experience any thrombotic event while using aspirin. The incidence may be as high as 30% of patients.[18,19] Practical reasons for the failure are noncompliance to therapy and use of nonsteroidal anti-inflammatory agents (NSAIDs) before the intake of aspirin, preventing access of aspirin to its catalytic site of action.[20] Other reasons for failure could be individual variations in metabolism of aspirin, polymorphism in COX-1, COX-2–mediated thromboxane A_2 production that is not inhibited by low-dose aspirin, thromboxane A_2 production by COX-2 in monocytes, endothelial cells and young platelets or agonists to the thromboxane receptor other than thromboxane A_2 such as the isoprostanes.[21,22] Because effective antiplatelet drugs other than aspirin are now available, aspirin monotherapy should be questioned in patients in whom aspirin resistance is clinically suspected and in patients showing side effects of aspirin. No specific clinical criteria exist for the diagnosis of aspirin resistance, and no diagnostic tests have been standardized although sub-optimal inhibitions of many platelet function tests have been described.[18,19]

Adenosine Diphosphate Receptor Antagonists

Ticlopidine and clopidogrel are two thienopyridines blocking the adenosine diphosphate receptor. Clopidogrel is better than ticlopidine because of a better safety profile and clopidogrel's lack of the serious life-threatening side effects of leukopenia and thrombocytopenia that can occur with ticlopidine. Clopidogrel is also more potent and better tolerated and can be administered as a loading dose. Ticlopidine might still be tried in patients not tolerating clopidogrel. The thienopyridines share many of the pharmacodynamic properties of aspirin. They produce dose-related, cumulative, and irreversible platelet inhibition. A loading dose of 300 mg of clopidogrel is used to achieve full inhibition within 2 to 4 hours, followed by a maintenance dose to inhibit the platelet pool regenerated daily. Unlike aspirin, however, the thienopyridines are prodrugs and need liver transformation to be active, they inhibit only approximately 50% of receptor activity, and, more importantly, they inhibit a different pathway to platelet activation.

Clopidogrel was evaluated in two large trials, in one as single therapy[23] and in the other as combined therapy with aspirin versus aspirin alone.[24] In the Clopidogrel versus Aspirin in Patients at Risk of Ischaemic Events (CAPRIE) trial, a total of 19,185 patients with recent ischemic stroke, recent MI, or symptomatic peripheral disease were randomized to aspirin, 325 mg/day, or clopidogrel, 75 mg/day.[23] Clopidogrel reduced the annual risk of ischemic stroke, MI, or vascular death during a follow-up of 1 to 3 years by 8.7% ($P = .043$). The risk was reduced by 23.8% ($P = .00028$) in patients with peripheral vascular disease, was reduced by 7.3% in patients with previous stroke, and was increased by 5.03% ($P = .66$) in patients with MI. Patients who appeared to derive special benefit with clopidogrel versus aspirin in the CAPRIE trial were those who had previously undergone coronary artery bypass grafting (CABG) (relative risk reduction [RRR], 22%); those with multiple previous ischemic events (RRR, 11%) and multiple vascular territory involvement (RRR, 22%); and those with diabetes (RRR, 12%) and hypercholesterolemia (RRR, 19%).

In the Clopidogrel in Unstable angina to prevent Recurrent Events (CURE) trial, 12,562 patients were randomized within 24 hours after the onset of a non–ST-elevation ACS to receive clopidogrel (300 mg bolus, 75 mg daily) or placebo in addition to aspirin 160 to 360 mg daily for 3 to 12 months.[24] The primary composite end point of cardiovascular death, nonfatal MI, or stroke occurred in 9.3% of patients in the clopidogrel group and 11.4% of patients in the placebo group (RR, 0.80; 95% CI, 0.72 to 0.90; $P < .001$). (Fig. 28.15.) Clopidogrel also reduced the rates of in-hospital severe ischemia and revascularization, the need for thrombolytic therapy or intravenous GP IIb/IIIa receptor antagonists, and the occurrence of heart failure. The benefits were apparent within a few hours of treatment initiation and increased throughout the follow-up period up to 1 year. The benefits were highly homogeneous among all secondary end points, subgroup analyses, and patients at low, medium, and high risk. Major bleeding occurred more frequently with clopidogrel than with aspirin alone (3.7% vs. 2.7%; RR, 1.38; $P = .001$), with no excess in life-threatening bleeding or hemorrhagic strokes. CABG performed within the first 5 days of stopping clopidogrel was associated with an increase in the risk of severe bleeding (9.6% vs. 6.3%; RR, 1.53; $P = .06$), but there was no excess when surgery was delayed for more than 5 days (4.4% vs. 5.3% with placebo). The CURE trial was mainly aimed at medical management, with no early use of percutaneous coronary intervention (PCI) or GPIIb/IIIa antagonists. Revascularization was performed during the initial admission in 23% of patients.

The Clopidogrel for Reduction of Events During Observation (CREDO) trial compared the efficacy of a 300 mg clopidogrel loading dose administered 3 to 24 hours preceding PCI with 75 mg of clopidogrel given at the time of the procedure, on a background of aspirin, with or without the planned use of a GPIIb/IIIa antagonist.[25] More than half the patients had an ACS at entry. Pretreatment reduced the relative risk of the composite of death, MI, or urgent target vessel revascularization at 28 days by 18.5% ($P = 0.23$). Interestingly, the loading dose had no benefit when given less than 6 hours before the procedure but was associated with a 38.6% reduction when given 6 to 24 hours before. The benefit of clopidogrel pretreatment was greater in patients treated with a GPIIb/IIIa antagonist, whether electively or as bailout therapy. At one year, long-term clopidogrel therapy was associated with a 26.9% reduction in the relative risk of death, MI, or stroke ($P = 0.02$).[256]

GPIIb/IIIa Receptor Blockers

Abciximab, eptifibatide, and tirofiban are the three GPIIb/IIIa antagonists approved for clinical use. Abciximab has a short plasma half-life of approximately 10 minutes but a biologic half-life that extends 6 to 12 hours because of the high affinity of the antibody for the receptor. Although receptor occupancy can persist for weeks after drug exposure, platelet aggregation progressively returns to normal within 12 to 24 hours. Abciximab also inhibits the vitronectin receptor ($\alpha v\beta 3$) on the endothelium and smooth muscle cell and CD11b/CD18 ($\alpha m\beta 2$) integrin on neutrophils and monocytes. The clinical relevance of the occupancy of these receptors involved in cell proliferation and leuko-

cyte activation, respectively, remains poorly defined. Eptifibatide and tirofiban have no special affinity for the receptor, and receptor occupancy parallels blood levels. The plasma and biologic half-life is approximately 2 hours, with 50% recovery of receptor occupancy and platelet aggregation within 4 hours after drug discontinuation and nearly 100% within 8 hours. Both eptifibatide and tirofiban are specific for binding the GPIIb/IIIa receptor.

Recommended doses were derived from clinical trials and may not be optimal in all clinical situations. Thus, abciximab is associated with a high level of inhibition of platelet aggregation early after the bolus administration, but the levels of inhibition after a few hours may fall; the acute effects of tirofiban and eptifibatide are more variable but become more predictable during steady-state administration.[26] The acute dosing problem was corrected with eptifibatide in the catheterization laboratory by injecting two boluses of 180 g/kg 10 minutes apart followed by a continuous infusion of 2.0 g/kg/min for 18 to 24 hours.[27]

The efficacy of GPIIb/IIIa antagonists to prevent complications associated with balloon dilatation and stent implantation has been documented in numerous trials involving patients in stable and unstable condition as well as stent and balloon interventions (see Chapter 36). Abciximab reduced the rates of death or MI by 50% to 80% and of the need for urgent target vessel revascularization by 30% to 70%, respectively. Eptifibatide in double-bolus injections combined with aspirin, heparin, and a thienopyridine reduced the 30-day end point of death, MI, or urgent target vessel revascularization by 35% ($P = .0034$).[27] In a head-to-head comparison trial, abciximab was significantly better than tirofiban in preventing complications associated with urgent or elective stent at 30 days,[28] but the gain was even long-term.[29]

The benefits of abciximab for the medical management of acute coronary syndromes outside the context of percutaneous interventions are more mitigated. In ST-segment elevation MI, abciximab improves prognosis when associated with half doses of tissue plasminogen activator and tenecteplase but causes excess bleeding.[30,31] The benefit was also marked in a primary angioplasty study when administered in the emergency department before PCI.[32] In non–ST-segment ACS, the drug is only effective in preselected patients who will undergo PCI within 20 to 24 hours[33]; however, it is not effective and may be deleterious in patients not undergoing PCI.[34] The Global Use of Strategies To Open occluded coronary arteries (GUSTO-IV) trial showed that the drug was ineffective and associated with an excess of events with medical therapy alone.[34] This lack of benefit was consistent across the subgroups investigated and, remarkably, in patients with elevated troponin T or I. On the other hand, the efficacy of tirofiban was documented in the Platelet Receptor Inhibition in Ischemic Syndrome Management in Patients Limited by Unstable Signs and Symptoms (PRISM-PLUS) trial[35] and of eptifibatide in the large Platelet IIb/IIIa in Unstable Angina: Receptor Suppression Using Integrilin Therapy (PURSUIT) trial.[36] PRISM-PLUS studied a global management strategy recommending coronary angiography on study drug infusion. Overall, 90% of patients underwent angiography, 31% angioplasty, 23% CABG, and 36% medical management. The risk of death or MI at 30 days was reduced by 30% ($P = .03$) with the combination of aspirin, unfractionated heparin, and tirofiban; among patients who underwent a percutaneous procedure, the risk reduction reached 44%. The Treatment of Angina with Aggrastat and Determine Cost of Therapy with an Invasive or Conservative Strategy (TACTICS) trial compared early invasive management strategy with early aggressive management applied 4 to 48 hours after admission; all patients in the trial received aspirin, unfractionated heparin, and tirofiban.[37] The trial showed the superiority of routine invasive management. The PURSUIT trial documented a 10% risk reduction in the rate of death or MI ($P = .042$) at 30 days with eptifibatide compared with placebo among 9461 randomized patients and a 31% reduction among the 13% of patients who underwent PCI on drug infusion.

Tirofiban and eptifibatide were especially interesting in patients with diabetes, patients who had previously undergone CABG, patients using aspirin before the events, and patients who underwent CABG after randomization. The benefit was present in patients randomized in a primary care hospital as well as in patients randomized in a tertiary care hospital.[38]

Numerous meta-analyses have defined modalities for the benefit of intravenous GPIIb/IIIa antagonist therapy in patients with an ACS. One by Boersma et al, performed before the results of GUSTO-IV were known, included the data from the CAPTURE, PURSUIT, and PRISM-PLUS studies.[39] The three trials altogether demonstrated a 34% reduction in the composite of death or nonfatal MI during pharmacologic therapy preceding PCI (if any) (OR, 0.66; 95% CI, 0.54 to 0.81) and an additional 41% reduction in PCI-related events (OR, 0.59; 95% CI, 0.44 to 0.81) in patients who underwent a procedure. Mortality was also reduced during medical therapy (OR, 0.50; 95% CI, 0.30 to 0.83). It was concluded that GP IIb/IIIa antagonist therapy conferred an early benefit during medical treatment and a larger secondary gain when PCI was performed during drug therapy.

A more recent meta-analysis performed by the same group of investigators involved 31,402 patients from six trials, including GUSTO-IV. The 30-day rate of death or MI was reduced from 11.8% with placebo to 10.8% with the GPIIb/IIIa antagonist (OR, 0.91; $P = .015$).[40] The odds ratios were 0.92 ($P = .03$) until PCI or 30-day follow-up, whichever came first, and 0.91 ($P = .027$) until the moment of either PCI or CABG, if any. The absolute benefit was largest in high-risk patients. Although there was a benefit in women with elevated troponin levels, a significant interaction occurred between gender and allocated treatment, with a treatment benefit in men but not in women.

A third meta-analysis looked specifically at the 6458 diabetic patients enrolled in the six trials. In these patients, the GPIIb/IIIa inhibitors reduced the 30-day mortality rate from 6.2% to 4.6% ($P < .007$).[41] The mortality rate at 30 days among the 1279 patients who underwent PCI was reduced from 4.0% to 1.2% (OR, 0.30; $P < .002$). A recent meta-analysis that included

29,570 patients showed a gradient in benefit that correlated with the revascularization management strategy used: In the total population, the rate of death or MI was reduced from 11.5% to 10.7% (OR, 0.91; $P = .02$); the reduction among patients undergoing PCI went from 12.7% to 10.7% (OR, 0.82; $P = .01$) and in patients managed medically went from 9.7% to 9.3% (OR, 0.95; $P = .27$).[42] Among patients undergoing intervention, the benefit was more pronounced (13.6% to 10.5%) if the procedure was performed during the infusion of the GPIIb/IIIa inhibitor (OR, 0.74; $P = .02$) than if revascularization occurred after drug discontinuation (12.37% to 10.9%) (OR, 0.87; $P = .17$).

The analysis of the relative benefit of GPIIb/IIIa antagonists by dichotomizing patients with or without PCI is problematic in all these trials because the decision to perform the procedure was made after randomization and could therefore have been influenced by the effects of the study drugs. Furthermore, the analyses assumed a class effect of the various GPIIb/IIa antagonists. Many observations, however, could suggest some drug-specific effects, such as the differential effects in the catheterization laboratory in the TARGET trial[28]; the absence of benefit of abciximab in the medical management of ACS[34]; the failure of lamifiban to show conclusive results despite a favorable pharmacokinetic profile[43]; and, importantly, the excess mortality observed with oral agents.[44]

It can be concluded that eptifibatide and tirofiban are associated with a significant but modest benefit in the medical management of patients with a high-risk non–ST-segment elevation and that the benefit is increased when PCI is performed under drug infusion. Abciximab should only be used in the catheterization laboratory after PCI has been chosen.

Unfractionated Heparin and Low-Molecular-Weight Heparins

Controlled trials have independently documented the efficacy of unfractionated heparin and of LMWHs in non–ST-segment ACS. A meta-analysis of 12 trials totaling 17,157 patients that compared an LMWH or UFH to placebo showed a short-term reduction at 7 days in the odds of MI or death of 0.53 (95% CI, 0.38 to 0.73; $P = .0001$) in favor of the anticoagulant.[45] The trials have generally showed reactivation of the disease after the discontinuation of the heparin or LMWH, resulting in an attenuation of the benefit after 1 month.[46,47]

Low-Molecular-Weight Heparins

Four trials have directly compared an LMWH to unfractionated heparin. Two of these trials, one with dalteparin in 1482 patients[48] and another with fraxiparin (nadroparin) in 2357 patients,[49] failed to show any advantage of the LMWH. The two trials that tested enoxaparin showed its superiority over UFH. In the Efficacy and Safety of Subcutaneous Enoxaparin in Non–Q-Wave Coronary Events (ESSENCE) trial, enoxaparin, 1 mg/kg administered twice daily for 48 hours to 8 days (median

2.6) in 3171 patients, reduced the composite outcome of death, MI, or recurrent angina by 16.2% at 14 days (16.6% vs. 19.8%; P = .019) and by 19% at 30 days (19.8% vs. 23.3%; P = .017).[50] The rate of death was unaffected and the rate of MI reduced by 29% (3.2% vs. 4.5%; P = .06) at 14 days and by 26% (3.9% vs. 5.2%) at 30 days (P = .08). In 3910 patients, the TIMI IIB trial showed a reduction in the composite end point of death, MI, or refractory ischemia requiring urgent revascularization from 16.6% to 14.2% at 14 days (P = .04) and from 19.6% to 17.3% at 43 days (P = .06).[51] Meta-analyses of all LMWH trials versus UFH showed no statistically significant difference in the odds of death or MI (OR, 0.88; 95% CI, 0.69 to 1.12; P = .34).[45,52] On the other hand, a combined analysis of the data from ESSENCE and TIMI IIB showed a statistically significant reduction in the rate of death or MI in favor of enoxaparin.[53] Massel and Cruickshank computed a putative enoxaparin versus placebo/control odds ratio with the odds of the pooled results of the enoxaparin/unfractionated heparin trials and the unfractionated heparin/placebo-controlled trials.[54] The analysis showed a nonsignificant reduction in the risk of death or AMI during treatment with the two enoxaparin trials compared with unfractionated heparin (P = .24) and a significant reduction of 18% at 43 days (P = .02).

Direct Thrombin Inhibitors

Hirudin has been investigated in three major trials. One involved patients with non–ST-segment ACS,[55] one patients with ST-segment elevation,[56] and one both ST-elevation and non–ST-elevation ACS.[57] The clinical experience showed a narrow margin between efficacy and bleeding that required down-titration of the drug in many trials. The efficacy results were not conclusive in patients with ST-segment elevation MI.[56,57] In non–ST-segment ACS trials, a statistically significant benefit over unfractionated heparin was consistently seen during the infusion of the drug, although this effect attenuated after drug discontinuation.[55,57] Although a meta-analysis of trials showed a statistically significant reduction in the risk of death or MI at 35 days (RR, 0.90; P = .015),[55] the drug did not receive approval for the specific indication except in patients with heparin-induced thrombocytopenia.

Bivalirudin, argatroban, efegatran, and inogatran have been evaluated in smaller trials in ACSs and in coronary angioplasty. A meta-analysis of 35,970 patients in 11 trials, including the hirudin trials, showed an overall reduction in the risk of death or MI at the end of the treatment period with direct antithrombin compared with unfractionated heparin (4.3% vs. 5.1%; OR, 0.85; 95% CI, 0.77 to 0.94; P = .001) and after 30 days (7.4% vs. 8.2%; OR, 0.91; 95% CI, 0.84 to 0.99; P = .02).[58] Only hirudin and bivalirudin contributed to the benefit in the meta-analysis. The meta-analysis of 6 trials, which included 4603 patients undergoing elective PCI and 1071 ACS patients, showed that bivalirudin was as effective as heparin and associated with significantly less major bleeding (OR 0.41, P = < 0.001).[58b] Bivalirudin, however, was associated with significantly more bleeding than unfractionated heparin when used as adjunctive therapy to

streptokinase in AMI.[58c] In this large trial involving 17,073 patients, mortality rates at 30 days were similar to bivalirudin and unfractionated heparin, but the rates of MI within the first 96 hours were less with bivalirudin. Recent trials have suggested that bivalirudin with planned or provisional abciximab could be a safe and effective alternative to low-dose heparin plus abciximab during PCI in stable patients.[58d]

Long-Term Anticoagulation

Prolonged anticoagulation with LMWH and coumadin has been evaluated in a attempt to prolong the benefit of anticoagulant past the acute phase and prevent reactivation of the disease. The administration of LMWH for up to 3 months after hospital discharge in general showed no consistent benefit (OR, 0.98; P = .80) but an excess risk of major bleeding (OR, 2.26; P < .0001).[45] The administration of dalteparin for 3 months following 5 days of open-labeled administration in the Fragmin during Instability in Coronary Artery Disease II (FRISC II) trial resulted in a significant reduction in rates of death, MI, and revascularization after 30 days (3.1% vs. 5.9%; P = .02) and 3 months (29.1% vs. 33.4%; P = .03), but not after 6 months.[59] Long-term administration of an LMWH after an ACS is not recommended except for selected patients waiting for a delayed intervention.

Results of trials with anticoagulants are more confounding because they vary with different levels of anticoagulation (target for home prothrombin monitoring, or *target INR*), the concomitant use or nonuse of aspirin, and likely by the countries where the investigations are performed. Countries with enthusiasm for the approach and with a careful monitoring system such as Scandinavian countries usually report better results. One study of primary prevention in high-risk persons showed that dose-adjusted coumadin to a low-intensity INR of 1.3 to 1.8 reduced the risk of ischemic heart disease to an extent similar to that of aspirin, 75 mg; coumadin prevented more selectively fatal events, and aspirin prevented more nonfatal MI; the combination was effective to prevent the two end points but increased the incidence of fatal strokes and minor bleeding.[60]

Many large studies have looked at the combination of coumadin and aspirin in the secondary prevention of MI. In two of these studies, no advantages emerged from the combination of aspirin with low doses of coumadin.[61, 62] Two other trials tested higher-intensity coumadin to an INR of 2.8 to 4.2 when the drug was used alone and to an INR of 2.0 to 2.5 when used in combination with aspirin. The two trials showed a superiority of the two coumadin regimens over aspirin alone. In one study of 999 patients, the rates of death, MI, or stroke were 9% with aspirin, 5% with coumadin alone (RR, 0.55; P = .048), and 5% with the combination (RR, 0.50; P = .03 vs. aspirin alone)[63]; in the other study of 3650 patients, these rates were 20.0%, 16.7% (RR, 0.81; P = .03), and 15.0% (RR, 0.71; P = .001 vs. aspirin alone), respectively.[64]

The Organization to Assess Strategies for Ischemic Syndromes 2 (OASIS-2) trial enrolled 3712 patients early after an episode of non–ST-segment elevation MI. The trial failed to show a significant gain with moderate-intensity coumadin to an INR of 2 to 2.5 in combination with aspirin over aspirin alone; a post-hoc analysis showed a significant gain in countries with good compliance and a trend to increased events in countries with poor compliance.[65] The Antithrombotics in the Prevention of Reocclusion In Coronary Thrombolysis 2 (APRICOT-2) trial was a study of late patency after successful thrombolysis in patients with an acute myocardial infarction.[66] Antithrombotic therapy with aspirin and coumadin to an INR to 2.6 reduced the 3-month incidence of reocclusion after successful fibrinolytic therapy by 40% compared with aspirin alone.

In aggregate, the data on oral anticoagulants suggest a benefit in a setting of good compliance and well-organized INR monitoring system. The benefit of the combination of aspirin and coumadin over coumadin alone has not been well validated. Coumadin to an INR of 2 combined with aspirin is associated with a twofold to threefold increase in the risk of minor and major bleeding without an increased risk of intracerebral hemorrhage.[67]

The use of coumadin in the setting of an ACS is rather limited for various reasons, including the lack of unanimity on the data, the complexity of treatment, and the risk of bleeding. This use is not likely to increase considering that other potentially effective drugs are emerging, including the combination of aspirin and clopidogrel and new oral anticoagulants such as factor Xa and thrombin inhibitors that do not require close monitoring.

New Antithrombotics

Numerous new drugs are under development and represent either an improvement in current drugs, new pharmacologic agents, or new combination therapy. These drugs are reviewed in Chapters 28 and 29. Antiplatelet drugs close to or under clinical investigation are a thromboxane receptor with a favorable pharmacokinetic profile and a non-thienopyridine P2Y12 receptor blocker. New anticoagulants include fondaparinux, the nematode anticoagulant peptide, ximelagatran, and activated protein C.

RISK STRATIFICATION AND TREATMENT

Non–ST-segment ACSs now account for more than two thirds of admissions to coronary care units. This population accounts for only a minority of persons consulting for chest pain (see Chapter 12) and is poorly representative of the much broader population at risk for vulnerable coronary lesions at a preclinical stage of the disease (see Chapter 5). The development of signs and symptoms of instability marks rapid progression of the disease and is a harbinger of a serious ischemic event in the short term that can irreversibly affect the function of the target organ and can be fatal. These patients need to be recognized because appropriate therapeutic measures can halt the evolution of the disease process in the short term. However, the disease process may continue to evolve, impairing prognosis for the months and years that follow. The disease is endemic and can recur in the

■ ■ ■

TABLE 31–1   MAIN DETERMINANTS OF PROGNOSIS IN CLINICAL PRACTICE

Determinants of short-term prognosis	
Confirming the diagnosis of ACS	Clinical pattern of pain
	ST-T ischemic changes
	Troponin T or I elevation
	Hemodynamic or electrical instability
Other major determinants	Older age
	Left-ventricular dysfunction
	Recent myocardial infarction
	Recurrent ischemia
	Diabetes
	Previous myocardial infarction
	Previous coronary artery bypass graft
	Previous aspirin use
	Presence of an intracoronary thrombus
	Depression
Determinants of long-term prognosis	Left-ventricular dysfunction
	Diabetes
	Extensive coronary artery disease
	Strongly positive provocative testing
	Elevated levels of C-reactive protein
	Elevated levels of the brain natriuretic peptide
	Depression

same patients. It requires specialized action. ACSs are therefore highly demanding for society and the health care system.

The sophistication achieved in risk stratification has permitted cost-effective discrimination of patients consulting for chest pain into low-, medium-, and high-risk categories. The evaluation is mainly based on clinical evaluation, the 12-lead ECG, and the determination of blood markers of cell necrosis. Table 31–1 summarizes the main determinants to be retained in clinical practice. The TIMI risk score has been well validated in many studies and permits very early stratification and discrimination of risk over a wide scale.

Beyond being essential to patient orientation, risk stratification is critical for treatment selection. It permits one to identify patients who will likely profit from intensive antithrombotic therapy and early invasive management. Table 31–2 emphasizes this aspect. It shows the relative benefit of enoxaparin over unfractionated heparin, of a GPIIb/IIIa antagonist versus no GPIIb/IIIa antagonists, and of early invasive versus an early conservative management strategy by troponin levels, ST-segment shift, and TIMI risk score. All observations concur to show that patients who profit from more intensive therapy are those with an abnormal-appearing ECG, troponin elevation, or a high TIMI score. Although most of these results were obtained from post-hoc analyses of clinical trials, they are now prospectively used in trials. Alternatively, the data show that patients with no high-risk features may not profit and may be harmed by an aggressive approach. Reasons for negative results could be a lack of power to detect a benefit in low-risk

■ ■ ■

TABLE 31–2   TROPONIN LEVELS AND CARDIAC EVENTS IN VARIOUS STUDIES

TRIALS	NO. OF PATIENTS	END POINT	CUT POINTS	EVENT RATES WHEN POSITIVE		EVENT RATES WHEN NEGATIVE	
				Control Group	Treated Group	Control Group	Treated Group
By Troponin Level							
Dalteparin vs. placebo (FRISC)	971	Death/MI 40 days	TnT ≥ 0.1 µg/L	14.2 *P* = .005	7.4	5.9 *P* = .68	8.9
Tirofiban vs. UFH (PRISM)	2222	Death/MI 30 days	TnT ≥ 1.0 g/µL	13.0 *P* = <.001	4.3	4.9 *P* = .5	5.7
Abciximab vs. placebo (CAPTURE)	1265	Death/MI 30 days	TnT > 0.1 µg/L	19.6 *P* = .001	5.8	4.9 *P* = 1.0	5.2
Lamifiban vs. placebo (PARAGON B)	1160	Death/MI 30 days	TnT ≥ 0.1 µg/L	19.0 *P* = .02	11.0	10.3 *P* = .75	9.6
Abciximab vs. placebo (GUSTO)	7707	Death/MI 30 days	TnT ≥ 0.1 µg/L	10.0 *P* = .9	10.0+	5.4 *P* = .23	6.1*
				10.0 *P* = .17	11.16†	5.4 *P* = .84	5.9†
Invasive vs. noninvasive (FRISC II)	2311	Death/MI 6 months	TnT ≥ 0.1 µg/L	13.4 *P* = .06	10.2	10.3 *P* = .15	8.4
Invasive vs. conservative (TACTICS)	1821	Death/MI 6 months	TnI ≥ 1.0 µg/L	12.6 *P* = .03	8.5	3.8 *P* = .65	4.4
By ST-Segment Shift							
Invasive vs. noninvasive (FRISC-II)	2311	Death/MI 6 months	Yes/no	15.5 *P* = .01	10.3	3.8 *P* = .76	8.4
Invasive vs. noninvasive (TACTICS)	2220	Death/MI/RI 6 months	Yes/no	26.3 *P* = .0004	16.4	15.3 *P* = .8	15.6
Abciximab vs. placebo (GUSTO-4)	7707	Death/MI 30 days	Yes/no	8.4 *P* = .9	8.5*	6.7 *P* = .82	6.9*
				8.4 *P* = .09	9.9†	6.7 *P* = .33	6.0†
By TIMI Score							
Tirofiban vs. UFH (PRISM)	1915	Death/MI/RI 7 days	0–2 3–5	28.5 *P* = .005	19.3	10.2 *P* = .3	8.2
Enoxaparin vs. UFH (TIMI IIB)	3910	Death/MI/RI 14 days	0–3 4–7	24.3 *P* = .0006	17.6	10.9 *P* = .74	11.4
Enoxaparin vs. UFH (ESSENCE)	3171	Death/MI/RI 14 days	0–2 3–7	18.1 *P* = .003	12.9	10.0 *P* = .41	8.7

*24-Hour perfusion.
†48-Hour perfusion.
MI, myocardal infarction; RI, recurrent infarction; TnI, troponin I; TnT, troponin T; UFH, unfractionated heparin.

patients, pathophysiologic mechanisms that are less directly related to thrombus activity, or an unfavorable risk/benefit ratio. The relation between risk and benefit was less apparent in the CURE trial: Patients with or without ST-segment shifts and with or without CK elevation showed similar relative risk reductions acutely and in the long term.[24] This observation illustrates the continuum in disease severity and the need to care about the tiny gap that may exist between a stable and a stabilized disease in order to prevent reactivation and recurrence of the syndrome.

Although high-performing, risk stratification remains an imperfect tool that needs much further sophistication. Thus, ischemic events still occur in 4% to 10% of patients with normal troponin levels, in 6% to 16% of patients without ST-segment changes, and in 8% to 11% of patients with a low TIMI risk score; these figures are greater than the absolute reductions in event rates with

treatment in the high-risk groups (Table 38–2). Clearly, the challenges of improved risk stratification and development of more-efficient therapy persist. A combination of ancillary and new markers is emerging as a more effective approach.[68] One could foresee risk-stratification algorithms in the near future that will combine a panel of markers, each one being specific for one of the many pathophysiologic steps involved in the cascade of events leading to ACSs and cell death, allowing individualized therapy.

This era is already at our door. In one study, the incidence of coronary restenosis during 6-month follow-up was not related to troponin T status (3% vs. 4.5%; *P* = .49) but was related to C-reactive protein status (7% vs. 2.3%; *P* = .03).[69] In other studies, elevated C-reactive protein levels predicted an impaired short- and long-term prognosis after PCI[70] and an increased risk of new, late ischemic events following CABG.[71] Antithrombotic therapy is less effective in these patients,[69] whereas observation studies have suggested that early statin therapy could be useful.[72]

Patients with Noncardiac Pain

The majority of patients consulting for chest pain do not experience an ACS (see Chapter 12). The likelihood of coronary artery disease is appreciated in these patients by various clinical criteria such as age, risk factors, and antecedents of cardiovascular disease and is helped by provocative testing as required. Appropriate cause-specific therapy is subsequently applied (see Chapters 12 and 50). Reassurance as to the cause of pain is often all that is needed. The consultation may be seen as a good opportunity to discuss risk factors, hormone therapy replacement (if applicable), and general lifestyle recommendations. Prophylactic therapy is based on age and on the risk factors, including blood pressure and lipid measurement. The control of blood factors and therapy with aspirin and statin have been effective measures for primary prevention. A meta-analysis of more than 51,000 subjects administered aspirin in four controlled primary prevention trials showed significant risk reduction, reaching 32% for nonfatal MI and 13% for any important vascular events, with no increases in risk of vascular death and nonfatal stroke but a significant 1.7-fold increase in the risk of hemorrhagic stroke.[73]

Patients with Atypical Angina and Stable Angina

Typical angina is recognized by the quality, location, and duration of pain and by factors that trigger and relieve, including rest or nitroglycerin. Special care is required to identify angina equivalents, such as inappropriate dyspnea, nausea, and fatigue. Atypical angina describes symptoms that meet two of the criteria of typical angina listed earlier. In these patients, the prevalence of underlying coronary artery disease and myocardial ischemia ranges from 20% to 50% and is higher when risk factors are present. In women and in the elderly, the symptoms may be more atypical, the initial manifestations more subtle, and the results of noninvasive testing less reliable. Unstable angina, by definition, has atypical features in terms of factors that trigger and relieve pain, the duration of pain, and the response to nitroglycerin. Diagnostic tests are indicated in these patients. Noninvasive testing is usually adequate for this purpose, but coronary angiography may be indicated in selected patients. Prophylactic aspirin is indicated in all patients with documented coronary artery disease as well as other preventive measures.

Low-Risk Patients with Acute Coronary Syndromes

The stratification of ACSs into a low-risk category implies stabilization of the clinical status, normal troponin values at first and second determination, and the absence of ST-T changes. This category typically applies to patients with new-onset effort angina and no progression in symptoms and patients with known coronary artery disease but atypical symptoms. The imperfections of risk stratification, however, should be remembered; a minority of these patients may not be at such low risk. These patients need to be stratified for the severity of the underlying coronary artery disease. This can be performed on an outpatient basis after having ruled out an acute syndrome. For this purpose, an exercise treadmill test can be done or a provocative method with visualization of the ischemic deficit with a nuclear scan or a two-dimensional echocardiography. Coronary angiography is often useful and allows correlation of functional deficits with angiographic anatomy. The first line of antithrombotic therapy for these patients is aspirin. Additional therapy is adjusted to the findings of risk stratification, including an assessment of left-ventricular function.

High-Risk Patients with Acute Coronary Syndromes

The high-risk patient is identified by the clinical features of evolving chest pain at rest or minimal exercise, elevation of troponin levels or ST-segment depression (or both), or significant T-wave inversion or pseudonormalization. The risk can be further scaled to other clinical characteristics that include those contained in the TIMI score more importantly, age and presence of diabetes mellitus. A depressed ejection fraction adds another important dimension to risk.

The patient with hemodynamic instability is at very high risk and needs urgent treatment, as does the patient with recurrent ischemia on medical treatment. Intra-aortic balloon counterpulsation to stabilize the coronary circulation and improve the hemodynamic situation is extremely useful in these patients. The procedure can be promptly done in the catheterization laboratory along with coronary angiography. It may also be done at the bedside if a catheterization laboratory is not immediately available.

In recent years, a number of interventions have independently been shown useful beyond the use of aspirin and unfractionated heparin (UHF) (see Fig. 31-1). These include:

- The combination of aspirin and enoxaparin as documented by the FRISC trial[47]
- The addition of tirofiban or eptifibatide to aspirin and UFH as showed by the PRISM-PLUS and PURSUIT trials, respectively[35,36]; enoxaparin advantageously substitutes unfractionated heparin in this combination as documented by the Antithrombotic Combination Using Tirofiban and Enoxaparin II (ACUTE II) and INTegrilin and Enoxaparin Randomised assessment of Acute Coronary Syndrome Treatment (INTERACT) trials[74,75]; abciximab is contraindicated except when PCI is performed
- The combination of aspirin-heparin and clopidogrel as conclusively documented by the CURE trial[24]
- An invasive management strategy on the background of pretreatment with aspirin and a LMWH pretreatment for many days corresponding to the FRISC II trial[59]

- An invasive management strategy on the background of pretreatment with tirofiban for a few hours or days corresponding to the TACTICS approach[38]

Enoxaparin and eptifibatide were investigated in the context of a medical management strategy. The PRISM-PLUS strategy used a strategy similar to the invasive arm of the TACTICS trial, with early angiography performed in nearly all patients and an intervention in the majority. On the other hand, the CURE strategy with clopidogrel targeted medical management, A total of 2658 patients had PCI during the study a median of 10 days after randomization.[76] About 25% of these patients received open-labelled clopidogrel before PCI and 80% after PCI in both study groups. Patients randomized to clopidogrel had fewer cardiovascular deaths, MI, or urgent revascularization from PCI to 30 days (4.5% versus 6.4%, P = 0.03), indicating that pretreatment with clopidogrel was protective against complications of PCI. Over all, after a mean follow-up of 9 months, there was a 31% reduction in the rate of death or MI (8.8% versus 12.6%, P = 0.002).

Evidence from clinical trials as well as current clinical experience and preferences all suggest that antithrombotic therapy and reperfusion procedures are complementary therapy in ACSs, the former intending the control of the pathophysiologic process and the latter intending relief of the obstructive of lesion and plaque remodeling. The optimal timing for interventions, however, remains unsettled. In ST-segment elevation, immediate urgent reperfusion is required to interrupt the ongoing cell necrosis. In non–ST-segment elevation ACSs, reperfusion can be done immediately, done within hours and days (the TACTICS trial strategy), done within days or weeks (the FRISC II strategy), or delayed for some time after hospital discharge. The latter approach is far from optimal from the perspective of patient rehabilitation and is associated with a risk of progression of the disease and a severe ischemic event in the interim period.[77]

On the other hand, the hazard of early interventions has always been recognized in clinical trials as well as in registry data. Recent data suggest that the early hazard could be overcome with modern medical and intervention treatment. Indeed, there was no excess in early events in the TACTICS trial with the combination of aspirin, heparin, tirofiban, and coronary angioplasty and stenting performed within 4 to 48 hours after admission.[38] Many centers used an immediate intervention approach in light of the high success rate of procedures to restore lumen patency of the culprit coronary artery lesion; this approach has not yet been validated in the

■ ■ ■

TABLE 31–3 ACC/AHA RECOMMENDATIONS FOR ANTIPLATELET AND ANTICOAGULATION THERAPY

Class I

1. Antiplatelet therapy should be initiated promptly. ASA should be administered as soon as possible after presentation and continued indefinitely. (*Level of evidence*: A)
2. Clopidogrel should be administered to hospitalized patients who are unable to take ASA because of hypersensitivity or major gastrointestinal intolerance. (*Level of evidence*: A)
3. In hospitalized patients in whom an early noninterventional approach is planned, clopidogrel should be added to ASA as soon as possible on admission and administered for at least 1 month (*Level of evidence*: A) and for up to 9 months (*Level of evidence*: B).
4. In patients for whom a PCI is planned, clopidogrel should be started and continued for at least 1 month (*Level of evidence*: A) and up to 9 months in patients who are not at high risk for bleeding (*Level of evidence*: B).
5. In patients taking clopidogrel in whom CABG is planned, if possible the drug should be withheld for at least 5 days, preferably for 7 days. (*Level of evidence*: B).
6. Anticoagulation with subcutaneous LMWH or intravenous unfractionated heparin (UFH) should be added to antiplatelet therapy with ASA and/or clopidogrel. (*Level of evidence*: A).
7. A platelet GPIIb/IIIa antagonist should be administered, in addition to ASA and heparin, to patients in whom catheterization and PCI are planned. The GPIIb/IIIa antagonist may also be administered just prior to PCI. (*Level of evidence*: A)

Class IIa

1. Eptifibatide or tirofiban should be administered, in addition to ASA and LMWH or UFH, to patients with continuing ischemia, an elevated troponin, or other high-risk features in whom an invasive management strategy is not planned. (*Level of evidence*: A)
2. Enoxaparin is preferable to UFH as an anticoagulant in patients with UA/NSTEMI, unless CABG is planned within 24 h. (*Level of evidence*: A)
3. A platelet GPIIb/IIIa antagonist should be administered to patients already receiving heparin, ASA, and clopidogrel in whom catheterization and PCI are planned. The GPIIb/IIIa antagonist may also be administered just prior to PCI. (*Level of evidence*: B)

Class IIb

1. Eptifibatide or tirofiban, in addition to ASA and LMWH or UFH, should be administered to patients *without* continuing ischemia who have no other high-risk features and in whom PCI is *not* planned. (*Level of evidence*: A)

Class III

1. Intravenous thrombolytic therapy in patients without acute ST-segment elevation, a true posterior MI, or a presumed new left bundle-branch block (LBBB). (*Level of evidence*: A) Abciximab administration in patients in whom PCI is not planned. (*Level of evidence*: A)

Definition of recommendations:
Class I: Conditions for which there is evidence and/or general agreement that a given procedure or treatment is useful and effective
Class II: Conditions for which there is conflicting evidence and/or a divergence of opinion about the usefulness/efficacy of a procedure or treatment
  Class IIa: Weight of evidence/opinion is in favor of usefulness/efficacy
  Class IIb: Usefulness/efficacy is less well established by evidence/opinion
Class III: Conditions for which there is evidence and/or general agreement that the procedure/treatment is not useful/effective and in some cases may be harmful
ASA, aspirin; CABG, coronary artery bypass graft; LMWH, low-molecular-weight heparin; PCI, percutaneous coronary intervention; UA/NSTEMI, unstable angina or non–ST-segment myocardial infarction.

context of the early hazard. Some data in the literature suggest that plaque stabilization for some hours before the procedure could be advantageous. This was the case in the TACTICS trial.[37] This was also the case in the PCI-CURE[76] and CREDO[25] studies. In the PCI-CURE trial, patients who received clopidogrel per randomization in the main trial for a mean of 10 days before PCI fared better than patients in the placebo group, who received clopidogrel within 24 hours before the intervention. In the CREDO trial, only patients who were pretreated for 6 hours or more before the intervention profited from the loading dose of clopidogrel. These were uncontrolled observations, however.

Observations from clinical trials also suggest that clopidogrel adds to the benefit of GPIIb/IIIa antagonists[25] and that GPIIb/IIIa antagonists add to the benefit of clopidogrel.[28,78] Another unanswered question is the optimal timing for the initiation of clopidogrel and of the GPIIb/IIIa antagonists. Many physicians are reticent to initiate clopidogrel therapy before knowing the coronary angiographic anatomy because of the excessive severe bleeding that can occur if the patient undergoes CABG within 5 days after the discontinuation of clopidogrel—not an unusual situation.[24] On the other hand, early treatment could be important to prevent early events, facilitate early PCI, and promote plaque passivation. A patient-based approach could be useful. The alert clinician can obtain some clues as to the coronary anatomy and therefore the likelihood for patient orientation to PCI or CABG, although such clues could be misleading. Thus, patients with deep T-wave inversion in the anterior lead are likely to have stenosis of left anterior descending coronary artery that will be amenable to PCI. Patients showing ST-segment elevation in the lead aVR are likely have severe three-vessel disease and to be candidates for CABG. Very unstable patients with diffuse ST-T changes might have left main artery disease.

Until more evidence is obtained, the best practice is likely the one that conforms to clinical trial designs and Guidelines recommendations (see Chapters 49 and 50). So far trials that have used a combination of aspirin, unfractionated heparin, and a GPIIb/IIIa antagonist have provided the best results in the context of early PCI. With planned medical management or delayed PCI, the combination of aspirin, enoxaparin, and clopidogrel has been highly successful. Recurrent ischemia on treatment is an indication to add a GPIIb/IIIa antagonist and to perform prompt angiography. Enoxaparin advantageously replaces unfractionated heparin when PCI or CABG is not immediately planned as well as with a GPIIb/IIIa antagonist. In any case, clopidogrel is indicated with stent implantation and with medical management. The duration of administration of clopidogrel may need clinical judgment beyond the recommendation based on the CURE trial, which showed an accrual benefit for up to 12 months. The patient with successfully dilated one-vessel disease may not need clopidogrel in the long term, whereas the patient with severe disease and partial correction could profit from clopidogrel for more than 1 year. The Guidelines of the European Society of Cardiology and of the American College of Cardiology/American Heart Association for the management of patients with unstable angina and non–ST-segment elevation myocardial infarction are presented in Chapters 49 and 50, respectively.

REFERENCES

1. Mallat Z, Benamer H, Hugel B, et al: Elevated levels of shed membrane microparticles with procoagulant potential in the peripheral circulating blood of patients with acute coronary syndromes. Circulation 2000;101:841–843.
2. Libby P, Simon DI: Inflammation and thrombosis: The clot thickens. Circulation 2001;103:1718–1720.
3. Michelson AD, Barnard MR, Krueger LA, et al: Circulating monocyte-platelet aggregates are a more sensitive marker of in vivo platelet activation than platelet surface P-selectin: Studies in baboons, human coronary intervention, and human acute myocardial infarction. Circulation 2001;104:1533–1537.
4. Henn V, Slupsky J, Grafe M, et al: CD40L on activated platelets triggers an inflammatory reaction of endothelial cells. Nature 1998;391:1047–1054.
5. Joyce DE, Gelbert L, Ciaccia A, et al: Gene expression profile of antithrombotic protein C defines new mechanisms modulating inflammation and apoptosis. J Biol Chem 2001;276:11199–11203.
6. Bhakdi S, Torzewski M, Klouche M, Hemmes M: Complement and atherogenesis: Binding of CRP to degraded, nonoxidized LDL enhances complement activation. Arterioscler Thromb Vasc Biol 1999;19:2348–2354.
7. Lagrand WK, Visser CA, Hermens WT, et al: C-reactive protein as a cardiovascular risk factor: More than an epiphenomenon? Circulation 1999;100:96–102.
8. von Hundelshausen P, Weber KS, Huo Y, et al: RANTES deposition by platelets triggers monocyte arrest on inflamed and atherosclerotic endothelium. Circulation 2001;103:1772–1777.
9. Welty-Wolf KE, Carraway MS, Ortel TL, Piantadosi CA: Coagulation and inflammation in acute lung injury. Thromb Haemost 2002;88:17–25.
10. Sambrano GR, Weiss EJ, Zheng YW, et al: Role of thrombin signalling in platelets in haemostasis and thrombosis. Nature 2001;413:74–78.
11. Montalescot G, Collet JP, Lison L, et al: Effects of various anticoagulant treatments on von Willebrand factor release in unstable angina. J Am Coll Cardiol 2000;36:110–114.
12. Witting JI, Bourdon P, Brezniak DV, et al: Thrombin-specific inhibition by slow cleavage of hirulog-1. Biochem J 1992;282:737–743.
13. Peter K, Schwartz M, Ylanne J, et al: Induction of fibrinogen binding and platelet aggregation as a potential intrinsic property of various glycoprotein IIb/IIIa (αIIb β3) inhibitors. Blood 1998;92:3240–3249.
14. Patrono C, Coller B, Dalen JE, et al: Platelet-Active Drugs. The relationships among dose, effectiveness, and side effects. Chest 2001;119:39S–63S.
15. Collaborative meta-analysis of randomised trials of antiplatelet therapy for prevention of death, myocardial infarction, and stroke in high-risk patients. BMJ 2002;324:71–86.
16. Garcia-Dorado D, Theroux P, Tornos P, et al: Previous aspirin use may attenuate the severity of the manifestation of acute ischemic syndromes. Circulation 1995;92:1743–1748.
17. Alexander JH, Harrington RA, Tuttle RH, et al: Prior aspirin use predicts worse outcomes in patients with non-ST elevation acute coronary syndromes. PURSUIT Investigator. Platelet IIb/IIIa in Unstable Angina: Receptor Suppression Using Integrilin Therapy. Am J Cardiol 1999;83:1147–1151.
18. Gum PA, Kottke-Marchant K, Poggio ED, et al: Profile and prevalence of aspirin resistance in patients with cardiovascular disease. Am J Cardiol 2001;88:230–235.
19. Eikelboom JW, Hirsh J, Weitz JI, et al: Aspirin-resistant thromboxane biosynthesis and the risk of myocardial infarction, stroke, or cardiovascular death in patients at high risk for cardiovascular events. Circulation 2002;105:1650–1655.
20. Catella-Lawson F, Reilly MP, Kapoor SC, et al: Cyclooxygenase inhibitors and the antiplatelet effects of aspirin. N Engl J Med 2001;345:1809–1817.

21. Cayatte AJ, Du Y, Oliver-Krasinski J, et al: The thromboxane receptor antagonist S18886 but not aspirin inhibits atherogenesis in apo E-deficient mice. Evidence that eicosanoids other than thromboxane contribute to atherosclerosis. Arterioscler Thromb Vasc Biol 2000;20:1724–1728.

22. Cipollone F, Ciabattoni G, Patrignani P, et al: Oxidant stress and aspirin-insensitive thromboxane biosynthesis in severe unstable angina. Circulation 2000;102:1007–1013.

23. CAPRIE Steering Committee: A randomized, blinded trial of clopidogrel versus aspirin in patients at risk of ischaemic events (CAPRIE). Lancet 1996;348:1329–1339.

24. Yusuf S, Zhao F, Mehta SR, Chrolavicius S, et al: Effects of clopidogrel in addition to aspirin in patients with acute coronary syndromes without ST-segment elevation. N Engl J Med 2001;345:494–502.

25. Steinhubl SR, Berger PB, Mann JT, et al: Early and sustained dual oral antiplatelet therapy following percutaneous coronary intervention. JAMA 2002;288:2411–2420.

26. Batchelor WB, Tolleson TR, Huang Y, et al: Randomized comparison of platelet inhibition with abciximab, tirofiban and eptifibatide during percutaneous coronary intervention in acute coronary syndromes: the COMPARE trial. Comparison Of Measurements of Platelet aggregation with Aggrastat, Reopro, and Eptifibatide. Circulation 2002;106:1470–1476.

27. The ESPRIT investigators: Novel dosing regimen of eptifibatide in planned coronary stent implantation (ESPRIT): A randomized, placebo-controlled trial. Lancet 2000;356:2037–2044.

28. Topol EJ, Moliterno DJ, Herrmann HC, et al: For the TARGET investigators. Comparison of two platelet glycoprotein IIb/IIIa inhibitors, tirofiban and abciximab, for the prevention of ischemic events with percutaneous coronary revascularization. N Engl J Med 2001;344:1888–1894.

29. Roffi M, Moliterno DJ, Meier B, et al: Impact of different platelet glycoprotein IIb/IIIa receptor inhibitors among diabetic patients undergoing percutaneous coronary intervention: Do Tirofiban and ReoPro Give Similar Efficacy Outcomes Trial (TARGET) 1-year follow-up. Circulation 2002;105:2730–2736.

30. The Assessment of the Safety and Efficacy of a New Thrombolytic Regimen (ASSENT)-3 Investigators. Efficacy and safety of tenecteplase in combination with enoxaparin, abciximab, or unfractionated heparin: The ASSENT-3 randomised trial in acute myocardial infarction. Lancet 2001;358:605–613.

31. The GUSTO V Investigators: Reperfusion therapy for acute myocardial infarction with fibrinolytic therapy or combination reduced fibrinolytic therapy and platelet glycoprotein IIb/IIIa inhibition: The GUSTO V randomised trial. Lancet 2001;357:1905–1914.

32. Montalescot G, Barragan P, Wittenberg O, et al: Platelet glycoprotein IIb/IIIa inhibition with coronary stenting for acute myocardial infarction. N Engl J Med 2001;344:1895–1903.

33. CAPTURE Investigators: Randomized placebo-controlled trial of abciximab before and during coronary intervention in refractory unstable angina: The CAPTURE study. Lancet 1997;349:1429–1435.

34. The GUSTO IV investigators: Randomized placebo controlled trial of abciximab before early coronary revascularization: The GUSTO IV-ACS randomized trial. Lancet 2001;357:1915–1924.

35. Platelet receptor inhibition in ischemic syndrome management in patients limited by unstable signs and symptoms (PRISM PLUS) study investigators: Inhibition of the platelet glycoprotein IIb/IIIa receptor with tirofiban in unstable angina and non-Q wave myocardial infarction. N Engl J Med 1998;338:1488–1497.

36. The platelet glycoprotein IIb/IIIa in unstable angina: Receptor suppression using integrilin therapy (PURSUIT) trial investigators. Inhibition of platelet glycoprotein IIb/IIIa with eptifibatide in patients with acute coronary syndromes. N Engl J Med 1998;339:436–443.

37. Cannon CP, Weintraub WS, Demopoulos LA, et al: For the TACTICS-TIMI 18 investigators. Comparison of early invasive and conservative strategies for patients with unstable coronary syndromes treated with the glycoprotein IIb/IIIa inhibitor tirofiban. N Engl J Med 2001;344:1879–1887.

38. Theroux P, Alexander J Jr, Dupuis J, et al: Upstream use of tirofiban in patients admitted for an acute coronary syndrome in hospitals with or without facilities for invasive management. PRISM-PLUS Investigators. Am J Cardiol 2001;87:375–380.

39. Boersma E, Akkerhuis KM, Theroux P, et al: Platelet glycoprotein IIb/IIIa receptor inhibition in non-ST-elevation acute coronary syndromes: Early benefit during medical treatment only, with additional protection during percutaneous coronary intervention. Circulation 1999;100:2045–2048.

40. Boersma E, Harrington RA, Moliterno DJ, et al: Platelet glycoprotein IIb/IIIa inhibitors in acute coronary syndromes: A meta-analysis of all major randomised clinical trials. Lancet 2002;359:189–198.

41. Roffi M, Chew DP, Mukherjee D, et al: Platelet Glycoprotein IIb/IIIa inhibitors reduce mortality in diabetic patients with non-ST-segment-elevation acute coronary syndromes. Circulation 2001;104:2767–2771.

42. Roffi M, Chew DP, Mukherjee D, et al: Platelet glycoprotein IIb/IIIa inhibition in acute coronary syndromes. Gradient of benefit related to the revascularization strategy. Eur Heart J 2002;23:1441–1448.

43. The Platelet IIb/IIIa Antagonist for the Reduction of Acute coronary syndrome events in a Global Organization Network (PARAGON)-B Investigators. Randomized, placebo-controlled trial of titrated intravenous lamifiban for acute coronary syndromes. Circulation 2002;105:316–321.

44. Chew DP, Bhatt DL, Sapp S, Topol EJ: Increased mortality with oral platelet glycoprotein IIb/IIIa antagonists. A meta-analysis of Phase III Multicenter Randomized Trials. Circulation 2001;103:201–206.

45. Eikelboom JW, Anand SS, Malmberg K, et al: Unfractionated heparin and low-molecular-weight heparin in acute coronary syndrome without ST elevation: A meta-analysis. Lancet 2000;355:1936–1942.

46. Theroux P, Waters D, Lam J, et al: Reactivation of unstable angina after the discontinuation of heparin. N Engl J Med 1992;327:141–145.

47. Fragmin during Instability in Coronary Artery Disease (FRISC) study group: Low-molecular-weight heparin during instability in coronary artery disease. Lancet 1996;347:561–568.

48. Klein W, Buchwald A, Hillis SE, et al: Fragmin in unstable coronary artery disease study: Comparison of low-molecular-weight heparin with unfractionated heparin acutely and with placebo for 6 weeks in the management of unstable coronary artery disease. Circulation 1997;96:61–68.

49. The FRAX.IS Study Group: Comparison to two treatment durations (6 days and 14 days) of a low molecular weight heparin with a 6-day treatment of unfractionated heparin in the initial management of unstable angina or non-Q wave myocardial infarction: FRAX.IS. Eur Heart J 1999;20:1553–1562.

50. Cohen M, Demers C, Gurfinkel EP, et al: For the efficacy and safety of subcutaneous enoxaparin in non-Q-wave coronary events Study Group. A comparison of low-molecular-weight heparin with unfractionated heparin for unstable coronary artery disease. N Engl J Med 1997;337:447–452.

51. Antman E, McCabe CH, Gurfinkel EP, et al: For the TIMI IIB Investigators. Enoxaparin prevents death and cardiac ischemic events in unstable angina/non-Q-wave myocardial infarction. Circulation 1999;100:1593–1601.

52. Cairns JA, Theroux P, Lewis HD Jr, et al: Antithrombotic agents in coronary artery disease. Chest 2001;119:228S–252S.

53. Antman EM, Cohen M, Radley D, et al: Assessment of the treatment effect of enoxaparin for unstable angina/non-Q-wave myocardial infarction. TIMI IIB-ESSENCE meta-analysis. Circulation 1999;100:1602–1608.

54. Massel D, Cruickshank MK: Enoxaparin in acute coronary syndromes: Evidence for superiority over placebo or untreated control. Am Heart J 2002;143:748–752.

55. OASIS-2 Investigators: Effects of recombinant hirudin (lepirudin) compared with heparin on death, myocardial infarction, refractory angina, and revascularisation procedures in patients with acute myocardial ischaemia without ST elevation: A randomised trial. Lancet 1999;353:429–438.

56. Hirudin in acute myocardial infarction: Thrombolysis and Thrombin Inhibition in Myocardial Infarction (TIMI) 9B trial. Circulation 1996;94:911–921.

57. The Global Use of Strategies to Open Occluded Coronary Arteries (GUSTO) IIa Investigators: Randomized trial of intravenous heparin versus recombinant hirudin for acute coronary syndromes. Circulation 1994;90:1631–1637.

58. Direct thrombin inhibitors in acute coronary syndromes: Principal results of a meta-analysis based on individual patients' data. Lancet 2002;359:294–302.

58b. Kong DF, Topol EJ, Bittl JA, et al: Clinical outcome of bivalirudin for ischemic heart disease. Circ 1999; 100:2049–2053.

58c. White H: Thrombin-specific anticoagulation with bivalirudin versus heparin in patients receiving fibrinolytic therapy for acute myocardial infarction: The HERO-2 randomized trial. Lancet 2001;358:1855–1863.

58d. Lincoff AM, Kleiman NS, Kottke-Marchant K, et al: Provisional abciximab versus low-dose heparin and abciximab during percutaneous revascularization: Results of the Comparison of Abciximab Complications with Hirulog for Ischemic Events Trial (CACHET). Am Heart J 2002;143:847–853.

59. Fragmin and revascularization during instability in coronary artery disease (FRISC II) Investigators. Lancet 1999;353:701–707.

60. The Medical Research Council's General Practice Research Framework. Thrombosis prevention trial: Randomised trial of low-intensity oral anticoagulation with warfarin and low-dose aspirin in the primary prevention of ischemic heart disease in men at increased risk. Lancet 1998;351:233–241.

61. Coumadin Aspirin Reinfarction Study (CARS) Investigators: Randomised double-blind trial of fixed low-dose warfarin with aspirin after myocardial infarction. Lancet 1997;350:389–396.

62. Fiore LD, Ezekowitz MD, Brophy MT, et al: Combination hemotherapy and mortality prevention (CHAMP) Study Group. Circulation 2002;105:557–563.

63. van Es RF, Jonker JJ, Verheugt FW, et al: Antithrombotics in the secondary prevention of events in coronary thrombosis-2 (ASPECT-2) Research Group. Aspirin and coumadin after acute coronary syndromes (the ASPECT-2 study): A randomised controlled trial. Lancet 2002;360:109–113.

64. Hurlen M, Abdelnoor M, Smith P, et al: Warfarin, aspirin, or both after myocardial infarction. N Engl J Med 2002;347:969–974.

65. The Organization to Assess Strategies for Ischemic Syndromes (OASIS-2) Investigators: Effects of long-term, moderate-intensity oral anticoagulation in addition to aspirin in unstable angina. J Am Coll Cardiol 2001;37:475–484.

66. Brouwer MA, van den Bergh PJ, Aengevaeren WR, et al: Aspirin plus coumarin versus aspirin alone in the prevention of reocclusion after fibrinolysis for acute myocardial infarction: Results of the Antithrombotics in the Prevention of Reocclusion In Coronary Thrombolysis (APRICOT)-2 Trial. Circulation 2002;106:659–665.

67. Brouwer MA, Vergheult FWA: Oral anticoagulation for acute coronary syndromes. Circulation 2002;105:1270–1274.

68. Sabatine MS, Morrow DA, de Lemos JA, et al: Multimarker approach to risk stratification in non-ST elevation acute coronary syndromes: Simultaneous assessment of troponin I, C-reactive protein, and B-type natriuretic peptide. Circulation 2002;105:1760–1763.

69. Heeschen C, Hamm CW, Bruemmer J, Simoons ML: Predictive value of C-reactive protein and troponin T in patients with unstable angina: A comparative analysis. CAPTURE Investigators. Chimeric c7E3 AntiPlatelet Therapy in Unstable angina REfractory to standard treatment trial. J Am Coll Cardiol 2000;35:1535–1542.

70. Chew DP, Bhatt DL, Robbins MA, et al: Incremental prognostic value of elevated baseline C-reactive protein among established markers of risk in percutaneous coronary interventions. Circulation 2001;104:992–997.

71. Milazzo D, Biasucci LM, Luciani N, et al: Elevated levels of C-reactive protein before coronary artery bypass grafting predict recurrence of ischemic events. Am J Cardiol 1999;84:459–461.

72. Walter DH, Fichtlscherer S, Britten MB, et al: Statin therapy, inflammation and recurrent coronary events in patients following coronary stent implantation. J Am Coll Cardiol 2001;38:2006–2012.

73. Hebert PR, Hennekens CH: An overview of the 4 randomized trials of aspirin therapy in the primary prevention of vascular disease. Arch Intern Med 2000;160:3123–3127.

74. Cohen M, Theroux P, Borzak S, et al: Randomized double-blind safety study of enoxaparin versus unfractionated heparin in patients with non-ST-segment elevation acute coronary syndromes treated with tirofiban and aspirin: The ACUTE II study. The Antithrombotic Combination Using Tirofiban and Enoxaparin. Am Heart J 2002;144:470–477.

75. Goodman SG, Fitchett D, Armstrong PW, et al: Randomized evaluation of the safety and efficacy of enoxaparin versus unfractionated heparin in high-risk patients with non—ST-segment elevation acute coronary syndromes receiving the glycoprotein IIb/IIIa inhibitor eptifibatide. Circ 2003;107:238–244.

76. Chen L, Chester MR, Redwood S, et al: Angiographic stenosis progression and coronary events in patients with "stabilized" unstable angina. Circulation 1995;91:2319–2324.

77. Mehta SR, Yusuf S, Peters RJ, et al: Effects of pretreatment with clopidogrel and aspirin followed by long-term therapy in patients undergoing percutaneous coronary intervention: The PCI-CURE study. Lancet 2001;358:527–533.

78. EPISTENT Investigators: Randomised placebo-controlled and balloon angioplasty-controlled trial to assess safety of coronary stenting with use of platelet glycoprotein IIb/IIIa blockade. Lancet 1998;352:87–92.

Treatment of Cardiovascular Inflammation

James T. Willerson

This chapter reviews the role of inflammation in initiating and sustaining various cardiovascular problems, including the conversion from stable to unstable coronary heart disease syndromes, vascular aneurysms, and congestive heart failure. The chapter identifies various interventions that may reduce inflammation in the coronary arteries and hearts in humans, including marked lipid lowering, weight loss, peroxisome proliferator activated receptor agonists (PPARs), aspirin, and monoclonal antibodies to vascular cell adhesion molecule (VCAM) and intercellular vascular adhesion molecule (ICAM). Additional work is needed to identify the best ways to prevent or modulate vascular and myocardial inflammation with the expectation that such interventions will lead to more effective treatment of atherosclerosis, heart failure, and vascular aneurysms.

Inflammation plays a major role in initiating and sustaining cardiovascular problems, including the conversion from stable to unstable coronary heart disease syndromes, the development of vascular aneurysm, and congestive heart failure.[1-5] Inflammation also serves as an important predictor of future adverse events following interventional procedures in coronary arteries.[6] However, inflammation may also serve to identify unstable or vulnerable atherosclerotic plaques, potentially allowing treatment of these entities prior to their fissuring or ulceration and the development of unstable angina and acute myocardial infarction.[7,8] This chapter discusses potential mechanisms responsible for vascular and myocardial inflammation, consequences of such inflammation, systemic markers identifying the presence of inflammation, and potential treatments of cardiovascular inflammation.

MECHANISMS RESPONSIBLE FOR INFLAMMATION

The response to injury in the vasculature and heart is inflammation. Atherosclerosis results from a response to injury of the endothelium followed by inflammation and the development of atherosclerosis (Fig. 32-1). Vascular injuries that lead to inflammation and contribute to atherosclerosis and coronary artery disease are shown in Table 32-1. Although this topic is discussed in detail in Chapter 7, it is important to recognize that vascular and myocardial infection from various pathogens results in vascular inflammation and almost certainly contributes to atherosclerosis and the development of acute coronary artery syndromes.[9-11] No single infection has yet

been identified as playing a major role in vascular injury, inflammation, and progression to atherosclerosis; instead, current evidence favors prior exposure to multiple pathogens.[12,13] However, a relatively common but yet-unidentified infection may play a major role in vascular infection and atherosclerosis.

Genetic predisposition is likely to lead to inflammation, impaired endothelial vascular repair, vascular infection, thrombosis, and vasoconstriction. The aging process itself is almost certainly associated with altered vascular and myocardial defense mechanisms, predisposing some persons to inflammation. The oxidation of total cholesterol and low-density lipoprotein (LDL) cholesterol leads to the production of oxidized radicals that promote vascular inflammation and the recruitment of macrophage-derived monocytes (Fig. 32-2).[14-17] Similarly, interventional injury, including angioplasty and stenting, causes endothelial inflammation, thrombosis, and fibroproliferation.

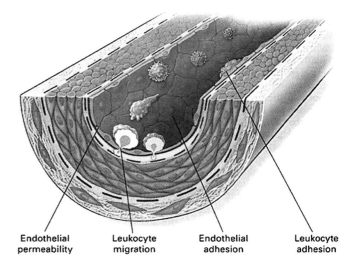

Endothelial permeability   Leukocyte migration   Endothelial adhesion   Leukocyte adhesion

FIGURE 32-1. The earliest changes that precede the formation of lesions of atherosclerosis take place in the endothelium. These changes include increased endothelial permeability to lipoproteins and other plasma constituents mediated by nitric oxide, prostacyclin, platelet-derived growth factor, angiotensin I, and endothelin; upregulation of leukocyte adhesion molecules, including L-selectin, integrins, and platelet-endothelial cell adhesion molecule 1; upregulation of endothelial adhesion molecules, including E-selectin, P-selectin, intercellular adhesion molecule 1, and vascular cell adhesion molecule 1; and migration of leukocytes into the artery wall, mediated by oxidized low-density lipoprotein, monocyte chemotactic protein 1, interleukin-8, platelet-derived growth factor, macrophage colony-stimulating factor, and osteopontin. (From Ross R: Atherosclerosis—An Inflammatory Disease. N Engl J Med 1999;340:117.)

RISK FACTORS FOR ATHEROSCLEROSIS

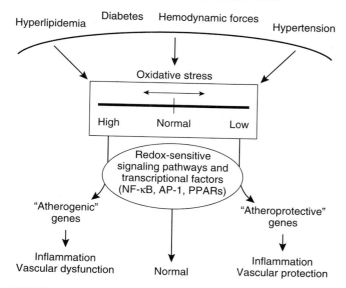

FIGURE 32–2. The association of atherosclerotic risk factors, oxidative stress, and redox-sensitive gene expression. Various risk factors for atherosclerosis, including hypertension, hyperlipidemia, diabetes, and vascular hemodynamic stresses (shear stresses), result in intracellular oxidative stress. The mechanisms by which these risk factors generate oxidative stress are not well characterized and may act synergistically. Various cellular processes are influenced by nutrition, and therapeutic interventions may regulate the relative level of intracellular oxidative stress. Relatively high levels of oxidative stress result in the induction of vascular inflammatory ("atherogenic") genes through redox-sensitive signaling pathways and activation of redox-sensitive transcription factors. Relatively lower levels of oxidative stress maintain a noninflammatory or vascular protective effect through induction of "atheroprotective" genes. Thus, intracellular oxidative stress resulting from an oxidative stress may act as a specific regulator in the signal transduction network to relay environmental and physical signals generated at the cell membrane to nuclear regulatory signals, leading to modulation of inflammatory gene expression. (From Kunsch C, Medford RM: Oxidative stress as a regulator of gene expression in the vasculature. Circ Res 1999;85:754.)

Inflammation causes the following:

- Smooth muscle cell proliferation and migration
- Lipid accumulation
- Endothelial dysfunction[17,18]

Immunologically mediated cellular injury leads to the activation of T cells; the development of antibodies to heat shock proteins; and antibodies to infectious agents, oxidized LDL cholesterol, and components of the inflammatory process itself.[19,20]

INFLAMMATION AND COMPLEX CORONARY HEART DISEASE LESIONS

Monocyte-derived macrophages and activated T cells are important to the development of unstable atherosclerotic plaques (Fig. 32–3).[21,22] Proteases released from macrophages after their entry into the arterial wall degrade collagen in the fibrous atherosclerotic plaque, leading to its weakening and fissuring, ulceration, or both, which causes abrupt thrombosis and dynamic vaso-

■ ■ ■

TABLE 32-1 PATHOGENESIS OF ACUTE CORONARY ARTERY DISEASE SYNDROMES

Infection with various pathogens
Genetic predisposition resulting from mutations and genetic polymorphisms leading to inflammation, impaired endothelial repair and stability, vascular infection, thrombosis, and/or vasoconstriction
Aging
Oxidized free radicals
Hyperlipidemia
Homocysteine
Diabetes
Smoking
Cocaine
Hypertension
Interventional Injury

constriction.[21,23,24] Unstable atherosclerotic plaques have thin fibrous caps, numerous inflammatory cells (primarily macrophages but also activated T cells) just beneath the fibrous cap or on its surface, and an adjacent lipid pool (Fig. 32–4).[25,26] Thus, the process of inflammation is pivotal in the conversion of stable to unstable coronary heart disease syndromes.

INFLAMMATION AND PROGRESSIVE CONGESTIVE HEART FAILURE

Considerable evidence indicates that inflammation and the accumulation of a selective mediator of inflammation, i.e., tumor necrosis factor α, may play a role in the progression of heart failure in experimental animal models and humans.[27-30] Tumor necrosis factor α is increased in the myocardium of patients with progressive heart failure.[29] Transgenic mice overexpressing tumor necrosis factor α experience dilated cardiomyopathy.[5] Tumor necrosis factor α has negative inotropic effects on ventricular function,[29] and this mediator is probably one of several that accumulate during inflammation and contribute to progressive congestive heart failure in selected persons.

SYSTEMIC MARKERS OF INFLAMMATION

Numerous studies have demonstrated that increases in serum C-reactive protein (CRP) identify risk of future vascular events, including myocardial infarction, cerebrovascular accidents, and death (see Chapter 16).[6,7,31-33] Elevations in serum CRP concentration identify patients with unstable angina and non–Q-wave myocardial infarction at increased risk for future acute coronary events.[33-36] Similarly, elevations in serum CRP predict patients at greater risk for restenosis after interventional procedures.[37]

Increases in serum troponin I, serum amyloid-like protein, fibrinogen, and interleukins-1, -2, -6, -8, and -18 have also been shown to identify patients with unstable

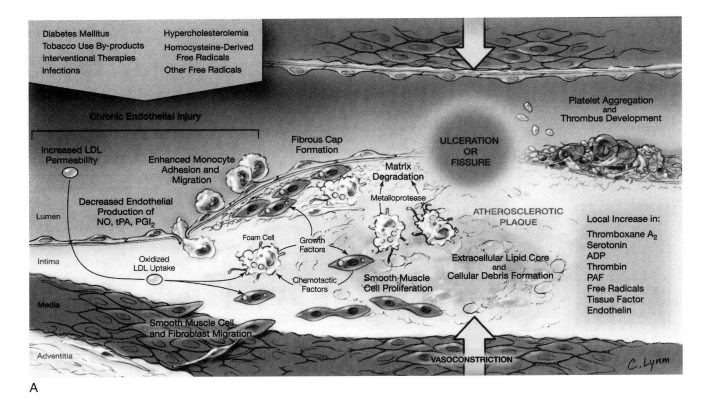

A

FIGURE 32–3. *A*, Chronic endothelial injury, inflammation, and oxidative stress are central to the development of atherosclerosis. Endothelial injury results from a variety of factors, including tobacco use, hypercholesterolemia, interventional therapy with angioplasty or coronary stents, and ulceration or fissuring of atherosclerotic plaques. At sites of endothelial injury, production of endothelial-derived substances (nitric oxide [NO], tissue-type plasminogen activator [t-PA], and prostacyclin [PGI₂]) is decreased, creating a prothrombotic environment characterized by increased platelet and leukocyte adhesion, increased permeability to plasma lipoproteins, myointimal hyperplasia, and vasoconstriction. Ulceration or fissuring of the atherosclerotic plaque results from degradation of collagen matrix in the fibrous cap by metalloproteases released from macrophages. Exposure of the subendothelium after plaque ulceration or fissuring leads to platelet adhesion and aggregation and local accumulation of largely platelet-derived mediators (thromboxane A₂, serotonin, adenosine diphosphate [ADP], thrombin, platelet-activating factor [PAF], oxygen-derived free radicals, tissue factor, and endothelin) that promote thrombus growth, fibroproliferation, and vasoconstriction. LDL, low-density lipoprotein. (From Lefkowitz RJ, Willerson JT: Prospects for cardiovascular research. JAMA 2001;285:583 by permission.) (*Figure continued on page 447.*)

angina and non–Q-wave myocardial infarction at increased risk for coronary events.[7,36–40] Thus, several systemic markers may be used to identify inflammation in patients with coronary heart disease and hence help identify an increased risk of future events.

In the case of CRP, more recent evidence has demonstrated that it is not only a marker of inflammation but also a contributor to the development of inflammation. Work from Pasceri et al and others has demonstrated that CRP amplifies the effects of other activators of inflammation (including endotoxin) and causes the expression of VCAM and ICAM at physiologically relevant concentrations in cultured vascular cells.[41–44] Others have demonstrated that CRP promotes tissue factor production by macrophages in culture and uptake of LDL cholesterol.[45]

TREATMENT OPTIONS

Studies have shown that marked reduction in total serum cholesterol and LDL cholesterol concentrations reduces the risk for future coronary events in patients with known coronary atherosclerosis.[46–48] More recent evidence from the Cholesterol and Recurrent Events (CARE) trial demonstrated that a statin such as pravastatin reduces total serum cholesterol, LDL cholesterol, and CRP concentrations (Fig. 32–5).[49] In the CARE study, which was directed at determining the influence of reduction in total cholesterol and LDL cholesterol in reducing future coronary events, reduction in serum CRP concentrations was identified months to years after the drug was begun. More recent studies have shown that a statin that reduces total cholesterol, LDL cholesterol, and CRP values improves endothelial function and reverses abnormal endothelial function within a few weeks.[50] Thus, marked reduction in total serum cholesterol and LDL cholesterol reduces inflammation and improves endothelial function, although this response is not immediate and may require weeks to months. Similar studies in experimental animal models have also shown that marked reduction in total serum cholesterol and LDL cholesterol reverses inflammation in atherosclerotic lesions.[51]

Ridker et al have shown that aspirin reduces the risk of myocardial infarction associated with higher serum CRP levels (Fig. 32–6).[52]

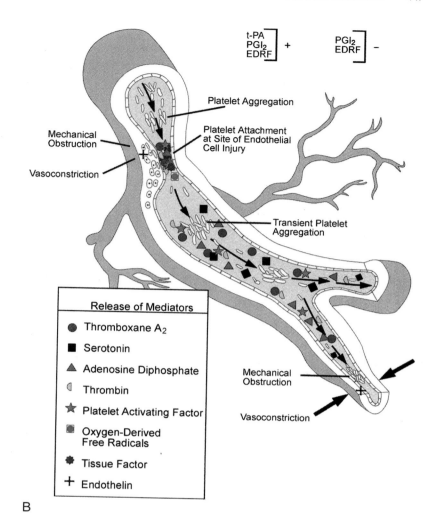

FIGURE 32–3, Cont'd. *B*, Schematic diagram suggests probable mechanisms responsible for the conversion from chronic coronary heart disease to acute coronary artery disease syndromes. In this scheme, endothelial injury, generally at sites of atherosclerotic plaques and usually of plaque ulceration or fissuring, is associated with platelet adhesion and aggregation and the release and activation of selected mediators, including thromboxane A_2, serotonin, adenosine diphosphate, platelet-activating factor, thrombin, oxygen-derived free radicals, and endothelin. Local accumulation of thromboxane A_2, serotonin, platelet-activating factor, thrombin, adenosine diphosphate, and tissue factor promotes platelet aggregation. Thromboxane A_2, serotonin, thrombin, and platelet-activating factor are vasoconstrictors at sites of endothelial injury. Therefore, the conversion from chronic stable to acute unstable coronary heart disease syndromes is usually associated with endothelial injury, platelet aggregation, accumulation of platelet- and other cell-derived mediators, further platelet aggregation, and vasoconstriction, with consequent dynamic narrowing of the coronary artery lumen. In addition to atherosclerotic plaque fissuring or ulceration, other reasons for endothelial injury include flow shear stress, hypertension, immune complex deposition and complement activation, infection, and mechanical injury to the endothelium as it occurs with coronary artery angioplasty and after heart transplantation. EDRF, endothelium-derived relaxing factor; PGI_2, prostaglandin I_2; t-PA, tissue-type plasminogen activator. (From Willerson JT, Cohn JN: Cardiovascular Medicine. Philadelphia: Churchill Livingstone, 2000.)

B

Appropriate treatment of an infection also reduces inflammation. Antimicrobial treatment directed at *Chlamydia pneumoniae* has been associated with improved endothelial function and reduced selected serum markers of inflammation, including E-selectin.[53]

Weight loss in postmenopausal obese females is associated with reductions in serum CRP concentration.[54] Available evidence suggests that estrogens may increase serum CRP concentrations in postmenopausal women,[55,56] but even more recent evidence suggests

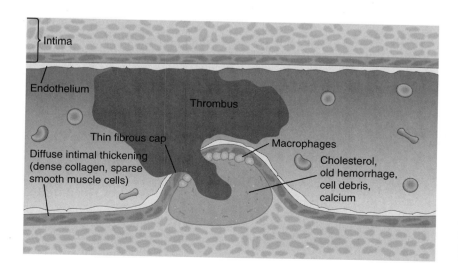

FIGURE 32–4. The morphologic appearance of the unstable atherosclerotic plaque shows a thin fibrous cap, numerous inflammatory cells underneath or on the surface of the atherosclerotic cap (or in both places), and an adjacent lipid pool.

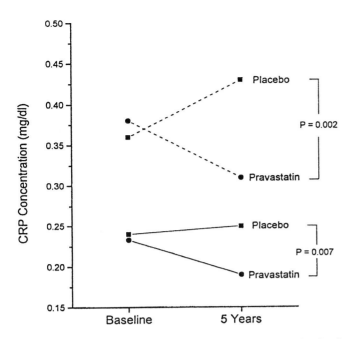

FIGURE 32–5. Median *(solid lines)* and mean *(dotted lines)* levels of C-reactive protein (CRP) at baseline and at 60 months, according to placebo or pravastatin assignment. (From Ridker PM, Rifai N, Pfeffer MA, et al: Long-term effects of pravastatin on plasma concentration of C-reactive protein. Circulation 1999;100:232.)

that, at least in some women, estrogen and progesterone therapy given together decrease serum CRP concentrations and other markers of inflammation.[54] Various drugs and antibodies targeting selected components of the

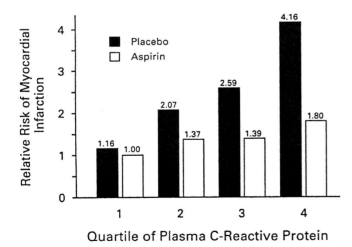

FIGURE 32–6. Relative risk of a first myocardial infarction associated with baseline plasma concentrations of C-reactive protein, stratified according to randomized assignment to aspirin or placebo therapy. Analyses are limited to events occurring before the unblinding of the aspirin component of the Physicians' Health Study. The reduction in the risk of myocardial infarction associated with the use of aspirin was 13.9% in the first (lowest) quartile of C-reactive protein values, 33.4% in the second quartile, 46.3% in the third quartile, and 55.7% in the fourth (highest) quartile. (From Ridker PM, Cushman M, Stampfer MJ, et al: Inflammation, aspirin, and the risk of cardiovascular disease in apparently healthy men. N Engl J Med 1997;336:973–979.)

inflammatory process have been investigated or are currently under investigation in acute ischemic conditions in humans. Pilot studies with methylprednisone in unstable angina,[57] with monoclonal antibodies to the CD18 subunit of the β_2 integrin adhesion receptors[58] and to tissue factor necrosis, and to a P-selectin glycoprotein ligand 1 in acute myocardial infarction did not show the expected benefit. A monoclonal antibody to the C5 component of the complement system failed to reduce infarct size.

EXPERIMENTAL ANIMAL MODELS

We have developed an experimental model in which macrophages are labeled with fluorescent microspheres and re-injected into apolipoprotein E–deficient mice in which the macrophages "home" to atherosclerotic plaques (Figs. 32-7 and 32-8).[59] In this model, monoclonal antibodies directed at VCAM and ICAM markedly diminish macrophage homing and inflammation in atherosclerotic plaques.[59] Selected PPARs, including troglitazone, could reduce macrophage homing to atherosclerotic plaques in patients undergoing thrombolysis or primary angioplasty, but reduced mortality in patients undergoing primary angioplasty.[59a, 60] Others have shown that selected PPAR agonists diminish inflammation.[61,62] The general effects of PPAR agonists are shown in Figure 32-9.

INFLAMMATION AS A DIRECT PREDICTOR OF UNSTABLE ATHEROSCLEROTIC PLAQUES

Casscells and Willerson hypothesized that inflammation in unstable atherosclerotic plaques results in temperature heterogeneity within the plaque.[25] We have shown that temperature heterogeneity exists in human carotid endarterectomy specimens and that the temperature heterogeneity correlates with inflammation (Fig. 32-10). Stefanadis and his colleagues confirmed these observations and showed acute myocardial infarction temperature heterogeneity in vivo in the coronary arteries of patients with recent unstable angina.[63] Thus, one may also use the presence of inflammation as an aid in identifying the unstable atherosclerotic plaque before it fissures or ulcerates, although this remains to be proved in additional patient studies. If this use of inflammation is verified in humans and if systems that identify vulnerable atherosclerotic plaques prior to their ulceration or fissuring are developed, it may become possible to treat plaques locally with antiproliferative, anti-inflammatory, and anti-thrombotic substances that rapidly improve inflammation; such agents might subsequently be followed by the administration of statins, aspirin, weight loss, and potentially other modifiers of inflammation with long-term benefit. Such local therapies may well include selected forms of gene therapy and possibly local heating of the unstable plaque itself.[64-69]

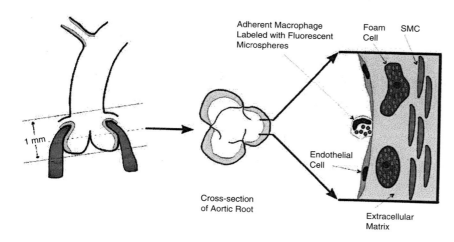

FIGURE 32–7. Schematic diagram of the study area depicting a labeled macrophage adhering to the plaque. (From Patel SS, Thiagarajan R, Willerson JT, et al: Inhibition of α_4 integrin and ICAM-1 markedly attenuate macrophage homing to atherosclerotic plaques in ApoE-deficient mice. Circulation 1998;97:78.) SMC, smooth muscle cells.

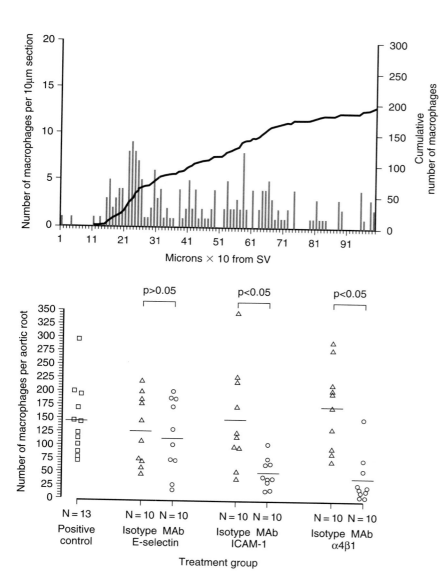

FIGURE 32–8. Inhibition of macrophage recruitment by antibody against α_4 or intercellular vascular adhesion molecule (ICAM)-1 but not by anti–E-selectin antibody. The group of mice that were not treated with antibody is labeled as *Positive Control*. Appropriate isotype-matched antibody was used for each specific antibody. Mean of each treatment group is indicated by a *bar*. Comparison of the seven treatment groups was performed with one-way ANOVA followed by Scheffé's test for post hoc pairwise comparisons. All analyses were done with SAS statistical programs; $P < .05$ was considered statistically significant. MAb, monoclonal antibody. (From Patel SS, Thiagarajan R, Willerson JT, et al: Inhibition of α_4 integrin and ICAM-1 markedly attenuate macrophage homing to atherosclerotic plaques in ApoE-deficient mice. Circulation 1998;97:80.)

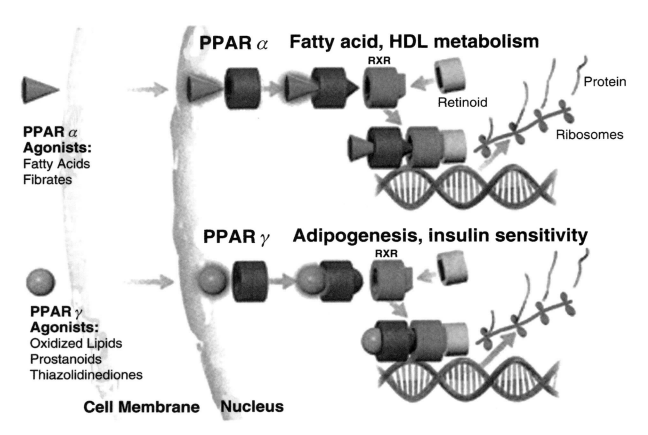

FIGURE 32–9. Peroxisome proliferator activated receptor (PPAR) pathways. Originally recognized as instigators of peroxisomal proliferation unique to rodents, PPARs are nuclear receptors for small lipophilic molecules that freely partition into cells. When these receptors bind their small ligand partner, they pair with another member of nuclear receptor family, retinoid X receptor (RXR). This heterodimeric transcription factor complex then binds to cognate sequences in promoter regions of target genes, altering their transcription. PPAR-α regulates the cassette of genes involved in lipoprotein metabolism, raising levels of apolipoprotein A$_1$, a major apolipoprotein of high-density lipoprotein (HDL). PPAR-γ regulates expression of genes involved in adipogenesis and insulin sensitivity. Kindreds with mutations that affect function of PPAR-γ develop an insulin resistance syndrome, including hypertension. (From Libby P: Current concepts of the pathogenesis of the acute coronary syndromes. Circulation 2001;104:365–372.)

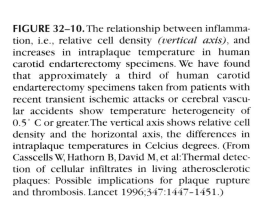

FIGURE 32–10. The relationship between inflammation, i.e., relative cell density *(vertical axis)*, and increases in intraplaque temperature in human carotid endarterectomy specimens. We have found that approximately a third of human carotid endarterectomy specimens taken from patients with recent transient ischemic attacks or cerebral vascular accidents show temperature heterogeneity of 0.5° C or greater. The vertical axis shows relative cell density and the horizontal axis, the differences in intraplaque temperatures in Celcius degrees. (From Casscells W, Hathorn B, David M, et al:Thermal detection of cellular infiltrates in living atherosclerotic plaques: Possible implications for plaque rupture and thrombosis. Lancet 1996;347:1447–1451.)

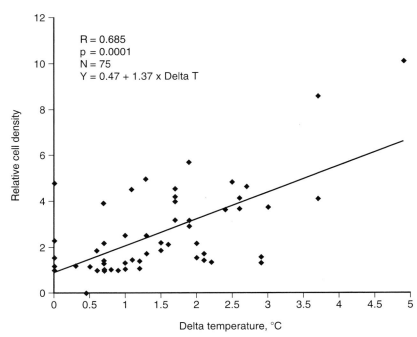

REFERENCES

1. Ross R: Atherosclerosis—An inflammatory disease. N Engl J Med 1999;340:115–126.

2. Falk E: Morphologic features of unstable atherothrombotic plaques underlying acute coronary syndromes. Am J Cardiol 1989;63:114E–120E.

3. Lendon CL, Davies MJ, Born GV, Richardson PD: Atherosclerotic plaque caps are locally weakened when macrophages density is increased. Atherosclerosis 1991;87:87–90.

4. Goodall S, Crowther M, Hemingway DM, et al: Ubiquitous elevation of matrix metalloproteinase-2 expression in the vasculature of patients with abdominal aneurysms. Circulation 2001;104:304–309.

5. Sivasubramanian N, Coker ML, Kurrelmeyer KM, et al: Left ventricular remodeling in transgenic mice with cardiac restricted overexpression of tumor necrosis factor. Circulation 2001;104:826–831.

6. Chew DP, Bhatt DL, Robbins MA, et al: Incremental prognostic value of elevated baseline C-reactive protein among established markers of risk in percutaneous coronary intervention. Circulation 2001;104:992–997.

7. Liuzzo G, Biasucci LM, Gallimore JR, et al: The prognostic value of C-reactive protein and serum amyloid a protein in severe unstable angina. N Engl J Med 1994;331:417–424.

8. Shah PK, Falk E, Badimon JJ, et al: Human monocyte-derived macrophages induce collagen breakdown in fibrous caps of atherosclerotic plaques: Potential role of matrix-degrading metalloproteinases and implications for plaque rupture. Circulation 1995;92:1565–1569.

9. Muhlestein JB, Horne BD, Carlquist JF, et al: Cytomegalovirus seropositivity and C-reactive protein have independent and combined predictive value for mortality in patients with angiographically demonstrated coronary artery disease. Circulation 2000;102:1917–1923.

10. Saikku P, Leionen M, Mattila K, et al: Serological evidence of an association of a novel Chlamydia, TWAR, with chronic coronary heart disease and acute myocardial infarction. Lancet 1988;2:983–985.

11. Grayston JT: Chlamydia in atherosclerosis. Circulation 1993;87:1408–1409.

12. Anderson JL, Carlquist JF, Muhlestein JB, et al: Evaluation of C-reactive protein, an inflammatory marker, and infectious serology as risk factors for coronary artery disease and myocardial infarction. J Am Coll Cardiol 1998;32:35–41.

13. Ridker PM, Hennekens CH, Stampfer MJ, et al: Prospective study of herpes simplex virus, cytomegalovirus, and the risk of future myocardial infarction and stroke. Circulation 1998;98:2796–2799.

14. Steinberg D, Parthasarathy S, Carew TE, et al: Beyond cholesterol: Modifications of low-density lipoprotein that increase its atherogenicity. N Engl J Med 1989;320:915–920.

15. Marui N, Offermann MK, Swerlick R, et al: Vascular cell adhesion molecule-1 (VCAM-1) gene transcription and expression are regulated through an antioxidant-sensitive mechanism in human vascular endothelial cells. J Clin Invest 1993;92:1866–1874.

16. Weber C, Erl W, Pietsch A, et al: Antioxidants inhibit monocyte adhesion by suppressing nuclear factor-kappa B mobilization and induction of vascular cell adhesion molecule-1 in endothelial cells stimulated to generate radicals. Arterioscler Thromb 1994;14:1665–1673.

17. Lehr HA, Hübner C, Menger MD, et al: Mechanisms and mediators of leukocyte/endothelium interaction during atherogenesis. Atheroscler Rev 1993;25:49–57.

18. Bhakdi S, Torzewski M, Klouche M, et al: Complement and atherosclerosis: Binding of CRP to degraded, nonoxidized LDL enhances complement activation. Arterioscler Thromb Vasc Biol 1999;19:2348–2354.

19. Serneri GGN, Abbate R, Gori AM, et al: Transient intermittent lymphocyte activation is responsible for the instability of angina. Circulation 1992;86:790–797.

20. Biasucci LM, Liuzzo G, Fantuzzi G, et al: Increasing levels of interleukin (IL)-1Ra and IL-6 during the first 2 days of hospitalization in unstable angina are associated with increased risk of in-hospital coronary events. Circulation 1999;99:2079–2084.

21. Libby P, Geng YJ, Aikawa M, et al: Macrophages and atherosclerotic plaque stability. Curr Opin Lipidol 1996;7:330–335.

22. Kockx MK, Knaapen MWM, Martinet W, et al: Expression of the uncoupling protein UCP-2 in macrophages of unstable human atherosclerotic plaques. Circulation 2000;102:II-12.

23. Hirsh PD, Hillis LD, Campbell WB, et al: Release of prostaglandins and thromboxane into the coronary circulation in patients with ischemic heart disease. N Engl J Med 1981;304:685–691.

24. Willerson JT, Golino P, Eidt J, et al: Specific platelet mediators and unstable coronary artery lesions. Experimental evidence and potential clinical implications. Circulation 1989;80:198–205.

25. Casscells W, Hathorn B, David M, et al: Thermal detection of cellular infiltrates in living atherosclerotic plaques: Possible implications for plaque rupture and thrombosis. Lancet 1996;347:1447–1451.

26. Davies MJ, Thomas T: The pathological basis and microanatomy of occlusive thrombus formation in human coronary arteries. Philos Trans R Soc Lond B Biol Sci 1981;294:225–229.

27. Spinale FG, Coker ML, Krombach SR, et al: Matrix metalloproteinase inhibition during the development of congestive heart failure: Effects on left ventricular dimensions and function. Circ Res 1999;85:364–376.

28. Kapadia S, Lee JR, Torre-Amione G, et al: Tumor necrosis factor gene and protein expression in adult feline myocardium after endotoxin administration. J Clin Invest 1995;96:1042–1052.

29. Torre-Amione G, Kapadia S, Lee J, et al: Expression and functional significance of tumor necrosis factor receptors in human myocardium. Circulation 1995;92:1487–1493.

30. Li YY, Feng YQ, Kadokami T, et al: Myocardial extracellular matrix remodeling in transgenic mice overexpressing tumor necrosis factor alpha can be modulated by anti-tumor necrosis factor alpha therapy. Proc Natl Acad Sci U S A 2000;97:12746–12751.

31. Ridker PM, Hennekens CH, Buring JE, et al: C-reactive protein and other markers of inflammation in the prediction of cardiovascular disease in women. N Engl J Med 2000;342:836–843.

32. Koenig W, Sund M, Froelich M, et al: C-reactive protein, a sensitive marker of inflammation, predicts future risk of coronary heart disease in initially healthy middle-aged men: Results from the MONICA (Monitoring trends and determinants in cardiovascular disease) Augsburg Cohort Study. 1984 to 1992. Circulation 1999;99:237–242.

33. Tracy R, Lemaitre R, Psaty B, et al: Relationship of C-reactive protein to risk of cardiovascular disease in the elderly: Results from the Cardiovascular Health Study and the Rural Health Promotion Project. Arterioscler Thromb Vasc Biol 1997;17:1121–1127.

34. Ridker PM, Glynn RJ, Hennekens CH: C-reactive protein adds to the predictive value of total and HDL cholesterol in determining risk of first myocardial infarction. Circulation 1998;97:2007–2011.

35. Maseri A: Inflammation, atherosclerosis, and ischemic events: Exploring the hidden side of the moon. N Engl J Med 1997;336:1014–1016.

36. Haverkate F, Thompson SG, Pyke SDM, et al: Production of C-Reactive protein and risk of coronary events in stable and unstable angina. Lancet 1997;349:462–466.

37. Buffon A, Liuzzo G, Biasucci LM, et al: Preprocedural serum levels of C-reactive protein predict early complications and late restenosis after coronary angioplasty. J Am Coll Cardiol 1999;34:1512–1521.

38. Ridker PM, Rifai N, Stampfer MJ, et al: Plasma concentration of interleukin-6 and the risk of future myocardial infarction among apparently healthy men. Circulation 2000;101:1767–1772.

39. Heeschen C, Hamm CW, Bruemmer J, et al: Predictive value of C-reactive protein and troponin T in patients with unstable angina: A comparative analysis: CAPTURE Investigators: Chimeric c7E3 Anti-Platelet Therapy in Unstable angina REfractory to standard treatment trial. J Am Coll Cardiol 2000;35:1535–1542.

40. Mallat Z, Corbaz A, Scoazec A, et al: Expression of interleukin-18 in human atherosclerotic plaques and relation to plaque instability. Circulation 2001;104:1598–1603.

41. Pasceri V, Willerson JT, Yeh ETH: Direct proinflammatory effect of C-reactive protein on human endothelial cells. Circulation 2000;102:2165–2168.

42. Pasceri V, Chang J, Willerson JT, Yeh ETH: Modulation of C-reactive protein-mediated monocyte chemoattractant protein-1 induction in human endothelial cells by anti-atherosclerosis drugs. Circulation 2001;103:2531–2534.

43. Yeh ETH, Anderson HV, Pasceri V, Willerson JT: C-Reactive protein: Linking inflammation to cardiovascular complications. Editorial. Circulation 2001;104:974–975.

44. Theroux P, Willerson JT, Armstrong P: Acute coronary syndromes. Fifty years of progress. Circulation 2000;102 (Suppl 4):2-13.

45. Zwaka TP, Hombach V, Torzewski J: C-reactive protein-mediated low density lipoprotein uptake by macrophages. Implications for atherosclerosis. Circulation 2001;103:1194-1197.

46. 4S Investigators: Randomised trial of cholesterol lowering in 4444 patients with coronary heart disease: The Scandinavian Simvastatin Survival Study (4S). Lancet 1994;344:1383-1389.

47. Shepherd J, Cobbe SM, Ford I, et al: Prevention of coronary heart disease with pravastatin in men with hypercholesterolemia. N Engl J Med 1995;333:1301-1307.

48. Sacks FM, Pfeffer MA, Moye LA, et al: The effect of pravastatin on coronary events after myocardial infarction in patients with average cholesterol levels. N Engl J Med 1996;335:1001-1009.

49. Ridker PM, Rifai N, Pfeffer MA, et al: Long-term effects of pravastatin on plasma concentration of C-reactive protein. Circulation 1999;100:230-235.

50. Dupuis J, Tardif JC, Cernacek P, Theroux P: Cholesterol reduction rapidly improves endothelial function after acute coronary syndromes: The RECIFE (reduction of cholesterol in ischemia and function of the endothelium) trial. Circulation 1999;99:3227-3233.

51. Fukumoto Y, Libby P, Rabkin E, et al: Statins alter smooth muscle cell accumulation and collagen content in established atheroma of Wantanabe heritable hyperlipidemic rabbits. Circulation 2001;103:993-999.

52. Ridker PM, Cushman M, Stampfer MJ, et al: Inflammation, aspirin, and the risk of cardiovascular disease in apparently healthy men. N Engl J Med 1997;336:973-979.

53. Anderson JL, Muhlestein JB, Carlquist J, et al: Randomized secondary prevention trial of azithromycin in patients with coronary artery disease and serological evidence for *Chlamydia pneumoniae* infection. The Azithromycin in Coronary Artery Disease: Elimination of Myocardial Infection with Chlamydia (ACADEMIC) Study. Circulation 1999;99:1540-1547.

54. Wakatsuki A, Okatani Y, Ikenoue N, Fukaya T: Effect of Medroxyprogesterone acetate on vascular inflammatory markers in postmenopausal women receiving estrogen. Circulation 2002;105:1436-1439.

55. Ridker PM, Hennekens CH, Rifai N, et al: Hormone replacement therapy and increased plasma concentration of C-reactive protein. Circulation 1999;100:713-716.

56. Cushman M, Legault C, Barrett-Connor E, et al: Effects of postmenopausal hormones on inflammation sensitive proteins: The Postmenopausal Estrogen/Progestin Interventions (PEPI) Study. Circulation 1999;100:717-722.

57. Azar RR, Rinfret S, Theroux P, et al: A randomized placebo-controlled trial to assess the efficacy of antiinflammatory therapy with methylprednisolone in unstable angina (MUNA trial). Eur Heart J 2000;21:2026-2032.

58. Baran KW, Nguyen M, McKendall GR, et al: Double-blind, randomized trial of an anti-CD18 antibody in conjunction with recombinant tissue plasminogen activator for acute myocardial infarction: Limitation of myocardial infarction following thrombolysis in acute myocardial infarction (LIMIT AMI) study. Circulation 2001;104: 2778-2783.

59. Patel SS, Willerson JT, Yeh ET-H: Inhibition of α_4 integrin and ICAM-1 markedly attenuate macrophage homing to atherosclerotic plaques in ApoE-deficient mice. Circulation 1998;97:75-81.

59a. Granger CB, Mahaffey KW, Weaver D, et al: Effect of pexelizumab, an anticomplement antibody, as adjunctive therapy to primary percutaneous coronary intervention in acute myocardial infarction: Complement inhibition in myocardial infarction treated with angioplasty (COMMA) trial Circulation: Submitted.

60. Pasceri V, Wu HD, Willerson JT, Yeh ET-H: Modulation of vascular inflammation *in vitro* and *in vivo* by Peroxisome Proliferator-Activated Receptor-γ activators. Circulation 2000;101:235-238.

61. Marx N, Sukhova GK, Collins T, et al: PPARα activators inhibit cytokine-induced vascular cell adhesion molecule-1 expression in human endothelial cells. Circulation 1999;99:3125-3131.

62. Marx N, Sukhova G, Murphy C, et al: Macrophages in human atheroma contain PPARγ: Differentiation-dependent PPARγ expression and reduction in MMP-9 activity through PPARγ activation in mononuclear phagocytes. Am J Pathol 1998;153:17-23.

63. Stefanadis C, Toutouzas K, Tsiamis E, et al: Increased local temperature in human coronary atherosclerotic plaques: An independent predictor of clinical outcome in patients undergoing a percutaneous coronary intervention. J Am Coll Cardiol 2001;37:1277-1283.

64. Zoldhelyi P, Chen Z-Q, Shelat HS, et al: Local gene transfer of tissue factor pathway inhibitor regulates intimal hyperplasia in atherosclerotic arteries. Proc Natl Acad Sci U S A 2001;98:4078-4083.

65. Shyue S-K, Tsai M-J, Liou J-Y, et al: Selective augmentation of prostacyclin production by combined prostacyclin synthase and cyclooxygenase-1 gene transfer. Circulation 2001;103:2090-2095.

66. Shelat HS, Liu T-J, Hickman-Bick D, et al: Growth suppression of human coronary vascular smooth muscle cells by gene transfer of the transcription factor E2F-1. Circulation 2001;103:407-414.

67. Zoldhelyi P, Eichstaedt H, Jax T, et al: The emerging clinical potential of cardiovascular gene therapy. Semin Intervent Cardiol 1999;4:151-165.

68. Zoldhelyi P, McNatt J, Shelat HS, et al: Thromboresistance of balloon-injured porcine carotid arteries after local gene transfer of human tissue factor pathway inhibitor. Circulation 2000;101:289-295.

69. Zoldhelyi P, McNatt J, Xu XM, et al: Prevention of arterial thrombosis by adenovirus-mediate transfer of cyclooxygenase gene. Circulation 1996;93:10-17.

Myocardial Cell Protection in Acute Coronary Syndromes

David Garcia-Dorado

LETHAL CELL INJURY DURING ISCHEMIA-REPERFUSION

In recent decades, the cellular and molecular mechanisms responsible for destabilization of atheromatous plaques associated with acute coronary syndromes have been intensively investigated. The determinants of plaque rupture, fissuring, and erosion and the factors modulating the formation and evolution of intracoronary thrombus secondary to plaque complication are increasingly better understood. Antithrombotic therapy and reperfusion therapy are highly effective in preventing ischemic events and attenuating their severity. Myocardial cell ischemia, however, is often present when patients consult or appear in-hospital despite antithrombotic therapy and reperfusion procedures. The consequences of such myocardial ischemia range from transient, reversible functional derangement to cell death and irreversible myocardial damage. Cell death can be massive or can occur repeatedly following symptomatic or nonsymptomatic episodes of ischemia resulting in pump failure of the heart, a major health problem.

This chapter discusses the mechanisms of myocardial cell death during ischemia-reperfusion and the strategies to prevent or limit the consequences of transient coronary occlusion on left-ventricular function.

PATHOPHYSIOLOGY OF MYOCARDIAL INJURY DURING TRANSIENT CORONARY OCCLUSION

Ischemia can be defined as a situation of insufficient blood flow to permit the oxidative phosphorylation required for maintaining adequate adenosine triphosphate (ATP) concentration and contractile function. Ischemia can result from increased oxygen demand, as in effort angina (high residual flow); decreased supply, as in acute myocardial infarction (low residual flow); or cardioplegic arrest (reduced work, hypothermia). Ischemia in acute coronary syndromes is generally the consequence of thrombotic obstruction of an epicardial coronary artery compromising distal flow. Flow deprivation has a component of *hypoxia*—reduced O^2 supply—and a component of *ischemia*—accumulation of metabolic by-products.

The consequences of low-flow ischemia are influenced by severity (magnitude of residual flow), duration, and basal physiologic conditions such as hemodynamic status and tissue temperature. The manifestations of ischemia are remarkably constant during the first few minutes of coronary flow reduction and consist of electrical instability and contractile failure.

Within the first 2 to 5 minutes of acute occlusion, segmental systolic expansion (dyskinesia) and wall thinning replace shortening and thickening[1] well before cells become significantly energy-depleted and changes in cytosolic composition (including acidosis) develop.[2]

Within a narrow range of flow reduction and ischemia, the adaptive response to contractile failure can reorient energy consumption to cell survival. An equilibrium is reached that allows survival of noncontractile segment, a phenomenon called *acute hibernation.*[3] Prolonged ischemia, however, usually results in cell necrosis that can be prevented with early reperfusion. Recovery of function is often delayed, a condition called *myocardial stunning.* The more prolonged the period of ischemia, the longer the period of stunning before complete functional recovery.

Stunning persists for more than 24 hours when reperfusion is performed after a 25-minute period of severe normothermic ischemia in laboratory animals and in humans.[4] Further delay in reperfusion is usually not compatible with cell survival because the number of dying cells grows exponentially as severe ischemia continues. Beyond 90 minutes, the area of necrosis involves most of the area at risk. A remarkable feature of incompletely reperfused infarcts is a clear abrupt demarcation between the areas of necrosis and the areas of normal myocardium. Infarct zones show continuous, compact, and irregular borders, and there is an absence of scattered necrotic cells within the normal areas of myocardium.[5] When necrosis is limited to only part of the area at risk, its spatial distribution is not homogeneous and involves mainly the subendocardial layers and the interface between the area at risk and the control adjacent myocardium. Reperfusion after periods of occlusion lasting 3 hours or more at best saves only few cardiomyocytes.[6,7] Even so, late reperfusion may still modify the physical properties and the histologic milieu of the necrotic area, attenuate infarct expansion and remodeling, and improve healing.[8]

Reperfusion can have multiple effects. It influences cardiomyocytes, coronary microvasculature, blood-borne cells within the infarct, and the interactions among the various cells. The effects on cardiomyocytes are most important and ultimately determine global cardiac performance. This chapter focuses mainly on cardiomyocyte death associated with ischemia-reperfusion, discussing the implication of other cell types when present.

Ischemia-Reperfusion and the Cardiomyocyte

The effects of ischemia at the cellular level have been studied mainly in vitro in cultures of freshly isolated cells from adult rats or rabbits submitted to conditions simulating ischemia (e.g., anoxia or metabolic inhibition plus acidosis, abnormal extracellular substrate composition). These effects have been subsequently validated when possible in intact and in situ hearts.

Cellular Changes Induced by Ischemia

Anaerobic Metabolism, Acidosis, and Contractile Failure   Depletion of cell energy and accumulation of ischemia by-products mainly affects cardiomyocytes (Fig. 33–1). Intracellular Po_2 falls within the first few minutes of ischemia with cessation of electron transport in the inner mitochondria membrane and extrusion of protons into the intermembrane space. The $[H^+]$ gradient in the inner mitochondrial membrane dissipates, and ATP synthesis ceases. Available ATP is hydrolyzed by the multiple ATPases involved in the contractile activity and in the maintenance of ionic homeostasis such as the sarcolemmal Na^+ pump. The concentrations of ADP and P_i rise as a consequence.

An important consequence of cell acidification is activation of alkalinizing sarcolemmal ion transport systems that introduce Na^+ into the cell, namely the Na^+/H^+ exchanger (NHE) and the Na^+/CO_3H^- (bicarbonate) symporter.[9,10] These two systems attenuate further intracellular acidosis but contribute to a cytosolic overload in Na^+. The inactivation of the sarcolemmal Na^+/K^+ ATPase pump that normally extrudes Na^+ entering cells during systolic depolarization contributes to this overload.

Na^+ overload has critical importance in cell injury: Na^+ is exchanged for Ca^{2+} by enhanced activity of the sarcolemmal Na^+/Ca^{2+} exchanger (NCX) with a coupling ratio of 1:3. The direction of the exchange and the net movement of positive charges are influenced by the intracellular and extracellular concentrations of Na^+ and Ca^{2+} and the transmembrane potential.[11] During diastole, forward NCX is an important mechanism for extruding Ca^{2+} that has entered the cell during systole. The reverse NCX transport is particularly important when cytosolic $[Na^+]_i$ is elevated, as in ischemia.[12]

Rigor Contracture and Ca2+ Overload   Cytosolic ATP concentration descends to values close to zero when ischemia progresses. At critically low concentrations of ATP, actin and myosin interact to form low-energy bonds by a mechanism largely Ca^{2+} independent, leading to the phenomenon known as *rigor contracture*.[13] Rigor contracture can generate active tension by mechanisms not

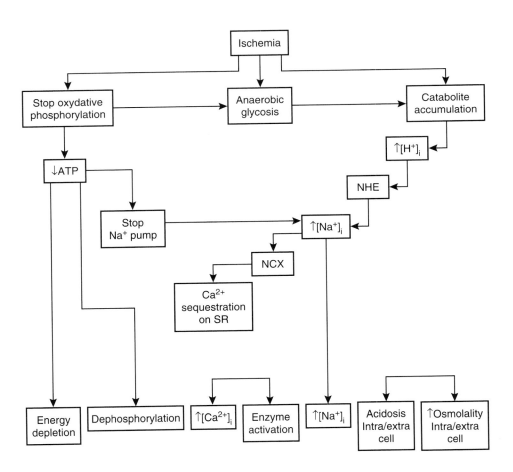

FIGURE 33–1. Principal alterations in the homeostasis of cardiomyocytes during myocardial ischemia. SR, sarcoplasmic reticulum.

perfectly understood and can shorten isolated cardiomyocytes to approximately 50% of the initial length in the absence of mechanical load. There is no contraction of intact heart in situ, but the heart becomes abruptly stiffer and left-ventricular end-diastolic pressure increases. Rigor usually occurs between 15 and 30 minutes after the onset of ischemia and is a reliable marker of severe ATP depletion and a hallmark of progression to ischemic injury. Complete exhaustion of ATP and a rise in $[Ca^{2+}]$ closely follow,[14] possibly because the exhaustion of ATP completely arrests Na^+ extrusion by Na^+/K^+ ATPase, accelerating Na^+ overload, NCX activity, and the loss of Ca^{2+} sequestration into the sarcoplasmic reticulum (SR). Increased $[Ca^{2+}]_i$ inactivates the numerous Ca^{2+}-dependent enzymes, including phospholipases, proteases, and phosphatases, thus initiating important intracellular signaling cascades. High $[Ca^{2+}]_i$ at the onset of reperfusion is an important determinant of hypercontracture (discussed later).

Cellular Edema Cell swelling during reversible ischemic injury is negligible because water influx is passively linked to Na^+ and anion influx and is favored by the colleidoncotic and osmotic gradients.[15,16] Loss of the control of intracellular volume is a hallmark of ischemic cell death (oncosis). The transmembrane osmotic driving force is reduced as the ischemic by-products leave the cell and accumulate in the confined extracellular space.

Cell-to-Cell Crosstalk During Ischemia The myocardium in normal conditions functions as a syncytium through gap junctions that allow fast propagation of cell depolarization to adjacent cells. Adult ventricular cardiomyocytes are connected to an average of nine neighboring cells through gap junctions, mainly distributed in the intercalated disks.

The electrical uncoupling that occurs shortly after the development of rigor contracture and the rise in Ca^{2+} is explained by an abrupt reduction in the conductance of gap junctions.[17] The onset of electrical uncoupling is associated with marked electrical instability manifested as frequent premature ventricular contractions and a high incidence of ventricular fibrillation (phase Ib of ischemic arrhythmias). This electrical instability is thought to be caused by spatial heterogeneities resulting from the coexistence of coupled and uncoupled areas within the ischemic area.[18]

Enzyme Activation and Cell Fragility Ischemia activates phosphatases and accelerates the fall in the phosphorylation potential secondary to ATP depletion. On the other hand, ischemia activates protein kinases that phosphorylate key proteins to initiate complex, interrelated intracellular signal cascades that are important for cell survival and function during ischemia-reperfusion (see later under the heading Myocardial Protection During Ischemia-Reperfusion: Endogenous and Pharmacologic Protection).

Nonlysosomal Ca^{2+}-dependent proteases, namely the calpain system, are activated during ischemia. Many structural proteins, including some maintaining sarcolemmal integrity such as spectrin (fodrin) and dystrophin, as well as contractile myofilaments and ion channels, are substrates for these proteases.[19] Because calpain activity is strongly dependent on pH with maximal activity at a neutral pH, concomitant intracellular acidosis constrains its role.

Activation of Ca^{2+}-dependent phospholipases, mainly of the PLA2 family, results in the hydrolysis of phospholipids. The loss of phospholipids and the detergent action of the amphipathic by-products of their hydrolysis (lysophospholipids) alters the composition and physical properties of cell membrane. Lysophospholipids accumulate in ischemic myocardium and may have many multiple effects on different protein systems in cardiomyocytes, including structural proteins, sarcolemmal channels, and gap junctions.[20,21] The action of PLA2 on certain phospholipids is of particular biologic importance, as in the case of arachidonic acid. Overall, PLA2 activation has been proposed as an important mechanism of sarcolemmal changes associated with ischemia.[22,23]

Alterations in Intracellular Signal Transduction Systems Recent studies have demonstrated that ischemia dramatically reduces the ability of cardiomyocytes and endothelial cells to synthesize cyclic guanosine monophosphate (cGMP) in response to NO or atrial natriuretic peptides (by soluble and membrane-bound guanylyl cyclases, respectively); this effect is mediated by acidosis during early ischemia and later by ATP depletion.[24]

Changes Occurring During Reperfusion

Reperfusion causes a very rapid (seconds) recovery of cell energy in cardiomyocytes accompanied by a burst of radical oxygen species (ROS). Reperfusion also modifies mitochondrial function, intracellular ion concentrations and water homeostasis, and produces secondary changes in the activities of many enzymes, gene expression, and protein synthesis.

Restoration of ATP Synthesis and Cation Homeostasis With O_2 being available, electron transport in the respiratory chain, H^+ extrusion and influx, and ATP synthesis are resumed in the inner mitochondrial membrane. Inadequate oxidation in damaged mitochondrias, however, may still generate large amounts of ROS.[25]

Although ATP or creatine phosphate concentrations need several hours to recover normal levels, free energy of exchange of ATP (the actual indicator of energy availability) is restored within seconds of O_2 restoration.

Dramatic changes in cation homeostasis involving H^+, Na^+, and Ca^2 appear within minutes of reperfusion (Fig. 33-2). The washout of extracellular H^+ and accelerated NHE and Na^+/CO_3H^- cotransport allows correction of the intracellular acidosis within 5 to 10 minutes.

Normalization of $[Na^+]_i$ is of crucial importance for the recovery of Ca^{2+} homeostasis.[26] Almost immediately upon restoration of O_2 availability, sarcolemmal Ca^{2+}

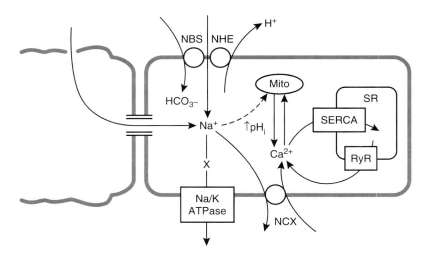

FIGURE 33–2. Mechanisms of cytosolic Na$^+$ and in Ca^{2+} overload during reperfusion. Na$^+$ enters the cell through ion transporters involved in correction of cytosolic acidosis and cannot be adequately extruded in the presence of impaired activity of the Na$^+$ pump (Na/K ATPase). Na$^+$ may also enter from neighboring cells via gap junctions and leads to Ca^{2+} overload by activating reverse-mode Na$^+$/Ca^{2+} exchange (NCX). Mito, mitochondria; NBS, Na$^+$-bicarbonate symporter; NCX, Na$^+$/Ca^{2+} exchanger; NHE, Na$^+$/H$^+$ exchanger; SR, sarcoplasmic reticulum.

ATPase sequesters Ca^{2+} into the SR. Cytosolic Ca^{2+} may also enter mitochondria once mitochondrial electronegative potential is restored. The rapid reduction in [Ca^{2+}]$_i$ may occur even if large amounts of Ca^{2+} are entering the cell simultaneously through reverse NCX.[27,28]

During early reperfusion after prolonged periods of ischemia, increased [Na$^+$]$_i$ and cell depolarization result in continuous reverse-mode operation of NCX. Na$^+$ extrusion through the Na$^+$/K$^+$ ATPase eventually resumes, and the trans-sarcolemmal Na$^+$ gradient recovers in cells surviving the initial phase of reperfusion. NCX operates in the forward mode during diastole in these cells and represents essential mechanisms for extrusion of Ca^{2+} and elimination of cell Ca^{2+} overload.

Uptake of large amounts of Ca^{2+} by SR during the first minutes of reoxygenation or reperfusion may trigger Ca^{2+} release that in turn elevates [Ca^{2+}]$_i$ and triggers Ca^{2+} reuptake. The resulting oscillations of [Ca^{2+}]$_i$ have been shown to contribute to the development of hypercontracture and to the genesis of reperfusion arrhythmias.[28]

Contractile Activation   During the initial seconds or few minutes after energy restoration, elevated [Ca^{2+}]$_i$ does not cause excessive contractile activation because of the presence of severe intracellular acidosis. Normally, diastolic [Ca^{2+}]$_i$ recovers faster than intracellular pH, which is delayed for several minutes.[10] The rapid

and wide Ca^{2+} oscillations that persist after correction of intracellular acidosis or late elevations in [Ca^{2+}]$_i$, however, may be associated with maximal contractile activation.[28]

Cell Swelling   With reperfusion after a prolonged period of ischemia, the osmolality and pH of the extracellular fluid are rapidly normalized, resulting in the generation of an important transmembrane osmotic gradient and an influx of additional Na$^+$ and other anions[29,30] and cell edema (Fig. 33–3).

Enzymatic Activation   The abnormalities in [Ca^{2+}]$_i$ may lead to activation of Ca^{2+}-dependent enzymes, in particular proteases and phospholipases. Although Ca^{2+} is already elevated before reperfusion, the activity of pH sensitive Ca^{2+}-activated enzymes can increase dramatically at the time of reperfusion because of correction of intracellular acidosis. This has been well studied in the case of calpain. Calpain has been suggested to cause damage to structural proteins during reperfusion and to contribute to sarcolemmal rupture and cell death.[31]

Mitochondrial Alterations   Although resumption of mitochondrial respiration and ATP production is a pre-

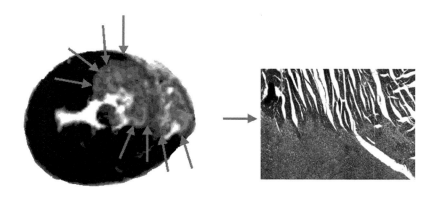

FIGURE 33–3. *Left,* Magnetic resonance imaging of the left ventricle of a pig submitted to 48 minutes of transient occlusion of the left descending coronary artery and 30 minutes of reperfusion. The gray scale reflects myocardial water content. Note severe edema of reperfused myocardium. *Right,* Low-magnification histologic section of the border zone between reperfused and normal myocardium. The *arrows* indicate the border.

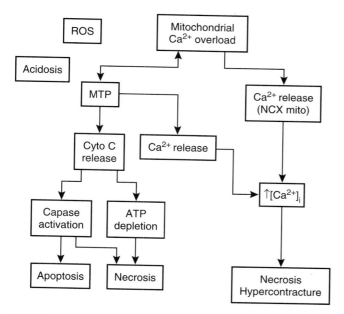

FIGURE 33–4. Mechanisms of mitochondrial-driven cell death. Mito, mitochondria; NCX, Na^+/Ca^{2+} exchanger; ROS, radical oxygen species.

requisite for cell recovery, the inability of mitochondria to synthesize ATP upon reperfusion does not seem to practically limit cell survival. During reperfusion, cell death occurs mostly in cells that have recovered metabolic competence.[32] However, mitochondria, which are the most important source of ROS during reperfusion, may contribute to derangements in $[Ca2+]_i$, and may release apoptotic and other harmful material (Fig. 33–4).

Upon restoration of the electronegative mitochondrial membrane potential, Ca^{2+} influx into mitochondria through the Ca^{2+} uniporter may contribute to normalization of $[Ca^{2+}]_i$. Increased Ca^{2+} concentration in mitochondrial matrix has potential adverse effects, however, including accelerated generation of ROS and opening of the mitochondrial transition pores,[33] which are megachannel pores allowing the free diffusion of molecules less than 1 kD between the mitochondrial matrix and the cytosol.

Mechanisms of Cell Death During Ischemia-Reperfusion

Sustained severe ischemia inevitably results in cardiomyocyte cell death. It is difficult to define the exact timing of cell death mainly because of the lack of a universally valid definition. Rupture of cell membranes, allowing the passage of large molecules, identifies cell death but may not be a prerequisite. For example, cells undergoing apoptosis may disassemble into apoptotic vesicles and be eventually engulfed by other cells without suffering sarcolemmal rupture. Ischemic cells can suffer massive proteolysis of structures essential for life (e.g., mitochondrial matrix) and DNA degradation before losing cell-membrane integrity. Cells can be thus irreversibly injured and committed to death before executing the apoptosis program or losing their sarcolemmal integrity.

Cell death in the following sections is defined as sarcolemmal rupture or apoptotic cell fragmentation.

Cardiomyocyte Cell Death During Ischemia Ischemic cell death, also known as oncosis, is characterized by loss of control of intracellular ion concentrations and water content, resulting in severe cell edema and loss of sarcolemmal integrity. Oncosis is a late phenomenon that is observed well after any benefit of reperfusion can be demonstrated for cell survival.

Ischemia can also induce apoptosis. Apoptotic cell death is the result of the execution of a well-conserved genetic program that includes the activation of specific enzyme systems, among which caspases play a major role, and eventually leads to intranucleosomal DNA cleavage, fragmentation of the cell without sarcolemmal rupture into vesicles that undergo phagocytosis by other cells. In contrast with necrotic cell death, apoptosis does not result in the release of intracellular contents such as enzymes and results in much less inflammatory reaction. The process requires energy but can occur under severe hypoxic conditions, and thus occurs during myocardial ischemia. In addition to its obvious role in cardiac development during embryogenesis, there is solid evidence that cardiomyocyte apoptosis occurs in many different contexts, including myocardial hypertrophy and hypertrophy regression, cardiomyopathy, heart failure, xenograft rejection, and ischemia-reperfusion.[34-36] During ischemia, the enhanced generation of ROS, severe ATP depletion, increased $[Ca^{2+}]_i$, and other alterations in cell homeostasis are potent stimuli for the initiation of apoptosis. It has been suggested that apoptosis could be the most important form of cell death during prolonged myocardial ischemia, particularly at the border between ischemic and normoxic myocardium. However, there are many limitations in the methods of quantification of apoptosis in reperfused myocardium. Studies show no important role of apoptosis in the genesis of cell death during the initial hours of acute myocardial ischemia, when reperfusion may still salvage myocardium at risk.[37]

Cell Death During Reperfusion Cardiomyocytes can die immediately after reperfusion or hours later. The following events occur upon the first few hours of reperfusion: sarcolemmal rupture, enzyme release, extensive contractile activation, abnormal cell shortening, and marked disruption of cell architecture resulting in a characteristic histopathologic pattern known as *contraction band necrosis*.[38,39] Delayed necrosis is due to either apoptosis or a toxicity associated with an inflammatory-like reaction induced by reperfusion.[34,40,41] Finally, restoration of coronary blood flow does not imply restoration of myocardial blood flow across the area at risk, and particular zones of myocardium may remain ischemic or become transient or permanently ischemic during the reperfusion period.[42]

Solid evidence shows that the immediate reperfusion damage is the most important mechanism for cell death when reperfusion is performed early enough to salvage myocardial cells.

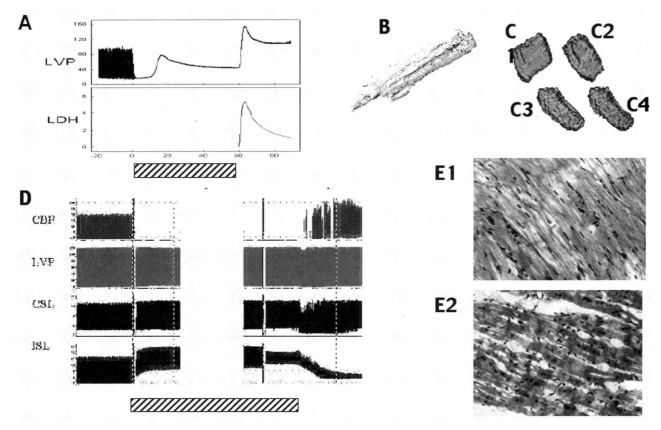

FIGURE 33–5. Role of cardiomyocyte hypercontracture in early lethal reperfusion injury. *A,* Left-ventricular pressure (LVP) and LDH release (LDH) in an isolated rat heart submitted to 80 minutes of transient coronary occlusion *(dashed bar).* Note cessation of contraction early during ischemia. The elevation of pressure during ischemia denotes rigor. Further elevation at the onset of reperfusion denotes hypercontracture and coincides with LDH release. In isolated cardiomyocytes *(B),* ischemia induces rigor contracture *(C,1).* Upon reperfusion, abrupt further shortening denotes hypercontracture *(C2-C4).* In the in situ pig heart *(D),* transient coronary occlusion *(dashed bar)* results in abolition of coronary blood flow (CBF) and expansion (upward shift) of the ischemic segment length (ISL) with compensatory changes in normal segment *(CSL).* Reperfusion is associated with an abrupt reduction in end-diastolic segment length, which has been shown to correlate with hypercontracture as manifested by contraction band necrosis *(E2).* A histologic view of control myocardium is provided for comparison *(E1).* CSL, Control segment length.

Contraction band necrosis is observed as early as 5 minutes after reflow to rapidly reach plateau and to remain unchanged thereafter.[43] The extent of contraction band necrosis correlates well with the magnitude of the reduction in the diastolic length of the reperfused myocardial segment and with the amount of enzyme release associated with reperfusion (Fig. 33-5).[44]

Cardiomyocyte hypercontracture is the main determinant of contraction band necrosis.[38,45] Maneuvers preventing hypercontracture in isolated cardiomyocytes limit contraction band necrosis in reperfused myocardium.[45] However, hypercontracture does not cause cell death in isolated cardiomyocytes despite extreme cell shortening and disruption of cell architecture,[32,46] indicating that hypercontracture requires other factors to cause sarcolemmal disruption. These factors include sarcolemmal and cytoskeletal fragility, cell swelling, and cell-to-cell and cell-to-matrix mechanical interactions (Fig. 33-6).[47]

Hypercontracture propagates with adjacent cells through gap junctions (see Fig. 33-6). Heptanol closes the gap junctions and prevents propagation of hypercontracture.[48] The Ca^{2+} rise in the adjacent cell is due to the passage of Na^+ that induces influx of extracellular Ca^{2+} via reverse Na^+/Ca^{2+}.[49] Propagation of hypercontracture never exceeds the limits of the area at risk, probably because cells without fragility can undergo hypercontracture without developing sarcolemmal disruption and massive Na^+ and Ca^{2+} influx.

The relevance of this mechanism of cell-to-cell interaction in the propagation of hypercontracture during reperfusion is supported by recent evidence that gap junction conductance and chemical coupling persist after the onset of rigor. This cell-to-cell propagation of hypercontracture to adjacent myocytes contributes to final infarct size and its geometry (Fig. 33-7).[48]

Many reports have stressed the potential relevance of apoptosis associated with transient ischemia.[50] During reperfusion, apoptosis may be triggered by free radicals (ROS, NO) from inside the cell or by mitochondrial injury (mitochondrial transition pore opening), or may

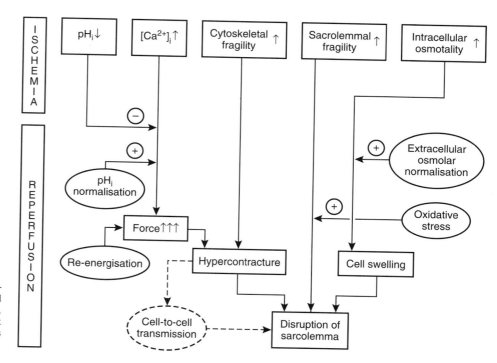

FIGURE 33–6. Schematic representation of changes leading to acute lethal reperfusion injury. (From Piper HM, Garcia-Dorado D, Ovize M: A fresh look on reperfusion injury. Cardiovasc Res 1998; 38: 291–300, with permission.)

be secondary to inflammatory cytokines in the inflammatory-like response.

The abnormal function of the respiratory chain in reperfused cardiomyocytes may produce ROS, mainly through superoxide anion (O_2) in excess of the normal production rate of approximately 1% of O_2 consumed. Oxidation of arachidonic acid may also contribute to ROS production.[25,51] The transformation of xanthine dehydrogenase in xanthine oxidase during ischemia provides a powerful source of O_2 during reperfusion in the cardiomyocytes of several species (but not in humans) and in the endothelial cells of most species (including humans).[51] Polymorphonuclear neutrophils (PMNs) infiltrating reperfused myocardium (see later) also are an important source of ROS.[41]

NO can have a dual action on apoptosis. NO can be protective or initiate apoptosis in relation with the concentration of NO and the molecular ambiance. NO is an extremely active but short-lived radical. Its concentration is mainly influenced by O_2 concentration because the two molecules react at diffusion-limited rates to produce peroxinitrite. Peroxinitrite is an extremely reactive radical that reacts with many biomolecules to release other highly toxic radicals, including the hydroxyl radical (HO·), and peroxinitrite can serve as a substrate for the regeneration of NO. Thus, NO can scavenge O_2 and become inactivated. At high concentrations, however, NO can initiate apoptosis by mechanisms that are cGMP-dependent and -independent, including opening of the mitochondrial transition pore. In reperfused myocardium,

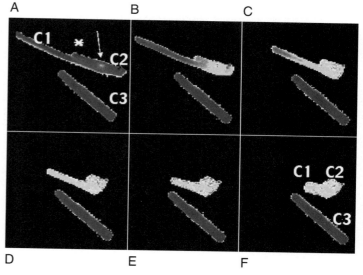

FIGURE 33–7. Propagation of hypercontracture induced by microinjection of extracellular buffer (*arrow*) in a pair of cardiomyocytes (C1 and C2) connected through an intercalated disc (*asterisk*). A third non-connected myocyte (C3) serves as control. Shading denotes cytosolic Ca^{2+} concentration (Fura-2 ratio). The time elapsed between A and E was 16 s. (From Ruiz-Meana et al: Propagation of cardiomycete hypercontracture by passage of Na^+ through gap junctions. Circ Res 1999; 85: 280–287, with permission.)

large amounts of NO can be produced by the polynuclear cells and by expression in cardiomyocytes and in the microvascular endothelial cells of the inducible form of the NO synthase (NOSi, or NOS2).[52]

Cardiomyocytes, endothelial cells, neutrophils, and platelets may release multiple cytokines in reperfused myocardium, including tumor necrosis factor α, interleukin-1, interleukin-6, platelet-activating factor, or tissue factor. Cytokines induce multiple important cellular effect through different pathways. For example, tumor necrosis factor α may induce apoptosis but upregulates nuclear factor kappa beta ($NF_{\kappa\beta}$), which has an anti-apoptotic effect.[53]

Several lines of evidence suggest that apoptosis unlikely plays an important role in cardiomyocyte cell death during reperfusion. First, the extension of myocardial necrosis is determined very early after the onset of reperfusion, before apoptosis can develop, and keeps remarkably constant during the following 24 to 72 hours.[43] Second, within reperfused infarcts, the mass of necrotic myocardium predicted by the total enzyme release correlates well with the histologic size of the infarct, which should not be the case in apoptosis, an enzymatically silent form of cell death. Recent studies in isolated cardiomyocytes and intact hearts have found an increased susceptibility of cardiomyocytes that have been re-energized after prolonged ischemia to undergo apoptosis in response to ROS or NO. A protective effect against apoptosis occurs only during the initial few hours of reperfusion, and its mechanism is unknown.[54,55] Some data suggest an important role of apoptosis in heart failure. Pathologic observations in patients with acute myocardial infarction are consistent with a secondary role of apoptosis in cardiomyocyte cell death in reperfused myocardium.[56]

Microvascular Dysfunction and Inflammatory-Like Reaction

Transient severe ischemia induces microvascular changes that may range from minimal alterations in endothelial cell function to cell death, depending mainly on the duration of ischemia. In endothelial cells, ATP depletion induced by ischemia proceeds more slowly than in cardiomyocytes, partly because of lesser dependence on aerobic glycolysis. Upon reperfusion, endothelial cells swell and develop some degree of contracture, which results in the formation of gaps between adjacent endothelial cells. As a result, the permeability of microvascular endothelium increases.[57] Important amounts of albumin and other proteins enter the interstitial space, causing interstitial edema.

Extravascular compression secondary to cardiomyocyte contracture and to interstitial and cellular edema can impair microvascular flow. After more prolonged ischemia, endothelial cells may die. Loss of microvascular integrity allows blood cell extravasation and intramyocardial hemorrhage.[58] These events, however, take place only in the core of areas of myocardial necrosis. Intramyocardial hemorrhage and no reflow secondary to severe endothelial injury thus appear to be epiphenomena of severe, lethal myocardial injury and not primarily responsible for cardiomyocyte cell death.

In addition to showing increased microvascular permeability, endothelial cells present more subtle changes that are important in the inflammatory reaction associated with ischemia-reperfusion. Reperfused endothelium releases a number of cytokines and very active molecules, including platelet-activating factor and interleukin-8, expresses cell surface adhesive molecules that mediate PMNs and platelet accumulation in reperfused myocardium, and critical elements of the complement system such as C5a.[41,59]

In reperfused myocardium, activated endothelial cells translocate to the cell surface constitutive P-selectin and inducible E-selectin, express tissue factor, and synthesize less NO (the availability of which is further reduced by increased O_2^- generation). PMNs attracted to the reperfused myocardium are first tethered to endothelium by interactions between P-selectin and E-selectin on endothelial cell surface and PSGL-1 and sialyl Lewis x on PMN surface, as well as by the interaction between L-selectin expressed by PMNs and the endothelial sialyl Lewis A. While rolling on endothelial surface, PMNs are activated by endothelial cytokines and translocate the CD11/CD18 integrin receptor to the cell surface, which interacts with endothelial intracellular adhesion molecule 1 (ICAM-1) and with the complement-derived protein iC3b in endothelial extracellular matrix, resulting in the firm adhesion of PMNs (Fig. 33–8). Adhered PMNs release ROS, NO, hypochlorous acid, and diverse proteolytic enzymes and can plug into capillaries and obstruct them (Fig. 33–9). Adhered PMNs also migrate across the endothelium by diapedesis (see Fig. 33–8), infiltrate myocardial tissue, and adhere to cardiomyocytes expressing ICAM-1.[59,41]

Although PMN accumulation in reperfused myocardium correlates well with infarct size, the demonstration of a causative role of PMNs in cell death remains elusive. Neutropenia and treatments aimed at preventing PMN accumulation have been deemed effective in limiting infarct size by some groups but not by others.[60] The beneficial effects against reperfusion injury of some therapies as L-arginine and adenosine have been imputed to reduce PMN accumulation. These drugs, however, have other effects that can explain a benefit as discussed later. Several lines of evidence suggest that in the context of transient coronary occlusion, the role of PMN infiltration in the genesis of cell death is marginal. Infiltration of PMNs into reperfused myocardium becomes significant only 1 to 2 hours after reperfusion, when the area of myocardial necrosis is very close to its final size. Observations on reperfusion periods as long as 72 hours have not shown significantly larger infarcts. The relationship that exists between the duration of ischemia and infarct size is similar in isolated rat hearts and in intact rats. Finally, genetic deletion of ICAM-1 and P-selectin impairs leukocyte trafficking in reperfused myocardium but do not modify infarct size 24 hours after reflow.[61]

Platelets accumulate in large amounts in reperfused myocardium. It has been suggested that these could originate from cyclic repetitive distal embolization of platelet aggregates forming at the site of the culprit

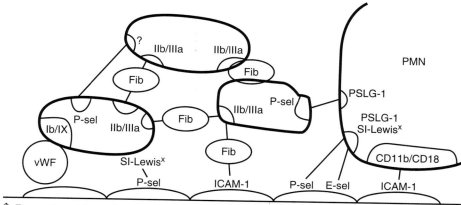

FIGURE 33–8. Leukocyte-platelet-endothelial cell interactions in response to activation of the endothelium in reperfused myocardium. See text for description. E-sel, E-selectin; ICAM-1, intracellular adhesion molecule 1; PMN, polymorphonuclear neutrophils; P-sel, P-selectin; PSGL-1, P-selectin glycoprotein ligant-1.

lesion. This explanation is highly unlikely, however, since prevention of cyclic aggregation with aspirin or inhibitors of platelet IIb/IIIa receptors has no effect on myocardial platelet content.[62] Platelet deposition in reperfused myocardium seems to depend on local adhesion through platelet receptors other than IIb/IIIa, such as Ib/IX or sialyl Lewis x. Platelets may also adhere to PMNs to form leukoplatelet aggregates (see Fig. 33–8). The consequences of platelet aggregation on myocardial cell death during reperfusion are not well known; detrimental, beneficial, and absent effects have been described.[63, 64] It has been suggested that platelets activated by ischemia and expressing P-selectin, but not inactive platelets, could have a detrimental effect.[65]

The complement system is activated during myocardial ischemia through still poorly understood mechanisms. Activation results in a cascade of proteolytic events and merging of activated elements that result in (1) the formation of anaphylatoxins (C3a, C5a), which increase vascular permeability and have vasodilatory and chemotactic properties, and (2) the assembly of the terminal attack complex that inserts into the membrane of target cells to form large pores that cause cell death.[41] However, complete assembly of the membrane attack complex has been documented in cardiomyocytes only after several hours of ischemia. Deposition of membrane attack complex is faster in reperfused myocardium, contributing to the increased microvascular permeability and the recruitment of PMNs. It has been suggested that reperfused cardiomyocytes have an impaired ability to remove complement elements from their surface. Some studies have shown that the complement system enhances PMN-mediated injury secondary to ischemia reperfusion, and monoclonal antibodies against different complement elements have been reported to limit infarct size. Studies in animals genetically deficient in complement elements have been described to exhibit fewer areas of no reflow and less necrosis than nondeficient animals.[41]

MYOCARDIAL PROTECTION DURING ISCHEMIA-REPERFUSION: ENDOGENOUS AND PHARMACOLOGIC PROTECTION

Ischemic preconditioning (PC) was originally defined as a paradoxical and dramatic protective effect of episodes of brief, sublethal myocardial ischemia against cell death caused by a subsequent episode of prolonged ischemia followed by reperfusion.[66] The existence of PC has been confirmed in all species of animal, including humans.[67] The characteristics of the ischemic episodes inducing protection were soon characterized.[68] The ischemia has to last a minimum of approximately 2 minutes, and one episode is generally sufficient, more than two conferring no additional protection. The protection is transient and disappears after approximately 2 hours. The concept of reconditioning was subsequently expanded to ischemic events other than cell death, such as stunning, arrhythmias, and microvascular dysfunction; the existence and relevance of the protection against functional disorders remains controversial, however.

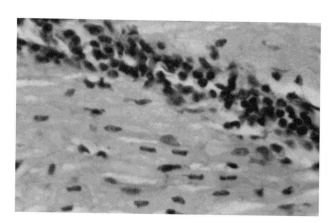

FIGURE 33–9. Neutrophils plugging a capillary vessel in reperfused myocardium (H&E × 600).

More recently, it was found that another wave of protection against cell death reappears a few hours after the first is gone, to last several additional hours before disappearing for good. This phenomenon has been called the *second window of PC*.[68] Finally, the concept of preconditioning was applied to phenomena other than myocardial ischemia such as ischemia at a distance and to diverse maneuvers such as rapid electrical pacing, stretch, and administration of various compounds.

It is important to distinguish pharmacologic preconditioning from pharmacologic pretreatment against ischemia-reperfusion. Pharmacologically induced preconditioning triggers the endogenous protective response characteristic of PC. The drug does not need to be present in myocardium during the lethal ischemic period to exert its effect. Pharmacologic pretreatment, on the other hand, targets the prevention and counteraction of one or more pathophysiologic mechanisms responsible for cell injury; to be effective, the drug then needs to be present during ischemia.

Mechanisms of Ischemic Preconditioning

Despite a huge research effort, the current understanding of the molecular mechanisms involved in the protective effect of preconditioning remains incomplete. A series of mediators and membrane receptors, and interactions between them, are involved in the initial transduction signals.[67] Stimulation of A1 and A3 adenosine receptors, δ and μ opioid receptors, B2 bradykinin receptors, and increased levels of ROS contribute to initiate preconditioning. Subsequent transduction signals involve activation and translocation of protein kinase C (PKC) and mitogen-activated protein kinase (MAPK). Mitochondria, more particularly the ATP-dependent K^+ channels, are implicated in the process. A relevant aspect in the signaling transduction cascade is its redundancy with involvement of multiple parallel pathways. The stimulation provided by parallel pathways could be additive, and preconditioning can occur when stimulation reaches a critical threshold. Several subthreshold stimuli could therefore elicit protection when acting in synergy. The field of investigation is complex since many pathways are animal species–dependent and can work in series in certain species and in parallel in others.[69,70]

The mechanisms involved in second window preconditioning seem to be partially concurrent with those identified in classic PC, particularly regarding the role of MAPK and PKC and of mitochondrial K^+_{ATP} channels. Increased NO availability secondary to induction of NOSi and enhanced expression of HSP70 and of other protective proteins seem to play an important role.[68]

In contrast with our knowledge of the triggers of PC, the links that exist between the initial events in the direct mechanisms preventing cardiomyocyte cell death are totally unknown. The very modest modifications observed in function, metabolism, and ionic changes as well as their time course could hardly explain the powerful protection that is observed at the time of reperfusion. The rate of ATP depletion during sustained ischemia is slightly delayed in certain models of preconditioned myocardium,[71] and in others it is unchanged despite a similar protection.[72] Furthermore, the onset of rigor contracture is not delayed and can even be accelerated by PC,[72] an observation difficult to reconcile with the absence of an effect of preconditioning on the interval of time during which reperfusion can be performed without inducing hypercontracture after rigor development.[73] PKC stimulation, which mimics PC in isolated cardiomyocytes, does not modify the time to rigor onset and the time course and magnitude of the rise in cytosolic Ca^{2+}.[12] The most reproducible finding with PC is a delay of 5 to 10 minutes in the time to intracellular acidosis.[71] Acidosis, however, is not deleterious, as it slows down ATP depletion during ischemia, prevents hypercontracture during reperfusion, and inhibits mitochondrial transition pore opening.[74] Although PC preserves cGMP, limits sarcolemmal or cytoskeletal fragility, improves Na^+ recovery, inhibits NHE, and reduces exchange through gap junction in the immediate reperfusion period,[67,43] its fundamental mechanism for preventing cell necrosis remains mysterious.

Because PC prevents cell death during ischemia-reperfusion but does not preserve cell energy during transient ischemia, the hypothesis that ischemic injury represents a deficit in energy is wrong. Prevention of energy depletion is not a prerequisite for myocardial protection.

Therapeutic Exploitation of Ischemic Preconditioning

PC protects the heart against ischemia associated with cardiac surgery during extracorporeal circulation, and is a practical method to improve myocardial tolerance to normothermic regional ischemia in minimally invasive surgery. In patients with an acute coronary syndrome, repetitive episodes of brief ischemia often precede sustained coronary occlusion. Although it is difficult to document a protective effect of this preceding ischemia, because of variable collateral circulation, ventricular dysfunction, comorbidities, and drug therapy, the available information suggests that pre-infarction angina may lessen the impact of prolonged ischemia on left-ventricular function and early survival.[75] Controlled induction of ischemia is generally not possible in these patients.

Pharmacologic Induction of Preconditioning

Adenosine, generated by ATP breakdown during brief episodes of ischemia and released into the interstitial space, contributes to PC by an agonist effect on the A1 and A3 adenosine receptors.[70,67] Exogenous adenosine also induces PC in several animal species, with the exception of rats.[69] As the clinical usefulness of adenosine is limited by side effects related to vasodilatation, various other agonists to the receptors have been tested.[67,76] Of interest, the A1 and A3 adenosine receptor agonists induce first and second window preconditioning by mechanisms involving K^+_{ATP} channels and NOS activity, respectively, opening a possibility of inducing long-lasting protection against transient ischemia.[69] The activation of A1 receptors by NOS is mediated via PLC and PI3, which in turn trigger the cascade reactions involving calcium/calmodulin and PKC. It has been suggested that the increase in interstitial adenosine concentration that is obtained with dipyridamole lowers the threshold for ischemic PC.[77]

Endogenous opioids constitute a broad group of neuropeptides involved in the modulation of many important biologic functions, such as perception of pain and pleasure, emotions, breathing, and movement. They are synthesized from three different pro-peptides into three different families, the enkephalins, endorphins, and dynorphins, that act on receptors of type δ, μ, and κ, respectively. Cardiomyocytes are able to synthesize compounds of each family.[78] The precise physiologic functions of each peptide have not been established. Morphine is a powerful δ^1 and μ (and κ) opioid receptor agonist, which probably exerts cardioprotective effect at concentrations used clinically for the control of pain.[79-81] The use of morphine and other exogenous opioids for inducing PC in high-risk patients is limited by drug side effects and problems related to their prolonged administration. Better understanding of the mechanisms for the side effects of opioids, such as respiratory depression, and of the molecular basis of tolerance might circumvent these limitations. The cardioprotective effects of opioids make relevant their acute use as analgesics in patients with an acute coronary syndrome.

Although stimulation of bradykinin B2 receptors elicits first and second window PC, no practical means of stimulating these receptors in patients is as yet available. Inhibitors of the angiotensin-converting enzyme (ACE) increase the levels of bradykinin because ACE is identical to kinase II, which degrades bradykinin into inactive metabolites. It has thus been suggested that ACE inhibitors could have protective effects against myocardial ischemia mediated through bradykinin. A lowering of the threshold for various stimuli to induce PC has also been shown with ACE inhibitors.[82] On the other hand, bradykinin is an agonist of NO production, and part of its cardioprotective effects can be mediated through increased NO availability.

Elucidation of the mechanism of preconditioning could help avoid the use of drugs that could inhibit it. One example is glibenclamide, which is widely used for the control of hyperglycemia in patients with type II diabetes. The drug blocks K^+_{ATP} channels and abolishes PC in most experimental models.[67] Clinical experience supports an adverse outcome in patients with an acute myocardial infarction given glibenclamide-related drugs[83]; an alternative therapy has been recommended in diabetic patients at risk for acute coronary syndromes.[84]

Pharmacologic Protection During Ischemia-Reperfusion

The success of cell protection drugs during ischemia-reperfusion can be influenced by many factors including safety, timing, and methods of administration. An important determinant of success is application of treatment at a time that is favorable for its effect. This requires knowledge of the mechanisms of cell death at various times of ischemia and of reperfusion, and of the effects of the various interventions. Accordingly, therapeutic strategies can be classified as acting before the onset of myocardial ischemia (pharmacologic pretreatment against ischemia) and during reflow or later (pharmacologic pretreatment against ischemia) and during reflow or later (pharmacologic protection against reperfusion injury). Furthermore, interventions need to be considered as acting during ischemia or during reperfusion as the severely ischemic myocardium is generally excluded from the circulation.

Pretreatment Against Ischemia

Until recently, effective treatments that could be administered safely in humans were lacking, although a large number of drugs had been shown to be protective against ischemia in isolated cells and in vitro preparations. The introduction of specific inhibitors of the NHE was a milestone in cell protection.

Inhibitors of NHE The hypothesis that NHE activity contributed to the genesis of Ca^{2+} overload during ischemia reperfusion was raised decades ago. It was initially proposed that normalization of pHi during initial reperfusion through NHE resulted in Na^+ overload and secondary NCX-mediated Ca^{2+} influx.[85] Early results with amiloride derivatives supported a role of NHE activity in ischemia-reperfusion injury. More specific molecules were subsequently produced, such as HOE694 and, more recently, HOE642 (cariporide), which definitively established the important role of NHE in cell death associated with ischemia-reperfusion and the potent protective effect of inhibition of the exchanger.[86,87] It soon became clear that the drug needed to be administered before ischemia occurred to obtain full benefit and that the protection afforded when given at the time of reperfusion was small or null.[86,88] The reason for the lack of benefit with NHE inhibition applied at the time of reperfusion is inadequate tissue concentrations during the first seconds of reflow. The intracoronary administration of the drug at the time of reperfusion could not circumvent the limitation.[86] Inhibition of NHE strikingly delays the progression of all indexes of ischemic injury including ATP depletion, rigor onset, and electrical uncoupling during ischemia.[86,89,90]

Despite these effects, the exact mechanisms of NHE action continue to be debated. Intracellular acidosis is influenced not only by the NHE antiporter but also by Na^+/CO_3H^+ and Na^+ lactate symporters. NHE does not modify the time course and severity of intracellular acidosis, and although most studies have shown a reduction in Na^+ overload, others have not.[91] On the other hand, NHE remains protective in the absence of effects on intracellular cation concentrations.[92] It has been suggested that NHE inhibitors could exert part of their effects at the mitochondrial level.[93]

Several clinical studies have evaluated NHE inhibition, most studies using cariporide. Phase II studies described a beneficial effect of cariporide in patients with anterior myocardial infarction undergoing percutaneous transluminal coronary angioplasty,[94] in the preservation of hearts for xenografts, and in cardioplegic arrest during extracorporeal circulation.[95] The largest study to date has been the GUARd During Ischemia Against Necrosis (GUARDIAN) trial, with more than 11,000 patients enrolled. Entry criteria were a non–ST-segment elevation acute coronary syndrome, a high-risk percutaneous coronary procedure, or high-risk bypass surgery. Patients were randomized to receive placebo or cariporide at 20, 80, or 120 mg every 8 hours for the period of risk.[96] The trial documented the safety of cariporide but failed to show its efficacy on primary end point of death or myocardial infarction, assessed after 36 days. The dose of 120 mg was associated with a 10% risk reduction ($P = .12$); this dose in the subset of patients undergoing bypass surgery resulted in a 25% risk reduction ($P = .03$) that was maintained after 6 months. The rate of Q-wave myocardial infarction was reduced by 32% across all entry diagnostic groups (2.6% vs. 1.8%, $P = .03$), but the rate of non–Q-wave myocardial infarction was reduced only in patients undergoing surgery (7.1% vs. 3.8%, $P = .005$). Several aspects of this trial deserve special attention. Although patients in the trial were appropriately treated before the ischemic event, the doses used were small, and the high dose (of approximately 1.6 mg/kg of body weight) was smaller than the one shown effective in most experimental studies (3 mg/kg). Furthermore, the benefit of the drug could not have emerged because it was diluted by a high number of patients with no events. Additional studies are needed with higher doses in patients at a higher risk for an event. Such a study, the Na^+/H^+ EXchange inhibition to Prevent coronary Events in acute cardiac conDITIONs (EXPEDITION) has been completed among patients undergoing CABG. The results should be known soon.

Enaporide was investigated in a Phase II study involving 900 patients with an acute ST-segment elevation myocardial infarction treated with a thrombolytic agent or primary percutaneous transluminal coronary angioplasty in the Enaporide in Acute Myocardial Infarction (ESCAMI) trial. The drug in the trial was mitrated after coronary occlusion which is not ideal for eliciting a benefit. No benefit was seen in the trial with any of the three dises tested.[97]

L-Arginine Supplementation Various experimental models have shown a protective effect of pretreatment with L-arginine against transient ischemia-induced cell death.[98] In humans, supplementation of L-arginine has consistently been associated with a benefit in patients with atherosclerosis, including patients with peripheral vascular disease and coronary artery disease.[99] The benefit was first believed to be related to improved endothelial function and microcirculation and reduced leukocyte infiltration through increased NO availability. More recently, it was shown that L-arginine conferred benefit in the absence of leukocytes and in the absence of an effect on coronary blood flow,[100,101] and that it attenuates the depletion of myocardial cGMP concentration at the onset of reper-

fusion.[100] Studies in cardiomyocytes and endothelial cells have shown that higher cGMP concentration protects against reoxygenation-induced hypercontracture.

L-arginine must be administered before the onset of ischemia to increase cGMP during the initial minutes of reperfusion. L-arginine supplementation can be administered chronically by different routes.[99] Whether prolonged L-arginine supplementation will provide a long-lasting protection against transient ischemia has not been established.

Temperature Infarct size is closely related to myocardial temperature, and elevated temperature has a large impact on the extent of necrosis. For example, average infarct size in the pig after 45 minutes of transient coronary occlusion is usually less than 10% of the area at risk when the myocardial temperature during ischemia is 35.5°C and 75% more when it is 38.5°C. The control of body temperature could therefore be simple way to help patients with ongoing myocardial ischemia. A trial is now ongoing evaluating systemic hypothermia in acute myocardial infarction.

Treatment to Prevent Reperfusion Injury

Early animal studies showed that restoration of blood flow after transient ischemia could be associated with dramatic noxious changes such as arrhythmias, enzyme release, or severe intramyocardial hemorrhage that were interpreted as reperfusion injury. These studies also documented generation of oxygen free radicals (ROS), thought to be important mediators of reperfusion injury. Much of the concerns were soon put aside with the unequivocal documentation of the clinical benefit of reperfusion therapy on survival. Although the benefit lessens as the time to reperfusion after the onset of symptoms grows longer, can still be beneficial and reperfusion is not harmful. Animal studies and a few human studies showed no benefit with anti-ROS therapies. Many then suggested that reperfusion injury was either nonexistent, an accelerated expression of preexistent injury, or clinically irrelevant. The plausibility of the latter hypothesis (reperfusion injury as a laboratory artifact) was supported by the paradox of frequent lethal reperfusion arrhythmias in laboratory animals but not in humans. It has been argued that phenomena such as transient ST-segment re-elevation at the time of reperfusion and rapid elevation of blood markers of necrosis by washout reflect preexisting ischemic damage uncovered by reperfusion.

This chapter does not attempt to make a case for the presence or absence of a reperfusion injury and its clinical significance. Reperfusion therapy is mandated in acute myocardial infarction, and measures that would prevent reperfusion injury would be meaningless without reperfusion. However, any additional measure that could save some of the myocardium following reperfusion would be a positive gain. Accordingly, reperfusion injury is herewith defined as an injury that can be prevented by interventions applied at the time of reperfusion.[102]

Prevention of Early Lethal Reperfusion Injury

The therapeutic strategies proposed to prevent immediate cell death (immediate lethal reperfusion injury) aim at prevention of hypercontracture, cell-to-cell spreading of hypercontracture, cell edema, and cell fragility.

Prevention of Hypercontracture Hypercontracture-related cell death does not occur immediately upon reflow but after a few minutes when the intracellular acidosis has been corrected because acidosis is a potent inhibitor of contractility. This small delay can allow drugs administered at the time of reperfusion to reach their target on time. Three basic strategies are available: acceleration of recovery of Ca^{2+} homeostasis, delaying correction of intracellular acidosis, and desensitization of cells to Ca^{2+}.

Therapeutic Strategies to Accelerate the Normalization of $[Ca^{2+}]i$ Approaches under investigation include limitation of additional Ca^{2+} influx at the onset of reperfusion and prevention of SR-mediated $[Ca^{2+}]_i$ oscillations.

The most direct way of limiting influx of extracellular Ca^{2+} during initial reperfusion is to inhibit reverse-mode operation of the sarcolemmal NCX. This method effectively limits cell death in isolated cardiomyocytes, in isolated hearts, and in all animal models of transient coronary occlusion.[27] No specific inhibitors currently can be applied in human. KB-R7943, initially described as highly selective for NCX[103], lacks this preferential effect in physiologic conditions.[104] An important feature of KB-R7943 is that it is quite selective in inhibiting cells operating under unidirectional ionic conditions, particularly when this direction is the reverse mode. This feature provides a relatively wide therapeutic window for blocking NCX-mediated $[Ca^{2+}]_i$ influx in cells with severe Na^+ overload when the exchanger operates in the reverse mode without interfering with extrusion of Ca^{2+} through forward-mode NCX in cells that have recovered the trans-sarcolemmal Na^+ gradient. NCX blockade is effective when applied at the time of reperfusion with alternate forward- and reverse-mode operation during diastole and depolarization, respectively.

Inhibition of oscillations of Ca^{2+} between cytosol and SR during initial reperfusion consistently prevents hypercontracture in isolated cardiomyocytes. This can be achieved by reducing influx of extracellular Ca^{2+} (as with NCX inhibition) or by interfering with SR sequestration or release of Ca^{2+}. This is achieved experimentally with thapsigargin (a blocker of Ca^{2+} ATPase of the SR) and ryanodine (a blocker of the SR Ca^{2+} release channels). Halothane, a volatile anesthetic, strongly inhibits Ca^{2+} oscillations and prevents hypercontracture when given at the time of re-energization,[26] but this effect is not clear in patients. Other volatile anesthetics have been shown to be cardioprotective, but their mechanisms of action can be different. Thus, isoflurane protects the myocardium through opening of K^+_{ATP} channel when administered before ischemia occurs.[105]

One of the possible mechanisms for the benefit of cGMP at the time of reperfusion could be a reduction of $[Ca^{2+}]_i$ oscillations.

Slowing Correction of Intracellular Acidosis The prevention of the correction of the acidosis during initial reperfusion protects against cell necrosis[9,45] but is difficult to achieve in vivo. The delay observed with NHE inhibition appears too weak to modify the time course of pHi normalization, probably because compensatory activation of $Na+/CO_3H^-$ and $H+/lactate$ cotransporters is predominant. On the other hand, the inhibition of $Na+/CO_3H^-$ failed to afford myocardial protection. Regional manipulation of pH is complex and difficult to apply.

Contractile Blockade The complete blockade of the contractile apparatus with 2,3-butendionemonoxyme during the initial minutes of reperfusion prevents hypercontracture in vitro and reduces infarct size in large animal models.[39,106,107] 2,3-Butendionemonoxyme has strong unspecific phosphatase activity and is highly toxic. These limitations could be eventually circumvented with less toxic agents, yet these agents will require in situ administration so as not to cause complete asystole. NO and cGMP can have a marked negative inotropic effect in the reperfused myocardium.

Stimulation of cGMP Synthesis cGMP synthesis is activated by the soluble form of guanylyl cyclase, of which NO is the most important agonist, or by activation of the membrane-bound form of the enzyme, as is the case with atrial natriuretic peptides.

Although not unanimously, experimental studies have described a benefit of NO donors and L-arginine, the NO synthase substrate, on myocardial ischemia-reperfusion injury.[100,101,108] The benefit was not confirmed by the Gruppo Italiano per lo Studio della Sopravivienza nell'Infarto miocardio (GISSI)-2 and International Study of Infarct Survival (ISIS)-3 trials in patients with acute myocardial infarction who randomly received a nitrate, an ACE inhibitor, or both, with no benefit shown over placebo. The time window to drug administration, however, was wide in the trial, up to 24 hours after symptom onset, and the crossover rates from placebo to nitrate were high, precluding definitive conclusions. A combined analysis of the two studies revealed a strong trend to benefit of nitrates on the end point of death or myocardial infarction, a trend that became statistically significant when patients receiving ACE inhibitors were excluded from the analysis.[109]

Part of the benefit of NO can at least be mediated through an increase in the cellular cGMP content of cardiomyocytes, which will attenuate reperfusion-induced hypercontracture. Soluble cGMP analogues can also prevent hypercontracture.[109] The mechanism of action of cGMP is not known but could be related to an effect of PKG on SR Ca^{2+}ATPase or ryanodine, or both, which attenuate Ca^{2+} oscillations. Cyclic GMP also desensitizes myofilaments to Ca^{2+}. Intravenous administration of

L-arginine increases cGMP concentration in reperfused myocardium and attenuates hypercontracture and myocardial necrosis in rats and pigs when administered before ischemia occurs.[101]

Direct activation of membrane guanylyl cyclase stimulates the L-arginine/NO pathway to cGMP synthesis independently of both NOS function and ROS production. Such stimulation at the time of reflow can increase myocardial cGMP content within the first minutes of reperfusion. The increase is dose-dependent and may normalize cellular cGMP content and increase it to several times above normal. Normalization of myocardial cGMP content was associated with less hypercontracture and cell death, but the benefit was lost with levels that were above normal.[101,110] Such effects do not occur in isolated cardiomyocytes, suggesting that the toxicity of high cGMP concentrations is related to microvascular endothelial cells.[23] Long half-life atrial natriuretic peptide–related drugs such as urodilatin stimulate the membrane-bound form of guanylyl cyclase with no or little hemodynamic changes. Urodilatin has the potential of being effective for cell protection in patients with acute myocardial infarction undergoing reperfusion therapy. A range of doses will need to be tested, considering the bimodal effect observed in experimental models.

Prevention of Cell-to-Cell Spread of Hypercontracture
The intracoronary injection of heptanol selectively blocks gap junctions in the myocardium. When injected during the initial minutes of reperfusion, heptanol limits infarct size and modifies infarct geometry by fractioning the areas of contraction-band necrosis without increasing the incidence of lethal arrhythmias.[86] Similar changes in infarct geometry have been obtained by interrupting the cell-to-cell spreading of necrosis with 2,3-butendionemonoxyme, which blocks the contractile apparatus as well as the gap junctions.[39] In the same line, gap-junction blockade with heptanol consistently reduces cell death during cerebral ischemia. The low specificity, toxic effects, and narrow therapeutic window of available gap-junction blockers, as well as the need for in situ application, currently preclude clinical evaluation. Selective blockage of gap-junction channels of cells with low pHi, high Ca^{2+}, and altered phosphorylation status of Cx43 might someday circumvent some of these problems. A more promising approach could be to interfere with the reverse-mode NCX transport of Ca^{2+} into the cell through gap-junction Na^+ exchange.[49]

Glucose-Insulin-Potassium
A therapeutic approach named *repolarizing solution* was initially proposed in 1963 by Sodi-Palarez from Mexico City. The merits of the solution have long been debated. More recent clinical trials and meta-analyses support the safety, efficacy, and favorable cost-benefit ratio of this treatment. One meta-analysis of trials performed before the thrombolytic era described a mortality reduction of 28% to 48% that was influenced by the time of onset and the dose.[111] The Estudios Cardiologicos Latinoamerica (ECLA) study confirmed these results in more than 400 patients treated within 24 hours of the onset of symptoms[112]; the bene-

fit occurred in patients receiving a high dose of glucose-insulin-potassium (GIK—25% glucose, 50 IU of insulin, and 80 mmol of KCl per liter) and in patients receiving reperfusion. The Diabetes and Insulin-Glucose Infusion in Acute Myocardial Infarction (DIGAMI) study also showed a benefit of the GIK infusion followed by subcutaneous insulin in 620 diabetic patients with an acute myocardial infarction treated within 24 hours; the discontinuation of benzoguanidines in this study in patients receiving insulin could have contributed to the benefit.[113]

The mechanisms for cell protection with the GIK infusion are not clear. Glucose and insulin improve the energetic status of reperfused myocardium, whereas insulin can trigger protective signal cascades and possesses anti-inflammatory effects.[114] The benefit observed with late treatment is particularly puzzling. One possible explanation could be that treatment protects against damage associated with recurrent ischemic events. In experimental models, GIK effectively reduced infarct size in rats when given at the time of reperfusion[115]; in another study, GIK had no effect when applied 15 minutes after reperfusion.[116]

Collectively, the available information suggests that GIK protects the myocardium against cell death following a transient coronary occlusion, preserves left-ventricular function, and improves survival. Three large trials are evaluating the potential of the GIK infusion: The ECLA-2 study, a study in Asia, and one of the Organization to Assess Strategies for Ischemic Syndromes (OASIS) trials.

Attenuation of Oxidative Stress
Superoxide dismutase (SOD) has been extensively investigated as an antioxidant and has been considered a standard. Different protein formulations have been evaluated by the metal content (Cu, Zn, or Mn) and method of production (human-recombinant) in a large array of models, with conflicting results.[41,117] SOD was conjugated with different molecules to prolong its short half-life (polyethylene glycol SOD, lethitin SOD); conjugated SOD did not improve results.[118,119] Studies testing different concentrations have also yielded negative results.[120] Data with SOD combined with other enzymes, mainly catalase were also conflicting.[121] The use of human-recombinant SOD did not help improve results.[122] Recombinant SOD administered to patients undergoing percutaneous transluminal coronary angioplasty during an acute myocardial infarction failed to produce any detectable beneficial effect or to preserve myocardial function.[123] Despite a recommendation to interrupt the investigation of SOD because of the large amount of inconclusive data,[124] additional studies are being performed, including some involving genetic manipulation to increase the availability of SOD (see later). Studies in transgenic animals suggest that this approach has a beneficial effect.[125,126] An important point to keep in mind is that SOD does not penetrate the cell and thus cannot prevent damage by intracellular ROS generated intracellularly.

Various other antioxidants, including allopurinol, ascorbic acid, and α-tocopherol, have been studied on a smaller scale and have yielded equally controversial results. Some of the investigated agents possess other potent effects unrelated to free radicals.[127] This is the case with Mg^{2+}, which is discussed later.

Attenuation of Inflammatory Response   The complexity of the inflammatory process and the numerous interactions involved between cells and mediators lend themselves to multiple possible interactions. A main target in myocardial infarction is leukocyte-mediated injury. Tested strategies have included inhibitors of cytokines and other mediators; modulation of intracellular transduction systems in inflammatory cells; blockade of adhesion molecules on platelets, leukocytes, and endothelium; and inhibitors of matrix metalloproteinases.

Inhibition of thrombin with hirudin, tissue factor with monoclonal antibodies, and platelet-activating factor with tulopafant also reduces neutrophil accumulation and infarct size in animal studies.[128] This approach is attractive because it interferes with coagulation and inflammation, the main pathophysiologic intravenates in acute coronary syndromes.

Interventions that interfere with activation of endothelial cells, neutrophils, and platelets, particularly activators of the NO/cGMP pathway (L-arginine, NO donors, atrial natriuretic-related peptides) and adenosine, are most promising to control microvascular and leukocyte-mediated injury. These drugs have other important direct effects on cardiomyocytes.

Pilot clinical studies with monoclonal antibodies against ICAM-1, CD11b/CD18,[129] and P-selectin showed no benefit, although some experimental results were interesting.[130] Reperfusion injury is not attenuated in ICAM-1/P-selectin knockout mice.[61]

Direct complement inhibition is a promising approach for limiting infarct size.[40,132] In the complement inhibition in myocardial infarction treated with angioplasty (CARDINAL-COMMA) trial, psxelizumab, an anti-C5 complement antibody, had no effects on infarct size assessed by CK-MB release, but a significant mortality reduction in patients undergoing primary PCI for acute myocardial infarction.[129b] The data suggest that psxelizumab protects against inflammation and delays necrosis and apoptosis.

Glycoprotein IIb/IIIa receptor blockers prevent microvascular embolization and no-reflow in the context of acute coronary interventions.[42] The hypothesis that they could also directly protect the myocardium by preventing myocardial platelet deposition[42] was not confirmed in one study in pigs in which lamifiban failed to reduce infarct size and platelet deposition in pigs submitted to intimal coronary injury and transient coronary occlusion.[62] Heparin and related glycosaminoglycans inhibit the complement cascade at various sites and could limit infarct size independently of the anticoagulant actions.[131] Heparin is widely used in patients with acute coronary syndromes, its potential cardioprotective effect may be relevant.

Aspirin in the ISIS-2 trial reduced mortality as much as streptokinase. This benefit is generally related to its antithrombotic effect. Studies have generally reported no direct cardioprotective effect of aspirin or other anti-inflammatory drugs and a possible trend toward adverse effects.[44,133] In one study, aspirin induced NO release by neutrophils[134]; in another in pigs, aspirin reduced infarct size when the infarct was induced by coronary intimal injury but not when it was induced by external coronary ligation.[43]

Other Treatments   Many therapeutic approaches proposed to limit lethal reperfusion injury have multiple or poorly understood actions. Among them, adenosine and magnesium have received particular attention.

Many experimental data support a benefit of adenosine to reduce infarct size beyond its effects on preconditioning. Administration of adenosine during the first 2 hours of reperfusion reduced cell death in dogs.[135] The adenosine receptor agonist AMP579 administered before reperfusion in rabbits also reduced infarct size, indicating that the effect is independent of preconditioning and leukocyte-mediated injury.[136] The mechanisms for the benefit are unknown; they could be related in part to modulation of Bcl-2 and Bax proteins. In the first Acute Myocardial Infarction Study of ADenosine (AMISTAD) study, which involved 236 patients with an acute myocardial infarction, adenosine administered within 6 hours of symptom onset reduced infarct size in patients with an anterior wall myocardial infarction as assessed with SPECT imaging with technetium sestamibi.[137] These findings were not confirmed in the second AMISTAD trial.

Magnesium interferes with many ion transport systems in cell membranes and organelles, modulates cytosolic Ca^{2+} concentration, and exerts vasodilator, antiarrhythmic, and antithrombotic actions.[138] In addition, magnesium may act as an ROS scavenger. The second Leicester Intravenous Magnesium Intervention (LIMIT-2) trial evaluated the effect of intravenous administration of Mg^{2+} for 24 hours starting before thrombolytic therapy in 2316 patents with suspected acute myocardial infarction and reported a reduction in all-cause and cardiac mortality and the incidence of left-ventricular failure[138b]. In the ISIS-4 trial, Mg^{2+} therapy initiated within 24 hours of infarction showed no benefit[138c] In the MAGnesium In Coronaries (MAGIC) Trial, neutral effects were observed with magnesium compared with placebo among 6208 patients with an acute myocardial infarction eligible or not for reperfusion.[138d]

Multiple other agents have been investigated in smaller trials with results not judged compelling enough to pursue the investigation. Some of them are prostacyclin, Fluosol, and poloxamer-188.[139,140]

Gene and Cell Therapy Against Myocardial Ischemia-Reperfusion Injury

The phenomenal progress in the field of molecular genetics and in the knowledge and understanding of the human genome are introducing a new era of revolutionary tools for research and therapy.

Transfected and genetically modified cells and animals increasingly serve cardiovascular research. Genes of interest are deleted, modified, or overexpressed. Sophisticated engineering allows gene-specific targeting of organs and mechanisms of interest. Examples within the field of myocardial protection are overexpression of the A1 adenosine receptor, heme oxygenase-1, Bcl-2, SOD, glutathione peroxidase, or heat shock protein 72 genes, all of them having a potential for reducing cell death associated with ischemia. Some limitations of transgenic models as research tools involve deletion of genes encoding critically important proteins, a situation that is usually incompatible with fetal development and life, and genetic modifications that often induce compensatory changes that obscure the interpretation of experiments.

Therapeutic tools are also being rapidly developed, although the progress in clinical applications are slower than expected with no clear documentation of efficacy in most situations. This situation may change rapidly.

Gene Therapy

The term *gene therapy* in prevention of cell death secondary to ischemia may only be used to describe a long-term treatment. The transgenic techniques that have been the most widely investigated in laboratory animals and in humans by direct intramyocardial gene transfer or through adenoviral vectors are those encoding various angiogenic growth factors such as vascular endothelial growth factor or fibroblast growth factor 4.[141] These are discussed in Chapter 37. A direct example of gene therapy against lethal ischemia-reperfusion injury is the transfection of human extracellular SOD.[142] This has been accomplished in rabbits using a recombinant replication–deficient adenovirus that overexpresses extracellular SOD with the liver as a target.[143] The genetic treatment administered for 3 days before a transient coronary occlusion increased the expression of the enzyme and reduced infarct size. The authors suggested that the discrepancies between their results and previous studies could be explained by the intravenous administration of SOD in the former, reflecting the pharmacokinetic limitations of exogenous enzyme delivery. Another encouraging example of gene therapy is adenoviral NOSe gene transfer.[142]

Cell Therapy and Prevention of Remodeling

The concept that cardiomyocytes cannot generate is now outdated. Recent reports suggest that it is possible to replace dead cardiomyocytes by exogenous or extracardiac cells (Chapter 45). One approach consists of the transplantation of potentially differentiable cells into the infarcted or peri-infarction area.[144,145] This was done successfully in mice using primitive bone marrow cells; convincing evidence showed that these cells infiltrated the area of necrosis, differentiated into cardiomyocytes, and became functional.[146] Autologous cell transplantation has been reported successful in one patient who received autologous cardiomyoblasts and is now being investigated in pilot clinical trials. However, skeletal muscle cells do not express CX43 and thus cannot be expected to be electrically coupled to adjacent host myocardium. The demonstration of cytokine-induced mobilization of primitive bone marrow cells that can find their way to the infarct area to differentiate into adult contracting cardiomyocytes is even more interesting. Bone marrow– derived pluripotent cells lack the immunologic and ethical problems of embryonic stem cells and can obviate the need for local injection.[146] Much research work is required to understand the mechanisms of primitive cell mobilization, sequestration, and differentiation, which should lead to a completely novel treatment strategy in patients with coronary heart disease.

CONCLUSIONS

The research in the field of cell protection is still flourishing and expanding as new therapeutic tagets and new drugs are emerging, such as the NHE exchanger, glucose-potassium-insulin solution, agonists to cGMP synthesis, and anti-inflammatory drugs. Even more promising are new Na^+/Ca^{2+} exchange inhibitors, mitochondria-directed treatments, and gene and cell therapy. Facing a promising and challenging future, one must remember that cell protection is now a concern in the practice of cardiology with reperfusion therapy and adjunctive antithrombotic therapy, β-blockers, ACE inhibitors, nitrates, hypoglycemics, and other measures related to preconditioning.

ACKNOWLEDGMENTS

The author thanks Gema Santos for her excellent secretarial work. Partially supported by a grant from the Spanish Ministry of Science and Technology: CICYT-SAF99/0102.

REFERENCES

1. Theroux P, Franklin D, Ross J, Kemper WS: Regional myocardial function during acute coronary artery occlusion and its modification by phamacologic agents in the dog. Circ Res 1974;35:896–908.
2. Jennings RB, Reimer KA, Hill ML, Mayer SE: Total ischemia in dog hearts, in vitro. Comparison of high energy phosphate production, utilization, and depletion, and of adenine nucleotide. Circ Res 1981;49:892–900.
3. Heusch G, Schulz R: Hibernating myocardium: A review. J Mol Cell Cardiol 1996;28:2359–2372.
4. Duncker DJ, Schulz R, Ferrari R, et al: "Myocardial stunning" remaining questions. Cardiovasc Res 1998;38:549–558.
5. Garcia-Dorado D, Theroux P, Desco M, et al: Cell-to-cell interaction: A mechanism to explain wave-front progression of myocardial necrosis. Am J Physiol 1989;256:H1266–1273.
6. García-Dorado D, Théroux P, Elízaga J, et al: Myocardial reperfusion in the pig model: Infarct size and duration of coronary occlusion. Cardiovasc Res 1987;21:537–544.
7. Reimer KA, Jennings RB: Effects of reperfusion on infarct size: experimental studies. Eur Heart J 1985;6:97–108.
8. Kim CB, Braunwald E: Potential benefits of late reperfusion of infarcted myocardium. The open artery hypothesis. Circulation 1993;88:2426–2436.
9. Piper HM, Balser C, Ladilov V, et al: The role of Na^+/H^+ exchange in ischemia-reperfusion. Basic Res Cardiol 1996;91:191–202.
10. Schäfer S, Ladilov V, Siegmund B, Piper HM: Importance of bicarbonate transport for protection of cardiomyocytes against reoxygenation injury. Am J Physiol 2000;278:H1457–H1463.

11. Blaustein MP, Lederer WJ: Sodium/calcium exchange: Its physiological implications. Physiol Rev 1999;79:763–854.

12. Ladilov YV, Balser-Schäfer C, Haffner S, et al: Pretreatment with PKC activator protects cardiomyocytes against reoxygenation-induced hypercontracture independently of Ca^{2+} overload. Cardiovasc Res 1999;43:408–416.

13. Allshire A, Piper HM, Cuthbertson KS, Cobbold PH: Cytosolic free Ca^{2+} in single rat heart cells during anoxia and reoxygenation. Biochem J 1987;244:381–385.

14. Steenbergen C, Murphy E, Watts JA, London RE: Correlation between cytosolic free calcium, contracture, ATP, and irreversible ischemic injury in perfused rat heart. Circ Res 1990;66:135–146.

15. García-Dorado D, Oliveras J: Myocardial edema: A preventable cause of reperfusion injury. Cardiovasc Res 1993;27:1555–1563.

16. Nishimura Y, Lemasters JJ: Glycine blocks opening of a death channel in cultured hepatic sinusoidal endothelial cells during chemical hypoxia. Cell Death Differ 2001;8:850–858.

17. Dekker LR, Coronel R, VanBavel E, et al: Intracellular Ca^{2+} and delay of ischemia-induced electrical uncoupling in preconditioned rabbit ventricular myocardium. Cardiovasc Res 1999;44:101–112.

18. Smith WT, Fleet WF, Johnson TA, et al: The Ib phase of ventricular arrhythmias in ischemic in situ porcine heart is related to changes in cell-to-cell electrical coupling. Experimental Cardiology Group, University of North Carolina. Circulation 1995;92:3051–3060.

19. Weinbrenner C, Baines CP, Liu GS, et al: Fostriecin, an inhibitor of protein phosphatase 2A, limits myocardial infarct size even when administered after onset of ischemia. Circulation 1998;98:899–905.

20. Yu L, Netticadan T, Xu YJ, et al: Mechanisms of lysophosphatidylcholine-induced increase in intracellular calcium in rat cardiomyocytes. J Pharmacol Exp Ther 1998;286:1–8.

21. Daleau P: Lysophosphatidylcholine, a metabolite which accumulates early in myocardium during ischemia, reduces gap junctional coupling in cardiac cells. J Mol Cell Cardiol 1999;31:1391–1401.

22. McHowat J, Liu S, Creer MH: Selective hydrolysis of plasmalogen phospholipids by Ca^{2+}-independent PLA2 in hypoxic ventricular myocytes. Am J Physiol 1998;274:C1727–C1737.

23. Cummings BS, McHowat J, Schnellmann RG: Phospholipase A(2)s in cell injury and death. J Pharmacol Exp Ther 2000;294:793–799.

24. Agulló L, Garcia-Dorado D, Escalona N, et al: Hypoxia and acidosis impair cyclic GMP synthesis in coronary endothelial cells. Am J Physiol 2002;286:H917–H925.

25. Dhalla NS, Elmoselhi AB, Hata T, Makino N: Status of myocardial antioxidants in ischemia-reperfusion injury. Cardiovasc Res. 2000;47:446–456.

26. Siegmund B, Ladilov YV, Piper HM: Importance of sodium for recovery of calcium control in reoxygenated cardiomyocytes. Am J Physiol 1994;267:H506–H513.

27. Inserte J, García-Dorado D, Ruiz-Meana M, et al: Inhibition of reverse mode of Na$^+$/CA^{2+} exchanger at the time of myocardial reperfusion limits hypercontracture and cell death. Cardiovasc Res 2002;55:739–748.

28. Siegmund B, Schlack W, Ladilov YV, et al: Halothane protects cardiomyocytes against reoxygenation-induced hypercontracture. Circulation 1997;96:4372–4379.

29. García-Dorado D, Oliveras J, Gili J, et al: Analysis of myocardial edema by magnetic resonance imaging early after coronary artery occlusion with or without reperfusion. Cardiovasc Res 1993;27:1462–1469.

30. García-Dorado D, Oliveras J: Myocardial edema: A preventable cause of reperfusion injury. Cardiovasc Res 1993;27:1555–1563.

31. Yoshida K, Inui M, Harada K, et al: Reperfusion of rat heart after brief ischemia induces proteolysis of calspectin(nonerythroid spectrin or fodrin) by calpain. Circ Res 1995;77:603–610.

32. Siegmund B, Koop A, Klietz T, et al: Sarcolemmal integrity and metabolic competence of cardiomyocytes under anoxia-reoxygenation. Am J Physiol 1990;258:H285–H291.

33. Halestrap AP: Calcium-dependent opening of a non-specific pore in the mitochondrial inner membrane is inhibited at pH values below 7. Implications for the protective effect of low pH against chemical and hypoxic cell damage. Biochem J 1991;278:715–719.

34. Bartling B, Holtz J, Darmer D: Contribution of myocyte apoptosis to myocardial infarction? Basic Res Cardiol 1998;93:71–84.

35. Chakrabarti S, Hoque ANE, Karmazyn M: A rapid ischemia-induced apoptosis in isolated rat hearts and its attenuation by the sodium-hydrogen exchange inhibitor HOE 642 (cariporide). J Mol Cell Cardiol 1997;29:3169–3174.

36. Szaboles M, Michler RE, Yang X, et al: Apoptosis of cardiac myocytes during cardiac allograft rejection. Relation to induction of nitric oxide synthase. Circulation 1996;94:1665–1673.

37. Labat-Moleur F, Guillermet C, Lorimier P, et al: TUNEL apoptotic cell detection in tissue sections: Critical evaluation and improvement. J Histochem Cytochem 1998;46:327–334.

38. Ganote CE: Contraction band necrosis and irreversible myocardial injury. J Mol Cell Cardiol 1983;15:67–73.

39. García-Dorado D, Théroux P, Durán JM, et al: Selective inhibition of the contractile apparatus. A new approach to the modification of infarct size, infarct composition and infarct geometry during coronary artery occlusion and reperfusion. Circulation 1992;85:1160–1174, H1266–H1273.

40. Vakeva AP, Agah A, Rollins SA, et al: Myocardial infarction and apoptosis after myocardial ischemia and reperfusion. Role of the terminal complement components and inhibition by anti-C5 therapy. Circulation 1998;97:2259–2267.

41. Park JL, Lucchesi BR: Mechanisms of myocardial reperfusion injury. Ann Thorac Surg 1999;68:1905–1912.

42. Rezkalla SH, Kloner RA: No-reflow phenomenon. Circulation 2002;105:656–662.

43. Garcia-Dorado D, Ruiz-Meana M, Padilla F, et al: Gap-Junction mediated intercellular communication in ischemic preconditioning. Cardiovasc Res 2002;55:456–465.

44. Barrabés JA, García-Dorado D, Oliveras J, et al: Intimal injury at a transiently occluded coronary artery increases myocardial necrosis. Effect of aspirin. Pflügers Arch Eur J Physiol 1996;432:663–670.

45. Piper HM, García-Dorado D, Ovize M: A fresh look on reperfusion injury. Cardiovasc Res 1998;38:291–300.

46. Ruiz-Meana M, García-Dorado D, González MA, et al: Effect of osmotic stress on sarcolemmal integrity of isolated cardiomyocytes following transient metabolic inhibition. Cardiovasc Res 1995;30:64–69.

47. Ganote CE, Vander Heide RS: Cytoskeletal lesions in anoxic myocardial injury: A conventional and high voltage electron microscopic and immunofluorescence study. Am J Pathol 1987;129:327–344.

48. García-Dorado D, Inserte J, Ruiz Meana M, et al: Gap junction uncoupler heptanol prevents cell-to-cell progression of hypercontracture and limits necrosis during myocardial reperfusion. Circulation 1997;96:3579–3586.

49. Ruiz-Meana M, García-Dorado D, Hofstaetter B, et al: Propagation of cardiomyocyte hypercontracture by passage of Na$^+$ through gap junctions. Circ Res 1999;85:280–287.

50. Olivetti G, Quaini F, Sala R, et al: Acute myocardial infarction in humans is associated with activation of programmed myocyte cell death in the surviving portion of the heart. J Mol Cell Cardiol 1996;28:2005–2016.

51. Semenza GL: Cellular and molecular dissection of reperfusion injury: ROS within and without. Circ Res 2000;86:117–118.

52. Piantadosi CA, Tatro LG, Whorton AR: Nitric oxide and differential effects of ATP on mitochondrial permeability transition. Nitric Oxide 2002;6:45–60.

53. Melo LG, Agrawal R, Zhang L, et al: Gene therapy strategy for long-term myocardial protection using adeno-associated virus-mediated delivery of heme oxygenase gene. Circulation 2002;105:602–607.

54. Taimor G, Hofstaetter B, Piper HM: Apoptosis induction by nitric oxide in adult cardiomyocytes via cGMP-signaling and its impairment after simulated ischemia. Cardiovasc Res 2000;45:588–594.

55. Inserte J, Taimor G, Hofstaetter B, et al: Influence of stimulated ischemia on apoptosis induction by oxidative stress in adult cardiomyocytes of rats. Am J Physiol Heart Circ 2000;278:H94–H99.

56. Saraste A, Pulkki K, Kallajoki M, et al: Apoptosis in human acute myocardial infarction. Circulation 1997;95:320–323.

57. Watanabe H, Kuhne W, Spahr R, et al: Macromolecule permeability of coronary and aortic endothelial monolayers under energy depletion. Am J Physiol 1991;260:H1344–H1352.

58. García-Dorado D, Théroux P, Solares J, et al: Determinants of hemorrhagic infarcts. Histologic observations from experiments including coronary occlusion coronary reperfusion and re-occlusion. Am J Pathol 1989;173:301–311.

59. Forman MB, Puett DW, Virmani R: Endothelial and myocardial injury during ischemia and reperfusion: Pathogenesis and therapeutic implications. J Am Coll Cardiol 1989;13:450–459.

61. Briaud SA, Ding ZM, Michael LH, et al: Leukocyte trafficking and myocardial reperfusion injury in ICAM-1/P-selectin-knockout mice. Am J Physiol Heart Circ Physiol 2001;280:H60–H67.

62. Barrabés JA, García-Dorado D, Ruiz-Meana M, et al: Lack of effect of glycoprotein IIb/IIIa blockade on myocardial platelet or polymorphonuclear leukocyte accumulation and on infarct size after transient coronary occlusion in pigs. J Am Coll Cardiol 2001;39: 157–165.

63. Seligmann C, Kupatt C, Becker BF, et al: Adenosine endogenously released during early reperfusion mitigates postischemic myocardial dysfunction by inhibiting platelet adhesion. J Cardiovasc Pharmacol 1998;32:156–163.

64. Heindl B, Zahler S, Welsch U, Becker BF: Disparate effects of adhesion and degranulation of platelets on myocardial and coronary function in postischaemic hearts. Cardiovasc Res 1998;38: 383–394.

65. Mirabet M, Garcia-Dorado D, Inserte J, et al: Platelets activated by transient coronary occlusion exacerbate ischemia-reperfusion injury in rat hearts. Am J Physiol 2002;283:H1134–H1141.

66. Murry CE, Jennings RB, Reimer KA: Preconditioning with ischemia: A delay of lethal cell injury in ischemic myocardium. Circulation 1986;74:1124–1136.

67. Schulz R, Cohen MV, Behrends M, et al: Signal transduction of ischemic preconditioning. Cardiovasc Res 2001;52:181–198.

68. Yellon DM, Baxter GF, García-Dorado D, et al: Ischaemic preconditioning: present position and future directions. Cardiovasc Res 1998;37:21–33.

69. Ganote CE, Armstrong S, Downey JM: Adenosine and A1 selective agonists offer minutesimal protection against ischaemic injury to isolated rat cardiomyocytes. Cardiovasc Res 1993;27:1670–1676.

70. Takano H, Bolli R, Black RG, et al: A(1) or A(3) adenosine receptors induce late preconditioning against infarction in conscious rabbits by different mechanisms. Circ Res 2001;88:520–528.

70a. Tanaka M, Brooks SE, Richard VJ, et al: Effect of anti-CD18 antibody on myocardial neutrophil accumulation and infarct size after ischemia and reperfusion in dogs. Circulation 1993;87:526–535.

71. Kida M, Fujiwara H, Ishida M, et al: Ischemic preconditioning preserves creatine phosphate and intracellular pH. Circulation 1991;84:2495–2503.

72. Kolocassides KG, Seymour AM, Galinanes M, Hearse DJ: Paradoxical effect of ischemic preconditioning on ischemic contracture? NMR studies of energy metabolism and intracellular pH in the rat heart. J Mol Cell Cardiol 1996;28:1045–1057.

73. Stern MD, Chien AM, Capogrossi MC, et al: Direct observation of the "oxygen paradox" in single rat ventricular myocytes. Circ Res 1985;56:899–903.

74. Koop A, Piper HM: Protection of energy status of hypoxic cardiomyocytes by mild acidosis. J Mol Cell Cardiol 1992;24: 55–65.

75. Ottani F, Galvani M, Ferrini D, et al: Prodromal angina limits infarct size. A role for ischemic preconditioning. Circulation 1995;91: 291–297.

76. Baxter GF, Marber MS, Patel VC, Yellon DM: Adenosine receptor involvement in a delayed phase of myocardial protection 24 hours after ischemic preconditioning. Circulation 1994;90:2993–3000.

77. Auchampach JA, Gross GJ: Adenosine A1 receptors, KATP channels, and ischemic preconditioning in dogs. Am J Physiol 1993;264:H1327–H1336.

78. Connor M, Christie MJ: Opioid receptors signaling mechanisms. Clin Exp Pharmacol 1999;26:493–499.

79. Miki T, Cohen MV, Downey JM: Opioid receptor contributes to ischemic preconditioning through protein kinase C activation in rabbits. J Mol Cell Cardiol 1998;186:3–12.

80. Schulz R, Gres P, Heusch G: Role of endogenous opioids in ischemic preconditioning but not in short-term hibernation in pigs. Am J Physiol Heart Circ Physiol 2001;280:H2175–H2181.

81. Fryer RM, Hsu AK, Eells JT, et al: Opioid-Induced second window of cardioprotection. Potential role of mitochondrial K ATP channels. Circ Res 1999;84:846–851.

82. Jaberansari MT, Baxter GF, Muller CA, et al: Energy metabolism in preconditioned and control myocardium: Effect of total ischemia. J Mol Cell Cardiol 1991;23:1449–1458.

83. Gustafsson I, Hildebrandt P, Seibaek M, et al: Long-term prognosis of diabetic patients with myocardial infarction: Relation to antidiabetic treatment regimen. The TRACE Study Group. Eur Heart J 2000;21:1937–1943.

84. Mocanu MM, Maddock HL, Baxter GF, et al: Glimepiride, a novel sulfonylurea, does not abolish myocardial protection afforded by either ischemic preconditioning or diazoxide. Circulation 2001; 103:3111–3116.

85. Steenbergen C, Murphy E, Levy L, London RE: Elevation in cytosolic free calcium concentration early in myocardial ischemia in perfused rat heart. Circ Res 1987;60:700–707.

86. García-Dorado D, González MA, Barrabés JA, et al: Prevention of ischemic rigor contracture during coronary occlusion by inhibition of Na^+/H^+ exchange. Cardiovasc Res 1997;35:80–89.

87. Klein HH, Pich S, Bohle RM, et al: Myocardial protection by Na^+-H^+ exchange inhibition in ischemic, reperfused porcine hearts. Circulation 1995;92:912–917.

88. Klein HH, Pich S, Bohle RM, et al: Na^+/H^+ exchange inhibitor cariporide attenuates cell injury predominantly during ischemia and not at onset of reperfusion in porcine hearts with low residual blood flow. Circulation 2000;102:1977–1982.

89. Ruiz-Meana M, Garcia-Dorado D, Lane S, et al: Persistence of gap junction communication during myocardial ischemia. Am J Physiol Heart Circ Physiol 2001;280:H2563–H2571.

90. Rodriguez-Sinovas A, García-Dorado D, Padilla F, et al: Pretreatment with the Na+/H+ exchange inhibitor caripode delays cell-to-cell electrical uncoupling during myocardial ischemia. Cardiovasc Res 2003 (in press).

91. Xiao XH, Allen DG: Role of Na^+/H^+ exchanger during ischemia and preconditioning in the isolated rat heart. Circ Res 1999;85:723–730.

92. Schafer C, Ladilov YV, Schafer M, Piper HM: Inhibition of NHE protects reoxygenated cardiomyocytes independently of anoxic Ca^{2+} overload and acidosis. Am J Physiol Heart Circ Physiol 2000;279:H2143–H2150.

93. Miura T, Liu Y, Goto M et al: Mitochondrial ATP-sensitive K^+ channels play a role in cardioprotection by Na^+H^+ exchange inhibition against ischemia-reperfusion injury. J Am Cll Cardiol 2001;37: 957–963.

94. Rupprecht HJ, vom Dahl J, Terres W, et al: Cardioprotective effects of the Na^+/H^+ exchange inhibitor cariporide in patients with acute anterior myocardial infarction undergoing direct PTCA. Circulation 2000;101:2902–2908.

95. Avkiran M, Marber MS: Na^+/H^+ exchange inhibitors for cardioprotective therapy: Progress, problems and prospects. J Am Coll Cardiol 2002;39:747–753.

96. Theroux P, Chaitman BR, Danchin N, et al: Inhibition of the sodium-hydrogen exchanger with cariporide to prevent myocardial infarction in high-risk ischemic situations. Main results of the GUARDIAN trial. Guard during ischemia against necrosis (GUARDIAN) Investigators. Circulation 2000;102: 3032–3038.

97. Zeymer U, Suryapranata H, Monassier JP, et al: The Na^+/H^+ exchange inhibitor eniporide as an adjunct to early reperfusion therapy for acute myocardial infarction. Results of the evaluation of the safety and cardioprotective effects of eniporide in acute myocardial infarction (ESCAMI) trial. J Am Coll Cardiol 2001;38:1644–1650.

98. Pabla R, Buda AJ, Flynn DM, et al: Nitric oxide attenuates neutrophil-mediated myocardial contractile dysfunction after ischemia and reperfusion. Circ Res 1996;78:65–72.

99. Lerman A, Burnett JC Jr, Higano ST, et al: Long-term L-arginine supplementation improves small-vessel coronary endothelial function in humans. Circulation 1998;97:2123–2128.

100. Agulló L, García-Dorado D, Inserte J, et al: L-Arginine limits myocardial cell death secondary to hypoxia-reoxygenation by a cGMP-dependent mechanism. Am J Physiol 1999;45:H1574–H1580.

101. Padilla F, Garcia-Dorado D, Agulló L, et al: L-Arginine administration prevents reperfusion-induced cardiomyocyte hypercontracture and reduces infarct size in the pig. Cardiovasc Res 2000;46: 412–420.

102. Scheel KW, Daulat G, Mass HJ, Williams SE: Intramural coronary collateral flow in dogs. Am J Physiol 1990;258:H679–H682.

103. Watano T, Harada Y, Harada K, Nishimura N: Effect of Na^+/Ca^{2+} exchange inhibitor, KB-R7943 on ouabain-induced arrhythmias in guinea-pigs. Br J Pharmacol 1999;127:1846–1850.

104. Kimura J, Watano T, Kawahara M, et al: Direction-independent block of bidirectional Na^+/Ca^{2+} exchange current by KB-R7943 in guinea-pig cardiac myocytes. Br J Pharmacol 1999;128: 969–974.

105. Piriou V, Chiari P, Knezynski S, et al: Prevention of isoflurane-induced preconditioning by 5-hydroxydecanoate and gadolinium:

Possible involvement of mitochondrial adenosine triphosphate-sensitive potassium and stretch-activated channels. Anesthesiology 2000;93:756–764.

106. Siegmund B, Klietz T, Schwartz P, Piper HM: Temporary contractile blockade prevents hypercontracture in anoxic-reoxygenated cardiomyocytes. Am J Physiol 1991;260:H426–H435.

107. Schlack W, Uebing A, Schäfer M, et al: Regional contractile blockade at the onset of reperfusion reduces infarct size in the dog heart. Pflug Arch Eur J Phy 1994;428:134–141.

108. Weyrich AS, Ma XL, Lefer AM: The role of L-arginine in ameliorating reperfusion injury after myocardial ischemia in the cat. Circulation 1992;86:279–288.

109. Hempel A, Friedrich M, Schluter KD, et al: ANP protects against reoxygenation-induced hypercontracture in adult cardiomyocytes. Am J Physiol 1997;273(1 Pt 2):H244–H249.

110. Inserte J, García-Dorado D, Agulló L, et al: Urodilatin limits acute reperfusion injury in the isolated rat heart. Cardiovasc Res 2000;45:351–359.

111. Fath-Ordoubadi F, Beatt KJ: Glucose-insulin-potassium therapy for treatment of acute myocardial infarction: An overview of randomized placebo-controlled trials. Circulation 1997;96: 1152–1156.

112. Diaz R, Paolasso EA, Piegas LS, et al: Metabolic modulation of acute myocardial infarction. The ECLA (Estudios Cardiologicos Latinoamerica) Collaborative Group. Circulation 1998;98: 2227–2234.

113. Malmberg K, Norhammar A, Wedel H, Ryden L: Glycometabolic state at admission: Important risk marker of mortality in conventionally treated patients with diabetes mellitus and acute myocardial infarction: Long-term results from the Diabetes and Insulin-Glucose Infusion in Acute Myocardial Infarction (DIGAMI) study. Circulation 1999;99:2626–2632.

114. Das UN: Possible beneficial action(s) of glucose-insulin-potassium regimen in acute myocardial infarction and inflammatory conditions: A hypothesis. Diabetologia 2000;3:1081–1082.

115. Jonassen AK, Aasum E, Riemersma RA, et al: Glucose-insulin potassium reduces infarct size when administered during reperfusion. Cardiovasc Drugs Ther 2000;6:615–623.

117. Downey JM, Omar B, Ooiwa H, McCord J: Superoxide dismutase therapy for myocardial ischemia. Free Radic Res Commun 1991;12(13 Pt 2):703–720.

118. Tamura Y, Chi L, Driscoll EM, et al: Superoxide dismutase conjugated to polyethylene glycol provides sustained protection against myocardial ischemia/reperfusion injury in canine heart. Circ Res 1988;63:944–959.

119. Nakajima H, Hangaishi M, Ishizaka N, et al: Lecithinized copper, zinc-superoxide dismutase ameliorates ischemia-induced myocardial damage. Life Sci 2001;69:935–944.

120. Watanabe BI, Premaratne S, Limm W, et al: High- and low-dose superoxide dismutase plus catalase does not reduce myocardial infarct size in a subhuman primate model. Am Heart J 1993;126:840–846.

121. Gallagher KP, Buda AJ, Pace D, et al: Failure of superoxide dismutase and catalase to alter size of infarction in comscious dogs after 3 hours of occlusion followed by reperfusion. Circulation 1986;73:1065–1076.

122. Matsuda M, Fujiwara H, Kawamura A, et al: Failure to reduce infarct size by intracoronary infusion of recombinant human superoxide dismutase at reperfusion in the porcine heart: Immunohistochemical and histological analysis. J Mol Cell Cardiol 1991;11:1287–1296.

123. Flaherty JT, Pitt B, Gruber JW, et al: Recombinant human superoxide dismutase (h-SOD) fails to improve recovery of ventricular function in patients undergoing coronary angioplasty for acute myocardial infarction. Circulation 1994;89:1982–1991.

124. Engler R, Gilpin E: Can superoxide dismutase alter myocardial infarct size? Circulation 1989;79:1137–1142.

125. Chen Z, Siu B, Ho YS, et al: Overexpression of MnSOD protects against myocardial ischemia/reperfusion injury in transgenic mice. J Mol Cell Cardiol 1998;30:2281–2289.

126. Wang P, Chen H, Qin H, et al: Overexpression of human copper, zinc-superoxide dismutase (SOD1) prevents postischemic injury. Proc Natl Acad Sci U S A 1998;95:4556–4560.

127. Tripathi Y, Hegde BM: Effect of N-acetylcysteine on myocardial infarct size following ischemia and reperfusion in dogs. Ind J Physiol Pharmacol 1998;42:50–56.

128. Erlich JH, Boyle EM, Labriola J, et al: Inhibition of the tissue factor-thrombin pathway limits infarct size after myocardial ischemia-reperfusion injury by reducing inflammation. Am J Pathol 2000;157:1849–1862.

129. Rusnak JM, Kopecky SL, Clements IP, et al: An anti-CD11/CD18 monoclonal antibody in patients with acute myocardial infarction having percutaneous transluminal coronary angioplasty (the FESTIVAL study). Am J Cardiol 2001;88:482–487.

129b. Granger CB, Mahaffey KW, Weaver WD, et al: Effect of pexelizumab, and anti-C5 complement antibody, as adjunctive therapy to primary percutaneous coronary intervention in acute myocardial infarction: complement inhibition in myocardial infarction treated with angioplasty (COMMA) trial. Circ (submitted).

130. Simpson PJ, Todd RF III, Mickelson JK, et al: Sustained limitation of myocardial reperfusion injury by a monoclonal antibody that alters leukocyte function. Circulation 1990;81:226–237.

131. Black SC, Gralinski MR, Friedrichs GS, et al: Cardioprotective effects of heparin or N-acetylheparin in an in vivo model of myocardial ischaemic and reperfusion injury. Cardiovasc Res 1995;29:629–636.

132. Lazar HL, Bao Y, Gaudiani J, et al: Total complement inhibition: An effective strategy to limit ischemic injury during coronary revascularization on cardiopulmonary bypass. Circulation 1999;100: 1438–1442.

133. Golino P, Ambrosio G, Villari B, et al: Endogenous prostaglandin endoperoxides may alter infarct size in the presence of thromboxane synthase inhibition: studies in a rabbit model of coronary artery occlusion reperfusion. J Am Coll Cardiol 1993;21: 493–501.

134. Lopez-Farre A, Riesco A, Digiuni E, et al: Aspirin-stimulated nitric oxide production by neutrophils after acute myocardial ischemia in rabbits. Circulation 1996;94:83–87.

135. Zhao ZQ, Budde JM, Morris C, et al: Adenosine attenuates reperfusion-induced apoptotic cell death by modulating expression of Bcl-2 and Bax proteins. J Mol Cell Cardiol 2001;33:57–68.

136. Xu Z, Yang XM, Cohen MV, Neumann T, et al: Limitation of infarct size in rabbit hearts by the novel adenosine receptor agonist AMP 579 administered at reperfusion. J Mol Cell Cardiol 2000;32: 2339–2347.

137. Mahaffey KW, Puma JA, Barbagelata NA, et al: Adenosine as an adjunct to thrombolytic therapy for acute myocardial infarction: results of a multicenter, randomized, placebo-controlled trial: The Acute Myocardial Infarction Study of ADenosine (AMISTAD) trial. J Am Coll Cardiol 1999;34:1711–1720.

138. Ravn HB: Pharmacological effects of magnesium on arterial thrombosis—mechanisms of action? Magnes Res 1999;12: 191–199.

138b. Woods KL, Fletcher S. Long-term outcome after intravenous magnesium sulphate in suspected acute myocardial infarction: the second Leicester Intravenous Magnesium Intervention Trial (LIMIT-2) Lancet. 1994 Apr 2;343(8901):816–9.

138c. ISIS-4: A randomised factorial trial assessing early oral captopril, oral mononitrate, and intravenous magnesium sulphate in 58,050 patients with suspected acute myocardial infarction. ISIS-4 (Fourth International Study of Infarct Survival) Collaborative Group. Lancet. 1995 Mar 18;345(8951):669–685.

138d. Early administration of intravenous magnesium to high-risk patients with acute myocardial infarction in the Magnesium in Coronaries (MAGIC) Trial: a randomised controlled trial. Lancet. 2002 Oct 19;360(9341):1189–1196.

139. O'Keefe JH, Grines CL, DeWood MA, et al: Poloxamer-188 as an adjunct to primary percutaneous transluminal coronary angioplasty for acute myocardial infarction. Am J Cardiol 1996;78: 747–750.

140. Schaer GL, Spaccavento LJ, Browne KF, et al: Beneficial effects of RheothRx injection in patients receiving thrombolytic therapy for acute myocardial infarction. Results of a randomized, double-blind, placebo-controlled trial. Circulation 1996;94:298–307.

141. Isner JM: Myocardial gene therapy. Nature 2002;415:234–239.

142. Abunasra HJ, Smolenski RT, Morrison K, et al: Efficacy of adenoviral gene transfer with manganese superoxide dismutase and endothelial nitric oxide synthase in reducing ischemia and reperfusion injury. Eur J Cardiothorac Surg 2001;20: 153–158.

143. Li Q, Bolli R, Qiu Y, et al: Gene therapy with extracellular super-oxide dismutase protects conscious rabbits against myocardial infarction. Circulation 2001;103:1893–1898.

144. Jiang Y, Jahagirdar BN, Reinhardt RL, et al: Pluripotency of mes-enchymal stem cells derived from adult marrow. Nature 2002;418:41–49.

145. Boheler KR, Czyz J, Tweedie D, et al: Differentiation of pluripotent embryonic stem cells into cardiomyocytes. Circ Res 2002;91:189–201.

146. Orlic D, Kajstura J, Chimenti S, et al: Transplanted adult bone mar-row cells repair myocardial infarcts in mice. Ann N Y Acad Sci 2001;938:221–229, discussion 229–230.

■ ■ ■ c h a p t e r **3 4**

Revascularization in Acute Coronary Syndromes: Which Patients and When?

Lars Wallentin

RATIONALE OF REVASCULARIZATION

The manifestations of ischemia in unstable coronary artery disease (CAD), i.e., unstable angina or non–ST-elevation myocardial infarction, are caused by a severe flow-limiting stenosis or occlusion of a coronary artery. Most cases show signs of myocardial infarction, which might be related as much to thrombotic occlusion at the culprit coronary lesion as to downstream embolization of thrombotic material from the lesion (Figs. 34–1 and 34–2).[1-3] The thrombotic component of the disease can be influenced by the modern treatment with platelet and thrombin inhibitors.[4-9] Despite such treatment, severe coronary stenoses[10,11] usually remain, which leads to a risk of recurrence with withdrawal of the initially intense antithrombotic therapy.[12-14] This is the rationale for early coronary angiography and revascularization. Elimination of the flow-limiting lesions by coronary percutaneous intervention or bypass grafting might be the ideal method for long-term stabilization. Although appealing from a mechanistic point of view, this approach has advantages and disadvantages that must be validated in prospective, randomized, multicenter trials.

Over the years, the enthusiasm for an early invasive approach has grown rapidly in centers with facilities for these procedures. Accordingly, large differences in the proportion of patients treated with early invasive procedures have developed between different centers and different countries, with potentially large consequences for patients.[15-18] The early randomized trials, performed in the 1980s and the beginning of the 1990s, could not demonstrate any advantages over the early invasive treatment.[19-22] These controversial results have repeatedly been reviewed, and the arguments pro and con have been scrutinized in many presentations.[23-26] The early trials were performed before the advent of intense antithrombotic treatment until and during the procedures and without the availability of stents and glycoprotein-IIb/IIIa inhibitors at percutaneous coronary interventions. In contrast, the two latest and largest trials, randomizing patients to an early invasive versus a selected invasive strategy and using intense antithrombotic treatment before and during the procedures as

well as coronary stenting, finally confirmed the benefits of the early invasive approach.[27-29] These two studies have provided a wealth of information on the pertinent issues of benefits, risks, costs, and the optimal timing of an early invasive strategy in different patient categories (Table 34–1). Therefore, this chapter mainly focuses on the results obtained in these two recent trials, which used modern percutaneous or surgical low-risk revascularization technologies after pretreatment with the currently recommended and evidence-based antithrombotic combination therapy.

OLDER RANDOMIZED TRIALS—THE CONTROVERSY

Recent decades have seen rapid development in the technology for revascularization for both coronary artery bypass surgery[30-33] and coronary angioplasty and stenting.[34-37] Initially, both revascularization methods were avoided in the acute phase of myocardial infarction and in unstable angina pectoris because of a raised risk of procedure-related complications.[38-42] With time, the use of direct revascularization for unstable CAD and acute myocardial infarction has increased.[5,43,44] Previously, the accepted indications for these methods were mainly severe incapacitating angina or severe ischemia because no protective effects regarding subsequent mortality or myocardial infarction could be demonstrated in randomized trials[19-22] or in registries.[16] Still, the use of early revascularization in unstable CAD grew rapidly, as did belief in the benefits of this management in centers that could easily employ the technology.[45] However, in centers and countries with limited resources for invasive procedures, patients were primarily treated conservatively.[16] Thus, the controversy over an invasive versus a noninvasive approach in unstable CAD continued,[23-26] which was also reflected in the ambiguous message in the contemporary treatment guidelines.[5]

The first evidence of a protective effect of early revascularization concerning re-infarction was shown by the 50% reduction in risk of myocardial infarction by

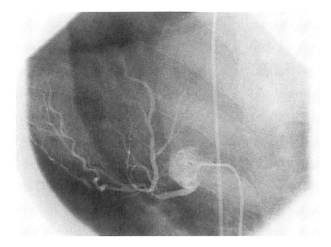

FIGURE 34–1. Coronary angiography in a patient with acute coronary syndrome: The left coronary artery shows severe stenosis and an intra-coronary filling defect as an indicator of plaque fissure, with a super-imposed thrombus.

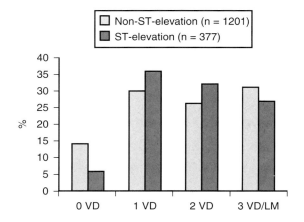

FIGURE 34–2. Extent of coronary artery disease and unstable coronary artery disease in the 1201 patients undergoing early routine coronary angiography in the FRISC II trial compared with 377 patients undergoing early routine coronary angiography in a simultaneous trial 4 days after thrombolysis for ST-elevation myocardial infarction. LMD, left main disease; VD, vessel diseased.

revascularization in patients with exercise-induced ischemia after ST-elevation myocardial infarction in the DANish trial in Acute Myocardial Infarction (DANAMI trial).[46] Thereafter, almost every trial of direct angioplasty in ST-elevation myocardial infarction has corroborated the protection from reinfarction by early revascularization in this patient category.[47,48] However, until 1999, no corresponding evidence was available concerning other acute coronary syndromes.

MODERN RANDOMIZED TRIALS—THE NEW EVIDENCE

The first large-scale, prospective, multicenter, random-ized trial of an early invasive versus a noninvasive strat-egy in unstable CAD, using modern antithrombotic

TABLE 34–1   ISSUES CONCERNING AN INVASIVE OR NONINVASIVE TREATMENT STRATEGY IN UNSTABLE CORONARY SYNDROMES

Benefits

Survival
Recurrent myocardial infarction
Late revascularization
Late readmission
Recurrent incapacitating angina
Need for anti-anginal medication
Quality of life

Risks

Procedure-related mortality
Procedure-related myocardial infarction
Procedure-related extra cardiac side effects and morbidity
Re-stenosis and recurring need for revascularisation
Recurrence of angina

Costs

Procedure-related costs
Length of hospital stay
Costs for medication
Costs for sick-leave and retirement pension

Patient Selection

Risk indicators in relation to benefits, risks, and cost
Risk scores
Optimal revascularization method
Optimal timing of revascularization

medication until the procedures and with frequent stent-ing at percutaneous procedures, was the Fragmin during Instability in Coronary Artery Disease (FRISC) II trial (Fig. 34–3).[27,28] This trial randomized 2247 patients with unstable angina or non–ST-elevation myocardial infarc-tion from all types of hospitals in three Scandinavian Countries. In the invasive arm, 96% of patients under-went coronary angiography within 7 days after admis-sion. In the noninvasive group, only 7% underwent coronary angiography over the same period because of the predefined indications (severe angina, severe ischemia before discharge exercise test, or myocardial infarction or re-infarction). The proportions of coronary angiography had increased to 99% and 52% after 6 months in the invasive and noninvasive strategy groups, respectively.

Within the first 10 days, 71% of the invasive group ver-sus 9% of the noninvasive group underwent revascular-ization; after 12 months, these proportions had increased to 78% and 43% (Fig. 34–4). In the invasive and noninva-sive strategy groups, respectively, 44% and 21% of the procedures were coronary angioplasty and 34% and 19% were coronary artery bypass surgery. Coronary artery bypass surgery was the recommended procedure and performed in 82% of patients with three-vessel or left main disease. Coronary angioplasty was recommended and performed in 83% of patients with one-vessel and 61% of patients with two-vessel disease. The angioplasty procedures were associated with stenting in 65% of cases but were associated with stenting in only 10% of cases involving glycoprotein-IIb/IIIa inhibition. One in-

FRISC II Study Design

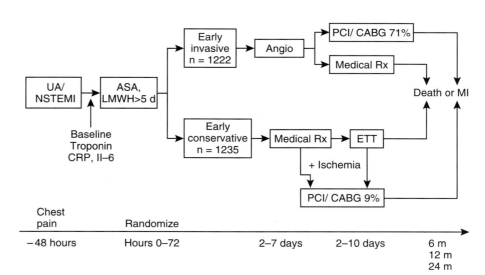

FIGURE 34–3. Design of the FRISC II trial. ASA, Aspirin; CABG, coronary artery bypass graft; CRP, C-reactive protein; ETT, Exercise treadmill test; LMWH, low-molecular-weight heparin; MI, myocardial infarction; NSTEMI, non–ST-elevation MI; PCI, percutaneous intervention; UA, unstable angina.

hospital fatality occurred among the percutaneous interventions. Also, coronary artery bypass procedures were associated with a low rate of complications and a mere 1.7% 30-day mortality rate. All patients were treated with aspirin and low-molecular-weight heparin from admission until the invasive procedures.

The results of the FRISC II trial showed that the invasive treatment strategy was associated with a 2.7% absolute reduction in the primary composite end point of myocardial infarction and death, a 2.3% absolute

decrease in myocardial infarction alone, and a 1% absolute reduction in mortality at the primary end point after 6 months (Table 34–2). The benefit of the early invasive approach was further strengthened during longer-term follow-up, with a significant 1.7% absolute reduction in mortality alone, a 3% absolute reduction in myocardial infarction alone, and a 3.7% absolute reduction in the composite of these events at 12 months (see Table 34–2; (Figs. 34-5, 34-6, 34-7). In the first year following discharge from the hospital, there was a substantial

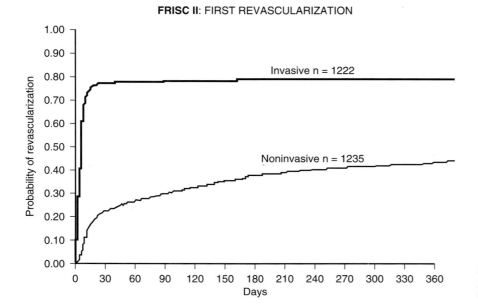

FIGURE 34–4. Proportion of revascularization procedures during the first year in the invasive and noninvasive arms of the FRISC II trial.

■ ■ ■

TABLE 34–2   RESULTS OF THE FRISC II TRIAL: DEATH AND/OR MYOCARDIAL INFARCTION (MI) AFTER 6 MONTHS IN THE INVASIVE AND THE NONINVASIVE GROUPS

	INVASIVE (n = 1222)	NONINVASIVE (n = 1235)	RISK RATIO (95% CI)	*P*
6 Months' Outcome				
Death and/or MI	113 (9.4%)	148 (12.1%)	0.78 (0.62–0.98)	0.031
MI	94 (7.8%)	124 (10.1%)	0.77 (0.60–0.99)	0.045
Death	23 (1.9%)	36 (2.9%)	0.65 (0.39–1.09)	0.10
12 Months' Outcome				
Death and/or MI	127 (10.4%)	174 (14.1%)	0.74 (0.60–0.92)	0.005
MI	105 (8.6%)	143 (11.6%)	0.74 (0.59–0.94)	0.015
Death	27 (2.2%)	48 (3.9%)	0.57 (0.36–0.90)	0.016
24 Months' Outcome				
Death and/or MI	146 (12.1%)	200 (16.3%)	0.74 (0.61–0.90)	0.003
MI	111 (9.2%)	156 (12.7%)	0.72 (0.57–0.91)	0.005
Death	45 (3.7%)	67 (5.4%)	0.68 (0.47–0.98)	0.038

FRISC II: DEATH OR MI DURING 12 MONTHS

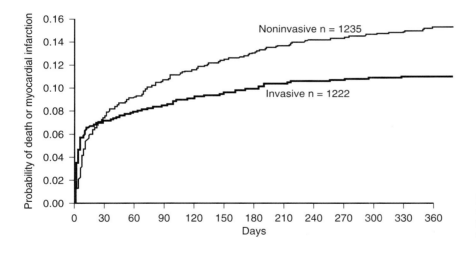

FIGURE 34–5. Probability of death or myocardial infarction in the invasive and noninvasive arms of the FRISC II trial. MI, myocardial infarction.

FRISC II: MORTALITY DURING 12 MONTHS

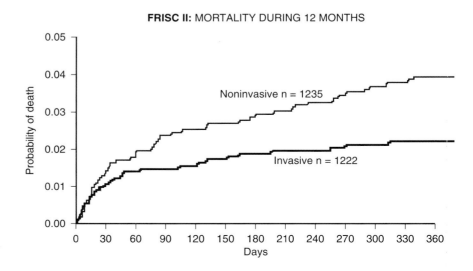

FIGURE 34–6. Mortality in the invasive and noninvasive arms of the FRISC II trial.

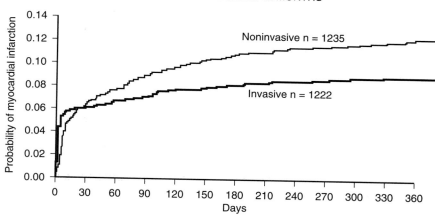

FIGURE 34–7. Myocardial infarction (MI) in the invasive and noninvasive arms of the FRISC II trial.

crossover to invasive treatment in the noninvasive arm. Thus, during the first 6 months, 37% in the invasive group underwent revascularization; during the remainder of the first year, 43% had crossed over to invasive treatment (see Fig. 34-4). Despite this development, there was, even during the second year, a lower risk of myocardial infarction in the early invasive group, leading to a 4.2% absolute reduction of death or myocardial infarction after 24 months (see Table 34-2). This trial was the first to provide clear evidence of the beneficial effects of an early invasive strategy in unstable CAD. So far, it is the only trial demonstrating reduced long-term mortality by an early invasive treatment in unstable coronary syndromes. This is the only available regimen that has been shown to improve long-term survival in acute coronary syndromes.

The Treat Angina with Aggrastat and Determine Cost of Therapy with an Invasive or Conservative Strategy/Thrombolysis in Myocardial Infarction 18 (TACTICS-TIMI 18) trial was the second large-scale, prospective, multicenter, randomized trial of an early invasive versus a noninvasive strategy in unstable CAD using modern antithrombotic medication with aspirin, heparin, and glycoprotein-IIb/IIIa inhibition and with an appropriate USE of coronary angioplasty and stenting (Fig. 34-8).[29]

This trial involved 2220 patients with unstable angina or non–ST-elevation myocardial infarction, of whom 83% were from the United States.

In the invasive arm, 97% of patients underwent coronary angiography before hospital discharge and at a median of 22 hours after admission. In the noninvasive group, there was also a high (51%) rate of early coronary angiography before hospital discharge because of any of the predefined indications: refractory angina, ischemia before discharge stress test, or myocardial infarction or re-infarction. Before hospital discharge, 60% of the invasive versus 36% of the noninvasive group underwent revascularization procedures: Two thirds were angioplasty procedures performed at a median of 25 hours after admission, and one third were coronary artery bypass procedures performed at a median of 89 hours after admission. Stenting was also used in 83% of the angioplasty procedures. The coronary artery bypass procedures were associated with a low rate of complications but a 3.6% 30-day mortality rate. All patients were treated with aspirin, unfractionated heparin, and the glycoprotein-IIb/IIIa inhibitor tirofiban from admission. During the angioplasty procedures, the glycoprotein inhibitor was used by 94% of the invasive group and by 59% of the conservative group.

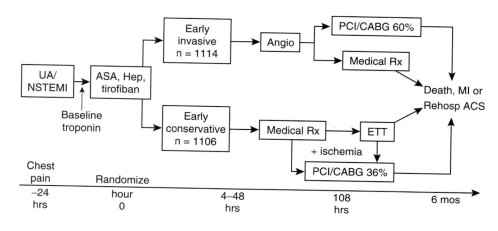

TACTICS-TIMI 18 STUDY DESIGN

FIGURE 34–8. Design of the TACTICS-TIMI 18 trial. ACS, acute coronary syndrome; Angio, angioplasty; ASA, Aspirin; CABG, coronary artery bypass graft; ETT, Exercise Treadmill Test; Hep, heparin; MI, myocardial infarction; NSTEMI, non–ST-elevation MI; PCI, percutaneous intervention; Rehosp, rehospitalization; UA, unstable angina.

The results showed that the invasive treatment strategy was associated with a 3.5% absolute reduction in the primary triple end point of death, myocardial infarction, or rehospitalization for acute coronary syndrome, a 2.2% absolute decrease in the composite of death or myocardial infarction, and a 2.1% decrease in myocardial infarction, but no difference (0.2% reduction) in mortality at the primary end point after 6 months (Table 34-3; Fig. 34-9). Being the second prospective randomized large-scale trial, this study provided the necessary confirmation of the benefits of an early invasive strategy, which thereby became a grade IA recommendation for treatment of non–ST-elevation acute coronary syndrome in the current guidelines for treatment of acute coronary syndromes.[44]

EXTENT OF CORONARY ARTERY LESIONS

At early coronary angiography in unstable CAD, the extent of major coronary lesions[11,49] is similar to what is observed in ST-elevation myocardial infarction[50,51] and in chronic stable angina (see Fig. 34-2).[52-54] Severe coronary lesions are more common in patients with signs of ischemia at entry (i.e., ST-segment depression)[55,56] (Fig. 34-10) or with signs of myocardial infarction (i.e., elevation of troponin—Fig. 34-11).[11,57,58] Accordingly, there is a rationale for a more aggressive treatment approach and a better effect of an early invasive treatment in these

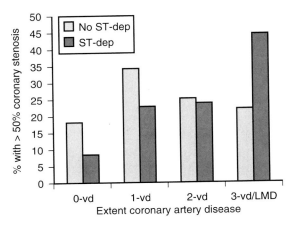

FIGURE 34–10. Extent of coronary artery disease (CAD) in relation to ST-depression in ECG at entry in patients with unstable coronary artery disease in the 1201 patients who underwent early routine coronary angiography in the FRISC II trial. LMD, Left Main Disease; vd, vessel diseased.

patient groups.[4,5] When troponin levels are elevated, more thrombotic material is present at the coronary lesion, which explains the higher risk of new myocardial damage and the better response to mechanical as well as to antithrombotic treatment.[11,57,59-61] Also, other risk

TABLE 34–3   RESULTS OF THE TACTICS TRIAL: DEATH AND/OR MYOCARDIAL INFARCTION (MI) AFTER 6 MONTHS IN THE INVASIVE AND THE NONINVASIVE GROUPS

	INVASIVE (n = 1106)	NONINVASIVE (n = 1114)	RISK RATIO (95% CI)	P
Death and/or MI	81 (7.3%)	77 (9.5%)	0.74 (0.54–1.00)	<0.05
MI	53 (4.8%)	76 (6.9%)	0.67 (0.46–0.96)	0.029
Death	37 (3.3 %)	39 (3.5 %)	0.93 (0.58–1.47)	0.74

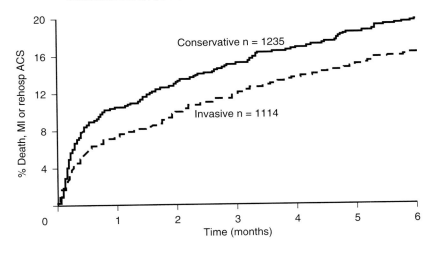

FIGURE 34–9. Death, myocardial infarction (MI), or rehospitalization because of acute coronary syndrome (ACS) in the invasive and conservative arms in the TACTICS trial.

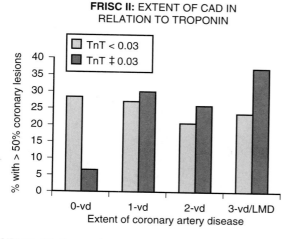

FIGURE 34–11. Extent of coronary artery disease (CAD) in relation to troponin-T (TnT) level at entry in patients with unstable coronary artery disease in the 1201 patients who underwent early routine coronary angiography in the FRISC II trial. LMD, Left Main Disease; vd, vessel diseased.

indicators—such as age (Fig. 34-12), diabetes, previous myocardial infarction, and previous angina—are associated with more severe CAD and thus with a larger benefit from early invasive treatment.[27-29] However, despite similar clinical disease characteristics, females show a consistently higher rate of nonsignificant coronary lesions and less three-vessel and left main disease than do male patients (Fig. 34-13).[62,63] This difference in the severity of coronary lesions contributes to the finding that female patients with unstable CAD experience less benefit of an early invasive strategy than men do.[63]

EFFECTS ON SURVIVAL

It is well established that revascularization with coronary artery bypass surgery is associated with improved sur-

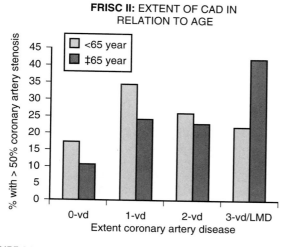

FIGURE 34–12. Extent of coronary artery disease (CAD) in relation to age in patients with unstable coronary artery disease in the 1201 patients who underwent early routine coronary angiography in the FRISC II trial. LMD, Left Main Disease; vd, vessel diseased.

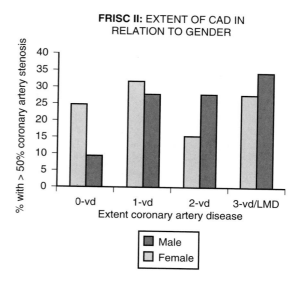

FIGURE 34–13. Extent of coronary artery disease (CAD) in relation to gender in patients with unstable coronary artery disease in the 1201 patients who underwent early routine coronary angiography in the FRISC II trial. LMD, Left Main Disease; vd, vessel diseased.

vival in patients with left main, three-vessel, or two-vessel disease involving the left anterior descending artery.[64,65] Also, exercise testing in patients with ischemia shows that revascularization with coronary artery bypass surgery is associated with improved survival.[46,64] Recent years have seen a series of comparisons between coronary artery bypass surgery and angioplasty in coronary multivessel disease, suggesting the same survival benefits when both methods can be applied.[66-69] In acute ST-elevation myocardial infarction, direct angioplasty is associated with better survival than a pharmacologic approach.[47,48] However, in non–ST-elevation myocardial infarction, early trials showed that an early invasive regimen confers no survival benefits and an even higher mortality rate.[20] In the Veterans Affairs Non–Q-Wave Infarction Strategies in Hospital (VANQWISH) trial, this higher mortality in the invasive group occurred in both those undergoing coronary angiography without later revascularization and those revascularized by coronary artery bypass surgery because of a surprisingly high (11.6% at 30 days) surgical mortality rate.[20] Of course, the lack of current appropriate antithrombotic treatment, with a combination of platelet and coagulation inhibition before and in association with diagnostic and therapeutic invasive procedures, might have contributed to the less favorable outcome in these older trials.

Despite the inherent hazards in all interventional procedures, not least coronary artery bypass surgery, the FRISC II trial showed a sustained reduction in mortality in the invasive group during the whole study period. Thus, despite the raised rate of early procedure-related myocardial infarctions, no early mortality hazard was detected in the invasive group. In the angioplasty cohort, there was only one early death. The 1.7% 30-day mortality rate in the cohort treated with coronary artery bypass surgery in the FRISC II trial was no different from what is observed in patients with chronic stable angina undergoing elective surgery.[70]

However, the TACTICS trial has revealed no corresponding mortality benefit so far. Most of the mortality benefit in the FRISC II trial was probably related to the coronary artery bypass surgery used in patients with left main and three-vessel disease who, according to previous experiences,[64,65,71] experience the highest mortality and the largest benefits of revascularization. Therefore the difference in mortality benefit between the two trials might be related to the higher 30-day mortality rate after coronary artery bypass surgery (3.6%) in the TACTICS trial. This difference in coronary artery bypass surgery complications might be related to the differences in pharmacologic pretreatment or in the time to procedures. Thus, the results of coronary artery bypass surgery in unstable CAD have been best when the surgery is performed after a few days of stabilization on intense antithrombotic and anti-ischemic treatment. Until further experiences have been obtained with other approaches, this should be the recommended approach in left main and three-vessel disease when pharmacologic treatment can bring about clinical stabilization.

EFFECTS ON MYOCARDIAL INFARCTION

It has become obvious that myocardial infarction often should be looked at as an indicator of an underlying disease process rather than as a final event.[72] Thus, spontaneous myocardial infarction usually is caused by a thrombotic occlusion of major coronary artery, leading to severe deterioration of coronary blood flow to an area of the myocardium.[1,73] In contrast, a myocardial infarction associated with coronary angioplasty and stenting usually is caused by distal embolization of material from the dilated lesion,[74] but still the procedure is associated with a substantial improvement of the coronary blood flow to a jeopardized area of the myocardium. The same exists with CABG with an early excess mortality but with better long term prognosis.[72]

It remains unclear whether the myocardial infarction associated with procedures are related to the procedure itself or to more severe underlying disease.[75,76] The immediate clinical consequences and the long-term prognosis of spontaneous and procedure-related myocardial infarction vary. It has been recommended that these events be separated in the reporting of clinical trials because their prevention might have different implications[72] since the MIs in the invasive and non-invasive arms might have different consequences.

In the FRISC II trial, there was a substantial 4.2% absolute and 26% relative reduction in the long-term (2 years) risk of myocardial infarction. However, during the in-hospital phase, there was a higher rate of myocardial infarctions in the invasive arm but a substantially lower risk of spontaneous myocardial infarction subsequently[28] (Fig. 34-14). The limited impact of the procedure-related compared with spontaneous myocardial infarctions was also supported by the lack of any early mortality hazard and the long-term benefit in survival conferred by the invasive treatment.

In the TACTICS trial, there was a difference in myocardial infarction but not in mortality over the first 6

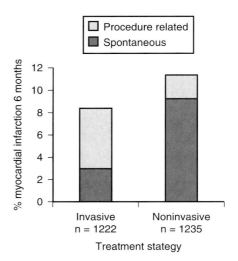

FIGURE 34–14. Spontaneous or procedure-related myocardial infarctions (MIs) during the first year in the invasive and noninvasive arms in the FRISC II trial.

months. The difference in event rate was manifested during the first few weeks and thereafter remained unchanged. One of the assets of the TACTICS trial was the use of the glycoprotein-IIb/IIIa inhibitor tirofiban in all patients during the initial 3 to 4 days and always until and during the early percutaneous invasive procedures. Thus, the early gain in terms of myocardial infarction in this trial probably was related to the use of the glycoprotein-IIb/IIIa inhibitor, which previously had been shown to substantially reduce myocardial infarctions at procedures.[6,10,72,77-79] The lack of later divergence of the event rates in the TACTICS trial might be explained by the high rate of early procedures in the noninvasive arm, leading to a small contrast (60% vs. 36%) in the proportion of patients undergoing revascularization.

Thus, early invasive treatment in unstable CAD substantially reduces the risk of late spontaneous myocardial infarction, recurrent angina, need for hospital readmission, and improves prognosis.

EFFECTS ON SYMPTOMS, LATE REVASCULARIZATION, AND READMISSION

Symptom relief is more rapid and more complete with an invasive rather than a pharmacologic approach in patients with chronic stable angina and with myocardial infarction.[48,80] Similarly, the FRISC II and TACTICS trials demonstrated fewer recurrences of unstable angina in the invasively managed cases of unstable CAD. In the FRISC II trial, there were fewer recurrences of angina, less need for anti-anginal medication, and fewer readmissions and late revascularizations during follow-up (Table 34-4). These benefits were substantiated by exercise tests after 3 months that showed better exercise tolerance, less limitation by anginal pain, and less ischemia

■ ▨ ■

TABLE 34–4 RESULTS OF THE FRISC II TRIAL: SYMPTOMS, READMISSION, AND MEDICATION DURING 6 MONTHS' FOLLOW-UP IN THE INVASIVE VERSUS THE NONINVASIVE GROUPS

	INVASIVE (n = 1106)	NONINVASIVE (n = 1114)	RISK RATIO (95% CI)	P
Angina	22 %	39 %	0.56 (0.50–0.64)	<0.001
CCS III–IV	3 %	7 %	0.38 (0.25–0.56)	<0.001
Readmission	31 %	49 %	0.62 (0.60–0.69)	<0.001
β-Blockade	74 %	84 %	0.88 (0.85–0.92)	<0.001
Long-acting nitrate	17 %	38 %	0.45 (0.39–0.53)	<0.001
Calcium antagonist	18 %	23 %	0.78 (0.67–0.92)	0.003

CCS, Canadian Cardiovascular Score.

compared with the noninvasive group (Fig. 34–15).[81] Furthermore, in the noninvasive group of the FRISC II trial, the average improvement in exercise tolerance and reduction in limiting chest pain and ischemia, which could be seen by comparing exercise tests at discharge and after 3 months, occurred entirely in patients who had undergone revascularization before the second test. In an extensive program, using SF-36 and other established quality-of-life forms, FRISC II trial also demonstrated that the invasive strategy was associated with improvements in all aspects of quality of life as evaluated after 6 and 12 months.[82] In the TACTICS trial, both treatment arms showed a substantial improvement in most aspects in quality of life after 6 months.[83] This better evolution in the TACTICS trial probably reflected the early crossover of 45% of patients to an invasive treatment in the conservative arm versus 65% in the invasive arm. Thus, in addition to an improvement in survival and reduced risk of myocardial infarction, early invasive treatment is also associated with better quality of life, and less need for readmission to the hospital. Approximately 60%

of primarily noninvasively treated patients will need coronary angiography within two years and 50% a revascularization procedure.

WHICH PATIENTS BENEFIT FROM EARLY INVASIVE TREATMENT?

Risk Stratification

It is a general observation that high-risk patients benefit the most from revascularization (Table 34–5). Most prognostic information is already available in the patient's history, with age, male gender, diabetes, previous myocardial infarction, previous severe angina, congestive heart failure, and medication for any of these conditions.[84,85] More severe manifestations of the disease like chest pain during the last 12 to 24 hours, recurrent episodes of pain despite pharmacologic treatment are associated with higher risk. Signs of ischemia (ST-segment depression) on the ECG at entry[86,87] or episodes of ST-depression during continuous monitoring are also related to a worse prognosis.[87-92] Left-ventricular dysfunction, as evaluated by any means, is another observation associated with impaired prognosis.[93,94]

Elevation of biochemical markers of myocardial infarction, i.e., troponin, is now a well-established indicator of increased risk.[95-100] Other biochemical markers of

■ ▨ ■

TABLE 34–5 RISK INDICATORS IN UNSTABLE CORONARY SYNDROME IDENTIFYING PATIENTS WITH HIGHER RISK AND A LARGER BENEFIT OF AN EARLY INVASIVE STRATEGY

Age
Metabolic dysfunction: diabetes mellitus, hypertension
Renal dysfunction: elevated creatinine or reduced clearance
Cardiac dysfunction: left-ventricular dysfunction, elevated B-type natriuretic peptide
Severe coronary artery disease: incapacitating angina, ST-segment depression
Previous myocardial infarction
Coronary thrombosis: ischemic episodes at rest, elevated troponin
Inflammation: elevation of C-reactive protein, fibrinogen, or interleukin-6

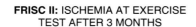

FRISC II: ISCHEMIA AT EXERCISE TEST AFTER 3 MONTHS

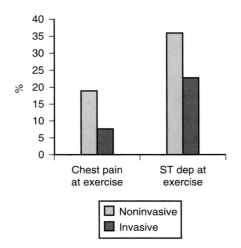

FIGURE 34–15. Signs of ischemia at a symptom-limited exercise test after 3 months in the invasive and noninvasive arms in the FRISC II trial. ST dep, ST depression.

inflammatory activity like C-reactive protein[101-103] and interleukin-6[104] are associated with impaired survival at short-and long-term follow-up. The combination of several of these risk indicators permits more accurate risk stratification than one marker alone. The combination of ST-segment depression as a probable indicator of severe coronary stenosis and elevated troponin as a marker of coronary thrombosis or myocardial infarction provides better prognostic information than either of these indicators alone.[105-108] The addition of a marker of inflammation will further improve risk stratification.[101-104,109]

Multivariate analyses of the various predictions have yielded risk scores of key factors[110,111] that can be readily applicable at hospital admission (see Table 34-5).

Risk Markers in Relation to the Effects of Invasive Treatment

The FRISC II[27,28] and the TACTICS[29] trials showed that the absolute risk reduction of subsequent coronary events was larger in patients at higher risk according to most of the risk indicators (Figs. 34-16 and 34-17). Thus, the invasive treatment was associated with greater relative and absolute benefits in patients older than 65 years and more so in patients older than 70 years. When the waiting list for interventions is long, the elderly patient should often have priority.

Patients with diabetes mellitus have a considerably higher risk of death and new myocardial infarction than nondiabetic patients.[112] The proportional risk reduction is similar in diabetic and nondiabetics, but the absolute risk reduction is larger in diabetic patients (see Figs. 34-16 and 34-17). This finding should be considered in view of previous studies that have described an enhanced risk of periprocedural complications at bypass surgery and less successful results at angioplasty in diabetic patients.[113] Patients with diabetes mellitus and unstable coronary syndrome thus also should be prioritized for early invasive procedures.

Similarly, patients with previous myocardial infarction or left-ventricular dysfunction are at higher risk but are among subgroups that benefit more from an invasive approach.[56] The FRISC II and the TACTICS trial demonstrated that almost all benefits of the invasive strategy were among patients with detectable blood troponin levels (Fig. 34-18). In the FRISC II trial, most (82%) of patients had detectable troponin I levels[114,115] (see Fig. 34-18). A linear relation exists between the level of troponin and mortality.[103,116] Thus, in the prioritization of patients for invasive procedures, any detectable troponin supports an invasive approach, the urgency of the procedure increasing the higher are the troponin levels. Patients with no detectable troponin are at very low risk and gain little if nothing from invasive procedures unless indicated by incapacitating symptoms of angina.

The relative risk reduction is within the same range in patients with and without elevated C-reactive protein and fibrinogen levels, resulting in a greater absolute risk

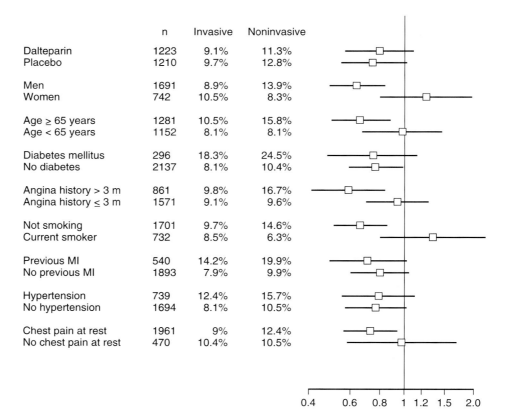

FIGURE 34–16. Death or myocardial infarction (MI) after 6 months in subgroups based on clinical baseline characteristics in the invasive and noninvasive arms in the FRISC II trial.

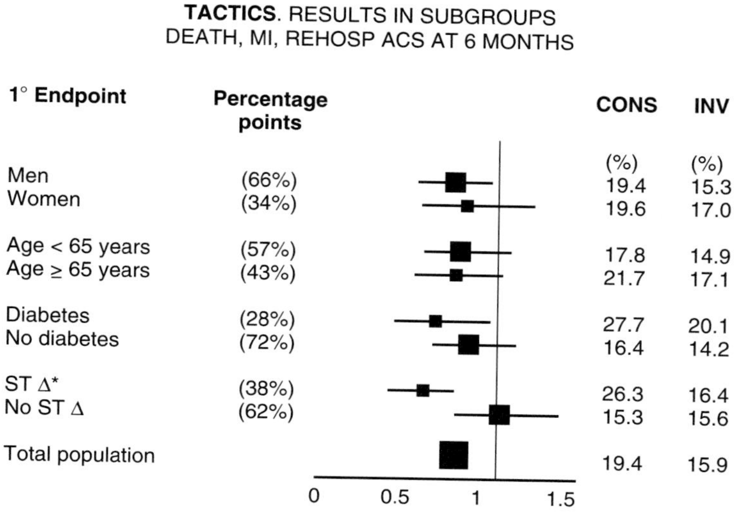

TACTICS. RESULTS IN SUBGROUPS
DEATH, MI, REHOSP ACS AT 6 MONTHS
1° Endpoint
Percentage points
CONS
INV
(%)
(%)
Men
(66%)
19.4
15.3
Women
(34%)
19.6
17.0
Age < 65 years
(57%)
17.8
14.9
Age ≥ 65 years
(43%)
21.7
17.1
Diabetes
(28%)
27.7
20.1
No diabetes
(72%)
16.4
14.2
ST Δ*
(38%)
26.3
16.4
No ST Δ
(62%)
15.3
15.6
Total population
19.4
15.9
0
0.5
1
1.5

FIGURE 34–17. Death, myocardial infarction (MI), or rehospitalization (REHOSP) because of acute coronary syndrome in subgroups based on clinical baseline characteristics in the invasive and noninvasive arms in the TACTICS trial. CONS, conservative strategy; INV, invasive strategy.

when these levels are elevated. In the FRISC II study, the initial level of interleukin-6 was a better marker of a higher mortality in the total population and of benefit of early invasive treatment (Fig. 34—19).[104]

Risk Scores in Relation to the Effects of Early Invasive Treatment

Using combinations of various markers, the TACTICS and the FRISC II trials demonstrated that the main benefit of invasive strategy occurred in patients with elevated troponin levels, especially in those who also demonstrated ST-segment depression. This categorization is modulated, however, by the other factors, such as age, diabetes, previous myocardial infarction, left-ventricular dysfunction, severity of previous and current symptoms, medication for angina, and markers of inflammatory activity (Fig. 34-20).[117]

Accordingly, risk scores were developed to account for these factors. Patients with high scores benefit most from invasive management with a gradient between benefit and the score (Fig. 34-21).[29] An early invasive treatment, with its inherent risk of complications, does not reduce risk in patients with lower risk scores. Yet, revascularization may still be performed in some of these patients with incapacitating symptoms. In these cases, the interventions are not urgent (Fig. 34-22).[27]

Stress Tests for Risk Stratification

Provocative testing is performed in patients stable on medical management to unveil a higher risk stratification.[55,118-122] Tests usually require that the patient has been free from episodes of chest pain and ECG signs of ischemia for at least 24 hours. Furthermore, there should be no indication from the biochemical markers of an ongoing myocardial infarction over the last 48 hours, implying in practice that the creatinine kinase MB levels are back to normal. Finally, the patient should have no signs of hemodynamic compromise or congestive heart failure.

FRISC II
% death or MI at 12 months
50
45
40
35
30
25
20
15
10
5
0
p = NS
p = 0.004
n = 439
n = 2088
TnI < 0.02
TnI ≥ 0.02
INV
CONS
TACTICS
% death, MI rehosp ACS 6 months
30
25
20
15
10
5
0
p = NS
P < 0.001
N = 414 396
463 495
TnI < 0.01
TnT ≥ 0.01
INV
CONS

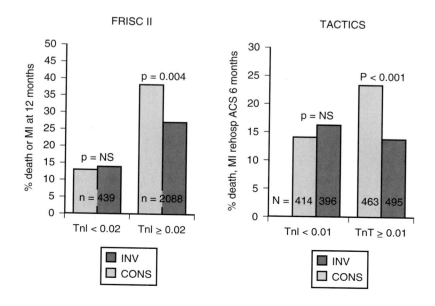

FIGURE 34–18. Effects of an early invasive strategy in relation to elevation of troponin in the FRISC II and TACTICS trials. ACS, acute coronary syndrome; CONS, conservative strategy; INV, invasive strategy; MI, myocardial infarction; TnI, troponin I; TnT, troponin T.

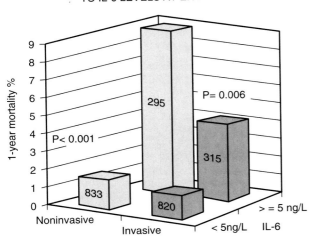

FRISC II 1-YEAR MORTALITY IN RELATION
TO IL-6 LEVELS AT ENTRY

FIGURE 34–19. 1-year mortality in the invasive and noninvasive arm in subgroups based on elevation of the interleukin-6 (IL-6) level at entry in the FRISC II trial.

The provocative test usually is performed on a treadmill according to the Bruce protocol or by bicycle ergometry in order to evaluate the occurrence of ischemia and also the exercise tolerance and limiting symptoms. Reversible ischemia is diagnosed by ST-segment deviations on continuous 12-lead ECG recordings and, if available, by the radionuclide scintigraphy. High risk is defined by either large or multiple areas of exercise-induced myocardial ischemia or low exercise tolerance because of ischemia or an inadequate blood pressure response to exercise. Low risk is defined by adequate exercise tolerance without any definite signs of exercise-induced ischemia. Accordingly, the intermedi-

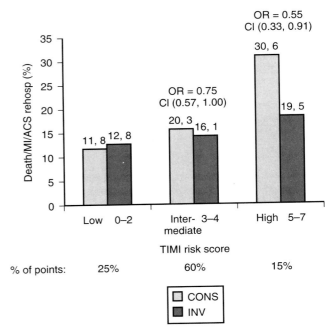

TACTICS: OUTCOME IN RELATION
TO TIMI UA RISK SCORE

FIGURE 34–21. Outcome in relation to the multivariate TIMI unstable angina (UA) risk score in the TACTICS trial. ACS, acute coronary syndrome; CI, confidence interval; CONS, conservative strategy; INV, invasive strategy; MI, myocardial infarction; OR, odds ratio.

ate group consists of patients with findings that are in between. In the high-risk category, early catheterization and revascularization are clearly indicated because the findings are highly associated with multivessel or left main CAD.[64,65] In the low-risk category, no early invasive procedures are usually indicated because the procedural risks are greater than the potential future benefits.[25,122] Decisions in the intermediate-risk category are supported by clinical judgment.

Coronary Angiography for Early Risk Stratification and Selection of Treatment

Coronary angiography often provides the most reliable information on risk stratification. It permits the characterization of the culprit lesion, the extent of CAD, the area at risk, and left-ventricular function. Among patients with ST-T changes or elevation of blood markers, 10% have left main disease, 25% three-vessel disease, 25% two-vessel disease, 25% one-vessel disease, and 15% no significant disease (see Fig. 34–2). Age, male gender, diabetes, previous myocardial infarction, previous severe angina, troponin, and a high risk stress test are associated with a higher incidence of left main and three-vessel disease (see Figs. 34–10 through 34–13). The relation between these risk indicators and the extent of CAD remains, however, not perfect as some patients with severe coronary lesions may not be identified by any of these risk indicators. Thus, from the perspective of individual patients, it could be preferable to obtain coronary

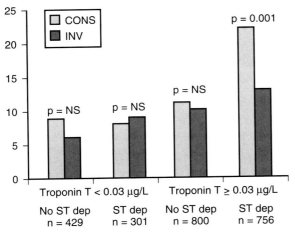

FRISC II: DEATH/MI AT 12 MONTHS IN RELATION
TO TROPONIN-T AND ST-DEPRESSION

FIGURE 34–20. Death or myocardial infarction (MI) after 12 months in subgroups based elevation of troponin and occurrence of ST-depression in ECG at entry in the invasive and noninvasive arms in the FRISC II trial. CONS, conservative strategy; INV, invasive strategy; p, p-value.

FRISC II: ANGINA IN SUBGROUPS AT 6 MONTHS

	n	Invasive	Noninvasive
Dalteparin	1189	22%	40%
Placebo	1162	29%	37%
Men	1632	19%	36%
Women	719	28%	44%
Age ‡°65 years	1224	21%	40%
Age < 65 years	1127	23%	38%
Diabetes mellitus	268	24%	41%
No diabetes	2083	22%	38%
Angina history > 3 m	822	25%	45%
Angina history † 3 m	1528	20%	35%
Smoker	713	24%	38%
Not smoking	1638	21%	39%
Previous MI	511	25%	38%
No previous MI	1840	21%	39%
Hypertension	706	25%	40%
No hypertension	1645	20%	38%
Chest pain at rest	1894	23%	39%
No chest pain at rest	456	16%	37%
TnT ‡°0.1 ug/L	1286	21%	35%
TnT < 0.1 ug/L	951	24%	43%
ST dep at inclusion	1050	22%	37%
No ST dep at inclusion	1257	22%	40%

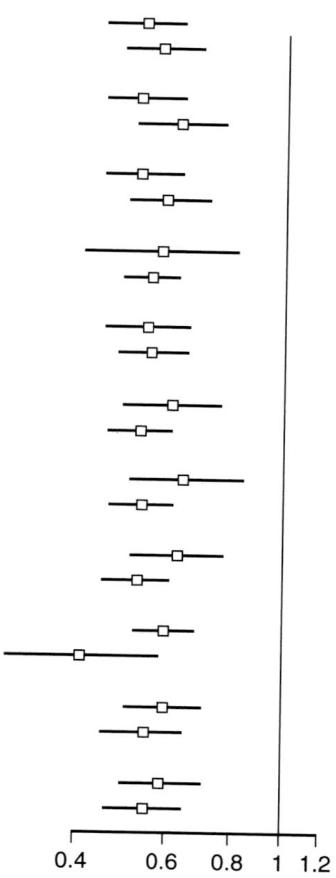

0.4   0.6   0.8   1 1.2

FIGURE 34–22. Symptoms of angina at 6 months in subgroups based on clinical baseline characteristics in the invasive and noninvasive arms in the FRISC II trial. MI, myocardial infarction; TnT, troponin T.

angiography and noninvasive risk indicators as a basis for a decision of early revascularization.

A possible disadvantage of such an approach is that all significant lesions identified at coronary angiography could be dilated and stented during the procedure regardless of other risk indicators. In the invasive arm of the FRISC II trial, the extent of CAD was not related to subsequent coronary events, what could suggest that the early invasive procedure reduces the risk associated with severe coronary lesions. These findings support a recommendation of routine early coronary angiography in the majority of patients with unstable CAD in order to identify severe coronary lesions that could be corrected by early revascularization. The markers of inflammatory activity do not correlate with the extent of underlying CAD but are nevertheless predictors of future mortality suggesting that various mechanisms could influence prognosis. Early intervention was also useful in these patients, indicating that alleviating ischemia and/or crushing the plaque can help.

Gender and Selection of Invasive Treatment

Unstable coronary artery syndromes are more frequent in men than in women. Approximately 70% of patients enrolled in clinical trials are men. Women have more frequently no CAD despite similar diagnostic criteria. When they have CAD, they are older than men[62,63] and have a similar extent of the disease.[63]

The FRISC II trial showed a significantly better benefit of the invasive strategy in men than in women. This could be partly explained by less frequent revascularization in women in the invasive group but less frequent CAD. Also, the associated with early coronary artery bypass surgery was higher in women particularly when they had diabetes or were older.[63] In contrast, the TACTICS trial showed no gender difference in benefit of the early invasive treatment.[29]

The discordance in results could be artificial since men had an unusually low periprocedural mortality rate for coronary artery bypass surgery, whereas women had an unusually high rate. The periprocedural risks associated with angioplasty procedures were similar in both genders. Leveling would give similar results. To properly evaluate women with unstable coronary syndromes, it seems preferable to employ the same angiographic indicators as are used in men. However, in the selection of the most appropriate treatment, the higher risk in women undergoing coronary bypass surgery should be considered.[63,123,124]

HOW DO PATIENTS BENEFIT FROM EARLY INVASIVE TREATMENT?

Complete Revascularization

Patients with unstable coronary syndromes demonstrate the same extent of CAD as patients with chronic stable angina and ST-elevation myocardial infarction, i.e., approximately 10% left main disease, 25% three-vessel, 25% two-vessel, 25% one-vessel, and 15% no significant CAD (see Fig. 34–2).[11,62] A culprit lesion with severe stenosis and signs of plaque rupture and intracoronary thrombus is usually identified.[49,125-127] Intracoronary thrombi are more common in patients with troponin elevation.[11,57,58] Approximately 25% of cases show a greater than 90% stenosis or total occlusion of the culprit artery with some collateral blood flow supplying the jeopardized myocardium.

Strategy for early revascularization procedures in patients with unstable coronary syndromes have evolved with time. Some years ago, angioplasty was restricted to the culprit lesions to avoid the hazards of multiple procedures. With the new catheterization materials, routine and effective platelet inhibition, the risks of multilesion and multivessel percutaneous coronary interventions have been substantially reduced.[128] The same holds true for CABG.[129] Therefore, the preferred strategy at the present time is complete revascularization. This strategy was used successfully in both the FRISC II and the TACTICS. It improves survival and survival without myocardial infarction provides more complete symptom relief, decreases readmission, late revascularization, and improves the cost/benefit ratio.

Coronary Stenting and Glycoprotein-IIb/IIIa Inhibition

Recruitment in the FRISC II trial was performed between 1996 and 1998 and in the TACTICS trial between 1998 and 1999 influencing best therapy. Thus, coronary stenting was available in both trials. Glycoprotein-IIb/IIIa platelet inhibition was however used in only 10% of interventions in the FRISC II trial but in all patients in the TACTICS trial. Coated stents to prevent restenosis were not then available.[130] Thus, in both the FRISC II and the TACTICS trials, percutaneous coronary intervention was the preferred technology for one-to two-vessel disease and was used in 80% of patients, whereas the majority of patients with three-vessel or left main stem disease had CABG.

Coronary Artery Bypass Surgery

The 30-day mortality rates were low, 1.7% in the FRISC II trial and 3.6% in the TACTICS trial. The higher surgical mortality rate in the TACTICS trial could be explained by differences in patients characteristics between the two trials. It could also be related to the timing of surgery, a median of 89 hours after the acute event in the TACTICS trial and of 8 days in the FRISC II trial. Very early bypass surgery in unstable coronary syndromes or acute myocardial infarction has been associated with higher mortality than in elective coronary artery bypass surgery.[20,42,43] This could be because of better plaque passivation, or healed myocardium. In the FRISC-II study, a combination treatment with aspirin, low-molecular-weight heparin, β-blockade, nitrates, and often angiotensin-converting enzyme inhibitors and statins was used up to the time of CABG. Therefore, antithrombotic pretreatment should be preferred when surgery is needed.[131,132] This holds true even if CABG is delayed for more than 7 days.

Antithrombotic Pretreatment

Older less successful studies of early revascularization in unstable coronary syndromes have used no adequate antithrombotic treatment before, during, or after the procedure. The VANQWISH trial,[20] in patients with non–ST-elevation myocardial infarction, did not routinely use continuous heparin infusion. Glycoprotein-IIb/IIIa inhibition, and clopidogrel were then unavailable.

Pretreatment with a low molecular weight heparin likely contributed to the low complication rate associated with early coronary artery bypass surgery in the FRISC-II trial[27], and with a glycoprotein-IIb/IIIa inhibitor with the low event rate associated with DCI in the TACTICS trial.[10,77,78,133,134] Myocardial infarction related to procedures has a negative impact on long term prognosis.

Bivalirudin has been approved as an alternative anticoagulant to unfractionated heparin during angioplasty procedures, Bivalirudin provides dose-related anticoagulant with smaller variation in activated partial thromboplastin time than with unfractionated heparin. In an angioplasty trial, the subgroup of patients with non–ST-elevation myocardial infarction, had greater benefit of bivalirudin and a lower risk of thrombotic events compared with unfractionated heparin.[135,136] As more data on the combination of bivalirudin with clopidogrel and glycoprotein-IIb/IIIa inhibitors become available, bivalirudin might replace unfractionated heparin during the acute phase of unstable CAD.[135,136]

Low-molecular-weight heparin is well-documented as effective treatment in the acute phase of unstable CAD. Unfractionated heparin was, however, used at the time of angioplasty and CABG in both the FRISC-2 and TACTICS trials. Recent registry observations have suggested that a low molecular weight heparin could be a valid substitute to unfractionated heparin.[137,138] It also seems that glycoprotein-IIb/IIIa inhibition can be combined with low-molecular-weight heparin with no excess bleeding and, possibly, better efficacy.[139,140]

WHEN SHOULD PATIENTS UNDERGO EARLY INVASIVE PROCEDURES?

In unstable CAD, the risk of new events is highest during the first hours and days after the acute event and tapers off over the following 2 to 3 months. In patients who have not undergone revascularization, 40% of new events occur during the first 2 weeks, 40% between 2 weeks and 6 months, and 20% between 6 and 12 months.[27,141] Thus, treatment should be applied early with aspirin, a low-molecular weight heparin or unfractionated heparin and, also, with a glycoprotein-IIb/IIIa antagonist if an intervention is contemplated.[4,5,44] A glycoprotein-IIb/IIIa antagonist with a short half-life is preferred.

With this pharmacologic approach, the diagnostic coronary angiography and associated catheter-based interventions can be performed within the initial 24 hours without undue risk.[29] In high-risk patients who cannot be adequately revascularized by angioplasty, the combination treatment with aspirin, low-molecular-weight or unfractionated heparin, and a glycoprotein-IIb/IIIa inhibitor with a short half-life should be continued until coronary bypass surgery is undertaken. The gains derived by reducing time to CABG is a delicate decision, weighing risk versus benefit, a delicate balance with the periprocedural risks that must be accounted for in terms of the timing of catheter-based and surgical revascularization.

SECONDARY PREVENTION

Before and after revascularization, patients with an acute coronary syndrome should be prescribed secondary preventive treatment with aspirin, β-adrenoceptor blockade, cholesterol lowering agents with statins, and angiotensin-converting enzyme inhibitors, unless contraindicated.[4,5] After percutaneous coronary interventions, which usually are associated with stenting, clopidogrel should be used for at least 1 month.[142] In patients with multivessel CAD or other indicators of a high risk of recurrence (e.g., diabetes mellitus, previous myocardial infarction, previous revascularization), prolonged treatment with clopidogrel in addition to aspirin seems prudent after bypass surgery as well as after percutaneous coronary interventions.[143]

COST EFFICACY

From a 1-year perspective, the FRISC II strategy of routine catheterization and, if appropriate, revascularization, was associated with higher costs than a strategy of invasive procedures only with severe ischemia or recurrent myocardial infarction.[144] However, the costs of the invasive strategy could have been shortened by performing invasive procedures within the first 48 hours after. The TACTICS trial detected no cost differences comparing routine early catheterization with a nonroutine catheterization strategy with earlier revascularization procedures.[145] Thus, considering that in 40% to 50% of patients there will be a need for revascularization within a year, the early invasive strategy is cost-effective, especially if performed without undue delay. This approach will be favored by patients because their initial hospital stay is shortened, the risk of new events and readmissions reduced, and quality and quantity of life improved.

REFERENCES

1. Theroux P, Fuster V: Acute coronary syndromes: Unstable angina and non-Q-wave myocardial infarction. Circulation 1998;97:1195-1206.
2. Falk E, Shah PK, Fuster V: Coronary plaque disruption. Circulation 1995;92:657-671.
3. Davies M: Stability and instability—Two faces of coronary atherosclerosis. Circulation 1996;94:2013-2020.
4. Bertrand ME, Simoons ML, Fox KA, et al: Management of acute coronary syndromes: Acute coronary syndromes without persistent ST segment elevation—Recommendations of the Task Force of the European Society of Cardiology. Eur Heart J 2000;21: 1406-1432.
5. Braunwald E, Antman EM, Beasley JW, et al: ACC/AHA guidelines for the management of patients with unstable angina and non-ST-segment elevation myocardial infarction. A report of the American College of Cardiology/American Heart Association Task Force on Practice Guidelines (Committee on the Management of Patients With Unstable Angina). J Am Coll Cardiol 2000;36:970-1062.
6. Boersma E, Harrington R, Moliterno D, et al: Platelet glycoprotein IIb/IIIa inhibitors in acute coronary syndromes. A meta-analysis of all randomised clinical trials that enrolled over 1000 patients. Lancet 2001;357:1905-1914.
7. Yusuf S, Zhao F, Mehta S, et al: The Clopidogrel in Unstable Angina to Prevent Recurrent Events Trial Investigators. Effects of clopidogrel in addition to aspirin in patients with acute coronary syndromes without ST-segment elevation. N Engl J Med 2001;345: 494-502.
8. Wallentin L: Low molecular weight heparin in unstable coronary artery disease. Expert Opin Investig Drugs 2000;9:581-592.
9. Cohen M: Update on the management of acute coronary syndromes. Cardiology 2000;93:210-219.
10. CAPTURE Investigators: Randomised placebo-controlled trial of abciximab before and during coronary intervention in refractory unstable angina—the CAPTURE Study. Lancet 1997;349: 1429-1435.
11. Lindahl B, Diderholm E, Lagerqvist B, et al: Mechanisms behind the prognostic value of troponin T in unstable coronary artery disease: A FRISC II substudy. J Am Coll Cardiol 2001;38:979-986.
12. Theroux P, Waters D, Lam J, et al: Reactivation of unstable angina after the discontinuation of heparin. N Engl J Med 1992;327: 141-145.
13. FRISC Study Group: Low-molecular-weight heparin during instability in coronary artery disease, Fragmin during Instability in Coronary Artery Disease (FRISC) study group. Lancet 1996;347:561-568.
14. TRIM Study Group: A low molecular weight, selective thrombin inhibitor, inogatran, vs heparin, in unstable coronary artery disease in 1209 patients. A double-blind, randomized, dose-finding study. Eur Heart J 1997;18:1416-1425.
15. Anderson HV, Gibson RS, Stone PH, et al: Management of unstable angina pectoris and non-Q-wave acute myocardial infarction in the United States and Canada (the TIMI III Registry). Am J Cardiol 1997;79:1441-1446.
16. Yusuf S, Flather M, Pogue J, et al: Variations between countries in invasive cardiac procedures and outcomes in patients with suspected unstable angina or myocardial infarction without initial ST elevation. OASIS (Organisation to Assess Strategies for Ischaemic Syndromes) Registry Investigators. Lancet 1998;352:507-514.
17. Scull GS, Martin JS, Weaver WD, Every NR: Early angiography versus conservative treatment in patients with non-ST elevation acute myocardial infarction: MITI Investigators. Myocardial Infarction Triage and Intervention. J Am Coll Cardiol 2000;35:895-902.
18. Michalis LK, Stroumbis CS, Pappas K, et al: Treatment of refractory unstable angina in geographically isolated areas without cardiac surgery. Invasive versus conservative strategy (TRUCS study). Eur Heart J 2000;21:1954-1959.
19. Scott SM, Deupree RH, Sharma GV, Luchi RJ: VA Study of Unstable Angina. 10-year results show duration of surgical advantage for patients with impaired ejection fraction. Circulation 1994;90(Part 2):120-123.
20. Boden WE, O'Rourke RA, Crawford MH, et al: Outcomes in patients with acute non-Q-wave myocardial infarction randomly assigned to an invasive as compared with a conservative management strategy. Veterans Affairs Non-Q-Wave Infarction Strategies in Hospital

(VANQWISH) Trial Investigators [see comments]. N Engl J Med 1998;338:1785-1792.

21. TIMI IIIB Investigators: Effects of tissue plasminogen activator and a comparison of early invasive and conservative strategies in unstable angina and non-Q-wave myocardial infarction. Results of the TIMI IIIB Trial. Circulation 1994;89:1545-1556.

22. Anderson HV, Cannon CP, Stone PH, et al: One-year results of the Thrombolysis in Myocardial Infarction (TIMI) IIIB clinical trial. A randomized comparison of tissue-type plasminogen activator versus placebo and early invasive versus early conservative strategies in unstable angina and non-Q wave myocardial infarction. J Am Coll Cardiol 1995;26:1643-1650.

23. Steg PG, Himbert D, Seknadji P: Revascularization of patients with unstable coronary artery disease: The case for early intervention. Am J Cardiol 1997;80:45E-50E.

24. Verheugt FW: Acute coronary syndromes: Interventions. Lancet 1999;353(Suppl 2): 16-19.

25. Boden WE: Avoidance of routine revascularization in the management of patients with non-ST-segment elevation acute coronary syndromes. Am J Cardiol 2000;86:42M-47M.

26. Pepine CJ: An ischemia-guided approach for risk stratification in patients with acute coronary syndromes. Am J Cardiol 2000;86: 27M-35M.

27. FRISC-II Investigators: Invasive compared with non-invasive treatment in unstable coronary-artery disease: FRISC II prospective randomised multicentre study. FRagmin and Fast Revascularisation during InStability in Coronary artery disease Investigators. Lancet 1999;354:708-715.

28. Wallentin L, Lagerqvist B, Husted S, et al: Outcome at 1 year after an invasive compared with a non-invasive strategy in unstable coronary-artery disease: The FRISC II invasive randomised trial. FRISC II Investigators. Fast Revascularisation during Instability in Coronary artery disease. Lancet 2000;356:9-16.

29. Cannon CP, Weintraub WS, Demopoulos LA, et al: Comparison of early invasive and conservative strategies in patients with unstable coronary syndromes treated with the glycoprotein IIb/IIIa inhibitor tirofiban. N Engl J Med 2001;344:1879-1887.

30. Stamou SC, Corso PJ: Coronary revascularization without cardiopulmonary bypass in high-risk patients: A route to the future. Ann Thorac Surg 2001;71:1056-1061.

31. Smith KM, Lamy A, Arthur HM, et al: Outcomes and costs of coronary artery bypass grafting: comparison between octogenarians and septuagenarians at a tertiary care centre. Canadian Medical Association Journal 2001;165:759-764.

32. Grover FL, Shroyer AL, Hammermeister K, et al: A decade's experience with quality improvement in cardiac surgery using the Veterans Affairs and Society of Thoracic Surgeons national databases. Ann Surg 2001;234:464-472; Discussion, 472-474.

33. Bourassa MG: Clinical trials of coronary revascularization: Coronary angioplasty vs. coronary bypass grafting. Curr Opin Cardiol 2000; 15:281-286.

34. Mercado N, Boersma E, Wijns W, et al: Clinical and quantitative coronary angiographic predictors of coronary restenosis: A comparative analysis from the balloon-to-stent era. J Am Coll Cardiol 2001;38:645-652.

35. Hofma SH, van Beusekom HM, Serruys PW, van Der Giessen WJ: Recent developments in coated stents. Curr Interv Cardiol Rep 2001;3:28-36.

36. Serruys PW, Kay IP: Benestent II, a remake of benestent I? Or a step towards the era of stentoplasty? Eur Heart J 1999;20:779-781.

37. Lincoff AM, Califf RM, Topol EJ: Platelet glycoprotein IIb/IIIa receptor blockade in coronary artery disease. J Am Coll Cardiol 2000;35:1103-1115.

38. Ross AM: The role of coronary angioplasty in the management of unstable angina pectoris. Am J Cardiol 1991;68:58C-60C.

39. Gunnar RM, Bourdillon PD, Dixon DW, et al: ACC/AHA guidelines for the early management of patients with acute myocardial infarction. A report of the American College of Cardiology/American Heart Association Task Force on Assessment of Diagnostic and Therapeutic Cardiovascular Procedures (subcommittee to develop guidelines for the early management of patients with acute myocardial infarction). Circulation 1990;82:664-707.

40. The American College of Cardiology/American Heart Association Task Force on Practice Guidelines (Committee on Management of Acute Myocardial Infarction): ACC/AHA Guidelines for the management of patients with acute myocardial infarction. J Am Coll Cardiol 1996;28:1328-1428.

41. Stomel RJ, Kovack PJ: Unstable angina: Clinical practice guidelines for diagnosis and management. Agency for Health Care Policy and Research. J Am Osteopath Assoc 1995;95:45-51.

42. ACC/AHA Guidelines and Indications for Coronary Artery Bypass Graft Surgery: A report of the American College of Cardiology/ American Heart Association Task Force on Assessment of Diagnostic and Therapeutic Cardiovascular Procedures (Subcommittee on Coronary Artery Bypass Graft Surgery). Circulation 1991; 83:1125-1173.

43. Eagle KA, Guyton RA, Davidoff R, et al: ACC/AHA Guidelines for Coronary Artery Bypass Graft Surgery: A Report of the American College of Cardiology/American Heart Association Task Force on Practice Guidelines (Committee to Revise the 1991 Guidelines for Coronary Artery Bypass Graft Surgery). American College of Cardiology/American Heart Association. J Am Coll Cardiol 1999;34:1262-1347.

44. Hamm CW, Bertrand M, Braunwald E: Acute coronary syndrome without ST elevation: Implementation of new guidelines. Lancet 2001;358:1533-1538.

45. de Feyter PJ, Serruys PW, Suryapranata H, et al: Coronary angioplasty early after diagnosis of unstable angina. Am Heart J 1987;114(Part 1):48-54.

46. Madsen JK, Grande P, Saunamaki K, et al: Danish multicenter randomized study of invasive versus conservative treatment in patients with inducible ischemia after thrombolysis in acute myocardial infarction (DANAMI). DANish trial in Acute Myocardial Infarction. Circulation 1997;96:748-755.

47. Michels KB, Yusuf S: Does PTCA in acute myocardial infarction affect mortality and reinfarction rates? A quantitative overview (meta-analysis) of the randomized clinical trials [see comments]. Circulation 1995;91:476-485.

48. Weaver WD, Simes RJ, Betriu A, et al: Comparison of primary coronary angioplasty and intravenous thrombolytic therapy for acute myocardial infarction: A quantitative review [see comments]. JAMA 1997;278:2093-2098.

49. Diver DJ, Bier JD, Ferreira PE, et al: Clinical and arteriographic characterization of patients with unstable angina without critical coronary arterial narrowing (from the TIMI-IIIA Trial). Am J Cardiol 1994;74:531-537.

50. GUSTO Angiographic Investigators: The effects of tissue plasminogen activator, streptokinase, or both on coronary-artery patency, ventricular function, and survival after acute myocardial infarction. N Engl J Med 1993;329:1615-1622.

51. GUSTO IIb Angioplasty Substudy Investigators: A clinical trial comparing primary coronary angioplasty with tissue plasminogen activator for acute myocardial infarction. The Global Use of Strategies to Open Occluded Coronary Arteries in Acute Coronary Syndromes. N Engl J Med 1997;336:1621-1628.

52. Gibbons RJ, Chatterjee K, Daley J, et al: ACC/AHA/ACP-ASIM guidelines for the management of patients with chronic stable angina: a report of the American College of Cardiology/American Heart Association Task Force on Practice Guidelines (Committee on Management of Patients With Chronic Stable Angina). J Am Coll Cardiol 1999;33:2092-2197.

53. Williams SV, Fihn SD, Gibbons RJ: Guidelines for the management of patients with chronic stable angina: Diagnosis and risk stratification. Ann Intern Med 2001;135:530-547.

54. Cianflone D, Ciccirillo F, Buffon A, et al: Comparison of coronary angiographic narrowing in stable angina pectoris, unstable angina pectoris, and in acute myocardial infarction. Am J Cardiol 1995;76:215-219.

55. Karlsson JE, Bjorkholm A, Nylander E, et al: ST-changes in ECG at rest or during exercise indicate a high risk of severe coronary lesions after an episode of unstable coronary artery disease. Int J Cardiol 1993;42:47-55.

56. Diderholm E, Andren B, Frostfeldt G, et al: ST depression in ECG at entry indicates severe coronary lesions and large benefits of an early invasive treatment strategy in unstable coronary artery disease. The FRISC II ECG substudy. Eur Heart J 2002;23:41-49.

57. Heeschen C, van Den Brand MJ, Hamm CW, Simoons ML: Angiographic findings in patients with refractory unstable angina according to troponin T status. Circulation 1999;100:1509-1514.

58. Jurlander B, Farhi ER, Banas JJ Jr, et al: Coronary angiographic findings and troponin T in patients with unstable angina pectoris. Am J Cardiol 2000;85:810-814.

59. Lindahl B, Venge P, Wallentin L: Troponin T identifies patients with unstable coronary artery disease who benefit from long-term

antithrombotic protection. Fragmin in Unstable Coronary Artery Disease (FRISC) Study Group. J Am Coll Cardiol 1997;29: 43–48.

60. Hamm C, Heeschen C, Goldmann B, et al: Benefit of abciximab in patients with refractory unstable angina in relation to serum troponin T levels. c7E3 Fab Antiplatelet Therapy in Unstable Refractory Angina (CAPTURE) Study Investigators. N Engl J Med 1999;340:1623–1629.

61. Morrow DA, Antman EM, Tanasijevic M, et al: Cardiac troponin I for stratification of early outcomes and the efficacy of enoxaparin in unstable angina: A TIMI-IIB substudy. J Am Coll Cardiol 2000;36:1812–1817.

62. Hochman JS, McCabe CH, Stone PH, et al: Outcome and profile of women and men presenting with acute coronary syndromes: A report from TIMI IIIB. TIMI Investigators. Thrombolysis in Myocardial Infarction. J Am Coll Cardiol 1997;30:141–148.

63. Lagerqvist B, Safstrom K, Stahle E, et al: Is early invasive treatment of unstable coronary artery disease equally effective for both women and men? FRISC II Study Group Investigators. J Am Coll Cardiol 2001;38:41–48.

64. Varnauskas E: Twelve-year follow-up of survival in the randomized European Coronary Surgery Study. N Engl J Med 1988;319: 332–337.

65. Yusuf S, Zucker D, Peduzzi P, et al: Effect of coronary artery bypass graft surgery on survival: Overview of 10-year results from randomised trials by the Coronary Artery Bypass Graft Surgery Trialists Collaboration [see comments] [published erratum appears in Lancet 1994;344:1446]. Lancet 1994;344:563–570.

66. Hamm CW, Reimers J, Ischinger T, et al: A randomized study of coronary angioplasty compared with bypass surgery in patients with symptomatic multivessel coronary disease. German Angioplasty Bypass Surgery Investigation (GABI). N Engl J Med 1994;331: 1037–1043.

67. Wahrborg P: Quality of life after coronary angioplasty or bypass surgery: 1-Year follow-up in the Coronary Angioplasty versus Bypass Revascularization Investigation (CABRI) trial. Eur Heart J 1999;20:653–658.

68. Henderson RA, Pocock SJ, Sharp SJ, et al: Long-term results of RITA-1 trial: clinical and cost comparisons of coronary angioplasty and coronary-artery bypass grafting. Randomised Intervention Treatment of Angina. Lancet 1998;352:1419–1425.

69. Berger PB, Velianou JL, Aslanidou Vlachos H, et al: Survival following coronary angioplasty versus coronary artery bypass surgery in anatomic subsets in which coronary artery bypass surgery improves survival compared with medical therapy. Results from the Bypass Angioplasty Revascularization Investigation (BARI). J Am Coll Cardiol 2001;38:1440–1449.

70. Brorsson B, Lindvall B, Bernstein S, Aberg T: CABG in chronic stable angina pectoris patients—Indications and outcomes (SECOR/SBU). Swedish Societies for Cardiology, Thoracic Radiology and Thoracic Surgery/Swedish Council for Technology Assessment in Health Care. Eur J Cardiothorac Surg 1997;12: 746–752.

71. Rahimtoola S, Fessler C, Grunkemeier G, Starr A: Survival 15 to 20 years after coronary bypass surgery for angina. J Am Coll Cardiol 1993;21:151–157.

72. ACC/ESC Committee for the Redefinition of Myocardial Infarction. Myocardial infarction redefined—A consensus document of the Joint European Society of Cardiology/American College of Cardiology. Eur Heart J 2000;21:1502–1513.

73. Falk E: Coronary thrombosis—Pathogenesis and clinical manifestations. Am J Cardiol 1991;68:28B–35B.

74. Simoons ML, van den Brand M, Lincoff M, et al: Minimal myocardial damage during coronary intervention is associated with impaired outcome. Eur Heart J 1999;20:1112–1119.

75. Tardiff BE, Califf RM, Tcheng JE, et al: Clinical outcomes after detection of elevated cardiac enzymes in patients undergoing percutaneous intervention. IMPACT-II Investigators. Integrilin (eptifibatide) to Minimize Platelet Aggregation and Coronary Thrombosis-II. J Am Coll Cardiol 1999;33:88–96.

76. Alexander JH, Sparapani RA, Mahaffey KW, et al: Association between minor elevations of creatine kinase-MB level and mortality in patients with acute coronary syndromes without ST-segment elevation. PURSUIT Steering Committee. Platelet Glycoprotein IIb/IIIa in Unstable Angina: Receptor Suppression Using Integrilin Therapy. JAMA 2000;283:347–353.

77. EPIC Investigators: Use of a monoclonal antibody directed against the platelet glycoprotein IIb/IIIa receptor in high-risk coronary angioplasty. The EPIC Investigators. N Engl J Med 1994;330: 956–961.

78. EPISTENT Investigators: Randomised placebo-controlled and balloon-angioplasty-controlled trial to assess safety of coronary stenting with use of platelet glycoprotein-IIb/IIIa blockade. Lancet 1998;352:87–92.

79. Boersma E, Akkerhuis KM, Theroux P, et al: Platelet glycoprotein IIb/IIIa receptor inhibition in non-ST-elevation acute coronary syndromes: Early benefit during medical treatment only, with additional protection during percutaneous coronary intervention. Circulation 1999;100:2045–2048.

80. RITA2 trial participants: Coronary angioplasty versus medical treatment for angina: The second randomised intervention treatment of angina. Lancet 1997;350:461–468.

81. Diderholm E, Andren B, Frostfeldt G, et al: Influence on ischemia and exercise tolerance by an early invasive strategy in unstable coronary artery disease. Submitted 2002.

82. Janzon M, Levin LA, Swahn E: Quality of life one year after invasive intervention in unstable coronary artery disease: Results from the FRISCII invasive trial. J Am Coll Cardiol 2001;37:360A.

83. Mahoney EM, Jurkovitz C, Spertus J, et al: Changes in Seattle angina questionnaire scores following treatment for acute coronary syndromes: A follow-up evaluation from the TACTICS-TIMI18 trial. Eur Heart J 2001;22:718.

84. Klein W, Hodl R, Kraxner W: Diagnosis and risk stratification in patients with acute coronary syndromes according to ESC guidelines. Thromb Res 2001;103(Suppl 1):57–61.

85. Solomon DH, Stone PH, Glynn RJ, et al: Use of risk stratification to identify patients with unstable angina likeliest to benefit from an invasive versus conservative management strategy. J Am Coll Cardiol 2001;38:969–976.

86. Nyman I, Areskog M, Areskog NH, et al: Very early risk stratification by electrocardiogram at rest in men with suspected unstable coronary heart disease. The RISC Study Group. J Intern Med 1993;234:293–301.

87. Holmvang L, Andersen K, Dellborg M, et al: Relative contributions of a single-admission 12 lead electrocardiogram and early 24 hour continous electrocardiographic monitoring for early risk stratification in patients with unstable coronary artery disease. Am J Cardiol 1999;83:667–674.

88. Andersen K, Eriksson P, Källström G, et al: Continuous vector cardiography predicts clinical events in patients with unstable coronary disease [Abstract]. Eur Heart J 1996;17:575.

89. Andersen K, Eriksson P, Dellborg M: Non-invasive risk stratification within 48 h of hospital admission in patients with unstable coronary disease. Eur Heart J 1997;18:780–788.

90. Patel D, Knight C, Holdright D, et al: Long-term prognosis in unstable angina. The importance of early risk stratification using continuous ST segment monitoring. Eur Heart J 1998;19:240–249.

91. Jernberg T, Lindahl B, Wallentin L: ST-segment monitoring with continuous 12-lead ECG improves early risk stratification in patients with chest pain and ECG nondiagnostic of acute myocardial infarction. J Am Coll Cardiol 1999;34:1413–1419.

92. Abrahamsson P, Andersen K, Grip L, et al: Early assessment of long-term risk with continuous ST-segment monitoring among patients with unstable coronary syndromes. Results from 1-year follow-up in the TRIM study. J Electrocardiol 2001;34:103–108.

93. Shaw LJ, Peterson ED, Kesler K, et al: A metaanalysis of predischarge risk stratification after acute myocardial infarction with stress electrocardiographic, myocardial perfusion, and ventricular function imaging. Am J Cardiol 1996;78:1327–1337.

94. de Lemos JA, Morrow DA, Bentley JH, et al: The prognostic value of B-type natriuretic peptide in patients with acute coronary syndromes. N Engl J Med 2001;345:1014–1021.

95. Ravkilde J, Hansen AB, Horder M, et al: Risk stratification in suspected acute myocardial infarction based on a sensitive immunoassay for serum creatine kinase isoenzyme MB. A 2.5-year follow-up study in 156 consecutive patients. Cardiology 1992;80:143–151.

96. Ohman EM, Armstrong PW, Christenson RH, et al: Cardiac troponin T levels for risk stratification in acute myocardial ischemia. GUSTO IIA Investigators. N Engl J Med 1996;335:1333–1341.

97. Lindahl B, Venge P, Wallentin L: Relation between troponin T and the risk of subsequent cardiac events in unstable coronary artery disease. The FRISC study group. Circulation 1996;93:1651–1657.

98. Luscher MS, Thygesen K, Ravkilde J, Heickendorff L: Applicability of cardiac troponin T and I for early risk stratification in unstable coronary artery disease. TRIM Study Group. Thrombin Inhibition in Myocardial ischemia. Circulation 1997;96:2578-2585.

99. Christenson RH, Duh SH, Newby LK, et al: Cardiac troponin T and cardiac troponin I: Relative values in short-term risk stratification of patients with acute coronary syndromes. GUSTO-IIa Investigators. Clin Chem 1998;44:494-501.

100. Newby LK, Christenson RH, Ohman EM, et al: Value of serial troponin T measures for early and late risk stratification in patients with acute coronary syndromes. The GUSTO-IIa Investigators. Circulation 1998;98:1853-1859.

101. Toss H, Lindahl B, Siegbahn A, Wallentin L: Prognostic influence of increased fibrinogen and C-reactive protein levels in unstable coronary artery disease. FRISC Study Group. Fragmin during Instability in Coronary Artery Disease. Circulation 1997;96:4204-4210.

102. Heeschen C, Hamm CW, Bruemmer J, Simoons ML: Predictive value of C-reactive protein and troponin T in patients with unstable angina: A comparative analysis. CAPTURE Investigators. Chimeric c7E3 AntiPlatelet Therapy in Unstable angina REfractory to standard treatment trial. J Am Coll Cardiol 2000;35:1535-1542.

103. Lindahl B, Toss H, Siegbahn A, et al: Markers of myocardial damage and inflammation in relation to long-term mortality in unstable coronary artery disease. FRISC Study Group. Fragmin during Instability in Coronary Artery Disease. N Engl J Med 2000;343:1139-1147.

104. Lindmark E, Diderholm E, Wallentin L, Siegbahn A: Relationship between interleukin 6 and mortality in patients with unstable coronary artery disease: Effects of an early invasive or noninvasive strategy. JAMA 2001;286:2107-2113.

105. Lindahl B, Andren B, Ohlsson J, et al: Risk stratification in unstable coronary artery disease. Additive value of troponin T determinations and pre-discharge exercise tests. FRISK Study Group [see comments]. Eur Heart J 1997;18:762-770.

106. Dellborg M, Andersen K: Key factors in the identification of the high-risk patient with unstable coronary artery disease: clinical findings, resting 12-lead electrocardiogram, and continuous electrocardiographic monitoring. Am J Cardiol 1997;80:35E-39E.

107. Jernberg T, Lindahl B, Wallentin L: The combination of a continuous 12-lead ECG and troponin T: A valuable tool for risk stratification during the first 6 hours in patients with chest pain and a non-diagnostic ECG. Eur Heart J 2000;21:1464-1472.

108. Nörgaard B, Andersen K, Dellborg M, et al: Admission risk assessment by cardiac troponin T in unstable coronary artery disease: Additional prognostic information from continous ST segment monitoring. J Am Coll Cardiol 1999;33:1519-1527.

109. Morrow DA, Rifai N, Antman EM, et al: C-reactive protein is a potent predictor of mortality independently of and in combination with troponin T in acute coronary syndromes: A TIMI IIA substudy. Thrombolysis in Myocardial Infarction. J Am Coll Cardiol 1998;31:1460-1465.

110. Boersma E, Pieper KS, Steyerberg EW, et al: Predictors of outcome in patients with acute coronary syndromes without persistent ST-segment elevation. Results from an international trial of 9461 patients. The PURSUIT Investigators. Circulation 2000;101:2557-2567.

111. Antman EM, Cohen M, Bernink PJ, et al: The TIMI risk score for unstable angina/non-ST elevation MI: A method for prognostication and therapeutic decision making. JAMA 2000;284:835-842.

112. McGuire DK, Emanuelsson H, Granger CB, et al: Influence of diabetes mellitus on clinical outcomes across the spectrum of acute coronary syndromes. Findings from the GUSTO-IIb study. GUSTO IIb Investigators. Eur Heart J 2000;21:1750-1758.

113. BARI Investigators: Influence of diabetes on 5-year mortality and morbidity in a randomized trial comparing CABG and PTCA in patients with multivessel disease: The Bypass Angioplasty Revascularization Investigation (BARI). Circulation 1997;96:1761-1769.

114. Venge P, Lindahl B, Wallentin L: New generation cardiac troponin I assay for the access immunoassay system. Clin Chem 2001;47:959-961.

115. Antman EM: Troponin measurements in ischemic heart disease: More than just a black and white picture. J Am Coll Cardiol 2001;38:987-990.

116. Antman EM, Tanasijevic MJ, Thompson B, et al: Cardiac-specific troponin I levels to predict the risk of mortality in patients with acute coronary syndromes. N Engl J Med 1996;335:1342-1349.

117. Diderholm E, Andren B, Frostfeldt G, et al: The prognostic and therapeutic implications of increased troponin levels and ST-depression in unstable coronary artery disease. Am Heart J 2002;143:760-767.

118. Theroux P, Waters DD, Halphen C, et al: Prognostic value of exercise testing soon after myocardial infarction. N Engl J Med 1979;301:341-345.

119. Theroux P, Waters DD, Moise A, et al: Exercise testing in the early period after myocardial infarction in the evaluation of prognosis. Cardiol Clin 1984;2:71-77.

120. Swahn E, Areskog M, Wallentin L: Early exercise testing after coronary care for suspected unstable coronary artery disease—safety and diagnostic value. Eur Heart J 1986;7:594-601.

121. Nyman I, Larsson H, Areskog M, et al: The predictive value of silent ischemia at an exercise test before discharge after an episode of unstable coronary artery disease. RISC Study Group. Am Heart J 1992;123:324-331.

122. Lindahl B, Andren B, Ohlsson J, et al: Noninvasive risk stratification in unstable coronary artery disease: Exercise test and biochemical markers. FRISC Study Group. Am J Cardiol 1997;80:40E-44E.

123. Hammar N, Sandberg E, Larsen FF, Ivert T: Comparison of early and late mortality in men and women after isolated coronary artery bypass graft surgery in Stockholm, Sweden, 1980 to 1989. J Am Coll Cardiol 1997;29:659-664.

124. Koch CG, Higgins TL, Capdeville M, et al: The risk of coronary artery surgery in women: A matched comparison using preoperative severity of illness scoring. J Cardiothorac Vasc Anesth 1996;10:839-843.

125. van den Brand MJ, van Miltenburg A, de Boer MJ, et al: Correlation between clinical course and quantitative analysis of the ischemia related artery in patients with unstable angina pectoris, refractory to medical treatment. Results of two randomized trials. The European Cooperative Study Group. Int J Card Imag 1994;10:177-185.

126. Uchida Y, Nakamura F, Tomaru T, et al: Prediction of acute coronary syndromes by percutaneous coronary angioscopy in patients with stable angina. Am Heart J 1995;130:195-203.

127. Dangas G, Mehran R, Wallenstein S, et al: Correlation of angiographic morphology and clinical presentation in unstable angina. J Am Coll Cardiol 1997;29:519-525.

128. Smith SC Jr, Dove JT, Jacobs AK, et al: ACC/AHA guidelines of percutaneous coronary interventions (revision of the 1993 PTCA guidelines)—executive summary. A report of the American College of Cardiology/American Heart Association Task Force on Practice Guidelines (committee to revise the 1993 guidelines for percutaneous transluminal coronary angioplasty). J Am Coll Cardiol 2001;37:2215-2238.

129. Morey SS: ACC/AHA revised guidelines for coronary bypass surgery. American College of Cardiology/American Heart Association. Am Fam Physician 2000;61:2881-2882, 2884.

130. Sousa JE, Costa MA, Abizaid A, et al: Lack of neointimal proliferation after implantation of sirolimus-coated stents in human coronary arteries: A quantitative coronary angiography and three-dimensional intravascular ultrasound study. Circulation 2001;103:192-195.

131. FRISC-II Investigators: Long-term low-molecular-mass heparin in unstable coronary-artery disease: FRISC II prospective randomised multicentre study. FRagmin and Fast Revascularisation during InStability in Coronary artery disease Investigators. Lancet 1999;354:701-707.

132. Husted S, Kher A: Acute and prolonged treatment with low-molecular-weight heparin therapy in patients with unstable coronary artery disease. Ann Med 2000;32(Suppl 1):53-59.

133. EPILOG Investigators: Platelet glycoprotein IIb/IIIa receptor blockade and low-dose heparin during percutaneous coronary revascularization. N Engl J Med 1997;336:1689-1696.

134. ESPRIT Investigators: Novel dosing regimen of eptifibatide in planned coronary stent implantation (ESPRIT)—A randomised, placebo-controlled trial. Lancet 2000;356:2037-2044.

135. Bittl JA, Strony J, Brinker JA, et al: Treatment with bivalirudin (Hirulog) as compared with heparin during coronary angioplasty for unstable or postinfarction angina. Hirulog Angioplasty Study Investigators. N Engl J Med 1995;333:764-769.

136. Bittl JA, Chaitman BR, Feit F, et al: Bivalirudin versus heparin during coronary angioplasty for unstable or postinfarction angina: Final report reanalysis of the Bivalirudin Angioplasty Study. Am Heart J 2001;142:952-959.

137. Rabah MM, Premmereur J, Graham M, et al: Usefulness of intravenous enoxaparin for percutaneous coronary intervention in stable angina pectoris. Am J Cardiol 1999;84:1391-1395.

138. Kereiakes DJ, Young J, Broderick TM, et al: Therapeutic adjuncts for immediate transfer to the catheterization laboratory in patients with acute coronary syndromes. Am J Cardiol 2000;86:10M-17M.

139. Kereiakes DJ, Kleiman NS, Fry E, et al: Dalteparin in combination with abciximab during percutaneous coronary intervention. Am Heart J 2001;141:348-352.

140. Kereiakes DJ, Grines C, Fry E, et al: Enoxaparin and abciximab adjunctive pharmacotherapy during percutaneous coronary intervention. J Invasive Cardiol 2001;13:272-278.

141. Piegas LS, Flather M, Pogue J, et al: The Organization to Assess Strategies for Ischemic Syndromes (OASIS) registry in patients with unstable angina. Am J Cardiol 1999;84:7M-12M.

142. Bertrand ME, Rupprecht HJ, Urban P, et al: Double-blind study of the safety of clopidogrel with and without a loading dose in combination with aspirin compared with ticlopidine in combination with aspirin after coronary stenting: The CLopidogrel ASpirin Stent International Cooperative study (CLASSICS). Circulation 2000;102:624-629.

143. Mehta SR, Yusuf S, Peters RJ, et al: Effects of pretreatment with clopidogrel and aspirin followed by long-term therapy in patients undergoing percutaneous coronary intervention: The PCI-CURE study. Lancet 2001;358:527-533.

144. Janzon M, Levin LA, Swahn E, FRISCII Investigators: Cost-effectiveness of early invasive treatment in unstable coronary artery disease: A one year follow-up from the FRISCII invasive trial. J Am Coll Cardiol 2001;37:376A.

145. Mahoney EM, Jurkovitz C, Chu H, et al: Length of stay for the treatment of acute coronary syndromes: International experience from the TACTICS-TIMI18 trial. Eur Heart J 2001;22:223.

chapter 35

Advantages and Hazards of Early Revascularization

Christopher P. Cannon

There are two general approaches to the use of cardiac catheterization and revascularization in unstable angina and non–ST-segment elevation myocardial infarction (MI). One is an *invasive* strategy, involving routine cardiac catheterization and revascularization with percutaneous coronary intervention (PCI) or coronary artery bypass graft (CABG) surgery depending on the coronary anatomy (Fig. 35-1). Alternatively a *conservative* approach can be undertaken, with initial medical management with catheterization and revascularization carried out only if the patient shows recurrent ischemia either at rest or on a noninvasive stress test. The latter also has been termed an *ischemia-guided* strategy.

Seven randomized trials have assessed these two general strategies, six before the advent of glycoprotein IIb/IIIa inhibition[1-5] and one afterward (Fig. 35-2).[6] The results of the trials now strongly favor the invasive strategy. Of the seven trials, one showed worse outcomes with an invasive strategy, two showed equivalent outcomes, and three showed improved outcomes with the invasive approach.

TIMI IIIB

In the TIMI (Thrombolysis in Myocardial Infarction) IIIB trial, 1473 patients were randomized to follow either an early invasive strategy with routine angiography 18 to 48 hours after randomization with revascularization as appropriate or an early conservative strategy with angiography and revascularization performed only for recurrent ischemia. All patients received intravenous heparin, aspirin, β-blockers, nitrates, and calcium antagonists as clinically indicated. The conservative strategy was truly an ischemia-guided strategy, with the indications for catheterization based on careful assessment for recurrent ischemia: ischemia at rest with electrocardiogram (ECG) changes, ST-segment depression on a Holter monitor, and a "high-risk" exercise thallium stress test. Despite this requirement for objective evidence of recurrent ischemia, 57% of patients required in-hospital coronary angiography, and 40% underwent in-hospital revascularization.[1]

No difference was seen in the rate of the primary end point, death, MI, or a strongly positive exercise test at 6 weeks, between the two strategies (16.2% for invasive versus 18.1% for conservative strategy; *P* = not significant).[1] Similarly, there was no difference in the incidence of death or MI at 6 weeks or 1 year (10.8% versus 12.2%; *P* = not significant) (see Fig. 35-2).[2] Subgroup analyses suggested a benefit of the early invasive strategy in elderly patients.[2] In a subsequent, more comprehensive analysis of risk, using the TIMI risk score,[7] there appeared to be a trend toward benefit of an invasive strategy.[8]

MATE

The results of TIMI IIIB were nearly duplicated in the smaller MATE (Medicine versus Angiography in Thrombolytic Exclusion) trial (see Fig. 35-1).[4] This latter trial evaluated an early invasive strategy, with time to cardiac catheterization approximately 7 hours after randomization in the invasive group. This trial showed equivalent long-term outcomes on death or MI (see Fig. 35-1). The investigators observed, however, a lower rate of in-hospital recurrent ischemia with the early invasive strategy.[4]

VANQWISH

The VANQWISH (VA Non–Q-Wave Infarction Strategies In-Hospital) trial compared invasive and conservative strategies in 920 patients with non–Q-wave MI (not unstable angina, but including approximately 15% of patients with non–ST-segment elevation MI). There was no significant difference in the primary end point of death or nonfatal MI during follow-up (approximately 2 years) (26.9% in the invasive arm versus 29.9% in the conservative arm; *P* = .35).[3] There were significantly more deaths in patients assigned to the invasive compared with the conservative strategy at hospital discharge (4.5% versus 1.3%; *P* = 0.007), however, a difference that remained significant at 1 year (see Fig. 35-1). There was an 11.6% peri–CABG surgery mortality in the invasive group, which explains about half of the early hazard of the early invasive group. When the investigators used the TIMI risk score to stratify patients, they found that even in this trial, the high-risk patients (score 5 to 7) had a significant *benefit* of the early invasive strategy.

FRISC II

The FRISC (FRagmin and Fast Revascularisation during InStability in Coronary Artery Disease) II trial randomized

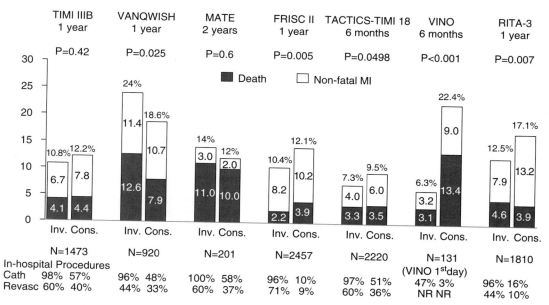

FIGURE 35–1. Results from the first six randomized trials of invasive versus conservative strategies in unstable angina and non–ST-segment eleva-tion myocardial infarction. The duration of follow-up is shown for each trial at the top, and the number of patients is shown at the bottom. The rate of cardiac catheterization during the initial hospitalization and the rates of revascularization (revasc) with percutaneous coronary intervention or coronary artery bypass graft surgery are shown. (Data from Anderson et al,[2] Boden et al,[3] McCollough et al,[4] FRagmin and Fast Revascularisation during InStability in Coronary Artery Disease investigators,[5] Cannon et al,[6] and Spacek et al.[13])

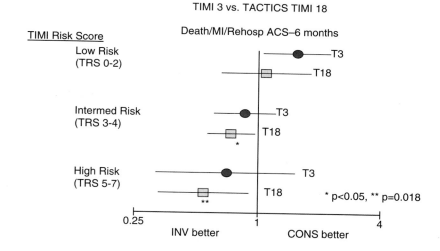

FIGURE 35–2. Comparison of event rates in the TIMI 3 versus TACTICS-TIMI 18 trials stratified by the TIMI risk score. (Data from Sabatine MS, Cannon CP, Murphy SA, et al: Implications of upstream glycopro-tein IIb/IIIa inhibition and stenting in the invasive management of UA/NSTEMI: A comparison of TIMI IIIB and TACTICS-TIMI 18. Circulation 2001;104 [suppl II]:II-549.)

2457 patients with unstable angina and non–ST-segment elevation MI.[5] Patients were included in the trial if they had chest pain within 48 hours, with either ST-segment or T-wave changes or positive serum markers. They received subcutaneous dalteparin in the hospital and were randomized to an invasive versus conservative strategy, with a second randomization to continued dal-teparin versus placebo after discharge. In the invasive arm, cardiac catheterization was to be carried out within 3 days of randomization and revascularization within 7 days; this strategy was a "delayed" invasive strategy. Criteria for catheterization in the conservative strategy were strict and required refractory angina despite maxi-

mal medical treatment or a positive ECG exercise test with greater than or equal to 0.3 mV ST-segment depres-sion. Thallium imaging was not done with the stress test-ing. Accordingly, with these strict criteria in the conservative strategy, only 9% of patients underwent revascularization during the first 7 days.[5]

The primary end point, death or MI at 6 months, was significantly lower in the invasive versus conservative group (9.4% versus 12.1%; $P = .031$).[5] At 1 year, there was a significant reduction in *mortality* in the invasive versus conservative groups (2.2% versus 3.9; $P = .016$) and of death or MI (10.4% versus 14.1; $P = .005$) (see Fig. 35–1).[9] Additional analyses showed greater benefit of the invasive strategy in higher risk groups identified by ST-segment depression on the admission ECG or troponin T greater than or equal to 0.01 ng/dL.[10,11] The 30-day mortality after CABG surgery was less than 2% in this study.[5]

The authors noted that there was an increase in early MI, likely periprocedural events, over the first 2 weeks. This increase was quickly erased, however, with a significant improvement in outcomes by 6 months and 1 year. In this trial, only 10% of patients had a glycoprotein IIb/IIIa inhibitor used for their PCI.

TACTICS-TIMI 18

The TACTICS (Treat Angina with Aggrastat and Determine Cost of Therapy with an Invasive or Conservative Strategy)-TIMI 18 trial was conducted in the current era. It was hypothesized that the two major advances in the field of unstable angina and non–ST-segment elevation MI—the use of glycoprotein IIb/IIIa inhibition and coronary stenting—would allow an early invasive strategy to be superior to a more conservative approach.[6] Patients were enrolled if they had a prolonged episode (>20 minutes) or recurrent episodes of angina at rest or with minimal effort) within the preceding 24 hours or if they had ST-segment or T-wave changes, elevated cardiac markers, or a history of documented coronary disease. All patients received aspirin, heparin, and the glycoprotein IIb/IIIa inhibitor tirofiban at the time of randomization for at least 48 hours, including 12 hours or more after PCI.

Patients in the early invasive strategy were to undergo coronary angiography 4 to 48 hours after randomization and revascularization when feasible based on coronary anatomy. Patients in the conservative strategy were treated medically and if stable underwent a predischarge exercise tolerance test (which included nuclear perfusion imaging or echocardiography in approximately 85% of patients). In the conservative group, patients underwent angiography and revascularization if they had recurrent angina at rest associated with ECG or enzyme changes or a positive stress test (≥0.1 mV ST depression). For PCI procedures in both treatment strategies, stents were used in 85% of patients.

The rate of the primary end point, death, MI, or rehospitalization for an acute coronary syndrome at 6 months, was reduced with the early invasive strategy, from 19.4% in the conservative group to 15.9% in the early invasive group (odds ratio [OR], 0.78; P = .025).[6] This reduction was seen after 7 days: 5.7% versus 3.9% in the conservative versus invasive groups (OR, 0.66; P = .039). Similarly at 30 days, the event rates were 10.5% for conservative versus 7.4% for invasive groups (OR, 0.67; P = .009). Death or nonfatal MI was reduced significantly at 30 days (7% to 4.7%; P = .02) and at 6 months (P = .0498). A reduction in MI (fatal or nonfatal) was noted at 7 days (OR, 0.59; P = .033), 30 days (OR, 0.51; P = .002), and 6 months (OR, 0.67; P = .029). The benefit of the early invasive strategy was consistent across the major subgroups, including men and women, younger and older patients, and in diabetics and nondiabetics.[6]

Risk Stratification

Using troponin, the prespecified secondary hypothesis of the trial, there was a significantly greater benefit in patients with positive troponin values compared with negative values.[6] In patients with a troponin T value greater than 0.01 ng/mL, there was a relative 39% risk reduction in the primary end point with the invasive versus conservative strategy (P < .001), whereas patients with a negative troponin value had similar outcomes with either strategy. Death or nonfatal MI also was significantly reduced with the invasive strategy in patients with troponin T values greater than 0.01 ng/mL. Similar results were obtained using a troponin T cutoff point of 0.1 ng/mL and with troponin I.[12]

The same findings of benefit were seen in patients with ST-segment changes on admission, with a 10% absolute benefit in the primary end point versus no benefit in patients without ST-segment changes on admission. Using the TIMI risk score, there was significant benefit of the early invasive strategy in intermediate-risk (score 3 to 4) and high-risk (score 5 to 7) patients, whereas low-risk (score 0 to 2) patients had similar outcomes when managed with either strategy.[6] The intermediate-risk and high-risk groups comprised 75% of the total population in the trial.

This study shows that among patients with unstable angina and non–ST-segment elevation MI and treated with the glycoprotein IIb/IIIa inhibitor tirofiban, an early invasive strategy was superior to a conservative strategy in reducing major cardiac events at 7 days, 30 days, and 6 months. This strategy using "upstream" glycoprotein IIb/IIIa inhibition with tirofiban combined with an early invasive strategy leads to excellent outcomes and could be considered the treatment of choice for most patients with unstable angina and non–ST-segment elevation MI.

VINO

The VINO (Value of First Day Angiography/Angioplasty In Evolving Non-ST Segment Elevation Myocardial Infarction: an Open Multicenter Randomized Trial) study[13] was a small study of 131 patients randomized in the Czech Republic to a strategy of early invasive strategy with first-day angiography (mean, 6 hours) after randomization compared with a conservative strategy, in which the mean time to angioplasty for the 55% of patients who required it was 61 days. The primary end point of death or MI at 6 months was reduced in the invasive group from 13.4% to 3.1% (P < .03).[13]

RITA-3 AND TRUCS

The final trial was the RITA-3 (Randomized Intervention Trial of Unstable Angina) study. This trial was conducted in the United Kingdom and focused on patients with unstable angina.[14] A total of 810 patients were randomized to an invasive versus a conservative strategy. In the two groups, angiography was carried out during the index hospitalization in 96% versus 16% of patients in the conservative versus invasive groups. The primary end point was death, MI, or refractory angina at 4 months. The results showed that this end point was 14.5% in the conservative group versus 9.6% in the invasive group ($P = .001$).[14] The end point of death or MI (using the standard European Society of Cardiology/American College of Cardiology definition) at 1 year was 17.1% in the conservative group versus 12.5% in the invasive group ($P = .007$).[14] This study showed that an early invasive strategy is superior to a conservative strategy. With the TRUCS (Treatment of Refractory Unstable angina in geographically isolated areas without Cardiac Surgery) trial, this is the fifth trial in a row to show the benefit of an invasive approach. The TRUCS trail compared invasive (on-site coronary angioplasty or emergency air ambulance for CABG) to conservative management in 140 patients.[15] At 30 days, death occurred in 11.1% of patients in the conservative arm and 2.6% ($P = .03$) of patients in the invasive arm, MI in 2.6% and 4.2% (NS), and the combined endpoint in 5.3% and 15.3% (NS). At 12 months, these events occurred in 3.9% and 12.5% ($P = .05$), and 3.9% and 4.2% (NS), and 17.1% and 23.6% (NS), respectively. Late readmission, coronary angioplasty, and bypass surgery were required as frequently in the two groups. The high mortality rates in this study are probably explained by enrollment of high-risk patients with refractory angina.

EARLY RISKS VERSUS BENEFITS

Benefit of the early invasive strategy of TACTICS-TIMI 18 may be explained by two components: (1) the early use of glycoprotein IIb/IIIa inhibition and (2) the early timing of revascularization. With regard to the use of glycoprotein IIb/IIIa inhibition, in the first four randomized trials conducted without glycoprotein IIb/IIIa inhibition,[1-5,9] the rate of MI tended to be higher in the invasive group over the first 2 weeks, consistent with an "early hazard" associated with coronary interventions. In contrast, in TACTICS-TIMI 18, we observed a significantly *lower* rate of MI and the composite end point at this early time point, an effect that may be attributable to well-documented protection afforded by glycoprotein IIb/IIIa inhibition.[16]

Another analysis examined the contribution of glycoprotein IIb/IIIa inhibition in improving outcomes in high-risk ACS patients: a comparison of the results from TIMI III with those from TACTICS-TIMI 18. In TIMI III and TACTICS-TIMI 18, inclusion and exclusion criteria were similar, but the medical treatment consisted of only aspirin, heparin, and anti-ischemic therapy. In TACTICS-TIMI 18, patients also received tirofiban. (In addition, stents were used in 85% of patients in TACTICS-TIMI 18 versus none in TIMI III.) The patients were stratified by the TIMI risk score.

An interesting pattern emerged: There was a consistently better outcome seen in the TACTICS-TIMI 18 trial compared with the TIMI III trial in each of the risk strata (see Fig. 35–2).[8] In low-risk patients, in TIMI III, the incidence of death, MI, or rehospitalization after 6 months was significantly worse among patients randomized to the invasive strategy arm, whereas in TACTICS-TIMI 18, event rates among low-risk patients were approximately the same for both treatment strategies. For intermediate-risk patients, outcomes for the invasive versus the conservative group were roughly equal in TIMI III, whereas they were significantly better for the invasive versus conservative strategy in TACTICS-TIMI 18. Although there was a trend for improved outcomes among high-risk patients treated invasively in the TIMI III trial, in TACTICS-TIMI 18, there was a dramatic 10% absolute reduction in events. These differences are consistent with the main hypothesis of the trial that the new advances in cardiology of coronary stenting and glycoprotein IIb/IIIa inhibition would improve the safety of the early invasive strategy and lead to an overall benefit compared with a conservative approach.

TIMING OF ANGIOGRAPHY

Cardiac procedures in the early invasive strategy were carried out approximately 2 to 3 days earlier than in the conservative strategy in TACTICS-TIMI 18 and 60 days earlier in VINO. Because the first several days are the highest risk period, and postrevascularization, event rates are generally low, the early revascularization in the invasive strategy seems to have prevented events that otherwise would have occurred over this early time period and contributed to the overall benefit of the early invasive strategy. The dramatic difference seen in VINO is consistent with the early benefit of an invasive strategy.

A remaining question is whether immediate angiography (i.e., within 2 to 4 hours) would be better than an early invasive approach (which was between 4 and 48 hours, average 22 hours, in TACTICS-TIMI 18). In nonrandomized data from TACTICS-TIMI 18, no significant difference was seen in outcomes, but the true answer to this question would come from a prospective trial of immediate versus early angiography. One such trial is in an early planning stage at the time of this writing.

CONSERVATIVE STRATEGIES

Among the prior studies, two conservative strategies were tested. In TIMI IIIB and the VANQWISH trial, the conservative strategy employed careful monitoring for ischemia, using stress testing with radionuclide or echocardiographic imaging in nearly all patients and ECG criteria greater than or equal to 0.1 mV for a positive test, which are consistent with the 1994 and 2000 unstable angina and non–ST-segment elevation MI guidelines.[17,18] This approach led to cardiac catheterization in these trials in approximately 50% of patients.

The conservative strategy in the FRISC II trial used more stringent criteria for ischemia, using only an ECG stress test and requiring greater than or equal to 0.3 mV of ST-segment depression as evidence of ischemia to warrant cardiac catheterization. As a result, only 10% of patients underwent cardiac catheterization during the initial hospitalization. This trial documented a significant benefit of the invasive strategy compared with this conservative strategy in the rate of death or MI and in 1-year mortality rate.[5] The small VINO trial also was conservative (mean time to angiography in the conservative arm was 61 days), and the investigators documented a dramatic reduction in death or MI. These two trials together document that a conservative strategy is inferior to an invasive strategy.

In contrast, the conservative strategy in TACTICS-TIMI 18 was less strict for evidence of recurrent ischemia that would permit angiography and is consistent with recommendations of the 1994 and 2000 unstable angina and non–ST-segment elevation MI guidelines.[18,19] It was important to test the outcomes of a more "selective invasive" strategy. In TACTICS-TIMI 18, the early invasive strategy was shown to be superior to this "optimized" conservative strategy, the selective invasive strategy.

COST-EFFECTIVENESS

Three analyses have been published on the cost-effectiveness of an invasive strategy. From the VANQWISH trial, overall the conservative strategy was better on efficacy, as was its cost-effectivess.[20] In the FRISC II trial, an estimated cost of approximately $150,000 per death was avoided, but no calculation of the expected cost per life-year saved was calculated.[21]

An analysis from TACTICS-TIMI 18 has shown that the overall strategy of early glycoprotein IIb/IIIa inhibition and an invasive strategy was cost-effective relative to a conservative strategy.[22] Estimated cost per life-year gained for the invasive strategy, based on projected life expectancy from the Framingham and Duke databases, was approximately $8000 to $15,000 depending on the assumptions used. In high-risk patients with a positive troponin value or ST-segment changes, these figures were $4000 to $10,000 per life-year saved. In patients with unstable angina and non–ST-segment elevation MI treated with the glycoprotein IIb/IIIa inhibitor tirofiban, the clinical benefit of an early invasive strategy is achieved with a small increase in cost, yielding favorable projected estimates of cost per life-year gained. These results provide further support for the broader use of an early invasive strategy employing early glycoprotein IIb/IIIa inhibition.

CONCLUSION

Based on the current evidence from seven randomized trials in unstable angina and non–ST-segment elevation MI, an early invasive strategy is superior to a conservative strategy in reducing major cardiac events. This benefit applied to most patients studied, notably patients at intermediate risk or high risk (especially patients with positive troponin values). In contrast, lower risk patients had similar outcomes with either strategy, meaning that either a conservative or an invasive strategy can be used in low risk patients. In general, an early hazard had been seen in the early trials, but in the one trial that included

upstream glycoprotein IIb/IIIa inhibition in combination with an early invasive approach, this was not seen. It is suggested that glycoprotein IIb/IIIa inhibition can be helpful in reducing events, especially in patients managed with an early invasive strategy. Accordingly, the 2002 American College of Cardiology/American Heart Association and the European Society of Cardiology guidelines for unstable angina and non–ST-segment elevation MI recommend with a class I recommendation and level of evidence A that glycoprotein IIb/IIIa inhibition be used in patients managed with an invasive strategy.

REFERENCES

1. TIMI IIIB investigators: Effects of tissue plasminogen activator and a comparison of early invasive and conservative strategies in unstable angina and non-Q-wave myocardial infarction: Results of the TIMI IIIB Trial. Circulation 1994;89:1545–1556.
2. Anderson HV, Cannon CP, Stone PH, et al, for the TIMI-IIIB investigators: One-year results of the Thrombolysis in Myocardial Infarction (TIMI) IIIB clinical trial: A randomized comparison of tissue-type plasminogen activator versus placebo and early invasive versus early conservative strategies in unstable angina and non-Q-wave myocardial infarction. J Am Coll Cardiol 1995;26:1643–1650.
3. Boden WE, O'Rourke RA, Crawford MH, et al, for the Veterans Affairs Non-Q-Wave Infarction Strategies in Hospital (VANQWISH) Trial investigators: Outcomes in patients with acute non-Q-wave myocardial infarction randomly assigned to an invasive as compared with a conservative strategy. N Engl J Med 1998;338:1785–1792.
4. McCullough PA, O'Neill WW, Graham M, et al: A prospective randomized trial of triage angiography in acute coronary syndromes ineligible for thrombolytic therapy: Results of the medicine versus angiography in thrombolytic exclusion (MATE) trial. J Am Coll Cardiol 1998;32:596–605.
5. FRagmin and Fast Revascularisation during InStability in Coronary Artery Disease investigators: Invasive compared with non-invasive treatment in unstable coronary-artery disease: FRISC II prospective randomised multicentre study. Lancet 1999;354:708–715.
6. Cannon CP, Weintraub WS, Demopoulos LA, et al: Comparison of early invasive and conservative strategies in patients with unstable coronary syndromes treated with the glycoprotein IIb/IIIa inhibitor tirofiban. N Engl J Med 2001;344:1879–1887.
7. Antman EM, Cohen M, Bernink PJ, et al: The TIMI risk score for unstable angina/non-ST elevation MI: A method for prognostication and therapeutic decision making. JAMA 2000;284:835–842.
8. Sabatine MS, Cannon CP, Murphy SA, et al: Implications of upstream GP IIb/IIIa inhibition and stenting in the invasive management of UA/NSTEMI: A comparison of TIMI IIIB and TACTICS-TIMI 18. Circulation 2001;104(suppl II):II-549.
9. Wallentin L, Lagerqvist B, Husted S, et al: Outcome at 1 year after an invasive compared with a non-invasive strategy in unstable coronary-artery disease: The FRISC II invasive randomised trial. FRISC II investigators. Fast Revascularisation during Instability in Coronary Artery Disease. Lancet 2000;356:9–16.
10. Laqerqvist B, Diderholm E, Lindahl B, et al: An early invasive treatment strategy reduces cardiac events regardless of troponin levels in unstable coronary artery disease (UCAD) with and without troponin-elevation: A FRISC II substudy. Circulation 1999;100(suppl I):I-497.
11. Diderholm E, Andren B, Frostfeldt G, et al: ST depression in ECG at entry identifies patients who benefit most from early revascularization in unstable coronary artery disease: A FRISC II substudy. Circulation 1999;100(suppl I):I-497–I-498.
12. Morrow DA, Cannon CP, Rifai N, et al, for the TACTICS-TIMI 18 investigators: Ability of minor elevations of troponin I and T to predict benefit from an early invasive strategy in patients with unstable angina and non-ST elevation myocardial infarction: Results from a randomized trial. JAMA 2001;286:2405–2412.

13. Spacek R, Widimsky P, Straka Z, et al: Value of first day angiography/angioplasty in evolving non-ST segment elevation myocardial infarction: An open multicenter randomized trial. The VINO Study. Eur Heart J 2002;23:230-238.

14. Fox KA: The Randomized Intervention Trial of Unstable Angina (RITA)-3 study. In European Society of Cardiology Congress, Berlin, 2002.

15. Michalis LK, Stroumbis CS, Pappas K, et al: Treatment of refractory unstable angina in geographically isolated areas without cardiac surgery. Invasive versus conservative strategy (TRUCS study). Em Heart J 2000;21:1954-1959.

16. Kong DF, Califf RM, Miller DP, et al: Clinical outcomes of therapeutic agents that block the platelet glycoprotein IIb/IIIa integrin in ischemic heart disease. Circulation 1998;98:2829-2835.

17. Braunwald E, Jones RH, Mark DB, et al: Diagnosing and managing unstable angina. Circulation 1994;90:613-622.

18. Braunwald E, Antman EM, Beasley JW, et al: ACC/AHA guidelines for the management of patients with unstable angina and non-ST segment elevation myocardial infarction: A report of the American College of Cardiology/American Heart Association Task Force on Practice Guidelines (Committee on the Management of Unstable Angina and Non-ST Segment Elevation Myocardial Infarction). J Am Coll Cardiol 2000;36:970-1056.

19. Braunwald E, Mark DB, Jones RH, et al: Unstable Angina: Diagnosis and Management. Clinical Practice Guideline No 10. Rockville, MD, Agency for Health Care Policy and Research and the National Heart, Lung, and Blood Institute, Public Health Service, U.S. Department of Health and Human Services, 1994.

20. Barnett PG, Chen S, Boden WE, et al: Cost-effectiveness of a conservative, ischemia-guided management strategy after non-Q-wave myocardial infarction: Results of a randomized trial. Circulation 2002;105:680-684.

21. Janzon M, Levin LA, Swahn E: Cost-effectiveness of an invasive strategy in unstable coronary artery disease: Results from the FRISC II invasive trial. The Fast Revascularisation during InStability in Coronary Artery Disease. Eur Heart J 2002;23:31-40.

22. Mahoney EM, Jurkovitz CT, Chu H, et al, for the Treat Angina with Aggrastat and Determine Cost of Therapy with an Invasive or Conservative Strategy (TACTICS)-TIMI 18 investigators: Cost and cost-effectiveness of an early invasive versus conservative strategy for the treatment of unstable angina and non-ST elevation myocardial infarction. JAMA 2002;288:1851-1858.

New Surgical and Percutaneous Revascularization Procedures

Ali E. Denktas
David R. Holmes, Jr.

The ultimate goal of coronary intervention is normal flow to the coronary bed. When complete revascularization is not feasible, the closest approach to achieving functionally complete revascularization should be chosen. This chapter reviews the newer modalities of surgical and percutaneous interventions.

SURGICAL ADVANCES

Coronary artery bypass surgery has revolutionized the approach to the patient with coronary artery disease. However, the need for hospitalization, the attendant perioperative mortality, and the morbidity associated with the rather extensive invasive nature of this approach has led to the development of less invasive methods such as percutaneous revascularization. On the other hand, to this date the surgical approach has been superior for the treatment of multivessel disease in terms of the repeat procedures and hospitalizations. There are also data regarding the decrease in mortality in diabetic patients who undergo coronary artery bypass grafting (CABG) versus percutaneous interventions.[1]

Surgery for coronary artery revascularization has also improved in recent years. Limited thoracotomy and beating-heart surgeries have been perfected. Now we are entering the era of robotics and endoscopic techniques for CABG.

Minimally Invasive Coronary Artery Bypass Surgery

Direct coronary artery bypass surgery on the beating heart is not a new concept. It was performed successfully in the 1980s.[2] The development of stabilizers (which allow the surgeon to work on the beating heart) and of limited access methods have revolutionized cardiac surgery for coronary artery disease. The initial experience with minimally invasive direct coronary artery bypass (MIDCAB) using mini left and right anterior thoracotomy and subxiphoid incisions was reported by Subramanian et al.[3] Their series showed no perioperative mortality and minimal morbidity. Twelve of the 18 patients underwent follow-up angiography that showed that 10 of the 12 grafts were patent. This procedure is most commonly performed through a 6- to 7-cm left

anterior thoracotomy incision in the fourth intercostal space.[4]

Although thoracoscopic internal mammary artery (IMA) harvest has been described, it is generally done under direct vision.[5,6] Once the IMA harvesting is complete, the stabilization device is placed before the anastomosis is performed. After the anastomosis, the wound is closed and the patient is extubated in the surgical suite. The patient is generally discharged on postoperative day 2 or 3.[4] The majority of experience with MIDCAB is limited to left anterior descending (LAD) revascularization. MIDCAB has also been used successfully in patients with multivessel disease.[7] To allow multiple vessels to be reached through a minimally invasive approach, a transabdominal approach has been proposed.[8] In selective patients, a hybrid procedure with MIDCAB for the revascularization of the LAD and PTCA or stent therapy for the non-LAD lesions approachable by the percutaneous approach has been advocated.[9-11]

There have been many reports on the outcomes of the MIDCAB IMA grafts.[12,13] The patency rates for conventional bypass grafting of the IMA to the LAD are 90% to 95%.[14] In the reported series with MIDCAB, the patency rates are similar, at 92% to 100%.[4] The results for short-term patency rates are encouraging and seem to be translating to good long-term outcomes.[4,13] Mack reported a single-center series with a 3-year major adverse cardiac and cerebral event rate of 7.5%. In a report by Mehran et al, the 1-year mortality rate after MIDCAB was 2.5%; the 1-year major adverse cardiac event (MACE) rate was 7.8%, but when only the cases after the initial 100 were considered, the 1-year MACE rate was 6%.[13] The MIDCAB procedure is a safe alternative to single-vessel conventional IMA-to-LAD bypass, with excellent results when performed by experienced operators.[13]

Lateral Thoracotomy Coronary Artery Bypass

Lateral thoracotomy coronary artery bypass is the performance of a single vein graft or radial artery graft bypass through a lateral thoracotomy. This procedure is typically performed for the circumflex system when the percutaneous approach is not possible and when the patient has a functioning IMA graft to the LAD.[4] This approach can be associated with decreased need for transfusions, less neuropsychologic changes, shorter duration of hospitalization and lower rate of postoperative atrial fibrillation than conventional bypass.[15] Although the existing series document good clinical outcomes, the overall experience with this approach is limited.[4]

Off-Pump Coronary Artery Bypass

CABG started as a beating-heart procedure.[16] Once cardiopulmonary bypass was developed, the enthusiasm for off-pump bypass was limited. Nevertheless, there have been reports of off-pump revascularization in large series performed in Argentina[2] and in Brazil.[17] Benetti et al reported a mortality rate of 1% and a morbidity of 4% in their series using multivessel off-pump coronary artery bypass (OPCAB).[2] Buffolo et al reported 1274 off-pump procedures with a 2.5% mortality rate.[17] With the introduction of MIDCAB, there has been a renewed interest in off-pump surgery. This procedure is usually performed via a median sternotomy approach, although alternative incisions have a role.

The reports from the current era using new stabilization techniques are encouraging.[18,19] In the report of Tasdemir et al of 2052 patients, the mortality rate was only 1.9%.[18] The presence of bronchial asthma, hypertension, poor quality of the left anterior descending artery, and ungrafted circumflex coronary artery disease were the early predictors of mortality. In 74% of patients, blood transfusions were not needed. In their review of the Medtronic Octopus (Medtronic, Minneapolis, MN), Hart et al reported the results of 1582 patients: 1% mortality, 2.6% conversion to cardiopulmonary bypass, and 1.2% myocardial infarction.[19]

Other reports have documented fewer blood transfusions, less renal dysfunction, and fewer microemboli with OPCAB compared with on-pump CABG.[20-25] In a retrospective study of 744 patients comparing multivessel OPCAB to CABG, with the mean number of distal anastomoses greater than three in both groups, Kshettry et al documented a decreased need for transfusions in patients undergoing OPCAB.[26] However, the groups showed no difference in mortality. It has been suggested that OPCAB is associated with less neurocognitive dysfunction.[27] In a small study, Diegeler et al randomized 40 patients into OPCAB or conventional CABG and analyzed the transient high-amplitude signals by transcranial Doppler and neurocognitive function pre- and post-operatively.[27] They showed significantly more microemboli in the conventional group as well as increased neurocognitive dysfunction.

The benefit of OPCAB is the elimination of cardiopulmonary bypass, shorter operating time, decreased need for transfusions, and decreased cost. Although the data are limited, there is a potential for less renal and cerebral injury. Off-pump coronary artery bypass still requires median sternotomy, can cause local ischemia, and may be associated with a postoperative increase in coagulability.[4] Nevertheless, as techniques improve and objective benefits are defined in clinical trials, OPCAB could become the procedure of choice.

Port-Access Coronary Artery Bypass

The Port-Access system (Heartport, Redwood City, CA) involves arterial and venous access to institute cardiopulmonary bypass and a catheter-based balloon system for aortic occlusion in cardioplegic delivery. With this system, cardioplegia is delivered either through the proximal port of the balloon catheter or through a percutaneously placed coronary sinus catheter. This system was designed to provide standard myocardial protection and allow for cardiac operations without a sternotomy. The major advantage of this method is the ability to perform multivessel revascularization on an arrested heart with a bloodless operative field. The downside is the need for longer cardiopulmonary bypass with increased incidence of neuropsychiatric complications.[28,29]

Port-Access coronary artery bypass surgery has been reported to have good initial results and excellent graft patency (100% for IMA, 97.7% overall).[30] In the first report of the Port-Access International Registry (PAIR), Galloway et al reported the data on 1063 patients (583 patients undergoing CABG, 55%) who underwent cardiac surgery with the Heartport system.[29] The operative mortality rate was 1% for patients undergoing CABG. The most common complication was atrial fibrillation (5.5%), followed by stroke (2.2%). There were no reoperations for the primary procedure, but 1.5% of patients required reoperation for other reasons. A more recent update of the Port-Access International Registry reported 3210 cases from 113 centers.[31] Of these patients, 1676 underwent Port-Access CABG. In a subset of patients with comprehensive data capture, the conversion rate to conventional sternotomy was 53 of 1547 (3.4%), mainly due to vascular injury and poor visualization. Of the patients undergoing CABG, only 0.5% required reoperation for the primary procedure and 3.6% required reoperation because of bleeding. In the United States cohort, the median length of stay was 4 days. It appears that in the near future, Port-Access cardiac surgery will have the potential to be used in the totally endoscopic coronary artery bypass (TECAB).[4]

Totally Endoscopic Coronary Artery Bypass

TECAB has been made possible by the introduction of the da Vinci robotic system (Intuitive Surgical, Mountain View, CA). This system provides full intracorporeal articulation, which facilitates placement of the device to stabilize the section of interest. This device also has slotted cleats to hold the silastic vessel loops, permitting temporary target-vessel occlusion. The new system also allows for irrigation of the site of anastomosis.[32] Despite these advances, lack of tactile sensation is inherent to all robotic surgical procedures. The first TECAB procedure was reported by Loulmet et al.[33] In their experience, two patients underwent TECAB with the left IMA anastomosed to the LAD. Both of the patients had an uneventful hospital course and were discharged on postoperative days 6 and 7, respectively. The angiographic examination before discharge showed patency of the anastomosis. In two other patients, the left IMA was harvested using the same robotic system but the anastomosis had to be performed using a mini-thoracotomy. There was interference between the arms of the system or between the arms and the body of the patient during the dissection for left IMA harvesting. Positioning of the left IMA at the beginning of the anastomosis was difficult in the absence of an assistant.

At the same time, Reichenspurner et al reported the use of the Zeus Robotic Surgical system (Computer Motion, Goleta, CA) in endoscopic harvesting and anastomosis of the left IMA.[34] Although this group added a mini-thoracotomy for patient safety and part of the procedure was done through this thoracotomy, the robotic assistance device was used for anastomosis.

Even though these reports are exciting, TECAB is still time-consuming, it requires extensive experience with video-assisted surgery, and the expense of the equipment is significant. Furthermore, only single-vessel grafts have been reported. With improvement in technology and further miniaturization of equipment, TECAB may become more widely applicable.

Ventriculocoronary Artery Bypass

Ventriculocoronary artery bypass is a novel experimental approach for myocardial revascularization. With this method, implantation of an L-shaped titanium tube into the left ventricle connects the LAD directly to the ventricular cavity (Fig. 36–1).[35] Of the 11 pigs that Tweeden et al included in their study, 10 had patent tubes at the end of 2 weeks. This approach needs to be further evaluated before any human use is attempted but may provide an alternative for patients with extensive prior bypass surgery with limited arterial or venous conduits available for bypass.

Transmyocardial Laser Revascularization

Transmyocardial laser revascularization (TMR) has been suggested as an alternative for patients with symptomatic end-stage coronary artery disease responding poorly to maximal medical treatment. Initially, the reptilian heart was taken as a model and the channels created

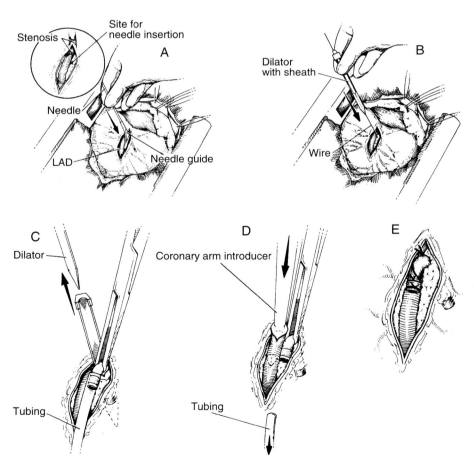

FIGURE 36–1. Ventriculocoronary bypass technique. *A*, Creation of the ventricle access tract. *B*, Introducer sheath with dilator. *C*, Seating of the device in ventricle. *D*, Introduction of device into coronary artery. *E*, Implanted device. (Adapted from Tweden KS, Eales F, Cameron JD, et al: Ventriculocoronary artery bypass [VCAB], a novel approach to myocardial revascularization. Heart Surg Forum 2000;3:47–54.)

were thought to remain open and provide the myocardium with blood from the ventricle. However, later studies proved these channels to be occluded.[36] The continued interest in these procedures came from the hypothesis that the local injury caused by the creation of these channels upregulates the local release of vascular endothelial growth factor (VEGF), which in turn increases the local neovascularization. Initial clinical trials of TMR in patients with refractory angina showed promising results. These trials, which were not blinded, showed a decrease in the angina class as well as an improvement in the exercise tolerance.

In a multicenter, nonrandomized, unblinded study, Horvath et al investigated a cohort of 200 patients before and after TMR. They showed significant improvement in the angina class as well as the number of reversible defects on radionuclide perfusion scans.[37] In another series of 268 patients, Vincent et al showed a decrease in the angina class and improvement in the quality of life but no improvement in survival.[38]

In the prospective Angina Treatments—Lasers and Normal Therapies In Comparison (ATLANTIC) trial, 182 patients were randomized to medical management or TMR. The TMR group showed a significant increase in exercise tolerance compared with the medical group.[39] Despite the improvement in somewhat subjective angina class, thallium scans did not show any improvement in the blood flow with TMR. Some reports trace the effectiveness of TMR partly to cardiac sympathetic denervation.[40-42] However, other reports dispute this theory.[43,44]

In another randomized prospective but unblinded study, Frazier et al concluded that TMR improved angina class, improved myocardial perfusion, and reduced the number of hospitalizations compared with medical treatment alone.[45]

Allen et al looked at 275 patients with refractory angina and coronary artery disease who could not be treated by percutaneous or surgical intervention. These authors randomized them to TMR or medical management. The 1-year follow-up showed improvement in angina and fewer cardiac-related hospitalizations, but neither survival nor myocardial perfusion had improved.[46]

In contradiction to these findings, Schofield et al found that TMR conferred no improvement in exercise time or mortality in their series of 188 patients. However, the decrease in the angina class was greater in the TMR group.[47] The Norwegian study also showed relief of symptoms but no benefit in survival or exercise time.[48]

Despite these somewhat conflicting results, there appeared to be a consensus that surgical TMR improves the angina class of patients with advanced coronary artery disease. This sparked interest in the use of percutaneous techniques for myocardial revascularization. In the studies of percutaneous transmyocardial revascularization (PTMR), the holmium:YAG laser was used with fluoroscopic or electromagnetic mapping.

The Potential Class Improvement From Intramyocardial Channels (PACIFIC) study was a multicenter randomized trial. However, as with previous TMR trials, it was unblinded. PTMR conferred improvements in exercise tolerance time and angina score but not in mortality or event-free survival.[49]

When the effectiveness of transmyocardial revascularization was tested in a randomized and blinded fashion in the Direct Myocardial Revascularization in Regeneration of Endocardial Channels (DIRECT) trial, there was a statistically significant improvement in all the groups, including the placebo arm, in the 6-month change in exercise duration, which was the primary end point of this study. The groups also showed no difference in the improvement in angina class. Single photon emission computed tomography (SPECT) showed no convincing evidence of improvement with PTMR. This study demonstrates the dramatic effect of placebo in these no-option patients because both the placebo and the TMR groups showed significant improvement. Although some authors have argued that there is a distinction between TMR and PTMR, the lack of placebo-controlled, blinded surgical trials to support this hypothesis makes it difficult to disregard the placebo effect, as seen in the DIRECT trial.

PERCUTANEOUS REVASCULARIZATION TECHNIQUES

Thrombectomy Devices

A significant number of patients presenting with acute coronary syndromes have a thrombus-containing lesion.[50] These lesions are associated with in-hospital and long-term adverse outcomes.[51] Thrombus-containing lesions are also associated with an increased rate of acute closure and the need for emergency bypass surgery after coronary interventions.[52] Multiple nonballoon devices have been used in patients with thrombus-containing lesions.

Transluminal extraction atherectomy (TEC) has been used successfully in thrombus-containing lesions.[53,54] Although some studies show less CK elevation after TEC compared with PTCA, distal embolization may not be prevented by TEC.[55] In the New Approaches to Coronary Interventions (NACI) trial, stand-alone TEC was one of the multivariate predictors of distal embolization and distal embolization was associated with a sixfold increase in in-hospital mortality.[56] With the advent of more powerful thrombus extraction devices, TEC use has decreased markedly.

Another device emerging for use in patients with thrombus-containing arteries is the Acolysis catheter, which uses ultrasound energy to dissipate the existing thrombus.[57] In experimental studies, therapeutic ultrasound was shown to require 20 times more energy to damage the vessel wall than what is necessary to lyse thrombi.[58] The use of coronary ultrasound thrombolysis has been reported in a small series of patients with acute myocardial infarction.[57] In the Analysis of Coronary Ultrasound Thrombolysis Endpoint (ACUTE) trial, 15 patients underwent coronary ultrasound thrombolysis. The ultrasound treatment achieved TIMI 3 flow in 87% of the patients without any adverse clinical events.[57] In the Acolysis registry, ultrasound thrombolysis was performed in 32 centers on 126 patients, procedural success was achieved in 98% of cases, and there were no major adverse clinical events.[59] The Acolysis during Treatment of Lesions Affecting SVGs (ATLAS) trial evaluated ultrasound thrombolysis in saphenous vein graft disease but was stopped prematurely because of higher postprocedural enzyme increase in the device arm.[60] Ultrasound atherectomy is a safe and effective method that can be used without serious adverse effects. However, the safety of its use in the vein graft disease is now in question.

Two devices use the Venturi effect to aspirate the thrombus. Hydrolyzer (Cordis Europa N.V., Roden, The Netherlands) is a 6-French double-lumen over-the-wire catheter that has an injection lumen and a large exhaust lumen with side holes at the tip (Fig. 36–2). Through the injection lumen, a saline/heparin solution is injected; this high-speed jet is directed over the side hole. With the reduction of pressure, thrombus is sucked through the side hole. In a small series by van den Bos et al, the device was successful but one of the seven patients experienced distal embolization.[61] In a larger study involving 31 patients, van Ommen et al were able to remove thrombus in 29 of 31 patients. Two of the 31 patients experienced distal embolization, one of which resulted in a non–Q-wave myocardial infarction.[62] There is limited experience with this system, which has not been approved by the FDA.

AngioJet (Possis Medical, Minneapolis) is a relatively new system that is used to macerate and aspirate thrombus. The retrogradely directed high-pressure saline jet creates a localized low-pressure zone; this is used to break down the thrombus, which is then aspirated through the proximal end of the catheter (Fig. 36–3).

The AngioJet catheter was used successfully to remove the thrombus compared with intracoronary urokinase infusion in the Vein Graft AngioJet Study (VEGAS 2) trial.[63] Although AngioJet thrombectomy achieved a better in-hospital MACE rate with much less bleeding and vascular complications, the 30-day MACE rate—which was the primary end point of the study—was not different in the urokinase group.

AngioJet has also been used safely and successfully in patients with acute myocardial infarction.[64] Nakagawa et al used the AngioJet catheter in 31 patients with acute or recent myocardial infarction and native coronary lesions.[64] TIMI flow improved significantly after the use of thrombectomy, and angiographic follow-up at 6 months showed a binary restenosis rate of 8% in stented and 29% in nonstented cases. At 1 year of clinical follow-up, no additional event was observed. VEGAS 1 and VEGAS 2 investigators also looked at the use of rheolytic thrombectomy in patients with acute myocardial infarction.[65] Thrombectomy significantly improved the TIMI flow in this study: Of the 70 patients included, 15% experienced distal embolization and the in-hospital mortality rate was 7% despite the fact that 16% of the patients experienced cardiogenic shock. The reported studies with the AngioJet catheter were done using the 5-French catheter, which can fit through an 8-French guiding catheter. With the advent of the new XMI catheter,

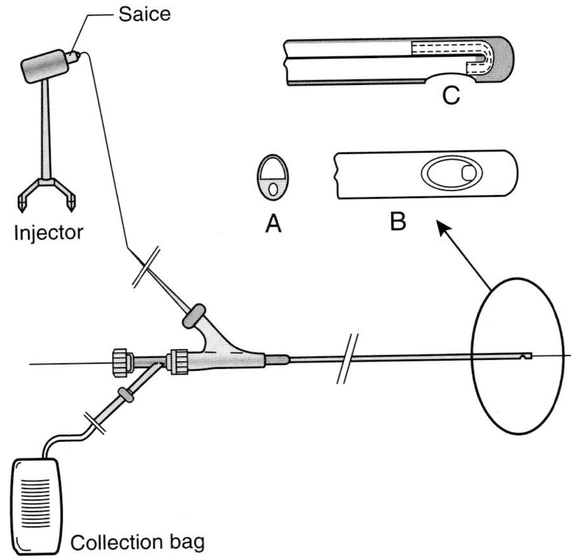

FIGURE 36–2. Double-lumen 6-French Hydrolyser. The contrast injector is connected to the hydrolyser. The removed material is collected in the collection bag. A, cross-section of the catheter body; B, view of the catheter tip from above; C, view from the side of the catheter tip. (Adapted from van Ommen VG, van den Bos AA, Pieper M, et al: Removal of thrombus from aortocoronary bypass grafts and coronary arteries using the 6Fr Hydrolyser. Am J Cardiol 1997;79:1012–1016.)

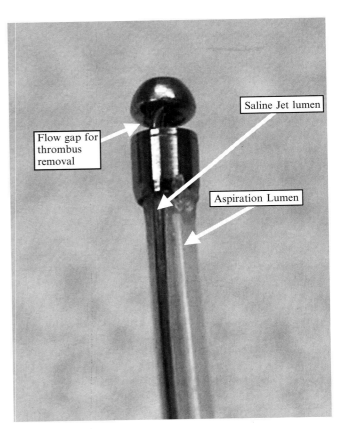

FIGURE 36–3. AngioJet catheter tip, showing the aspiration lumen, flush lumen, and the gap where the thrombus is aspirated.

which can be used through a 6-French catheter, the clinical utility of rheolytic thrombectomy may increase. The studies with this new catheter in the setting of acute myocardial infarction are yet to be reported.

Despite the promising results of rheolytic thrombectomy, it has some pitfalls. The AngioJet catheter can hemolyze red blood cells, resulting in occasional hemoglobinuria.[66] Acute increase in the ST segments also occurs and is thought to be due to hemolysis and local hyperkalemia. Bradycardia is also thought to be related to hemolysis and local increase in adenosine.[66,67] Vessel injury, although rare, can occur if the catheter is used in smaller vessels, where it is occlusive.[68] Distal embolization can occur with AngioJet use and has been reported in clinical trials.[66] Fortunately, the prevalence of Q-wave infarction resulting from the AngioJet catheter is rare.[66]

The X-SIZER catheter (EndiCOR Medical, San Clemente, CA) is a newly developed device for soft tissue and thrombus removal from the coronary arteries or saphenous vein grafts. This device has a helical cutter assembly connected to an external vacuum source. The device consists of a 5.5-French over-the-wire catheter with a helical cutter at the tip and a battery drive unit at the proximal end. The catheter lumen is connected to a vacuum bottle (Fig. 36–4). The device can be used through an 8-French catheter system over standard coronary wires.

The feasibility and safety of this catheter have been tested in a multicenter trial.[69] Eighty-five patients with angiographic appearance of thrombus and a reference vessel diameter of greater than 3 mm were included in this study. Of these 85 patients, 18 had saphenous vein graft lesions. In 84% of patients, the X-SIZER was successfully deployed to the target lesion; final procedural success was 93% after the use of balloons or stents, or both. Technical failure was mainly due to an inability to negotiate the coronary artery because of the physical characteristics of the catheter. In one patient, a thrombus fragment dislodged forward, causing an increase in creatine kinase. Two side branch occlusions occurred because of thrombus dislodgement. There was also a vessel perforation in a saphenous vein graft after balloon dilatation following X-SIZER use. However, coronary flow and thrombus burden improved significantly after X-SIZER use. With improved design, the next generation

of X-SIZER devices might show improved technical success. The advantages of this system are its ease of setup and lack of need to buy additional equipment. However, more data are needed before it can be used clinically. Two trials are underway that use this device: the X-SIZER for Treatment of Thrombus and Atherosclerosis in Coronary Interventions Trial (X-TRACT) in the United States and the X-SIZER in AMI Patients for Negligible Embolization and Optimal ST Resolution (XAMINE ST) trial in Europe.

Although generally safe and effective, thrombectomy devices may not completely prevent distal embolization. Another approach to prevent distal embolization, especially in the degenerated saphenous venous graft, is the distal protection device.

Distal Protection Devices

Distal embolization of particulate matter, including plaque debris and thrombus, complicate percutaneous coronary and peripheral interventions, especially in the setting of saphenous vein grafts. This often results in diminished blood flow to the distal vascular bed and is associated with periprocedural end-organ ischemia and infarction, as demonstrated by serum cardiac enzyme elevation.[70] Periprocedural myocardial infarction is associated with a worse prognosis, particularly when it is large. This is particularly a problem in saphenous vein graft interventions. Hong et al studied 1056 consecutive patients with angiographically successful percutaneous coronary intervention of 1693 saphenous vein graft lesions. One-year mortality was significantly increased in patients with periprocedural CK-MB elevation, even among patients without any apparent procedure-related or in-hospital complication.[71]

A number of distal protection devices that aim to reduce or eliminate distal embolization during percutaneous coronary and carotid interventions are under development (Table 36–1).

The PercuSurge GuardWire (Medtronic, Santa Rosa, CA) is the only distal protection device approved for use. It is an occlusion thrombectomy device that consists of a wire containing a central lumen that communicates with a low-pressure distal occlusion balloon incorporated into the tip (Fig. 36–5). This wire serves both as a

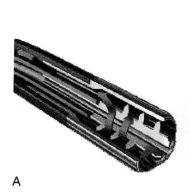

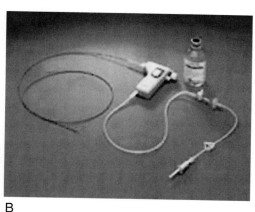

A   B

FIGURE 36–4. X-SIZER catheter, showing the helical cutter at the tip (A) and the system (B). The only required assembly is hooking the suction catheter to the bottle.

■ ■ ■
TABLE 36–1 DISTAL PROTECTION DEVICES UNDER DEVELOPMENT

Balloon Occlusion Devices

PercuSurge GuardWire (Medtronic, Santa Rosa, CA)

Filter Devices

AngioGuard (Cordis Corp., Minneapolis, MN)
FilterWire EX (Boston Scientific Corp., Natick, MA)
Mednova Neuroshield (MedNova Inc., Galway, Ireland)
AccuNet (Guidant Corp., Indianapolis, IN)

Catheter Occlusion Devices

Parodi Anti-Embolism Catheter (ArteriA Medical Science, Inc., San Francisco, CA)

---

guidewire and as a distal protection device. A dial-up inflation device attached to the end of the wire allows one to dial the desired distal balloon size to achieve total occlusion of the vessel, thus preventing any debris from going downstream during the percutaneous intervention. Once the intervention is completed, the aspiration catheter is used to remove the debris before the distal balloon is deflated and antegrade flow to the distal vessel is restored.

The safety and efficacy of this device was initially evaluated in 103 patients from seven sites and resulted in a 4.3% MACE rate.[72] In 95% of the cases, visible material was recovered; 81% of the material was under 96 µm in size.[72] After these encouraging results, the Saphenous Vein Graft Angioplasty Free of Emboli, Randomized (SAFER) trial was conducted in the United States.[73] Forty-seven sites enrolled 551 patients before the trial was stopped. Patients with lesions (50% to 100%) in saphenous vein grafts 3 to 6 mm in diameter, more than 5 mm from the ostium, 20 mm from the distal anastomosis, and of at least TIMI-I flow at baseline were included. Patients with ongoing myocardial infarction, depressed left-ventricular ejection fraction, and chronic renal insufficiency were excluded. Patients who were scheduled for atherectomy were also excluded. The primary end point

was major adverse clinical events at the index hospitalization. The PercuSurge system led to a 50% reduction in the primary end point of major adverse clinical events during the index hospitalization (17.3% vs. 8.8%; $P = .003$). This benefit was also present at 30 days (19.8% vs. 9.9%). The PercuSurge system use was also associated with a significantly less no-reflow phenomenon (94.2% vs. 98.1%). These results were independent of the use of glycoprotein-IIb/IIIa inhibitors.

This trial was stopped by the data safety monitoring board, and FDA approval was granted. Currently, PercuSurge is the only distal protection device in the United States available for clinical use. The superiority of this device over other devices under development is its ability to prevent any particle from going downstream. However, this also prevents visualization of the lesion during the intervention. Furthermore, the distal vascular bed remains ischemic throughout the inflation of the distal balloon. For these reasons, filter devices have been proposed as a next class of distal protection devices.

AngioGuard (Cordis Corp., Minneapolis, MN) is an example of such a device that has received approval for marketing in Europe. This is an angioplasty guidewire that has a filter at the distal end, which can expand to 6 mm to capture the embolic debris (Fig. 36–6). At the end of the procedure, the filter is collapsed and the particulate material is retrieved. The AngioGuard device has multiple 100 µm holes to allow for distal perfusion during the procedure. This may be particularly important in patients with reduced left-ventricular function and in patients in whom a vein graft supplies a large amount of myocardium. On the other hand, it has been suggested that the incomplete occlusion of the vessel allows for the passage of some particulate material downstream. In fact, in the SAFE trial, 80% of the material captured was less than 100 µm in size. However, the clinical significance of such small particulate matter is unclear and is difficult to determine unless these distal protection devices are compared head to head.

The initial experience with the AngioGuard Emboli Capture Guidewire has been published.[74] The investiga-

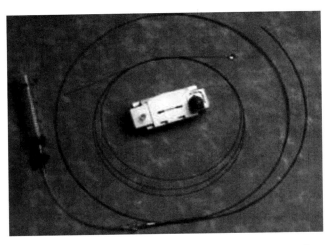

FIGURE 36–5. PercuSurge GuardWire system (Medtronic, Santa Rosa, CA).

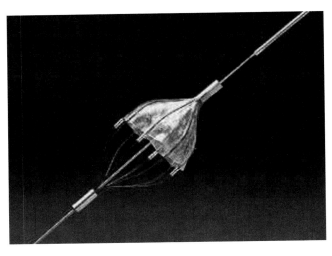

FIGURE 36–6. AngioGuard filter wire system.

tors reported their experience on 26 patients (15 native coronary artery and 11 vein graft interventions). Their success rate was 96.2%, and in only one patient were they unable to pass the guidewire. They reported no adverse events related to the device. Two patients were found to have a periprocedural myocardial infarction. This study shows the feasibility of the AngioGuard system but does not provide evidence of the clinical effectiveness of the device compared with the standard of care. The definition of standard of care in emboli-prone lesions, especially in vein grafts, is now debatable since the results of the SAFER trial have become known. Some might argue that the effectiveness of the newer distal protection devices should be compared with the PercuSurge Guard wire system.

The FilterWire EX (Boston Scientific Corp., Natick, MA) is another filter device currently under clinical investigation (Fig. 36–7). It consists of a microporous polyurethane net, with 80 μm pore size, attached to a self-expanding nitinol ring attached to a 0.0014-inch guidewire. When withdrawn into the restraining sheath, the system is 3.8-French. The feasibility of this device was reported in 41 patients undergoing saphenous vein graft intervention.[75] The procedural success rate was 98%, and the only in-hospital complication was an increase in CK-MB to greater than eight times normal in two patients (4.9%). This device is in its early stages of development and is not yet available for clinical use.

The MedNova NeuroShield (MedNova, Galway, Ireland) is a filter that is mounted on the distal tip of a 0.014-inch guidewire. Its use requires both a delivery catheter and a retrieval catheter. The filter contains a preshaped nitinol expansion system that facilitates fluoroscopic visualization, accurate deployment, and wall apposition. The filter guidewire is placed within the delivery catheter and is passed through the target stenosis, the delivery catheter is withdrawn, and the filter is deployed; after vascular intervention is completed, the retrieval catheter is used to envelop the filter. Then, the entire device and its embolic contents are withdrawn. A feasibility study was done in five centers and included 29 patients.[76] The device was successfully deployed in all patients, but three patients experienced non–ST-segment elevation myocardial infarction (CK-MB was three times the upper limit of normal) and one procedure was complicated by no-reflow and myocardial infarction. The data are still preliminary for this device, and larger studies are needed.

The clinical significance of distal embolization with small amounts of particulate material is uncertain, but the clinical consequence of large infarcts that may occur because of distal embolization in degenerated vein graft intervention is obvious. The currently available devices are not perfect, but with improvement of their design and ease of use, they offer to be promising new tools with a high potential for distal embolization.

Cutting Balloon Angioplasty

The cutting balloon (CB) (Interventional Technologies, San Diego, CA) is a newer device with microblades longitudinally affixed to the surface of the balloon (Fig. 36–8). The CB is a noncompliant balloon that achieves efficient lumen enlargement by creating a controlled dissection within the vessel wall. Slow low-pressure inflations of 4 to 10 atmospheres are recommended. The CB was recently approved in the United States and is available in 10 and 15 mm at various balloon sizes. CB use has been advocated for high-pressure balloon–resistant lesions, ostial lesions, small-vessel angioplasty, and in-stent restenotic lesions. When inflated, the blades are exposed and incise the stenotic tissue.

Some investigators have successfully used the CB in the treatment of in-stent restenosis (ISR).[77–79] Muramatsu et al compared the CB with PTCA in 47 patients with ISR.[79] The authors observed a higher acute gain and a lower late loss in the lumen area by intravenous ultrasonosgraphy. The restenosis rate at 6 months of follow-up was lower in the CB group (59% vs. 24%). In a randomized pilot study, Chevalier et al reported that CB achieved a higher acute gain. However, at 9 months of follow-up, the rates of target vessel late revascularization were not statistically significant (20% vs. 12% with CB).[80] On the other hand, Mizobe et al showed that CB was associated with a lower TLR rate at 6 months (3.8% vs. 28%).[81] In a study of 258 lesions, Adamian et al compared CB with rotational atherectomy (RA) and PTCA alone for ISR.[82] At 1 year of follow-up, the TLR rate was lower with CB.[82]

In a nonrandomized study of 519 patients, Lauer et al compared PTCA to CB angioplasty for the treatment of ISR. CB was associated with less late loss, greater net gain, and a reduced TLR rate (16.3% vs. 39.1%). In this study, the use of CB was the only predictor of freedom from future ISR.[83]

The use of CB in the treatment of ISR in conjunction with brachytherapy is an emerging concept. Together with the good acute and long-term results, another advantage of CB is the ability to accurately position the CB without much "watermelon seeding," thus limiting the length of the injured segment. Studies of CB combined with vascular brachytherapy for the treatment of ISR are yet to be reported.

Ostial lesions with high elastic recoil still present a problem for percutaneous interventions. Stenting of

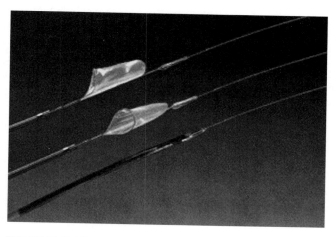

FIGURE 36–7. FilterWire EX (Boston Scientific Corp., Natick, MA).

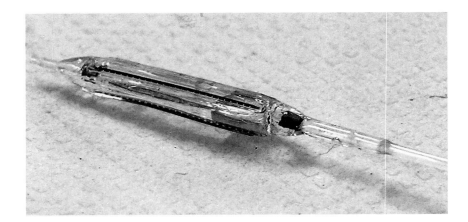

FIGURE 36–8. Cutting balloon with micro-blades affixed to the surface of the balloon.

both native and saphenous vein grafts have been promising. However, before a stent is deployed, adequate angioplasty is needed. Kurbaan et al reported a small series of patients who had undergone unsuccessful high-pressure balloon angioplasty in whom the CB produced satisfactory results and facilitated the deployment of stents.[84] CB angioplasty has also been used without stenting for ostial lesions and has shown better results than PTCA.[85] This approach may be used to prevent plaque shift to another major branch in some vessels.[86]

Small-vessel angioplasty is still challenging, with high restenosis rates even after the use of stents.[87] CB angioplasty has been effectively used for small-vessel interventions.[88] In an early trial, CB angioplasty was compared with PTCA in vessels smaller than 3 mm. At 6 months of angiographic follow-up, CB angioplasty achieved a lower angiographic restenosis (27% vs. 47%).[88] The 9-month event-free survival rate was also better with CB angioplasty (72% vs. 49%). Izumi et al reported the largest comparison of CB with PTCA in small vessels.[89] Achieving lower inflation pressures with CB, the investigators reported a lower restenosis angiographic follow-up at 3 months (25.2% vs. 41.5%), especially for vessels smaller than 2.25 mm (24.2% vs. 49.2%). The 1-year clinical follow-up showed a lower event rate with the CB angioplasty (27.2% vs. 39.0%). The impact of drug-eluting stents on intervention for small vessels remains to be determined. Until then, CB may be an alternative to stenting in small vessels except for bailout situations.

Drug-Eluting Stents

Despite improvements in interventional cardiology with the advent of stenting, ISR remained the Achilles heel of stenting. The reason for restenosis after balloon angioplasty is elastic recoil and neointimal hyperplasia. Stents have taken care of the elastic recoil problem, but the neointimal hyperplasia was not reduced and in fact increased by stent implantation.[90] Intracoronary brachytherapy has offered some hope, but the prevention of ISR remained a challenge. In an attempt to prevent restenosis, drug-eluting stents have been developed. A number of companies have developed this new technology (Table 36–2).

Sirolimus (rapamycin) is one of the substances currently being investigated in clinical trials. It is a natural macrolide antibiotic and is a potent immunosuppressive agent developed by Wyeth-Ayerst Laboratories (Philadelphia). Sirolimus has been used to prevent renal transplant rejection.[91] Sirolimus binds to an intracellular protein (FK506-binding protein) and elevates p27 levels, which in turn inhibits cyclin/cyclin-dependent kinase (CDK) complexes and causes cell cycle arrest in the late G1 phase.[92] Sirolimus selectively targets smooth muscle cells and inhibits smooth muscle cell proliferation and migration.[93,94]

Implantation of sirolimus-coated stents in de novo lesions was shown to be effective in limiting neointimal formation.[95] In 30 patients with angina, sirolimus-coated stents with slow and fast release were implanted. Fast-release stents released sirolimus in less than 15 days, whereas slow-release stents released the drug for more than 28 days. At 4 months' intravascular ultrasound follow-up, lumen loss was minimal. No patient reached greater than 50% vessel narrowing, and only three patients experienced greater than 15% intimal hyperplasia. There was no edge stenosis and stent thrombosis, and there were no adverse effects at 8 months of clinical follow-up. There was no difference between the slow-release and fast-release groups. Another 15 patients in the Netherlands underwent implantation of the slow-release drug-eluting stents. In the long-term (12 months) follow-up of the 30 patients from Brazil and the 6-month follow-up of the 15 patients from the Netherlands, there was no restenosis by binary defini-

■ ■ ■

TABLE 36–2 DRUGS IN DEVELOPMENT FOR DRUG-ELUTING STENTS

Cordis/JJIS	Sirolimus
Guidant	Actinomycin D
AVE/Medtronic	Antisense
Cook	Taxol
BSC	Paclitaxel (Taxol)
Biodivysio	Dexamethasone, Batimastat, Angiopeptin
Tamai	Tranilast

tion. There was again minimal in-stent or in-lesion late lumen loss.[96]

After these encouraging experiences, the randomized double-blind study with the sirolimus-eluting Bx Velocity (Cordis Corp., Minneapolis, MN) balloon expandable stent in the treatment of de novo native coronary artery lesions (RAVEL) study included 238 patients. This study compared sirolimus-eluting and bare Bx Velocity stents in patients with single de novo lesions in native coronary arteries less than 18 mm in length and 2.5 to 3.5 mm in diameter. The restenosis rate was 0% in the drug-eluting stent group and 26% in the bare stent group.[97] The event-free survival rate at 210 days was 96.7% in the sirolimus group and 72.9% in the control group. None of the patients in the sirolimus group required re-intervention, and there were no deaths in this group. The sirolimus-eluting stents were beneficial regardless of vessel size. Even in the diabetic subgroup (44 patients, 19 of whom were given the sirolimus-eluting stent), the restenosis rate was 0% and the diameter stenosis remained at 16% versus the 38% in the control group. No edge restenosis or late thrombosis was observed. A larger yet similar study that includes 1101 patients with de novo lesions in native coronary arteries and compares the sirolimus-eluting Bx Velocity stent with the bare metal Bx Velocity stent (SIRIUS trial). The results presented at the Transcatheter Cardiovascular Therapeutic (TCT)-2002 meeting showed a striking reduction in the 8-month rates of in-stent stenosis (3% versus 35%, $P<0.001$) with the drug-eluting sten.[97b]

Another drug that has been shown to inhibit smooth muscle cell migration and proliferation is paclitaxel. Paclitaxel (Taxol), extracted from the Pacific yew tree *Taxus brevifolia*, exerts its antineoplastic effects by interfering with cell microtubule function. Paclitaxel interferes with cell replication at stages G_0/G_1 and G_2/M.[98,99] Systemic administration of paclitaxel causes a significant reduction of neointimal proliferation in rats at blood concentrations 100 times lower than antineoplastic levels.[100] Because drug-eluting stents allow targeting of specific vascular beds with high local drug concentrations and minimal systemic effects, paclitaxel has been tried with and without the polymeric coating in drug-eluting stents.[101,102] The highly lipophilic character of paclitaxel makes it very suitable for this purpose. The results of the first clinical studies have been reported. The TAXUS I study was a prospective, randomized, double-blind trial done in three centers in Germany. In this trial, paclitaxel was eluted through a customized polymer carrier on the NIRx (Boston Scientific Corp., Natick, MA) stent. The TAXUS I trial included 61 patients with de novo lesions up to 12 mm in length. The primary end point of this study was 30-day major adverse events, which was not different among the groups. However, both groups experienced MACE rates of 0% because of the outstanding performance of the control group. At 6 months of follow-up, the binary restenosis rate was 10% in the bare stent group and 0% in the paclitaxel-eluting stent group.[103]

The role of different polymers to control the release of drugs has been a topic of discussion. Several manufacturers do not use the polymeric coating for paclitaxel-eluting stents. In the Asian paclitaxel-eluting stent clinical trial (ASPECT), the stent used was the paclitaxel-coated Supra G stent (Cook, Bloomington, IN), which did not have a polymeric coating.[104] This study included 177 patients with de novo lesions and a reference vessel diameter of greater than 2.5 mm and a lesion length of less than 15 mm. These were mainly type A or B1 lesions. In three treatment groups, the uncoated Supra G stent was tested against the low-dose-density and high-dose-density paclitaxel-coated Supra G stents. The primary end point of this study was restenosis at 6 months. The patients in the control group had significantly greater loss in mean lumen diameter than the patients in the coated-stent groups. The binary restenosis rate was 4% in the high-dose density group and 12% in the low-dose density group in contrast with the 27% rate in the bare stent group. Although 139 patients were treated with aspirin and ticlopidine or clopidogrel after the procedure, 37 patients were given aspirin and cilostazol (12 high-dose, 15 low-dose, 10 control) and 1 patient received no antiplatelet therapy. The subgroup of patients with high-dose paclitaxel who received cilostazol instead of thienopyridine antiplatelet drugs experienced a higher MACE rate.

Another Cook-funded trial also showed a significant decrease in the restenosis rate (3% vs. 21%) with the paclitaxel coated V-Flex Plus stent (Cook, Bloomington, IN) and was known as the EvaLUation of pacliTaxel-Eluting Stent (ELUTES) clinical trial.[105] Similar to the case with the ASPECT trial, patients had type A or B1 lesions that were less than 15 mm in length in native 2.75 to 3.5 mm vessels. No late thromboses were associated with the target lesion in the study (all patients received clopidogrel for 3 months). Despite excellent results with binary restenosis, the event-free survival rate at 6 months was not different between the groups (89% in both groups) (Table 36–3).

The debate regarding the coating of the stent with polymer is still ongoing. The idea behind the coating is the controlled release of the drug. On the other hand, proponents of the bare stent with drug attached directly to the steel surface raise concerns over the potential of polymer itself stimulating neointimal formation. Both the ASPECT and ELUTES trials used non–polymer-coated stents with good results. The TAXUS trials are using polymer coating for controlled release of the paclitaxel, also with good results. It is hoped that the issue of coating will be resolved when the results of these trials become available.

Another issue regarding drug-eluting stents is the length and composition of the antiplatelet regimens. In the RAVEL trial, patients received up to 8 weeks of clopidogrel or ticlopidine. In the ELUTES trial, patients were given 3 months of aspirin and clopidogrel. In the TAXUS I trial, patients received 6 months of antiplatelet therapy. In the ASPECT trial, although patients were supposed to get 1 to 6 months of antiplatelet therapy, 37 of 177 patients received cilostazol instead of thienopyridine antiplatelet drugs and experienced high rates of thrombosis. There is no consensus regarding the duration of antiplatelet therapy after the placing of drug-eluting

■ ■ ■

TABLE 36–3 KEY COMPARISONS OF THE MAJOR DRUG-ELUTING STENT TRIALS (MOST EFFECTIVE TREATMENT ARMS)

	RAVEL N = 120	TAXUS I N = 31	ASPECT N = 60 (HIGH-DOSE)	ELUTES N = 50 (HIGH-DOSE)
Late loss (mm)	– 0.01	0.36	0.29	0.10
Change in diameter stenosis (%)	< 1%	13%	10%	14%
MACE better than control	Yes	No	No	No
Binary restenosis	0%	0%	4%	3%
Thrombosis	0%	0%	5%	0%

MACE, major adverse cardiac event.

stents. Nevertheless, the data seem to support a course of clopidogrel for 2 to 6 months.

Despite the encouraging results of these recent trials with drug-eluting stents, there is still concern about the long-term effect and the potential for late thrombosis as well as the effects of the stent design. Recently the SCORE trial was terminated early because of high MACE rate. This study was a European randomized, multicenter study initiated by Quanam Medical (Santa Clara, CA) before the company was purchased by Boston Scientific Corp.. The study was stopped after 300 of the anticipated 400 patients were enrolled. The Quanam QuaDS-QP2 stent used in this study used a paclitaxel-impregnated polymer and was laid in slabs which were placed along the length of the stent. The design of the stent, polymer coating, or the protocol violations in this study might have contributed to the adverse outcome.

There was a case report from Italy of a patient who had late total occlusion seven months after the implantation of a Quanam paclitaxel-eluting stent which occurred while the patient was taking aspirin but shortly after the discontinuation of ticlopidine.[106] The patient had a follow-up angiogram at six-months after the stent implantation which did not show intimal hyperplasia. This lack of intimal hyperplasia, together with the time course of the event being shortly after the discontinuation of ticlopidine, suggests a thrombotic occlusion. With this in mind, the duration of double antiplatelet therapy with aspirin and a thienopyridine should be considered for long-term use for the patients receiving drug-eluting stents. The mechanism of the stent thrombosis might have been delayed re-endothelialization after the stent implantation. Whether or not the design of the stent had anything to do with this is debatable. Nevertheless, long-term follow-up results of the drug-eluting stent studies will shed light on this problem.

The future of drug-eluting stents involves testing them in in-stent restenosis, bifurcation disease, small vessels and left main coronary artery stenting. The stent versus surgery trials in multivessel disease may have to be redone with the advent of the drug-eluting stents.

Using the Coronary Veins as Arterial Conduits

Interventional cardiology has made important strides within the last few decades, but not all the lesions are approachable by conventional techniques. Newer strategies are required for complete revascularization using the catheter-based approach. Atherosclerosis is not observed in the cardiac veins and their proximity to the respective coronary arteries makes them suitable conduits for newer methods of revascularization. The heart has two interconnected venous systems, the lesser and the greater systems. These systems communicate with each other through a complex network.[107] This system can therefore be used as a conduit for arterial revascularization without rendering the heart devoid of its venous drainage. The interest in the cardiac veins for coronary perfusion is quite old.[108] Initial attempts to use retroperfusion of the heart through connecting arterial conduits to the coronary sinus (Beck I and Beck II procedures) were associated with high (>25%) mortality and with the development of coronary artery bypass surgery, the enthusiasm for this procedure faded.[107] Later on, in selected patients, surgeons have used selective coronary venous bypass grafting by anatomizing to a specific vein that drains the targeted ischemic area.[109,110] Sometimes the coronary veins bypassed were inadvertently mistaken for the neighboring coronary artery.[111] The results were not as successful as standard bypass operations, but this might have been an effective therapy for patients with severe angina pectoris and no further options for revascularization.

Coronary veins have also been used for temporary support for the jeopardized myocardium. These methods are synchronized retroperfusion of the coronary sinus, synchronized suction and retroperfusion, and pressure-controlled intermittent coronary sinus occlusion. In synchronized retroperfusion, arterial blood is retrogradely infused into the coronary sinus in an ECG gated fashion so that the coronary sinus is perfused in diastole and the venous blood is permitted to drain in systole. This method has been tested in dogs for safety and efficacy and was shown not to damage the coronary sinus.[112]

There was also no evidence of myocardial edema or hemolysis.

This method has been used in the setting of PTCA.[113] In a study involving 30 patients Kar et al showed that coronary sinus retroperfusion was associated with a lower angina score, delayed onset of angina during balloon inflations, and decreased left ventricular dysfunction during balloon inflations. It was also used both as a bridge to coronary bypass surgery[114] and successfully in patients with unstable angina or evolving myocardial infarction to relieve ischemia.[115] The patients experienced relief of symptoms with improvement in the ST segment changes and wall motion in the ischemic zone.[115] The use of synchronized retroperfusion has not gained much support with the increased use of coronary stents decreasing the abrupt closure or threatened closure cases and the need for a specialized retroperfusion system as well as the need for experienced operators for the use of this system.

The other method proposed for retroperfusion through the coronary veins is selective synchronized suction and retroperfusion. In this method the regional coronary vein is cannulated and the venous drainage in systole is augmented by suction. This approach was tested on a limited number of patients undergoing percutaneous coronary intervention.[116] Since the clinical data on the use of this system are extremely limited and the use of stents made interventions on a variety of anatomical subsets much easier by decreasing the need for prolonged inflations, the use of selective synchronized suction and retroperfusion has not gained much popularity.

In patients with severe coronary artery disease who are unwilling to go for coronary artery bypass surgery or in whom general anesthesia poses a great risk and the revascularization options are limited to percutaneous techniques, new investigational methods might offer hope in the future. Despite improvements in the cardiac surgery and coronary intervention techniques, some patients still remain not good candidates for both sur-

gery and PCI. The use of coronary veins as bypass conduits is not a new concept as described above. However, the use of percutaneous techniques in creating arteriovenous conduits and using coronary veins supplying arterial blood to the ischemic area is an emerging technique. Two different procedures have been described to achieve this goal, percutaneous in situ coronary venous arterialization and percutaneous in situ coronary artery bypass (PICAB). Percutaneous in situ coronary venous arterialization (PICVA) involves creating an arteriovenous communication between the coronary artery and the adjacent vein and a proximal blocking device is deployed into the vein to prevent retrograde flow of arterial blood (Fig. 36–9). This procedure might offer an alternative method of treatment for patients with chronic total occlusion of the coronary artery with viable myocardium in the territory supplied by that coronary artery. The first successful PICVA procedure in humans was recently reported.[116] This patient had a chronic total occlusion of the left anterior descending coronary artery with an apical infarct and surrounding ischemia. The attempts to cross the total occlusion were unsuccessful and because of the diffuse disease in the distal LAD, it was deemed unsuitable for bypass surgery.[117] In this patient, the communication was created between the LAD and the anterior interventricular vein which remained functional at the 3-month follow-up angiogram. At 12-month clinical follow-up the patient remained free of angina. Although this first case is encouraging, there have been other unsuccessful attempts to achieve cardiac venous arterialization.[117] Furthermore, the durability of the arteriovenous channel is unknown. As the technique is perfected this procedure may offer an alternative to the so-called "no-option" patients. The long-term goal in developing these techniques is to perform in situ bypass in patients with good distal targets.

Percutaneous in situ coronary artery bypass (PICAB) involves creating two channels between the artery and the adjacent vein proximal and distal to the narrowed

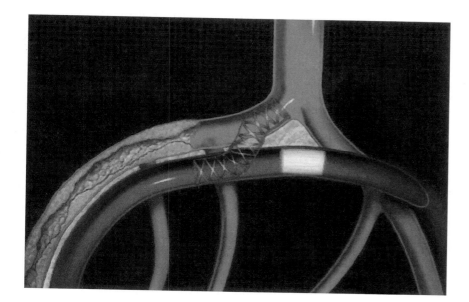

FIGURE 36–9. Percutaneous in situ coronary venous arterialization. (From Oesterle SN, Reifart N, Hauptmann E, et al: Percutaneous in situ coronary venous arterialization: Report of the first human catheter-based coronary artery bypass. Circulation 2001;103:2539–2543.)

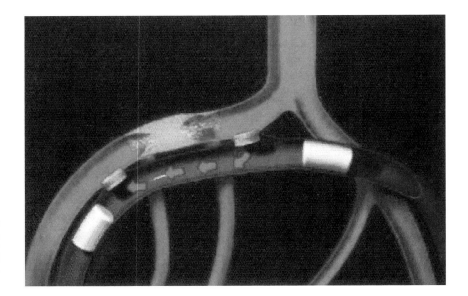

FIGURE 36–10. Percutaneous in situ coronary artery bypass. (From Oesterle SN, Reifart N, Hauptmann E, et al: Percutaneous in situ coronary venous arterialization: Report of the first human catheter-based coronary artery bypass. Circulation 2001;103:2539–2543.)

arterial segment (Fig. 36–10). Deployment of blocking devices in the vein proximal and distal to the anastomosis sites isolates the segment of the vein and allows it to function as a bypass conduit. There are no clinical data available for this procedure as yet and the clinical studies with this procedure can be done after the safety and feasibility of the technique is shown in the PICVA trials.

CONCLUSIONS

Coronary revascularization continues to evolve rapidly. Some of this evolution has resulted from the introduction and widespread dissemination of interventional techniques, which have been widely embraced by the patients because they are less invasive than surgery. Such competition has been good for the field and has provided more options for patient care. The evolution continues, fueled by the demographics of patient population and the changing creative technology so that we can continue to identify optimal approaches to this large group of patients.

REFERENCES

1. Detre KM, Guo P, Holubkov R, et al: Coronary revascularization in diabetic patients: A comparison of the randomized and observational components of the Bypass Angioplasty Revascularization Investigation (BARI). Circulation 1999;99:633–640.
2. Benetti FJ, Naselli G, Wood M, et al: Direct myocardial revascularization without extracorporeal circulation. Experience in 700 patients. Chest 1991;100:312–316.
3. Subramanian VA: Clinical experience with minimally invasive reoperative coronary bypass surgery. Eur J Cardiothorac Surg 1996;10:1058–1062.
4. Mack MJ: Coronary surgery: Off-pump and port access. Surg Clin North Am 2000;80:1575–1591.
5. Nataf P, Lima L, Regan M, et al: Thoracoscopic internal mammary artery harvesting: technical considerations. Ann Thorac Surg 1997;63:S104–S106.
6. Nataf P, Lima L, Regan M, et al: Minimally invasive coronary surgery with thoracoscopic internal mammary artery dissection: Surgical technique. J Cardiovasc Surg 1996;11:288–292.
7. Watanabe G, Misaki T, Kotoh K, et al: Multiple minimally invasive direct coronary artery bypass grafting for the complete revascularization of the left ventricle. Ann Thorac Surg 1999;68:131–136.
8. Subramanian VA, Patel NU: Transabdominal minimally invasive direct coronary artery bypass grafting (MIDCAB). Eur J Cardiothorac Surg 2000;17:485–487.
9. Cohen HA, Zenati M, Smith AJ, et al: Feasibility of combined percutaneous transluminal angioplasty and minimally invasive direct coronary artery bypass in patients with multivessel coronary artery disease. Circulation 1998;98:1048–1050.
10. De Canniere D, Jansens JL, Goldschmidt-Clermont P, et al: Combination of minimally invasive coronary bypass and percutaneous transluminal coronary angioplasty in the treatment of double-vessel coronary disease: Two-year follow-up of a new hybrid procedure compared with "on-pump" double bypass grafting. Am Heart J 2001;142:563–570.
11. Riess FC, Schofer J, Kremer P, et al: Beating heart operations including hybrid revascularization: Initial experiences. Ann Thorac Surg 1998;66:1076–1081.
12. Mack MJ, Magovern JA, Acuff TA, et al: Results of graft patency by immediate angiography in minimally invasive coronary artery surgery. Ann Thorac Surg 1999;68:383–389; discussion 389–390.
13. Mehran R, Dangas G, Stamou SC, et al: One-year clinical outcome after minimally invasive direct coronary artery bypass. Circulation 2000;102:2799–2802.
14. Berger PB, Alderman EL, Nadel A, et al: Frequency of early occlusion and stenosis in a left internal mammary artery to left anterior descending artery bypass graft after surgery through a median sternotomy on conventional bypass: Benchmark for minimally invasive direct coronary artery bypass. Circulation 1999;100: 2353–2358.
15. Stamou SC, Bafi AS, Boyce SW, et al: Coronary revascularization of the circumflex system: Different approaches and long-term outcome. Ann Thorac Surg 2000;70:1371–1377.
16. Kolessov VI: Mammary artery–coronary artery anastomosis as method of treatment for angina pectoris. J Thorac Cardiovasc Surg 1967;54:535–544.
17. Buffolo E, de Andrade CS, Branco JN, et al: Coronary artery bypass grafting without cardiopulmonary bypass. Ann Thorac Surg 1996;61:63–66.
18. Tasdemir O, Vural KM, Karagoz H, et al: Coronary artery bypass grafting on the beating heart without the use of extracorporeal circulation: Review of 2052 cases. J Thorac Cardiovasc Surg 1998;116:68–73.
19. Hart JC, Spooner TH, Pym J, et al: A review of 1,582 consecutive Octopus off-pump coronary bypass patients. Ann Thorac Surg 2000;70:1017–1020.
20. Ascione R, Lloyd CT, Underwood MJ, et al: On-pump versus off-pump coronary revascularization: Evaluation of renal function. Ann Thorac Surg 1999;68:493–498.

21. Yokoyama T, Baumgartner FJ, Gheissari A, et al: Off-pump versus on-pump coronary bypass in high-risk subgroups. Ann Thorac Surg 2000;70:1546-1550.

22. Gerritsen WB, van Boven WJ, Driessen AH, et al: Off-pump versus on-pump coronary artery bypass grafting: Oxidative stress and renal function. Eur J Cardiothorac Surg 2001;20:923-929.

23. Al-Ruzzeh S, George S, Yacoub M, et al: The clinical outcome of off-pump coronary artery bypass surgery in the elderly patients. Eur J Cardiothorac Surg 2001;20:1152-1156.

24. Bowles BJ, Lee JD, Dang CR, et al: Coronary artery bypass performed without the use of cardiopulmonary bypass is associated with reduced cerebral microemboli and improved clinical results. Chest 2001;119:25-30.

25. BhaskerRao B, VanHimbergen D, Edmonds HL Jr, et al: Evidence for improved cerebral function after minimally invasive bypass surgery. J Cardiovasc Surg 1998;13:27-31.

26. Kshettry VR, Flavin TF, Emery RW, et al: Does multivessel, off-pump coronary artery bypass reduce postoperative morbidity? Ann Thorac Surg 2000;69:1725-1730; discussion 1730-1731.

27. Diegeler A, Hirsch R, Schneider F, et al: Neuromonitoring and neurocognitive outcome in off-pump versus conventional coronary bypass operation. Ann Thorac Surg 2000;69:1162-1166.

28. Subramanian VA, Patel N: New minimal access approaches to multivessel coronary artery bypass grafting without pump. Curr Cardiol Rep 1999;1:311-312.

29. Galloway AC, Shemin RJ, Glower DD, et al: First report of the Port Access International Registry. Ann Thorac Surg 1999;67:51-56; discussion 57-58.

30. Ribakove GH, Miller JS, Anderson RV, et al: Minimally invasive port-access coronary artery bypass grafting with early angiographic follow-up: Initial clinical experience. J Thorac Cardiovasc Surg 1998;115:1101-1110.

31. Ribakove GH, Gossi EA, Steinberg BM, et al: Port-access minimally invasive CABG: Techniques and results. J Card Surg 2000;15:296-302.

32. Falk V, Diegeler A, Walther T, et al: Total endoscopic off-pump coronary artery bypass grafting. Heart Surg Forum 2000;3:29-31.

33. Loulmet D, Carpentier A, d'Attellis N, et al: Endoscopic coronary artery bypass grafting with the aid of robotic assisted instruments. J Thorac Cardiovasc Surg 1999;118:4-10.

34. Reichenspurner H, Boehm DH, Gulbins H, et al: Robotically assisted endoscopic coronary artery bypass procedures without cardiopulmonary bypass. J Thorac Cardiovasc Surg 1999;118:960-961.

35. Tweden KS, Eales F, Cameron JD, et al: Ventriculocoronary artery bypass (VCAB), a novel approach to myocardial revascularization. Heart Surg Forum 2000;3:47-54.

36. Fisher PE, Khomoto T, DeRosa CM, et al: Histologic analysis of transmyocardial channels: Comparison of CO2 and holmium:YAG lasers. Ann Thorac Surg 1997;64:466-472.

37. Horvath KA, Cohn LH, Cooley DA, et al: Transmyocardial laser revascularization: Results of a multicenter trial with transmyocardial laser revascularization used as sole therapy for end-stage coronary artery disease. J Thorac Cardiovasc Surg 1997;113:645-653; discussion 653-654.

38. Vincent JG, Bardos P, Kruse J, et al: End stage coronary disease treated with the transmyocardial CO2 laser revascularization: A chance for the "inoperable" patient. Eur J Cardiothorac Surg 1997;11:888-894.

39. Burkhoff D, Schmidt S, Schulman SP, et al: Transmyocardial laser revascularisation compared with continued medical therapy for treatment of refractory angina pectoris: A prospective randomised trial. ATLANTIC Investigators. Angina Treatments—Lasers and Normal Therapies in Comparison. Lancet 1999;354:885-890.

40. Al-Sheikh T, Allen KB, Straka SP, et al: Cardiac sympathetic denervation after transmyocardial laser revascularization. Circulation 1999;100:135-140.

41. Kwong KF, Kanellopoulos GK, Nickols JC, et al: Transmyocardial laser treatment denervates canine myocardium. J Thorac Cardiovasc Surg 1997;114:883-889; discussion 889-890.

42. Arora RC, Hirsch GM, Hirsch K, et al: Transmyocardial laser revascularization remodels the intrinsic cardiac nervous system in a chronic setting. Circulation 2001;104:I115-I120.

43. Minisi AJ, Topaz O, Quinn MS, et al: Cardiac nociceptive reflexes after transmyocardial laser revascularization: Implications for the neural hypothesis of angina relief. J Thorac Cardiovasc Surg 2001;122:712-719.

44. Hirsch GM, Thompson GW, Arora RC, et al: Transmyocardial laser revascularization does not denervate the canine heart. Ann Thorac Surg 1999;68:460-468; discussion 468-469.

45. Frazier OH, March RJ, Horvath KA: Transmyocardial revascularization with a carbon dioxide laser in patients with end-stage coronary artery disease. N Engl J Med 1999;341:1021-1028.

46. Allen KB, Dowling RD, Fudge TL, et al: Comparison of transmyocardial revascularization with medical therapy in patients with refractory angina. N Engl J Med 1999;341:1029-1036.

47. Schofield PM, Sharples LD, Caine N, et al: Transmyocardial laser revascularisation in patients with refractory angina: A randomised controlled trial. Lancet 1999;353:519-524.

48. Aaberge L, Nordstrand K, Dragsund M, et al: Transmyocardial revascularization with CO2 laser in patients with refractory angina pectoris. Clinical results from the Norwegian randomized trial. J Am Coll Cardiol 2000;35:1170-1177.

49. Oesterle SN, Sanborn TA, Ali N, et al: Percutaneous transmyocardial laser revascularisation for severe angina: The PACIFIC randomised trial. Potential Class Improvement From Intramyocardial Channels. Lancet 2000;356:1705-1710.

50. Gotoh K, Minamino T, Katoh O, et al: The role of intracoronary thrombus in unstable angina: Angiographic assessment and thrombolytic therapy during ongoing anginal attacks. Circulation 1988;77:526-534.

51. Singh M, Reeder GS, Ohman EM, et al: Does the presence of thrombus seen on a coronary angiogram affect the outcome after percutaneous coronary angioplasty? An Angiographic Trials Pool data experience. J Am Coll Cardiol 2001;38:624-630.

52. Ambrose JA, Almeida OD, Sharma SK, et al: Angiographic evolution of intracoronary thrombus and dissection following percutaneous transluminal coronary angioplasty (the Thrombolysis and Angioplasty in Unstable Angina [TAUSA] trial). Am J Cardiol 1997;79:559-563.

53. Annex BH, Larkin TJ, O'Neill WW, et al: Evaluation of thrombus removal by transluminal extraction coronary atherectomy by-percutaneous coronary angioscopy. Am J Cardiol 1994;74:606-609.

54. Kaplan BM, Larkin T, Safian RD, et al: Prospective study of extraction atherectomy in patients with acute myocardial infarction. Am J Cardiol 1996;78:383-388.

55. Al-Shaibi KF, Goods CM, Jain SP, et al: Does transluminal extraction atherectomy reduce distal embolization in saphenous vein grafts? [Abstract]. Circulation 1995;92:I-329.

56. Moses JW, Moussa I, Popma JJ, et al: Risk of distal embolization and infarction with transluminal extraction atherectomy in saphenous vein grafts and native coronary arteries. NACI Investigators. New Approaches to Coronary Interventions. Catheter Cardiovasc Interv 1999;47:149-154.

57. Rosenschein U, Roth A, Rassin T, et al: Analysis of coronary ultrasound thrombolysis endpoints in acute myocardial infarction (ACUTE trial). Results of the feasibility phase. Circulation 1997;95:1411-1416.

58. Rosenschein U, Frimerman A, Laniado S, et al: Study of the mechanism of ultrasound angioplasty from human thrombi and bovine aorta. Am J Cardiol 1994;74:1263-1266.

59. Brosh D, Bartorelli A, Cribier A, et al: Percutaneous transluminal therapeutic ultrasound for high-risk thrombus containing lesions in native coronary arteries. Catheter Cardiovasc Interv 2002;55:43-49.

60. Rosenschein U, Brosh D, Halkin A: Coronary ultrasound thrombolysis: From acute myocardial infarction to saphenous vein grafts and beyond. Curr Interv Cardiol Rep 2001;3:5-9.

61. van den Bos AA, van Ommen V, Corbeij HM: A new thrombosuction catheter for coronary use: Initial results with clinical and angiographic follow-up in seven patients. Cathet Cardiovasc Diagn 1997;40:192-197.

62. van Ommen VG, van den Bos AA, Pieper M, et al: Removal of thrombus from aortocoronary bypass grafts and coronary arteries using the 6Fr Hydrolyser. Am J Cardiol 1997;79:1012-1016.

63. Kuntz RE, Baim DS, Cohen DJ, et al: A trial comparing rheolytic thrombectomy with intracoronary urokinase for coronary and vein graft thrombosis (the vein graft AngioJet study). Am J Cardiol 2002;89:326-330.

64. Nakagawa Y, Matsuo S, Kimura T, et al: Thrombectomy with AngioJet catheter in native coronary arteries for patients with acute or recent myocardial infarction. Am J Cardiol 1999;83: 994-999.

65. Silva JA, Ramee SR, Cohen DJ, et al: Rheolytic thrombectomy during percutaneous revascularization for acute myocardial infarction: Experience with the AngioJet catheter. Am Heart J 2001;141: 353-359.

66. Whisenant BK, Baim DS, Kuntz RE, et al: Rheolytic thrombectomy with the Possis AngioJet? Technical considerations and initial clinical experience. J Invasive Cardiol 1999;11:421-426.

67. Henry TD, Murad BB, Wahlberg MD, et al: Mechanism of heart block with the AngioJet® catheter [Abstract]. Circulation 1997;96:I-527.

68. Henry TD, Setum CM, Wilson GJ, et al: Preclinical Evaluation of a Rheolytica Catheter for percutaneous coronary artery/saphenous vein graft thrombectomy. J Invasive Cardiol 1999;11:475-484.

69. Ischinger T: Thrombectomy with the X-SIZER catheter system in the coronary circulation: Initial results from a multi-center study. J Invasive Cardiol 2001;13:81-88.

70. Califf RM, Abdelmeguid AE, Kuntz RE, et al: Myonecrosis after revascularization procedures. J Am Coll Cardiol 1998;31:241-251.

71. Hong MK, Mehran R, Dangas G, et al: Creatine kinase–MB enzyme elevation following successful saphenous vein graft intervention is associated with late mortality. Circulation 1999;100:2400-2405.

72. Gerckens MR, Staberock M, Grube E: Clinical experiences with the PercuSurge GuardWire—a new system for prevention of peripheral embolism in catheter interventions or degenerated coronary venous bypasses. Z Kardiol 2000;89:316-322.

73. Baim DS: The SAFER Trial: Evaluation of the clinical safety and efficacy of the PercuSurge GuardWire in saphenous vein graft intervention. Presented at TCT, Washington, D.C., 2000.

74. Grube E, Gerckens U, Yeung AC, et al: Prevention of distal embolization during coronary angioplasty in saphenous vein grafts and native vessels using porous filter protection. Circulation 2001;104:2436-2441.

75. Stone GW, Ramee S, Almany S, et al: Safety and efficacy of distal protection during saphenous vein graft intervention with the EPI FilterWireEX(tm)—first report from the U.S. phase I feasibility study [Abstract]. Circulation 2001;104:II-623.

76. Savage MP, O'Shaughnessy CS, Farhat NM, et al: Distal protection during intervention in aged vein grafts using a novel filter-guidewire: Initial experience with the MedNova Cardioshield [Abstract]. Circulation 2001;104:II-778.

77. Albiero R, Nishida T, Karvouni E, et al: Cutting balloon angioplasty for the treatment of in-stent restenosis. Catheter Cardiovasc Interv 2000;50:452-459.

78. Freitas Junior JO, Berti SL, Bonfa JG, et al: Cutting balloon angioplasty for intrastent restenosis treatment. Arq Bras Cardiol 1999;72:615-620.

79. Muramatsu T, Tsukahara R, Ho M, et al: Efficacy of cutting balloon angioplasty for in-stent restenosis: An intravascular ultrasound evaluation. J Invasive Cardiol 2001;13:439-444.

80. Chevalier B, Royer T, Guyon P, et al: Treatment of instent restenosis: Short and midterm results of a pilot study between balloon and cutting balloon [Abstract]. J Am Coll Cardiol 1999;33:63A.

81. Mizobe M, Oohata K, Osada T: The efficacy of cutting balloon for in-stent restenosis: Compared with conventional balloon angioplasty [Abstract]. Circulation 1999;100:I-308.

82. Adamian M, Colombo A, Briguori C, et al: Cutting balloon angioplasty for the treatment of in-stent restenosis: A matched comparison with rotational atherectomy, additional stent implantation and balloon angioplasty. J Am Coll Cardiol 2001;38:672-679.

83. Lauer B, Schmidt E, Stellbring S, et al: Cutting balloon angioplasty for treatment of in-stent restenosis [Abstract]. Circulation 2000;102:II-365.

84. Kurbaan AS, Kelly PA, Sigwart U: Cutting balloon angioplasty and stenting for aorto-ostial lesions. Heart 1997;77:350-352.

85. Muramatsu T, Tsukahara R, Ho M, et al: Efficacy of cutting balloon angioplasty for lesions at the ostium of the coronary arteries. J Invasive Cardiol 1999;11:201-206.

86. Colombo A, Adamian M: Cutting balloon angioplasty of ostial coronary lesions: Do we need the stent support? J Invasive Cardiol 1999;11:231-232.

87. Kastrati A, Schomig A, Dirschinger J, et al: A randomized trial comparing stenting with balloon angioplasty in small vessels in patients with symptomatic coronary artery disease. ISAR-SMART Study Investigators. Intracoronary Stenting or Angioplasty for Restenosis Reduction in Small Arteries. Circulation 2000; 102:2593-2598.

88. Ergene O, Seyithanoglu BY, Tastan A, et al: Comparison of angiographic and clinical outcome after cutting balloon and conventional balloon angioplasty in vessels smaller than 3 mm in diameter: A randomized trial. J Invasive Cardiol 1998;10:70-75.

89. Izumi M, Tsuchikane E, Funamoto M, et al: Final results of the CAPAS trial. Am Heart J 2001;142:782-789.

90. Kuntz RE, Baim DS: Prevention of coronary restenosis: The evolving evidence base for radiation therapy. Circulation 2000; 101:2130-2133.

91. Groth CG, Backman L, Morales JM, et al: Sirolimus (rapamycin)-based therapy in human renal transplantation: Similar efficacy and different toxicity compared with cyclosporine. Sirolimus European Renal Transplant Study Group. Transplantation 1999;67:1036-1042.

92. Abizaid A, Dangas G, Costa M, et al: Sirolimus-coated stent prevents neointimal proliferation. Curr Interv Cardiol Rep 2001;3:1-4.

93. Poon M, Marx SO, Gallo R, et al: Rapamycin inhibits vascular smooth muscle cell migration. J Clin Invest 1996;98: 2277-2283.

94. Marx SO, Jayaraman T, Go LO, et al: Rapamycin-FKBP inhibits cell cycle regulators of proliferation in vascular smooth muscle cells. Circ Res 1995;76:412-417.

95. Sousa JE, Costa MA, Abizaid A, et al: Lack of neointimal proliferation after implantation of sirolimus-coated stents in human coronary arteries: A quantitative coronary angiography and three-dimensional intravascular ultrasound study. Circulation 2001;103:192-195.

96. Sousa JE, Costa MA, Abizaid AC, et al: Sustained suppression of neointimal proliferation by sirolimus-eluting stents: One-year angiographic and intravascular ultrasound follow-up. Circulation 2001;104:2007-2011.

97. Morice MC, Serruys PW, Sousa JE, et al: Randomized comparison of a sirolimus-eluting stent with a standard stent for coronary circulation. N Engl J Med 2002;346:1773-1780.

97b. Leon MB: Results of the SIRIUS study with the sirolimus-eluting stent. Paris Course on Revascularization PCR). Paris, France, Oct 2002.

98. Axel DI, Kunert W, Goggelmann C, et al: Paclitaxel inhibits arterial smooth muscle cell proliferation and migration in vitro and in vivo using local drug delivery. Circulation 1997;96:636-645.

99. Wani MC, Taylor HL, Wall ME, et al: Plant antitumor agents. VI. The isolation and structure of Taxol, a novel antileukemic and antitumor agent from *Taxus brevifolia*. J Am Chem Soc 1971;93: 2325-2327.

100. Sollott SJ, Cheng L, Pauly RR, et al: Taxol inhibits neointimal smooth muscle cell accumulation after angioplasty in the rat. J Clin Invest 1995;95:1869-1876.

101. Drachman DE, Edelman ER, Seifert P, et al: Neointimal thickening after stent delivery of paclitaxel: Change in composition and arrest of growth over six months. J Am Coll Cardiol 2000;36:2325-2332.

102. Heldman AW, Cheng L, Jenkins GM, et al: Paclitaxel stent coating inhibits neointimal hyperplasia at 4 weeks in a porcine model of coronary restenosis. Circulation 2001;103:2289-2295.

103. Grube E, Silber SM: Taxus I: Prospective, randomized, double-blind comparison of Nirx(tm) stents coated with paclitaxel in a polymer carrier in de-novo coronary lesions compared with uncoated controls [Abstract]. Circulation 2001;104:II-462.

104. Park S-J, Ho DS, Raizner AE, et al: The clinical effectiveness of paclitaxel/coated coronary stents for the reduction of restenosis in the ASPECT trial [Abstract]. Circulation 2001;104:II-464.

105. Gershlick AH, Descheerder I, Chevalier B, et al: Local drug delivery to inhibit coronary artery restenosis. Data from the ELUTES (EvaLUation of pacliTaxel Eluting Stent) clinical trial [Abstract]. Circulation 2001;104:II-416.

106. Liistro F, Colombo A: Late acute thrombosis after paclitaxel eluting stent implantation. Heart 2001;86:262-264.

107. Keelan PC, Kantor B, Gerber TC, et al: Bypass without the surgeon: The coronary veins as arterial conduits. Curr Interv Cardiol Rep 2000;2:11-19.

108. Pratt F: The nutrition of the heart through the vessels of Thebesius and the coronary veins. Am J Physiol 1893;1:86-103.

109. Park SB, Magovern GJ, Liebler GA, et al: Direct selective myocardial revascularization by internal mammary artery–coronary vein anastomosis. J Thorac Cardiovasc Surg 1975;69:63-72.

110. Benedict JS, Buhl TL, Henney RP: Cardiac vein myocardial revascularization. An experimental study and report of 3 clinical cases. Ann Thorac Surg 1975;20:550-557.

111. Hochberg M, Roberts A, Parsonnet V: Selective arterialization of coronary veins: Clinical experience of 55 American heart surgeons. In Steinkopff MW, Darmstadt V (eds): Clinics of CSI. Springer-Verlag, New York, 1986, pp 195-201.

112. Drury JK, Yamazaki S, Fishbein MC, et al: Synchronized diastolic coronary venous retroperfusion: Results of a preclinical safety and efficacy study. J Am Coll Cardiol 1985;6:328-335.

113. Kar S, Drury JK, Hajduczki I, et al: Synchronized coronary venous retroperfusion for support and salvage of ischemic myocardium during elective and failed angioplasty. J Am Coll Cardiol 1991;18:271-282.

114. Kar S, Nordlander R: Coronary veins: An alternate route to ischemic myocardium. Heart Lung 1992;21:148-157.

115. Barnett JC, Freedman RJ, Touchon RC, et al: Coronary venous retroperfusion of arterial blood for the treatment of acute myocardial ischemia. Cathet Cardiovasc Diagn 1993;28:206-213.

116. Boekstegers P, Giehrl W, von Degenfeld G, et al: Selective suction and pressure-regulated retroinfusion: An effective and safe approach to retrograde protection against myocardial ischemia in patients undergoing normal and high risk percutaneous transluminal coronary angioplasty. J Am Coll Cardiol 1998;31:1525-1533.

117. Oesterle SN, Reifart N, Hauptmann E, et al: Percutaneous in situ coronary venous arterialization: Report of the first human catheter-based coronary artery bypass. Circulation 2001;103:2539-2543.

chapter 37

Pharmacologic Revascularization

Michael J. B. Kutryk
Duncan J. Stewart

PROBLEM

Ischemic heart disease is the major cause of death in adults in most developed and many developing countries and is now the most common cause of death worldwide. Effective revascularization strategies for coronary artery disease (CAD) involve either percutaneous revascularization techniques, such as balloon angioplasty and stenting, or coronary artery bypass graft (CABG) surgery. The long-term success of both of these approaches is limited by the development over time of native vessel narrowing and graft occlusions. Despite continued advances in the prevention and treatment of CAD, there are still many patients who are not candidates for conventional treatments. Therapeutic angiogenesis, in the form of the administration of growth factor protein or gene therapy, has emerged as a promising new method of treatment for patients with CAD.

HISTORICAL PERSPECTIVE

The modern era of proangiogenesis therapy was presaged by the pioneering work of Vineberg[1] at McGill University in Montreal, Canada. The original Vineberg procedure, developed in 1945, was one of many surgical treatments implemented early in the twentieth century as a means of augmenting the blood supply to ischemic myocardium. Vineberg envisioned enhanced collaterization by the creation of a "third coronary artery" with the implantation of a systemic artery into the myocardium.[1,2] The internal mammary artery (IMA) was thought ideal because it serves no tissues exclusively, is easily accessible surgically, carries a high flow, and tends to be free of atherosclerosis. Vineberg hoped that the implanted artery would sprout branches that would join with the intramyocardial portion of the native microcirculation, which consists of (1) the terminal arterioles and (2) the intramyocardial sinusoidal spaces, neither of which develop atherosclerosis.

On the basis of experimental works,[2-5] Vineberg initiated clinical series. The first patient underwent a Vineberg operation in 1950; however, the procedure was not widely accepted until the introduction of coronary arteriography in 1958 provided objective proof of IMA implantation. In the following years, many medical centers adopted the Vineberg procedure. In the latter part of the 1960s, surgeons abandoned the Vineberg procedure in favor of CABG surgery, a direct revascularization procedure. There has been renewed interest in the Vineberg procedure with advances in molecular biology and the introduction of adjunct growth factors to induce neoangiogenesis.[6]

MECHANISMS OF VASCULAR DEVELOPMENT

This section briefly reviews the mechanisms of vascular growth and development, with a focus on the mechanisms relevant to the postnatal revascularization of damaged or ischemic tissues. Three terms commonly are used to describe this process: *vasculogenesis, angiogenesis*, and *arteriogenesis*.

Angiogenesis

The term *angiogenesis*, first used by Hertig in 1935 to describe the growth of blood vessels in the placenta, was reintroduced by Folkman[7] in 1972 to describe neovascularization accompanying solid tumor growth. Angiogenesis is the process by which new capillaries are formed and differentiate from preexisting postcapillary microvascular networks. The process involves the enlargement of blood vessels, which subsequently extend sprouts (sprouting angiogenesis)[8] or become divided by intervascular pillars of periendothelial cells or by transendothelial cell bridges (intussusception),[9] which then separate into individual capillaries (Fig. 37-1). This process results in newly developed endothelial microvessels, most of which resemble capillaries (diameter of 5 to 8 μm). The involvement of periendothelial cells (pericytes in small vessels; smooth muscle cells in large vessels) is important to complete the angiogenic process. Periendothelial cells stabilize nascent vessels by inhibiting endothelial cell proliferation and migration and stimulating extracellular matrix production and the formation of a basement membrane, protecting fragile endothelial lined vessels against traumatic rupture and regression.

The initiation of angiogenesis, the angiogenic switch, depends on a dynamic balance between proangiogenic and antiangiogenic factors in the immediate environment of endothelial cells.[10] The principal angiogenic growth factors are reviewed here; the reader is referred to other reviews for a detailed discussion of the antiangiogenic factors.[11,12] A balance in favor of angiogenic factors results in new vessel formation, whereas the

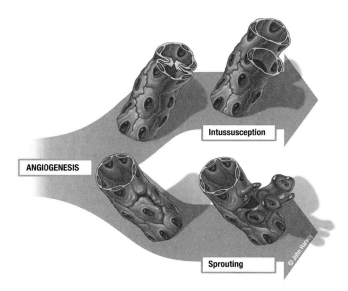

FIGURE 37–1. Two mechanisms of new capillary formation during angiogenesis. Intussusception involves the division of an existing vessel into two vessels by transendothelial cell bridges. New vessels also may arise de novo from existing blood vessels by sprouting angiogenesis.

prevalence of antiangiogenic factors shifts the equilibrium to vessel quiescence or vessel regression.[10] Although the exact mechanisms by which new vessels are formed are not fully understood, angiogenesis is thought to involve a series of events, including (1) activation of endothelial cells and inhibition of endothelial cell apoptosis, ensuring endothelial cell survival within a preexisting vessel; (2) vasodilation of the parent vessel mediated by nitric oxide (NO); (3) degradation of the basement membrane and extracellular matrix; (4) migration of activated endothelial cells from the parent vessel directed by chemotactic factors liberated from fibroblasts, monocytes, platelets, mast cells, and neutrophils toward the site where angiogenesis is required; (5) proliferation of endothelial cells in the newly forming vessels; (6) redifferentiation of these endothelial cells back to a quiescent phenotype with lumen formation; (7) recruitment of pericytes along the newly formed vascular structures; (8) formation of a new basement membrane by the newly organized endothelial cells and pericytes; and (9) remodeling of the neovascular network, with maturation and stabilization of the blood vessels (Fig. 37–2).

Angiogenesis is initiated in response to hypoxia or ischemia, and endothelial cell activation is the first process to take place in physiologic or pathophysiologic angiogenesis. Hypoxia induces increased levels of a family of hypoxia-inducible transcription factors (HIFs) including HIF-1β (or the aryl hydrocarbon-receptor nuclear translocator), HIF-1α, and HIF-2α. HIFs mediate the response to hypoxia by binding to specific DNA sequences, the hypoxia-response promoter elements, which regulate the transcription of an array of genes crucial to the cellular response to hypoxia, including several genes that regulate angiogenesis.[13]

Angiogenesis is tightly linked to inflammation and blood coagulation. Leukocytes and platelets are rich sources of angiogenic growth factors and express several adhesion, chemoattractant, and activator molecules that govern their emigration from the bloodstream. Membrane adhesion proteins, including integrins, also play an important role in the process of angiogenesis. Integrins are heterodimeric cell surface receptors composed of two noncovalently associated transmembrane glycoproteins (α and β) that mediate attachment of cells to their foundation but also are involved in intracellular signal transduction.[14-17] Endothelial cells express many different integrins, and their interaction with various extracellular matrix molecules is required to prevent rapid apoptosis, a phenomenon called *anoikis*.[18] The integrin receptors $\alpha_v\beta_3$ and $\alpha_v\beta_5$ are expressed during in vivo angiogenesis and are markers of the angiogenic phenotype of endothelial cells.[19,20] $\alpha_v\beta_3$ is a receptor for many proteins with an exposed Arg-Gly-Asp tripeptide component, including vitronectin, fibronectin, fibrinogen, laminin, collagen, thrombospondin, osteopontin, and

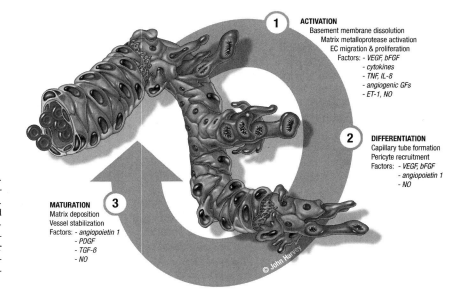

FIGURE 37–2. Sequential events in angiogenesis. (1) Activation—basement membrane disintegration opens the way for endothelial cell migration. (2) Differentiation—cords of cells proliferate and define a new vascular channel. (3) Maturation—cessation of cell migration and proliferation coincides with the recruitment of perivascular support cells with the formation of a new basement membrane and vessel maturation and stabilization.

von Willebrand factor. Although the $\alpha_v\beta_3$ receptor is not widely expressed, it is prominent on cytokine-activated endothelial cells or smooth muscle cells.[21] Many angiogenic cytokines have been shown to increase the expression of the α_v and β_3 subunits on endothelial cells.[22-25] It has been shown that blocking antibodies or antagonistic peptides to $\alpha_v\beta_3$-integrin, which interrupt the $\alpha_v\beta_3$-mediated adhesion to extracellular matrix proteins, leads to the inhibition of tumor-induced and growth factor–induced angiogenesis by selectively inducing apoptosis of endothelial cells in newly formed blood vessels.[14,19,26-28] Newer data suggest that there is a functional cross-talk between integrin-mediated and growth factor–mediated signaling and that endothelial cell survival and proliferation in response to vascular endothelial growth factor (VEGF) may require the association of one of its receptors with $\alpha_v\beta_3$ (Fig. 37-3).[29,30]

Basement membrane degradation, extracellular matrix invasion, and capillary lumen formation also are essential components of the angiogenic process, all of which depend on a cohort of proteases and protease inhibitors. Although many enzymatic systems have been implicated in extracellular proteolysis, many of the enzymes belong to one of two families, the serine proteases, in particular, the plasminogen activator (PA)/plasmin system, and the matrix metalloproteases (MMPs). Plasminogen activators u-PA and t-PA convert the ubiquitous plasma protein plasminogen to plasmin. Plasmin activates certain MMPs, has a broad trypsin-like activity, and degrades proteins such as fibronectin, laminin, and the protein core of proteoglycans.[31-33]

Subsequent steps in angiogenesis, including endothelial cell migration, proliferation, and new vessel formation and maturation, result in the formation of a functional vascular conduit (Fig. 37-4; see also Fig. 37-2).[15,34-36] NO seems to play a crucial role in mediating many of these processes, including terminating the proliferative actions of growth factors and promoting the formation of vascular tubes.[37-40] In the setting of coronary ischemia, NO is required for the full activity of VEGF.[40] Some groups have suggested that NO is a downstream mediator of the angiogenic effects of VEGF.[41] The crucial role of normal endothelial function in angiogenesis and neovascularization is reviewed in detail later. Another crucial step in the stabilization and maturation of the newly formed neovessel is the attraction of pericytes and the formation of the nascent vascular media. Secretion of platelet-derived growth factor seems to be particularly important in this regard.[42] In turn, the action of transforming growth factor-β (TGF-β) is thought to spur the differentiation and maturation of pericytes into smooth muscle cells[36] and promote the resynthesis of basement membrane and other extracellular matrix components that are crucial for the establishment of the competence and integrity of the developing neovessel. The glycoprotein angiopoietin-1 (Ang-1) and its tyrosine receptor kinase Tie-2 function to stabilize the immature endothelial cell network by promoting pericyte-endothelial interactions and the reconstitution of a competent basement membrane[36] and play an important role in the organization and maturation of neovessels (discussed later) (see Fig. 37-4).

Vasculogenesis

The process of vasculogenesis is distinct from that of angiogenesis. Vasculogenesis is the process of in situ formation of blood vessels from endothelial progenitor cells or angioblasts. Initially, mesenchymal cells differentiate in situ into early hemangioblasts that form cellular aggregates (blood islands), in which the inner cell population differentiates into hematopoietic precursors, and the

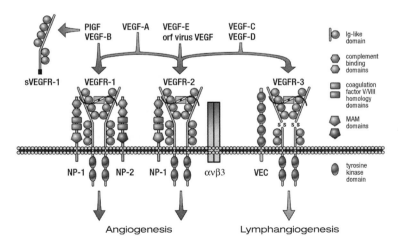

FIGURE 37–3. The currently known growth factors and receptors of the VEGF family. The three signaling tyrosine-kinase receptors of the VEGF family (VEGFR-1, VEGFR-2, and VEGFR-3), the soluble VEGFR-1 receptor, the accessory isoform-specific receptors neuropilin-1 (NP-1) and neuropilin-2 (NP-2), the integrin receptor $\alpha_v\beta_3$, and VE-cadherin are shown with their major structural features. Ligand binding induces receptor signal transduction leading to various responses. VEGFR-1 and VEGFR-2 mediate angiogenesis, whereas VEGFR-3 is also involved in lymphangiogenesis. NRP-1 and NP-2 bind to specific COOH-terminal sequences present only on VEGFs that bind to VEGFR-1 or VEGFR-2 or both. $\alpha_v\beta_3$ integrin and VE-cadherin have been found complexed with activated VEGFR-2. VE-cadherin also associates with an activated VEGFR-3 complex. sVEGFR-1, soluble VEGFR-1; VEC, VE cadherin; NP-1, neuropilin-1; NP-2, neuropilin 2; MAM, meprin, A5 antigen, protein tyrosine phosphatase μ. (See Chen and colleagues[282] for explanations of the various structural motifs of the neuropilins.) (Modifed from[283] Veikkola T, Karkkainen M, Claesson-Welsh L, et al: Regulation of angiogenesis via vascular endothelial growth factor receptors. Cancer Res 2000;60:203–212.)

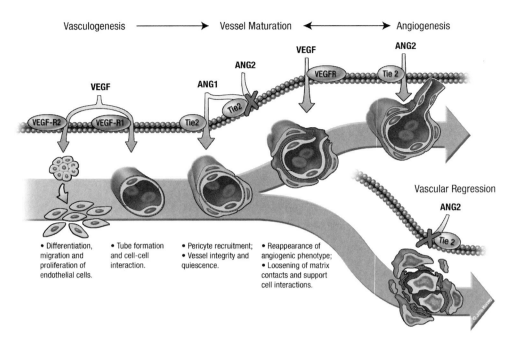

FIGURE 37–4. Coordinated and complementary angiogenic activities of VEGF and the angiopoietins. VEGF, angiopoietin-1, and angiopoietin 2 bind to receptor thymidine kinases (RTKs) that have similar cytoplasmic signaling domains. Binding of the ligands to their receptors elicits downstream signals with distinctive cellular responses. Only VEGF binding to the VEGF-R2 receptor sends a classic proliferative signal. VEGF binding to VEGF-R1 elicits endothelial cell-cell interactions and capillary tube formation. Ang-1 binding to the Tie2 RTK recruits and likely maintains association of periendothelial support cells (pericytes, smooth muscle cells, myocardiocytes), thus stabilizing a newly formed blood vessel. Ang-2 binds and blocks Tie2 activation in endothelial cells. In the absence of VEGF, this leads to endothelial cell apoptosis and vascular regression. With high concentrations or with prolonged exposure, Ang-2 behaves as an agonist of Tie-2, allowing endothelial cell activation and contributing directly to the maturation and stabilization of newly formed blood vessels. (Modified from Hanahan D: Signaling vascular morphogenesis and maintenance. Science 1997;277:48–50.)

outer cell population gives rise to the primitive endothelial cells that generate a functioning vascular labyrinth.[44-46] The primitive vascular plexus subsequently develops into a complex, interconnecting network of mature blood vessels.

Until more recently, vasculogenesis was considered restricted to embryonic development, whereas angiogenesis, recognized to occur in the embryo as well, was considered to be solely responsible for neovascularization in the adult. The demonstration that bone marrow–derived endothelial precursor cells circulate in the peripheral blood[47,48] and can incorporate into areas of neovascularization in the adult revised this paradigm. It now is accepted that neovascularization in the adult occurs by angiogenesis and vasculogenesis.

Efficient neovascularization depends on two distinct processes—endothelial cell activation and proliferation and vessel differentiation. These processes must occur in harmony for functioning vessels to arise, but opposite biologic actions seem to be required. It is paradoxical that an angiogenic growth factor such as VEGF stimulates the migration and proliferation of endothelial cells in the initiation of the angiogenic response and directs endothelial cell capillary tube formation leading to complex three-dimensional vascular structures. How can the same mediator at one time stimulate endothelial cell mitosis and at another promote their differentiation and quiescence? The answer may relate to complex interactions between the myriad of mediators that normally par-

ticipate in this process. Although VEGF and fibroblast growth factor (FGF) may regulate basement membrane disintegration and leukocyte and precursor cell recruitment, proliferation, and adhesion, the presence of Ang-1 may be required for cell differentiation, maturation, and establishment of a mature vessel (see Fig. 37–3). The interdependence of angiogenic factors also is exemplified by FGF and NO. In the presence of NO, the action of FGF may switch from one that causes endothelial cell activation to one responsible for differentiation.[39] Such a paradigm would suggest that effective strategies of therapeutic angiogenesis would require the orchestration of the expression of many factors, all at appropriate time points in the process to achieve efficient neovascularization (see Fig. 37–4).[49]

Arteriogenesis

The importance of the collateral coronary circulation has long been known,[34,50-55] and the mechanisms governing the recruitment, growth, and proliferation of collateral vessels differ from those regulating angiogenesis and vasculogenesis. Acute occlusion of a large-or medium-sized artery often results in the recruitment of preexisting arteriolar connections that can bypass the site of occlusion. Although not requiring new vessel formation, the subsequent growth and proliferation of these collateral vessels occur through a process called *arteriogenesis*. Collateral vessels also may be produced de novo, however, by angiogenesis or vasculogenesis and subsequently organized into arterial channels, possibly by the action of maturation factors such as Ang-1. Regardless of their origins, collateral arteries are able to mature into large conductance arteries, which can restore blood flow efficiently to ischemic territories. Adequate development of these collaterals may take days to weeks to compensate for critical stenoses of the nutrient branches of the coronary tree. Genetic factors likely are responsible for the variable number of preexisting intracoronary connections and their capacity to grow and contribute to the well-recognized interspecies and intraspecies variability.[56,57] An important stimulator of arteriogenesis is increased shear stress that leads to changes within the newly recruited artery, which to a large extent are transduced by the endothelium.[58,59] The most important change is the activation of the endothelium. This activation results in the increased expression of many genes, partially via a protein that binds to the shear stress responsive element that is present in the promoter of many of these genes, including nitric oxide synthase (NOS), platelet-derived growth factor, and monocyte chemoattractant protein (MCP-1).[60] Adhesion molecules also are up-regulated, allowing for the adhesion and invasion of monocytes and platelets, which also are potent producers of growth factors. The process of arteriogenesis does not seem to require hypoxia as a physical stimulus.[61]

OVERVIEW OF VASCULAR GROWTH FACTORS

The existence of biologic mediators of vascular growth was first hypothesized in the 1970s with the discovery of a tumor factor that was found to be mitogenic for endothelial cells.[62] This factor subsequently was identified as a member of the FGF family.[63] It soon became evident that tumor biology could be applied in a practical way to common disease processes, such as peripheral vascular disease and CAD. A wide variety of angiogenic proteins have been identified (Table 37-1). The most extensively studied and best-characterized angiogenic growth factors are members of the VEGF and FGF families. More recently, attention has focused on the angiopoietin family, which includes Ang-1 to Ang-4.

Fibroblast Growth Factor

In 1984, Shing and colleagues[64] discovered a tumor-derived factor with a high affinity for heparin. The purified protein had a molecular mass of 14,800 Da and stimulated the proliferation of capillary endothelial cells[65] and subsequently was identified as bFGF. The FGF family consists of 22 structurally similar compounds, of which FGF-1 and FGF-2 (also called *acidic* [aFGF] and *basic* [bFGF] based on their isoelectric points) are best described.[36,49,66,67] The members of the FGF family possess a high degree of homology and share important features, including (1) an ability to bind heparin with high affinity; (2) an ability to bind high-affinity receptors possessing tyrosine kinase activity,

which subsequently initiates intracellular signaling pathways responsible for inducing cell division (modulated by attachment to the low-affinity receptor); and (3) an ability to bind to a low-affinity, high-capacity receptor that represents a site that modulates the activity and function of the high-affinity receptor with cell surface heparin sulfate proteoglycans.[68-70] The aFGF and bFGF proteins are single-chain, heparin-binding polypeptides of 154 and 146 amino acids.[63,71] In contrast to other members of the FGF family, which have signal sequences and are secreted through standard secretory pathways, aFGF and bFGF do not have signal sequences and are not secreted by classic mechanisms.

The FGFs have been shown to modulate many intracellular and extracellular activities that are necessary for angiogenesis, including (1) the up-regulation of proteases that are essential in the modulation of the extracellular matrix, (2) the activation of kinases that regulate intracellular signaling pathways that are important to cell replication, (3) the signaling of molecules involved in cell-cell interactions and interactions related to capillary tubule formation, and (4) the inhibition of endothelial cell apoptosis. Their ability to act directly on smooth muscle cells has led to the hypothesis that FGF compounds are better suited for larger vessel formation.[15,36,72]

Lessons from Transgenic Mice

aFGF and bFGF knockout mice are viable and fertile.[73] Although bFGF-deficient mice show a range of relatively mild phenotypic defects, which include a change in the number of neurons present in the cerebral cortex, a delay in the healing of epithelial wounds, and hypotension,[74-76] aFGF-deficient mice are phenotypically normal.[73] These findings may suggest that other growth factors, either other members of the FGF family or unrelated compounds, might be providing a compensatory signal. If this is the case, there is a remarkable degree of redundancy among various FGF family members or between multiple growth factor signaling pathways. An alternate explanation is that aFGF and bFGF play a limited role in normal vascular development and that only by studying the null mice in the appropriate pathologic state would marked differences become apparent.

Vascular Endothelial Growth Factor

In 1989, Ferrera and Henzel[77] and Plouet and colleagues[78] independently reported the purification and sequencing of an endothelial cell–specific mitogen, which they called *VEGF* and *vasculotropin*. The VEGF family of endothelial selective mitogens and their tyrosine kinase receptors subsequently have been shown to play a central role in physiologic and pathologic angiogenesis (see Fig. 37-4). The VEGF family currently includes six known members, VEGF (VEGF-A, VEGF-1), placental growth factor (PlGF), VEGF-B, VEGF-C (VEGF-2), VEGF-D, and orf virus VEGF (VEGF-E). The family members are dimeric glycoproteins, all of which contain a characteristic pattern of eight regularly spaced cysteine residues, the so-called cystine knot motif, and all

■ ■ ■

TABLE 37–1 ANGIOGENIC PROTEIN

ANGIOGENIC PROTEIN	ENDOTHELIAL CELL SPECIFIC
Acidic fibroblast growth factor (aFGF)	No
Basic fibroblast growth factor (bFGF)	No
Fibroblast growth factor 3 (FGF-3)	No
Fibroblast growth factor 4 (FGF-4)	No
Fibroblast growth factor 5 (FGF-5)	No
Fibroblast growth factor 6 (FGF-6)	No
Fibroblast growth factor 7 (FGF-7)	No
Fibroblast growth factor 8 (FGF-8)	No
Fibroblast growth factor 9 (FGF-9)	No
Angiogenin 1	Yes
Angiogenin 2	Yes
Hepatocyte growth factor/scatter factor (HGF/SF)	No
Platelet-derived growth factor (PDE-CGF)	Yes
Transforming growth factor-α (TGF-α)	No
Transforming growth factor-β (TGF-β)	No
Tumor necrosis factor-α (TNF-α)	No
Vascular endothelial growth factor 121 (VEGF 121)	Yes
Vascular endothelial growth factor 145 (VEGF 145)	Yes
Vascular endothelial growth factor 165 (VEGF 165)	Yes
Vascular endothelial growth factor 189 (VEGF 189)	Yes
Vascular endothelial growth factor 206 (VEGF 206)	Yes
Vascular endothelial growth factor B (VEGF-B)	Yes
Vascular endothelial growth factor C (VEGF-C)	Yes
Vascular endothelial growth factor D (VEGF-D)	Yes
Vascular endothelial growth factor E (VEGF-E)	Yes
Vascular endothelial growth factor F (VEGF-F)	Yes
Placental growth factor	Yes
Angiopoietin-1	No
Angiopoietin-2	No
Thrombospondin (TSP)	No
Proliferin	Yes
Ephrin-A1 (B61)	Yes
E-selectin	Yes
Chicken chemotactic and angiogenic factor (cCAF)	No
Leptin	Yes
Heparin affinity regulatory peptide (HARP)	No
Heparin	No
Granulocyte colony-stimulating factor	No
Insulin-like growth factor	No
Interleukin-8	No
Thyroxine	No
Sphingosine 1-phosphate	No

Modified from[281] Hamaway AH, Lee LY, Crystal RG, et al: Cardiac angiogenesis and gene therapy: A strategy for myocardial revascularization. Curr Opin Cardiol 1999;14:515–522.

contain a secretory signal sequence, which directs active secretion of VEGF from intact cells. The first identified and the best-studied member of the group is VEGF (VEGF-A), a soluble mitogen mapped to chromosome 6p21.3, which plays a role in nearly all angiogenic processes.[79-83] VEGF was described independently by many different groups using a variety of different assays. For many years, this protein was referred to variably as vascular permeability factor or vasculotropin. Alternative splicing from a single gene gives rise to six different isoforms of VEGF comprising 121, 145, 165, 183, 189, and 206 amino acids in humans. These isoforms differ with regard to the expression of exons 6 and 7 of the VEGF gene, which encode independent heparin binding domains. The various isoforms differ in their mitogenicity, chemotactic properties, protein trafficking, signal transduction, growth factor interactions, receptor binding characteristics, and heparin and heparin-sulfate proteoglycan binding. The shortest VEGF form, $VEGF_{121}$, lacks exons 6 and 7, and does not bind to heparin. $VEGF_{165}$ includes the peptide encoded by exon 7, $VEGF_{145}$ includes the peptide encoded by exon 6, and $VEGF_{189}$ includes both exons.[84] $VEGF_{183}$, similar to $VEGF_{189}$, contains both exons; however, it has an 18-bp deletion in the exon 6A–encoded region of VEGF.[85,86] The 165 and 121 isoforms are the predominant forms. $VEGF_{165}$ is the most potent stimulator of endothelial cell division, 50-fold to 100-fold more potent than $VEGF_{121}$. $VEGF_{165}$ and $VEGF_{145}$ are secreted, whereas $VEGF_{183}$ and $VEGF_{189}$ are predominantly cell-anchored proteins that promote increased vascular permeability but require extracellular cleavage or release by heparin or plasmin to promote mitogenic activity. Because $VEGF_{121}$ lacks heparin-binding ability and it is not anchored to the extracellular matrix when secreted, it may be more available for exerting a paracrine effect. The greater mitogenic potency of $VEGF_{165}$ may be conferred by its neuropilin-1 binding region, which is encoded by exon 7 of the VEGF gene (see Fig. 47-3).[87]

VEGF-B has similar endothelial mitogenic potency to VEGF and is expressed primarily in developing myocardium and in developing muscle, bone, pancreas, adrenal gland, and smooth muscle cells.[88] The expression of VEGF-B is not regulated by hypoxia, and its biologic half-life is unusually long (>8 hours). VEGF-B is coexpressed and heterodimerizes with VEGF.

VEGF-C stimulates the migration and proliferation of endothelial cells in vitro and in vivo.[89] In adults, it is expressed in the heart, placenta, lung, kidney, muscle, ovary, and small intestine. VEGF-C regulates lymphangiogenesis and may be involved in the development of the venous system.[90-93]

VEGF-D is mitogenic for endothelial cells[94] and is expressed in the lung, heart, and small intestine and in lesser amounts in the pituitary, kidney, liver, and skin.[95] The structural similarities between VEGF-C and VEGF-D suggest similar functions; however, their expression patterns differ, and the role for VEGF-D in angiogenesis is unknown.

A gene encoding a VEGF homologue has been discovered in the genome of the orf viruses, a parapoxvirus that infects sheep, goats, and humans. The lesions induced by orf virus infection show extensive proliferation of the vascular endothelium and blood vessel dilation. Two different variants of the viral VEGF are known, and they are unique in that they bind only to one of the known VEGF receptors.[96,97]

The VEGF homologues are ligands for a set of tyrosine kinase receptors, VEGFR-1 (Flt-1), VEGFR-2 (KDR/Flk-1), and VEGFR-3 (FLT-4) (see Fig. 37-3). In adult tissues, VEGFR-1 and VEGFR-2 localize to vascular endothelial cells, whereas VEGFR-3 is expressed mainly in the lymphatic endothelium. The ligand specificities of the VEGF receptors differ: VEGFR-1 binds VEGF, VEGF-B, and PlGF; VEGFR-2 binds VEGF, VEGF-C, VEGF-D, and the orf virus VEGF; and VEGFR-3 binds VEGF-C and VEGF-D. Ligand binding induces receptor dimerization and subsequent autophosphorylation and transphosphorylation, leading to the initiation of signal transduction cascades.

Neuropilin-1 (NP-1) and neuropilin-2 (NP-2), which are cell surface glycoproteins that control axon guidance during embryonic development, have been identified as isoform-specific receptors for $VEGF_{165}$ and several members of the VEGF family. They have short intracellular domains and are unlikely to function as independent receptors; no responses to $VEGF_{165}$ were observed when cells expressing NP-1 and no other VEGF receptors were stimulated with $VEGF_{165}$. NP-1 seems to function as an enhancer of VEGFR-2 activity in the presence of $VEGF_{165}$ and is probably the result of complex formation between VEGFR-2 and NP-1 (see Fig. 37-3).[98,99] The related NP-2 receptor also behaves as an isoform-specific VEGF receptor that binds $VEGF_{165}$, but in contrast to NP-1, it also is able to bind $VEGF_{145}$.[100] PlGF binds to NP-1

and NP-2,[100,101] and VEGF-B also is able to bind NP-1 (see Fig. 37-3).[102]

The expression of VEGF is highly regulated by oxygen tension, which provides a physiologic feedback mechanism to accommodate insufficient tissue oxygenation by promoting blood vessel formation. The transcription of the VEGF gene under hypoxic conditions is mediated by a family of HIFs (HIF-1α, HIF-1β, and HIF-2α), which bind to hypoxia-responsive elements in the VEGF promoter.[103] Hypoxia also induces the up-regulated expression of a RNA-binding protein (HuR). HuR stabilizes the VEGF mRNA through interaction with sequences in the 3′ untranslated region.[104-107] Hypoxia also up-regulates VEGFR-2 expression in endothelial cells,[108,109] which is consistent with an autocrine loop. In contrast, in a neonatal rat model of hyperoxia-induced retinopathy, Alon and associates[110] showed that hyperoxia-induced down-regulation of VEGF expression in the neonatal rat retina leads to the regression of retinal capillaries via selective apoptosis of endothelial cells.[110] This apoptotic effect on endothelial cells could be prevented by the intraocular injection of VEGF.

The mechanisms by which VEGF mediates apoptotic signaling gradually are becoming understood. VEGF has been shown to induce the expression of antiapoptotic proteins, such as Bcl-2,[111,112] A1,[111] survivin, and XIAP.[113] VEGF also has been shown to promote endothelial cell survival by activation of the phosphatidylinositol 3 (PI-3) kinase/Akt pathway. The survival effect of VEGF depends on the binding of VEGF on VEGFR-2.[114] VEGFR-1-specific ligands do not promote survival of endothelial cells.[114] These findings suggest that VEGFR-2 and the PI-3 kinase/Akt signal transduction pathway are crucial elements in the promotion of endothelial cell survival mediated by VEGF. The downstream second messenger pathways mediating the antiapoptotic effects of VEGF include Akt-dependent activation of endothelial NOS (eNOS), resulting in enhanced NO synthesis.[115,116] The PI-3 kinase/Akt pathway also up-regulates the transcription of survivin[117] and can inhibit the p38 mitogen activated protein kinase.[118]

The inhibition of VEGF has been shown to lead to endothelial cell apoptosis and vessel regression in several models of tumor angiogenesis.[119-122] The effect seems to be selective, with the abrupt withdrawal of VEGF leading to the selective apoptosis of only endothelial cells in immature tumor vessels, devoid of periendothelial cells, with resultant vessel regression.[120] Mature tumor vessels with recruited pericytes seem to be resistant to VEGF withdrawal–induced apoptosis and regression.[120]

VEGFR-1 and VEGFR-2 can be activated by the same ligand; however, their downstream signaling pathways lead to different cellular responses. VEGFR-2 activation is required for the determination of the fate of endothelial and hematopoietic cells, their migration, and proliferation[114,123] and generally is regarded as the VEGF receptor that transduces signals required for angiogenesis. VEGFR-1 activation may play a role in the regulation of endothelial cell migration and adhesion and blood vessel organization.[124,125] VEGFR-3 principally mediates lymphangiogenesis (see Fig. 37-3).[126]

In general, VEGF expression in adults is low.[127] The female reproductive organs are one exception, including the ovarian follicle, where it may be involved in embryo implantation, endometrial vascularization, and development of the corpus luteum.[128] Expression is increased in pathologic states associated with increased vascularity, such as arthritis and tumor growth, and may be a protective response in myocardial ischemia.[66] Among patients with CAD, VEGF concentrations have been found to be elevated in atherosclerotic lesions, particularly in lesions with increased collaterals,[50,129] suggesting a possible role of intraplaque angiogenesis in the progression of the atheromatous lesion.

There are two features of VEGF that distinguish it from the FGF family of angiogenic growth factors. First, receptors for VEGF are found predominantly, but not exclusively, on vascular endothelial cells, resulting in a specific target organ effect, whereas the FGFs serve as ligands for other cell types, including smooth muscle cells and fibroblasts. Second, the terminal amino acid sequence allows for secretion from cells. This feature allows for the delivery of the DNA sequence encoding VEGF, with its subsequent transcription and translation, which leads to greater and more sustained tissue concentrations when compared with protein delivery alone.[130] The effects of FGF and VEGF on neovascularization may be synergistic, however.[59]

Lessons from Transgenic Mice

Four alternatively transcribed isoforms of VEGF have been identified in the mouse ($VEGF_{115}$, $VEGF_{120}$, $VEGF_{164}$, and $VEGF_{188}$).[131] Targeted inactivation of even a single VEGF-A allele in the mouse (haploinsufficiency) results in embryonic lethality with marked abnormalities in blood vessel development at around 9 days of gestation, attesting to the importance of VEGF in embryonic development.[132,134] In heterozygous VEGF-deficient mice, the lumen of the dorsal aorta was reduced, less angiogenic sprouting of vessels was observed, large abnormal thoracic blood vessels were apparent, and only an irregular plexus of enlarged capillaries was present in the yolk sac and placenta. The early embryonic lethality of haploinsufficient mice prevents the production of embryos homozygous for the null allele by germline breeding. This limitation was circumvented when completely embryonic stem cell–derived embryos were made by the aggregation of homozygous VEGF-A-deficient stem cells with tetraploid embryos.[132,134] The resulting homozygote embryos showed more severe vascular defects. Homozygous embryos, similar to heterozygotes, died at midgestation (E9.5) owing to cardiovascular dysfunction. Although endothelial cell development was delayed in heterozygous VEGF-A-deficient mice, it was not entirely aborted. Precise VEGF concentration gradients seem to be required for correct lumen formation, sprouting, and angiogenesis.

A critical concentration dependence for VEGF-A is supported by studies involving excess VEGF in developing avian embryos. Exogenously administered VEGF in a Japanese quail embryo resulted in a hyperperfused network of vessels, the development of vessels in areas normally avascular,[135] and severe malformations of the heart and venous system.[136] Retrovirally induced overexpression of VEGF-A in the chick developing limb bud resulted in local increases of vascular density with no other abnormalities.[137] A twofold to threefold overexpression of VEGF-A in mice has been shown to result in severe abnormalities in heart development and embryonic lethality at E12.5-E14.[138] The mutant embryos displayed an attenuated compact layer of myocardium, overproduction of trabeculae, defective ventricular septation, and abnormalities in remodeling of the outflow tract of the heart. Aberrant development of the coronary artery tree was characterized by the formation of oversized epicardial vessels. These results confirm that embryonic survival requires a narrow window of VEGF-A expression.

Mice lacking $VEGF_{164}$ and $VEGF_{188}$ developed ischemic cardiomyopathy and died less than 14 days after birth of heart failure resulting from impaired postnatal myocardial angiogenesis.[139] A fraction of these mice died shortly after birth, presumably because of a cardiomyopathy, increased vascular fragility, and hemorrhage into several organs. In wild-type mice, the number of capillaries and coronary vessels increased during the first 3 postnatal weeks to match the increasing metabolic demands of the hypertrophying cardiomyocytes. The capillary density did not change in $VEGF_{164}$-deficient and $VEGF_{188}$-deficient mice, resulting in larger intercapillary and myocyte-to-capillary ratios and impaired oxygen delivery. Hearts from animals deficient in $VEGF_{164}$ and $VEGF_{188}$ also contained fewer coronary vessels and reduced smooth muscle coverage, suggesting significantly impaired pericyte and smooth muscle cell recruitment. $VEGF_{115}$ and $VEGF_{120}$ can rescue the defective embryonic vascular development of heterozygous VEGF-A–deficient embryos but seem to be insufficient to produce a functional vasculature in a homozygous form. The severe angiogenic defects seen in mice deficient in $VEGF_{164}$ and $VEGF_{188}$ illustrate the functional complementarity of the VEGF isoforms in angiogenesis.

Mice expressing only $VEGF_{164}$ were born at a normal mendelian frequency, were fertile, and produced litters of normal size. Mice expressing only $VEGF_{188}$ were underrepresented at birth, indicating that a fraction died in utero. Surviving mice expressing only $VEGF_{188}$ gained less weight than normal mice, and breeding pairs were less fertile and had smaller litter sizes.[140]

In contrast to VEGF-A knockout mice, mice lacking the VEGF-B gene were healthy and fertile.[141] The hearts from these animals were reduced in size, however, and displayed vascular dysfunction after coronary occlusion and impaired recovery from experimentally induced myocardial ischemia, suggesting a role for VEGF-B in the vascular adaptation to ischemia-reperfusion.

Gene knockout studies have revealed distinct vasculogenic and angiogenic roles for the VEGF receptors during embryonic development. Disruption of any of the three VEGFR genes leads to embryonic lethality; however, the phenotypes of the embryos are distinct. Embryos with targeted null mutations of the VEGFR-2 show the most dramatic phenotype, with a complete failure of vasculogenesis, endothelial cell differentiation, and hematopoiesis.[142] VEGFR-2 null mice die between embryonic day 8.5 and 9.5 with defects in blood island formation and lack of organized blood vessels in either the yolk sac or the embryo proper.[142] Although VEGFR-2 does not seem to be required for hemangioblast formation (endothelial/hematopoietic precursor cells),[143,144] it seems to be essential for subsequent VEGF-directed hemangioblast migration to appropriate environments in the developing embryo, and in the absence of VEGFR-2 signaling, hemangioblasts rapidly disappear.

Homozygous VEGFR-1 knockout mice display an embryonic lethal phenotype, with endothelial cell hyperproliferation in embryonic and extraembryonic locations and the formation of enlarged, poorly organized blood vessels.[124] This observation has led to the suggestion that VEGFR-1 signaling pathways may regulate normal endothelial cell-cell or cell-matrix interactions during vascular development. The increase in endothelial cell numbers has been shown to be a result of an alteration in cell fate determination among mesenchymal cells, leading to increased hemangioblast commitment.[145] When only the tyrosine kinase domain of VEGFR-1 is deleted, however, leaving the ligand binding extracellular moiety and the transmembrane domain intact, embryos develop normal vessels and survive.[146] One of the proposed explanations for this finding is that during embryogenesis, VEGFR-1 regulates the amount of free VEGF available for vascular development. In the absence of VEGFR-1, there would be an excess of free VEGF available to VEGFR-2. It seems that coordinated expression of VEGFR-1 and VEGFR-2 is essential for controlled early vascular development.

Disruption of VEGFR-3 leads to a defective remodeling of the primary vascular plexus and cardiovascular failure after embryonic day 9.5, whereas endothelial cell differentiation, formation of primitive vascular networks, and vascular sprouting occur normally.[147] This phenotype suggests that VEGFR-3 is required for maturation of the primary vascular plexus into a hierarchy of large and small vessels. Although VEGFR-3 has a high affinity for the VEGF-C isoform implicated in lymphangiogenesis, mice null for functional VEGFR-3 show that early in development it has a function in regulating vascular development and only later becomes restricted mostly to the lymphatic system.

Targeted disruption of the mouse *NP1* gene causes severe abnormalities in the peripheral nervous system and cardiovascular failure.[148] Transgenic mice in which *NP1* and *NP2* were targeted died at embryonic day 8.5,[149] at which time their yolk sacs were totally avascular. Mice deficient for *NP2* but heterozygous for *NP1* (NP1[+/-] NP2[-/-]) or deficient for *NP1* and heterozygous for *NP2* (NP1[-/-] NP2[+/-]) survived to embryonic day 10 to 10.5. The yolk sacs showed a lack of large collecting vessels, absence of branching arteries and veins, large avascular spaces between the blood vessels, and a less dense capillary network. The embryos displayed blood vessels heterogeneous in size, large avascular regions in the head and trunk, and blood vessel sprouts that were not connected with the circulation. These results show that the neuropilins are crucial early genes in embryonic vessel development and that *NP1* and *NP2* are required for normal vasculogenesis in the developing embryo.

Angiopoietins

The angiopoietins represent a relatively new family of closely related angiogenic growth factors first described in 1996.[150,151] Five members of the angiopoietin family have been identified to date. Ang-1 is a 70-kDa glycoprotein that induces tyrosine phosphorylation of Tie-2, a cell membrane receptor, in endothelial cells.[150] Ang-1 also interacts through Tie-1, a structural homologue of the membrane receptor Tie-2. Ang-1 activation of the Tie-2 receptor inhibits endothelial cell apoptosis[152,153] and induces endothelial cell migration and capillary tube formation,[152] but in contrast to VEGF stimulation, does not have a mitogenic effect on endothelial cells.[154] The Ang-1 effect on survival of endothelial cells depends on the activation of the PI-3 kinase/Akt pathway.[117,155,156] Ang-1-mediated activation of Akt up-regulates the antiapoptotic protein survivin, whereas it has no effect on the transcription of Bcl-2. Early in development (embryonic day 9 to 11), Ang-1 is found most prominently in the heart myocardium closely associated with the endocardium. Later in development, Ang-1 is distributed much more widely, being found in the mesenchymal and smooth muscle cells surrounding most blood vessels in close association with endothelial cells. In the adult, Ang-1 also is found in the liver and lung[157] and in many other organs at lower levels. Ang-1–Tie-2 interactions are believed to play an important homeostatic role in the postnatal vasculature, maintaining the normal quiescent state of the endothelium and the low permeability to extravasation plasma components characteristic of the endothelial layer (see Fig. 37–4).[157-159]

Ang-2 is unique among ligands of receptor tyrosine kinases in that it seems to act as a natural antagonist of Ang-1 activation of endothelial cell Tie-2, blocking its stabilizing function.[176] It may loosen cell-cell junctions and cell-matrix interactions, increasing the plasticity of the capillary structure and rendering endothelial cells more responsive to other angiogenic stimuli, such as VEGF (see Fig. 37–4).[157,160,161,169] In contrast to the expression pattern of Ang-1, Ang-2 is not readily detected in the developing heart, but it is abundant in the dorsal aorta and major aortic branches, specifically in the smooth muscle layer immediately beneath the vessel endothelium. In the adult, Ang-2 is found in the ovary, placenta, and uterus, which are the three predominant sites of vascular remodeling.[154]

More recently, two other ligands of Tie-2 have been identified, Ang-3 and Ang-4. Ang-3 and Ang-4 bind to Tie-2 but not to Tie-1.[162,163] Ang-4, similar to Ang-1, is an agonist for Tie-2, whereas Ang-3, similar to Ang-2, is an antagonist.[163] Ang-3 is a secreted protein with 45.1% and 44.7% identity with human Ang-1 and Ang-2, respectively.[162,164] In the adult, it is expressed in the adrenal gland, placenta, thyroid gland, heart, and small intestine,[162] whereas Ang-4 is expressed primarily in human lung.[163] The angiopoietins seem to act in a complementary and coordinated fashion with VEGF, increasing the complexity and maturity of the vasculature[165]; however, much still needs to be learned about the developmental and physiologic roles of the different isoforms of angiopoietins.

In vitro studies have shown that hypoxia up-regulates Ang-2 expression and down-regulates Ang-1.[166-168] In a corneal micropocket model of angiogenesis, Asahara and colleagues[169] showed that exogenous coadministration of Ang-1 with VEGF produced larger and more numerous blood vessels than VEGF alone. Evidence has suggested that Ang-2 also might have biphasic actions under circumstances of low oxygen tension, initially blocking Ang-1 activity by acting as a Tie-2 antagonist, allowing endothelial cell activation in response to VEGF and other cytokines and later contributing directly to the stabilization and maturation of newly formed blood vessels, as a partial or full Tie-2 agonist.[170] In high concentrations, Ang-2 has been shown to initiate Tie-2 signaling and to inhibit extracellular apoptosis.[171] These observations have important implications because Ang-2 seems to be the dominant isoform in proangiogenic conditions. It seems that the action of Ang-2 at the Tie-2 receptor is subject to complex regulation such that at the onset of the angiogenic response, it mainly acts to inhibit the tonic homeostatic influence of Ang-1 and to increase endothelial plasticity in response to VEGF; however, at later stages, it may promote signaling directly via Tie-2 and participate in the formation of capillary tubes and their stabilization and maturation (see Fig. 37–4), in a manner identical to Ang-1. Ang-2, by virtue of its dual actions, may the more effective isoform for proangiogenesis therapy. A report has shown that Ang-2, in the presence of endogenous VEGF, was highly effective to induce capillary growth and enlargement in the transient ocular microvessel network (pupillary membrane) of the eye.[172]

Lessons from Transgenic Mice

Mouse embryos homozygous for Ang-1 or Tie-2 gene disruption appear grossly abnormal by embryonic day 11 and die by embryonic day 12.5. The most prominent defect in these embryos involves the heart, which has noticeably less complex ventricular infoldings and an almost collapsed endocardial lining. The heart is devoid of trabeculae and consists of a simple open ventricle lined with a poorly adherent endocardial layer. Tie-2[-/-] and Ang-1[-/-] mice also show deficiencies in vessel branching with fewer and simpler vessels, a poorly organized subendothelial matrix, loosening of endothelial cell contacts with the basement membrane, and a generalized lack of perivascular cells, although the total number of endothelial cells seems unaffected.[151,173-175] These results suggest that Ang-1 and Tie-2 are important for the later steps of the angiogenic process, the remodeling and the maturation of the newly formed vascular system and have a stabilizing effect on the capillaries.

Transgenic overexpression of Ang-2 during embryogenesis also leads to a lethal phenotype similar to that seen in embryos lacking either Ang-1 or Tie-2 consistent with a role for Ang-2 as a natural antagonist for Tie-2.[176] Tie-1 knockout mice die immediately after birth from respiratory failure and edema attributed to a lack of vessel integrity, suggesting a role for Tie-1 in the control of fluid exchange across capillaries.[174]

ENDOTHELIAL FUNCTION AND ANGIOGENESIS

Angiogenesis is a highly complex process involving a myriad of interrelated signaling pathways. Ultimately, these complex influences converge on a single cell type that is of much greater importance than any other in this response, specifically the endothelial cell. Endothelial cells are sufficient at least for the initiation of angiogenesis and the formation of capillary-like networks, and most in vitro model systems of angiogenesis are composed solely of this cell type. Endothelial-derived factors may be of particular importance in the angiogenic cascade, and several have been implicated in various ways in the modulation of endothelial cell growth and differentiation (e.g., NO[177] and endothelin[178]). By far the most evidence points to NO as an essential component of efficient postnatal angiogenesis.[37]

Role of Nitric Oxide in In Vitro Models

Although earlier studies suggested an antiangiogenic effect of NO, more recent reports have shown consistently that NO plays an obligatory role as a downstream mediator of the angiogenic response to many different growth factors. This role first was identified by Ziche and colleagues,[179,180] who showed that capillary-like network formation in three-dimensional fibrin matrices was prevented by the addition of inhibitors of NOS and that VEGF up-regulated NO production in vitro. The same group also showed that NO mediated endothelial cell proliferation in cardiac venular endothelial cells.[181] Other groups, including our own, have shown a similar role for NO as a downstream mediator of response to basic FGF,[39,182] TGF-β,[183] and more recently Ang-1 (K. Tiechert-Kuliszewska, unpublished observations). NO may represent a final common pathway for angiogenesis shared by many different signaling molecules.

Less is known about the mechanisms by which NO contributes to angiogenesis. It is doubtful that NO mediates all effects of VEGF because VEGF and other endothelial cell growth factors act through receptor tyrosine kinases, which initiate a multitude of signal transduction cascades, including PI-3 kinase/Akt, mitogen-activated protein kinases, and protein kinase C. Although some of these pathways can lead to increased NOS activity or expression,[38,184-186] there is ample evidence that they also result directly in endothelial cell proliferation, growth, and migration. More likely, NO plays an important role in modulating the direct cellular responses to angiogenic factors. We have suggested that capillary-like tube formation may be an important example of this cooperative interaction and that the induction of increased NO release alters the endothelial cell "genetic program" in response to angiogenic growth factor from one of activation to one of differentiation.[39]

Role of Nitric Oxide in In Vivo Angiogenesis

Although cell culture model systems are useful in identifying mechanisms of new vessel formation, they are an oversimplification of the angiogenic process that occurs in intact systems. Ziche and colleagues[187] showed that postcapillary endothelial cell mobilization and growth and in vivo angiogenesis induced by VEGF were blocked by the NOS inhibitior L-NMMA and by the guanylate cyclase inhibitor LY 83583, indicating that NO is a downstream imperative of VEGF. The development of transgenic mouse models with targeted disruption of the NOS isoforms[177] is a tremendous advance for the elucidation of the role of NO in developmental and postnatal angiogenesis. Many reports have confirmed an important defect in postnatal angiogenesis in ischemic[188,189] and nonischemic models in eNOS-deficient animals, consistent with a role for endothelium-derived NO in neovascularization in vivo. Some questions remain about its relevance in vasculogenesis and angiogenesis in embryonic development because this must occur normally for viable eNOS$^{-/-}$ pups to be born, and although postnatal angiogenesis is reduced, it is not abolished. Although eNOS$^{-/-}$ can breed successfully, their litter sizes are much smaller than wild-type animals (approximately two pups per litter), possibly because of a high rate of embryonic lethality. Of pups that survive, there is a significant incidence of developmental defects of the heart[190] and extremities.[191] These resemble defects induced by administration of thalidomide (an angiogenesis inhibitor) during pregnancy and certain human syndromes of congenital heart disease (i.e., Holt-Oram syndrome). These observations suggest that an abnormality in cardiovascular development may underlie the high in utero loss of eNOS-deficient animals. That some normal vascular development can occur in some eNOS$^{-/-}$ animals is not surprising given the redundancy that is often inherent in mechanisms controlling key developmental steps, and this is a major limitation of nonconditional knockout approaches.

Endothelial Dysfunction

Given the crucial role of endothelium-derived NO in the angiogenic response, it follows that in states of endothelial dysfunction, characterized by reduced NO bioavailability,[192] there would be reduced potential for new blood vessel formation. In animal models of endothelial dysfunction induced by hypercholesterolemia, it has been shown that neovascularization and collateral vessel formation in the ischemic hind limb is markedly reduced.[193] Similar defects have been identified in aging mice,[194] another model of endothelial dysfunction. These observations have particular relevance for clinical studies of proangiogenic therapy because patients with occlusive CAD, especially patients with extensive and diffuse involvement, often have multiple risk factors and exhibit marked endothelial dysfunction. The population that is most in need of collateral vessels seems to be the least able to generate these. As such, therapeutic angiogenic strategies need to take into consideration ways of reducing endothelial dysfunction and increasing NO bioavailability in this population. This can be accomplished by aggressive treatment of risk factors, especially reduction in plasmid lipids using potent agents such as the statins. In addition to their beneficial effects of

endothelial function by lowering cholesterol levels, these agents may have direct effects on the expression and activity of endothelial NOS and may influence endothelial cell survival and angiogenesis by stimulating the PI-3 kinase/Akt pathway.[195] Another class of pharmacologic agents having direct impact on endothelial function is the angiotensin-converting enzyme inhibitors. These drugs not only inhibit the generation of angiotensin II, but also prevent the breakdown of bradykinin, an important endogenous stimulator of basal NO release.[196] Angiotensin-converting enzyme inhibitors have been shown to improve endothelial dysfunction in animal and clinical studies. Increased neovascularization and collateral vessel formation in response to quinapril was reported in the rabbit ischemic hind limb model.[197] Although this is likely a class effect, similar benefit was not observed with captopril.[198] This benefit is most likely a result of the ability of this agent to reduce MMP activity by virtue of its sulfhydryl groups and directly inhibit an important step in the angiogenic cascade.[198]

GROWTH FACTOR–INDUCED MYOCARDIAL ANGIOGENESIS

The identification of many of the key proteins that regulate blood vessel growth has opened the door for their use in proangiogenesis therapies. The promise of biologic revascularization of ischemic myocardium in patients who are unable to undergo conventional procedures has spurred tremendous interest, and many proangiogenesis strategies currently are being evaluated clinically.

Preclinical Studies

The most consistent limitation to progress in angiogenesis research has been the availability of simple, reliable, reproducible, and quantitative assays of the angiogenic response.[199] Standard animal models include the hamster cheek pouch, the rabbit ear chamber, the chick embryo chorioallantoic membrane, the iris and avascular cornea of the rodent eye, the rat and rabbit hind limb, and the dog and pig myocardial ischemia models. Although each model has limitations, investigations using these models have helped in the understanding of the link between growth factors and new vessel formation.

The angiogenic growth factors first used for the purpose of stimulating angiogenesis were members of the FGF family. Baffour and coworkers[200] administered FGF-2 in daily intramuscular doses of 1 or 3 µg to rabbits with acute hind limb ischemia. At the completion of 14 days of treatment, angiography and necropsy measurement of capillary density in the lower limb showed evidence of augmented collateral vessel formation compared with control. FGF-1 was used to treat rabbits in which the acute effects of surgically induced hind limb ischemia were allowed to subside for 10 days before the initiation of a 10-day course of daily 4-mg intramuscular injections.[201] At 30 days after the induction of ischemia, animals treated with FGF-1 showed angiographic and hemodynamic evidence of collateral development superior to that of placebo-treated animals. Salvage of infarcted myocardium by the administration of FGF-2 was shown by Yanagisawa-Miwa and colleagues.[202] They administered FGF-2 intra-arterially at the time of coronary occlusion in a dog model of myocardial infarction. A second bolus was given 6 hours later. The systolic function was greater and the infarct size smaller in the treated animals compared with controls. Blood vessel density also was higher in the infarct zone in the FGF-treated animals.

Evidence that VEGF could stimulate angiogenesis in vivo first was obtained from experiments using the rat and rabbit cornea[203,204] and the chick chorioallantoic membrane models.[73,205] The demonstration that VEGF could be used to achieve angiogenesis that was "therapeutic" first was reported by Takeshita and associates.[206] They administered $VEGF_{165}$ as a single intra-arterial bolus to the internal iliac artery of rabbits in which the ipsilateral femoral artery was excised to induce hind limb ischemia. Statistically significant augmentation of angiographically visible collateral vessels and histologically identified capillaries was seen with the administration of doses of 500 to 1000 µg of VEGF. Hind limb blood flow and distal perfusion pressure also were better in the treated animals. Similar dose-dependent results were observed with a 10-day administration of VEGF by an intramuscular route initiated 10 days after the induction of hind limb ischemia.[207]

Since these pioneering experiments, abundant data have been collected in animal models to support the potential utility of recombinant protein therapy for therapeutic myocardial angiogenesis[208-219] and to provide the proof of principle necessary for the initiation of studies employing genes encoding angiogenic factors.

Clinical Trials of Proangiogenesis Therapy

Until more recently, human angiogenic experiments have been limited predominantly to small series in which mainly VEGF or FGF, protein or gene, have been administered.[72,220-238] Delivery strategies have included intracoronary, epicardial, or direct myocardial injection of VEGF or bFGF protein or genetic material. The genetic material can be delivered as naked plasma DNA or in a viral vector.

Schumacher and colleagues[222] were the first to report on therapeutic angiogenesis in human myocardium. In this phase I, randomized, blinded study, 40 patients undergoing CABG surgery with a left internal mammary artery graft and a left anterior descending artery stenosis distal to the anastomosis site were enrolled. Patients were assigned randomly to direct intramyocardial injection of aFGF or denatured protein control near the distal nongrafted segment. At 3 months, the investigators observed increased "coronary blush," a surrogate measure of collateral formation, among FGF-injected patients compared with placebo-injected patients. This effect persisted to 3 years and was associated with improved echocardiographic ejection fraction and functional class.[223] Similar positive results were seen in small trials using FGF therapy reported by Sellke and colleagues,[72]

Laham and colleagues,[224,227] Unger and colleagues,[225] and Udelson and colleagues[226] (Table 37-2).

Six small studies evaluated VEGF delivery to ischemic myocardium (Table 37-3). Protein therapy, performed with varying doses of intracoronary recombinant human VEGF, was studied by Henry and associates[228] and Hendel and coworkers.[229] DNA coding for VEGF has been delivered as naked plasmid DNA[230-232,235,238] or using an adenoviral vector.[233,234] The results of these small trials were promising and suggested that VEGF protein and DNA were effective for the production of new blood vessels.

Collectively, these phase I and II studies described the experience of 318 patients without blinded outcome assessment. Although data from these studies cannot be used to make conclusions concerning efficacy, they firmly established the feasibility and safety of different methods of gene transfer, and they have set the stage for larger randomized trials.

Only three relatively large, randomized, double-blind, placebo-controlled studies have been performed in humans. The FIRST (FGF-2 Initiating Revascularization Support Trial) recruited 337 patients with angina who were considered suboptimal for traditional revascularization.[239] In a double-blind, placebo-controlled manner, participants were randomized to placebo or one of three doses of intracoronary recombinant bFGF protein (0.3, 3, and 30 µg/kg). Efficacy was evaluated at 90 and 180 days by exercise tolerance test, myocardial nuclear perfusion imaging, Seattle Angina Questionnaire (SAQ), and Short-Form 36 questionnaire. At 90 days, there was no difference between groups in the primary end point of exercise treadmill times. Recombinant bFGF administration reduced angina symptoms as measured by the angina frequency score of the SAQ (overall, $P = .035$) and the physical component summary scale of the Short-Form 36 (pairwise, $P = .033$, all FGF groups versus placebo). None of the differences were significant at 180 days because of continued improvement in the placebo group. Adverse events were similar across all groups except for hypotension, which occurred with higher frequency in the 30-µg/kg bFGF group.

The VIVA (VEGF in Ischemia for Vascular Angiogenesis) trial involved a patient cohort similar to that of the FIRST with evidence of a reversible perfusion defect on nuclear scans.[240] Patients (n = 178) were assigned randomly to two doses of VEGF (17 or 50 ng/kg) or placebo. VEGF protein was administered as a 20-minute intracoronary infusion during coronary angiography, followed by three 4-hour intravenous infusions on days 3, 6, and 9. Although no improvement was seen in the primary end point of treadmill score at 60 days, mean Canadian Cardiovascular Society (CCS) anginal class was significantly lower for the high-dose group compared with the placebo group at 120 days (1.6 ± 0.1 vs. 2.1 ± 0.1, $P = .04$).

The objectives of the AGENT (Angiogenic GENe Therapy) trial were to evaluate the safety and anti-ischemic effects of the intracoronary administration of Ad5-FGF4 in patients with angina.[241] A total of 79 patients with chronic stable angina CCS class 2 or 3 underwent double-blind randomization (1:3) to placebo (n = 19) or to one of five ascending doses of Ad5-FGF4

TABLE 37–2 CLINICAL TRIALS OF FIBROBLAST GROWTH FACTOR DELIVERY

PARAMETER	SCHUMACHER ET AL (1998)[222]	LAHAM ET AL (1999)[224]	UNGER ET AL (2000)[225]	LAHAM ET AL (2000)[227]	SELKE ET AL (1998)[72]	FIRST 2002[239]	AGENT 2002[241]
N	40	24	25	66	8	337	79
Design	RDB	RDB	RDB	Observational	Observational	RDB	RDB
Placebo-controlled	Yes	No	Yes	No	No	Yes	Yes
Thoracotomy	Yes	Yes	No	No	Yes	No	No
Agent	aFGF protein	bFGF protein	bFGF protein	bFGF protein	bFGF protein	bFGF protein	FGF-4 DNA
Vector	None	Heparin/alginate microcapsules	None	None	Heparin/alginate microcapsules	None	Adenovirus
Dose	70 mg	10/100 µg	3–100 µg/kg	0.33–48 µg/kg	10/100µg	200 µg	3.2×10^8 to 3.2×10^{10} viral particles
Delivery	Intramyocardial	Epicardial fat implantation	Intracoronary	IC/IV	Epicardial fat implantation	Intracoronary	Intracoronary
End point	DSA	Clinical/MPI	GXT	MPI	MPI	GXT/MPI/QOL	GXT
Result	Positive	Positive	Safe	Positive	Safe	Negative	Negative

DSA, digital subtraction angiography; GXT, graded exercise stress test; IC, intracoronary; IV, intravascular; MPI, myocardial perfusion imaging; QOL, quality of life; RDB, randomized, double-blind.

PARAMETER	HENDEL ET AL (2000)[235]	HENRY ET AL (1998)[228]	VALE ET AL (2001)[232]	SYMES ET AL (1999)[231]	HENDEL ET AL (2000)[229]	ROSENGART ET AL (1999)[233]	LOSORDO ET AL (1998)[230]	VALE ET AL (2001)[237]	LOSORDO ET AL (2002)[238]	VIVA 2001[240]
N	30	15	30	20	14	21	5	6	19	178
Design	Observational	Observational	Observational	Observational	Observational	Observational	Observational	Randomized	Randomized	RDB
Placebo-controlled	No	No	No	No	No	No	No	Yes	Yes	Yes
Thoracotomy	No	No	Yes	Yes	No	Yes	Yes	No	No	No
Agent	VEGF-C DNA	rhVEGF protein	$VEGF_{165}$ DNA	$rhVEGF_{165}$ DNA	rhVEGF protein	$VEGF_{121}$ DNA	$VEGF_{165}$ DNA	VEGF-C DNA	VEGF-C DNA	rhVEGF protein
Vector	Plasmid	None	Plasmid	Plasmid	None	Adenovirus	Plasmid	Plasmid	Plasmid	None
Dose	0.2/0.8/2.0 mg	0.005/0.017/ 0.05/ 0.167 µg/kg	125/250/ 500 µg	125/250 µg	0.005/0.017/ 0.05/ 0.167 µg/kg	1000 µg	125 µg	200 µg	200/800/ 2000 µg	17/50 ng/kg/min
Delivery	Intramyocardial	Intracoronary	Intramyocardial	Intramyocardial	Intracoronary	Intramyocardial	Intramyocardial	Intramyocardial	Intramyocardial	IC/IV
End point	Clinical/GXT/ MPI/NOGA	MPI	Clinical/GXT/ MPI	Clinical/MPI/ angiography	MPI	Clinical/MPI/ angiography/ GXT	Clinical/MPI/ angiography	Clinical/GXT/ MPI/NOGA	Clinical/GXT/ MPI/NOGA	Clinical/GXT/ angiography
Result	Positive	Positive	Positive	Positive	Positive	Positive	Safety	Positive	Positive	Negative

GXT, graded exercise stress test; IC, intracoronary; IV, intravascular; MPI, myocardial perfusion imaging; NOGA, NOGA electromechanical mapping; RDB, randomized, double blind.

(from 3.3×10^8 to 3.3×10^{10} viral particles in half-log increments; n = 60). Safety evaluations were performed at each visit, and exercise treadmill testing was done at baseline and at 4 and 12 weeks. Single intracoronary administration of Ad5-FGF4 seemed to be safe and well tolerated with no immediate adverse events. Transient, asymptomatic elevations in liver enzymes occurred in two patients in lower dose groups, and fever of less than 1 day's duration occurred in three patients in the highest dose group. Serious adverse events during follow-up (mean, 311 days) were not different between placebo and Ad5-FGF4 groups. Improvement in exercise time was not significantly different between placebo and FGF-treated groups at either 4 or 12 weeks' follow-up. A protocol-specified, subgroup analysis showed a significant improvement in exercise time in patients with a baseline exercise treadmill testing less than or equal to 10 minutes at 4 weeks (1.6 minutes versus 0.6 minutes, $P = .01$, n = 50) and 12 weeks (1.86 minutes versus 1.27 minutes, $P = .01$, n = 50) in the Ad5-FGF4–treated group compared with placebo. These results show evidence of favorable anti-ischemic effects with Ad5-FGF4 compared with placebo with a satisfactory safety profile.

Although none of these trials were unable to show efficacy by their primary end point, several factors may account for the lack of effect. In the three trials, delivery was accomplished via an intracoronary or intravenous route. It is unclear if this method provides adequate tissue levels to stimulate and maintain angiogenesis. This is particularly true for bFGF protein, given the poor specificity for target endothelium. Dose-ranging studies for FGF and VEGF suggest a dose-dependent response.[225,229] It is possible that injection into myocardium or pericardial fat is necessary for clinically relevant dose delivery and transfection rates as evidenced by several preclinical and clinical studies.[224,242] The AGENT trial provided the most encouraging results to date and was closest to meeting its primary end point. This is possibly an indication that gene therapy may offer the advantage of prolonged production and release of angiogenic proteins after a single administration.

Issues of Study Design

The previous clinical experience with proangiogenesis studies highlighted many issues that investigators must consider in planning future controlled trials to assess the effectiveness of protein or gene therapies, including (1) selection of the optimal factor, (2) protein or gene therapy, (3) determination of appropriate end points to be studied, (4) quantification and resultant objectification of the results, (5) assurance of adequate controls, (6) selection of patients to be included, (7) determination of the mechanisms of any observed clinical effects, and (8) assessment of complications (potential, actual, local, systemic, immediate, and long-term).

Choice of Optimal Therapeutic Agent

The success of proangiogenic therapy for myocardial ischemia depends on the choice of the best factor or combinations of factor. To date, the greatest experience has been with VEGF or FGF. Although there are substantive preclinical data to support their use, there are limited data of their relative efficacy, compared with each other or with other factors. Although the endothelial selective VEGF is perhaps the most crucial factor in vascular development, its use in proangiogenic therapy is thought to result in fragile capillary-like structures that lack mature basement membrane, exhibit high permeability, and may be prone to regression.[243] FGF may have an advantage because by acting on endothelial and smooth muscle cells, it may produce larger and more competent arterial vessels containing a medial layer.[15,36,72] The angiopoietins, by virtue of their actions at later stages of the angiogenesis cascade, offer promise as therapeutic "arteriogenesis" agents[160]; however, there are currently only limited data on their efficacy in preclinical ischemic models, and there is no experience in clinical trials. Combinations of angiogenic factors (e.g., VEGF and Ang-1) may be necessary for an optimal response; however, the experience with such strategies is limited. Another way of harnessing the potential benefits of multiple angiogenic factors is to use a "master switch" gene, such as HIF-1α, which regulates the expression of more than 40 HIF genes.[244] Studies on the safety and efficacy of HIF-1α gene therapy for ischemic peripheral and coronary vascular diseases are under way; however, no data are currently available. Many other angiogenetic factors are also in various stages of preclinical and clinical evaluation, including erythropoietin[245] and Del-1, a novel transcription factor that is involved in the poorly understood process of vascular remodeling.[246] The results of these studies are anticipated with great interest.

Protein versus Gene Therapy

Delivery of growth factors to the heart can be accomplished through the use of single or multiple doses of recombinant protein or by a gene transfer approach, and each strategy has its limitations. Potential advantages for the use of proteins include the ability to adjust their dose and be able to define a therapeutic window between efficacy and toxicity. This allows withdrawal of treatment if and when necessary. Arguments against the use of protein for therapeutic angiogenesis are (1) the considerable cost involved in producing significant quantities of pyrogen-free materials, (2) the appearance of secondary effects (prolonged administration of bFGF is associated with a decrease in arterial pressure, moderate thrombocytopenia, and moderate anemia), and (3) the requirement for repeated or prolonged administration of protein because of a short half-life. Local perivascular delivery via myocardial injection, pericardial fat implantation of coated microspheres, or pericardial instillation has been attempted to address the last-mentioned limitation.[247-249] Delivery strategies for protein have been studied more thoroughly in experimental models. In a pig model, tissue and myocardial distribution of labeled bFGF was determined at 1 hour and 24 hours after intracoronary or intravenous delivery by measuring ^{125}I-bFGF–specific activity.[242-250] At 1 hour, total cardiac activity was 0.88 with intracoronary delivery, which decreased significantly to 0.05 at 24 hours. Cardiac-specific activity with intravenous administration was lower at 1 hour (0.26), which also decreased significantly to 0.04 by 24 hours. Intracoronary but not intravenous delivery resulted in higher deposition in ischemic than normal myocardium. Intrapericardial delivery resulted in a cardiac-specific activity of 1.45 after 1 hour, which increased to 2.98 by 24 hours.[250] The 1-hour cardiac-specific activity was highest with intramyocardial delivery at 4.31, which decreased to 2.30 by 24 hours. The study showed that intrapericardial and intramyocardial delivery results in a more favorable myocardial distribution of growth factor than intracoronary or intravenous delivery. Additional data from the study indicated that intrapericardial delivery was limited to the epicardial layers and required a normal pericardium.

In contrast to protein delivery, gene therapy can result in the prolonged secretion of growth product by host cells, offering sustained local protein levels after a single administration. The potential for uptake of vector and gene expression at distant sites with unwanted effects in nontarget tissues is of concern, however. There are many means to deliver genes coding for angiogenic products. The simplest is through the delivery of naked plasmid DNA. Injection of naked DNA into myocardium has been shown to result in growth factor expression for a considerable period, without incorporation into host DNA.[247,251] The presence of a secretory signal on the genes being tested must be considered, however. In contrast to VEGF, the common forms of FGF (aFGF and bFGF) lack a secretory signal sequence, and clinical trials of FGF gene transfer have required the modification of the FGF gene[252] or use of a member of the FGF gene family with a signal sequence.[253] Facilitated means of gene delivery also have been studied. Liposomal encapsulation has been tested; however, current techniques are associated with low in vivo transfection efficiencies and toxicity resulting from proinflammatory actions. Retrovirus encapsulation and delivery allows for effective and long-term gene expression through DNA incorporation into the genome; however, the potential for activation of retroviral genes in the host DNA is of concern. The use of adenoviral vectors is an effective means of enhancing in vivo transfection efficiency; however, it is associated with an immune response that can lead to destruction of the vector or a significant systemic inflammatory response,[254] which can result in morbidity and even mortality, as was shown with the death of an 18-year-old volunteer in a phase I clinical trial.[255] At this time, there is insufficient evidence on which to make any strong statements on the relative superiority of one approach versus another based on the current clinical trials. In the near future, trials using intramyocardial injection of plasmid DNA or adenoviral vectors containing the VEGF gene will be completed, and it is hoped that the results will be positive. These data will provide much needed insight into these important questions.

Efficacy End Points

The choice of efficacy end points for clinical trials on therapeutic angiogenesis is an area of uncertainty. The ideal end point for angiogenesis trials should have the following characteristics: (1) It should address the primary hypothesis and represent a direct marker of efficacy, (2) it should be clinically meaningful, (3) it should be easily measured and not be prohibitively costly to perform or analyze, (4) it should provide insight into mechanisms, and (5) it should lend itself to statistical analysis. The end points for trials of angiogenesis can be considered either clinical (angina status, functional capacity, or quality of life) or physiologic (improved myocardial perfusion, improvement in vessel collateralization, improvement in global or regional wall motion).

Although objective end points, such as death, myocardial infarction, and repeat revascularization, are more reliable, they require larger numbers of patients for adequate statistical power. Results from several trials in patients with no therapeutic options indicate a mortality rate over 2 years of follow-up of approximately 5%. A prohibitively large study population would be required to show a reduction in mortality. Of the surrogate clinical assessments, exercise stress testing has been most widely used, in part because of regulatory requirements. The advantages of employing exercise testing as a clinical end point for angiogenesis trials is that it is readily available and clinically meaningful. Depending on the methodology used, the results can be quantitative (rate pressure product, time to ST-segment depression), and the findings are reproducible.[256] The disadvantages of using exercise testing as an end point are that comorbidities (peripheral vascular disease, chronic obstructive lung disease, arthritis) may limit exercise performance, day-to-day variability exists, and the reasons for test termination still may be subjective.

Changes in CCS score and response to the SAQ also have been used as clinical end points in angiogenesis trials. The advantages of these types of assessments are that they are sensitive, highly relevant clinically, easy to interpret, fairly reproducible (especially the SAQ), and familiar to most clinicians (i.e., the CCS score is used in clinical practice). The disadvantages of these assessments are that they are more subjective than exercise stress testing, making blinding necessary; the CCS score requires observer input; changes in the SAQ are not easily interpreted because of lack of familiarity by clinicians; and the placebo effects are substantial (approximately 40% in the DIRECT [DMR in Regeneration of Endomyocardial Channels Trial]). The advantages of using the MOS SF-36 or Health Utility Index are that they are broadly applicable, they are sensitive to change, and normal values have been established for various disease states. Disadvantages of these types of analyses as end points are that they are considered to be softer end points, they are more subjective, and the changes are not easily interpreted.

A problem common to all clinical end points is that they are prone to placebo effects. These may be of a surprising magnitude, especially in trials involving innovative new therapies for which the investigators and the patients have considerable hope and enthusiasm, as was borne out in the DIRECT, FIRST, and VIVA trial. The issue of placebo effect must be addressed by adequate trial design if clinical end points are to be meaningful. An additional problem with clinical end points is that small changes may be undetected but still be clinically meaningful (the so-called basement effect). Although clinical end points are employed in trials of myocardial angiogenesis, physiologic assessments are preferred as primary end points. Several physiologic end points have been considered, including single-photon emission computed tomography (SPECT) myocardial perfusion imaging, magnetic resonance imaging (MRI), and positron emission tomography (PET). The advantages of nuclear scintigraphy are that it is sensitive to changes after revascularization, it is reproducible, and wall motion can be assessed. There are concerns, however, over the adequacy of the spatial resolution obtainable with nuclear imaging. MRI has enormous potential and provides excellent spatial resolution and information on structure, function, and flow. Although MRI is gaining greater acceptance with time, prohibitive cost and restrictive availability limit its use. PET is more sensitive than SPECT in measuring coronary flow reserve. PET is the only way to measure absolute blood flow. Limitations of PET are poor spatial resolution, lack of widespread availability, and cost.

Potential Complications

The delivery of angiogenic factors can produce many unwanted effects, some of which are potentially serious. These are reviewed briefly.

Hypotension. The risks associated with therapeutic angiogenesis include risks that are related to the particular growth factor employed and risks specific to the strategies employed for the promotion of angiogenesis. Administration of either VEGF or bFGF recombinant proteins may lead to hypotension[257,258] owing to their ability to up-regulate NOS and release NO.[259,260] Hypotension has been reported with FGF protein therapy in clinical trials for peripheral vascular angiogenesis[261] and in the FIRST,[239] which examined myocardial angiogenesis. Significant hypotension also limited the dose of VEGF protein used in the VIVA trial. This complication has never been described after gene transfer of VEGF or bFGF in either preclinical animal studies or clinical trials regardless of the vector or transgene. The absence of this complication with the use of gene therapy is likely the result of lower circulating levels of gene product compared with that with recombinant protein therapy.

Increased Vessel Permeability and Edema. VEGF first was described as a factor secreted by tumors that augmented vascular permeability. The potent permeability-enhancing effects have raised concerns over the safety of its use for therapeutic angiogenesis. These safety concerns have been fueled by results obtained from the study of transgenic mice engineered to overexpress VEGF[158] and lethal permeability-enhancing consequences of adenoviral gene transfer of VEGF in mice.[159] Evidence of enhanced permeability in humans has been limited to transient lower extremity edema in patients with critical limb ischemia after VEGF gene transfer,[161] and this appears to be a problem only with VEGF-A and its homologues.[262]

Abnormal Vascularization and Vascular Malformations. Preclinical data show the development of angiomas in mice[263,264] or rats[265] treated with transduced myoblasts or excessive doses of plasmid DNA, both expressing VEGF. Preclinical and clinical studies of gene therapy suggest that levels that have been investigated for therapeutic angiogenesis are not associated with hemangioma formation. There are safety issues concerning the potential to stimulate unintended neovascularization in nontarget tissues. Mitigating this possibility are data that suggest angiogenesis occurs in response to a cytokine only under appropriate conditions. Receptors for FGF and VEGF are up-regulated when tissues become ischemic,[266-269] and it would be expected that ischemic tissue would respond more sensitively to the biologic effects of FGF and VEGF than would normal tissues. This concept was supported by a study in which normal and ischemic canine myocardium was exposed to high local levels of aFGF protein administered with an epicardial sponge over a prolonged time.[270] In this study, only ischemic myocardium had an angiogenic response. Although the high threshold for neovascularization in normal tissue is reassuring, there is still concern about patients who have coexistent conditions in which cytokine receptors are abnormally up-regulated, such as diabetic retinopathy and malignant tumors.

Retinopathy. The concerns over the potential exacerbation of proliferative or hemorrhagic retinopathy with angiogenic growth factors is based on animal studies[271,272] and on the demonstration of high VEGF levels in the ocular fluid of patients with active proliferative retinopathy.[273,274] Clinical follow-up of patients with serial funduscopic examinations have not shown any evidence of new retinopathy, despite the high percentage of patients treated for vascular disease who previously were diagnosed with retinopathy.[275]

Neoplasia. The identification of angiogenesis as a target for the inhibition of the growth of tumors by Adamis and colleagues[274] and the subsequent introduction of antiangiogenic therapy for the treatment of malignancies raised concerns that there may be a potential for angiogenesis therapy to trigger the growth of existent but unrecognized tumors. FGF is a mitogen that stimulates a wide variety of cell types, and it may stimulate tumor cell growth directly. Although VEGF acts primarily on vascular endothelium, many nonendothelial tumor cells have been found to possess low levels of functional VEGF receptors.[276] In addition to the potential for direct effects of the angiogenic agents on tumor cell proliferation, there is evidence to suggest that solid tumors require an angiogenic stimulus to supply nutrients required for growth beyond a critical size. In the prevascular phase, a tumor rarely grows larger than a few millimeters in diameter. Without neovascularization, the primary mass of cancerous cells depends solely on diffusion for oxygen and nutrients. Neovascularization greatly improves oxygenation and the removal of waste products, permitting the tumor to grow. The development of new vessels increases the opportunity for malignant cells to enter the circulation, and newly formed capillaries have a discontinuous basement membrane and are penetrated more easily by tumor cells than are mature vessels. Based on these observations, it has been theorized that the induction of angiogenesis may contribute indirectly to the growth of dormant tumors. The available published data regarding this potential complication are reassuring, although limited to a few patients with a relatively short follow-up.

Accelerated Atherosclerosis. Animal data suggest that the administration of angiogenic cytokines might enhance atherosclerosis. When administered via a single intraperitoneal injection to apolipoprotein-E–deficient, cholesterol-fed mice, recombinant human VEGF protein enhanced atheroslerotic plaque progression.[277] Similar results were reported with the administration of recombinant human VEGF to cholesterol-fed rabbits. Moulton and coworkers[278] observed that when hypercholesterolemic mice were treated with inhibitors of angiogenesis, atherosclerotic plaque area in these animals was reduced significantly. Other studies have shown, however, a protective effect of VEGF treatment in models of arterial injury[279] and atherosclerosis (DJ Stewart et al, unpublished results), and there is still room for debate on these issues.[280] In most angiogenesis trials, the exposure to endothelial growth factors is typically relatively brief (<2 weeks), whereas atherosclerosis progression occurs over a much more extended period. It is possible, however, that this therapy will lead to instability of vascular lesions and increase the chance of plaque rupture and cardiac events, although the limited data available from clinical trials of proangiogenesis therapy to date do not support this. Careful monitoring of patients in future trials will be required.

FUTURE RESEARCH

Current animal studies are focusing on the mechanisms of angiogenesis, examining in particular the roles of different compounds and the local and host factors that govern their effectiveness. The action of angiogenic factors in the milieu of CAD is also an area of active research. The results of animal studies and early results of clinical trials suggest that delivery of a cocktail of angiogenic factors might be more effective than delivery of a single agent and may mimic more closely the physiologic angiogenic response. Finally, stem and progenitor cell transplantation may allow for the development of all components required for new myocardium and functioning vascular network and may provide a feasible therapy in the future.

SUMMARY

Exciting and promising options are being explored for the treatment of CAD. The discovery and study of vascular growth factors has led to much insight on the complex mechanistic processes of vascular development cogent to a wide variety of disease processes. This research has pooled resources from many disciplines, including molecular sciences, oncology, and vascular biology. Although still in its infancy, advances in the understanding of the endothelial organ and the insights gained from clinical studies are likely to provide a wealth of therapeutic options for modern diseases.

REFERENCES

1. Vineberg AM: Formation of a third coronary artery by internal mammary article implant. Geriatrics 1953;8:579-595.
2. Vineberg AM: The development of an anastomosis between the coronary vessels and a transplanted internal mammary artery. Can Med Assoc J 1946;55:117-119.
3. Vineberg AM, Jewitt BL: Development of an anastomosis between the coronary vessels and a transplanted internal mammary artery. J Thorac Surg 1949;18:839-850.
4. Vineberg AM: Development of anastomosis between the coronary vessels and a transplanted internal mammary artery. J Thorac Surg 1949;18:839-850.
5. Vineberg AM, Niloff PH: The value of surgical treatment of coronary artery occlusion by implantation of the internal mammary coronary artery into the ventricular myocardium: An experimental study. Surg Gynecol Obstet 1950;91:551-561.
6. Johnson WD, Chekanov VS, Kipshidze N: Vineberg procedure combined with therapeutic angiogenesis: Old wine in a new bottle. Ann Thorac Surg 2001;72:1438-1448.
7. Folkman J: Anti-angiogenesis: New concept for therapy of solid tumors. Ann Surg 1972;175:409-416.
8. Risau W: Mechanisms of angiogenesis. Nature 1997;386:671-674.
9. Patan S, Munn LL, Jain RK: Intussusceptive microvascular growth in a human colon adenocarcinoma xenograft: A novel mechanism of tumor angiogenesis. Microvasc Res 1996;51:260-272.
10. Hanahan D, Folkman J: Patterns and emerging mechanisms of the angiogenic switch during tumorigenesis. Cell 1996;86:353-364.
11. Sledge GW Jr, Miller KD: Angiogenesis and antiangiogenic therapy. Curr Probl Cancer 2002;26:1-60.
12. Cao Y: Endogenous angiogenesis inhibitors and their therapeutic implications. Int J Biochem Cell Biol 2001;33:357-369.
13. Wang GL, Semonza GI: Purification and characterization of hypoxia inducible factor 1. J Biol Chem 1995;270:1230-1237.
14. Brooks PC, Montgomery AM, Rosenfeld M, et al: Integrin alpha v beta 3 antagonists promote tumor regression by inducing apoptosis of angiogenic blood vessels. Cell 1994;79:1157-1164.
15. Tomanek RJ, Schatteman GC: Angiogenesis: New insights and therapeutic potential. Anat Rec 2000;261:126-135.
16. Hynes RO, Bader BL, Hodivala-Dilke K: Integrins in vascular development. Braz J Med Biol Res 1999;32:501-510.
17. Eliceiri BP, Cheresh DA: The role of av integrins during angiogenesis: Insights into potential mechanisms of action and clinical development. J Clin Invest 1999;103:1227-1230.
18. Meredith JE Jr, Fazeli B, Schwartz MA: The extracellular matrix as a cell survival factor. Mol Biol Cell 1993;4:953-961.
19. Brooks PC, Clark RAF, Cheresh DA: Requirement of vascular integrin $\alpha_v \beta_3$ for angiogenesis. Science 1994;264:569-571.
20. Friedlander M, Brooks PC, Shaffer RW, et al: Definition of two angiogenic pathways by distinct α_v integrins. Science 1995;270:1500-1502.
21. Varner JA, Brooks PC, Cheresh DA: The integrin $\alpha_v \beta_3$: Angiogenesis and apoptosis. Cell Adhes Commun 1996;3:367-374.
22. Basson CT, Kocher O, Basson MD, et al: Differential modulation of vascular cell integrin and extracellular matrix expression in vitro by TGF-β1 correlates with reciprocal effects on cell migration. J Cell Physiol 1992;153:118-128.
23. Swerlick RA, Brown EJ, Xu Y, et al: Expression and modulation of the vitronectin receptor on human dermal microvascular endothelial cells. J Invest Dermatol 1992;99:715-722.
24. Sepp NT, Li L-J, Lee KH, et al: Basic fibroblast growth factor increases expression of the $\alpha_v \beta_3$ integrin complex on human microvascular endothelial cells. J Invest Dermatol 1994;103:295-299.

25. Senger DR, Ledbetter SR, Claffey KP, et al: Stimulation of endothelial cell migration by vascular permeability factor/vascular endothelial growth factor through cooperative mechanisms involving the $\alpha_v\beta_3$ integrin, osteopontin, and thrombin. Am J Pathol 1996;149:293-305.

26. Brooks PC, Strömblad S, Klemke R, et al: Antiintegrin $\alpha_v\beta_3$ blocks human breast cancer growth and angiogenesis in human skin. J Clin Invest 1995;96:1815-1822.

27. Drake CJ, Cheresh DA, Little CD: An antagonist of integrin $\alpha_v\beta_3$ prevents maturation of blood vessels during embryonic neovascularization. J Cell Sci 1995;108:2655-2661.

28. Hammes H-P, Brownlee M, Jonczyk A, et al: Subcutaneous injection of a cyclic peptide antagonist of vitronectin receptor-type integrins inhibits retinal neovascularization. Nat Med 1996;2:529-533.

29. Soldi R, Mitola S, Strasly M, et al: Role of $\alpha_v\beta_3$ integrin in the activation of vascular endothelial growth factor receptor-2. EMBO J 1999;18:882-892.

30. Byzova TV, Goldman CK, Pampori N, et al: A mechanism for modulation of cellular responses to VEGF: Activation of the integrins. Mol Cell 2000;6:851-860.

31. Dvorak HF: Tumours: Wounds that do not heal: Similarities between tumour stroma generation and wound healing. N Engl J Med 1986;315:1650-1659.

32. Haas TL, Madri JA: Extracellular matrix-driven matrix metalloproteinase production in endothelial cells: Implications for angiogenesis. Trends Cardiovasc Med 1999;9:70-77.

33. Mignatti P, Rifkin DB: Plasminogen activators and matrix metalloproteinases in angiogenesis. Enzyme Protein 1996;49:117-137.

34. Buschmann I, Schaper W: The pathophysiology of the collateral circulation. J Pathol 2000;190:338-342.

35. Henry TD: Therapeutic angiogenesis. BMJ 1999;318:1536-1539.

36. Griffioen A, Molema G: Angiogenesis: Potentials for pharmacologic intervention in the treatment of cancer, cardiovascular diseases, and chronic inflammation. Pharm Rev 2000;52:237-268.

37. Cooke JP, Losordo DW: Nitric oxide and angiogenesis. Circulation 2002;105:2133-2135.

38. Fukumura D, Jain RK: Role of nitric oxide in angiogenesis and microcirculation in tumors. Cancer Metastasis Rev 1998;17:77-89.

39. Babaei S, Teichert-Kuliszewska K, Monge JC, et al: Role of nitric oxide in the angiogenic response in vitro to basic fibroblast growth factor. Circ Res 1998;82:1007-1015.

40. Goligorsky MS, Budzikowski AS, Tsukahara H, Noiri E: Co-operation between endothelin and nitric oxide in promoting endothelial cell migration and angiogenesis. Clin Exp Pharmacol Physiol 1999;26:269-271.

41. Matsunaga T, Warltier DC, Weihrauch DW, et al: Ischemia-induced coronary collateral growth is dependent on vascular endothelial growth factor and nitric oxide. Circulation 2000;102:3098-3103.

42. Ziche M, Morbidelli L: Nitric oxide and angiogenesis. J Neurooncol 2000;50:139-148.

43. Gendron RL: A plasticity for blood vessel remodeling is defined by pericyte coverage of the preformed endothelial network and is regulated by PDGF-B and VEGF. Surv Ophthalmol 1999;44:184-185.

44. Flamme I, Frolich T, Risau W: Molecular mechanisms of vasculogenesis and embryonic angiogenesis. J Cell Physiol 1997;173:206-210.

45. Risau W, Sariola H, Zerwes HG, et al: Vasculogenesis and angiogenesis in embryonic-stem-cell–derived embryoid bodies. Development 1988;102:471-478.

46. Nicosia RF, Villaschi S: Autoregulation of angiogenesis by cells of the vessel wall. Int Rev Cytol 1999;185:1-43.

47. Asahara T, Murohara T, Sullivan A, et al: Isolation of putative progenitor endothelial cells for angiogenesis. Science 1997;275:965-967.

48. Asahara T, Masuda H, Takahashi T, et al: Bone marrow origin of endothelial progenitor cells responsible for postnatal vasculogenesis in physiological and pathological neovascularization. Circ Res 1999;85:221-228.

49. Asahara T, Bauthers C, Zheng LP: Synergistic effect of vascular endothelial growth factor and basic fibroblast growth factor on angiogenesis in vivo. Circulation 1995;92(Suppl):II365-371.

50. Fleisch M, Billinger M, Eberli FR, et al: Physiologically assessed coronary collateral flow and intracoronary growth factor concentrations in patients with 1- to 3-vessel coronary artery disease. Circulation 1999;100:1945-1950.

51. Sasayama S, Fujita M: Recent insights into coronary collateral circulation. Circulation 1992;85:1197-1204.

52. Charney R, Cohen M: The role of the coronary collateral circulation in limiting myocardial ischemia and infarct size. Circulation 1993;126:937-945.

53. Ito W, Arras M, Scholz D: Angiogenesis but not collateral growth is associated with ischemia after femoral artery occlusion. Am J Physiol 1997;273:H2155-H2165.

54. Jones MK, Wang H, Peskar BM: Inhibition of angiogenesis by non-steroidal anti-inflammatory drugs: Insight into mechanisms and implications for cancer growth and ulcer healing. Nat Med 1999;5:1418-1423.

55. Cohen M, Rentrop KP: Limitations of myocardial ischemia by collateral circulation during sudden controlled coronary artery occlusion in human subjects: A prospective study. Circulation 1986;74:469.

56. Marcus ML, Chilian WM, Kanatsuka H, et al: Understanding the coronary circulation through studies at the microvascular level. Circulation 1990;82:1-7.

57. Schaper W: Control of coronary angiogenesis. Eur Heart J 1995;16(Suppl C):66-68.

58. Langille BL: Arterial remodeling: Relation to hemodynamics. Can J Physiol Pharmacol 1996;74:834-841.

59. Gloe T, Sohn HY, Meininger GA, Pohl U: Shear-stress induced release of bFGF from endothelial cells is mediated by matrix interaction via integrin alpha V beta 3. J Biol Chem 2002;277:23453-23458.

60. Ballermann BJ, Daardik A, Eng E, Liu A: Shear stress and the endothelium. Kidney Int 1998;67(Suppl):S100-108.

61. Deindl E, Buschmann I, Hoefer IE, et al: Role of ischemia and of hypoxia-inducible genes in arteriogenesis after femoral artery occlusion in the rabbit. Circ Res 2001;89:779-786.

62. Folkman J, Merier E, Abernathy C, Williams G: Isolation of a tumor factor responsible for angiogenesis. J Exp Med 1971;133:275-288.

63. Burgess WH, Maciag T: The heparin-binding (fibroblast) growth factor family of proteins. Ann Rev Biochem 1989;58:575-606.

64. Shing Y, Folkman J, Sullivan R, et al: Heparin affinity: Purification of a tumor-derived capillary endothelial cell growth factor. Science 1984;223:1296-1299.

65. Shing Y, Folkman J, Haudenschild C, et al: Angiogenesis is stimulated by a tumor-derived endothelial cell growth factor. J Cell Biochem 1985;29:275-287.

66. Gerwins P, Skoldenberg E, Claesson-Welsh L: Function of fibroblast growth factors and vascular endothelial growth factors and their receptors in angiogenesis. Crit Rev Oncol Hematol 2000;34:185-194.

67. Smallwood PM, Munoz-Sanjuan I, Tong P, et al: Fibroblast growth factor (FGF) homologous factors: New members of the FGF family implicated in nervous system development. Proc Natl Acad Sci U S A 1996;93:9850-9857.

68. Yayon A, Klagsbrun M, Esko J, et al: Cell surface heparin-like molecules required for binding of basic fibroblast growth factor to its high affinity receptor. Cell 1991;64:841-848.

69. Moscatelli D: Metabolism of receptor-bound and matrix-bound basic fibroblast growth by bovine capillary endothelial cells. J Cell Biol 1988;107:753-759.

70. Brown KJ, Hendry IA, Parish CR: Acidic and basic fibroblast growth factor bind with differing affinity to the same heparan sulfate proteoglycan on BALB/c3T3 cells: Implications for potentiation of growth factor action by heparin. J Cell Biochem 1995;58:6-14.

71. Slavin J: Fibroblast growth factors: At the heart of angiogenesis. Cell Biol Int 1995;19:431-418.

72. Sellke FW, Laham RJ, Edelman ER, et al: Therapeutic angiogenesis with basic fibroblast growth factor: Technique and early results. Ann Thorac Surg 1998;65:1540-1544.

73. Miller DL, Ortega S, Bashayan O, et al: Compensation by fibroblast growth factor 1 (FGF1) does not account for the mild phenotypic defects observed in FGF2 null mice. Mol Cell Biol 2000;20:2260-2268.

74. Dono R, Texido G, Dussel R, et al: Impaired cerebral cortex development and blood pressure regulation in FGF-2-deficient mice. EMBO J 1998;17:4213-4225.

75. Ortega S, Ittmann M, Tsang SH, et al: Neuronal defects and delayed wound healing in mice lacking fibroblast growth factor 2. Proc Natl Acad Sci U S A 1998;95:5672-5677.

76. Zhou M, Sutliff RL, Paul RJ, et al: Fibroblast growth factor 2 control of vascular tone. Nat Med 1998;4:201-207.

77. Ferrera N, Henzel WJ: Pituitary follicular cells secrete a novel heparin-binding growth factor specific for vascular endothelial cells. Biochem Biophys Res Commun 1989;161:851-855.

78. Plouet J, Schilling J, Gospodarowicz D: Isolation and characterization of a newly identified endothelial cell mitogen produced by AtT-20 cells. EMBO J 1989;8:3801–3806.

79. Neufeld G, Cohen T, Gengrinovitch S, Poltorak Z: Vascular endothelial growth factor (VEGF) and its receptors. FASEB J 1999;13:9–22.

80. Tischer E, Mitchell R, Hartman T, et al: The human gene for vascular endothelial growth factor: Multiple protein forms are encoded through alternative exon splicing. J Biol Chem 1991;266: 11947–11954.

81. Keyt BA, Berleau LT, Nguyen HV, et al: The carboxyl-terminal domain (111-165) of vascular endothelial growth factor is critical for its mitogenic potency. J Biol Chem 1996;271:7788–7795.

82. Zachary I: Vascular endothelial growth factor. Int J Biochem Cell Biol 1998;30:1169–1174.

83. Ferrara N: Molecular and biological properties of vascular endothelial growth factor. J Mol Med 1999;77:527–543.

84. Robinson CJ, Stringer SE: The splice variants of vascular endothelial growth factor (VEGF) and their receptors. J Cell Sci 2001;114: 853–865.

85. Lei J, Jiang A, Pei D: Identification and characterization of a new splicing variant of vascular endothelial growth factor: VEGF183. Biochim Biophys Acta 1998;1443:400–406.

86. Jingjing L, Srinivasan B, Roque RS: Ectodomain shedding of VEGF183, a novel isoform of vascular endothelial growth factor, promotes its mitogenic activity in vitro. Angiogenesis 2001;4: 103–112.

87. Veikkola T, Alitalo K: VEGFs, receptors and angiogenesis. Semin Cancer Biol 1999;9:211–220.

88. Olofsson B, Pajusola K, Kaipainen A, et al: Vascular endothelial growth factor B, a novel growth factor for endothelial cells. Proc Natl Acad Sci U S A 1996;93:2576–2581.

89. Taipale J, Makinen T, Arighi E, et al: Vascular endothelial growth factor receptor-3. Curr Top Microbiol Immunol 1999;237:85–96.

90. Joukov V, Pajusola K, Kaipainen A, et al: A novel vascular endothelial growth factor, VEGF-C, is a ligand for the Flt4 (VEGFR-3) and KDR (VEGFR-2) receptor tyrosine kinases. EMBO J 1996;15: 290–298.

91. Kukk E, Lymboussaki A, Taira S, et al: VEGF-C receptor binding and pattern of expression with VEGFR-3 suggest a role in lymphatic vascular development. Development 1996;122:3829–3837.

92. Kaipainen A, Korhonen J, Mustonen T, et al: Expression of the fms-like tyrosine kinase 4 gene becomes restricted to lymphatic endothelium during development. Proc Natl Acad Sci U S A 1995;92:3566–3570.

93. Lymboussaki A, Partanen TA, Olofsson B, et al: Expression of the vascular endothelial growth factor C receptor VEGFR-3 in lymphatic endothelium of the skin and in vascular tumors. Am J Pathol 1998;153:395–403.

94. Achen MG, Jeltsch M, Kukk E, et al: Vascular endothelial growth factor D (VEGF-D) is a ligand for the tyrosine kinases VEGF receptor 2 (Flk1) and VEGF receptor 3 (Flt4). Proc Natl Acad Sci U S A 1998;95:548–553.

95. Avantaggiato V, Orlandini M, Acampora D, et al: Embryonic expression pattern of the murine figf gene, a growth factor belonging to platelet-derived growth factor/vascular endothelial growth factor family. Mech Dev 1998;73:221–224.

96. Ogawa S, Oku A, Sawano A, et al: A novel type of vascular endothelial growth factor: VEGF-E (NZ-7 VEGF) preferentially utilizes KDR/Flk-1 receptor and carries a potent mitotic activity without heparin binding domain. J Biol Chem 1998;273:31273–31282.

97. Wise LM, Veikkola T, Mercer AA, et al: Vascular endothelial growth factor (VEGF)-like protein from orf virus NZ2 binds to VEGFR2 and neuropilin-1. Proc Natl Acad Sci U S A 1999;96:3071–3076.

98. Soker S, Takashima S, Miao HQ, et al: Neuropilin-1 is expressed by endothelial and tumor cells as an isoform specific receptor for vascular endothelial growth factor. Cell 1998;92:735–745.

99. Whitaker GB, Limberg BJ, Rosenbaum JS: VEGFR-2 and neuropilin-1 form a receptor complex that is responsible for the differential signaling potency of VEGF$_{165}$ and VEGF$_{121}$. J Biol Chem 2001; 25520–25531.

100. Gluzman-Poltorak Z, Cohen T, Herzog Y, Neufeld G: Neuropilin-2 and neuropilin-1 are receptors for 165-amino acid long form of vascular endothelial growth factor (VEGF) and of placenta growth factor-2, but only neuropilin-2 functions as a receptor for the 145 amino acid form of VEGF. J Biol Chem 2000;275: 18040–18045.

101. Migdal M, Huppertz B, Tessler S, et al: Neuropilin-1 is a placenta growth factor-2 receptor. J Biol Chem 1998;273:22272–22278.

102. Makinen T, Olofsson B, Karpanen T, et al: Differential binding of vascular endothelial growth factor B splice and proteolytic isoforms to neuropilin-1. J Biol Chem 1999;274:21217–21222.

103. Forsythe JA, Jiang BH, Iyer NV, et al: Activation of vascular endothelial growth factor gene transcription by hypoxia-inducible factor 1. Mol Cell Biol 1996;16:4604–4613.

104. Dor Y, Keshet E: Ischemia driven angiogenesis. Trends Cardiovasc Med 1997;7:289–294.

105. Levy AP, Levy NS, Goldberg MA: Post-transcriptional regulation of vascular endothelial growth factor by hypoxia. J Biol Chem 1996;271:2746–2753.

106. Levy NS, Chung S, Furneaux H, Levy AP: Hypoxic stabilization of vascular endothelial growth factor mRNA by the RNA-binding protein HuR. J Biol Chem 1998;273:6417–6423.

107. Levy AP, Levy NS, Wegner S, Goldberg MA: Transcriptional regulation of the rat endothelial growth factor gene by hypoxia. J Biol Chem 1995;270:13333–13340.

108. Waltenberger J, Maayr U, Pentz S, Hombach V: Functional upregulation of the vascular endothelial growth receptor KDR by hypoxia. Circulation 1996;94:1647–1654.

109. Li J, Brown LF, Hibberd MG, et al: VEGF, flk-1, flt-1 expression in a rat myocardial infarction model of angiogenesis. Am J Physiol 1996;270:H1803–H1811.

110. Alon T, Hemo I, Itin A, et al: Vascular endothelial growth factor acts as a survival factor for newly formed retinal vessels and has implications for retinopathy of prematurity. Nat Med 1995;1: 1024–1028.

111. Gerber HP, Dixit V, Ferrara N: Vascular endothelial growth factor induces expression of the antiapoptotic proteins Bcl-2 and A1 in vascular endothelial cells. J Biol Chem 1998;273: 13313–13316.

112. Nor JE, Christensen J, Mooney DJ, Polverini PJ: Vascular endothelial growth factor (VEGF)-mediated angiogenesis is associated with enhanced endothelial cell survival and induction of Bcl-2 expression. Am J Pathol 1999;154:375–384.

113. Tran J, Rak J, Sheehan C, et al: Marked induction of the IAP family antiapoptotic proteins survivin and XIAP by VEGF in vascular endothelial cells. Biochem Biophys Res Commun 1999;264: 781–788.

114. Gerber HP, McMurtrey A, Kowalski J, et al: Vascular endothelial growth factor regulates endothelial cell survival through the phosphatidylinositol 3′-kinase/Akt signal transduction pathway: Requirement for Flk-1/KDR activation. J Biol Chem 1998;273: 30336–30343.

115. Dimmeler S, Fleming I, Fisslthaler B, et al: Activation of nitric oxide synthase in endothelial cells by Akt-dependent phosphorylation. Nature 1999;399:601–605.

116. Fulton D, Gratton JP, McCabe TJ, et al: Regulation of endothelium-derived nitric oxide production by the protein kinase Akt. Nature 1991;399:597–601.

117. Papapetropoulos A, Fulton D, Mahboubi K, et al: Angiopoeitin-1 inhibits endothelial cell apoptosis via the Akt/survivin pathway. J Biol Chem 2000;275:9102–9105.

118. Gratton JP, Morales-Ruiz M, Kureishi Y, et al: Akt down-regulation of p38 signaling provides a novel mechanism of vascular endothelial growth factor–mediated cytoprotection in endothelial cells. J Biol Chem 2001;276:30359–30365.

119. Benjamin LE, Keshet E: Conditional switching of vascular endothelial growth factor (VEGF) expression in tumors: Induction of endothelial cell shedding and regression of hemangioblastoma-like vessels by VEGF withdrawal. Proc Natl Acad Sci U S A 1997;94:8761–8766.

120. Benjamin LE, Golijanin D, Itin A, et al: Selective ablation of immature blood vessels in established human tumors follows vascular endothelial growth factor withdrawal. J Clin Invest 1999;103: 159–165.

121. Jain RK, Safabakhsh N, Sckell A, et al: Endothelial cell death, angiogenesis, and microvascular function after castration in an androgen-dependent tumor: Role of vascular endothelial growth factor. Proc Natl Acad Sci U S A 1998;95:10820–10825.

122. Shaheen RM, Davis DW, Liu W, et al: Antiangiogenic therapy targeting the tyrosine kinase receptor for vascular endothelial growth factor receptor inhibits the growth of colon cancer liver metastasis and induces tumor and endothelial cell apoptosis. Cancer Res 1999;59:5412–5416.

123. Waltenberger J, Claesson-Welsh L, Siegbahn A, et al: Different signal transduction properties of KDR and Flt1, two receptors for vascular endothelial growth factor. J Biol Chem 1994;269:26988–26995.

124. Fong GH, Rossant J, Gertsenstein M, Breitman ML: Role of the Flt-1 receptor tyrosine kinase in regulating the assembly of vascular endothelium. Nature 1995;376:66–70.

125. Fong GH, Klingensmith J, Wood CR, et al: Regulation of flt-1 expression during mouse embryogenesis suggests a role in the establishment of vascular endothelium. Dev Dyn 1996;207:1–10.

126. Jeltsch M, Kaipainen A, Joukov V, et al: Hyperplasia of lymphatic vessels in VEGF-C transgenic mice. Science 1997;276:1423–1425.

127. Shalaby F, Rossant J, Yamaguchi TP, et al: Failure of blood-island formation and vasculogenesis in Flk-1-deficient mice. Nature 1995;376:62–66.

128. Shweiki D, Itin A, Neufeld G, et al: Patterns of expression of vascular endothelial growth factor (VEGF) and VEGF receptors in mice suggest a role in hormonally regulated angiogenesis. J Clin Invest 1993;91:2235–2243.

129. Inoue M, Itoh H, Ueda M, et al: Vascular endothelial growth factor (VEGF) expression in human coronary atherosclerotic lesions: Possible pathophysiological significance of VEGF in progression of atherosclerosis. Circulation 1998;98:2108–2116.

130. Isner JM, Pieczek A, Schainfield R: Clinical evidence of angiogenesis following arterial gene transfer of phVEGF165. Lancet 1996;348:370–374.

131. Sugihara T, Wadhwa R, Kaul SC, Mitsui Y: A novel alternatively spliced form of murine vascular endothelial growth factor, VEGF 155. J Biol Chem 1998;273:3033–3038.

132. Carmeliet P, Ferreira V, Breier G, et al: Abnormal blood vessel development and lethality in embryos lacking a single VEGF allele. Nature 1996;380:435–439.

133. Ferrara N, Carver-Moore K, Chen H, et al: Heterozygous embryonic lethality induced by targeted inactivation of the VEGF gene. Nature 1996;380:439–442.

134. Nagy A, Rossant J: Chimaeras and mosaics for dissecting complex mutant phenotypes. Int J Dev Biol 2001;45:577–582.

135. Drake CJ, Little CD: Exogenous vascular endothelial growth factor induces malformed and hyperfused vessels during embryonic neovascularization. Proc Natl Acad Sci U S A 1995;92:7657–7661.

136. Feucht M, Christ B, Wilting J: VEGF induces cardiovascular malformation and embryonic lethality. Am J Pathol 1997;151:1407–1416.

137. Flamme I, von Reutern M, Drexler HC, et al: Overexpression of vascular endothelial growth factor in the avian embryo induces hypervascularization and increased vascular permeability without alterations of embryonic pattern formation. Dev Biol 1995;171:399–414.

138. Miquerol L, Langille BL, Nagy A: Embryonic development is disrupted by modest increases in vascular endothelial growth factor gene expression. Development 2000;127:3941–3946.

139. Carmeliet P, Ng YS, Nuyens D, et al: Impaired myocardial angiogenesis and ischemic cardiomyopathy in mice lacking the vascular endothelial growth factor isoforms VEGF164 and VEGF188. Nat Med 1999;5:495–502.

140. Stalmans I, Ng Y-S, Rohan R, et al: Arteriolar and venular patterning in retinas of mice selectively expressing VEGF isoforms. J Clin Invest 2002;109:327–336.

141. Bellomo D, Headrick JP, Silins GU, et al: Mice lacking the vascular endothelial growth factor-B gene (Vegfb) have smaller hearts, dysfunctional coronary vasculature, and impaired recovery from cardiac ischemia. Circ Res 2000;86:E29–35.

142. Shalaby F, Rossant J, Yamaguchi TP, et al: Failure of blood island formation and vasculogenesis in Flk-1-deficient mice. Nature 1995;376:62–66.

143. Schuh AC, Faloon P, Hu Q-L, et al: In vitro hematopoietic and endothelial potential of flk-1−/− embryonic stem cells and embryos. Proc Natl Acad Sci U S A 1999;96:2159–2164.

144. Hidaka M, Stanford WL, Bernstein A: Conditional requirement for the Flk-1 receptor in the in vitro generation of early hematopoietic cells. Proc Natl Acad Sci U S A 1999;96:7370–7375.

145. Fong G-H, Zhang L, Bryce D-M, Peng J: Increased hemangioblast commitment, not vascular disorganization, is the primary defect in flt-1 knock-out mice. Development 1999;126:3015–3025.

146. Hiratsuka S, Minowa O, Kuno J, et al: Flt-1 lacking the tyrosine kinase domain is sufficient for normal development and angiogenesis in mice. Proc Natl Acad Sci U S A 1998;95:9349–9354.

147. Dumont D, Jussila L, Taipale J, et al: Cardiovascular failure in mouse embryos deficient in VEGF receptor-3. Science 1998;282:946–949.

148. Kitsukawa T, Shimizu M, Sanbo M, et al: Neuropilin-semphorin III/D-mediated chemorepulsive signals play a crucial role in peripheral nerve projection in mice. Neuron 1997;19:995–1005.

149. Takashima S, Kitakaze M, Asakura M, et al: Targeting of both mouse neuropilin-1 and neuropilin-2 genes severely impairs developmental yolk sac and embryonic angiogenesis. Proc Natl Acad Sci U S A 2002;99:3657–3662.

150. Davis S, Aldrich TH, Jones PF, et al: Isolation of angiopoietin-1, a ligand for the Tie2 receptor by secretion-trap expression cloning. Cell 1996;87:1161–1169.

151. Suri C, Jones PF, Patan S, et al: Requisite role of angiopoietin-1, a ligand for the Tie2 receptor, during embryonic angiogenesis. Cell 1996;87:1171–1180.

152. Kwak HJ, So JN, Lee SJ, et al: Angiopoietin-1 is an apoptosis survival factor for endothelial cells. FEBS Lett 1999;448:249–253.

153. Hayes AJ, Huang WQ, Mallah J, et al: Angiopoietin-1 and its receptor Tie-2 participate in the regulation of capillary-like tubule formation and survival of endothelial cells. Microvasc Res 1999;58:224–237.

154. Witzenbichler B, Maisonpierre PC, Jones P, et al: Chemotactic properties of angiopoietin-1 and -2 ligands for the endothelial-specific receptor tyrosine kinase Tie2. J Biol Chem 1998;273:18514–18521.

155. Fujikawa K, de Aos Scherpenseel I, Jain SK, et al: Role of PI 3-kinase in angiopoietin-1-mediated migration and attachment-dependent survival of endothelial cells. Exp Cell Res 1999;253:663–672.

156. Kim I, Kim HG, So JN, et al: Angiopoietin-1 regulates endothelial cell survival through the phosphatidylinositol 3′-kinase/Akt signal transduction pathway. Circ Res 2000;86:24–29.

157. Davis S, Yancopoulos GD: The angiopoietins: Yin and yang in angiogenesis. Curr Top Microbiol Immunol 1999;237:173–185.

158. Thurston G, Suri C, Smith K, et al: Leakage-resistant blood vessels in mice transgenically overexpressing angiopoietin-1. Science 1999;286:2511–2514.

159. Thurston G, Rudge JS, Ioff E, et al: Angiopoietin-1 protects the adult vasculature against plasma leakage. Nat Med 2000;6:460–463.

160. Hanahan D: Signaling vascular morphogenesis and maintenance. Science 1997;277:48–50.

161. Baumgartner I, Rauh G, Pieczek A, et al: Lower-extremity edema associated with gene transfer of naked DNA vascular endothelial growth factor. Ann Intern Med 2000;132:880–884.

162. Kim I, Kwak HJ, Ahn JE, et al: Molecular cloning and characterization of a novel angiopoietin family protein, angiopoietin-3. FEBS Lett 1999;443:353–356.

163. Valenzuela DM, Griffiths J, Rojas J, et al: Angiopoietins 3 and 4: Diverging gene counterparts in mice and humans. Proc Natl Acad Sci U S A 1999;96:1904–1909.

164. Nishimura M, Miki T, Yashima R, et al: Angiopoietin-3, a novel member of the angiopoietin family. FEBS Lett 1999;448:254–256.

165. Thurston G, Suri C, Smith K, et al: Leakage-resistant blood vessels in mice transgenically overexpressing angiopoietin-1. Science 1999;286:2511–2514.

166. Mandriota SJ, Pepper MS: Regulation of angiopoietin-2 mRNA levels in bovine microvascular endothelial cells by cytokines and hypoxia. Circ Res 1998;83:852–859.

167. Enholm B, Paavonen K, Ristimaki A, et al: Comparison of VEGF, VEGF-B, VEGF-C and Ang-1 mRNA regulation by serum, growth factors, oncoproteins and hypoxia. Oncogene 1997;14:2475–2483.

168. Oh H, Takagi H, Suzuma K, et al: Hypoxia and vascular endothelial growth factor selectively up-regulate angiopoietin-2 in bovine microvascular endothelial cells. J Biol Chem 1999;274:15732–15739.

169. Asahara T, Chen D, Takahashi T, et al: Tie2 receptor ligands, angiopoietin-1 and angiopoietin-2 modulate VEGF-induced postnatal neovascularization. Circ Res 1998;83:233–240.

170. Teichert-Kuliszewska K, Maisonpierre PC, Jones N, et al: Biological action of angiopoietin-2 in a fibrin matrix model of angiogenesis is associated with activation of Tie2. Cardiovasc Res 2001;49:659–670.

171. Kim I, Kim JH, Moon SO, et al: Angiopoietin-2 at high concentration can enhance endothelial cell survival through the

phosphatidylinositol 3'-kinase/Akt signal transduction pathway. Oncogene 2000;19:4549–4552.

172. Lobov IB, Brooks PC, Lang RA: From the cover: Angiopoietin-2 displays VEGF-dependent modulation of capillary structure and endothelial cell survival in vivo. Proc Natl Acad Sci U S A 2002;99:11205–11210.

173. Dumont DJ, Gradwohl G, Fong GH, et al: Dominant-negative and targeted null mutations in the endothelial receptor tyrosine kinase, tek, reveal a critical role in vasculogenesis of the embryo. Genes Dev 1994;8:1897–1909.

174. Sato TN, Tozawa Y, Deutsch U, et al: Distinct roles of the receptor tyrosine kinases Tie-1 and Tie-2 in blood vessel formation. Nature 1995;376:70–74.

175. Puri MC, Rossand J, Alitalo K, et al: The receptor tyrosine kinase TIE is required for the integrity and survival of vascular endothelial cells. EMBO J 1995;376:70–74.

176. Maisonpierre PC, Suri C, Jones PF, et al: Angiopoietin-2, a natural antagonist for Tie2 that disrupts in vivo angiogenesis. Science 1997;277:55–60.

177. Murohara T, Witzenbichler B, Spyridopoulos I, et al: Role of endothelial nitric oxide synthase in endothelial cell migration. Arterioscler Thromb Vasc Biol 1999;19:1156–1161.

178. Goliogorsky MS, Budzikowski AS, Tsukahara H, Noiri E: Co-operation between endothelin and nitric oxide in promoting endothelial cell migration and angiogenesis. Clin Exp Pharmacol Physiol 1999;26:269–271.

179. Hood JD, Meininger CJ, Ziche M, Granger HJ: VEGF upregulates ecNOS message, protein, and NO production in human endothelial cells. Am J Physiol 1998;274(3 Pt 2):H1054–H1058.

180. Ziche M, Morbidelli L, Masini E, et al: Nitric oxide mediates angiogenesis in vivo and endothelial cell growth and migration in vitro promoted by substance P. Clin Invest 1994;94:2036–2044.

181. Morbidelli L, Chang CH, Douglas JG, et al: Nitric oxide mediates mitogenic effect of VEGF on coronary venular endothelium. Am J Physiol 1996;270(1 Pt 2):H411–H415.

182. Kostyk SK, Kourembanas S, Wheeler EL, et al: Basic fibroblast growth factor increases nitric oxide synthase production in bovine endothelial cells. Am J Physiol 1995;269:H1583–H1589.

183. Inoue N, Venema RC, Sayegh HS, et al: Molecular regulation of the bovine endothelial cell nitric oxide synthase by transforming growth factor–beta 1. Arterioscler Thromb Vasc Biol 1995;15:1255–1261.

184. Kroll J, Waltenberger J: VEGF-A induces expression of eNOS and iNOS in endothelial cells via VEGF receptor-2 (KDR). Biochem Biophys Res Commun 1998;252:743–746.

185. Kroll J, Waltenberger J: A novel function of VEGF receptor-2 (KDR): Rapid release of nitric oxide in response to VEGF-A stimulation in endothelial cells. Biochem Biophys Res Commun 1999;65:636–639.

186. Shizukuda Y, Tang S, Yokota R, Ware JA: Vascular endothelial growth factor–induced endothelial cell migration and proliferation depend on a nitric oxide–mediated decrease in protein kinase C delta activity. Circ Res 1999;5:247–256.

187. Ziche M, Morbidelli L, Choudhuri R, et al: Nitric oxide synthase lies downstream from vascular endothelial growth factor–induced but not basic fibroblast growth factor–induced angiogenesis. J Clin Invest 1997;99:2625–2634.

188. Lee PC, Salyapongse AN, Bragdon GA, et al: Impaired wound healing and angiogenesis in eNOS-deficient mice. Am J Physiol 1999;277:H1600–H1608.

189. Mashimo H, Goyal RK: Lessons from genetically engineered animal models: IV. Nitric oxide synthase gene knockout mice. Am J Physiol 1999;277:G745–G750.

190. Lee TC, Zhao YD, Courtman DW, Stewart DJ: Abnormal aortic valve development in mice lacking endothelial nitric oxide synthase. Circulation 2000;101:2345–2348.

191. Hefler LA, Reyes CA, O'Brien WE, Gregg AR: Perinatal development of endothelial nitric oxide synthase-deficient mice. Biol Reprod 2001;64:666–673.

192. Li H, Forestermann U: Nitric oxide in the pathogenesis of vascular disease. Am J Pathol 2000;190:244–254.

193. Van Belle E, Rivard A, Chen D, et al: Hypercholesterolemia attenuates angiogenesis but does not preclude augmentation by angiogenic cytokines. Circulation 1997;96:2667–2674.

194. Rivard A, Fabre JE, Silver M, et al: Age-dependent impairment of angiogenesis. Circulation 1999;99:111–120.

195. Brouet A, Sonveaux P, Dessy C, et al: Hsp90 and caveolin are key targets for the proangiogenic nitric oxide–mediated effects of statins. Circ Res 2001;89:866–873.

196. Silvestre JS, Bergaya S, Tamarat R, et al: Proangiogenic effect of angiotensin-converting enzyme inhibition is mediated by the bradykinin B(2) receptor pathway. Circ Res 2001;89:678–683.

197. Fabre JE, Rivard A, Magner M, et al: Tissue inhibition of angiotensin-converting enzyme activity stimulates angiogenesis in vivo. Circulation 1999;99:3043–3049.

198. Volpert OV, Ward WF, Lingen MW, et al: Captopril inhibits angiogenesis and slows the growth of experimental tumors in rats. J Clin Invest 1996;98:671–679.

199. Auerbach R, Auerbach W, Polakowski I: Assays for angiogenesis: A review. Pharmacol Ther 1991;51:1–11.

200. Baffour R, Berman J, Garb JL, et al: Enhanced angiogenesis and growth of collaterals by in vivo administration of recombinant basic fibroblast growth factor in a rabbit model of acute lower limb ischemia: Dose-response effect of basic fibroblast growth factor. J Vasc Surg 1992;16:181–191.

201. Pu LQ, Sniderman AD, Brassard R, et al: Enhanced revascularization of the ischemic limb by angiogenic therapy. Circulation 1993;88:208–215.

202. Yanagisawa-Miwa A, Uchida Y, Nakamura F, et al: Salvage of infarcted myocardium by angiogenic action of basic fibroblast growth factor. Science 1992;257:1401–1403.

203. Levy AP, Tamargo R, Brem H, Nathans D: An endothelial cell growth factor from the mouse neuroblastoma cell line NB41. Growth Factors 1989;2:9–19.

204. Connolly DT, Heuvelman DM, Nelson R, et al: Tumor vascular permeability factor stimulates endothelial cell growth and angiogenesis. J Clin Invest 1989;84:1470–1478.

205. Leung DW, Cachianes G, Kuang WJ, et al: Vascular endothelial growth factor is a secreted angiogenic mitogen. Science 1989;246:1306–1309.

206. Takeshita S, Zheng LP, Brogi E, et al: Therapeutic angiogenesis: A single intraarterial bolus of vascular endothelial growth factor augments revascularization in a rabbit ischemic hind limb model. J Clin Invest 1994;93:662–670.

207. Takeshita S, Pu LQ, Stein LA, et al: Intramuscular administration of vascular endothelial growth factor induces dose-dependent collateral artery augmentation in a rabbit model of chronic limb ischemia. Circulation 1994;90:II228–II234.

208. Banai S, Jaklitsch MT, Shou M, et al: Angiogenic-induced enhancement of collateral blood flow to ischemic myocardium by vascular endothelial growth factor in dogs. Circulation 1994;89:2183–2189.

209. Unger EF, Banai S, Shou M, et al: Basic fibroblast growth factor enhances myocardial collateral flow in a canine model. Am J Physiol 1994;266:H1588–H1595.

210. Hariawala MD, Horowitz JR, Esakof D, et al: VEGF improves myocardial blood flow but produces EDRF-mediated hypotension in porcine hearts. J Surg Res 1996;63:77–82.

211. Pearlman JD, Hibberd MG, Chuang ML, et al: Magnetic resonance mapping demonstrates benefits of VEGF-induced myocardial angiogenesis. Nat Med 1995;1:1085–1089.

212. Sellke FW, Li J, Stamler A, et al: Angiogenesis induced by acidic fibroblast growth factor as an alternative method of revascularization for chronic myocardial ischemia. Surgery 1996;120:182–188.

213. Harada K, Grossman W, Friedman M, et al: Basic fibroblast growth factor improves myocardial function in chronically ischemic porcine hearts. J Clin Invest 1994;94:623–630.

214. Sellke FW, Wang SY, Friedman M, et al: Basic FGF enhances endothelium-dependent relaxation of the collateral-perfused coronary microcirculation. Am J Physiol 1994;267:H1303–H1311.

215. Harada K, Friedman M, Lopez JJ, et al: Vascular endothelial growth factor administration in chronic myocardial ischemia. Am J Physiol 1996;270:H1791–H1802.

216. Lopez JJ, Edelman ER, Stamler A, et al: Basic fibroblast growth factor in a porcine model of chronic myocardial ischemia: A comparison of angiographic, echocardiographic and coronary flow parameters. J Pharmacol Exp Ther 1997;282:385–390.

217. Lopez JJ, Edelman ER, Stamler A, et al: Angiogenic potential of perivascularly delivered aFGF in a porcine model of chronic myocardial ischemia. Am J Physiol 1998;274:H930–H936.

218. Shou M, Thirumurti V, Rajanayagam S, et al: Effect of basic fibroblast growth factor on myocardial angiogenesis in dogs with mature collateral vessels. J Am Coll Cardiol 1997;29:1102–1106.

219. Lazarous DF, Shou M, Stiber JA, et al: Adenoviral-mediated gene transfer induces sustained pericardial VEGF expression in dogs: Effect on myocardial angiogenesis. Cardiovasc Res 1999;44:294–302.

220. Baumgartner I, Pieczek A, Manor O, et al: Constitutive expression of phVEGF165 after intramuscular gene transfer promotes collateral vessel development in patients with critical limb ischemia. Circulation 1998;97:1114–1123.

221. Lazarous DF, Unger EF, Epstein SE, et al: Basic fibroblast growth factor in patients with intermittent claudication: Results of a phase I trial. J Am Coll Cardiol 2000;36:1239–1244.

222. Schumacher B, Pecher P, von Specht BU, Stegmann T: Induction of neoangiogenesis in ischemic myocardium by human growth factors: First clinical results of a new treatment for coronary heart disease. Circulation 1998;97:645–650.

223. Pecher P, Schumacher BA: Angiogenesis in ischemic human myocardium: Clinical results after 3 years. Ann Thorac Surg 2000;69:1414–1419.

224. Laham RJ, Sellke FW, Edelman ER, et al: Local perivascular delivery of basic fibroblast growth factor in patients undergoing coronary bypass surgery: Results of a phase I randomized, double-blind, placebo-controlled trial. Circulation 1999;100:1865–1871.

225. Unger EF, Goncalves L, Epstein SE, et al: Effects of a single intracoronary injection of basic fibroblast growth factor in stable angina pectoris. Am J Cardiol 2000;85:1414–1419.

226. Udelson JE, Dilsizian V, Laham RJ, et al: Therapeutic angiogenesis with recombinant fibroblast growth factor-2 improves stress and rest myocardial perfusion abnormalities in patients with severe symptomatic chronic coronary artery disease. Circulation 2000;102:1605–1610.

227. Laham RJ, Chronos NA, Leimbach M, et al: Results of a phase I open label dose escalation study of intracoronary and intravenous basic fibroblast growth factor (rFGF-2) in patients (pts) with severe ischemic heart disease: 6 months follow-up [abstract]. J Am Coll Cardiol 2000;35(Suppl A):73.

228. Henry TD, Rocha-Singh K, Isner JM, et al: Results of intracoronary recombinant human vascular endothelial growth factor (rhVEGF) administration trial [abstract]. J Am Coll Cardiol 1998;31(Suppl A):65A.

229. Hendel RC, Henry TD, Rocha-Singh K, et al: Effect of intracoronary recombinant human vascular endothelial growth factor on myocardial perfusion: Evidence for a dose-dependent effect. Circulation 2000;101:118–121.

230. Losordo DW, Vale PR, Symes JF, et al: Gene therapy for myocardial angiogenesis: Initial clinical results with direct myocardial injection of phVEGF165 as sole therapy for myocardial ischemia. Circulation 1998;98:2800–2804.

231. Symes JF, Losordo DW, Vale PR, et al: Gene therapy with vascular endothelial growth factor for inoperable coronary artery disease. Ann Thorac Surg 1999;68:830–836.

232. Vale PR, Symes JF, Esakof DD, et al: Direct myocardial gene transfer of VEGF165 in patients with end-stage coronary artery disease: 12-month results of a phase I/II clinical trial [abstract]. J Am Coll Cardiol 2001;37(Suppl A):285A.

233. Rosengart TK, Lee LY, Patel SR, et al: Six-month assessment of a phase I trial of angiogenic gene therapy for the treatment of coronary artery disease using direct intramyocardial administration of an adenovirus vector expressing the VEGF121 cDNA. Ann Surg 1999;230:466–470.

234. Rosengart TK, Lee LY, Patel SR, et al: Angiogenesis gene therapy: Phase I assessment of direct intramyocardial administration of an adenovirus vector expressing VEGF121 cDNA to individuals with clinically significant severe coronary artery disease. Circulation 1999;100:468–474.

235. Hendel RC, Vale PR, Losordo DW, et al: The effects of VEGF-2 gene therapy on rest and stress myocardial perfusion: Results of serial SPECT imaging [abstract]. Circulation 2000;102 (Suppl):II-769.

236. Fortuin FD Jr, Vale P, Losordo DW, et al: Direct myocardial gene transfer of vascular endothelial growth factor-2 (VEGF-2) naked DNA via thoracotomy relieves angina pectoris and increases exercise time: One-year follow-up of a completed dose-escalating phase 1 study [abstract]. J Am Coll Cardiol 2001;37(Suppl A):285A–286A.

237. Vale PR, Losordo DW, Milliken CE, et al: Randomized, single-blind, placebo-controlled pilot study of catheter-based myocardial gene transfer for therapeutic angiogenesis using left ventricular electromechanical mapping in patients with chronic myocardial ischemia. Circulation 2001;103:2138–2143.

238. Losordo DW, Vale PR, Hendel RC, et al: Phase 1/2 placebo-controlled, double blind, dose-escalating trial of myocardial vascular endothelial growth factor 2 gene transfer by catheter delivery in patients with chronic myocardial ischemia. Circulation 2002;105:2012–2018.

239. Simons M, Annex BH, Laham RJ, et al: Pharmacological treatment of coronary artery disease with recombinant fibroblast growth factor-2: Double-blind, randomized, controlled clinical trial. Circulation 2002;105:788–793.

240. Henry TD, Annex B, Azrin M, et al: Double blind placebo controlled trial of recombinant human vascular endothelial growth factor, the VIVA Trial. J Am Coll Cardiol 2001;33:384A.

241. Grines CL, Watkins MW, Helmer G, et al: Angiogenic gene therapy (AGENT) trial in patients with stable angina pectoris. Circulation 2002;105:1291–1297.

242. Laham RJ, Rezaee M, Garcia L: Tissue and myocardial distribution of intracoronary, intravenous, intrapericardial and intramyocardial ^{124}I-labeled basic fibroblast growth factor (bFGF) favor intramyocardial delivery [abstract]. J Am Coll Cardiol 1999;35(Suppl A):10A.

243. Thurston G: Complementary actions of VEGF and angiopoietin-1 on blood vessel growth and leakage. J Anat 2002;200:575–580.

244. Semenza GL: HIF-1 and tumor progression: Pathophysiology and therapeutics. Trends Mol Med 2002;8(4 Suppl):S62–S67.

245. Jaquet K, Krause K, Tawakol-Khodai M, et al: Erythropoietin and VEGF exhibit equal angiogenic potential. Microvasc Res 2002;64:326.

246. Hidai C, Zupancic T, Penta K, et al: Cloning and characterization of developmental endothelial locus-1: An embryonic endothelial cell protein that binds the $\alpha_v\beta_3$ integrin receptor. Genes Dev 1998;12:21–33.

247. Rosengart TK, Patel SR, Crystal RG: Therapeutic angiogenesis: Protein and gene therapy delivery strategies. J Cardiovasc Risk 1999;6:29–40.

248. Simons M, Bonow RO, Chronos NA, et al: Clinical trials in coronary angiogenesis: issues, problems, consensus: An expert panel summary. Circulation 2000;102:E73–E86.

249. Laham RJ, Garcia L, Baim DS, et al: Therapeutic angiogenesis using basic fibroblast growth factor and vascular endothelial growth factor using various delivery strategies. Curr Interv Cardiol Rep 1999;1:228–233.

250. Laham RJ, Rezaee M, Post M, et al: Intracoronary and intravenous administration of basic fibroblast growth factor: Myocardial and tissue distribution. Drug Metab Dispos 1999;27:821–826.

251. Anderson ED, Mourich DV, Leong JA: Gene expression in rainbow trout (Oncorhynchus mykiss) following intramuscular injection of DNA. Mol Mar Biol Biotechnol 1996;5:105–113.

252. Tabata H, Silver M, Isner JM: Arterial gene transfer of acidic fibroblast growth factor for therapeutic angiogenesis in vivo: Critical role of secretion signal in use of naked DNA. Cardiovasc Res 1997;35:470–479.

253. Giordano FJ, Ping P, McKirnan MD, et al: Intracoronary gene transfer of fibroblast growth factor-5 increases blood flow and contractile function in an ischemic region of the heart. Nat Med 1996;2:534–539.

254. McElvaney NG: Is gene therapy in cystic fibrosis a realistic expectation? Curr Opin Pulm Med 1996;2:466–471.

255. Somia N, Verma IM: Gene therapy: Trials and tribulations. Nat Rev Genet 2000;1:91–99.

256. Myers J, Froelicher VF: Exercise testing: Procedures and implementation. Cardiol Clin 1993;11:199–213.

257. Hariawala M, Horowitz JR, Esakof D, et al: VEGF improves myocardial blood flow but produces EDRF-medicated hypotension in porcine hearts. J Surg Res 1996;63:77–82.

258. Horowitz JR, Rivard A, van der Zee R, et al: Vascular endothelial growth factor/vascular permeability factor produces nitric oxide–dependent hypotension. Arterioscler Thromb Vasc Biol 1997;17:2793–2800.

259. van der Zee R, Murohara T, Luo Z, et al: Vascular endothelial growth factor (VEGF) vascular permeability factor (VPF)

augments nitric oxide release from quiescent rabbit and human vascular endothelium. Circulation 1997;95:1030-1037.

260. Murohara T, Asahara T, Silveer M, et al: Nitric oxide synthase modulates angiogenesis in response to tissue ischemia. J Clin Invest 1998;101:2567-2578.

261. Lazarous DF, Unger EF, Epstein SE, et al: Basic fibroblast growth factor in patients with intermittent claudication: Results of a phase I trial. J Am Coll Cardiol 2000;36:1339-1344.

262. Isner JM, Vale PR, Symes JF, Losordo DW: Assessment of risks associated with cardiovascular gene therapy in human subjects. Circ Res 2001;89:389-400.

263. Springer ML, Chen AS, Kraft PE, et al: VEGF gene delivery to muscle: Potential role of vasculogenesis in adults. Mol Cell 1998;2:549-558.

264. Lee RJ, Springer ML, Blanco-Bose WE, et al: VEGF gene delivery to myocardium: Deleterious effects of unregulated expression. Circulation 2000;102:898-901.

265. Schwartz ER, Speakman MT, Patterson M, et al: Evaluation of the effects of intramyocardial injection of DNA expressing vascular endothelial growth factor (VEGF) in a myocardial infarction model in the rat—angiogenesis and angioma formation. J Am Coll Cardiol 2000;35:1323-1330.

266. Brown LF, Detmar M, Claffey K, et al: Vascular permeability factor/vascular endothelial growth factor: A multifunctional angiogenic cytokine. EXS 1997;79:233-269.

267. Masumura M, Murayama N, Inoue T, Ohno T: Selective induction of fibroblast growth factor-1 mRNA after transient focal ischemia in the cerebral cortex of rats. Neurosci Lett 1996;213:119-122.

268. Detmar M, Brown LF, Berse B, et al: Hypoxia regulates the expression of vascular permeability factor/vascular endothelial growth factor (VPF/VEGF) and its receptors in human skin. J Invest Dermatol 1997;108:263-268.

269. Takami K, Kiyota Y, Iwane M, et al: Upregulation of fibroblast growth factor–receptor messenger RNA expression in rat brain following transient forebrain ischemia. Exp Brain Res 1993;97:185-194.

270. Banai S, Jaklitsch MT, Casscells W, et al: Effects of acidic fibroblast growth factor on normal and ischemic myocardium. Circ Res 1991;69:76-85.

271. Okamoto N, Tobe T, Hackett SF, et al: Animal model: Transgenic mice with increased expression of vascular endothelial growth factor in the retina: A new model of intraretinal and subretinal neovascularization. Am J Pathol 1997;151:281-291.

272. Baffi J, Byrnes G, Chan CC, Csaky KG: Choroidal neovascularization in the rat induced by adenovirus mediated expression of vascular endothelial growth factor. Invest Opthamol Vis Sci 2000;41:3582-3589.

273. Aiello LP, Avery RL, Arrigg PG, et al: Vascular endothelial growth factor in ocular fluids of patients with diabetic retinopathy and other retinal disorders. N Engl J Med 1994;331:1480-1487.

274. Adamis AP, Miller JW, Bernal M-T, et al: Increased vascular endothelial growth factor levels in the vitreous of eyes with proliferative diabetic retinopathy. Am J Ophthalmol 1994;118:445-450.

275. Vale PR, Rauh G, Wuensch DI, et al: Influence of vascular endothelial growth factor on diabetic retinopathy [abstract]. Circulation 1998;17:I-353.

276. Herold-Mende C, Steiner HH, Andl T, et al: Expression and functional significance of vascular endothelial growth factor receptors in human tumor cells. Lab Invest 1999;79:1573-1582.

277. Celletti FL, Waugh JM, Amabile PG, et al: Vascular endothelial growth factor enhances atherosclerotic plaque progression. Nat Med 2001;7:425-429.

278. Moulton KS, Heller E, Konerding MA, et al: Angiogenesis inhibitors endostatin and TNP-470 reduce intimal neovascularization and plaque growth in apolipoprotein E-deficient mice. Circulation 1999;99:1726-1732.

279. Van Belle E, Maillard L, Tio FO, Isner JM: Accelerated endothelialization by local delivery of recombinant human vascular endothelial growth factor reduces in-stent intimal formation. Biochem Biophys Res Commun 1997;235:311-316.

280. Freedman SB, Isner JM: Therapeutic angiogenesis for coronary artery disease. Ann Intern Med 2002;136:54-71.

281. Hamaway AH, Lee LY, Crystal RG, Rosengart TK: Cardiac angiogenesis and gene therapy: A strategy for myocardial revascularization. Curr Opin Cardiol 1999;14:515-522.

282. Chen H, Chedotal A, He Z, et al: Neuropilin-2, a novel member of the neuropilin family, is a high affinity receptor for the semaphorins Sema E and Sema IV but not Sema III. Neuron 1997;19:547-559.

283. Veikkola T, Karkkainen M, Claesson-Welsh L, Alitalo K: Regulation of angiogenesis via vascular endothelial growth factor receptors. Cancer Res 2000;60:203-212.

The Patient with Disabling Angina Not Amenable to Revascularization Procedures

Udho Thadani

The number of patients with disabling angina who are not amenable to revascularization has grown considerably in recent years. A majority of these patients have undergone at least one coronary artery bypass procedure and percutaneous coronary interventions and are not suitable candidates for a further percutaneous coronary intervention or repeat coronary bypass surgery. Others have diffuse coronary artery disease or are at very high risk for a revascularization procedure because of comorbid conditions.

A patient with disabling angina not amenable to revascularization is one who remains symptomatic despite optimal medical treatment with β-blockers, calcium channel blockers, and regimens and formulations of long-acting nitrates that do not produce tolerance.[1-9] It must be recognized that in some patients, (1) triple therapy with β-blockers, calcium channel blockers, and nitrates may not be superior to treatment with two agents[10,11] and (2) adjustment of doses of a class of drug or changing to a different drug in the same class or withdrawal of a medication may help relieve anginal symptoms.[4,7,12,13]

It is also assumed that comorbid conditions such as anemia, thyrotoxicosis, arrhythmias, and other comorbid conditions that may aggravate angina and myocardial ischemia are absent or, if present, are adequately treated before disabling angina is diagnosed.

In addition to receiving antianginal drugs, all patients with disabling angina must abstain from smoking and should be treated with daily aspirin,[14] lipid-lowering agents (especially statins),[15,16] and angiotensin-converting enzyme inhibitors.[17,18] These drugs are known to reduce serious adverse clinical outcomes in patients with coronary artery disease. Whether these agents decrease angina frequency or improve exercise tolerance in patients with disabling angina has not been adequately studied.

Patients with disabling angina experience angina with minimal activity or at rest. Many of these patients are hospitalized with unstable angina on multiple occasions. Several therapies have been used or are recommended in addition to standard antianginal drugs, aspirin, statins, and angiotensin-converting enzyme inhibitors to relieve angina and reduce adverse clinical outcomes. Noninvasive procedures, such as enhanced external counterpulsation (EECP) and transcutaneous nerve stimulation (TENS), and invasive procedures, such as spinal-cord stimulation (SCS) and to a lesser extent transmyocardial laser revascularization (TMLR), are gaining popularity.

Percutaneous transmyocardial laser revascularization (PTMLR), gene therapy, and other therapeutic modalities remain experimental. The use of many of these treatment modalities in patients with disabling angina is not based on well-designed placebo- or sham-controlled trials. The published data and options to treat these patients are discussed in this chapter.

BEPRIDIL

Bepridil, a nonspecific calcium channel blocker, exerts potent anti-anginal and anti-ischemic effects.[3,6,7,19] A study showed that in patients with stable angina, a combination of bepridil and propranolol was superior to propranolol alone.[20] Bepridil was shown to be superior to diltiazem in another study.[21] Overall, published data suggest that bepridil increases exercise duration and reduces angina frequency more than other calcium channel blockers in patients with stable angina.[3,7] Unfortunately, bepridil prolongs the QT interval and can cause torsades de pointes in 1% to 2% of treated patients.[3,7] This is a major concern in patients with hypokalemia and in the presence of drugs that also prolong the QT interval.[3] There are no controlled trials with bepridil in patients with disabling angina who remain symptomatic despite maximal medical treatment and are not candidates for a revascularization procedure.[3] However, personal experience in several such patients suggests that bepridil is effective when other calcium channel blockers are not. Bepridil in place of other calcium channel blockers should be tried only in patients who remain symptomatic despite optimal medical treatment with β-blockers, other calcium channel blockers, and nitrates and those who are not candidates for revascularization.

UNFRACTIONATED AND LOW-MOLECULAR-WEIGHT HEPARIN, ANTIPLATELET AGENTS, AND THROMBOLYTIC AGENTS

In patients with acute coronary syndrome, subcutaneous low-molecular-weight heparin plus aspirin reduces composite adverse clinical outcomes (death, myocardial infarction, and refractory angina) compared with aspirin plus intravenous unfractionated heparin.[22,23] In patients with stable angina, however, intravenous unfractionated heparin did not increase treadmill exercise duration.[24] Treatment with subcutaneous low-molecular-weight heparin for several weeks increased exercise duration and exercise time to ischemia and reduced angina frequency in other studies.[25,26]

No placebo-controlled, double-blind trials have studied long-term treatment with either unfractionated or low-molecular-weight heparin in patients with disabling angina.

Recently published results of the CURE trial[27] in patients with acute coronary syndrome (unstable angina or non–ST-segment elevation myocardial infarction) showed that treatment with clopidogrel plus aspirin for up to 11 months reduced the composite end point of death, myocardial infarction, and stroke compared with placebo plus aspirin therapy. No data suggest that antiplatelet agents, including aspirin and clopidogrel, reduce angina frequency or improve exercise performance in patients with disabling angina. At present, data do not support the routine prolonged use of unfractionated or low-molecular-weight heparin or antiplatelet agents (other than aspirin or perhaps clopidogrel) to manage disabling angina.

In open trials with intermittent but prolonged administration of urokinase, relief of angina in patients with refractory angina was reported.[28,29] However, these studies were not placebo-controlled and, given the risks of increased bleeding with urokinase and other thrombolytics, these agents cannot be recommended to manage disabling angina.[30]

OTHER MEDICAL THERAPIES OF UNPROVEN VALUE

Chelation Therapy

Chelation therapy with EDTA has been used to treat patients with peripheral vascular disease and those with known coronary artery disease.[30] However, placebo-controlled studies have failed to confirm that chelation therapy improves exercise performance in patients with intermittent claudication and those with stable angina pectoris.[31-33] No good published data suggest that chelation therapy is beneficial in patients with disabling angina.[30]

Enhanced External Counterpulsation

EECP mimics the principles of intra-aortic balloon pump counterpulsation in that EECP augments coronary blood flow in diastole and facilitates left-ventricular emptying in systole.[34-38] The EECP device currently marketed for clinical use consists of three paired pneumatic cuffs that are applied to the lower extremities.[38-42] The cuffs are sequentially inflated by applying 250 to 300 mm Hg of external pressure during diastole.[38] This increases venous return to the heart, with a resultant increase in cardiac output. An increase in aortic distention and pressure increases coronary blood flow in diastole.[38] The cuffs are deflated simultaneously in systole, reducing

peripheral resistance to flow and thus providing left-ventricular unloading and easier emptying in systole.[38]

The EECP device has been in use for several years, but previous devices were cumbersome and difficult to use.[38] The newer device is operator- and patient-friendly and has been approved by the Device Committee of the Food and Drug Administration (FDA) for clinical use. The approval has led to a wider use of the device in patients whose cases are considered refractory to conventional therapy and are poor candidates for revascularization procedures.[36,41,42] Whether such a practice is justified is open to question because of the lack of adequately designed studies in this group of patients.

Mechanism of Action of Enhanced External Counterpulsation

The exact mechanism by which EECP improves and maintains improvement in patients with stable angina remains unclear,[35,36,41] although various mechanisms—including an increase in collateral blood flow to the ischemic areas,[37] improvement in diastolic filling,[43] and neovascularization (angiogenesis) in the ischemic areas—have been proposed but not proven (Table 38-1).

Clinical Studies with Enhanced External Counterpulsation

Treatment requires 1-hour sessions, five times a week, for a total of 35 sessions[36,38,41]; although EECP is non-invasive, it is expensive. Earlier studies with EECP, which were uncontrolled and used small numbers of patients, showed an improvement in stress perfusion imaging[37] associated with an increase in treadmill exercise duration compared with baseline and an improvement in exercise hemodynamics compared with pretreatment (Table 38-2).[43] In a single-center, open study of 50 patients, stress perfusion imaging improved after treatment in 75% of patients.[37] In one of the studies, the lowest response rate was noted in patients with the most extensive disease and the fewest proximally patent conduits, including both native coronary arteries and bypass grafts.[34,35] These uncontrolled studies also reported that

■ ■ ■

TABLE 38–1   POSSIBLE MECHANISMS OF ACTION OF ENHANCED EXTERNAL COUNTERPULSATION (EECP)

Acute hemodynamic improvement mimicking the effects of intra-aortic balloon counterpulsation; increased coronary flow in diastole and improved systolic left-ventricular emptying and increased cardiac output (however, one would expect that the effects should last only during the treatment period of one hour each day)
Increased collateral blood flow (unproven)
Increased angiogenesis (unproven)
Increased endothelial cell production of nitric oxide and prostacyclin (unproven)

patients treated with EECP continued to show an improvement in myocardial perfusion and angina frequency for up to 5 years.[40]

The only controlled study to evaluate EECP was the MUlticenter STudy of Enhanced External Counter-Pulsation (MUST-EECP).[38] Effects of active EECP treatment on exercise-induced electrocardiographic myocardial ischemia, total exercise duration, and anginal episodes were compared with sham EECP. Only patients with stable exertional angina with Canadian Cardiovascular Society (CCS) classes I to III were considered for the study. Patients were excluded for the following reasons: unstable angina, a recent acute coronary syndrome, a myocardial infarction or bypass surgery within the previous 3 months, a history of heart failure, a left-ventricular ejection fraction less than 30%, hypertension with blood pressure greater than 180/100 mm Hg, a history of phlebitis or severe peripheral vascular disease, warfarin therapy, atrial fibrillation, and frequent ventricular premature beats. A total of 500 patients were screened, of whom 139 were randomized. All had evidence of electrocardiographic myocardial ischemia (ST-segment depression) during treadmill exercise in addition to exercise-induced angina. The ages ranged from 21 to 81 years. Patients received either active EECP with inflation pressures of 300 mm Hg or sham EECP with an inflation pressure of 75 mm Hg.

Of the 139 patients randomized, exercise data were available in only 115 patients. There were more patients in the active treatment group (n = 14) than the inactive treatment group (n = 4) who did not complete the study. The results failed to confirm that EECP improved total treadmill exercise duration.[38] Improvement in exercise duration was 42 ± 11 seconds in the active EECP group and 26 ± 12 seconds in the sham-EECP group ($P > .3$). However, time to stress-induced myocardial ischemia (1 mm ST-segment depression) increased significantly in the active treatment group compared with the sham-treated group (37 ± 11 seconds vs. –4 ± 12 seconds, $P = .01$), and there was also a decrease in angina frequency and improvement in functional class but no change in the sublingual nitroglycerin consumption in the active treatment group compared with the sham-treated group.

One of the drawbacks of the study regarding the evaluation of angina frequency was that patients were not asked to keep an anginal diary or an account of daily activities throughout the study. They were asked to remember whether they had any anginal attacks in the 24 hours preceding each treatment session.[38] More patients in the active EECP group experienced adverse events compared with the sham-treated EECP group (55% vs. 26%; $P < .001$). Device-related adverse experiences occurred in 33% of active EECP group members compared with 15% of sham-treated group members; paresthesias (2% vs. 1%), edema and swelling of legs (2% vs. 0%), skin abrasion, bruise, and blisters (13% vs. 2%), and pain in the back or legs (20% vs. 7%) were other findings in the active versus sham-EECP groups. The same investigators published a substudy in 71 patients on quality-of-life measures 12 months after treatment.[39] They reported a significant health-related quality-of-life improvement for up to 12 months after the completion of treatment with EECP.[39]

The EECP device was approved on the basis of this single trial in patients with stable angina. The approved indications included not only stable angina but also those unstable angina not responsive to conventional therapy. Subsequent to the approval of the device, registry data were prospectively collected.

The international EECP patient registry[41] reported the safety and benefit of EECP treatment in 548 patients with a history of heart failure.[42] At 6 months' follow-up, the procedure was well tolerated compared with patients without heart failure. However, significantly fewer patients with heart failure completed the course of EECP, and exacerbation of heart failure was more frequent, although angina class improved in 68% of patients with comparable quality-of-life benefit in the heart failure cohort.[42] At 6 months' follow-up, patients with congestive heart failure maintained their reduction in angina frequency but were significantly more likely to have experienced major adverse cardiac events (death, myocardial infarction, and revascularization).

In a 1996 report of 2289 consecutive patients enrolled in an EECP consortium, EECP was found to be safe and well tolerated with a 4.0% rate of adverse experiences.[36]

■ ▨ ■

TABLE 38–2 CLINICAL STUDIES* WITH ENHANCED EXTERNAL COUNTERPULSATION (EECP) AND OUTCOMES

STUDY DESIGN	OUTCOME
Open-label studies with baseline as control[34,37,38]	Increase in exercise duration Improvement in stress thallium perfusion imaging Reduction in angina Canadian Cardiovascular Class (CCC) functional class by 1 or 2 grades Lower response rate in patients with extensive disease and with poor conduits
MUST EECP–sham-controlled trial in stable angina[38]	No improvement in exercise duration Increase in exercise time to electrocardiographic myocardial ischemia (ST-segment depression) Reduction in angina frequency but not nitroglycerine consumption
Registry data with baseline as control in patients presumably refractory to conventional treatment[36,41]	Improvement in CCS functional class by 1 or 2 grades Local complications rate of 4% Safe in patients with heart failure

*Double-blind, sham-controlled studies in patients with disabling angina who are not candidates for a revascularization procedure have not been performed.

Angina class improved in 74% of patients with limiting angina (CCS functional class III to IV); patients who were most impaired at baseline demonstrated the greatest improvement, with 39.5% of patients in CCS classes III and IV improving two or more classes.[36] It is of interest that patients with CCS functional classes I and II, as well as III and IV, were included in the registry and that the results in the two groups were compared.

The registry data were updated (Fig. 38–1) and presented at the annual meeting of the American College of Cardiology in 2002 and showed marked improvement in functional class over time in the majority of patients. EECP's beneficial effects on psychosocial functions have been reported.[44]

It is unclear from the publications of the registry data whether all patients were on maximal medical treatment and whether they were candidates for revascularization. The reasons for treatment with EECP were diverse, including angina refractory to medical and surgical therapy, patient or physician preference, and poor candidates for surgery due to lack of graft material or targets or operative risk. During the study, only 0.2% of patients worsened by one CCS class.[41] The majority of the patients limited by their angina (CCS functional class II to IV) either improved their angina class (1531, or 73.4%, of patients) or remained unchanged in functional class after EECP (554, or 26.5%, of patients). Angina class improved by two or more functional classes in 48.5% of pretreatment angina class IV patients and in 34.9% of pretreatment functional class III patients. It is unclear whether any of the patients included in the registry had an acute coronary syndrome at the time of the study. In previous studies, patients with unstable and acute coronary syndrome were excluded.

Review of the published data leaves one to doubt whether the EECP treatment can be routinely recommended in patients with disabling angina who are not candidates for revascularization. No specific data have been published in this group of patients, and no controlled trials have been conducted. The only sham-controlled trial reported was in patients with stable angina, and that study failed to show an objective improvement in exercise tolerance, although there was an increase in time to ischemic threshold and a reduction in anginal episodes. Registry data are observational, not sham-controlled. Given a high rate of placebo response in patients with angina pectoris, it remains speculative whether EECP is effective in patients with disabling angina whose conditions are refractory to maximal medical therapy and who are not candidates for revascularization.

Thus, EECP treatment cannot be routinely recommended in patients with disabling angina whose conditions are refractory to maximum medical therapy and who are not candidates for revascularization. If the patient is very symptomatic, such therapy may be tried with the caveat that complete relief of angina or a reduction in anginal attacks might be a placebo effect during and after EECP. Such an approach may be justified if there are no other alternatives. However, before we accept routine EECP to treat patients with disabling angina who are not candidates for revascularization, adequately powered, sham-controlled studies need to be conducted to evaluate the effects of treatment on angina attacks, exercise tolerance, and the incidence of death and myocardial infarction.

Neuromodulation (Spinal Cord Stimulation and Other Neurologically Based Therapies)

Several procedures have been used, some of which have been abandoned because of high complication rates.

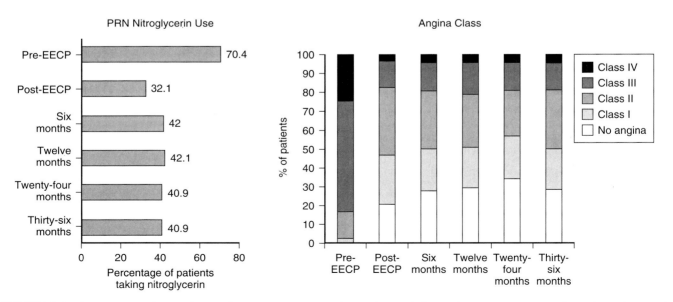

FIGURE 38–1. Changes in Canadian Cardiovascular Score (CCS) angina class and as-needed nitroglycerin use over time after enhanced external counterpulsation (EECP). Observational data before and 6 months, 12 months, 24 months, and 36 months after EECP therapy. Data reflect patients who completed the prescribed course of treatment and in whom follow-up information was available. From the international EECP patient registry (IEPR); database was frozen on 02/05/02 (IEPR newsletter, volume 4, issue 2, March 2002).

Acupuncture

Acupuncture has been used to treat intractable pain including refractory angina.[45] Unfortunately, no sham-controlled studies have been published and the procedure is not widely used in the Western Hemisphere.

Thoracic Epidural Anesthesia

Anesthesiologists have used thoracic epidural anesthesia (TEDA) to control pain.[45] Although successful, the procedure produces only temporary relief of pain and requires repeated administration of the local anesthetic; thus, this modality is not widely used.

Stellate Ganglion Block

Temporary left stellate ganglion block relieves angina. Permanent destruction of the left ganglion with relief of refractory angina has been documented in case reports.[46] No controlled series have been published.

Transcutaneous Nerve Stimulation

For TENS, electrodes are applied to the chest, one in the dermatome with the highest intensity of projected or referred pain and the other in the contralateral dermatome.[47-48] The stimulus intensity is adjusted to just below the individual's pain threshold. TENS leads to high-frequency stimulation of large non-nociceptive myelinated type A fibers and inhibits the impulse through smaller, unmyelinated type C fibers, thereby reducing the activation of central pain receptors. Studies from Scandinavia show that TENS improved exercise performance and reduced electrocardiographic myocardial ischemia during exercise or pacing and reduced lactate production during pacing-induced ischemia.[47-52] Sympathetic discharge also was reduced.[50] No sham-controlled trials have been reported, although in a presentation at the American College of Cardiology in 2002, the lead investigator suggested a possible placebo effect.[49]

TENS units have been used successfully to treat refractory angina, and data suggest that this mode of therapy reduces myocardial ischemia and delays the onset of angina. However, the procedure is not widely used because of local skin complications of the device and the only support for using TENS to reduce angina frequency in patients with disabling angina has come from case reports.[51-55]

Spinal Cord Stimulation

SCS is primarily used in the Scandinavian countries, with few cases being performed in Europe, the United States, and other parts of the world.[56-69]

Procedure and Mechanism of Action

Low-voltage electric stimulation of the spinal cord inhibits the sensation of pain (Table 38-3). The sensation of stimuli is perceived as paresthesia. The dural space

■ ■ ■

TABLE 38–3   MECHANISM OF ACTION OF SPINAL-CORD STIMULATION (SCS)

- Paresthesia in the area of referred pain
- Direct inhibition of sensory pathway carrying pain stimuli
- Reduction of myocardial ischemia
- Increase in pain threshold
- Reduction of sympathetic activity
- Reduction of myocardial oxygen demand

is opened, and an electrode is placed at the level of the T_4 and T_5 vertebra; a lead is placed at the T_1 and T_2 level.[57-59] During the procedure, the field of paresthesia produced is noted in the awake patient, and this should be in the area of referred pain. The stimulation device is connected to the lead and implanted under the skin in the abdomen or left lower thorax, and the patient is left with a small scar. The current applied varies from 2 to 7 volts, at rates of 30 to 90 Hz and a pulse width of 210 to 450 μJEK. The patient has a simple control mechanism and can turn the device on or off and can increase or decrease the amplitude of the current depending on the pain's intensity. The mechanism by which pain is alleviated is either direct inhibition of sensory pathways carrying the pain stimuli or a reduction of myocardial ischemia.[69]

Clinical Studies

Improvement in exercise duration and an increase in time to ST-segment depression and a reduction of total ischemic burden with SCS compared with controls has been well documented (Table 38–4).[57-60] Lactate production was also reduced during pacing-induced angina and SCS. Unfortunately, it is difficult to perform a placebo-controlled trial because the stimulation produces paresthesia. There has been a concern that abolition of pain with SCS may lead to myocardial ischemia not perceived by the patient and that a prolonged episode of silent ischemia may lead to myocardial infarction. Studies under controlled pacing conditions show that the pain threshold is diminished but not abolished[65,69] and that higher pacing rates are required to produce angina.[65,69] Under conditions of exercise-induced increase in heart rate, the patient still perceives anginal pain despite SCS, though at a higher heart rate.[69]

Holter monitoring studies in 19 patients showed a marked reduction of ischemic episodes and relief of symptoms during SCS compared with pre-SCS baseline values.[63] No ventricular ectopy was induced by SCS.[63] Studies have also have shown that SCS exerts antianginal effects and reduces myocardial oxygen demand. Myocardial ischemia is pacified but not abolished, and pain threshold is increased during SCS stimulation.[63,65,69]

In a recent trial in patients with stable angina pectoris and CCS class III and IV angina, 104 patients were either randomized to coronary bypass surgery or to SCS treatment. Relief of symptoms was experienced by 80% of patients in the coronary bypass surgery group and 84%

■ ▥ ■

TABLE 38–4 CLINICAL STUDIES WITH SPINAL-CORD STIMULATION (SCS)

STUDIES*	RESULTS
Open trials[57-62]	Marked reduction in angina frequency, improvement in exercise tolerance
Holter monitor data compared with baseline data[63]	Reduction of ischemic episodes and angina frequency
SCS compared with coronary bypass surgery in patients with Canadian Cardiovascular Score (CCS) class III and IV angina[68]	Similar reduction of angina frequency
	Greater increase in maximum workload and reduction in exercise-induced ischemia with coronary bypass surgery
	Higher mortality in the coronary bypass group

*Double-blind sham-controlled studies in patients with disabling angina who are not candidates for a revascularization procedure have not been performed.

of patients in the SCS group.[68] There was a marked reduction in angina frequency in both groups. There was a greater increase in maximum work performed in the surgical group than in the SCS group, and patients achieved a higher rate pressure product and had less ST-segment depression in the coronary artery bypass group.[68] Mortality in the coronary bypass surgical group was high compared with the SCS group (seven patients vs. one patient), with similar rates of nonfatal myocardial infarction (seven patients vs. seven patients).

In a retrospective analysis of patients treated with SCS,[65] 103 of the 517 patients had died by 23 months but had previously experienced a reduction in angina frequency. This was an observational study and not a controlled trial; therefore, results must be interpreted with caution.

The following conclusions can be derived from the published data. The SCS procedure in experienced hands is safe and relieves angina. However, only a relatively small number of patients have been treated with SCS. There are no placebo-controlled trials, and it remains to be proven whether SCS is effective because of a marked placebo effect that has been documented in patients with angina. The reason for the infrequent use of SCS to treat refractory angina, according to a lead proponent of SCS, is that the procedure is performed by neurologists whereas patients with disabling angina or no option angina are treated by cardiologists, who do not receive any monetary gain for a procedure they do not perform themselves.

The reported safety of the procedure is reassuring, and SCS may be offered to patients with disabling angina despite maximal therapy who are not candidates for revascularization, even if the procedure were to produce a placebo-derived beneficial effect.

Sympathectomy

In patients with intractable angina, sympathectomy has been tried with success but the procedure is associated with significant morbidity and an increased mortality. For these reasons, the procedure has been essentially abandoned.[65,68]

Transmyocardial Laser Revascularization

The concept of creating transmyocardial channels to increase myocardial blood flow and oxygen supply goes back to an observation in reptiles, in whom a network of channels in the myocardium communicates directly with the ventricular cavity. In humans, there are no communications between the ventricular cavity and the myocardium. The concept to increase myocardial blood flow via ventriculocoronary anastomosis (sinusoidal network) was proposed by Wearn and colleagues in 1933.[70] Subsequently, successful channels were created by direct myocardial punctures in animals and with lasers in humans in 1988.[71]

Two types of laser devices have been used to create intramyocardial channels, the CO_2 laser and homium:YAG laser. It has been claimed that more channels remain patent after the CO_2 laser device than after use of the homium:YAG laser procedure, and the lesions created by the two procedures are histologically different.

Through a lateral thoracotomy, under direct vision but without cardioplegia or cardiopulmonary bypass, 10 to 50 (average, 24) laser channels are created in the left ventricle. The epicardial openings either close spontaneously or with light direct compression.

Mechanism of Action

It has been proposed that transmyocardial channels remain open after transmyocardial laser revascularization (TMLR) and may lead to angiogenesis (Table 38–5).[72] Unfortunately, many of the channels close soon after the procedure and there are few objective data to support increased angiogenesis.[73,74] One autopsy study showed microinfarcts in the areas around the TMLR channels, with evidence of local fibrosis and cardiac denervation.[74] The exact mechanism by which TMLR relieves angina remains speculative, although cardiac denervation remains a likely mechanism.[74,75]

■ ▥ ■

TABLE 38–5 PROPOSED MECHANISM OF ACTION OF TRANSMYOCARDIAL LASER REVASCULARIZATION

- Exact mechanism unknown
- Increased blood flow to the myocardium via laser channels (most of the channels close spontaneously with time)?
- Neovascularization (angiogenesis)? (unproven)
- Cardiac denervation (likely)

Clinical Studies

TMLR has been performed only in patients who are not candidates for revascularization and have viable but ischemic myocardium. TMLR with CO_2 lasers and homium:YAG lasers was approved by the Device Committee of the FDA for clinical use in nonoption patients (i.e., patients who are not candidates for revascularization or who are at very high risk because of comorbid conditions).

Initial open uncontrolled trials in patients with refractory angina reported significant improvement in anginal symptoms and myocardial perfusion on thallium imaging in more than 75% of patients over a 12-month follow-up period after TMLR compared with baseline observations (Table 38-6).[72,75-79] Uncontrolled open studies have confirmed these observations for up to 3 to 5 years of observations.[72,75-79] However, these studies were observational and not randomized or sham-controlled.[75] Improvement in myocardial perfusion reported in earlier studies is questionable because of lack of reproducibility during sequential studies.[80]

Schofield et al compared TMLR with CO_2 laser plus continued medical treatment to medical treatment alone in 188 patients with CCS class III or IV angina.[81] Patients were randomly assigned to a treatment group. At 12 months, this study failed to show a statistical difference in exercise capacity or 12-minute walking distance between the two groups. The perioperative mortality rate was high in the TMLR group (5%), but the mortality at 12 months was similar in the two groups. Regarding subjective symptoms, there was a significant improvement in angina CCS functional class and a significant decrease in need for anti-anginal medications and fewer hospitalizations in the laser group. This trial failed to show an objective improvement in exercise duration, which was the primary end point of the study.[81]

In the Norwegian randomized trial, TMLR CO_2 laser plus optimal medical treatment was compared with optimal medical treatment in 100 patients with New York Heart Association class III and IV angina.[82,83] The angina class improved at 12 months,[82] an improvement still present at 3 to 5 years.[83] Hospitalizations for unstable angina were reduced by 55% in the TMLR group after 3 to 5 years but not at 12 months.[83] Treatment for heart failure increased after TMLR, but there were no differences in mortality or the incidence of myocardial infarction in the TMLR group compared with medical group.[83]

Frazier et al randomized 182 patients, with many patients in CCS angina functional class IV (69%), to either medical treatment plus TMLR CO_2 procedure or medical treatment.[84] At 12 months, there was a significant improvement in angina functional class, quality of life, and single-photon emission computed tomographic thallium imaging. There was also a marked reduction in rehospitalization for unstable angina in the TMLR group compared with the medical group (2% vs. 59%). However, survival rates at 12 months were similar. The perioperative mortality rate of the TMRL procedure was 3%. There was a high crossover rate to TMRL in the medically treated group.

In another study, TMLR plus continued medical treatment versus medical treatment alone in 275 patients with refractory angina showed a significant improvement in CCS angina functional class, a higher rate of cardiac event–free survival, a decrease in cardiac-related hospital admissions, and a higher rate of freedom from treatment failure.[85] In the TMLR plus continuous medical treatment group, despite an improvement in quality of life, myocardial perfusion did not differ between the two groups as assessed by thallium imaging. There was a high crossover rate from the medical group to TMLR therapy.

TMLR with homium:YAG laser plus medical treatment was compared with medical treatment in 182 patients with CCS functional class[86] III or IV angina. There were

■■■

TABLE 38–6   CLINICAL TRIALS WITH TRANSMYOCARDIAL LASER REVASCULARIZATION (TMLR)*

TRIAL	OUTCOME
Open, uncontrolled reports	Improvement in anginal symptoms
	Improvement in myocardial perfusion in >75% of patients
CO_2 laser plus medical treatment vs. medical treatment[83]	No difference in exercise capacity or 12-minute walk test
	Significant reduction in angina frequency
	Periprocedural mortality (5%)
	No difference in mortality at 12 months
CO_2 laser plus medical treatment vs. medical treatment[84,85]	Improvement in Canadian Cardiovascular Score (CCS) angina class and quality-of-life score
	Improvement in thallium perfusion
	Periprocedural mortality 3%
	No difference in mortality at 12 months
	High crossover rate in medical group
CO_2 laser plus medical treatment vs. medical treatment[82a,82b]	Improvement in New York Heart Association (NYHA) angina class
	Reduction in hospitalizations for unstable angina by 55% at 3–5 years' follow-up
	Increased incidence of heart failure; no difference in mortality or incidence of myocardial infarctiont at 3–5 years
Homium:YAG laser plus medical treatment vs. medical treatment[85]	No difference in myocardial perfusion or ejection fraction or mortality at 12 months
	Significant increase in exercise duration and angina functional class

*There are no sham-controlled trials with TMLR in patient with disabling angina and who are not candidates for revascularization.

no differences in myocardial perfusion or ejection fraction between the two groups as measured by echocardiography and dipyramidole thallium scanning. The mortality rates were also similar at 12 months. There was a significant increase in exercise duration and an improvement in angina functional class after TMRL therapy.

TMLR as a treatment option was approved after the TMLR procedure was documented to improve CCS angina functional class compared with medical therapy. No sham-controlled studies have been conducted.

Review of the published data with CO_2 or homium:YAG TMLR show conflicting results: Some studies show an improvement in myocardial perfusion and others show no improvement. Similarly, the effects of TMLR on exercise duration in different studies have shown either no improvement or a significant increase. The only consistent finding of all the studies has been an improvement in CCS angina functional class by one or two grades. None of the studies has shown a mortality benefit. The controversy has been discussed in several publications.[75,79-81] Perioperative morbidity and mortality of the procedure remain sources of major concern.[87]

Thus, caution is warranted in interpreting the data, especially in the absence of a placebo group. A high rate of symptomatic improvement and in functional class in patients with angina has been reported with placebo treatment in drug trials[7,19] and in a recent sham-controlled interventional trial with percutaneous TMLR.[88] The Vineberg procedure (implantation of the internal mammary artery directly into the myocardium) was in vogue in the early 1960s but was subsequently proven to be ineffective and abandoned. Thus, routine use of TMLR cannot be recommended in patients with refractory angina who are not candidates for revascularization because of the high initial perioperative morbidity and mortality related to TMLR.[75,86] Sham-controlled trials are needed to prove that TMLR is superior to continued medical therapy.

It has been argued that a sham-controlled study is unethical with TMLR because a thoracotomy is required and such a procedure will not be acceptable to the patient, the surgeon, or the FDA. Therefore, in patients who remain highly symptomatic despite maximal medical therapy, TMLR may be an option even if the response may be due to a placebo effect of the procedure because, in all of the published studies, angina CCS functional class has improved. However, it must be recognized that many of these refractory patients improve with time with continued optimal medical therapy.[89] A sham-controlled trial is therefore needed before TMLR can be accepted as a routine therapy in patients with disabling angina who are not candidates for revascularization.

Percutaneous Transmyocardial Laser Revascularization

Acceptance of TMLR to treat patients with no option angina has led to a wider use of the device.[76-78] However, TMLR requires expertise and is associated with significant perioperative mortality and morbidity.[87] To avoid periprocedural complications, percutaneous catheters were designed, and it became feasible to perform laser myocardial revascularization via the retrograde femoral arterial approach, creating laser channels from the cavity of the left ventricle into the myocardium.[90]

Clinical Studies

Initial open-label studies showed encouraging results (Table 38-7).[90,91] In the Potential Angina Class Improvement from Intramyocardial Channels (PACIFIC) trial, 221 patients with CCS class III or IV angina that was refractory to medical treatment and not suitable for revascularization were randomized to PTMRL plus medical treatment or to medical treatment alone.[92] At 12 months, there was a significant increase in total exercise duration and an improvement in angina class score and quality of life, but the mortality was similar in the two groups. The incidence of myocardial infarction was not evaluated. In another study of 330 patients with CCS class II to IV

■ ▪ ■

TABLE 38–7   TRIAL RESULTS OF PERCUTANEOUS TRANSMYOCARDIAL LASER REVASCULARIZATION (PTMLR)

TRIALS	RESULTS
Open-label uncontrolled reports[89,90]	Reduction in angina frequency
PTMLR plus medical treatment vs. medical treatment in Canadian Cardiovascular Score angina class III and IV[91]	Significant increase in exercise duration and an improvement in angina CCS functional class and quality-of-life measurements at 12 months
PTMLR plus medical treatment vs. medical treatment in CCS class II-IV refractory angina[92]	Mortality similar in two groups Increase in exercise duration and improvement in angina functional class No difference in mortality at 12 months
PTMLR plus medical treatment vs. medical treatment in patients with refractory angina and occluded coronary arteries[93]	Similar improvements in functional class and exercise duration at 6 months No differences in mortality or myocardial infarction rates
PTMR plus medical treatment vs. Sham procedure plus medical treatment[87]	Trial stopped prematurely at 6 months; No difference in mortality, exercise duration, CCS angina functional class, quality-of-life indices, ischemic threshold, mortality and myocardial infarction incidence

refractory angina, medical treatment with PTMLR plus medical treatment led to an improvement in exercise tolerance and to improvement in angina class and quality of life.[92] Again, there was no difference in mortality in the two groups.

These two trials were not sham-controlled. Given the known placebo effect in patients with angina, Leon and workers[88] conducted a sham-controlled study. In this double-blind randomized trial—the Direct myocardial revascularization In Regeneration of Endomyocardial Channel Trial (DIRECT)—298 patients were randomized to PTMLR with creation of 20 to 25 channels, a low PTMLR procedure with creation of 10 to 15 channels, or a sham (placebo) procedure with no laser channels created. The trial was stopped prematurely at 6 months because there was a similar increase in treadmill exercise duration among the three groups. Furthermore, time to stress-induced electrocardiographic ischemia (1 mm ST-segment depression) and time to onset of angina were also similar among the three groups. There was a similar reduction in CCS angina class and improvement in quality-of-life indices in the three groups. The incidence of death and myocardial infarction was also similar.

The results of this sham-controlled trial were completely divergent from the previously reported uncontrolled open trials and randomized trials that compared with medical treatment in that there was no objective or subjective improvement in the PTMLR group over the sham-treated group. The DIRECT trial highlights the importance of a placebo-treated group to evaluate PTMLR or any other device or surgical procedure and clearly documents a marked placebo response even in very symptomatic patients with coronary artery disease.

In another randomized, single-blind trial, PTMLR with homium:YAG laser plus maximum medical therapy (n = 71) was compared with maximum medical therapy (n = 70) in patients with refractory angina caused by one or more total coronary occlusions.[94] Percutaneous coronary intervention was attempted in all patients, but the procedure was unsuccessful. Patients were heavily sedated and did not know whether they were subsequently treated with PTMLR or not. At 6 months, angina class improved by two or more classes in 49% of patients treated with PTMLR and in 37% of those assigned to maximum medical therapy (P = .33). The median increase in exercise duration from baseline to 6 months was 64 seconds with PTMLR versus 52 seconds with maximum medical treatment (P = .73). There were no differences in 6-month rates of death (8.6% vs. 8.8%), myocardial infarction (4.3% vs. 2.9%) or any type of revascularization (4.3% vs. 5.3%) in the PTMLR and maximum medical therapy groups, respectively (P = NS for all). These observations confirm published data with drug trials in patients with stable angina, in whom an objective improvement in exercise performance and a marked reduction in angina frequency during placebo therapy has been consistently reported. PTMLR remains an investigative device and is not approved for clinical use by the FDA.

The results of the DIRECT trial[88] and single-blind PTMRL trial[94] raise a major concern with the widely accepted results of the previously discussed TMLR procedure with CO_2 and homium:YAG devices, which were not sham-controlled.[81-86]

Intra-Aortic Balloon Pump Counterpulsation

Intra-aortic balloon pump counterpulsation (IABPCP) increases coronary blood flow in diastole and improves left-ventricular systolic emptying. IABPCP is effective in controlling angina and reducing myocardial ischemia in patients with refractory unstable angina. This mode of treatment is used as a bridge prior to coronary bypass surgery or during cardiac catheterization and percutaneous coronary interventions in hemodynamically compromised patients. However, the device increases the risk of local complications and limb ischemia with prolonged use.[95] There is no role for IABPCP in patients with disabling angina who are not candidates for revascularization because it may be difficult to wean a patient from IABPCP, which may result in serious local ischemic complications requiring local vascular surgery or even amputation of the leg.[95]

NEWER PROMISING BUT UNPROVEN TREATMENTS

Dietary Supplementation with Arginine

In a 2000 report[96] concerning patients with stable angina of CCS class II or III, a food bar enriched with D-arginine and a combination of other nutrients increased total exercise duration, improved quality of life, but had no effect on electrocardiographic manifestations of ischemia. Arginine also led to improvement in flow medicated brachial-artery vasodilation. These observations confirm previous reports showing beneficial effects of L-arginine on exercise tolerance and endothelial function in patients with stable coronary artery disease.[97,98]

These observations are of interest; placebo-controlled trials in patients with disabling angina are needed to see if arginine and other nutrient supplements alleviate angina in this group.

Metabolic Modulators (See Chapter 27)

Inhibition of oxidative phosphorylation and substrate utilization from fatty acid and oxidation to glucose ameliorates experimental myocardial ischemia.[99] Studies in patients with stable angina that used trimetazidine[99] and ronalozine[100] have shown an improvement in exercise duration and reduction in myocardial ischemia compared with placebo. Whether these agents are useful in patients with refractory angina is unknown.

Angiogenic Gene Therapy (See Chapter 37)

In patients with coronary artery disease, collateral blood vessels are often visible during angiography and these vessels open in response to chronic myocardial ischemia. However, collateral blood flow is inadequate in many patients with disabling angina, especially during period of increased myocardial oxygen demand. Stimulation of angiogenesis presents an attractive and additional or alternative approach for the treatment of coronary artery disease.[101] In animal models of myocardial ischemia, an increase in coronary collateral formation has been reported with continuous administration of agents into the left coronary artery and with intracoronary gene transfer of fibroblast growth factor (FGF) and adenovirus-mediated gene transfer of the complementary deoxyribonucleic acid and for vascular endothelial growth factor (VEGF).[102-104] Encouraging results were reported in phase I and pilot studies with VEGF and fibroblast growth factor.[105-112]

Direct injection of FGF protein in the myocardium at the time of coronary bypass graft surgery resulted in angiographic evidence of enhanced collateral formation.[109,111]

In a randomized double-blind trial, low and high doses of recombinant VEGF, administered intravenously, were compared with placebo in 178 patients with stable angina who were not suitable for revascularization.[112] At 60 days, there was a likewise, increase in exercise duration after VEGF and placebo, a primary end point of the study. Likewise, there were likewise, improvements in angina functional class and no difference in myocardial perfusion after VEGF therapy compared with placebo. At 120 days, there was an improvement in angina functional class but no significant increase in exercise duration after VEGF therapy compared with placebo.

In another study, different doses of a single intracoronary injection of FGF-2 were compared with placebo in a randomized double-blind study involving 337 patients.[113] At 90 days, there was an increase in exercise duration in both the active and the placebo groups, with no statistical difference between the FGF and placebo groups. This was the primary end point of the study. FGF-2 also did not improve myocardial perfusion. FGF-2 administration conferred an improvement in angina functional class at 90 days but not at 180 days.

These two double-blind, placebo-controlled trials failed to show beneficial effects of intravenous VEGF or of FGF-2 administered intravenously and in the coronary artery. These findings directly contrast with the beneficial results reported in open studies.[114-116]

It has been suggested that gene therapy may be superior to protein therapy because the vascular endothelium or myocardium, or both, can incorporate genes, allowing sustained production of angiogenic protein. Open-label studies in humans have produced beneficial effects.[117] However, none of these studies was placebo-controlled.[117] In a 2001 report of 79 patients with coronary artery disease, safety and anti-ischemic effects of different doses of intracoronary AD5-FGF4 were assessed in patients with exercise-induced chronic stable angina of CCS class II or III.[117] The total exercise duration was increased by 1.3 minutes after gene therapy compared with an increase of 0.7 minutes with placebo (P = NS). The study was not powerful enough to evaluate the dose-response effects. Subgroup analysis showed a significant increase in exercise duration in patients with baseline exercise duration of 10 minutes or less. However, the significance of this finding remains questionable and needs prospective evaluation (it is currently being studied in the Berlex gene therapy trial).

Placebo-controlled studies with gene therapy are not available in patients with disabling angina who are not candidates for revascularization, and the results of ongoing studies in this group of patients are eagerly awaited. Concerns of increased atherosclerosis and the possibility of neoplasms secondary to gene therapy remain a concern.[104,116]

Thus, in the absence of placebo-controlled studies involving patients with refractory angina, gene therapy remains experimental.

Percutaneous in Situ Coronary Venous Arterialization

Percutaneous in situ coronary venous arterialization (PICVA) redirects arterial blood flow from an occluded coronary artery to the adjacent vein, thereby arterializing the vein and providing retroperfusion to the ischemic myocardium.[118-120] An isolated report of PICVA in a patient with CCS class IV angina, in whom medical treatment had failed and who was not a good candidate for coronary bypass surgery or percutaneous intervention, resulted in complete relief of angina, increased perfusion to the ischemia area, and an increase in angina-free walking.[119]

Sham-controlled trials are needed before this procedure can be used to treat patients with disabling angina.[30]

LAST-RESORT THERAPY

If all options fail and the patient continues to be disabled with angina, cardiac transplantation should be considered as an option provided there is no concomitant cerebrovascular disease or another comorbid condition that shortens survival. Long-term symptom-free survival is good in selected patients after transplantation. Donor hearts are scarce, and cardiac transplantation is usually offered only to younger patients with refractory angina who have no other comorbid conditions. Accelerated coronary atherosclerosis of the transplanted graft, however, remains a concern.

Best-Available Options for Treating Disabling Angina

Increasing numbers of patients who are not candidates for revascularization are presenting with disabling angina.[121] One must optimize antianginal therapy and use aggressive lipid-lowering therapy in all such patients. Patients must be advised to stop smoking.

Many patients improve with maximal medical therapy. A trial of bepridil in selected patients instead of other calcium channel blockers is justified provided there are no contraindications and the patient is made aware of the risk of possible torsades de pointes.

No large placebo-controlled trials have studied EECP, SCS, or TMLR in patients with disabling angina. In placebo-controlled trials, PTMLR and VEGF and FGF-2 protein therapy were not superior to sham (placebo) therapy. This raises a major concern in accepting the results of TMLR trials, which were not sham-controlled. In symptomatic patients, SCS and EECP are reasonable options even if the effects may be due in part to a placebo effect. SCS has more convincing documented physiologic effects and clinical benefit and should be considered as an option of choice in patients with disabling angina.

REFERENCES

1. Thadani U: Assessment of "optimal" beta-blockade in treating patients with angina pectoris. Acta Med Scand Suppl 1985;694:179-187.
2. Task Force of the European Society Cardiology: Management of stable angina pectoris: Recommendations of the Task Force of the European Society Cardiology. Eur Heart J 1997;18:394-413.
3. Asirvathan S, Sebastian C, Thadani U: Choosing the most appropriate treatment for table angina safety: Safety considerations. Drug Safety 1998;19:23-44.
4. Thadani U: Treatment of stable angina. Curr Opin Cardiol 1999;14:349-358.
5. ACC/AHA/ACP-ASIM Guidelines for the management of patients with chronic stable angina: Executive summary and recommendations. Circulation 1999;99:2829-2848.
6. Opie LH: First line drugs in chronic stable angina: The case for newer, long-lasting calcium channel blocking agents. J Am Coll Cardiol 2000;36:1967-1971.
7. Thadani U: Selective L-type, t-Type, and non specific calcium channel blockers for stable angina pectoris [Editorial]. Am Heart J 2002, in press.
8. Thadani U: Nitrate tolerance, rebound and their clinical relevance in stable angina pectoris, unstable angina and heart failure. Cardiovasc Drugs Ther 1996;10:735-742.
9. Heidenreich PA, McDonald KM, Hastie T, et al: Meta-analysis of trials comparing β-blockers, calcium antagonists, and nitrates for stable angina. JAMA 1999;281:1927-1936.
10. Tolins M, Weir EK, Chesler E, Pierpont GL: Maximal drug therapy is not necessarily optimal in chronic angina pectoris. Am Coll Cardiol 1984;4:1051-1057.
11. Thadani U: Combination therapy. Am Coll Cardiol Curr J Rev 1997;6:24-25.
12. Dunselman P, van Kempen L, Bouwens L, et al: Value of the addition of amlodipine to atenolol in patients with angina pectoris despite adequate beta blockade. Am J Cardiol 1998;81:128-132.
13. Knight CJ, Fox K, on behalf of the centralized European studies in angina research (CESAR) investigators: Amlodipine versus diltiazem as additional antianginal treatment to atenolol. Am J Cardiol 1998;81:133-136.
14. Fuster V, Dyken ML, Vokonas PS, Hennekens C: Aspirin as a therapeutic agent in cardiovascular disease. Circulation 1993;87:659-675.
15. Pitt B, Waters D, Brown WV, et al: Aggressive lipid-lowering therapy compared with angioplasty in stable coronary artery disease. N Engl J Med 1999;341:70-76.
16. Vaughan CJ, Gotto AM, Basson CT: The evolving role of statins in the management of atherosclerosis. J Am Coll Cardiol 2000;35:1-10.
17. Pepine C: Rationale for ACE inhibition as anti-ischemic therapy. Eur Heart J 1998;19:G34-G40.
18. The Heart Outcomes Prevention Evaluation Study Investigators: Effects of an angiotensin-converting-enzyme inhibitor, ramapril, on cardiovascular events in high-risk patients. N Engl J Med 2000;342:145-153.
19. Shapiro W, Dibianco R, Thadani U: Comparative efficacy of 200, 300, and 400 mg of bepridil for chronic, stable angina pectoris. Am J Cardiol 1985;55:36C-42C.
20. Frishman WH, Crawford MW, Dibianco R, et al: Combination propranolol-bepridil therapy in stable angina pectoris. Am J Cardiol 1985;55:43C-49C.
21. Singh BN: Comparative efficacy and safety of bepridil and diltiazem in chronic stable angina pectoris refractory to diltiazem. The Bepridil Collaborative Study Group. Am J Cardiol 1991;68:306-312.
22. Cohen M, Demers C, Gurfinkel EP, et al for the ESSENCE investigators: A comparison of low molecular-weight heparin with untraditional heparin for unstable coronary artery disease. N Engl J Med 1997;337:447-452.
23. The FRISC II Investigators: Invasive compared with non-invasive treatment in unstable coronary artery disease. FRISC II prospective randomized multicenter study fragmin and fast revascularization during instability in coronary artery disease Investigators. Lancet 1999;354:780-786.
24. Fragasso G, Piatti PM, Monti L, et al: Acute effects of heparin administration on the ischemic threshold of patients with coronary artery disease. J Am Coll Cardiol 2002;39:413-419.
25. Melandri G, Semprini F, Cervi V, et al: Benefit of adding low molecular weight heparin to the conventional treatment of stable angina pectoris: A double-blind randomized, placebo-controlled trial. Circulation 1993;88:2517-2523.
26. Quyyami AA, Diodati JG, Lakatos E, et al: Angiogenic effects of low molecular weight heparin in patients with stable coronary artery disease: A pilot study. J Am Coll Cardiol 1993;22:635-641.
27. The Clopidogrel in Unstable Angina to Prevent Recurrent Events Trial Investigators: Effects of clopidogrel in addition to aspirin in patients with acute coronary syndromes without ST-segment elevation. N Engl J Med 2001;345:494-502.
28. Schoebel FC, Leschke M, Jax TX, et al: Chronic-intermittent urokinase therapy in patients with end-stage coronary artery disease and refractory angina pectoris: A pilot study. Clin Cardiol 1996;19:115-120.
29. Leschke M, Schoebel FC, Mecklenbeck W, et al: Long-term intermittent urokinase therapy in patients with end-stage coronary artery disease and refractory angina pectoris: A randomized dose-response trial. J Am Coll Cardiol 1996;27:575-584.
30. Kim MC, Kini A, Sharma SK: Refractory angina pectoris. J Am Coll Cardiol 2002;39:923-934.
31. Ernst E: Chelation therapy for coronary heart disease: An overview of all clinical investigations. Am Heart J 2000;140:139-141.
32. Knudson ML, Wyse DG, Gailbraith PD, et al: Chelation therapy for ischemic heart disease: A randomized controlled trial. JAMA 2002;287:481-486.
33. American Heart Association: AHA statement on chelation therapy. In: Heart and Stroke A-Z Guide. Dallas, American Heart Association, 2000.
34. Lawson WE, Hui JC, Soroff HS, et al: Efficacy of enhanced external counterpulsation in the treatment of angina pectoris. Am J Cardiol 1992;70:859-862.
35. Lawson WE, Hui JC, Zheng ZS, et al: Improved exercise tolerance following enhanced external counterpulsation: Cardiac or peripheral effect? Cardiology 1996;87:271-275.
36. Lawson WE, Hui JC, Lang G, et al: Treatment benefit in the enhanced external counterpulsation consortium. Cardiology 2000;94:31-35.
37. Masuda D, Nohara R, Hirai T, et al: Enhanced external counterpulsation improved myocardial perfusion and coronary flow reserve in patients with chronic stable angina; evaluation by (13) N-ammonia positron emission tomography. Eur Heart J 2001;22:1451-1458.
38. Arora R, Chou T, Jain D, et al: The Multicenter Study of Enhanced External CounterPulsation (MUST-EECP): Effect of EECP on exercise-induced myocardial ischemia and anginal episodes. J Am Coll Cardiol 1999;33:1833-1840.
39. Arora R, Chou T, Jain F, et al: Effects of external counter pulsation on health-related quality of life continue 12 months after treatment. A substudy of multicenter study of enhanced external counter pulsation. J Invest Med 2002;50:25-32.
40. Lawson WE, Hui JC, Cohn PF: Long-term prognosis of patients with angina treatment with enhanced external counterpulsation: Five-year follow-up study. Clin Cardiol 2000;23:254-258.
41. Barsness G, Feldman AM, Holmes DR, et al: The International EECP Patient Registry (IEPR): Design, methods, baseline characteristics, and acute results. Clin Cardiol 2001;24:435-442.
42. Lawson WE, Kennaed ED, Holubkou R, et al: Benefit and safety of enhanced external counter pulsation in treating coronary artery disease patients with history of congestive heart failure. Cardiology 2001;96:78-84.
43. Urano H, Ikeda H, Ueno T, et al: Enhanced external counterpulsation improves exercise tolerance, reduces exercise-induced myocardial ischemia and improves left ventricular diastolic filling

in patients with coronary artery disease. J Am Coll Cardiol 2001;37:93-99.

44. Springer S, Fife A, Lawson W, et al: Psychosocial effects of enhanced external counterpulsation in the angina patient: A second study. Psychosomatics 2001;42:124-132.

45. Bueno EA, Mamtani R, Frishman WH: Alternative approaches to the medical management of angina pectoris. Acupuncture, electrical nerve stimulation, and spinal cord stimulation. Heart Dis 2001;3:236-241.

46. Chester M, Hammond C, Leach A: Long-term benefits of stellate ganglion block in severe chronic refractory angina. Pain 2000;87:103-105.

47. Chester M, Hammond C, Leach A: Transcutaneous electrical stimulation in severe angina pectoris. Eur Heart J 1982;3:297-302.

48. Mannheimer C, Carlsson CA, Emanuelson H, et al: The effects of transcutaneous electric stimulation in patients with severe angina pectoris. Circulation 1985;71:308-316.

49. Mannheimer C, Carlsson CA, Vedin A, Wilhelmsson C: Transcutaneous electrical nerve stimulation (TENS) in angina pectoris. Pain 1986;26:291-300.

50. Emanuelsson H, Mannheimer C, Waagstein F, Wilhelmsson C: Catecholamine metabolism during pacing-induced angina pectoris and the effect of transcutaneous electrical nerve stimulation. Am Heart J 1987;114:1360-1366.

51. Mannheimer C, Emanuelsson H, Waagstein F, Wilhemsson C: Influence of naloxone on the effects of high frequency transcutaneous electrical nerve stimulation in angina pectoris induced by atrial pacing. Br Heart J 1989;62:36-42.

52. Magarian GJ, Leikam B, Palac R: Transcutaneous electrical nerve stimulation (TENS) for treatment of severe angina pectoris refractory to maximal medical and surgical management—a case report. Angiology 1990;41;408-411.

53. West PD, Colquhoun DM: TENS in refractory angina pectoris. Three case reports. Med J Aust 1993;158:448-449.

54. Borjesson M, Eriksson P, Dellborg M, et al: Transcutaneous electrical nerve stimulation in unstable angina pectoris. Coronary Artery Dis 1997;8:543-550.

55. Borjesson M: Visceral chest pain in unstable angina pectoris and effects of transcutaneous electrical nerve stimulation. Herz 1999;24:114-125.

56. Murphy DF, Giles KE: Dorsal column stimulation for pain relief from intractable angina pectoris. Pain 1987;28:365-368.

57. Mannheimer C, Augustinsson LE, Carlsson CA, et al: Epidural spinal electrical stimulation in severe angina pectoris. Br Heart J 1988;49:46-61.

58. Sanderson JE, Brooksby P, Waterhouse D, et al: Epidural spinal electrical stimulation for severe angina: A study of its effects on symptoms, exercise tolerance and degree of ischaemia. Eur Heart J 1992;13:628-633.

59. Harke H, Ladleif HU, Rethage B, Grosser KD: Epidural spinal cord stimulation in therapy-resistant angina pectoris. Anaesthetist 1993;42:557-563.

60. Mannheimer C, Augustinsson LE, Eliasson T: Spinal cord stimulation in severe angina pectoris. Reduced ischemia and increased quality of life. Lakartidningen 1994;91:3257-3261.

61. Jacques L, Napoleon MS, Gagnon RM, et al: Epidural stimulation in the treatment of refractory angina. Ann Chir 1994;48:764-767.

62. Hautvast RW, DeJongste MJ, Staal MJ, et al: Spinal cord stimulation in chronic intractable angina pectoris: A randomized, controlled efficacy study. Am Heart J 1998;137:1114-1120.

63. Hautvast RWM, Brower J, DeJonste MJL, Lie KI: Effect of spinal cord stimulation on heart rate variability and myocardial ischemia in patients with chronic intractable angina pectoris: A prospective ambulatory electrocardiographic study. Clin Cardiol 1998;21:33-38.

64. Greco S, Auriti A, Fiume D, et al: Spinal cord stimulation for the treatment of refractory angina pectoris: A two-year follow up. Pacing Clin Electrophysiol 1999;22:26-32.

65. Norrsell H, Eliasson T, Augustinsson LE, Mannheimer C: Spinal cord stimulation in angina pectoris—what is the current situation? Lakartidningen 1999;96:1430-1432, 1435-1437.

66. Barolat G, Sharan AD: Future trends in spinal cord stimulation. 2000;22:279-284.

67. Latif OA, Nedeljkovic SS, Stevenson LW: Spinal cord stimulation for chronic intractable angina pectoris: A unified theory on its mechanism. Clin Cardiol 2001;24:533-541.

68. Mannheimer C, Eliasson T, Augustinsson LE, et al: Electrical stimulation versus coronary artery bypass surgery is severe angina pectoris: The ESBY study. Ciruculation 1998;37:1157-1163.

69. Murray S, Collins PD, James MA: Neurostimulation treatment for angina pectoris. Heart 2000;83:217-220.

70. Wearn JT, Mettier SR, Klumpp TG, et al: The nature of the vascular communications between the coronary arteries and the chambers of the heart. Am Heart J 1933;9:143-164.

71. Okada M, Ikuta H, Shimizu K, et al: Alternative method of myocardial revascularization by laser: Experimental and clinical study. Kobe J Med Sci 1986;32:151-161.

72. Horvath KA, Cohn LH, Cooley DA, et al: Transmyocardial laser revascularization: Results of a multicenter trial with transmyocardial laser revascularization used as sole therapy for end-stage coronary artery disease. J Thorac Cardiovasc Surg 1997;113:645-654.

73. Cherian SM, Bobryshev YV, Liang H, et al: Ultrastructural and immunohistochemical analysis of early myocardial changes following transmyocardial laser revascularization. J Car Surg 2000;15: 341-346.

74. Al-Sheikh T, Allen KB, Straka SP, et al: Cardiac sympathetic denervation after transmyocardial laser revascularization. Circulation 1999;13;100:135-140.

75. Lange RA, Hillis LD: Transmyocardial laser revascularization. N Engl J Med 1999;341:1074-1076.

76. Burns SM, Sharples LD, Tait S, et al: The transmyocardial laser revascularization international registry report. Eur Heart J 1999; 20:31-37.

77. Nagele H, Stubbe H, Niendaber C, Rodiger W: Results of transmyocardial laser revascularization in non-revascularizable coronary artery disease after 3 years follow up. Eur Heart J 1998;19: 1525-1530.

78. Horvath KA, Aranki SF, Cohn LH, et al: Sustained angina relief 5 years after transmyocardial laser revascularization with a CO_2 laser. Circulation 2001;104:181-184.

79. Bridges CR: Myocardial laser revascularization: The controversy and the data. Ann Thor Surg 2000;69:655-662.

80. Burkhoff D, Jones JW, Becker LC: Variability of myocardial perfusion defects assessed by thallium-201 scintigraphy in patients with coronary artery disease not amenable to angioplasty or bypass surgery. J Am Coll Cardiol 2001;38:1033-1039.

81. Schofield PM, Sharples LD, Caine N, et al: Transmyocardial laser revascularization in patients with refractory angina: A randomized controlled trial. Lancet 1999;353:519-524.

82. Aaberge L, Nordstrand K, Dragsund M, et al: Transmyocardial revascularization with CO_2 laser refractory angina pectoris clinical results from the Norwegian Randomized trial. J Am Coll Cardiol 2000;35:1170-1177.

83. Aaberge L, Rootwelt K, Blomhoff S, et al: Continued symptomatic improvement three to five years after transmyocardial revascularization with CO_2 laser. J Am Coll Cardiol 2002;39:1588-1593.

84. Frazier OH, March RJ, Horvath KA: Transmyocardial revascularization with a carbon dioxide laser in patients with end-stage coronary artery disease. N Engl J Med 1999;341:1021-1028.

85. Allen KB, Dowling RD, Fudge TL, et al: Comparison of transmyocardial revascularization with medical therapy in patients with refractory angina. N Engl J Med 1999;341:1029-1036.

86. Burkoff D, Schmidt S, Schulman SP, et al: The Angina Treatments—Lasers and Normal Therapies In Comparison Investigators (ATLANTIC). Transmyocardial laser revascularization compared with continued medical therapy for treatment of refractory angina pectoris: A prospective randomized trial. Lancet 1999;354: 885-890.

87. Hughes GC, Landolfo KP, Lowe JE, et al: Perioperative morbidity after transmyocardial laser revascularization: Incidence and risk factors for adverse events. J Am Coll Cardiol 1999;33: 1021-1026.

88. Leon MB, Bain DS, Moses JW, et al: Direct laser myocardial revascularization with Biosense™ LV electromechanical mapping in patients with refractory myocardial ischemia: Final results of a blind randomized clinical trial. J Am Coll Cardiol 2001;38: 595-596.

89. Grambow DW, Topol EJ: Effect of maximal medical therapy on refractionness of unstable angina pectoris. Am J Cardiol 1992;70:557-560.

90. Kornowski R, Bhargava B, Leon MB: Percutaneous transmyocardial laser revascularization: An overview. Cath Cardiov Interv 1999;47:354-359.

91. Lauer B, Junghans U, Stahl F, et al: Catheter-based percutaneous myocardial revascularization in patients with end-stage coronary artery disease. J Am Coll Cardiol 1999;34:1663–1670.

92. Oesterle SN, Sanborn TA, Ali N, et al: Percutaneous transmyocardial laser revascularisation for severe angina: The Potential Class Improvement From Intramyocardial Channels (PACIFIC) randomized trial. Lancet 2000;356:1705–1710.

93. Perin E: Eclipse PTMR system study: Late breaking trials. Presented at American College of Cardiology, March 20, 2000, Anaheim, CA.

94. Stone GW, Teirstein PS, Rubensteinet R, et al: A prospective, multicenter randomized trial of percutaneous transmyocardial laser revascularization in patients with nonrecanalizable chronic total occlusions. J Am Coll Cardiol 2002;39:1581–1587.

95. Makhoul RG, Cole CW, McCann RJ: Vascular complications of the intra-aortic balloon pump. An analysis of 436 patients. Am Surg 1993;59:564–569.

96. Blum A, Hathaway L, Mincemoyer R, et al: Oral L-arginine in patients with coronary artery disease on medical management. Circulation 2000;101:2160–2164.

97. Ceremuzynski L, Chaniec T, Herbaszynska-Cedro K: Effect of supplemental oral L-arginine on exercise capacity in patients with stable angina pectoris. Am J Cardiol 1997;80:331–333.

98. Lerman A, Burnett JC Jr, Higano ST, et al: Long-term L-arginine supplementation improves small-vessel coronary endothelial function in humans. Circulation 1998;97:2123–2128.

99. Kantor PF, Lucien A, Kozak R, et al: The antianginal drug trimetazidine shifts cardiac energy metabolism from fatty acid oxidation to glucose oxidation by inhibiting mitochondrial long-chain 3-ketoacyl coenzyme A thiolase. Circ Res 2000;86:580–588.

100. Anderson JR, Khou S, Nawarskas JJ: Ranolazine: A potential new treatment for chronic stable angina. Heart Dis 2001;3:263–269.

101. Takeshita S, Zheng LP, Brogi E, et al: Therapeutic angiogenesis. J Clin Invest 1994;93:662–670.

102. Lopez JJ, Laham RJ, Stamler A, et al: VEGF administration in chronic myocardial ischemia in pigs. Cardiovasc Res 1998;40:272–281.

103. Sato K, Lathan RJ, Pearlman JD, et al: Efficacy of intracoronary versus mitravenous FGF-2 in a pig model of chronic myocardial ischemia. Ann Thorac Surg 2000;70:2115–2118.

104. Kontos CD, Annex BH: Angiogenesis. Curr Atheroscler Rep 1999;1:165–171.

105. Losordo DW, Vale PR, Symes JF, et al: Gene therapy for myocardial angiogenesis: Initial clinical results with direct myocardial injection of ph VEGF 165 as sole therapy for myocardial ischemia. Circulation 1998;98:2800–2804.

106. Schumacher B, Pecher P, von Specht BU, et al: Induction of neoangiogenesis in ischemic myocardium by human growth factors: First clinical results of a new treatment of coronary heart disease. Circulation 1998;7:645–650.

107. Rosengart TK, Lee LY, Patel SR, et al: Angiogenesis gene therapy: Phase I assessment of direct intramyocardial administration of an adenovirus vector expressing VEGF121 cDNA to individuals with clinically significant severe coronary artery disease. Circulation 1999;100:468–474.

108. Rosengart TK, Lee LY, Patel SR, et al: Angiogenesis gene therapy: phase I assessment of direct intramyocardial administration of an adenovirus vector expressing VEGF121 cCNA to individuals with clinically significant severe coronary artery disease. Circulation 1999;100:468–474.

109. Laham RJ, Selke FW, Edelman ER, et al: Local perivascular delivery of basic fibroblast growth factor in patients undergoing coronary bypass surgery: Results of a phase I randomized, double-blind, placebo-controlled trial. Circulation 1999;100:1865–1871.

110. Udelson JE, Dilsizian J, Laham RJ, et al: Therapeutic angiogenesis with recombinant fibroblast growth factor-2 improves stress and rest myocardial perfusion abnormalities in patients with severe symptomatic chronic coronary artery disease. Circulation 2000;102:1605–1610.

111. Rosengart TK, Lee LY, Patel SR, et al: Six-month assessment of a phase I trial of angiogenic gene therapy for the treatment of coronary artery disease using direct intramyocardial administration of an adenovirus vector expressing the VEGF121 cDNA. Ann Surg 1999;230:466–470.

112. Henry TD, Annex, BH, Azrin MA, et al: Final results of the VIVA trial of rhVEGF for human therapeutic angiogenesis. Circulation 1999;100(Suppl I):476.

113. Simons M, Annex BH, Laham RJ, et al: Pharmacologist treatment of coronary artery disease with recombinant fibroblast growth factor-2 (rFGF-2): Double-blind, randomized controlled clinical trial. Circulation 2002;105:788–793.

114. Ware JA: Too many vessels? Not enough? The wrong kind? The VEGF debate continues. Nat Med 2001;7:425–429.

115. Henry TD, Rocha-Singh K, Isner JM, et al: Intracoronary administration of recombinant human vascular endothelial growth factor to patients with coronary artery disease. Am Heart J 2001;142:872–880.

116. Epstein SE, Kornowski R, Fuchs S, Dvorak HF: Angiogenesis therapy. Amidst the hype, the reflected potential for serious side effects. Circulation 2001;04:115–119.

117. Grines CL, Watkins MW, Helmer G, et al: Angiogenic gene therapy (AGENT) trial in patients with stable angina pectoris. Circulation 2002;05:1291–1297.

118. Kay EB, Suxuki A: Coronary venous retroperfusion for myocardial revascularization. Ann Thorac Surg 1975;9:63–72.

119. Oesterle SN, Reifart N, Hauptmann E, et al: Percutaneous in situ coronary venous arterialization: Report of the first human catheter-based coronary artery bypass. Circulation 2001;03:2539–2543.

120. Fitzgerald PJ, Hayase M, Yeung AC, et al: New approaches and conduits: In situ venous arterialization and coronary artery bypass. Curr Interv Cardiol Rep 1999;1:127–137.

121. Mukherjee D, Bhatt D, Roe MT, et al: Direct myocardial revascularization and angiogenesis: How many patients might be eligible? Am J Cardiol 1999;4:598–600.

■ ■ ■ chapter 3 9

The Elderly, Women, and Patients with Diabetes Mellitus

Darren K. McGuire
L. Kristin Newby
Mimi Sengupta Biswas
Judith S. Hochman

The recent guidelines published by the American College of Cardiology and the American Heart Association (ACC/AHA) for the management of patients with acute coronary syndromes (ACS), which include non–ST-segment elevation myocardial infarction (MI) and unstable angina, have identified several groups of patients that warrant special consideration in the management of ACS,[1,2] including the elderly, women, and patients with diabetes. This chapter reviews the considerations for each of these patient groups when they present with ACS.

THE ELDERLY

Epidemiology

The definition of *elderly* varies among different studies. As the population has aged, the criteria for elderly have largely shifted from age greater than 65 years to greater than 75 years. The elderly represent the fastest growing segment of the population in developed countries. In 1998, 1 in 35 Americans was older than age 75 years,[3] and in 2000, 1 in 17 Americans was older than age 75 (Table 39-1).[4] By 2050, it is projected that 1 in 12 will be older than age 75. The prevalence of coronary heart disease increases with age (Fig. 39-1). The elderly account for approximately 10% of all patients with ACS,[5] 60% of all deaths from MI, and greater than $10 billion in health care costs annually in the United States.[6,7] As the population ages, the worldwide burden of cardiac disease carried by the elderly segment of the population also will increase dramatically.

Despite the aging of the population and the accompanying increasing burden of coronary artery disease (CAD), much less is known about diagnosis and management of elderly patients with ACS and of the effects of secondary prevention strategies in this age group. In part, this decreased knowledge relates to the failure of

randomized clinical trials to enroll meaningful numbers of elderly participants and to the lack of systematic study of symptoms and signs of acute coronary disease in the elderly.[8]

Several unique pathophysiologic features of aging and of CAD in the elderly make them prone to more atypical presentations of unstable angina or MI. In addition, these properties and comorbidities render the elderly at higher risk for adverse outcomes after ACS, more likely to suffer side effects of routine medical therapies, and more likely to have complications of revascularization. Despite these observations, where evidence exists, the elderly in general derive as great or greater absolute benefit from most standard therapies for ACS even if relative treatment effects are lower. The complication rates and outcomes after revascularization are improving.

Given these complexities in the face of a growing elderly population, clinicians must understand better the

■ ■ ■

TABLE 39-1   PROJECTED 2000 U.S. POPULATION AND PROPORTION DISTRIBUTION BY AGE

AGE (YR)	POPULATION
Total	274,634,000
< 1	3,795,000
1–4	15,192,000
5–14	39,977,000
15–24	38,077,000
25–34	37,233,000
35–44	44,659,000
45–54	37,030,000
55–64	23,961,000
65–74	18,136,000
≥ 75	16,574,000

Adapted from Anderson RN, Rosenberg HM: Age standardization of death rates: Implementation of the year 2000 standard. National Vital Statistics Reports, vol 47. Hyattsville, MD, National Center for Health Statistics, 1998, pp 1–17.

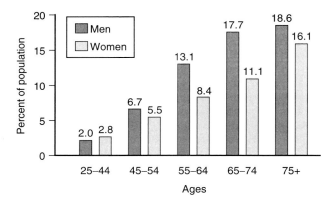

FIGURE 39–1. Estimated prevalence of coronary heart disease by age and sex: United States: 1988-1994. (From American Heart Association: American Heart Association heart and stroke 2001 statistical update, 2001.)

manifestations of coronary disease in the elderly and of their response to evidence-based therapies previously tested primarily in younger populations. Based on the data available, the ACC/AHA unstable angina guidelines make the following class I recommendations regarding management of the elderly with ACS[1,2]:

1. Decisions on management should reflect consideration of general health, comorbidities, cognitive status, and life expectancy.
2. Attention should be paid to altered pharmacokinetics and sensitivity to hypotensive drugs.
3. Intensive medical and interventional management of ACS may be undertaken but with close observation for adverse effects of these therapies.

Pathophysiology

The process of aging includes the development of atherosclerosis over time, resulting in an increased burden of coronary and cerebrovascular disease in the elderly compared with younger patients. The TIMI (Thrombolysis in Myocardial Infarction) III registry collected data on more than 800 patients older than age 75 years from among more than 3300 patients with non–ST-segment elevation ACS.[5] Coronary angiography was used less frequently in the elderly than in younger patients (relative risk, 0.65; $P < .001$), and when performed, the elderly had much more extensive disease (relative risk of multivessel disease, 2.0; $P < .001$). In the PURSUIT (Platelet Glycoprotein IIb/IIIa in Unstable Angina: Receptor Suppression Using Integrilin Therapy) clinical trial database, only 38% of 506 patients older than age 80 underwent angiography, but 72% of those who did had multivessel CAD.[9] Of 1324 patients between the ages of 70 and 80 years, 57% underwent angiography, and 68% had multivessel CAD.[9] In the 6557 patients younger than age 70, the corresponding figures were a 67% angiography rate and 33% rate of multivessel CAD.

In addition to a greater atherosclerotic burden, the elderly have decreased vascular compliance and more systolic hypertension resulting in increased afterload. Cardiac compliance is decreased because of ventricular

hypertrophy and fibrosis as a result of the aging process and unrecognized prior infarction, which is more common in the elderly than in younger patients.[10] These features result in a greater prevalence of systolic and, in particular, diastolic dysfunction among the elderly,[11,12] which in part contribute to their more atypical presentations of acute cardiac ischemia, especially dyspnea.

Physiologic changes of aging lead to changes in drug distribution and metabolism and alterations in response to anti-ischemic and antithrombotic medications in the elderly. The pharmacokinetics and pharmacodynamics of drugs frequently used to treat ACS are altered relative to younger populations.[13] As a result of diminished cardiac compliance and vascular tone and decreased β-adrenergic and baroreceptor responses, particular caution is warranted with the use of β-blockers and drugs that elicit a hypotensive response, such as angiotensin-converting enzyme (ACE) inhibitors and nitrates. Granger and colleagues[14] showed that after adjustment for other confounding factors, the elderly seem to be more sensitive to the effects of heparin anticoagulation therapy.

Lower volumes of distribution and age-related decreases in renal and hepatic function may lead to increased levels of many medications.[13] Renal insufficiency associated with aging can lead to increased plasma levels of drugs such as atenolol or small-molecule glycoprotein IIb/IIIa inhibitors, which depend on renal clearance of the unchanged parent drug. The effects of polypharmacy in the elderly in the setting of alterations in metabolism and competition for hepatic metabolic pathways and altered renal clearance are not well understood. Polypharmacy is increasingly a consideration because 25% of older patients experience an adverse drug reaction, and 3% to 10% of all hospitalizations among the elderly are the result of an adverse drug reaction.[15]

Clinical Presentation

Elderly patients with ACS often present with atypical symptoms that may lead to delayed diagnosis and intervention. Dyspnea, confusion, fatigue, and abdominal pain are frequently presenting symptoms of acute coronary ischemia in the elderly.[16] Although typical presentations of MI occur, they are much less frequent than in younger patients. Delayed recognition of atypical ischemic symptoms by patients and health care providers, greater prevalence of baseline electrocardiogram abnormalities (e.g., bundle-branch blocks and left ventricular hypertrophy) that obscure ischemic changes in the ST segment,[17] and social and physical isolation lead to delays in presentation and treatment of the elderly with ACS.

The elderly are more prone to bradyarrhythmias and tachyarrhythmias, which may complicate presentations with ACS. In addition, comorbidities, including age-related renal insufficiency, chronic obstructive pulmonary disease, and cerebrovascular disease, contribute to higher morbidity and mortality rates with ACS and may make medical therapy more complicated.

Compared with younger patients in the TIMI III registry, the risk of death after ACS in the elderly was 3.76-fold increased and for (re)MI, 2.02-fold increased.[5] In models derived from clinical trial databases, for acute ST-segment elevation MI and non–ST-segment elevation ACS, age is the strongest predictor of short-term mortality and is a strong predictor of the composite of death or MI.[18-20]

Clinical Management

Despite their higher risk and greater potential for benefit from proven medical therapies, the elderly frequently do not receive treatments that have been shown to be effective in clinical trials. In part, this situation relates to patient preference, higher risk for side effects, and greater likelihood of contraindications related to comorbidities, including impaired cognitive status. Rates of use of aspirin, β-blockers, and ACE inhibitors among the elderly remain low even among ideal candidates for these beneficial therapies, however. Krumholz and colleagues[21] showed that among Medicare patients older than age 65, the use of ACE inhibitors in ideal candidates at discharge after acute MI was only 45%. Similarly, among ideal MI patients 65 years or older in the Cooperative Cardiovascular Project database, only 50% were discharged on a β-blocker.[22] Among ACS patients randomized in the GUSTO IIb trial, the odds ratio for discharge use of aspirin was 0.85 (0.73 to 1.00) for patients aged 65 to 75 years and 0.76 (0.62 to 0.93) for patients older than 75 years relative to patients younger than 65 years.[23] In that study, patients older than age 75 were more likely to receive β-blockers and ACE inhibitors than younger patients, which may have been related to the higher likelihood of hypertension and diabetes among the elderly.

As detailed by Lee and colleagues,[8] the elderly continue to be underenrolled in phase III clinical trials designed to assess the efficacy and safety of medical interventions in this population. Much of clinical practice in the management of ACS requires the extrapolation of results from studies in younger patients to treatment in the elderly. Increased efforts to include the elderly in clinical trials and to improve the application of evidence-based therapy to optimize outcome and minimize risk in this high-risk group are indicated.

Antiplatelet Therapy

The beneficial effect of aspirin in the management of patients with ACS and in secondary prevention after these events has been shown. Although as previously noted, the elderly are at higher risk for adverse cardiovascular events, they derive similar or greater absolute benefit from aspirin therapy compared with younger patients. In the Antiplatelet Trialists meta-analysis of the effectiveness of aspirin in placebo-controlled studies, among 14,335 patients age 65 or older, the absolute benefit from aspirin therapy was 45 deaths, MIs, or strokes prevented per 1000 patients treated ($P < .0001$).[24] This benefit was greater than that for patients younger than 65 (32 events prevented/1000 patients treated, also highly significant). No data were available for the subset older than 75, but there is no reason to expect that the benefit would be less.

The CURE (Clopidogrel in Unstable Angina to Prevent Recurrent Ischemic Events) trial compared more potent oral antiplatelet therapy, clopidogrel (a thienopyridine derivative that inhibits platelet aggregation and activation via interaction with the platelet ADP receptor), combined with aspirin versus aspirin alone for treatment of patients with ACS.[25] Nearly half of the patients randomized in this trial were older than 65. Although at higher baseline risk, in the elderly cohort of 6208 patients, the absolute risk reduction (2%) associated with combination clopidogrel and aspirin therapy versus aspirin (13.3% versus 15.3%) was similar to that for patients younger than 65 (5.4% versus 7.6%).[25] Results were not reported for patients older than 75. The findings of CURE are particularly noteworthy since the population overall had a low rate of revascularization, which may be more reflective of clinical practice in the care of the elderly with ACS.

In addition to oral antiplatelet therapy in the treatment of ACS, intravenous inhibitors of the platelet glycoprotein IIb/IIIa receptor, eptifibatide and tirofiban, are effective in reducing the risk of death or (re)MI.[26-28] Although only small proportions of patients in phase III clinical trials of these agents were older than 75, the treatment benefits observed were not different by age subgroups. PRISM and PRISM-PLUS (Platelet Receptor Inhibition in Ischemic Syndrome Management in Patients Limited by Unstable Angina Signs and Symptoms), which investigated the use of tirofiban for treatment of ACS, revealed similar, favorable risk ratios for treatment with tirofiban across all age subgroups.[27,28]

Detailed analyses of the associations of age with outcome were carried out in the PURSUIT trial of eptifibatide for treatment of ACS.[9] In this trial, 2904 patients older than age 70 were randomized; 506 were 80 or older. In that study, for every 10-year increase in age, there was a 97% increase in the odds of death at 30 days and a 33% increase in the odds of death or MI. As age increased, there was an increased risk of bleeding with glycoprotein IIb/IIIa therapy, but there was no statistically significant interaction of age with the effect of therapy. Among 2938 patients between ages 70 and 79, the absolute reduction in death or MI was 1.8% and was similar to the 1.5% absolute reduction in the overall trial population, although the relative risk reduction was smaller. In the 506 patients age 80 or older, there was a higher 30-day death or MI rate among eptifibatide-treated compared with placebo-treated patients (29.3% versus 23.7%), which coupled with the increased bleeding rate suggests caution in using these drugs in the very elderly.

Antithrombotic Therapy

Antithrombotic therapy is a cornerstone of management of ACS. Intravenous unfractionated heparin combined with aspirin has been shown to be more effective than aspirin alone in treatment of patients with unstable angina.[29] Data are limited, however, on the efficacy of this therapy, specifically in the elderly. Caution in the use of intravenous unfractionated heparin is warranted in the elderly because the risk for bleeding with antithrombotic therapy increases with age. It seems that the elderly may have increased sensitivity to the anticoagulant effects of heparin even after adjusting for weight and other confounders.[14]

Low-molecular-weight heparins have been shown to be effective in treating non–ST-segment elevation ACS. In a pooled analysis of the TIMI 11B and Efficacy and Safety of Subcutaneous Enoxaparin in Non–Q-Wave Coronary Events (ESSENCE) trials, enoxaparin was shown to be modestly more effective than unfractionated heparin in preventing the occurrence of death or (re)MI at 43 days in short-term follow-up (odds ratio 0.82 [0.69 to 0.97]).[30] As in other trials, the experience with these agents in patients older than age 75 was limited. In both studies, subgroup analyses revealed greater treatment effects among patients older than 65 than the younger cohorts.[31,32]

Angiotensin-Converting Enzyme Inhibitors

As with other medical therapies, ACE inhibitors are underused in elderly patients, including patients who seem to be ideal candidates. In one report, the odds ratio for the use of ACE inhibitors in ideal candidates aged 75 to 84 years was 0.75 (0.66 to 0.85) relative to patients younger than 65.[21] In the older than 65 cohort, only 8% were classified as ideal candidates, however. As with many earlier trials in ACS and acute MI, age greater than 75 was an exclusion criterion to most trials of ACE inhibitors. The results of these trials should be extrapolated with caution to the elderly, particularly given the increasing prevalence of renal dysfunction and susceptibility to hypotension.

The results of the HOPE (Heart Outcomes Prevention Evaluation) study support the contention that, in the absence of contraindications, ACE inhibitor therapy should be prescribed for elderly patients for secondary prevention after ACS. The HOPE study randomized 5128 patients age 65 or older to either ramipril or placebo with follow-up over a mean of 4.5 years.[33] For the primary end point of death, MI, or stroke and for MI alone, among patients older than 65, the point estimate of the odds ratio of treatment effect with ramipril was even greater than in younger patients.[33,34]

β-Blockers

Most trials of β-blocker therapy after ACS have not enrolled patients older than age 75. Adjusted analyses in large administrative databases have shown, however, relative risk reductions with β-blocker use at discharge (14% lower risk of mortality at 1 year) similar to reductions that have been shown in clinical trials of younger and lower risk populations.[22] As noted earlier, β-blockers are underused in the elderly. β-Blockers are indicated for use in elderly patients with ACS acutely and long term after considering comorbidities and side effects in selecting, initiating, and titrating these agents.

Lipid-Lowering Therapy

The ACC/AHA guidelines for the management of patients with unstable angina and non–ST-segment elevation acute MI recommend as a class I indication the prescription of lipid-lowering therapy and diet after discharge in patients with low-density lipoprotein (LDL) cholesterol greater than 130 mg/dL.[1,2] Similarly the National Cholesterol Education Program–Adult Treatment Panel III recommendations include discharge prescription of statin therapy for ACS patients with LDL cholesterol greater than or equal to 130 mg/dL.[35] These recommendations are based largely on extrapolation from large trials of lipid-lowering therapy in secondary prevention, however, all of which excluded patients older than age 75. Despite these limitations in the data, in patients between 65 and 75 years old enrolled in these randomized trials, the use of statin therapy was associated with similar relative risk reductions and larger absolute reductions compared with younger patients.[36,37] Only randomized trials of statin therapy in older patients can confirm their safety and efficacy in the older-than-75 population. Until then, the National Cholesterol Education Program guidelines for cholesterol lowering in the elderly recommend the use of statin therapy similar to in younger populations unless life expectancy is less than 2 years.[38]

Revascularization

As with trials of medical therapy, patients older than 75 generally have been excluded from randomized clinical trials of coronary revascularization strategies. Although the use of angiography and coronary revascularization is lower in the elderly, and their risks (for mortality and morbidity) from these procedures are higher,[39,40] preliminary observational data suggest they may derive substantial benefit from percutaneous coronary intervention and bypass surgery when appropriate (Peterson ED, Alexander KP, personal communication). The ACC/AHA guidelines for bypass surgery and percutaneous coronary intervention recommend that while awaiting further data, age alone should not be used as the sole criterion when considering revascularization procedures.[41,42]

Comparisons of early invasive treatment with early conservative management of patients with ACS have shed some additional light on the effectiveness of invasive strategies in the elderly with non–ST-segment elevation ACS. Two large, multicenter randomized trials have addressed early conservative versus invasive strategies on the background of contemporary antithrombotic and antiplatelet therapy—the FRISC II trial with a background of low-molecular-weight heparin (dalteparin) therapy[43] and the TACTICS (Treat Angina with Aggrastat and Determine Cost of Therapy with an Invasive or Conservative Strategy) trial on a background of glycoprotein IIb/IIIa inhibitor therapy with tirofiban.[44] Although neither FRISC II nor TACTICS addressed specifically the issue of invasive versus conservative strategies in the elderly (≥75 years old), their findings in populations older than age 65 are of interest.

FRISC II randomized 2457 patients with unstable angina or non–ST-segment elevation MI to either early conservative care or angiography with revascularization within 7 days.[43] All patients received open-label dalteparin during the first 5 days or until percutaneous revascularization was accomplished (planned within 7 days of randomization). In this study, the median age in the invasive arm was 66 years, and the oldest patient was 84 years. At 1 year, there was a 1.7% absolute and 43% relative reduction in mortality and a 3.7% absolute and 26% relative reduction in death or MI in the invasive group compared with the conservative group.[45] By subgroup analysis, the point estimate of the odds ratio for death or MI at 1 year for early invasive versus conservative care was 0.63 (0.48 to 0.83) for the group age 65 or older (n = 1490), which was more favorable than for patients younger than 65 (n = 1013; OR 0.93 [0.85 to 1.33]).[45]

Similarly, in TACTICS, 2220 patients with non–ST-segment elevation ACS were randomized to an early invasive strategy with angiography within 4 to 48 hours and revascularization as appropriate or to an early conservative strategy, reserving catheterization for objective evidence of recurrent ischemia or after positive stress test.[44] In this study, 43% of the patients enrolled were at least 65 years old. The main study analysis showed an odds ratio for 6-month death or MI of 0.78 (0.26 to 0.97) for the invasive versus conservative strategy. As expected, the 6-month death or MI rate was higher among the 65 or older age group, but similar to the results of the FRISC II subgroup analysis; the point estimate of the odds ratio in this group was more favorable than for patients younger than 65.

The results of these analyses support consideration of early invasive strategies in older patients, although further study of the older-than-75 population is needed to confirm that these results can be extrapolated to more extremes of age. Patient preferences often determine the initial strategy.

Conclusions

The elderly are the fastest growing segment of the population, and in the developed world, they carry a great, ever-increasing burden of CAD and its sequelae. They represent one of the most understudied groups of patients with acute ischemic heart disease, however. Special conditions of aging leave the elderly at higher risk of adverse outcomes and adverse side effects and complications from standard medical and interventional treatment for ACS. These therapies have been tested mostly in younger populations. Enhanced inclusion of the elderly in clinical trials is imperative to generate the evidence base to treat these patients most appropriately. Until such evidence can be generated, cautious extrapolation from available studies is warranted, taking into account the special pathophysiologic considerations of the aging process and the preferences of the elderly for treatment.

WOMEN

Epidemiology

Cardiovascular disease is the leading cause of death and a major contributor to disability in women.[6] The disease incidence in women lags behind men by 10 years for total cardiovascular disease and longer for more serious clinical events, such as MI and sudden death.[46] Because of the higher proportion of women in the aging population, each year more women die of cardiovascular disease than men.[6] More importantly, although the death rate from cardiovascular disease in men has declined steadily, the rate has remained relatively constant for women (Fig. 39-2).[6]

Compared with men, women have an increased prevalence of several important cardiovascular disease risk factors, including advanced age, hypertension, diabetes, obesity, and sedentary lifestyle,[47-49] and the relative weight of these risks may be different in women compared with men (Table 39-2).[50] Diabetes is a more powerful risk factor in women, increasing CHD risk threefold to sevenfold compared with a twofold to threefold increase in risk in men.[47] With respect to dyslipidemia, low high-density lipoprotein (HDL) is a stronger risk factor for women than elevated LDL.[51] Increased triglycerides also may be an independent risk factor for CAD in women.[52] Coronary heart disease rates in women after menopause are two to three times those of women the same age before menopause.[6]

Tobacco abuse has emerged as an especially important concern among women. Although the overall prevalence of smoking is declining in the United States, rates are dropping more slowly in women compared with men.[53] Among middle-aged women with ACS, tobacco use accounts for more than half of the risk,[54] and similarly important, an adverse interaction has been observed between cigarette smoking and use of oral contraceptive pills.[55] In addition, although the newer, lower dose oral contraceptive pill formulations have not been associated with increased risk of MI in nonsmokers,[56] there remains an exponentially increased risk of MI and stroke in women older than age 35 who smoke and take oral contraceptive pills.[57]

ACS episodes, including non–ST-segment elevation MI and unstable angina, are a common complication of cardiovascular disease among women, with 46% of hospital admissions of patients of all ages with ACS accounted for by women.[58] Despite the prevalence of cardiovascular

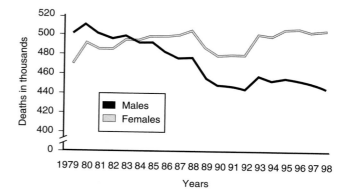

FIGURE 39–2. Cardiovascular disease mortality trends for men and women (United States: 1979–1998). (From American Heart Association: American Heart Association heart and stroke 2001 statistical update, 2001.)

■ ▒ ■

TABLE 39–2 RELATIVE IMPACT OF CORONARY RISK FACTORS ON CORONARY ARTERY DISEASE BY SEX

RISK FACTOR	MEN: RELATIVE RISK (95% CI)	WOMEN: RELATIVE RISK (95% CI)
Hypertension	1.4 (1.2–1.5)	1.4 (1.2–1.6)
High cholesterol level	1.5 (1.3–1.7)	1.1 (1.0–1.3)
Diabetes mellitus	2.0 (1.7–2.5)	2.2 (1.8–2.6)
Overweight	1.3 (1.1–1.5)	1.3 (1.1–1.5)
Smoking	1.4 (1.2–1.6)	1.7 (1.4–2.0)

CI, confidence interval.

disease and incidence of ACS among women, most knowledge regarding the effectiveness of diagnostic and therapeutic methods for cardiovascular disease is based on studies in men. Information about optimal treatment for primary and secondary risk modification is also sparse when compared with that for men.[8] This paucity of information is due to a combination of factors, including the exclusion of women from many randomized clinical trials directly by excluding women of childbearing age or indirectly via exclusion of the elderly. Until additional evidence becomes available specifically to guide the management of ACS among women, the current ACC/AHA ACS guidelines recommend that women with ACS should be managed in a manner similar to men (class I recommendation).[1,2]

Pathophysiology

Because women develop cardiovascular disease later in life than men, the pathophysiology of ACS in women can be explained in part by the mechanisms underlying ACS in the elderly, as discussed elsewhere in this chapter. In addition, the pathophysiologic consequences of the prevalent comorbidities associated with cardiovascular disease in women, such as diabetes and hypertension, play a role in ACS.

Although not completely understood, the pathophysiology of ACS in women is thought to be influenced uniquely by the reproductive hormonal milieu, especially with regard to the menopausal state, hormone replacement therapy (HRT), and oral contraceptive pills. Endogenous and exogenous estrogen can complex with estrogen receptors distributed throughout multiple organ systems to affect gene expression with a wide range of effects.[59] Estrogen may be chronically protective against the development and progression of atherosclerosis by inhibiting the response of blood vessels to injury via estrogen-mediated changes in vascular gene expression. Acutely, estrogen increases vasodilation via effects on nitric oxide,[59] which may be beneficial in the setting of ACS. Other potentially favorable effects of estrogen during and after an ACS episode are activation of endothelial nitric oxide synthase, inhibition of intimal hyperplasia and smooth muscle migration, promotion of angiogenesis, and antioxidant effects.[59,60] Estrogen also is associated with favorable effects on fibrinogen, plasma viscosity, plasminogen activator inhibitor-1, tissue plasminogen activator, insulin sensitivity, homocysteine, and

measures of platelet aggregation and endothelial cell activation.[61]

Estrogen also may influence cardiovascular disease via effects on other organ systems. In the liver, changes in apolipoprotein gene expression in response to endogenous or exogenous estrogen result in a reduction in LDL cholesterol and lipoprotein (a) concentrations and elevation of HDL cholesterol and triglyceride concentrations.[62] The addition of progesterone to estrogen replacement therapy attenuates the HDL-raising effect.[62]

Other effects of estrogen may adversely affect the risk for and consequences of ACS. Hepatic expression of the genes for several coagulation and fibrinolytic proteins is influenced by estrogen, producing potentially prothrombotic effects.[59] In addition, HRT is associated with increased C-reactive protein concentrations, which is an important consideration regarding the role of inflammation in the pathogenesis of ACS.[63] Further research is needed to elucidate fully the clinical significance of these biologic mechanisms and how they interface together to influence cardiovascular disease.

Clinical Presentation

Women with ACS are more likely than men to present with atypical symptoms, such as referred pain in the jaw, neck, shoulder, or other location. Nausea, vomiting, fatigue, and dyspnea also are common primary symptom complaints among women with ACS, in addition to the traditional substernal chest pain during an ACS episode.[64,65] The reasons for the disparity in ACS symptoms are unclear but are likely due to advanced age, lower activity level, and comorbid conditions (especially diabetes) contributing to the more frequent occurrence of such atypical presentations.[65]

Women are more likely to present later in the course of symptoms compared with men and more likely to have hypertension, tachycardia, and heart failure at the time of presentation. The type of coronary ischemic event may be influenced by sex, as seen in the GUSTO IIb trial, in which women more often presented with ACS and men more often with ST-segment elevation MI. In that same study, among the patients presenting with ACS, more women than men presented with unstable angina.[66]

Data on outcomes after ACS in women versus men are varied, depending on the type of ACS. In a large prospective observational study of ACS, the GUARANTEE (Global

Unstable Angina Registry and Treatment Evaluation) study, Scirica and colleagues[67] showed that although women were less likely to qualify for and undergo revascularization procedures compared with men, they experienced a similar incidence of adverse outcomes while in the hospital, including recurrent angina, MI, or death, despite different epidemiologic profiles and less evidence of CAD by invasive and noninvasive tests. In general, women with ACS are older; have a stronger family history of heart disease; have more comorbidity, such as diabetes mellitus and hypertension; and are more likely to have a history of congestive heart failure.[67] They are less likely than their male counterparts to have had a prior MI or prior cardiac procedures or to be currently smoking.[66,68] After adjustment for these and other differences in baseline characteristics and comorbidity, the outcome for men and women with ACS seems to be similar.[69-71] Higher rates of atypical symptoms and nondiagnostic electrocardiogram findings in women make the diagnosis of ACS more difficult than in men, unless cardiac markers, such as troponin, are elevated. Approximately one third of women diagnosed with unstable angina who underwent angiography in two large clinical trials had no obstructive coronary stenosis.[66,69] These women may have had other ischemic causes of chest pain (i.e., coronary spasm or syndrome X) or may have had gastrointestinal or other pathology.

Clinical Management

Few data are available specifically to guide therapeutic decision making for women presenting with ACS, largely as a result of the systematic underrepresentation of women in clinical trials.[8] In limited subgroup analyses from randomized trials, consistent treatment effects in women compared with men have been observed for most available ACS therapies.[36,72] Despite these data, women presenting with ACS tend to be evaluated less intensively, referred to a specialist less often, and less commonly treated with standard therapies.[73,74]

Much (but not all) of the difference shown in these studies can be attributed to differences in baseline characteristics.[75] Even after statistical adjustment for these differences, however, the use of evidence-based therapies is suboptimal (Fig. 39-3).[67,68] The reasons for such practice patterns are unclear, and the ACC/AHA guidelines have addressed this by specifically recommending similar treatment for men and women.[1,2]

Antiplatelet Therapy

The benefit of aspirin in the management of women with ACS and in secondary prevention after these events is supported by existing data, yet aspirin continues to be prescribed less frequently in women compared with

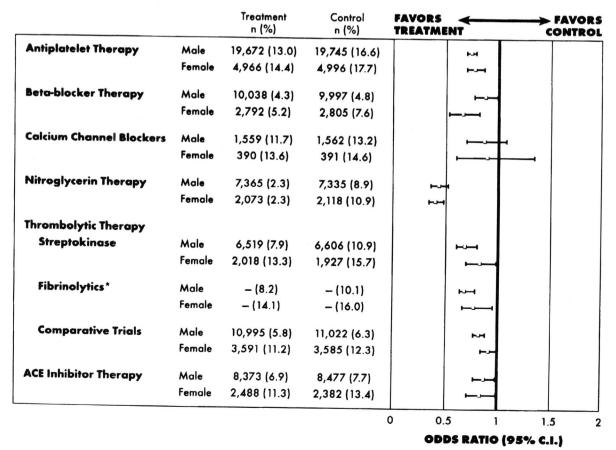

FIGURE 39-3. Proportional effects of treatment strategies on morbidity and mortality in women versus men from randomized controlled trials.

men during and after ACS episodes.[67] A meta-analysis of randomized trials of aspirin documented that among men (n = 39,417) and women (n = 9,962) with prior vascular disease, aspirin versus placebo treatment provided similar absolute risk reduction of subsequent events in women (3.3%) compared with men (3.6%).[24] Subgroup analysis in ISIS-2 (Second International Study of Infarct Survival) suggested that aspirin was equally effective in women and men for acute MI, with an absolute risk reduction of 2.5% versus placebo in women and 2.7% versus placebo in men.[76] The use of aspirin among women during and after ACS is a class I recommendation in the current ACC/AHA guidelines for ACS.[1,2]

The CURE trial evaluated the effect of the early and long-term use of clopidogrel compared with placebo in addition to usual therapy (including aspirin) in patients with ACS.[25] In the subgroup analysis of the 4836 women, the absolute risk reduction from combination therapy versus aspirin alone (10.7% to 9.5%) was similar to that for men (11.9% to 9.1%). Clopidogrel should be considered for all women with ACS, especially when a conservative management strategy is planned.

Improved outcomes have been shown with the use of glycoprotein IIb/IIIa antagonists in the setting of ACS in men and women. Two trials showed improved outcomes associated with the glycoprotein IIb/IIIa antagonist tirofiban in the setting of ACS,[27,28] with no evidence of a differential treatment effect by sex observed in either trial. In the PRISM-PLUS (Platelet Receptor Inhibition in Ischemic Syndrome Management in Patients Limited by Unstable Angina Signs and Symptoms) study, 506 of 1915 (26%) patients were women, and they had a similar absolute risk reduction of

the primary composite end point compared with men (5.6% versus 4.7%).[28] The PURSUIT trial showed improved clinical outcomes associated with the glycoprotein IIb/IIIa antagonist eptifibatide compared with placebo among patients with ACS.[26] In a subset analysis by sex, there was a suggestion of no treatment benefit associated with eptifibatide among women. In subjects enrolled in North America, where a more aggressive therapeutic strategy was used, women and men seemed to derive similar benefit from treatment with eptifibatide. There was no difference in the efficacy of eptifibatide in women versus men in an angioplasty trial, showing that this agent is effective in women.[77]

The role of glycoprotein IIb/IIIa antagonists for women with ACS has been clarified further by a meta-analysis of 31,402 patients in six placebo-controlled randomized trials (Fig. 39–4).[78] There was a significant interaction between sex and treatment effect. Higher risk women with ACS confirmed by troponin release derived a benefit from glycoprotein IIb/IIIa antagonists similar to men with troponin release, however. Women without troponin release or without troponin data available seemed to have adverse outcomes with these agents, in contrast to men. The reason for the adverse effect is unclear but may be explained in part by a higher rate of misdiagnosis of ACS in women, as noted in the preceding section. The current ACC/AHA guidelines do not distinguish treatment recommendations for the use of glycoprotein IIb/IIIa in patients with ACS, and these agents should be considered for women presenting with definite ACS, especially when accompanied by high-risk clinical features, troponin release, or planned percutaneous coronary intervention.

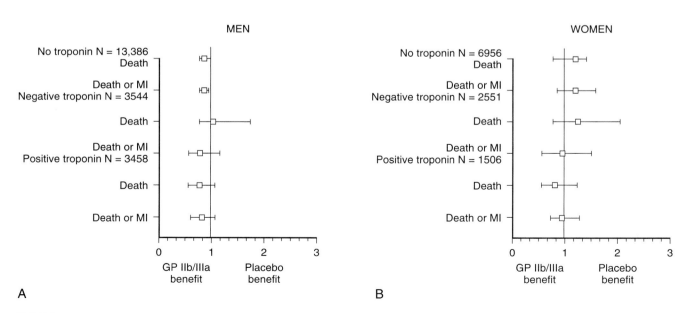

FIGURE 39–4. *A* and *B,* Meta-analysis of six clinical trials of glycoprotein IIb/IIIA antagonists in acute coronary syndromes (N = 31,402). Efficacy results according to sex and the baseline cardiac troponin level in men and women. Data represent outcome at 30 days. Odds ratios and corresponding 95% confidence intervals are presented. Troponin data were available for all troponin groups. Negative troponin is defined as troponin T or I less than 0.1 μg/L. Positive troponin is defined as troponin T or I greater than 0.1 μg/L. (Data derived from Boersma E, Harrington RA, Moliterno DJ, et al: Platelet glycoprotein IIb/IIIa inhibitors in acute coronary syndromes: Meta-analysis of all major randomised clinical trials. Lancet 2002;359:189–198.)

Antithrombotic Therapy

Despite major innovations in antithrombotic therapy, intravenous unfractionated heparin remains the most commonly used agent in the treatment of ACS. Large multicenter trials have shown that low body weight, older age, and female sex are independently associated with higher activated partial thromboplastin times.[14,79] Despite widespread use of unfractionated heparin, uncertainties remain regarding the optimal dosing strategy, especially in women. In an observational analysis from the GUSTO IIb trial database in ACS, female sex was an independent predictor for supratherapeutic activated partial thromboplastin time and increased risk for bleeding, along with older age and lower body weight.[14] Current ACC/AHA guidelines regarding unfractionated heparin dosing are the same for women and men and recommend an initial heparin bolus of 60 to 70 U/kg (5000 U maximum) followed by a continuous infusion at a rate of 12 to 15 U/kg/hr (1000 U/hr maximum) for a target activated partial thromboplastin time of 50 to 70 seconds.[1,2] Because female sex is associated with higher activated partial thromboplastin time, it is prudent to select the lower dose range for the heparin bolus and infusion (60 U/kg and 12 U/kg/hr).

Two phase III randomized trials, TIMI 11B (3910 patients, 46% female) and ESSENCE (3171 patients, 44% female), independently showed superiority of enoxaparin, a low-molecular-weight heparin, over unfractionated heparin in reducing a composite end point of death and serious cardiac ischemic events among patients with ACS.[31,32] Likewise, the FRIC (FRagmin in Unstable Coronary Artery Disease) study showed the beneficial effects associated with dalteparin, another low-molecular-weight heparin.[80] None of these trials reported a differential treatment effect according to sex in low-molecular-weight heparin with regards to safety or efficacy, and low-molecular-weight heparin should be considered an acceptable alternative to unfractionated heparin in the treatment of women with ACS.

Angiotensin-Converting Enzyme Inhibitors

Several trials have evaluated the effect of various ACE inhibitors during and after acute coronary ischemic events.[81-84] ACE inhibitors, including lisinopril, captopril, trandolapril, and ramipril, were associated with improved survival, with prespecified subgroup analyses in women showing results similar to the overall trial populations. Since there were significant numbers of patients enrolled in these trials with non–ST-segment elevation events, ACE inhibitors should be considered for all women with ACS in the absence of contraindications.

For long-term secondary prevention, ACE inhibitors are particularly beneficial, with no evidence of a difference in response based on sex. This statement is supported by data from the SAVE (Survival And Ventricular Enlargement) trial, which evaluated the effect of captopril in patients with asymptomatic left ventricular dysfunction after MI. Long-term administration of captopril was associated with an improvement in survival and reduced morbidity and mortality resulting from major

cardiovascular events in men and women.[85] More recently, in the HOPE study, 9297 patients (26.7% women) with or at high risk for cardiovascular disease were randomly assigned ramipril versus placebo to evaluate the effect on cardiovascular outcomes.[33] Ramipril was associated with a reduced risk for all outcomes assessed, including the primary composite of cardiovascular death, MI, and stroke. These benefits were observed in the setting of prevalent treatment with antiplatelet agents, β-blockers, and modest use of lipid-lowering therapy. There was no difference in the treatment effect according to sex.[33,34]

β-Blockers

Evidence for the beneficial effects of β-blockers in patients with ACS is based on limited randomized trial data, and recommendations are based on the benefit seen primarily among patients with acute MI, along with extrapolation from experience with other ischemic syndromes. Several randomized clinical trials evaluating β-blockers in ACS have reported analyses by sex and have shown consistently clinical benefits associated with β-blockers among the subset of women.[76,86,87] On average, subgroup analyses of β-blocker trials have shown an estimated 30% reduction in mortality in women.[75] Based on the accumulated data, the current ACC/AHA guidelines for ACS recommend β-blockers for all patients in the absence of contraindications as a class I recommendation.[1,2]

Lipid-Lowering Therapy

There is strong evidence to support the use of pharmacologic interventions in women with hyperlipidemia, particularly women with established coronary heart disease and patients with multiple cardiac risk factors. In the CARE (Cholesterol And Recurrent Events) study that included patients with recent MI and nonelevated LDL, treatment with pravastatin was associated with significant reduction of all end points (MI, cardiac death, and revascularization) compared with placebo.[88] Among women in the study, the treatment benefit tended to emerge earlier and to be greater in magnitude compared with the results observed in men. Likewise, the Scandinavian Simvastatin Survival Study (4S) assigned patients with CAD and hyperlipidemia to treatment with simvastatin or placebo and showed similar risk reduction for major coronary events in men and women.[89] Based on the accumulated data, the National Cholesterol Education Program–Adult Treatment Panel III report suggested treating men and women equally with respect to dyslipidemia, using statins as the first-line lipid-lowering drug.[35]

The effect of early statin treatment after ACS has been evaluated. In the MIRACL (Myocardial Ischemia Reduction with Aggressive Cholesterol Lowering) randomized clinical trial, treatment with atorvastatin, started within the first 24 to 96 hours after an ACS event and maintained for 4 months, was associated with improved cardiovascular prognosis by decreasing the combined risk of death (any cause), nonfatal MI, resuscitated cardiac arrest, and worsening angina with new objective evidence of ischemia requiring urgent hospitalization.[90] Sex analyses from the MIRACL trial have not been reported. These findings have been supported by observational analyses from two large cardiovascular databases, both of which suggested improved mortality over 6 months to 1 year after acute coronary ischemic events associated with statin prescription at hospital discharge.[91,92] These effects seem to be similar among women and men in both observational studies.

In contrast to the situation with statins, the seemingly beneficial effects of estrogen therapy on lipoprotein concentrations have not translated into improved clinical outcomes when evaluated in randomized clinical trials.[62,93] Similarly, estrogen therapy was not associated in improvements in angiographic end points, despite the favorable effects on lipoprotein profiles reported.[94] In light of the clear benefits from statin treatment and the emerging evidence of increased risk with HRT in women with documented CAD, the National Cholesterol Education Program guidelines no longer recommend HRT as first-line lipid-lowering therapy in women.[35]

Hormone Modulation

The potential role of HRT during and after ACS has not been evaluated systematically in randomized trials but has been addressed in at least one observational study. Data from the Coumadin Aspirin Reinfarction Study (CARS) were used to evaluate the association of HRT initiation among postmenopausal women shortly after MI with clinical outcomes. In those analyses, HRT was associated with an increased risk of the composite of cardiac death, MI, or unstable angina during follow-up.[95]

The role of HRT for long-term risk modification is similarly unclear. A series of epidemiologic observations suggesting benefit associated with HRT have been challenged by more recent results from randomized clinical trials. The Heart and Estrogen/Progestin Replacement Study (HERS), the first large-scale, randomized, clinical outcome trial of HRT for secondary prevention of death and MI in postmenopausal women, failed to show a beneficial effect of HRT on the primary outcome of cardiovascular death or MI after 4 years of follow-up.[93] The overall null effect was composed of an excess risk for death and MI in the first year of HRT with a trend toward fewer MIs with HRT in the third to fourth years but similar death rates.[93] Patients who participated in HERS are being followed an additional 2 years to determine whether the nonsignificant trends toward benefit observed at the end of HERS persisted or increased with time.[61] The ongoing Woman's Health Initiative (WHI) randomized trial will extend the evaluation of HRT in the setting of primary prevention for cardiovascular disease, evaluating opposed and unopposed estrogen.[96] In preliminary analyses, the WHI investigators already have observed, however, the same types of early hazard observed in HERS.[97] Similarly the results of the Women's Estrogen for Stroke Trial (WEST), which included women with documented cerebrovascular disease, showed the same pattern of early adverse outcomes in the secondary

prevention of stroke as was documented for CAD in the HERS trial.[98]

The Estrogen Replacement and Atherosclerosis (ERA) trial, which evaluated HRT in postmenopausal women with documented CAD, showed no benefit of HRT on angiographic progression of disease, in contrast to prior observational angiographic end point studies and consistent with the HERS findings.[94]

Although selective estrogen-receptor modulators have shown beneficial effects on some surrogate marers of CAD, it is not known whether this will translate into a clinical benefit.[60] The Raloxifene Use for The Heart (RUTH) trial currently is testing the effect of the selective estrogen-receptor modulator raloxifene on cardiovascular end points in more than 10,000 postmenopausal women with documented coronary heart disease.[99] Until randomized trials with adequate clinical outcomes are completed, these agents should not be used solely for prevention of CAD-related outcomes. Although potential benefits are intriguing, the selective estrogen-receptor modulators also carry some of the same risks as HRT, including increased incidence of deep vein thrombosis.

The accumulated data suggest no net cardiovascular benefit and a possible early increased risk of atherothrombotic events when HRT is initiated in women with documented atherosclerosis. The AHA/ACC guidelines for ACS recommend that postmenopausal women who receive HRT may continue, but that HRT should not be initiated for the secondary prevention of coronary events, with the caveat that there may be other indications for HRT in postmenopausal women (e.g., prevention of flushing, osteoporosis).[1,2] Likewise, in a position statement on HRT, the AHA recommends that the decision to continue or stop HRT in women with cardiovascular disease who have been undergoing long-term HRT should be based on established noncoronary benefits and risks and patient preferences.[60] Ongoing trials may offer additional insights (Table 39–3).

■ ▦ ■

TABLE 39–3   ONGOING STUDIES OF HORMONE REPLACEMENT THERAPY AND CORONARY HEART DISEASE

Angiographic End Point Trials

Estrogen and Bypass Graft Atherosclerosis Regression Trial (EAGER)
Women's Lipid Lowering Heart Atherosclerosis Trial (WELLHEART)
Women's Atherosclerosis Vitamin/Estrogen Trial (WAVE)

Primary Prevention Trials

Women's Health Initiative (WHI)
Women's International Study of long Duration Oestrogen after Menopause (WISDOM)

Secondary Prevention Trials

HERS follow-up study
Estrogen in the Prevention of ReInfarction Trial (ESPRIT)

Adapted from Mosca L, Collins P, Herrington DM, et al: Hormone replacement therapy and cardiovascular disease: A statement for healthcare professionals from the American Heart Association. Circulation 2001;104:499–503.

Risk Stratification

Current recommendations for noninvasive testing in women are the same as in men after ACS.[1,2] Although standard electrocardiogram exercise testing is thought to be less predictive of CAD in women than in men, most studies that have evaluated the diagnostic performance of noninvasive tests have failed to account for sex-specific differences in prevalence of disease or for confounding factors in ACS in women.[75,100] Although exercise testing among women may have limitations of specificity, normal test results are a good indicator that flow-limiting CAD is unlikely.[75] To enhance specificity, the addition of imaging techniques to functional testing is especially useful among women. For nuclear imaging, technetium agents are superior to thallium-201 owing to a reduction in breast tissue attenuation artifact with the former.[101] Stress echocardiography (dobutamine or exercise) is also an accurate and cost-effective technique for CAD detection in women.[102]

Revascularization

Female sex is an independent predictor of a lower likelihood of undergoing coronary angiography for patients with ACS, even after adjusting for differences in baseline characteristics.[66-69] Because coronary angiography is a prerequisite for percutaneous or surgical revascularization, as expected, women in these studies had a lower rate of revascularization. When catheterization is performed in women and CAD is found, sex-based differences in referral for revascularization tend to disappear.[73,103]

Women undergoing revascularization tend to have smaller artery size, advanced age, and increased comorbidity, which are thought to contribute to worse outcomes observed in some studies among women compared with men after percutaneous and surgical revascularization,[43,104,105] but other studies have failed to confirm these adverse outcomes among women undergoing coronary revascularization.[69,106,107]

Early invasive treatment of ACS in the FRISC II (Fragmin and Fast Revascularization during InStability in Coronary Artery Disease) trial, which randomized patients to early invasive versus conservative management of ACS, found no difference in MI or death at 12 months among women in the invasive and noninvasive groups, in contrast to the favorable effect in the invasively treated group of men.[43,108] This result was partly attributable to a higher bypass surgery–related mortality in women than in men observed in the study. Also, the selection of the invasive procedure (percutaneous coronary intervention versus coronary artery bypass graft surgery) was not based on randomization and could have resulted in a concentration of high-risk factors in women chosen for surgery. The FRISC II investigators concluded that the final evaluation of the efficacy of an early invasive strategy in women with ACS would have to await their long-term follow-up and the outcomes of other similar ongoing trials.

Similarly, in TACTICS, 1463 men and 757 women with ACS were randomized to an early invasive strategy with angiography within 4 to 48 hours and revascularization if appropriate versus a conservative strategy in which catheterization would be done only for signs or symptoms of recurrent ischemia.[44] The point estimates for the primary end point of death, nonfatal MI, or rehospitalization for ACS within 6 months for the invasive versus the conservative strategy were similar for men (15.3% versus 19.4%) compared with women (17.0% versus 19.6%), indicating that in subgroup analysis, the invasive strategy was better regardless of sex.

Angiographic success and late outcomes of percutaneous coronary intervention are similar in women and men as observed in several studies. A review of 3000 patients from the Mayo Clinic with unstable angina who underwent percutaneous coronary intervention reported that women had similar early and late results as men.[106] The BARI (Bypass Angioplasty Revascularization Investigation) trial, comprising 1829 patients with unstable angina, including 489 women, compared percutaneous transluminal coronary angioplasty and coronary artery bypass graft surgery and found that revascularization results were better in women than in men after adjustment for baseline differences, with a lower relative risk of death in women (relative risk, 0.6; $P = .003$).[107] Candidacy for percutaneous transluminal coronary angioplasty should be determined using the same clinical decision algorithm for women and men.

Clinical trials databases, registries, and population studies all reported similar graft patency and long-term survival benefits in women and men who have surgical revascularization.[105,107] The rates of perioperative death and complications (MI, stroke, and heart failure) are greater for women, but this disparity disappears when baseline factors, such as age and heart failure, are considered. Coronary artery bypass graft surgery provides excellent relief of symptoms and comparable survival benefits in women; concern about increased mortality should not influence referral for surgery in appropriate women.

Conclusions

Widespread underuse and delayed initiation of established treatments for ACS and preventive therapies for CAD have been documented in women. Established therapies for acute and chronic ischemia have been shown to benefit women; these interventions should be emphasized in clinical practice (see Fig. 39-4). The ACC/AHA's current recommendations for the management of ACS stress equality in treatment between the sexes unless contraindications exist. Available data suggest that aggressive secondary prevention practices should be similarly implemented.

PATIENTS WITH DIABETES MELLITUS

Epidemiology

Diabetes is prevalent among patients with ACS, present in 20% to 35% of patients.[109,110] The proportion of ACS patients who have diabetes is increasing and likely will continue to do so because the population has become more sedentary and overweight, and developing countries continue to evolve toward Western diet and activity patterns.[110] The global prevalence of diabetes is expected to double from the present estimate of 150 million people affected worldwide to an expected 300 million patients with diabetes by 2025.[111]

Diabetes is a complex metabolic disease that is associated with a twofold to sixfold increased risk for developing CAD, which accounts for 80% of deaths among patients with diabetes.[112, 113] When CAD develops, diabetes is associated with a doubling of the incidence of ACS and significantly worse short-term and long-term cardiovascular risk (Fig. 39–5).[109,113,114]

The increasing prevalence of diabetes worldwide, along with its concomitant cardiovascular risk, constitutes a global health crisis. Efforts aimed at understanding the cardiovascular pathophysiology underlying diabetes along with the development and application of more effective therapies for this high-risk group of patients are important clinical objectives.

Pathophysiology

A variety of basic pathophysiologic mechanisms have been proposed to explain the adverse influence of diabetes on coronary disease and clinical outcomes after ACS, including differences in atherosclerotic disease development, distribution, and progression[115,116]; metabolic perturbations[117,118]; autonomic neuropathy[119]; endothelial dysfunction[120]; derangements in the proteofibrinolytic system and platelet effects[121]; and exaggerations of inflammatory processes.[122] These abnormalities, individually or in aggregate, likely contribute to the adverse outcomes associated with ACS in diabetic patients.

Congestive heart failure complicating ACS is common among patients with diabetes and has been reported as the most common cause of death in this population.[123,124] Potential mechanistic explanations for this failure, which includes systolic and diastolic dysfunction, include a diseased myocardium beyond the infarct area with impairment of compensatory hyperkinesis, metabolic perturbations associated with the diabetic state, and impaired myocardial flow reserve.[117,124]

The second most cited cause of death in patients with diabetes is myocardial reinfarction,[124] most likely resulting from a combination of factors, such as more extensive coronary atherosclerosis, instability of atheromatous lesions, inflammatory burden within the atheroma, and the prothrombotic state associated with diabetes.[125,126] Despite advances in the management of ACS, including advances in antiplatelet and antithrombotic therapies, which are particularly effective among patients with diabetes, the incremental risk associated with diabetes after ACS persists.[109,114] This excess risk is likely due to unidentified characteristics associated with the diabetic condition that adversely affect clinical outcomes and predispose patients to recurrent ischemic events. A better understanding of these factors should lead to the development and application of more effective therapies for patients with diabetes having an ACS episode.

Clinical Presentation

Patients with diabetes tend to have characteristics associated with worse outcomes in the setting of cardiovascular complications. They are more likely to be female, to be older, to have more diffuse coronary disease, to have more congestive heart failure, and to have worse cardiovascular risk profiles.[109,114] Patients with diabetes tend to present with atypical symptoms of ACS, which may

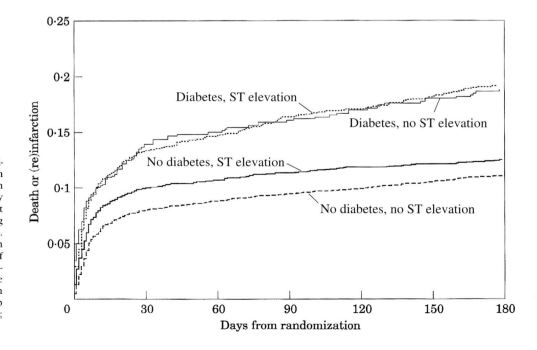

FIGURE 39–5. Kaplan-Meier estimate of the probability of death or (re)myocardial infarctio within 6 months after acute coronary syndrome, according to ST sement status on presentation among patients with and without diabetes. (From McGuire DK, Emanuelsson H, Granger CB, et al: Influence of diabetes mellitus on clinical outcomes across the spectrum of acute coronary syndromes: Findings from the GUSTO-IIb study. GUSTO IIb investigators. Eur Heart J 2000; 21:1750-1758.)

delay presentation to the hospital and may result in further delays in diagnosis and therapy.[127] Even after comprehensive statistical adjustment for recorded confounding variables, diabetes still imparts a markedly increased mortality risk after ACS,[109,114] suggesting that there are likely other characteristics of the diabetic condition that adversely affect clinical outcomes and predispose patients to recurrent ischemic events, as discussed previously.

Clinical Management

Few studies specifically have addressed the effect of current medical therapies for ACS in diabetic patients. Subgroup analyses of clinical trials allow examination of the impact of current therapies in this high-risk population. With rare exception, these analyses have suggested consistent treatment effects in patients with diabetes compared with the population in general. Despite the accumulated evidence showing the favorable risk/benefit profiles of these therapies, they continue to be underused in the high-risk population of diabetic patients during and after ACS events.[128] A principal focus of diabetic treatment should include optimal use of available therapies.

Antiplatelet Therapy

Aspirin is effective in the treatment of patients with ACS. Although few data have been reported regarding the specific influence of aspirin among the diabetic patients during and after ACS, results from several studies provide ample evidence to support the necessity of aspirin therapy for diabetic patients with ACS. In the ISIS-2 randomized trial that included patients within 24 hours of the onset of symptoms of suspected MI, the benefit of ASA was proved among a population that included 1289 (7.5%) patients with diabetes.[76] Subsequent long-term studies have shown the benefit of aspirin in diabetic patients with CAD or at risk for ischemic heart disease.[24,129] Based on these data, aspirin should remain a first-line therapy during and after ACS episodes in patients with diabetes.

Clopidogrel seems to be particularly beneficial among patients with diabetes, as suggested by subset analyses from the CAPRIE (Clopidogrel versus Aspirin in Patients at Risk of Ischemic Events) study of long-term risk prevention[130] and the CURE study, testing clopidogrel as an adjunct to conventional therapy for ACS that included aspirin.[25] The use of clopidogrel should be considered in the acute setting along with aspirin and other standard therapy for patients with diabetes presenting with ACS, especially when an early conservative approach or percutaneous coronary intervention is performed. There is excess risk of bleeding with coronary artery bypass graft surgery within 5 days of clopidogrel, however. After ACS, clopidogrel combined with aspirin seems to be acceptably safe and is associated with continued clinical benefit 9 months post-ACS.[25] Clopidogrel is also the therapy of choice for long-term treatment of patients with diabetes and cardiovascular disease who are intolerant to aspirin therapy.[130]

The effectiveness of the small-molecule glycoprotein IIb/IIIa receptor antagonists (eptifibatide, tirofiban) has been shown in many clinical trials involving patients with ACS.[26,28] Both drugs seem to be particularly beneficial among patients with diabetes. Given the safety, efficacy, and consistent estimates of treatment effect across reported trials, along with the high-risk features prevalent in diabetic patients, eptifibatide or tirofiban should be considered for every diabetic patient presenting with ACS with concomitant high-risk clinical features. These agents should be administered if an invasive strategy is planned.[20,78]

Antithrombotic Therapies

The hypercoagulable state associated with diabetes may limit the efficacy of antithrombotic therapies, and more aggressive dosing strategies or more potent antithrombotic therapies may be of particular benefit in these patients. Several antithrombin drugs, including unfractionated heparin, hirudin, bivalirudin, and low-molecular-weight heparins, have shown favorable clinical effects among the diabetic population in subset analyses of large-scale clinical trials of ACS. Patients with diabetes seem to require higher heparin doses than nondiabetic patients to achieve a therapeutic activated partial thromboplastin time.[79]

One major clinical concern regarding the use of antithrombin therapies in patients with diabetes is the risk for bleeding complications, especially ocular bleeding in the setting of diabetic retinopathy. Subset analyses from large-scale clinical trials of thrombolytic and antithrombin therapy have not supported these theoretical concerns, however.[114,131] No study has shown a significant differential treatment effect of these drugs according to diabetes status. Overall the clinical effect of systemic anticoagulation among diabetic patients seems to be at least as favorable as that observed among patients without diabetes. The biologic considerations of hypercoagulability and ocular bleeding risk remain theoretical, and antithrombin therapy is indicated for patients with diabetes presenting with ACS.

Angiotensin-Converting Enzyme Inhibitors

ACE inhibitors are highly effective among diabetic patients with acute coronary ischemic events.[132] A retrospective analysis of the GISSI-3 (Gruppo Italiano per lo Studio della Sopravvivenza nell'Infarto Miocardico) study suggested that most, if not all, of the 6-month mortality benefit resulting from treatment with lisinopril versus placebo was observed among the subset of patients with diabetes.[133] Similar results were observed in subset analyses of the CONSENSUS-II (Cooperative New Scandinavian Enalapril Survival Study II) and TRACE (Trandolapril Cardiac Evaluation) study databases.[134,135] Although the overall CONSENSUS II trial was negative with regard to the effect of intravenous enalapril during acute MI on mortality, the diabetic cohort assigned to ACE inhibitor therapy exhibited a significant improvement in outcomes at 6 months compared with placebo. These effects were of similar magnitude to those noted in the GISSI-3 study.

Observations of long-term primary and secondary cardiovascular risk prevention among patients with diabetes associated with ACE inhibitors underscore the important clinical benefit of this class of drugs when continued long-term. Most notably, the UKPDS (United Kingdom Prospective Diabetes Study) and the HOPE trial each showed significant clinical benefit compared with placebo for patients randomized to treatment with the ACE inhibitors captopril and ramipril (Fig. 39–6).[136,137] In the HOPE study, the beneficial effect was much greater than that expected from blood pressure control alone, suggesting favorable pleiotropic effects of ramipril. In aggregate, the data support the short-term and long-term use of ACE inhibitors in patients with diabetes after ACS regardless of whether congestive heart failure or hypertension is present.

β-Blockers

β-Blockers are among the most widely studied medications in the setting of acute ischemic events and are among the most effective therapies for patients with diabetes and ACS.[138,139] Reported studies consistently have suggested an average twofold greater reduction in mortality risk for diabetic compared with nondiabetic patients treated with β-blockers after ACS (Fig. 39–7).

Despite these compelling data, β-blockers continue to be underprescribed for patients with diabetes during or after ACS.[140] Because of historical concerns regarding impaired glucose metabolism, worsening of dyslipidemia, and masking of hypoglycemic symptoms, many clinicians are hesitant to prescribe β-blockers for patients with diabetes. These (largely hypothetical) concerns are well addressed, however, with an abundance of clinical outcomes data that show the benefit of β-blockers among patients with diabetes. β-Blocker therapy should be used in the absence of other contraindications in all patients with diabetes during and after an episode of ACS.

Lipid-Lowering Therapy

Diabetes is associated with a high prevalence of dyslipidemia, with a pattern that is particularly atherogenic and associated with incremental cardiovascular risk.[118] Typically, modest elevations of total and LDL cholesterol exist along with high triglycerides, low HDL cholesterol, and elevations of small, dense LDL subtype. Four large-scale secondary prevention studies, including a total of more than 5500 patients with diabetes, comparing hydroxymethylglutaryl-coenzyme A reductase inhibitors (statins) with placebo showed the long-term benefit of lipid-lowering therapy with statins among patients with diabetes (Fig. 39–8).[88,141-143] These data support the use of statin therapy as the primary treatment for dyslipidemia associated with diabetes mellitus in patients with ACS.[35]

Whether initiation of lipid-lowering therapy, especially with a statin, for patients with diabetes and hyperlipidemia is necessary during the index hospitalization

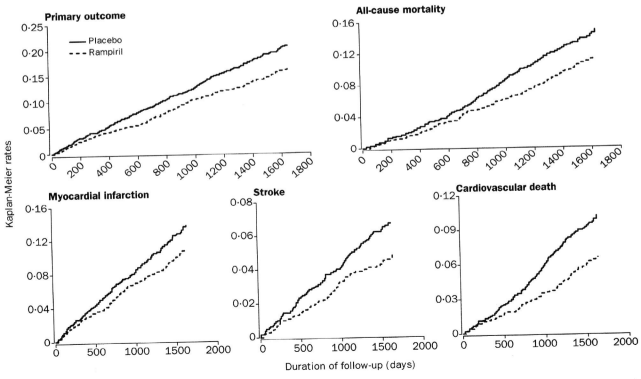

FIGURE 39–6. Kaplan-Meier curves for participants in the Heart Outcomes Prevention Evaluation trial with diabetes. (From Heart Outcomes Prevention Evaluation Study investigators: Effects of ramipril on cardiovascular and microvascular outcomes in people with diabetes mellitus: Results of the HOPE study and MICRO-HOPE substudy. Lancet 2000;355:253–259.)

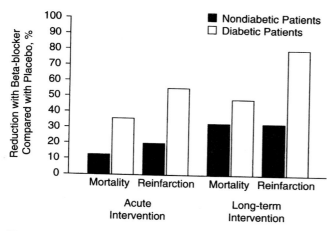

FIGURE 39–7. Effect of β-blocker therapy on mortality and reinfarction rates in patients with and without diabetes after myocardial infarction, expressed as percentage reduction compared with patients receiving placebo. (From Kendall MJ, Lynch KP, Hjalmarson A, Kjekshus J: Beta-blockers and sudden cardiac death. Ann Intern Med 1995;123: 358–367.)

(acutely or subacutely) or is simply an important objective during longitudinal follow-up remains to be determined. Even if early initiation of statin therapy is not associated directly with improved clinical outcomes, the increased compliance associated with medications initiated before index hospital discharge makes it a reasonable consideration, especially among the diabetic population with such a high prevalence of dyslipidemia.[144] Based on the existing data, the National Cholesterol Education Program–Adult Treatment Panel III report suggested that ACS patients with LDL cholesterol greater than 130 mg/dL should be discharged on lipid-lowering drug therapy and recommended clinical judgment at lower levels; the guidelines do not address acute initiation.[35]

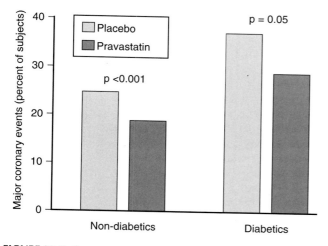

FIGURE 39–8. Occurrence of major coronary heart disease events during a 5-year median follow-up period in nondiabetic (n = 3573) and diabetic (n = 586) subjects randomized to placebo or pravastatin in the CARE trial. (From Garg A, Grundy SM: Diabetic dyslipidemia and its therapy. Diabetes Rev 1997;5:425–433.)

Glycemic Management

There is an association between the degree of hyperglycemia on hospital presentation for ACS and adverse long-term clinical outcomes.[145] Because there are a paucity of data addressing the acute and long-term effect of hypoglycemic therapies on important cardiovascular complications, however, substantial uncertainty remains regarding the optimal glycemic control strategy among patients with diabetes and cardiovascular disease.[146]

The selection of the therapies used to control blood glucose during and after an ACS episode may influence outcomes as much as or more than the intensity of glycemic control achieved. Many biologically plausible mechanisms for either clinical benefit or harm from the currently available hypoglycaemic medications have been proposed.[147,148]

Acute Phase Glycemic Control with Insulin. The myocardium is a metabolic omnivore, preferentially metabolizing free fatty acids (FFA) under physiologic conditions.[149] Under conditions of ischemia, however, the myocardium shifts to anaerobic metabolism using glucose as the primary substrate.[150] This is an insulin-dependent metabolic adjustment and is markedly impaired in patients with diabetes as a result of relative or absolute insulin deficiency. Insulin promotes glucose oxidation, which is known to be beneficial in the presence of ischemia and likely reduces infarct size and postischemic contractile dysfunction.[151] Increased concentration of circulating nonesterified FFA owing to high sympathetic activity is seen with acute myocardial ischemia.[149] FFA oxidation is potentially detrimental in the setting of myocardial ischemia because of an increased myocardial oxygen demand and a direct inhibition of glucose oxidation. Increased FFA metabolism during ischemia results in accumulation of toxic FFA metabolites, which may exacerbate membrane damage, provoke arrhythmias, and increase mechanical dysfunction.

In the setting of acute cardiac ischemia, insulin has been shown to decrease FFA concentrations.[152] Insulin also has been associated with acute improvements in parameters of coagulation, including decreased production of thromboxane A_2 and decreased plasminogen activator inhibitor-1 activity, and it may influence positively the high reinfarction rate linked to this patient group.[153] Glycemic control with insulin after acute MI was associated with a trend toward lower in-hospital mortality and significantly lower 1-year mortality compared with oral insulin-providing agents.[154] Given these observations, it is plausible that exogenous insulin administration in the ACS setting could improve outcomes. Critically ill ACS patients, including patients mechanically ventilated for pulmonary edema or shock and especially patients who undergo coronary artery bypass graft surgery, may derive particular benefit. Reduction of elevated glucose to less than 100 mg/dL by insulin in patients in a surgical intensive care unit, largely post–cardiac surgery, resulted in reduced in-hospital mortality in a randomized trial.[155] Although there is no direct evidence for reduction of the short-term event rate in ACS with tight control by insulin, the other supportive data suggest that in-hospital tight glycemic control is indicated.

Glucose, Insulin, and Potassium   The use of insulin for ACS first was described in 1963 by Sodi-Pallares and colleagues[156] with the intention of facilitating potassium flux in the ischemic myocardium, so-called polarizing therapy. After decades of investigation, this combination of glucose, insulin, and potassium has become known as GIK therapy, and the focus of attention has shifted from the polarizing effects to the effects mediated by insulin. The accumulated data on the effects of GIK for ACS have been reviewed.[148,157] In a meta-analysis of published studies evaluating GIK therapy, which included 1932 predominantly nondiabetic patients, a proportional mortality rate reduction of 28% was observed, or 49 lives saved per 1000 patients treated.[157] The insulin dosing in this scheme is severalfold higher than that required for glycemic control, and the clinical effects are most likely due to extraglycemic effects of insulin. In the meta-analysis by Fath-Ordoubadi and Beatt,[157] the treatment effect of GIK was enhanced when the analysis was restricted to the studies using high-dose intravenous GIK regimens.

Chronic Phase Glycemic Control After Acute Coronary Syndrome.   Long-term aggressive metabolic control has been associated with improvements in microvascular complications of diabetes.[158] Although several studies have supported the clinical benefit or absence of pernicious effects of currently available therapies,[158,159] especially in the acute setting of ACS,[154,159] findings from other studies have underscored the uncertainties that exist with regard to the optimal level of glycemic control and effects of the available drugs or drug combinations on macrovascular disease.[160-162] Analyses from two large cardiovascular databases independently suggested improved outcomes associated with insulin-sensitizing therapy (metformin or thiazolidinedione or both) compared with insulin-providing therapy (insulin or sulfonylurea or both).[163,164] The ongoing BARI 2D randomized trial, sponsored by the U.S. National Heart, Lung, and Blood Institute, will prospectively evaluate this issue.

Given the existing uncertainty regarding the role of hypoglycemic therapy and the lack of clinical outcomes data regarding the available therapies during and after ACS episodes, a primary goal of therapy in these patients should focus on using therapies that have been shown to improve clinical outcomes. Although glycemic control is an important clinical objective, until better data are available regarding the clinical impact of current hypoglycemic strategies, it would be prudent to redirect some of the focus of therapy from achievement of tight glycemic control to aggressive modification of cardiovascular risk during and after ACS episodes. A hemoglobin A_{1c} of 7% should be targeted according to current guidelines of the American Diabetes Association.[165]

Revascularization

Clinical practice guidelines from the ACC/AHA presently recommend similar approaches to the patient with or without diabetes regarding invasive versus conservative management of ACS.[1,2] For the overall population, the results of the FRISC II study and the TACTICS-TIMI 18 study have swung the pendulum in the direction of more liberal use of early invasive strategies with revascularization, either percutaneous or surgical, as determined necessary.[43,44] The early invasive approach seems to be most advantageous among higher risk patients, including patients older than 65, patients with ST-segment depression associated with the presentation, and patients with elevated serum markers of myocardial necrosis, as outlined by the ACC/AHA guidelines. Patients with diabetes who present with these high-risk characteristics should

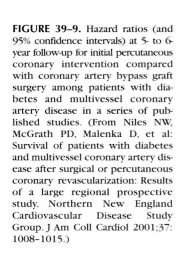

FIGURE 39–9. Hazard ratios (and 95% confidence intervals) at 5- to 6-year follow-up for initial percutaneous coronary intervention compared with coronary artery bypass graft surgery among patients with diabetes and multivessel coronary artery disease in a series of published studies. (From Niles NW, McGrath PD, Malenka D, et al: Survival of patients with diabetes and multivessel coronary artery disease after surgical or percutaneous coronary revascularization: Results of a large regional prospective study. Northern New England Cardiovascular Disease Study Group. J Am Coll Cardiol 2001;37: 1008–1015.)

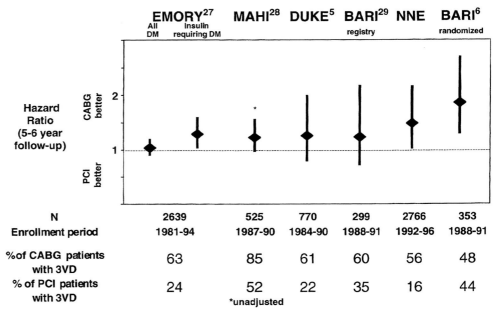

	EMORY[27]		MAHI[28]	DUKE[5]	BARI[29]	NNE	BARI[6]
	All DM	Insulin requiring DM			registry		randomized
N	2639		525	770	299	2766	353
Enrollment period	1981-94		1987-90	1984-90	1988-91	1992-96	1988-91
%of CABG patients with 3VD	63		85	61	60	56	48
% of PCI patients with 3VD	24		52	22	35	16	44

*unadjusted

be treated similarly as patients without diabetes. An early invasive strategy for such patients is supported by the diabetes subgroup findings from FRISC II and TACTICS-TIMI 18.[43,44]

When it is determined that revascularization is indicated, the optimal procedure remains to be defined. Analyses from several studies have suggested superiority of surgical versus percutaneous revascularization for patients with diabetes who have multivessel CAD (Fig. 39-9).[115,166] Given the selective entry criteria for these trials, inherent limitations in subgroup analyses, and advances in percutaneous and surgical therapies that have occurred in the interim, the validity and generalizibility of these observations have yet to be confirmed. Notably, BARI preceded the use of stents and glycoprotein IIb/IIIa antagonists. Few data exist comparing these revascularization options among diabetic patients with ACS, and the choice of surgical versus percutaneous revascularization remains grounded in clinical decision making on a case-by-case basis.

Conclusions

A review of the existing literature supports a clinical approach to patients with diabetes and ACS similar to the overall population.[1,2] For most evidence-based therapies available for the treatment of ACS, patients with diabetes tend to derive a greater magnitude of benefit compared with the nondiabetic population, in keeping with the increased clinical risk associated with diabetes. Despite improvements in outcomes after ACS over the past few decades, the mortality gradient between patients with and without diabetes remains, even after adjusting for prognostically important differences in the patient populations. The basis for these worse outcomes is incompletely understood, and continued efforts at defining the pathophysiology and developing more effective therapies is an important objectives of clinical and research pursuits.

REFERENCES

1. Braunwald E, Antman EM, Beasley JW, et al: ACC/AHA guidelines for the management of patients with unstable angina and non-ST-segment elevation myocardial infarction. A report of the American College of Cardiology/American Heart Association Task Force on Practice Guidelines (Committee on the Management of Patients With Unstable Angina). J Am Coll Cardiol 2000;36:970-1062.
2. Braunwald E, Antman EM, Beasley JW, et al: ACC/AHA guidelines for the management of patients with unstable angina and non-ST-segment elevation myocardial infarction: executive summary and recommendations. A report of the American College of Cardiology/American Heart Association task force on practice guidelines (committee on the management of patients with unstable angina). Circulation 2000;102:1193-1209.
3. Centers for Disease Control and Prevention, and National Health Vital Statistics System: US life tables. National Vital Statistics Reports, vol. 48. Hyattsville, MD, National Center for Health Statistics, 1998.
4. Anderson RN, Rosenberg HM: Age standardization of death rates: Implementation of the year 2000 standard. National Vital Statistics Reports, vol. 47. Hyattsville, MD, National Center for Health Statistics, 1998, pp 1-17.
5. Stone P, Thompson B, Anderson V, et al: Influence of race, sex, and age on management of unstable angina and non-Q-wave myocardial infarction. The TIMI III Registry. JAMA 1996;275:1104-1112.
6. American Heart Association: American Heart Association Heart and Stroke 2001 Statistical Update. Dallas, Texas, American Heart Association, 2000, pp 745-747.
7. National Center of Health Statistics: Plan and operation of the Third National Health And Nutrition Examination Survey, 1988-94. Vital Health Statistics, 1994.
8. Lee PY, Alexander KP, Hammill BG, et al: Representation of elderly persons and women in published randomized trials of acute coronary syndromes. JAMA 2001;286:708-713.
9. Hasdai D, Holmes DR Jr, Criger DA, et al: Age and outcome after acute coronary syndromes without persistent ST-segment elevation. Am Heart J 2000;139:858-866.
10. Nadelmann J, Frishman WH, Ooi WL, et al: Prevalence, incidence and prognosis of recognized and unrecognized myocardial infarction in persons aged 75 years or older: The Bronx Aging Study. Am J Cardiol 1990;66:533-537.
11. Aronow WS, Ahn C, Kronzon I: Prognosis of congestive heart failure in elderly patients with normal versus abnormal left ventricular systolic function associated with coronary artery disease. Am J Cardiol 1990;66:1257-1259.
12. Lakatta EG, Gerstenblith G, Weisfeldt ML: The aging heart: Structure, function, and disease. In Braunwald E (ed): Heart Disease, 5th ed. Philadelphia, WB Saunders, 1997, pp 1687-1703.
13. Stein B, Kupersmith J: Principles and practice of pharmacotherapy. In Kupersmith J, Deedwania PC (eds): The Pharmacologic Management of Heart Disease. Baltimore, Williams & Wilkins, 1997, pp 3-38.
14. Granger CB, Hirsh J, Califf RM, et al, for the GUSTO-I Investigators: Activated partial thromboplastin time and outcome after thrombolytic therapy for acute myocardial infarction: Results from the GUSTO-I Trial. Circulation 1996;93:870-878.
15. Chrischilles EA, Segar ET, Wallace RB: Self-reported adverse drug reactions and related resource use: A study of community-dwelling persons 65 years of age and older. Ann Intern Med 1992;117:634-640.
16. Bayer AJ, Chadha JS, Farag RR, Pathy MS: Changing presentation of myocardial infarction with increasing old age. J Am Geriatr Soc 1986;34:263-266.
17. Karlson BW, Herlitz J, Pettersson P, et al: One-year prognosis in patients hospitalized with a history of unstable angina pectoris. Clin Cardiol 1993;16:397-402.
18. Lee KL, Woodlief LH, Topol EJ, et al, for the GUSTO-I Investigators: Predictors of 30-day mortality in the era of reperfusion for acute myocardial infarction: Results from an international trial of 41,021 patients. Circulation 1995;91:1659-1668.
19. Boersma E, Pieper KS, Steyerberg EW, et al: Predictors of outcome in patients with acute coronary syndromes without persistent ST-segment elevation: Results from an international trial of 9461 patients. The PURSUIT Investigators. Circulation 2000;101:2557-2567.
20. Antman EM, Cohen M, Bernink PJ, et al: The TIMI risk score for unstable angina/non-ST elevation MI: A method for prognostication and therapeutic decision making. JAMA 2000;284:835-842.
21. Krumholz HM, Vaccarino V, Ellerbeck EF, et al: Determinants of appropriate use of angiotensin-converting enzyme inhibitors after acute myocardial infarction in persons > or = 65 years of age. Am J Cardiol 1997;79:581-586.
22. Krumholz HM, Radford MJ, Wang Y, et al: National use and effectiveness of beta-blockers for the treatment of elderly patients after acute myocardial infarction: National Cooperative Cardiovascular Project. JAMA 1998;280:623-629.
23. Alexander KP, Peterson ED, Granger CB, et al: Potential impact of evidence-based medicine in acute coronary syndromes: Insights from GUSTO-IIb. Global Use of Strategies to Open Occluded Arteries in Acute Coronary Syndromes trial. J Am Coll Cardiol 1998;32:2023-2030.
24. Antiplatelet Trialists' Collaboration: Collaborative overview of randomised trials of antiplatelet therapy: I. Prevention of death, myocardial infarction, and stroke by prolonged antiplatelet therapy in various categories of patients. BMJ 1994;308:81-106.
25. Yusuf S, Zhao F, Mehta SR, et al: Effects of clopidogrel in addition to aspirin in patients with acute coronary syndromes without ST-segment elevation. N Engl J Med 2001;345:494-502.
26. PURSUIT Trial Investigators: Inhibition of platelet glycoprotein IIb/IIIa with eptifibatide in patients with acute coronary syndromes. The PURSUIT Trial Investigators. Platelet Glycoprotein

IIb/IIIa in Unstable Angina: Receptor Suppression Using Integrilin Therapy. N Engl J Med 1998;339:436–443.

27. Platelet Receptor Inhibition in Ischemic Syndrome Management (PRISM) Study Investigators: A comparison of aspirin plus tirofiban with aspirin plus heparin for unstable angina. Platelet Receptor Inhibition in Ischemic Syndrome Management (PRISM) Study Investigators. N Engl J Med 1998;338:1498–1505.

28. Platelet Receptor Inhibition in Ischemic Syndrome Management in Patients Limited by Unstable Angina Signs and Symptoms (PRISM-PLUS) Study investigators: Inhibition of the platelet glycoprotein IIb/IIIa receptor with tirofiban in unstable angina and non-Q-wave myocardial infarction. Platelet Receptor Inhibition in Ischemic Syndrome Management in Patients Limited by Unstable Signs and Symptoms (PRISM-PLUS) Study Investigators. N Engl J Med 1998;338:1488–1497.

29. Oler A, Whooley MA, Oler J, Grady D: Adding heparin to aspirin reduces the incidence of myocardial infarction and death in patients with unstable angina: A meta-analysis. JAMA 1996;276:811–815.

30. Antman EM, Cohen M, Radley D, et al: Assessment of the treatment effect of enoxaparin for unstable angina/non-Q-wave myocardial infarction: TIMI 11B-ESSENCE meta-analysis. Circulation 1999;100:1602–1608.

31. Cohen M, Demers C, Gurfinkel EP, et al, for the Efficacy and Safety of Subcutaneous Enoxaparin in Non-Q-Wave Coronary Events Study Group. A comparison of low-molecular-weight heparin with unfractionated heparin for unstable coronary artery disease. N Engl J Med 1997;337:447–452.

32. Antman EM, McCabe CH, Gurfinkel EP, et al: Enoxaparin prevents death and cardiac ischemic events in unstable angina/non-Q-wave myocardial infarction: Results of the thrombolysis in myocardial infarction (TIMI) 11B trial. Circulation 1999;100:1593–1601.

33. Heart Outcomes Prevention Evaluation Study Investigators: Effects of an angiotensin-converting-enzyme inhibitor, ramipril, on cardiovascular events in high-risk patients. N Engl J Med 2000;342:145–153.

34. Dagenais GR, Yusuf S, Bourassa MG, et al: Effects of ramipril on coronary events in high-risk persons: Results of the Heart Outcomes Prevention Evaluation Study. Circulation 2001;104:522–526.

35. Expert Panel on Detection, Evaluation, and Treatment of High Blood Cholesterol in Adults: Executive Summary of the Third Report of the National Cholesterol Education Program (NCEP) Expert Panel on Detection, Evaluation, and Treatment of High Blood Cholesterol in Adults (Adult Treatment Panel III). JAMA 2001;285:2486–2497.

36. Miettinen TA, Pyorala K, Olsson AG, et al: Cholesterol-lowering therapy in women and elderly patients with myocardial infarction or angina pectoris: Findings from the Scandinavian Simvastatin Survival Study (4S). Circulation 1997;96:4211–4218.

37. Lewis SJ, Moye LA, Sacks FM, et al: Effect of pravastatin on cardiovascular events in older patients with myocardial infarction and cholesterol levels in the average range: Results of the Cholesterol And Recurrent Events (CARE) trial. Ann Intern Med 1998;129:681–689.

38. Grundy SM, Cleeman JI, Rifkind BM, Kuller LH: Cholesterol lowering in the elderly population. Coordinating Committee of the National Cholesterol Education Program. Arch Intern Med 1999;159:1670–1678.

39. Batchelor WB, Anstrom KJ, Muhlbaier LH, et al: Contemporary outcome trends in the elderly undergoing percutaneous coronary interventions: Results in 7,472 octogenarians. National Cardiovascular Network Collaboration. J Am Coll Cardiol 2000;36:723–730.

40. Alexander KP, Anstrom KJ, Muhlbaier LH, et al: Outcomes of cardiac surgery in patients > or = 80 years: Results from the National Cardiovascular Network. J Am Coll Cardiol 2000;35:731–738.

41. Smith SC Jr, Dove JT, Jacobs AK, et al: ACC/AHA guidelines of percutaneous coronary interventions (revision of the 1993 PTCA guidelines)—executive summary: A report of the American College of Cardiology/American Heart Association Task Force on Practice Guidelines (committee to revise the 1993 guidelines for percutaneous transluminal coronary angioplasty). J Am Coll Cardiol 2001;37:2215–2238.

42. Eagle KA, Guyton RA, Davidoff R, et al: ACC/AHA guidelines for coronary artery bypass graft surgery: Executive summary and recommendations: A report of the American College of

Cardiology/American Heart Association Task Force on Practice Guidelines (Committee to revise the 1991 guidelines for coronary artery bypass graft surgery). Circulation 1999;100:1464–1480.

43. FRagmin and Fast Revascularisation during InStability in Coronary artery disease (FRISC II) investigators: Invasive compared with non-invasive treatment in unstable coronary-artery disease: FRISC II prospective randomised multicentre study. Lancet 1999;354:708–715.

44. Cannon CP, Weintraub WS, Demopoulos LA, et al, for the TACTICS-Thrombolysis In Myocardial Infarction 18 investigators: Comparison of early invasive and conservative strategies in patients with unstable coronary syndromes treated with the glycoprotein IIb/IIIa inhibitor tirofiban. N Engl J Med 2001;344:1879–1887.

45. Wallentin L, Lagerqvist B, Husted S, et al: Outcome at 1 year after an invasive compared with a non-invasive strategy in unstable coronary-artery disease: The FRISC II invasive randomised trial. FRISC II Investigators. Fast Revascularisation during Instability in Coronary artery disease. Lancet 2000;356:9–16.

46. Stokes J 3rd, Kannel WB, Wolf PA, et al: The relative importance of selected risk factors for various manifestations of cardiovascular disease among men and women from 35 to 64 years old: 30 years of follow-up in the Framingham Study. Circulation 1987;75:V65–V73.

47. Manson JE, Spelsberg A: Risk modification in the diabetic patient. In Manson JE, Ridker PM, Gaziano JM, Hennekens CH (eds): Prevention of Myocardial Infarction. New York, Oxford University Press, 1996, pp 241–273.

48. Kuczmarski RJ, Flegal KM, Campbell SM, Johnson CL: Increasing prevalence of overweight among US adults. The National Health And Nutrition Examination Surveys, 1960 to 1991. JAMA 1994;272:205–211.

49. Behavioral risk factor surveillance, 1986–1990. MMWR Morb Mortal Wkly Rep 1991;40:1–23.

50. Yusuf HR, Giles WH, Croft JB, et al: Impact of multiple risk factor profiles on determining cardiovascular disease risk. Prev Med 1998;27:1–9.

51. Manolio TA, Pearson TA, Wenger NK, et al: Cholesterol and heart disease in older persons and women: Review of an NHLBI workshop. Ann Epidemiol 1992;2:161–176.

52. LaRosa JC: Triglycerides and coronary risk in women and the elderly. Arch Intern Med 1997;157:961–968.

53. Surveillance for selected tobacco-use behaviors—United States, 1900–1994. MMWR Morb Mortal Wkly Rep 1994;43:1–43.

54. Willett WC, Green A, Stampfer MJ, et al: Relative and absolute excess risks of coronary heart disease among women who smoke cigarettes. N Engl J Med 1987;317:1303–1309.

55. Acute myocardial infarction and combined oral contraceptives: Results of an international multicentre case-control study. WHO Collaborative Study of Cardiovascular Disease and Steroid Hormone Contraception. Lancet 1997;349:1202–1209.

56. Colditz GA: Oral contraceptive use and mortality during 12 years of follow-up: The Nurses' Health Study. Ann Intern Med 1994;120:821–826.

57. Salonen JT, Puska P, Tuomilehto J: Physical activity and risk of myocardial infarction, cerebral stroke and death: A longitudinal study in Eastern Finland. Am J Epidemiol 1982;115:526–537.

58. National Center of Health Statistics: Detailed diagnoses and procedures: National Hospital Discharge Survey, 1996. Hyattsville, MD, National Center for Health Statistics, 1998.

59. Mendelsohn ME, Karas RH: The protective effects of estrogen on the cardiovascular system. N Engl J Med 1999;340:1801–1811.

60. Mosca L, Collins P, Herrington DM, et al: Hormone replacement therapy and cardiovascular disease: A statement for healthcare professionals from the American Heart Association. Circulation 2001;104:499–503.

61. Mosca L: The role of hormone replacement therapy in the prevention of postmenopausal heart disease. Arch Intern Med 2000;160:2263–2272.

62. Postmenopausal Estrogen/Progestin Interventions (PEPI) Trial Writing Group: Effects of estrogen or estrogen/progestin regimens on heart disease risk factors in postmenopausal women. The Postmenopausal Estrogen/Progestin Interventions (PEPI) Trial. JAMA 1995;273:199–208.

63. Cushman M, Legault C, Barrett-Connor E, et al: Effect of postmenopausal hormones on inflammation-sensitive proteins: The

Postmenopausal Estrogen/Progestin Interventions (PEPI) Study. Circulation 1999;100:717–722.

64. Douglas PS, Ginsburg GS: The evaluation of chest pain in women. N Engl J Med 1996;334:1311–1315.

65. Willich SN, Lowel H, Lewis M, et al: Unexplained gender differences in clinical symptoms of acute myocardial infarction. J Am Coll Cardiol 1993;21(suppl A):238A.

66. Hochman JS, Tamis JE, Thompson TD, et al: Sex, clinical presentation, and outcome in patients with acute coronary syndromes. Global Use of Strategies to Open Occluded Coronary Arteries in Acute Coronary Syndromes IIb Investigators. N Engl J Med 1999;341:226–232.

67. Scirica BM, Moliterno DJ, Every NR, et al: Differences between men and women in the management of unstable angina pectoris (The GUARANTEE Registry). The GUARANTEE investigators. Am J Cardiol 1999;84:1145–1150.

68. Stone PH, Thompson B, Anderson HV, et al: Influence of race, sex, and age on management of unstable angina and non–Q-wave myocardial infarction: The TIMI III registry. JAMA 1996;275:1104–1112.

69. Hochman JS, McCabe CH, Stone PH, et al: Outcome and profile of women and men presenting with acute coronary syndromes: A report from TIMI IIIB. TIMI investigators. Thrombolysis in Myocardial Infarction. J Am Coll Cardiol 1997;30:141–148.

70. Roger VL, Farkouh ME, Weston SA, et al: Sex differences in evaluation and outcome of unstable angina. JAMA 2000;283:646–652.

71. Kim C, Schaaf CH, Maynard C, Every NR: Unstable angina in the myocardial infarction triage and intervention registry (MITI): Short- and long-term outcomes in men and women. Am Heart J 2001;141:73–77.

72. Welty FK, Mittleman MA, Healy RW, et al: Similar results of percutaneous transluminal coronary angioplasty for women and men with postmyocardial infarction ischemia. J Am Coll Cardiol 1994;23:35–39.

73. Steingart RM, Packer M, Hamm P, et al: Sex differences in the management of coronary artery disease. Survival And Ventricular Enlargement investigators. N Engl J Med 1991;325:226–230.

74. Ayanian JZ, Epstein AM: Differences in the use of procedures between women and men hospitalized for coronary heart disease. N Engl J Med 1991;325:221–225.

75. Fetters JK, Peterson ED, Shaw LJ, et al: Sex-specific differences in coronary artery disease risk factors, evaluation, and treatment: Have they been adequately evaluated? Am Heart J 1996;131:796–813.

76. ISIS-2 (Second International Study of Infarct Survival) Collaborative Group: Randomised trial of intravenous streptokinase, oral aspirin, both, or neither among 17,187 cases of suspected acute myocardial infarction. ISIS-2. Lancet 1988;2:349–360.

77. Fernandes LS, Tcheng JE, Kleiman NS, et al: Eptifibatide is as effective in women as in men: Lessons from the ESPRIT trial. Circulation 2000;102(suppl):II-785.

78. Boersma E, Harrington RA, Moliterno DJ, et al: Platelet glycoprotein IIb/IIIa inhibitors in acute coronary syndromes: Meta-analysis of all major randomised clinical trials. Lancet 2002;359:189–198.

79. Wali A, Hochman JS, Berkowitz S, et al: Failure to achieve optimal anticoagulation with commonly used heparin regimens: A review of GUSTO II. J Am Coll Cardiol 1998;31(suppl A):79A.

80. Klein W, Buchwald A, Hillis SE, et al: Comparison of low-molecular-weight heparin with unfractionated heparin acutely and with placebo for 6 weeks in the management of unstable coronary artery disease. Fragmin in unstable coronary artery disease study (FRIC). Circulation 1997;96:61–68.

81. Gruppo Italiano per lo Studio della Sopravvivenza nell'infarto Miocardico: GISSI-3: Effects of lisinopril and transdermal glyceryl trinitrate singly and together on 6-week mortality and ventricular function after acute myocardial infarction. Lancet 1994;343:1115–1122.

82. ISIS-4 Collaborative Group: ISIS-4: Randomized factorial trial assessing early oral captopril, oral mononitrate, and intravenous magnesium sulphate in 58,050 patients with suspected acute myocardial infarction. Lancet 1995;345:669–685.

83. Kober L, Torp-Pedersen C, Carlsen JE, et al: A clinical trial of the angiotensin-converting-enzyme inhibitor trandolapril in patients with left ventricular dysfunction after myocardial infarction. Trandolapril Cardiac Evaluation (TRACE) Study Group. N Engl J Med 1995;333:1670–1676.

84. Acute Infarction Ramipril Efficacy (AIRE) Study investigators: Effect of ramipril on mortality and morbidity of survivors of acute myocardial infarction with clinical evidence of heart failure. Lancet 1993;342:821–828.

85. Pfeffer MA, Braunwald E, Moye LA, et al, on behalf of the SAVE investigators: Effect of captopril on mortality and morbidity in patients with left ventricular dysfunction after myocardial infarction: Results of the survival and ventricular enlargement trial. The SAVE Investigators. N Engl J Med 1992;327:669–677.

86. Beta-Blocker Heart Attack Trial Research Group: A randomized trial of propranolol in patients with acute myocardial infarction: 1. Mortality results. JAMA 1982;247:1707–1714.

87. ISIS-1 (First International Study of Infarct Survival) Collaborative Group: Randomised trial of intravenous atenolol among 16,027 cases of suspected acute myocardial infarction. Lancet. 1986;2:57–66.

88. Sacks FM, Pfeffer MA, Moye LA, et al: The effect of pravastatin on coronary events after myocardial infarction in patients with average cholesterol levels. Cholesterol and Recurrent Events Trial investigators. N Engl J Med 1996;335:1001–1009.

89. Scandinavian Simvastatin Survival Study Group: Randomised trial of cholesterol lowering in 4444 patients with coronary heart disease: The Scandinavian Simvastatin Survival Study (4S). Lancet 1994;344:1383–1389.

90. Schwartz GG, Olsson AG, Ezekowitz MD, et al: Effects of atorvastatin on early recurrent ischemic events in acute coronary syndromes: The MIRACL study: A randomized controlled trial. JAMA 2001;285:1711–1718.

91. Stenestrand U, Wallentin L: Early statin treatment following acute myocardial infarction and 1-year survival. JAMA 2001;285:430–436.

92. Aronow HD, Topol EJ, Roe MT, et al: Effect of lipid-lowering therapy on early mortality after acute coronary syndromes: An observational study. Lancet 2001;357:1063–1068.

93. Hulley S, Grady D, Bush T, et al: Randomized trial of estrogen plus progestin for secondary prevention of coronary heart disease in postmenopausal women. Heart and Estrogen/progestin Replacement Study (HERS) Research Group. JAMA 1998;280:605–613.

94. Herrington DM, Reboussin DM, Brosnihan KB, et al: Effects of estrogen replacement on the progression of coronary-artery atherosclerosis. N Engl J Med 2000;343:522–529.

95. Alexander KP, Newby LK, Hellkamp AS, et al: Initiation of hormone replacement therapy after acute myocardial infarction is associated with more cardiac events during follow-up. J Am Coll Cardiol 2001;38:1–7.

96. Women's Health Initiative Study Group: Design of the Women's Health Initiative clinical trial and observational study. Control Clin Trials 1998;19:61–109.

97. Nelson HD, Humphrey LL, Nygren P, et al: Postmenopausal hormone replacement therapy: Scientific review. JAMA 2002;288:872–881.

98. Viscoli CM, Brass LM, Kernan WN, et al: A clinical trial of estrogen-replacement therapy after ischemic stroke. N Engl J Med 2001;345:1243–1249.

99. Mosca L, Barrett-Connor E, Wenger NK, et al: Design and methods of the Raloxifene Use for The Heart (RUTH) study. Am J Cardiol 2001;88:392–395.

100. Morise AP, Diamond GA: Comparison of the sensitivity and specificity of exercise electrocardiography in biased and unbiased populations of men and women. Am Heart J 1995;130:741–747.

101. Shaw LJ, Miller DD, Romeis JC, et al: Gender differences in the noninvasive evaluation and management of patients with suspected coronary artery disease. Ann Intern Med 1994;120:559–566.

102. Marwick TH, Anderson T, Williams MJ, et al: Exercise echocardiography is an accurate and cost-efficient technique for detection of coronary artery disease in women. J Am Coll Cardiol 1995;26:335–341.

103. Maynard C, Litwin PE, Martin JS, Weaver WD: Gender differences in the treatment and outcome of acute myocardial infarction: Results of the Myocardial Infarction Triage and Intervention Registry. Arch Intern Med 1992;152:972–976.

104. Kelsey SF, James M, Holubkov AL, et al: Results of percutaneous transluminal coronary angioplasty in women. 1985–1986 National Heart, Lung, and Blood Institute's Coronary Angioplasty Registry. Circulation 1993;87:720–727.

105. Fisher LD, Kennedy JW, Davis KB, et al: Association of sex, physical size, and operative mortality after coronary artery bypass in the Coronary Artery Surgery Study (CASS). J Thorac Cardiovasc Surg 1982;84:334-341.

106. Keelan ET, Nunez BD, Grill DE, et al: Comparison of immediate and long-term outcome of coronary angioplasty performed for unstable angina and rest pain in men and women. Mayo Clin Proc 1997;72:5-12.

107. Jacobs AK, Kelsey SF, Brooks MM, et al: Better outcome for women compared with men undergoing coronary revascularization: A report from the bypass angioplasty revascularization investigation (BARI). Circulation 1998;98:1279-1285.

108. Lagerqvist B, Safstrom K, Stahle E, et al: Is early invasive treatment of unstable coronary artery disease equally effective for both women and men? FRISC II Study Group investigators. J Am Coll Cardiol 2001;38:41-48.

109. Malmberg K, Yusuf S, Gerstein HC, et al, for the OASIS Registry investigators: Impact of diabetes on long-term prognosis in patients with unstable angina and non-Q-wave myocardial infarction: Results of the OASIS (Organization to Assess Strategies for Ischemic Syndromes) Registry. Circulation 2000;102:1014-1019.

110. Sprafka JM, Burke GL, Folsom AR, et al: Trends in prevalence of diabetes mellitus in patients with myocardial infarction and effect of diabetes on survival. The Minnesota Heart Survey. Diabetes Care 1991;14:537-543.

111. King H, Aubert RE, Herman WH: Global burden of diabetes, 1995-2025: Prevalence, numerical estimates, and projections. Diabetes Care 1998;21:1414-1431.

112. Wingard DL, Barrett-Connor E: Heart disease and diabetes. In Harris M (ed): Diabetes in America, 2nd ed. Bethesda, MD, National Institutes of Health, 1995, pp 429-456.

113. Haffner SM, Lehto S, Ronnemaa T, et al: Mortality from coronary heart disease in subjects with type 2 diabetes and in nondiabetic subjects with and without prior myocardial infarction. N Engl J Med 1998;339:229-234.

114. McGuire DK, Emanuelsson H, Granger CB, et al: Influence of diabetes mellitus on clinical outcomes across the spectrum of acute coronary syndromes: Findings from the GUSTO-IIb study. GUSTO IIb investigators. Eur Heart J 2000;21:1750-1758.

115. BARI investigators: Influence of diabetes on 5-year mortality and morbidity in a randomized trial comparing CABG and PTCA in patients with multivessel disease. The Bypass Angioplasty Revascularization Investigation (BARI). Circulation 1997;96:1761-1769.

116. Barsness GW, Peterson ED, Ohman EM, et al: Relationship between diabetes mellitus and long-term survival after coronary bypass and angioplasty. Circulation 1997;96:2551-2556.

117. Rodrigues B, McNeill JH: The diabetic heart: Metabolic causes for the development of a cardiomyopathy. Cardiovasc Res 1992;26:913-922.

118. Garg A, Grundy SM: Diabetic dyslipidemia and its therapy. Diabetes Rev 1997;5:425-433.

119. Scherrer U, Sartori C: Insulin as a vascular and sympathoexcitatory hormone: Implications for blood pressure regulation, insulin sensitivity, and cardiovascular morbidity. Circulation 1997;96:4104-4113.

120. McVeigh GE, Brennan GM, Johnston GD, et al: Impaired endothelium-dependent and independent vasodilation in patients with type 2 (non-insulin-dependent) diabetes mellitus. Diabetologia 1992;35:771-776.

121. Jokl R, Colwell JA: Arterial thrombosis and atherosclerosis in diabetes. Diabetes Rev 1997;5:316-330.

122. Pickup JC, Mattock MB, Chusney GD, Burt D: NIDDM as a disease of the innate immune system: Association of acute-phase reactants and interleukin-6 with metabolic syndrome X. Diabetologia 1997;40:1286-1292.

123. Zarich SW, Nesto RW: Diabetic cardiomyopathy. Am Heart J 1989;118:1000-1012.

124. Stone PH, Muller JE, Hartwell T, et al, for the MILIS Study Group: The effect of diabetes mellitus on prognosis and serial left ventricular function after acute myocardial infarction: Contribution of both coronary disease and diastolic left ventricular dysfunction to the adverse prognosis. The MILIS Study Group. J Am Coll Cardiol 1989;14:49-57.

125. Gilpin E, Ricou F, Dittrich H, et al: Factors associated with recurrent myocardial infarction within one year after acute myocardial infarction. Am Heart J 1991;121:457-465.

126. Moreno PR, Murcia AM, Palacios IF, et al: Coronary composition and macrophage infiltration in atherectomy specimens from patients with diabetes mellitus. Circulation 2000;102:2180-2184.

127. Nesto RW, Phillips RT: Silent myocardial ischemia: Clinical characteristics, underlying mechanisms, and implications for treatment. Am J Med 1986;81:12-19.

128. Lim LL, Tesfay GM, Heller RF: Management of patients with diabetes after heart attack: A population-based study of 1982 patients from a heart disease register. Aust N Z J Med 1998;28:334-342.

129. Steering Committee of the Physicians' Health Study Research Group: Final report on the aspirin component of the ongoing Physicians' Health Study. N Engl J Med 1989;321:129-135.

130. CAPRIE Steering Committee: A randomised, blinded, trial of clopidogrel versus aspirin in patients at risk of ischaemic events (CAPRIE). Lancet 1996;348:1329-1339.

131. Mahaffey K, Granger C, Toth C, et al: Diabetic retinopathy should not be a contraindication to thrombolytic therapy for acute myocardial infarction: Review of ocular hemorrhage incidence and location in the GUSTO-I trial. J Am Coll Cardiol 1997;30:1606-1610.

132. Nesto RW, Zarich S. Acute myocardial infarction in diabetes mellitus: Lessons learned from ACE inhibition. Circulation 1998;97:12-15.

133. Zuanetti G, Latini R, Maggioni AP, et al: Effect of the ACE inhibitor lisinopril on mortality in diabetic patients with acute myocardial infarction: Data from the GISSI-3 study. Circulation 1997;96:4239-4245.

134. Swedberg K, Held P, Kjekshus J, et al: Effects of the early administration of enalapril on mortality in patients with acute myocardial infarction: Results of the Cooperative New Scandinavian Enalapril Survival Study II (CONSENSUS II). N Engl J Med 1992;327:678-684.

135. Gustafsson I, Torp-Pedersen C, Kober L, et al: Effect of the angiotensin-converting enzyme inhibitor trandolapril on mortality and morbidity in diabetic patients with left ventricular dysfunction after acute myocardial infarction. Trace Study Group. J Am Coll Cardiol 1999;34:83-89.

136. UK Prospective Diabetes Study Group: Tight blood pressure control and risk of macrovascular and microvascular complications in type 2 diabetes: UKPDS 38. UK Prospective Diabetes Study Group. BMJ 1998;317:703-713.

137. Heart Outcomes Prevention Evaluation Study investigators: Effects of ramipril on cardiovascular and microvascular outcomes in people with diabetes mellitus: Results of the HOPE study and MICRO-HOPE substudy. Lancet 2000;355:253-259.

138. Kendall MJ, Lynch KP, Hjalmarson A, Kjekshus J: Beta-blockers and sudden cardiac death. Ann Intern Med 1995;123:358-367.

139. Kjekshus J, Gilpin E, Cali G, et al: Diabetic patients and beta-blockers after acute myocardial infarction. Eur Heart J 1990;11:43-50.

140. Younis N, Burnham P, Patwala A, et al: Beta blocker prescribing differences in patients with and without diabetes following a first myocardial infarction. Diabet Med 2001;18:159-161.

141. Haffner SM: The Scandinavian Simvastatin Survival Study (4S) subgroup analysis of diabetic subjects: Implications for the prevention of coronary heart disease. Diabetes Care 1997;20:469-471.

142. Long-term Intervention with Pravastatin in Ischaemic Disease (LIPID) Study Group: Prevention of cardiovascular events and death with pravastatin in patients with coronary heart disease and a broad range of initial cholesterol levels. N Engl J Med 1998;339:1349-1357.

143. Heart Protection Study Collaboration Group. MRC/BHF heart protection study of cholesterol lowering with simvastatin in 20,536 high-risk individuals: a randomized placebo-controlled trial. Lancet 2002;630:7-22.

144. Muhlestein JB, Horne BD, Bair TL, et al: Usefulness of in-hospital prescription of statin agents after angiographic diagnosis of coronary artery disease in improving continued compliance and reduced mortality. Am J Cardiol 2001;87:257-261.

145. Malmberg K, Norhammar A, Wedel H, Ryden L: Glycometabolic state at admission: Important risk marker of mortality in conventionally treated patients with diabetes mellitus and acute myocardial infarction: Long-term results from the Diabetes and Insulin-Glucose Infusion in Acute Myocardial Infarction (DIGAMI) study. Circulation 1999;99:2626-2632.

146. Stern MP: The effect of glycemic control on the incidence of macrovascular complications of type 2 diabetes. Arch Fam Med 1998;7:155-162.

147. Rao SV, Bethel MA, Feinglos MN: Treatment of diabetes mellitus: Implications of the use of oral agents. Am Heart J 1999;138:S334-337.

148. Malmberg K, McGuire DK: Diabetes and acute myocardial infarction: The role of insulin therapy. Am Heart J 1999;138:S381-386.

149. Oliver MF, Opie LH: Effects of glucose and fatty acids on myocardial ischaemia and arrhythmias. Lancet 1994;343:155-158.

150. Opie LH: Glucose and the metabolism of ischaemic myocardium. Lancet 1995;345:1520-1521.

151. Lopaschuk GD, Wambolt RB, Barr RL: An imbalance between glycolysis and glucose oxidation is a possible explanation for the detrimental effects of high levels of fatty acids during aerobic reperfusion of ischemic hearts. J Pharmacol Exp Ther 1993;264:135-144.

152. McDaniel HG, Papapietro SE, Rogers WJ, et al: Glucose-insulin-potassium induced alterations in individual plasma free fatty acids in patients with acute myocardial infarction. Am Heart J 1981;102:10-15.

153. Jain SK, Nagi DK, Slavin BM, et al: Insulin therapy in type 2 diabetic subjects suppresses plasminogen activator inhibitor (PAI-1) activity and proinsulin-like molecules independently of glycaemic control. Diabet Med 1993;10:27-32.

154. Malmberg K: Prospective randomised study of intensive insulin treatment on long term survival after acute myocardial infarction in patients with diabetes mellitus. DIGAMI (Diabetes Mellitus, Insulin Glucose Infusion in Acute Myocardial Infarction) Study Group. BMJ 1997;314:1512-1515.

155. Van den Berghe G, Wouters P, Weekers F, et al: Intensive insulin therapy in critically ill patients. N Engl J Med 2001;345:1359-1367.

156. Sodi-Pallares D, Bisteni A, Medrano G: The polarizing treatment of acute myocardial infarction. Dis Chest 1963;43:424-432.

157. Fath-Ordoubadi F, Beatt KJ: Glucose-insulin-potassium therapy for treatment of acute myocardial infarction: An overview of randomized placebo-controlled trials. Circulation 1997;96:1152-1156.

158. UK Prospective Diabetes Study (UKPDS) Group: Intensive blood-glucose control with sulphonylureas or insulin compared with conventional treatment and risk of complications in patients with type 2 diabetes (UKPDS 33). Lancet 1998;352:837-853.

159. Jollis JG, Simpson RJ Jr, Cascio WE, et al: Relation between sulfonylurea therapy, complications, and outcome for elderly patients with acute myocardial infarction. Am Heart J 1999;138:S376-380.

160. UK Prospective Diabetes Study (UKPDS) Group: Effect of intensive blood-glucose control with metformin on complications in overweight patients with type 2 diabetes (UKPDS 34). Lancet 1998;352:854-865.

161. Meinert CL, Knatterud GL, Prout TE, Klimt CR: A study of the effects of hypoglycemic agents on vascular complications in patients with adult-onset diabetes: II. Mortality results. Diabetes 1970;19(suppl):789-830.

162. Abraira C, Colwell JA, Nuttall FQ, et al: Veterans Affairs Cooperative Study on glycemic control and complications in type II diabetes (VA CSDM): Results of the feasibility trial. Veterans Affairs Cooperative Study in Type II Diabetes. Diabetes Care 1995;18:1113-1123.

163. McGuire DK, Newby LK, Bhapkar MV, et al: Diabetes doubles the risk of death among patients presenting with acute coronary syndromes: Insight from SYMPHONY, a large international trial. J Am Coll Cardiol 2001;37(suppl A):372A.

164. Lavasani F, Muhlestein JB, Horne BD, et al: Metformin versus other oral agents: Does the choice of discharge diabetic medications predict mortality? Results from a registry of 1428 diabetic patients. J Am Coll Cardiol 2001;37:299A.

165. American Diabetes Association: Standards of medical care for patients with diabetes mellitus. Tenn Med 2000;93:419-429.

166. Niles NW, McGrath PD, Malenka D, et al: Survival of patients with diabetes and multivessel coronary artery disease after surgical or percutaneous coronary revascularization: Results of a large regional prospective study. Northern New England Cardiovascular Disease Study Group. J Am Coll Cardiol 2001;37:1008-1015.

Coronary Artery Spasm

Hirofumi Yasue

Angina pectoris is a clinical syndrome caused by transient myocardial ischemia resulting from an imbalance between myocardial oxygen demand and supply. Classic or effort angina is characterized by the following: (1) The attack is induced by exertion and relieved by rest or nitroglycerin administration, and (2) the attack is associated with transient ST-segment depression on the electrocardiogram (ECG).[1] This form of angina has been well known for more than 200 years since its description by Heberden, and its pathogenesis has been explained by increased myocardial oxygen demand in the presence of fixed organic stenosis of epicardial coronary arteries. This concept was based on the fact that most patients with angina were found to have severe and extensive atherosclerotic narrowing in their coronary arteries. β-Adrenergic blocking agents, which reduce myocardial oxygen demand, have been used widely to treat angina. The efficacy of nitroglycerin has been attributed chiefly to its venodilatory effect, which results in pooling of blood in the venous system leading to decreased myocardial work, rather than to its direct effect on the coronary arteries.[2]

In 1959, Prinzmetal and colleagues[3] described a new form of angina pectoris that differed sharply from the classic angina and named it "variant form of angina pectoris." The characteristics of this syndrome were as follows: (1) The attack occurred at rest and was not provoked by exertion, and (2) the attack was associated with ST-segment elevation on the ECG. Because the attack occurred at rest and was not induced by exercise, an increase in myocardial oxygen demand could not explain the pathogenesis of this form of angina. Prinzmetal and colleagues[3] postulated that increased tonus in a vessel with atherosclerotic narrowing might lead transiently to critically diminished blood supply to an area of myocardium. This syndrome drew little attention among cardiologists at that time, however, probably because it was usually not induced by exercise in the daytime, and the concept of increased myocardial oxygen demand in the presence of fixed organic stenosis of coronary arteries as a cause of angina pectoris prevailed.[1]

After the introduction of coronary angiography and its widespread use, spasm of an epicardial coronary artery or coronary spasm was documented angiographically during the attack of variant angina at several institutions in the early 1970s.[4-7] Coronary spasm was established as the cause of variant angina.[7] With the introduction of ambulatory ECG monitoring for myocardial ischemia and its widespread use, many cases of variant angina have been reported, particularly in Japan.[8,9] It is now known that coronary spasm plays an important role in the pathogenesis not only of variant angina, but also of ischemic heart disease in general, including effort angina, unstable angina, acute myocardial infarction, and sudden death.[9-13] Variant angina is only one aspect of the wide spectrum of myocardial ischemic syndromes caused by coronary spasm.[10] Angina caused by coronary spasm now is usually called *coronary (vaso) spastic angina*, and the name *variant angina* is less often used.[13]

CORONARY CONSTRICTION AND SPASM

Similar to all blood vessels, coronary arteries are able to contract and relax via various mechanisms. Coronary constriction is a normal phenomenon and not necessarily pathologic. Under certain disease conditions, coronary constriction becomes more dominant than in healthy individuals, however, and may contribute to symptoms such as angina pectoris.[14] The degree of coronary constriction may differ considerably in different syndromes and different patients. In certain patients, coronary constriction may be only slightly increased, and no symptoms may occur at rest; however, the increased coronary tone may alter significantly the threshold for angina during exercise in these patients.[15,16] The fact that most coronary lesions are eccentric may explain why diseased segments also are able to relax and constrict to various stimuli.

Coronary constriction may be so severe that myocardial ischemia occurs even at rest in some patients with angiographically normal coronary arteries. Under such conditions, a near-total or total occlusion or severe diffuse constriction of the coronary artery can be shown. Some authors have emphasized the difference between increased constriction and total occlusion of a coronary artery and have restricted the expression *coronary spasm* to the latter condition.[17] Increased constriction contributes, however, to a varied spectrum of ischemic heart disease, and the same patients may have different degrees of coronary constriction at different times. The difference between hyperconstriction and total occlusion is gradual, and the distinction between coronary spasm and hyperconstriction is artificial.[14,18] Hyperconstriction usually involves the entire coronary artery, although the degree of constriction may differ among segments of the artery, resulting in total occlusion in some cases.

We define *coronary spasm* as an abnormal contraction of an epicardial coronary artery resulting in myocardial ischemia.[9,13] With this definition, there are no limits on the degree of lumen diameter reduction required to diagnose coronary spasm since ischemia must accompany the changes of vessel size.

PREVALENCE OF CORONARY SPASM

There are not enough data on the prevalence of coronary spasm in Eastern and Western countries, probably because it is difficult to examine coronary spasm systematically at the time of coronary angiography. The prevalence rate also may vary depending on the interest and eagerness on the part of the investigators. Bertrand and coworkers[19] reported in 1982 in 1089 consecutive patients undergoing coronary angiography that coronary spasm was provoked by ergonovine in 205 patients with recent myocardial infarction and in 155 patients who complained of chest pain. Coronary spasm has been said to become less frequent in Western countries. This change is probably due to the facts that calcium antagonists, which are specifically effective in suppressing coronary spasm, have been used widely for chest pain and hypertension and better nitrate regimens have been developed and used. Also, many cardiologists now are not as interested in coronary spasm, and provocation tests for it are performed less often.[20] Coronary spasm is still prevalent and provocation tests for it are performed routinely at many institutions in Japan[21] and perhaps in Korea.[22] A survey on the prevalence of coronary spasm at multiple institutions in Japan showed that coronary spasms were documented in 180 (43%) of 422 consecutive patients with angina pectoris who underwent coronary angiography.[21] There also seems to be a racial difference in the prevalence of coronary spasm between Japanese and whites. A report showed a major racial difference in coronary constrictor response between Japanese and whites.[23]

The prevalence has become less frequent also in Japan probably for the same reasons as in Western countries. Perhaps cardiologists now are interested only in patients in need of angioplasty or stenting and do not want to be bothered with coronary spasm.[20] Some cardiologists may consider the provocation test for coronary spasm too cumbersome and time-consuming to be done in the busy invasive-interventional laboratory. Many cardiologists may think that a trial of calcium antagonists is as helpful as a provocation test in the evaluation of possible spasm.[20]

CLINICAL MANIFESTATIONS

Circadian Variation

Coronary spasm occurs most often at rest, particularly from midnight to early morning (Fig. 40-1).[3-13] Although Prinzmetal and colleagues[3] emphasized that variant angina is not induced by exercise, an attack of variant angina or coronary spasm often can be induced by mild exercise in the early morning.[15,24] It is usually not induced in the afternoon, however, even by strenuous exercise. There is a circadian variation in the exercise capacity in patients with coronary spasm.[15] It is now known that attacks of all forms of ischemic heart disease, including acute myocardial infarction and sudden death, occur most often in the early morning.[25] This timing may be related at least partially to the fact that the tone of an epicardial coronary artery is increased in the early morning, whereas it is decreased in the afternoon.[15]

The causes of the circadian variation of coronary spasm remain to be elucidated. Because coronary spasm can be induced by intracoronary injection of acetylcholine (ACh),[26] the neurotransmitter of the parasympathetic nervous system, changes in the activity of the autonomic nervous system may be involved in the circadian variation of coronary spasm.[27] Coronary spasm also can be induced by stimulation of α-adrenergic receptors.[5] Circadian variations of the production of various hormones, including vasopressin, melatonin, growth hormone, insulin, and cortisol, also may be related to the circadian variation of coronary spasm.

Symptoms and Electrocardiogram Changes

The commonly associated manifestations of myocardial ischemia resulting from coronary spasm are chest pain and ST-segment changes on the ECG. Chest pain is similar in quality to that of stable effort angina but is often more severe and prolonged, accompanied by a cold sweat, nausea or vomiting, and sometimes syncope. Myocardial ischemia resulting from coronary spasm often occurs without accompanying symptoms.[13,28] The incidence of silent myocardial ischemia caused by coronary spasm is more than two times higher than that of symptomatic ischemia (see Fig. 40-1).[13]

The ECG changes that occur during a coronary spasm attack include ST-segment elevation or ST-segment depression or both; peaking or increase in amplitude of the T wave; a delay in the peak and an increase in the height and width of the R wave, resulting in fusion of R

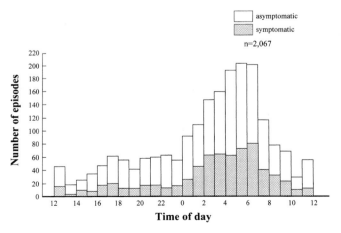

FIGURE 40-1. Diurnal distribution of ischemic episodes in patients with variant angina. The attacks occur most often from midnight to early morning. The number of asymptomatic attacks was larger than that of symptomatic attacks. (From Yasue H, Kugiyama K: Coronary spasm: Clinical features and pathogenesis. Intern Med 1997;36:760.)

wave with T wave; and a decrease in magnitude or disappearance of the S wave (Fig. 40-2). The negative U wave also may appear at the beginning or near the end of the attack and usually is associated with ST-segment changes in the anterolateral leads. It may be the only ECG change that occurs during a mild attack when spasm is not severe and does not occlude the coronary artery completely.

Total or subtotal occlusion of a major coronary artery by spasm results in ST-segment elevation in the leads that represent the area of myocardium supplied by the artery (Fig. 40-3). The ST-segment elevation usually is accompanied by reciprocal ST-segment depression in the opposite leads. It is important to record ECGs in multiple leads. The magnitude of ST-segment elevation varies and corresponds roughly to the degree of acute myocardial ischemia. As the attack proceeds, the magnitude of ST-segment elevation increases and, in association with an increase in magnitude and widening of the R wave in the same lead, may form a *monophasic curve* at the peak of the attack (see Fig. 40-2). This monophasic curve is usually not seen during acute myocardial infarction and is characteristic of a severe attack of coronary spasm occluding the proximal segment of a major coronary artery. The ST-segment elevation appears in the leads corresponding to the distribution of one major coronary artery. The leads in which ST-segment elevation appears are usually the same during each attack in the same patient, indicating that spasm usually appears at the same coronary artery in the same patient. ST-segment

elevation commonly occurs, however, in the anterior leads during one attack and in the inferior leads in another in the same patients. There are also patients in whom ST-segment elevation occurs simultaneously in the anterior and inferior leads (Figs. 40-4 and 40-5). These are patients with simultaneous multivessel coronary spasm, and the attacks often result in ventricular tachycardia or fibrillation or both (see Fig. 40-4).[28,29] There is not much difference in the incidence of ST-segment elevation between the anterior leads and inferior leads. The ECG may be unchanged at the beginning of an attack or when the attack is mild. Occasionally, pseudonormalization of a previously depressed ST segment may appear (see Fig. 40-2).

Coronary spasm also may cause ST-segment depression instead of elevation in the leads that represent the distribution area of the spasm artery. The ST-segment depression indicates less severe (nontransmural or subendocardial) myocardial ischemia than does ST-segment elevation, which represents transmural myocardial ischemia. The ST-segment depression occurs when (1) spasm of a major artery is less severe (subtotal or diffuse) (see Fig. 40-3), (2) a major artery receiving collaterals is completely occluded, or (3) a small artery is completely occluded.[18] The direction and extent of ST-segment change may vary from one episode to another, and ST-segment elevation and depression can occur in the same patient or in the same lead within minutes or hours.[10]

Various forms of arrhythmia often appear during attacks of coronary spasm associated with ST-segment

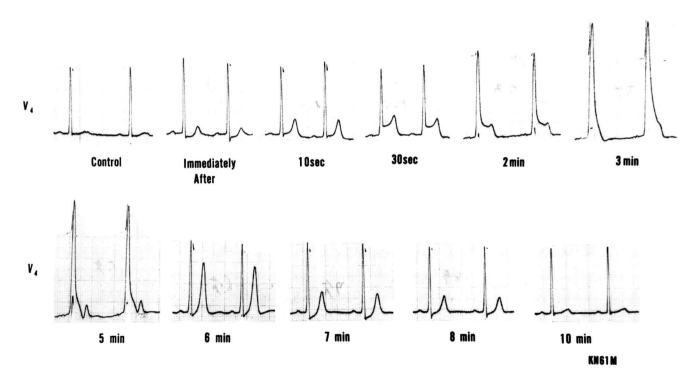

FIGURE 40-2. Electrocardiogram changes during an attack of exercise-induced coronary spasm. At the beginning of the attack, ST-segment depression and peaking of the T wave appeared. As the attack proceeded, ST-segment elevation and increase in amplitude and widening of the R wave occurred, resulting in a monophasic curve at the peak of the attack. The ST-segment depression and peaking of the T wave again appeared near the end of the attack. There is a pseudonormalization of ST segment during transition from ST-segment depression to ST-segment elevation. Times indicate after the end of exercise.

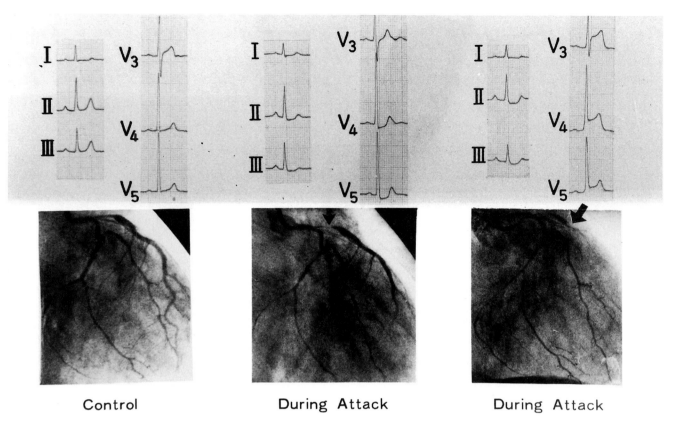

FIGURE 40–3. Coronary angiograms and corresponding electrocardiograms during attacks with either ST-segment elevation or ST-segment depression in the chest leads. During the attack with ST-segment elevation, spasm totally occluded the left anterior descending artery at the proximal segment as shown by the *arrow* on the right. During the attack with ST-segment depression, spasm subtotally occluded the same artery at the same segment as shown by the *arrow* in the center. The left panel shows the control. (From Yasue H, Omote S, Takizawa A, et al: Comparison of coronary arteriographic findings during angina pectoris associated with ST segment elevation or depression. Am J Cardiol 1981;47:539.)

elevation, including ventricular arrhythmias, such as ventricular premature contractions or ventricular tachycardia, bradyarrhythmias, atrioventricular block, and supraventricular arrhythmias (see Fig. 40-4). Ventricular fibrillation also may appear rarely.

Ventricular arrhythmias appear more often when ST-segment elevation occurs in the anterior leads. Bradyarrhythmias appear more frequently when ST-segment elevation occurs in the inferior leads. The high degrees of bradyarrhythmias often are associated with hypotension and sometimes with syncope. Lethal arrhythmias, such as ventricular tachycardia, ventricular fibrillation, and complete atrioventricular block, may appear particularly during an attack of multivessel spasm (see Fig. 40-4).[12,28,29] There is a good correlation between the incidence of arrhythmia and the degree of ST-segment elevation.

Coronary Angiographic and Hemodynamic Changes

Coronary spasm has been thought to occur at a site of organic stenosis of a major coronary artery.[3] Coronary spasm appears in angiographically normal arteries, however, and arteries with organic stenosis.[13,28-31] Of the 179 patients with coronary spasm at our institution,[13]

126 (71%) had normal or near-normal coronary arteries. Spasm may be diffuse or diffuse and focal[32] and may migrate from site to site. Spasm occurs not only at one large coronary artery, but also at two or three large arteries separately or simultaneously in the same patients. Multivessel spasm was shown in 93 (52%) patients (Fig. 40-6), and 77 (83%) of these patients had normal or near-normal coronary arteries.[13]

Patients with multivessel coronary spasm have the following characteristics: (1) Most of them have angiographically normal coronary arteries; (2) they are resistant to treatment and often require larger amounts of calcium antagonists to suppress the attacks, which often recur on cessation of calcium antagonists; and (3) they are more likely to have lethal arrhythmias, such as ventricular tachycardia or ventricular fibrillation, and are more likely to experience sudden death.[13]

There is no consistent increase in heart rate, blood pressure, or dP/dt before the onset of ST-segment elevation. The most typical and early hemodynamic pattern observed in the initial phase of coronary spasm is a reduction of positive and negative peak dP/dt and elevation of end-diastolic pressure of the left ventricle.[10] These hemodynamic changes occur before the appearance of ST-segment elevation. Subjective symptoms always follow ST-segment and hemodynamic changes. Myocardial ischemia not only alters the contractile

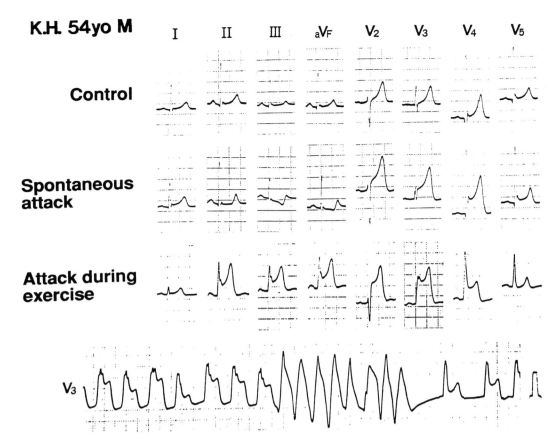

FIGURE 40–4. Electrocardiogram changes during the attacks of multivessel coronary spasm. During the spontaneous attack, ST-segment elevation appeared in the chest leads (leads V_{2-5}), and ST-segment depression appeared in the inferior leads (leads II, II, and aVF). During the attack induced by exercise, ST-segment elevation appeared in the anterior and the inferior leads (leads II, III, aVF, and V_{2-4}). Ventricular tachycardia also appeared during the attack as shown at the bottom.

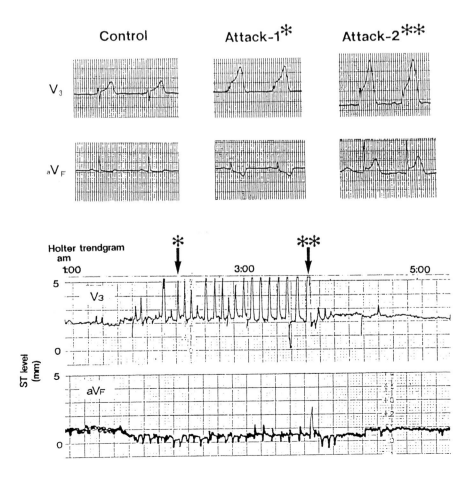

FIGURE 40–5. Ambulatory monitoring of electrocardiogram during spontaneous attacks of variant angina. Recurrent attacks appeared from 1:00 to 5:00 AM as shown by the ST trendgram in the bottom. Real-time electrocardiograms are shown in the upper panel. *Attack-1* was associated with ST-segment elevation in the anterior lead with reciprocal ST-segment depression in the inferior lead. *Attack-2* was associated with ST-segment elevation in the anterior and the inferior leads, indicating simultaneous multivessel coronary spasm.

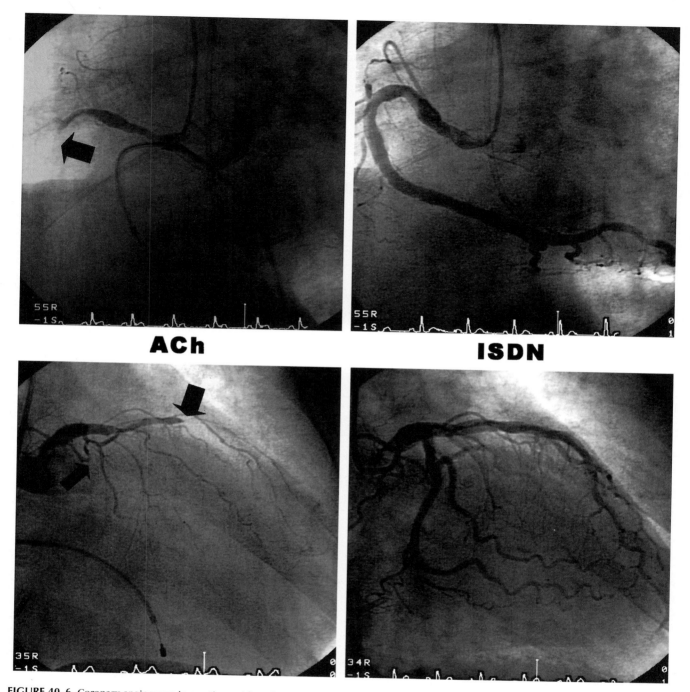

ACh

ISDN

FIGURE 40–6. Coronary angiograms in a patient with multivessel coronary spasm. Injection of acetylcholine (ACh) into the right coronary artery *(top left)* and the left coronary artery *(bottom left)* induced spasm in each of the arteries separately. Spasm appeared in all three major arteries (right coronary artery, left anterior descending artery, and left circumflex artery) as indicated by the *arrow*. Spasm was reversed after intracoronary injection of isosorbide dinitrate (ISDN) *(top right* and *bottom right)*. There was no significant organic stenosis in the arteries.

properties of the heart, but also impairs ventricular relaxation. The combination of incomplete myocardial relaxation and depressed contractility leads to elevated ventricular filling pressure. The appearance of wall motion abnormalities is the most sensitive marker of myocardial ischemia, and this can be detected easily by echocardiograms (Fig. 40–7).[22,33,34] The appearance of wall motion abnormalities of the left ventricle during the attack also has been shown by ventriculography.[6]

Precipitating Factors

Several triggers may precipitate coronary spasm and can be divided into physiologic factors and pharmacologic agents. Coronary spasm occurs most often at rest, most often from midnight to early morning. In the early morning, it may be induced by mild exercise.[15] Persistent physical or mental stress, especially the latter, may precipitate coronary spasm, particularly at rest,[13,35] as will

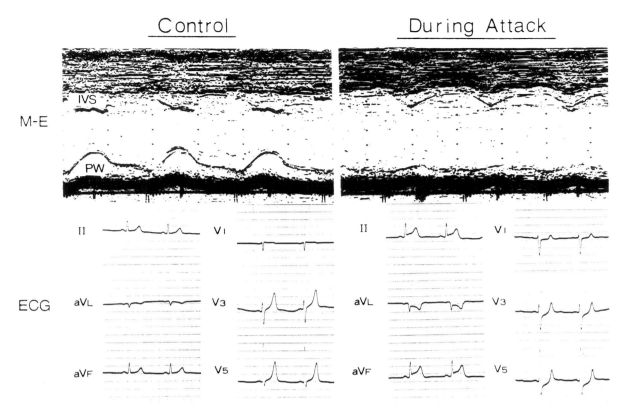

FIGURE 40–7. M-mode echocardiograms *(top)* and electrocardiograms *(bottom)* during an attack of coronary spasm. Marked reduction of motion and systolic thickening of the posterior wall appeared in the echocardiograms during the attack associated with ST-segment elevation in the inferior leads *(right panel)*. The *left panel* shows the control findings. (From Fujii H, Yasue H, Okumura K, et al: Hyperventilation-induced simultaneous multivessel coronary spasm in patients with variant angina: An echocardiographic and arteriographic study. J Am Coll Cardiol 1988;12:1184.)

exposure to cold,[36] Valsalva maneuver, and hyperventilation.[34,37-39] Magnesium deficiency also is associated with coronary spasm.[39,40] Spasm itself often induces spasm, creating a vicious cycle.[13]

Pharmacologic agents include catecholamines (epinephrine, norepinephrine, isoproterenol, dopamine, dobutamine),[5,41,42] parasympathomimetic agents (acetylcholine, methacholine, pilocarpine),[26,27] anticholinesterase agents (neostigmine),[43] ergonovine,[22,44-46] serotonin,[47] histamine,[48] β-adrenergic blocking agents,[26,49] withdrawal from long-term exposure to nitroglycerin,[50] cocaine,[51] nicotine,[52,53] and alcohol.[54,55] The daily use of alcohol is particularly important to note. Heavy drinking after stressful situations often induces coronary spasm, usually not immediately but after several hours, when blood levels of alcohol normalize. Coronary spasm occurring on withdrawal from chronic exposure to industrial nitrates was reported in the early 1970s.[50]

All aforementioned factors or agents may induce coronary spasm as a single provocative trigger. When several of these factors are combined, however, the likelihood of coronary spasm is higher.[13]

Coronary Spasm and Coronary Thrombosis

Coronary thrombosis causes acute coronary syndromes, including acute myocardial infarction, unstable angina,

and ischemic sudden death.[56-58] Coronary spasm also may be involved in the pathogenesis of acute coronary syndromes.[10-13] Plasma levels of fibrinopeptide A, a marker of thrombin generation, are increased after attacks of coronary spasm,[59,60] and there is a circadian variation in the occurrence of myocardial infarction that parallels that of attacks of coronary spasm (Fig. 40-8).[60] Plasma levels of plasminogen activator inhibitor 1 also show a similar circadian variation.[61] Platelets also are activated after attacks of coronary spasm but not after episodes of stable exertional angina (Fig. 40-9).[62] These findings indicate that coronary spasm can trigger coronary thrombosis and may play an important role in the pathogenesis of acute coronary syndromes.[10-13] Angioscopic studies have also shown that intracoronary thrombi can be found in patients with variant angina.[63]

DIAGNOSIS OF CORONARY SPASM

The diagnosis of coronary spasm can be difficult. In contrast to stable effort angina, which is reproducibly induced by exercise, coronary spastic angina is usually not induced by exercise, especially in the afternoon, and occurs mainly at rest, between midnight and early morning.[13,15] The attacks are transient, and may last only a few seconds, in an unpredictable pattern. Ambulatory monitoring of ECGs is crucial to detect ST-segment shifts (see

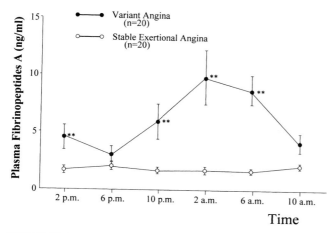

FIGURE 40–8. Circadian variation of plasma levels of fibrinopeptide A in patients with variant angina and patients with stable exertional angina. Plasma levels of fibrinopeptide A are increased and show marked circadian variation with a peak appearing from midnight to early morning in patients with variant angina. In contrast, the levels are not increased and do not show a circadian variation in patients with stable exertional angina. $*P < .05$, $**P < .01$, difference of the levels between patients with variant angina and patients with stable effort angina at each sampling time. (From Ogawa H, Yasue H, Oshima S, et al: Circadian variation of plasma fibrinopeptide A level in patients with variant angina. Circulation 1989;80:1617.)

Fig. 40–5),[8] but may not be diagnostic if no attacks occur during the monitoring period.

This has led to the use of provocation tests for diagnosis. These tests afford an opportunity to induce an episode of coronary spasm at selected times with adequate patient monitoring, when the patient is in a unit or a laboratory well equipped for appropriate documentation and treatment. Several provocative tests for coronary spasm have been developed. Of these, the ergonovine and ACh tests are used most often.[19,22,26,29,44-46] Coronary arteries prone to spasm are hypersensitive to ergonovine and ACh. Ergonovine is an ergot alkaloid that stimulates α-adrenergic and serotoninergic receptors. Intravenous administration of this agent at incremental

doses from 0.05 to 0.40 mg is used. Because of the risk of multifocal spasm, the intracoronary injection of smaller doses, ranging from 10 to 80 μg, is preferred in most institutions. The spasm will then involve only the coronary artery and will be relieved by the intracoronary injection of nitroglycerin.

ACh is injected intracoronary at doses of 10 to 100 μg.[26,29] Since Ach has a short effect, the induced spasm usually disappears spontaneously within 2 to 3 minutes without the need for nitrate administration. This approach allows provocation of spasm separately in the left and right coronary arteries and is useful to show multivessel spasm (see Fig. 40–6).[29] The intracoronary injection of ACh often induces bradyarrhythmias, particularly when injected into the right coronary artery. It is therefore necessary to insert a pacemaker in stand-by during the test.

Coronary spasm also can be induced by hyperventilation, which causes respiratory alkalosis.[37-39] The sensitivity of this test is 65%, and the specificity is 100%.[38] Indeed, an ischemic attack provoked by hyperventilation is almost diagnostic of a vasospastic disease. The method of provocation can induce multifocal spasm. Histamine,[48] epinephrine,[5] dopamine,[41] dobutamine,[42] serotonin,[47] exercise in the morning,[15,24] and the cold pressor test[36] all can induce coronary spasm, but none of these tests is as sensitive as ergonovine or ACh.

There are circadian, daily, monthly, and yearly variations in the attack of coronary spasm,[13] and the sensitivity of the tests is related to disease activity. The sensitivity is high when disease activity is high, whereas it is low when disease activity is low. A false-negative test often may be obtained in patients with established coronary spasm when disease activity is low.

Although the provocation tests for coronary spasm by ergonovine or ACh are usually safe, complications may occur, including various arrhythmias, hypertension, hypotension, abdominal cramps, nausea, vomiting, and other nonspecific complications. Rarely, serious complications, such as ventricular fibrillation, myocardial infarction, and death, may occur.[12,28] The tests should be

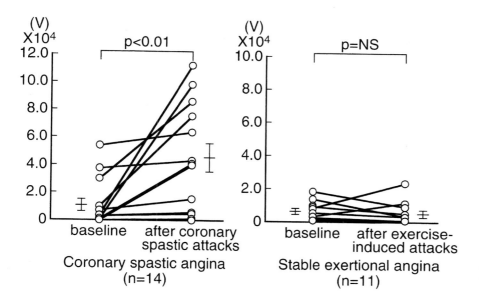

FIGURE 40–9. Platelet aggregation after attacks in patients with coronary spastic angina and patients with stable exertional angina. In patients with coronary spastic angina, the number of small-sized platelet aggregates increased significantly after the attacks *(right)*. The number did not change after the attacks in patients with stable exertional angina *(left)*. (From Miyamoto S, Ogawa H, Soejima H, et al: Formation of platelet aggregates after attacks with coronary spastic angina pectoris. Am J Cardiol 2000;85:494.)

conducted only by qualified physicians in a setting where appropriate resuscitation and other measures can be applied promptly.

The diagnosis of coronary spasm must be made on the basis of coronary angiographic findings during the attack. It is neither possible nor necessary to perform coronary angiography during the attack in every patient. Angina pectoris relieved promptly by sublingual administration of nitroglycerin may be diagnosed as coronary spastic angina without angiographic evidence when one of the following characteristics is present:

1. Attacks occurring at rest or induced by exercise in the morning but not in the afternoon.
2. Attacks associated with transient ST-segment elevation on the ECG.
3. Attacks induced by hyperventilation.
4. Attacks suppressed by calcium antagonists but not by β-blockers.

RISK FACTORS FOR CORONARY SPASM

Coronary spasm is mostly a disease of middle-aged and older men and postmenopausal women.[13,53] The disease occurs less often in young men and of premenopausal women, at least in the Japanese population. Age, low-density lipoprotein cholesterol, hypertension, diabetes mellitus, and smoking all are known as significant risk factors for coronary atherosclerosis, but only age and smoking are significant risk factors for coronary spasm.[52,53] Cigarette smoking is significantly more frequent among patients with coronary spastic angina than among patients with stable effort angina.[53] These facts suggest that the pathogenesis of coronary spasm may differ from that of coronary atherosclerosis, which is closely related to abnormalities of lipid metabolism. Cigarette smoking is a crucial risk factor for coronary spasm and may contribute to the high prevalence of coronary spasm among Japanese.[53] In addition to cigarette smoking and other environmental factors, genetic factors may also be involved in the pathogenesis of coronary spasm, as described in the next section.

MECHANISMS OF CORONARY SPASM

The exact mechanisms by which coronary spasm occurs remain to be elucidated.

Endothelial Dysfunction and Oxidative Stress

The vascular endothelium, once believed to be a simple passive barrier between circulating blood and surrounding tissues, has been recognized as a multifunctional organ whose integrity is essential to normal vascular physiology. Its dysfunction is a crucial factor in the pathogenesis of vascular disease.[64]

ACh causes vasodilation by releasing endothelium-derived relaxing factor in normal vessels, whereas it causes vasoconstriction when the endothelium is removed or damaged.[65] Endothelium-derived relaxing factor has been shown to be identical with nitric oxide (NO) or closely related substances.[66]

In humans, intracoronary infusion of ACh induces coronary vasodilation in young healthy subjects, whereas it causes vasoconstriction in patients with coronary atherosclerosis.[67,68] Coronary arteries in patients with coronary spastic angina are particularly hypersensitive to the vasoconstrictor effect of intracoronary injection of ACh, resulting in spasm (see Fig. 40–6).[26,29] Intracoronary injection of ACh is used as a provocative test for coronary spasm.[26,29] Ergonovine, serotonin, and histamine are all endothelium-dependent vasodilators by releasing NO.

Nitrates, including nitroglycerin, are endothelium-independent vasodilators and cause vasodilation by being converted into NO in vivo, which stimulates soluble guanylate cyclase, and an increase in cyclic guanosine monophosphate (GMP).[66] The coronary arteries in patients with coronary spasm are hypersensitive to the vasodilator effect of nitrates (Fig. 40–10),[32,69,70] suggesting a deficiency in endogenous NO activity.[69-71] The hypersensitivity to the vasoconstrictor effects of ACh and to the vasodilator response to nitrates extends to the entire coronary tree in patients with coronary spasm.[32,69,70]

NO is synthesized from L-arginine by way of NO synthase (NOS), and NO synthesis specifically is blocked by L-monomethyl-arginine (L-NMMA).[66] The coronary artery diameter decreases in response to intracoronary infusion of L-NMMA in control subjects, whereas it does not change significantly in patients with coronary spasm.[70] These observations indicate that NO is released in the basal state and is involved in the regulation of basal vascular tone in normal humans and a deficiency in NO activity in patients with spasm.[70] There is a significant inverse correlation between the response to L-NMMA and to nitroglycerin (i.e., the smaller the response to L-NMMA, the larger the response to nitroglycerin), indicating that the hypersensitivity to

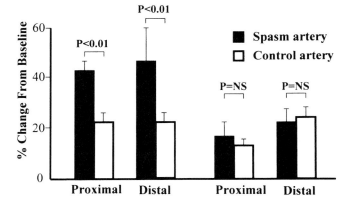

FIGURE 40–10. Percent change of coronary artery diameter in patients with coronary spastic angina *(solid bars)* and in controls *(open bars)* at the proximal and distal segments in response to nitroglycerin and diltiazem. Spasm arteries are supersensitive to nitroglycerin but not to diltiazem compared with control arteries. (From Kugiyama K, Yasue H, Okumura K, et al: Nitric oxide activity is deficient in spasm arteries of patients with coronary spastic angina. Circulation 1996;94:266.)

nitroglycerin is related to a deficiency in endogenous NO activity in patients with coronary spasm.[70,71] NO-mediated, flow-dependent dilatation is also impaired in patients with coronary spasm.[72]

Since NO suppresses the production of endothelin 1 and angiotensin II, which are potent vasoconstrictors of vascular smooth muscle cells, a deficiency in NO may enhance the synthesis of these potent vasoconstrictors.[73,74] Intimal thickening and hyperplasia are present in the coronary arteries involved in spasm.[75,76] This deficiency in NO activity can be due to decreased production or increased degradation.

Polymorphisms of eNOS Gene

Endothelial NO is synthesized by endothelial NOS, which is constitutively expressed in the endothelium.[66] In one study, we observed that polymorphisms of Glu298Asp in exon 7 and T^{-786} C in the 5′ flanking region of the eNOS gene were significantly more frequent in patients with coronary spasm.[77,78] These findings strongly suggest that the eNOS gene polymorphisms compromise the endothelial NO synthesis and predispose patients with these alleles to spasm. The NO polymorphisms, however, were found in only one third of patients, suggesting that other genes or factors may be involved in the pathogenesis of coronary spasm. The NO deficiency involves in general peripheral arteries as well as coronary arteries.[79-84]

Oxidative Stress

Oxygen free radicals degrade NO and cause vasoconstriction.[66] Basal and ACh-induced endothelial dysfunction in coronary arteries is improved by intracoronary injection of antioxidants, such as vitamin C or glutathione, in patients with coronary spastic angina.[82-84] Plasma levels of vitamin E, another antioxidant, are low in these patients, and the administration of vitamin E suppresses spasm in some patients.[85,86] Coronary spasm rarely occurs in premenopausal women except when they smoke[13]; estrogens by their antioxidant activity suppress attacks in postmenopausal women.[87] In premenopausal women, cyclic variations in disease activity can be present in relation with plasma levels of estrogens.[81] Coronary spasm can be associated with a polymorphism of the gene for paraoxonase I, which has an antioxidant effect.[89] An infusion of vitamin C can improve the brachial artery endothelial dysfunction in smokers.[90,91] Extracts from cigarette smoke suppress the Ach-induced, endothelium-dependent relaxation, and the suppression is prevented by antioxidants in isolated arteries.[92,93] All of these findings indicate that smoking degrades NO by way of oxygen radicals. Multiple regression analyses revealed that smoking, endothelial NOS, and paraoxonase I polymorphisms are strong risk factors for coronary spasm.[52,53,77,78,89]

Taken together, these findings indicate that endothelial dysfunction or deficiency of endothelial NO activity resulting from decreased NO release or increased NO degradation by oxygen radicals may play an important role in the pathogenesis of coronary spasm. Some controversies, however, still exist on the presence of endothelial dysfunction in patients with coronary spasm, as some investigators reported no endothelial NO deficiency or dysfunction in patients with spasm.[94,95]

Hypercontractility of Coronary Smooth Muscle

Contraction and relaxation of vascular smooth muscle are regulated by myosin light chain (MLC) kinase (MLCK) and myosin light chain phosphatase (MLCP) through phosphorylation and dephosphorylation of MLC.[96] The classic pathway through which contracting stimuli induce MLC phosphorylation is an increase in free intracellular Ca^{2+} concentration. The complex of Ca^{2+} and calmodulin activates MLCK, leading to increased MLC phosphorylation.[96] Coronary spasm may be regarded as hypercontraction of coronary smooth muscle triggered by an increase of intracellular Ca^{2+}. Calcium antagonists, which block the entry of Ca^{2+} into cells, are highly effective in suppressing coronary spasm.[9,24,46]

It has shown that Ca^{2+}-independent regulation also occurs through the inhibition of MLCP and that the level of MLC is determined by a balance between MLC phosphorylation by MLCK and dephosphorylation by MLCP.[96-99] Accumulating evidence now indicates that small GTPase RhoA, and its downstream effector ROCK/Rho-kinase, inhibit MLCP, leading to augmentation of MLC phosphorylation and to Ca^{2+} sensitization in response to vasoconstrictor stimuli.[96-99] RhoA/Rho-kinase pathway also has been shown to activate the transcription of genes encoding proteins for a contractile phenotype of smooth muscle.[100] Studies showed that RhoA/Rho-kinase activity is enhanced in the rat arteries with hypertension and vasospasm.[101,102]

Shimokawa and others[95,102] developed pig models of coronary spasm and showed that Rho-kinase activity is enhanced in smooth muscle cells of coronary arteries involved in spasm in these animals. They also showed that specific inhibitors of Rho-kinase relieved coronary spasm in this model. Enhanced Ca^{2+} sensitization via enhanced Rho/Rho-kinase activity and increased intracellular Ca^{2+} likely play a crucial role in the genesis of coronary spasm. The precise mechanisms by which the activity of Rho/Rho-kinase pathway is increased remain to be elucidated. Studies show that cGMP-dependent protein kinase inhibits RhoA-induced Ca^{2+} sensitization in vascular smooth muscles.[101-104] L-NAME, an inhibitor of NOS, increases Rho/Rho-kinase activity in the coronary and cerebral arteries of rats.[107,108] These new findings link the activity of RhoA/Rho-kinase to endothelial NO and are consistent with the clinical observations of hypersensitivity of spastic arteries to vasoconstrictor agonists and to nitrates.

Magnesium

Magnesium is an endogenous calcium antagonist, and infusion of magnesium suppresses hyperventilation-induced attacks in patients with coronary spasm.[39] Magnesium deficiency is present in 45% of patients with variant angina, and it may be related to the pathogenesis of coronary spasm in some patients.[40, 55]

TREATMENT

Acute Attack

The acute episodes of coronary spasm usually can be relieved promptly by the sublingual administration of nitroglycerin. Sublingual administration of isosorbide dinitrate may be used for the same purpose. In refractory spasm, intravenous or intracoronary injection of the drug may be necessary. Nitrates are converted in vivo to NO, which in turn activates soluble guanylate cyclase and leads to the formation of cGMP.[66] Nitrates are similar to NO, and the administration of nitrates is a replacement therapy for deficiency of endogenous endothelial NO in patients with coronary spasm. Coronary arteries involved in spasm are specifically supersensitive to nitrates, including nitroglycerin.[32,69,70]

Prevention of Coronary Spasm

Although the sublingual administration of nitroglycerin or isosorbide dinitrate rapidly relieves the attack, the duration of action of these drugs is short (<1 hour). For the prevention of attack, long-acting drugs are needed. In parallel with the elucidation of the mechanism of the attack of variant angina, new types of drugs that meet this requirement have been developed, calcium antagonists.

Calcium antagonists inhibit inflow of Ca^{2+} into the smooth muscle cell through voltage-sensitive Ca^{2+} channels, causing vasodilation.[9] The appearance of this class of drug is epoch-making not only in the treatment of coronary spasm, but also in the elucidation of the pathogenesis of ischemic heart disease and hypertension. The efficacy of these drugs against the attack of coronary spasm is often dramatic.

There are three major classes of calcium antagonists: (1) phenylalkylamines, of which verapamil is the prototype; (2) dihydropyridines, of which nifedipine is the prototype; and (3) benzodiazepines, of which diltiazem is the prototype. They belong to chemically heterogeneous groups, but they all are potent peripheral and coronary vasodilators with individual differences in their proclivity to depress sinoatrial and atrioventricular nodal functions or myocardial contractility. In addition to these prototypical drugs, many second-generation calcium antagonists are available, and these are mainly dihydropyridine derivatives. These agents differ in potency, tissue specificity, and pharmacokinetics and are potent vasodilators owing to greater vascular selectivity than seen with first-generation calcium antagonists.

Timing of the administration of these drugs is important because coronary spasm attacks usually occur from midnight to early morning. These drugs should be given before going to bed at night. Doses should be increased gradually in the individual patient, paying attention to the side effects. If the attacks do not occur in the daytime, there is no need to administer these drugs in the daytime. The attacks of coronary spasm often disappear for a certain period of time even after the withdrawal of calcium antagonists when they have been completely suppressed for several days by these drugs. There is no rebound reactivation following the discontinuation of calcium antagonists when used for the management of vasospasm.

Attacks of coronary spasm often disappear spontaneously. In individual patients there may be specific months or seasons for manifestation or relapse. Calcium antagonists may therefore be prescribed during certain periods, but not during others. In patients with multivessel coronary spasm, calcium antagonists should not be withdrawn, however, even when symptomatic attacks occur rarely because silent myocardial ischemia is often detected,[13] and there is a danger of sudden death from lethal arrhythmias in these patients.[12,13,28]

Long-acting nitrates (oral or transdermal) also are useful for preventing coronary spasm. The potency of nitrates is reduced by nitrate tolerance, however. In clinical practice, intermittent therapy with a nitrate-free window of at least 8 hours has been recommended. In general, when used in a dosing schedule that is designed to limit tolerance, nitrates should be combined with calcium antagonists for maximal benefit to control coronary spasm. Nicorandil, a nitrate and potassium channel activator, is also effective in suppressing coronary spasm.

For refractory coronary spasm, larger doses and combinations of different classes of calcium antagonists with nitrates may be necessary. Antioxidants such as vitamin C and E and estrogen in postmenopausal women also may have beneficial effects on coronary spasm.[82,83,85-87] Because contraction of vascular smooth muscle is under the dual control of intracellular Ca^{2+} and RhoA/Rho-kinase activity, it may be possible in the future that inhibitors of RhoA/Rho-kinase pathway may prove useful for the treatment and prevention of coronary spasm.[95]

General Measures

Because patients with coronary spasm have endothelial dysfunction,[70,72] the elimination or control of the factors that may impair endothelial function or increase oxidative stress, particularly smoking, is important. Elimination or control of all risk factors for coronary atherosclerosis is also necessary with a diagnosis of vasospastic disease. Drinking alcohol may induce attacks of coronary spasm usually not immediately but several hours after drinking in susceptible patients. Strenuous exercise in the daytime also may induce attacks between midnight and early morning.[13] Emotional stress is an important substratum for attacks, and anger or fear may induce the attacks. The attacks often disappear without any medications when the patients are hospitalized probably because they are shielded from social stress. Magnesium, which is an endogenous calcium antagonist, must be supplied when magnesium deficiency is documented.[39] Drugs that may induce coronary spasm must be avoided. Such drugs include catecholamines, muscarinic agonists, ergot alkaloids, prostaglandins, alcohol, and propranolol. Antioxidants such as vitamins C and E are recommended. In postmenopausal women with refractory coronary spasm, estrogen replacement therapy may be considered, weighing in the decision the adverse effects that are present when coronary atherosclerotic disease is present.[87,109]

PROGNOSIS

The natural history of variant angina or coronary spasm is generally characterized by periods of recurrent attacks lasting 3 to 6 months alternating with periods during which the patient is asymptomatic. Long-term survival is usually good as long as patients receive calcium antagonists and avoid smoking.[110-112]

The predictors of prognosis are the number of coronary arteries with significant organic stenosis, use of calcium antagonists, and presence of multivessel coronary spasm.[111] In many patients, the attacks tend to diminish with time after a few months of recurrent attacks. There is still no definitive answer to the question of how long the administration of calcium antagonists should be continued. I believe that patients with multivessel coronary spasm should receive calcium antagonists indefinitely because these patients often have lethal arrhythmias (ventricular tachycardia, ventricular fibrillation, high-degree atrioventricular block, or asystole) and are at high risk of sudden death,[12,13,28,29] even though they may be asymptomatic for some time. Such patients also require larger amounts of calcium antagonists to suppress the attacks. They should be supervised closely.

REFERENCES

1. Friedberg CK: Some comments and reflections on changing interests and new developments in angina pectoris. Circulation 1972;46:1037.
2. Parker JO: Nitrate therapy in stable angina pectoris. N Engl J Med 1987;316:1635.
3. Prinzmetal M, Kennamer R, Merlis R, et al: Angina pectoris: 1. A variant form of angina pectoris. Am J Med 1959;27:375.
4. Oliva PB, Potts DE, Pluss RG: Coronary arterial spasm in Prinzmetal angina: Documentation by coronary arteriography. N Engl J Med 1973;288:745.
5. Yasue H, Touyama M, Kato H, et al: Prinzmetal's variant form of angina as a manifestation of alpha-adrenergic receptor-mediated coronary artery spasm: Documentation by coronary arteriography. Am Heart J 1976;91:148.
6. Endo M, Hirosawa K, Kaneko N, et al: Prinzmetal's variant angina: Coronary arteriogram and left ventriculogram during angina attack induced by methacholine. N Engl J Med 1976;294:252.
7. Hillis LD, Braunwald E: Coronary artery spasm. N Engl J Med 1978;299:695.
8. Araki H, Koiwaya Y, Nakagaki O, et al: Diurnal distribution of ST-segment elevation and related arrhythmias in patients with variant angina: A study by ambulatory ECG monitoring. Circulation 1983;67:995.
9. Yasue H, Omote S, Takizawa A, et al: Coronary arterial spasm in ischemic heart disease and its pathogenesis: A review. Circ Res 1983;52(Suppl I):147.
10. Maseri A, Severi S, Nes MD, et al: "Variant" angina: One aspect of a continuous spectrum of vasospastic myocardial ischemia: Pathogenetic mechanisms, estimated incidence and clinical and

11. Maseri A, L'Abbate A, Baroldi G, et al: Coronary spasm as a possible cause of myocardial infarction: A conclusion derived from the study of "preinfarction" angina. N Engl J Med 1978;299:1271.
12. Nakamura M, Takeshita A, Nose Y: Clinical characteristics associated with myocardial infarction, arrhythmias, and sudden death in patients with vasospastic angina. Circulation 1987;75:1110.
13. Yasue H, Kugiyama K: Coronary spasm: Clinical features and pathogenesis. Intern Med 1997;36:760.
14. Lüscher TF, Pepine CJ: Coronary spasm and atherosclerosis. In Fuster V, Ross R, Topol EJ (eds): Atherosclerosis and Coronary Artery Disease. Philadelphia, Lippincott-Raven, 1996, p 657.
15. Yasue H, Omote S, Takizawa A, et al: Circadian variation of exercise capacity in patients with Prinzmetal's variant angina: Role of exercise-induced coronary arterial spasm. Circulation 1979;59:938.
16. Maseri A, Chierchia S, Kaski JC: Mixed angina pectoris. Am J Cardiol 1985;56:30E.
17. Maseri A, Davies G, Hackett D, et al: Coronary artery spasm and vasoconstriction: The case for a distinction. Circulation 1990;81:1983.
18. Yasue H, Omote S, Takizawa A, et al: Comparison of coronary arteriographic findings during angina pectoris associated with ST elevation or depression. Am J Cardiol 1981;47:539.
19. Bertrand ME, LaBlanche JM, Tilmant PY, et al: Frequency of provoked coronary arterial spasm in 1089 consecutive patients undergoing coronary arteriography. Circulation 1982;65:1299.
20. Hamilton JK, Pepine CJ: A renaissance of provocative testing for coronary spasm? J Am Coll Cardiol 2000;35:1857.
21. Yasue H, Kugiyama K: Coronary spasm: clinical features and pathogenesis. Intern Med 1997;36:760-765.
22. Song JK, Park SW, Kang DH, et al: Safety and clinical impact of ergonovine stress echocardiography for the diagnosis of coronary vasospasm. J Am Coll Cardiol 2000;35:1850.
23. Pristipino C, Beltrame JF, Finocchiaro ML, et al: Major racial differences in coronary constrictor response between Japanese and Caucasians with recent myocardial infarction. Circulation 2001;101:1102.
24. Yasue H, Omote S, Takizawa A, et al: Exertional angina pectoris caused by coronary arterial spasm: Effects of various drugs. Am J Cardiol 1979;43:647.
25. Muller JE, Stone PH, Turi ZG, et al: Circadian variation in the frequency of onset of acute myocardial infarction. N Engl J Med 1985;313:1315.
26. Yasue H, Horio Y, Nakamura N, et al: Induction of coronary artery spasm by acetylcholine in patients with variant angina: Possible role of the parasympathetic nervous system in the pathogenesis of coronary artery spasm. Circulation 1986;74:955.
27. Yasue H, Touyama M, Shimamoto M, et al: Role of autonomic nervous system in the pathogenesis of Prinzmetal's variant form of angina. Circulation 1974;50:534.
28. Myerburg RJ, Kessler KM, Mallon SM, et al: Life-threatening ventricular arrhythmias in patients with silent myocardial ischemia due to coronary artery spasm. N Engl J Med 1992;326:1451.
29. Okumura K, Yasue H, Horio Y, et al: Multivessel coronary spasm in patients with variant angina: A study with intracoronary injection of acetylcholine. Circulation 1988;77:535.
30. Onaka H, Hirota Y, Shimada S, et al: Clinical observation of spontaneous anginal attacks and multivessel spasm in variant angina pectoris with normal coronary arteries: Evaluation by 24-hour 12 lead electrocardiography with computer analysis. J Am Coll Cardiol 1996;27:38.
31. Selzer A, Langston M, Ruggeroli C, et al: Clinical syndromes of variant angina with normal coronary arteriogram. N Engl J Med 1976;295:1343.
32. Okumura K, Yasue H, Matsuyama K, et al: Diffuse disorder of coronary artery vasomotility in patients with coronary spastic angina: Hyperreactivity to the constrictor effects of acetylcholine and the dilator effects of nitroglycerin. J Am Coll Cardiol 1996;27:45.
33. Distante A, Rovai D, Picano E, et al: Transient changes in left ventricular mechanics during attacks of Prinzmetal's angina: An M-mode echocardiographic study. Am Heart J 1984;107:465.
34. Fujii H, Yasue H, Okumura K, et al: Hyperventilation-induced simultaneous multivessel coronary spasm in patients with variant

angina: An echocardiographic and arteriographic study. J Am Coll Cardiol 1988;12:1184.

35. Yeung AC, Vekshtein VI, Krantz DS, et al: The effect of atherosclerosis on the vasomotor response of coronary arteries to mental stress. N Engl J Med 1991;325:1551.

36. Raizner AE, Chahine RA, Ishimori T, et al: Provocation of coronary artery spasm by the cold pressor test: Hemodynamic, arteriographic and quantitative angiographic observations. Circulation 1980;62:925.

37. Yasue H, Nagao M, Omote S, et al: Coronary arterial spasm and Prinzmetal's variant form of angina induced by hyperventilation and Tris-buffer infusion. Circulation 1978;58:56.

38. Nakao K, Ohgushi M, Yoshimura M, et al: Hyperventilation as a specific test for diagnosis of coronary artery spasm. Am J Cardiol 1997;80:545.

39. Miyagi H, Yasue H, Okumura K, et al: Effect of magnesium on anginal attack induced by hyperventilation in patients with variant angina. Circulation 1989;79:597.

40. Goto K, Yasue H, Okumura K, et al: Magnesium deficiency detected by intravenous loading test in variant angina pectoris. Am J Cardiol 1990;65:709.

41. Crea F, Chierchia S, Kaski JC, et al: Provocation of coronary spasm by dopamine in patients with active variant angina pectoris. Circulation 1986;74:262.

42. Kawano H, Fujii H, Motoyama T, et al: Myocardial ischemia due to coronary artery spasm during dobutamine stress echocardiography. Am J Cardiol 2000;85:26.

43. Yamabe H, Yasue H, Okumura K, et al: Coronary spastic angina precipitated by the administration of an anticholinesterase drug. Am Heart J 1990;120:211.

44. Schroeder JS, Bolen JL, Quint RA, et al: Provocation of coronary spasm with ergonovine maleate: New test with results in 57 patients undergoing coronary arteriography. Am J Cardiol 1977;40:487.

45. Curry RC Jr, Pepine CJ, Sabom MB, et al: Similarities of ergonovine-induced and spontaneous attacks of variant angina. Circulation 1979;59:307.

46. Theroux P, Waters DD, Affaki GS, et al: Provocative testing with ergonovine to evaluate the efficacy of treatment with calcium antagonists in variant angina. Circulation 1979;60:504.

47. McFadden EP, Clarke JG, Davies GJ, et al: Effect of intracoronary serotonin on coronary vessels in patients with stable angina and patients with variant angina. N Engl J Med 1991;324:648.

48. Matsuyama K, Yasue H, Okumura K, et al: Effects of H1-receptor stimulation on coronary arterial diameter and coronary hemodynamics in humans. Circulation 1990;81:65.

49. Kugiyama K, Yasue H, Horio Y, et al: Effects of propranolol and nifedipine on exercise-induced attack in patients with variant angina: Assessment by exercise thallium-201 myocardial scintigraphy with quantitative rotational tomography. Circulation 1986;74:74.

50. Lange RL, Reid MS, Tresch DD, et al: Nonatherosclerotic ischemic heart disease following withdrawal from chronic industrial nitroglycerin exposure. Circulation 1972;46:666.

51. Pitts WR, Lange RA, Cigarroa JE, et al: Cocaine-induced myocardial ischemia and infarction: Pathophysiology, recognition, and management. Progr Cardiovasc Dis 1997;40:65.

52. Sugiishi M, Takatsu F: Cigarette smoking is a major risk factor for coronary spasm. Circulation 1993;87:76.

53. Takaoka K, Yoshimura M, Ogawa H, et al: Comparison of the risk factors for coronary artery spasm with those for organic stenosis in a Japanese population: Role of cigarette smoking. Int J Cardiol 2000;72:121.

54. Takizawa A, Yasue H, Omote S, et al: Variant angina induced by alcohol ingestion. Am Heart J 1984;107:25.

55. Miwa K, Igawa A, Miyagi Y, et al: Importance of magnesium deficiency in alcohol-induced variant angina. Am J Cardiol 1994;73:813.

56. Fuster V, Badimon L, Badimon JJ, Chesebro JH: The pathogenesis of coronary artery disease and the acute coronary syndromes. N Engl J Med 1992;326:242.

57. Theroux P, Fuster V: Acute coronary syndromes: Unstable angina and non-Q wave myocardial infarction. Circulation 1998; 97:1195.

58. Libby P: Current concepts of the pathogenesis of the acute coronary syndromes. Circulation 2001;104:365.

59. Oshima S, Yasue H, Ogawa H, et al: Fibrinopeptide A is released into the coronary circulation after coronary spasm. Circulation 1990;82:2222.

60. Ogawa H, Yasue H, Oshima S, et al: Circadian variation of plasma fibrinopeptide A level in patients with variant angina. Circulation 1989;80:1617.

61. Masuda T, Yasue H, Ogawa H, et al: Plasma plasminogen activator inhibitor activity and tissue plasminogen activator levels in patients with unstable angina and those with coronary spastic angina. Am Heart J 1992;124:314.

62. Miyamoto S, Ogawa H, Soejima H, et al: Formation of platelet aggregates after attacks with coronary spastic angina pectoris. Am J Cardiol 2000;85:494.

63. Etsuda H, Mizuno K, Arakawa K, et al: Angioscopy in variant angina: Coronary artery spasm and intimal injury. Lancet 1993;342:1322.

64. Rubanyi GM: The role of endothelium in cardiovascular homeostasis and diseases. J Cardiovasc Pharmacol 1993;22:S1.

65. Furchgott RF, Zawadzki JV: The obligatory role of endothelial cells in the relaxation of arterial smooth muscle by acetylcholine. Nature 1980;288:373.

66. Moncada S, Palmer RM, Higgs EA: Nitric oxide: Physiology, pathophysiology, and pharmacology. Pharmacol Rev 1991;43:109.

67. Ludmer PL, Selwyn AP, Shook TL, et al: Paradoxical vasoconstriction induced by acetylcholine in atherosclerotic coronary arteries. N Engl J Med 1986;315:1046.

68. Yasue H, Matsuyama K, Matsuyama K, et al: Responses of angiographically normal human coronary arteries to intracoronary injection of acetylcholine by age and segment: Possible role of early coronary atherosclerosis. Circulation 1990;81:482.

69. Kugiyama K, Ohgushi M, Sugiyama S, et al: Supersensitive dilator response to nitroglycerin but not to atrial natriuretic peptide in spastic coronary arteries in coronary spastic angina. Am J Cardiol 1997;79:606.

70. Kugiyama K, Yasue H, Okumura K, et al: Nitric oxide activity is deficient in spasm arteries of patients with coronary spastic angina. Circulation 1996;94:266.

71. Moncada S, Rees DD, Schulz R, et al: Development and mechanism of a specific super-sensitivity to nitrovasodilators after inhibition of vascular nitric oxide synthesis in vivo. Proc Natl Acad Sci U S A 1991;88:2166.

72. Kugiyama K, Ohgushi M, Motoyama T, et al: Nitric oxide-mediated flow-dependent dilation is impaired in coronary arteries in patients with coronary spastic angina. J Am Coll Cardiol 1997;30:920.

73. Boulanger C, Lüscher TF: Release of endothelin from the porcine aorta: Inhibition by endothelium-derived nitric oxide. J Clin Invest 1990;85:587.

74. Takemoto M, Egashira K, Usui M, et al: Important role of tissue angiotensin-converting enzyme activity in the pathogenesis of coronary vascular and myocardial structural changes induced by long-term blockade of nitric oxide synthesis in rats. J Clin Invest 1997;99:278.

75. Suzuki H, Kawai S, Aizawa T, et al: Histological evaluation of coronary plaque in patients with variant angina: Relationship between vasospasm and neointimal hyperplasia in primary coronary lesions. J Am Coll Cardiol 1999;33:198.

76. Miyao Y, Kugiyama K, Kawano H, et al: Diffuse intimal thickening of coronary arteries in patients with coronary spastic angina. J Am Coll Cardiol 2000;36:432.

77. Yoshimura M, Yasue H, Nakayama M, et al: A missense Glu298Asp variant in the endothelial nitric oxide synthase gene is associated with coronary spasm in the Japanese. Hum Genet 1998;103:65.

78. Nakayama M, Yasue H, Yoshimura M, et al: T-786→C mutation in the 5'-flanking region of the endothelial nitric oxide synthase gene is associated with coronary spasm. Circulation 1999;99:2864.

79. Motoyama T, Kawano H, Kugiyama K, et al: Flow-mediated, endothelium-dependent dilatation of the brachial arteries is impaired in patients with coronary spastic angina. Am Heart J 1997;133:263.

80. Hamabe A, Takase B, Uehata A, et al: Impaired endothelium-dependent vasodilation in the brachial artery in variant angina pectoris and the effect of intravenous administration of vitamin C. Am J Cardiol 2001;87:1154.

81. Moriyama Y, Tsunoda R, Harada M, et al: Nitric oxide-mediated vasodilatation is decreased in forearm resistance vessels in patients with coronary spastic angina. Jpn Circ J 2001;65:81.

82. Kugiyama K, Motoyama T, Hirashima O, et al: Vitamin C attenuates abnormal vasomotor reactivity in spasm coronary arteries in

patients with coronary spastic angina. J Am Coll Cardiol 1998;32:103.

83. Hirashima O, Kawano H, Motoyama T, et al: Improvement of endothelial function and insulin sensitivity with vitamin C in patients with coronary spastic angina: Possible role of reactive oxygen species. J Am Coll Cardiol 2000;35:1860.

84. Kugiyama K, Miyao Y, Sakamoto H, et al: Glutathione attenuates coronary constriction to acetylcholine in patients with coronary spastic angina. Am J Physiol Heart Circ Physiol 2001;280:H264.

85. Miwa K, Miyagi Y, Igawa A, et al: Vitamin E deficiency in variant angina. Circulation 1996;94:14.

86. Motoyama T, Kawano H, Kugiyama K, et al: Vitamin E administration improves impairment of endothelium-dependent vasodilation in patients with coronary spastic angina. J Am Coll Cardiol 1998;32:1672.

87. Kawano H, Motoyama T, Hirai N, et al: Estradiol supplementation suppresses hyperventilation-induced attacks in post-menopausal women with variant angina. J Am Coll Cardiol 2001;37:735.

88. Kawano H, Motoyama T, Ohgushi M, et al: Menstrual cyclic variation of myocardial ischemia in pre-menopausal women with variant angina. Ann Intern Med 2001;135:977.

89. Itoh A, Yasue H, Yoshimura M, et al: Paraoxonase gene Gln192Arg (Q192R) polymorphism is associated with coronary artery spasm. Hum Genet 2002;110:89–94.

90. Kugiyama K, Yasue H, Ohgushi M, et al: Deficiency in nitric oxide bioactivity in epicardial coronary arteries of cigarette smokers. J Am Coll Cardiol 1996;28:1161.

91. Motoyama T, Kawano H, Kugiyama K, et al: Endothelium-dependent vasodilation in the brachial artery is impaired in smokers: Effect of vitamin C. Am J Physiol 1997;273:H1644.

92. Ohta Y, Kugiyama K, Sugiyama S, et al: Impairment of endothelium-dependent relaxation of rabbit aortas by cigarette smoke extract: Role of free radicals and attenuation by captopril. Atherosclerosis 1997;131:195.

93. Sugiyama S, Kugiyama K, Ohgushi M, et al: Supersensitivity of atherosclerotic artery to constrictor effect of cigarette smoke extract. Cardiovasc Res 1998;38:508.

94. Egashira K, Katsuda Y, Mohri M, et al: Basal release of endothelium-derived nitric oxide at site of spasm in patients with variant angina. J Am Coll Cardiol 1996;27:1444.

95. Shimokawa H: Cellular and molecular mechanisms of coronary artery spasm—lessons from animal models. Jpn Circ J 2000;64:1.

96. Somlyo AP, Somlyo AV: Signal transduction and regulation in smooth muscle. Nature 1994;372:201.

97. Kimura K, Ito M, Amano M, et al: Regulation of myosin phosphorylation by Rho and Rho-associated kinase (Rho kinase). Science 1996;273:245.

98. Narumiya S: The small GTPase Rho: Cellular functions and signal transduction. J Biochem 1996;120:215.

99. Somlyo AP, Somlyo AV: Signal transduction by G-proteins, Rho-kinase and protein phosphatase to smooth muscle and non-muscle myosin II. J Physiol 2000;522:177.

100. Halyko AJ, Solway J: Molecular mechanisms of phenotypic plasticity in smooth muscle cells. J Appl Physiol 2001;90:358.

101. Uehata M, Ishizaki T, Satoh H, et al: Calcium sensitization of smooth muscle mediated by a Rho-associated protein kinase in hypertension. Nature 1997;389:990.

102. Sato M, Tani E, Fujikawa H, et al: Involvement of Rho-kinase–mediated phosphorylation of myosin light chain in enhancement of cerebral vasospasm. Circ Res 2000;87:195.

103. Kandabashi T, Shimokawa H, Miyata K, et al: Inhibition of myosin phosphatase by upregulated Rho-kinase plays a key role for coronary artery spasm in a porcine model with interleukin-1beta. Circulation 2000;101:1319.

104. Sauzeau V, Jeune HL, Cario-Toumaniantz C, et al: Cyclic GMP-dependent protein kinase signaling pathway inhibits RhoA-induced Ca^{2+} sensitization of contraction in vascular smooth muscle. J Biol Chem 2000;275:2172.

105. Sawada N, Itoh H, Yamashita J, et al: cGMP-dependent protein kinase phosphorylates and inactivates RhoA. Biochem Biophys Res Commun 2000;280:798.

106. Lincoln TM, Dey N, Sellak H: cGMP-dependent protein kinase signaling mechanisms in smooth muscle: From the regulation of tone to gene expression. J Appl Physiol 2001;91:1421.

107. Chrissobolis S, Sobey CG: Evidence that Rho-kinase activity contributes to cerebral vascular tone in vivo and is enhanced during chronic hypertension: Comparison with protein kinase C. Circ Res 2001;88:774.

108. Ikegaki I, Hattori T, Yamaguchi T, et al: Involvement of Rho-kinase in vascular remodeling caused by long-term inhibition of nitric oxide synthesis in rats. Eur J Pharmacol 2001;427:69.

109. Grady D, Harrington D, Bittner V, et al: Cardiovascular outcomes during 6.8 years of hormone therapy: Heart and Estrogen/progestin Replacement Study/follow up (HERS-II). JAMA 2002;288:49–57.

110. Waters DD, Miller D, Szlachcic J, et al: Factors influencing the long-term prognosis of treated patients with variant angina. Circulation 1983;68:258.

111. Yasue H, Takizawa A, Nagao M, et al: Long-term prognosis for patients with variant angina and influential factors. Circulation 1988;78:1.

112. Bory M, Pierron F, Panagides D, et al: Coronary artery spasm in patients with normal or near normal coronary arteries: Long-term follow-up of 277 patients. Eur Heart J 1996;17:1015.

The Patient with Chest Pain Despite Normal Coronary Angiography

Richard O. Cannon III

Despite the multitude of noninvasive tests available to detect myocardial ischemia and select patients for coronary angiography, many patients are found at cardiac catheterization to have normal-appearing coronary arteries or, at most, minimal luminal irregularities of arterial segments. A report from the WISE (Women's Ischemia Syndrome Evaluation) study[1] confirmed observations made in the 1970s[2]: Fewer than half the women who undergo cardiac catheterization because of symptoms of chest pain have angiographic evidence of clinically significant coronary artery disease. For patients with smooth coronary arteries by angiography, the prognosis is no different than that of the general population.[3,4] For patients with luminal irregularities, increased risk of myocardial infarction has been reported in these registries because of the thrombogenic potential of atherosclerotic arteries, regardless of the magnitude of obstruction to blood flow.

Despite being told of a benign prognosis, many patients with chest pain despite normal coronary angiograms continue to report symptoms, with considerable impact on quality of life and employment. As a result, health care resources continue to be used, including repeat hospitalizations and coronary angiography.[5,6] Many cardiologists conclude that in the absence of coronary artery disease or spasm or organic heart disease demonstrable by echocardiography or cardiac catheterization, the pain must be noncardiac, likely esophageal or psychogenic in origin. This belief is supported by atypical features of pain common to this patient population, including variability in circumstances that provoke pain, marked severity and persistence of pain, atypical location or radiation patterns, and inconsistent or brief responses to anti-ischemic therapy.

Despite a considerable volume of research into the cause of symptoms and abnormal noninvasive testing in this patient population that has been so problematic to cardiologists, a consensus on the pathophysiology of the syndrome has yet to emerge. This lack of consensus is likely due to multiple causes for symptoms, some—if not most—likely to be noncardiac, and conflicting data and interpretations of data in studies in which considerable efforts have been expended to make the patient population under study as homogeneous as possible. In addition, a multitude of treatments have been proposed, which may be effective in investigators' hands but not as effective in community practice. As a result, many patients seek multiple cardiologists for symptom relief,

with the inevitable duplication of noninvasive and invasive testing.

SHORT HISTORY OF CARDIOVASCULAR SYNDROME X

In 1967, two groups reported series of patients with angina-like chest pain despite normal coronary angiograms and noted not only a female predominance, but also the common occurrence of ST-segment depression during treadmill exercise testing consistent with inducible myocardial ischemia.[7,8] Shortly after these reports, investigators at the Montreal Heart Institute determined no hemodynamic evidence of ischemia during rapid atrial pacing in 10 patients with chest pain, normal coronary angiograms, and ST-segment depression during pacing stress (group X).[9] They concluded that the ST-segment changes in these patients, although ischemic in appearance, did not indicate the actual presence of myocardial ischemia during stress. In an editorial that accompanied this article, Kemp[10] introduced the term *syndrome X* to denote the uncertain cause of chest pain in these patients. Today, not only is usage of the term *syndrome X* confusing to physicians and patients, but also the cardiovascular syndrome X (commonly defined as patients with angina-like chest pain and ST-segment depression during exercise despite normal coronary angiograms) commonly is confused with the metabolic syndrome X of insulin resistance.

CORONARY FLOW DYNAMICS AND SYNDROME X

In the 1980s and 1990s, several groups examined the possibility of abnormal coronary flow responsiveness as a mechanism for ischemia presumably responsible for chest pain symptoms and ST-segment depression during exercise in patients with syndrome X, reporting limited coronary flow responses to pacing stress or to microvascular dilators, such as papaverine, dipyridamole, and adenosine.[11] A coronary microvascular cause for symptoms is appealing because small arteries (especially arterioles) within the myocardium regulate the coronary flow response to stress so that the metabolic needs of the myocardium are matched closely by appropriate perfusion and oxygen delivery to permit augmented cardiac work. In this regard, Inobe and coworkers[12] reported that 14 of 26 syndrome X patients had reversible defects on exercise thallium-201 perfusion imaging; 7 of these 14 patients also had reversible perfusion defects during adenosine thallium-201 imaging. At cardiac catheterization, these 14 patients had less of an increase in great cardiac vein blood flow in response to adenosine and to dobutamine stress compared with the other 12 patients. Rosen and colleagues[13] found no differences, however, in the myocardial perfusion response to dipyridamole measured by positron emission tomography in 29 syndrome X patients compared with 20 age-matched and sex-matched controls.

A growing list of abnormalities have been described in a series of patients with syndrome X to account for coronary microvascular dysfunction, including altered autonomic tone,[14,15] insulin resistance (syndrome X[2]?),[16-18] enhanced ion transport across cell membranes,[19] increased endothelin-1 release,[20,21] and estrogen deficiency.[22] More recently, subsets of patients with chest pain and normal coronary angiograms have been reported to have abnormal coronary endothelium-dependent coronary blood flow responsiveness to acetylcholine as determined by intracoronary Doppler measurements of flow velocity and quantitative angiography, findings consistent with reduced nitric oxide bioactivity. Egashira and coworkers[23] reported that 9 patients with syndrome X had less of a coronary flow response to acetylcholine compared with 10 patients whose exercise tests were negative. Coronary flow responses to the endothelium-independent vasodilator papaverine were similar for the two groups. Zeiher and coworkers[24] reported that 13 patients with chest pain and normal-appearing left anterior descending (LAD) coronary arteries who had reversible thallium-201 defects in this territory during exercise had less of an increase in LAD flow in response to acetylcholine than 14 patients with normal scans in the LAD territory. No mention was made regarding the frequency of ischemic-appearing ST-segment depression in patients with and patients without exercise-induced reversible thallium perfusion defects, and the incidence of syndrome X in this study is unknown. Hasdai and associates[25] reported that 7 patients with chest pain and "near-normal" coronary angiograms who had LAD-territory technetium-99m sestimibi perfusion defects (with the isotope injected after intracoronary infusion of acetylcholine) had an actual decrease in LAD flow in response to this agonist, consistent with endothelial dysfunction. In contrast, 13 other patients in this study without LAD-territory perfusion defects after intracoronary acetylcholine infusion had increased LAD flow. This publication did not report the incidence of exercise-induced ST-segment depression or reversible perfusion defects during exercise nuclear imaging for the study participants. For this study, the relationship between coronary endothelial dysfunction and exercise-induced indices of myocardial ischemia is unknown.

Interpretation of studies investigating coronary blood flow responses to acetylcholine is limited by the direct constrictor effects on smooth muscle, which can be shown in normal vascular tissue with sufficiently high concentrations of this agonist. Animals given nitric oxide synthase inhibitors, blocking synthesis of nitric oxide by the endothelium, have normal coronary blood flow responses to exercise, likely resulting from redundant dilator mechanisms in the coronary circulation activated during stress.[26] Accordingly the causal relationship between endothelial dysfunction and inducible myocardial ischemia in patients with normal coronary angiograms remains a matter of dispute.

IS SYNDROME X ASSOCIATED WITH MYOCARDIAL ISCHEMIA?

Although studies support the paradigm that abnormal coronary microvascular dilator responsiveness to stress may precipitate myocardial ischemia, other studies since the Montreal Heart Institute report in 1973 have questioned the existence of myocardial ischemia in patients with chest pain despite normal coronary angiograms, including the subset with syndrome X, based on their ischemic-appearing exercise test. Camici and colleagues[27] found no metabolic evidence of myocardial ischemia by analysis of coronary sinus metabolites of carbohydrate and fatty acid metabolism in 12 women with syndrome X during rapid atrial pacing. Nihoyannopoulos and coworkers[28] reported normal left ventricular systolic function by echocardiography immediately after exercise and during rapid atrial pacing in 18 patients with syndrome X despite experiencing chest pain with ischemic-appearing ST-segment depression during these stresses. Rosano and coworkers[29] performed pH monitoring of coronary sinus blood before and during rapid atrial pacing in 14 patients with chest pain and normal coronary angiograms; 11 patients had ischemic-appearing ST-segment depression during exercise and 6 had reversible perfusion defects on exercise thallium scintigraphy. During pacing, despite chest pain provoked in 11 of the 14 patients, only 3 patients showed declines in coronary sinus pH that approached the magnitude of reduction in pH measured in patients with coronary artery disease subjected to pacing stress.

We evaluated 70 consecutive patients with angina-like chest pain and normal coronary angiograms, 22 of whom had syndrome X by virtue of ischemic-appearing ST-segment depression during exercise.[30] Thirteen patients had reversible perfusion defects during exercise by thallium scintigraphy, abnormalities consistent with myocardial ischemia. The findings of thallium scintigraphy were not related, however, to the presence of ST-segment depression during exercise testing. The results of exercise testing and dobutamine stress echocardiography from these 70 patients were compared with those of 26 normal volunteers. We used the transesophageal route for imaging to maximize the number of ventricular segments visualized and the quality of images for assessment of contractility. Dobutamine infused in stepwise increments to 40 µg/kg/min induced chest pain in 59 patients but in none of the control subjects. Ischemic-appearing ST-segment depression developed in 22 patients (19 with syndrome X) and in 2 controls. Wall motion abnormalities occurred in none of the patients or controls. No differences were observed in transmural contractile response to dobutamine between patients and control subjects. Of the 70 patients with chest pain despite normal coronary angiograms, the quantitative myocardial contractile response to dobutamine was virtually identical in the 22 patients with syndrome X and the 48 patients without ischemic-appearing ST-segment depression during infusion. Despite the frequent provocation of characteristic chest pain and, in the syndrome X subset, ischemic-appearing ST-segment depression, patients with chest pain and normal coronary angiograms do not show concomitant regional wall motion abnormalities and show a quantitatively normal myocardial contractile response to dobutamine.

Despite these studies and others questioning ischemia in syndrome X, the controversy continues. Maseri and associates[31] proposed that patchy or diffuse microvascular constriction (or absence of appropriate vasodilation) may produce myocardial ischemia during stress that does not affect myocardial contractility because of compensatory vasodilation of adjacent arterioles.[31] The same group measured lipid hydroperoxides and conjugated dienes—molecules generated on reoxygenation of ischemic tissue—as metabolic markers of ischemia in arterial and great cardiac vein blood, based on their previous observations in patients with coronary artery disease.[32] Samples were drawn before and after rapid atrial pacing in nine patients with chest pain and normal coronary angiograms; seven patients had ischemic-appearing ST-segment depression during exercise stress, and five had reversible perfusion defects on exercise thallium scintigraphy. These measurements compared with those of five patients with mitral valve disease who underwent this study and served as controls. Levels of these molecules were higher in great cardiac vein blood than arterial blood before pacing in patients, whereas the reverse was true in controls. In patients, but not controls, great cardiac venous levels of these molecules increased after pacing (160 beats/min or heart rate at development of ST-segment depression for 3 minutes), which induced ST-segment depression and chest pain in all but one patient.

Buchthal and coworkers[33] from the WISE study reported that 7 of 35 women with chest pain and normal coronary angiograms who underwent nuclear magnetic resonance spectroscopy had findings compatible with myocardial ischemia during handgrip exercise. This conclusion was based on reduction in spectral signals from phosphate of creatine phosphate relative to the phosphates of ATP that was similar to the decline in the ratio of these high-energy phosphate spectra recorded in patients with coronary artery disease. Results of treadmill exercise testing (i.e., identification of who had syndrome X in this group) were not reported. The frequency of exercise-induced thallium perfusion defects and abnormal brachial artery endothelial testing (flow-mediated dilation) was similar, however, for the 7 women with reduction in the ratio of high-energy phosphate spectra as for the 28 women with lesser reduction (or actual increases) in these spectra.

The debate continues. The studies cited suggest, however, that noninvasive testing may not identify reliably the subset of patients who have stress-induced myocardial ischemia as a cause of chest pain symptoms and that specialized testing may be required to make this important distinction. For such testing to be clinically useful, investigators must show that patients identified as having abnormal coronary endothelial function and inducible myocardial ischemia by abnormal phosphorous-31 spectra or lipid peroxidation products in cardiac venous blood during stress respond to specific therapies or have a different natural history to their disorder than patients who do not have these abnormalities.

DOES ST-SEGMENT DEPRESSION ALWAYS INDICATE ISCHEMIA?

Although the ischemic-appearing ST-segment depression during exercise has convinced many clinicians that patients with syndrome X must have myocardial ischemia during stress, ischemic-appearing ST-segment depression may be observed occasionally in healthy subjects. In this regard, Toivonen and coworkers[34] noted that 10 of 30 healthy young physicians (including 6 of 9 women) on emergency duty had 1 mm or greater ST-segment depression on electrocardiogram monitoring when alerted by an alarm. Autonomic nervous system effects on repolarization during stress may cause changes in the electrocardiogram that mimic the ST-segment depression of myocardial ischemia.

SENSITIVE HEART

The observation that patients with chest pain and normal coronary angiograms, whether or not they are defined as having syndrome X based on their exercise electrocardiogram, commonly experience their characteristic chest pain during the performance of diagnostic cardiac catheterization has led several groups to consider abnormal cardiac pain perception as a fundamental abnormality in this patient population.[35-39] We found that in 36 patients with chest pain and normal coronary angiograms, characteristic chest pain could be provoked in 86% by electrical stimulation (right ventricular pacing) at a heart rate 5 beats faster than their resting heart rate, with the pain worsened by increasing the stimulus intensity.[36] In more than half of the same patients, pain could be provoked by simply injecting contrast media into the left coronary artery. In contrast, pain responses to right ventricular pacing or contrast media injection were seen in only 2 of 42 patients with coronary artery disease and in none of the 10 patients with valvular heart disease asymptomatic for chest pain. Other potent stimuli for pain provocation in syndrome X patients are dipyridamole and adenosine infusion.[37,38]

It is unknown whether heightened intracardiac pain sensitivity shown in patients with chest pain and normal coronary angiograms represents one extreme of the normal "bell curve" distribution of visceral sensory function or is indicative of a true abnormality in visceral sensory function. These patients may represent the opposite end of the cardiac pain spectrum from the subgroup of patients with coronary artery disease who have *silent ischemia*. Similar observations of exaggerated visceral pain sensitivity had been made within the esophagus of patients with chest pain and normal or near-normal coronary angiograms and may explain why elevated esophageal pressures and acid reflux, generally unrecognized by healthy subjects, cause chest pain in some patients.[40] Additionally, exaggerated visceral pain sensitivity has been shown within the rectum, sigmoid colon, and small intestines of patients with irritable bowel syndrome.[41] Patients with "sensitive hearts" may represent one manifestation of chronic pain associated with heightened visceral pain sensitivity. The mechanism of exaggerated visceral pain sensitivity may be neurophysiologically linked to whatever is responsible for anxiety and panic disorders commonly noted with patients with chest pain and normal coronary angiograms.[42,43]

MANAGEMENT OF PATIENTS WITH CHEST PAIN AND NORMAL CORONARY ANGIOGRAMS

Perhaps the most frustrating aspect of the syndrome of chest pain despite normal coronary angiograms, including the syndrome X subset, is the management of chest pain symptoms, recognized in the earliest reports in the literature. Numerous therapies have been reported to be successful in clinical trials generally including small numbers of patients, including nitrates,[44] β-blockers,[45] calcium channel blockers,[46] angiotensin-converting enzyme inhibitors,[47] aminophylline,[48] estrogen replacement therapy,[49] and L-arginine.[50] We considered the possibility that patients with chest pain and normal coronary angiograms, including the syndrome X subset, have a chronic pain syndrome resulting from abnormal cardiac pain sensitivity. We assessed the impact of drug therapy useful in the management of chronic pain syndromes in a clinical trial.[51] Sixty consecutive patients underwent baseline testing then participated in a randomized, double-blind, placebo-controlled trial of clonidine, 0.1 mg twice daily; imipramine, 50 mg nightly with morning placebo; or placebo twice daily (treatment phase) compared with an identical period of twice-daily placebo for all patients (placebo phase). Half of these patients had been hospitalized more than once because of chest pain symptoms, and 18 (30%) had undergone multiple cardiac catheterizations, with repeat demonstration of normal coronary arteries. The average duration of symptoms was more than 4 years. Baseline testing showed that 22% of patients had ischemic-appearing ST-segment depression during treadmill exercise and fulfilled criteria for syndrome X, 41% had esophageal dysmotility, and 63% fulfilled criteria for one or more lifetime psychiatric diagnoses (in particular, panic disorder). Of patients, 87% had their characteristic chest pain provoked by right ventricular electrical stimulation or intracoronary adenosine infusion, and 41% had their characteristic chest pain provoked by administration of edrophonium, infusion of hydrochloric acid, or intraesophageal balloon distention during esophageal motility testing. The prevalence of abnormal cardiac or esophageal pain sensitivity was similar for men and women and for patients with and patients without psychiatric diagnoses.

During the treatment phase, patients who received imipramine showed a statistically significant 52% reduction in chest pain episodes, as opposed to no change in chest pain frequency in the placebo group, when the treatment phase was compared with the placebo phase of the study. The symptom benefit of imipramine was noted equally in men and in women. The response to imipramine did not depend on results of cardiac (i.e., whether or not patients had syndrome X), esophageal, or psychiatric testing at baseline or on changes in psychiatric profile as assessed at baseline, after the placebo phase, and after the treatment phase of the study. Reassessment of cardiac sensitivity to right ventricular electrical stimulation while on treatment showed significant improvement in chest pain responses compared with baseline chest pain responses in the imipramine group. We concluded that imipramine improves chest pain symptoms in patients with chest pain and normal coronary angiograms, including patients with syndrome X, probably because of a visceral analgesic effect of this drug.

NONPHARMACOLOGIC APPROACHES TO PAIN MANAGEMENT

Despite many studies reporting therapeutic success with a variety of medications in reducing chest pain symptoms, the clinical experience has been that pain relief is often not sustained over time, and patients commonly are prescribed a large number of drugs, with associated side effects. Nonpharmacologic approaches may be of symptom benefit in this patient population. In this regard, Eriksson and colleagues[52] randomized 26 women with syndrome X to two exercise training groups (cycle ergometry for 30 minutes at 50% peak workload three times a week for 8 weeks) or to no exercise training. In the exercise groups, peak capacity improved by 34%, and onset of chest pain was delayed by 100% from pretraining values. Cunningham and coworkers[53] reported that 3 months' training in transcendental meditation reduced chest pain frequency and severity and improved quality of life assessed by questionnaires in nine postmenopausal women with syndrome X. This treatment also improved the time to ST-segment depression and maximum ST-segment depression during treadmill exercise testing compared with baseline values. Cognitive behavioral therapy with clinical psychologists has been reported to be of value in reducing symptoms and improving quality of life.[54] For patients resistant to these pharmacologic and nonpharmacologic approaches, transcutaneous electrical nerve stimulation or spinal cord stimulation may be of symptom benefit.[55-58]

APPROACH TO PATIENT MANAGEMENT

The management recommendations that follow are predicated on determination of normal cardiac pressures and angiograms during cardiac catheterization, a normal echocardiogram showing absence of myocardial or valvular disease, no evidence of coronary artery spasm (absence of characteristic ST-segment changes during spontaneous episodes of chest pain or negative ergonovine challenge), and no gastroesophageal source of symptoms. Given this constellation of findings, the patient should be reassured that he or she has a chest pain syndrome that poses no increased cardiovascular morbidity or mortality risk over that of the general population. For patients with luminal irregularities on coronary angiography or "nonsignificant" coronary artery disease, the risk of subsequent coronary events is higher than that of patients with entirely smooth coronary arteries, and these patients should undergo aggressive risk factor management and begin daily aspirin.

All patients should be started on a regular exercise program to improve their stamina (many are severely deconditioned) and to encourage a positive attitude regarding their health status. Efforts should be made to discontinue all unnecessary medications. In some, this approach is sufficient to alleviate symptoms, and no further evaluation is necessary. Should symptoms persist, empirical trials of anti-ischemic therapy, angiotensin-converting enzyme inhibitors, L-arginine, estrogen replacement therapy, or tricyclic antidepressants (coupled with a β-blocker to block anticholinergic effects of this therapy) may be required.

At present, there is no widely available or accepted test to determine whether or not patients have an ischemic cause for symptoms. Greater experience with stress nuclear magnetic resonance spectroscopy at specialized centers may resolve this dilemma in the future. Should exercise and therapeutic trials fail to control chest pain symptoms, referral to a pain clinic may be necessary for a multidisciplinary approach to pain management.

REFERENCES

1. Sharaf BL, Pepine CJ, Kerensky RA, et al: Detailed angiographic analysis of women with suspected ischemic chest pain (pilot phase data from the NHLBI-sponsored Women's Ischemia Syndrome Evaluation [WISE] Study Angiographic Core Laboratory). Am J Cardiol 2001;87:937.
2. Kennedy JW, Killip T, Fisher LD, et al: The clinical spectrum of coronary artery disease and its surgical and medical management, 1974-1979: The Coronary Artery Surgery Study. Circulation 1982;68(Suppl 3):III-16.
3. Kemp HG, Kronmal RA, Vliestra RE, et al: Seven year survival of patients with normal or near normal angiograms: A CASS registry study. J Am Coll Cardiol 1986;7:479.
4. Kemp HG, Kronmal RA, Vliestra RE, et al: Seven year survival of patients with normal or near normal coronary arteriograms: A CASS registry study. J Am Coll Cardiol 1986;7:479.
5. Ockene IS, Shay MJ, Alpert JS, et al: Unexplained chest pain in patients with normal coronary arteriography: A follow-up study of functional status. N Engl J Med 1980;303:1249.
6. Isner JM, Salem DN, Banas JS, et al: Long-term clinical course of patients with normal coronary angiography: Follow-up study of 121 patients with normal or nearly normal coronary arteriograms. Am Heart J 1981;102:645.
7. Likoff W, Segal BL, Kasparian H: Paradox of normal selective coronary arteriograms in patients considered to have unmistakable coronary heart disease. N Engl J Med 1967;276:1063.
8. Kemp HG, Elliott WC, Gorlin R: The anginal syndrome with normal coronary arteriography. Trans Assoc Am Physicians 1967;80:59.
9. Arbogast R, Bourassa MG: Myocardial function during atrial pacing in patients with angina pectoris and normal coronary arteriograms: Comparison with patients having significant coronary artery disease. Am J Cardiol 1993;32:257.
10. Kemp HG: Left ventricular function in patients with the anginal syndrome and normal coronary arteriograms. Am J Cardiol 1973;32:375.
11. Cannon RO, Camici PG, Epstein SE: Pathophysiological dilemma of syndrome X. Circulation 1992;85:883.
12. Inobe Y, Kugiyama K, Morita K, et al: Role of adenosine in pathogenesis of syndrome X: Assessment with coronary hemodynamic measurements and thallium-201 myocardial single-photon emission computed tomography. J Am Coll Cardiol 1996;28:890.
13. Rosen SD, Uren NG, Kaski JC, et al: Coronary vasodilator reserve, pain perception and sex in patients with syndrome X. Circulation 1994;90:50.
14. Rosano GMC, Ponikowski P, Adamopoulos D, et al: Abnormal autonomic control of the cardiovascular system in syndrome X. Am J Cardiol 1994;73:1174.
15. Frobert O, Molgaard H, Botker HE, et al: Autonomic balance in patients with angina and a normal coronary angiogram. Eur Heart J 1995;16:1356.
16. Chauhan A, Foote J, Petch MC, et al: Hyperinsulinemia, coronary artery disease and syndrome X. J Am Coll Cardiol 1994;23:364.
17. Swan J, Walton C, Godsland IF, et al: Insulin resistance syndrome as a feature of cardiological syndrome X in non-obese men. Br Heart J 1994;71:41.
18. Botker HE, Moller N, Schmitz O, et al: Myocardial insulin resistance in patients with syndrome X. J Clin Invest 1997;100:1919.
19. Gaspardone A, Ferri C, Crea F, et al: Enhanced activity of sodium-lithium countertransport in patients with cardiac syndrome X: A potential link between cardiac and metabolic syndrome X. J Am Coll Cardiol 1998;32:2031.
20. Kaski JC, Elliott PM, Salomone O, et al: Concentration of circulating plasma endothelin in patients with angina and normal coronary angiograms. Br Heart J 1995;74:620.
21. Lanza GA, Luscher TF, Pasceri V, et al: Effects of atrial pacing on arterial and coronary sinus endothelin-1 levels in syndrome X. Am J Cardiol 1999;84:1187.
22. Rosano GM, Collins P, Kaski JC, et al: Syndrome X in women is associated with oestrogen deficiency. Eur Heart J 1995;16:610.
23. Egashira K, Inou T, Hirooka Y, et al: Evidence of impaired endothelium-dependent coronary vasodilation in patients with angina pectoris and normal coronary angiograms. N Engl J Med 1993;328:1659.
24. Zeiher AM, Krause T, Shachinger V, et al: Impaired endothelium-dependent vasodilation of coronary resistance vessels is associated with exercise-induced myocardial ischemia. Circulation 1995;91:2345.
25. Hasdai D, Gibbons RJ, Holmes DR Jr, et al: Coronary endothelial dysfunction in humans is associated with myocardial perfusion defects. Circulation 1997;96:3390.
26. Altman JD, Kinn J, Duncker DJ, et al: Effect of inhibition of nitric oxide formation on coronary blood flow during stress in the dog. Cardiovasc Res 1994;28:119.
27. Camici PG, Marraccini P, Lorenzoni R, et al: Coronary hemodynamics and myocardial metabolism in patients with syndrome X: Response to pacing stress. J Am Coll Cardiol 1991;17:1461.
28. Nihoyannopoulos P, Kaski JC, Crake T, et al: Absence of myocardial dysfunction during stress in patients with syndrome X. J Am Coll Cardiol 1991;18:1463.
29. Rosano GM, Kaski JC, Arie S, et al: Failure to demonstrate myocardial ischaemia in patients with angina and normal coronary arteries: Evaluation by continuous coronary sinus pH monitoring. Eur Heart J 1997;17:1175.
30. Panza JA, Laurienzo JM, Curiel RV, et al: Investigation of the mechanism of chest pain in patients with angiographically normal coronary arteries using transesophageal dobutamine stress echocardiography. J Am Coll Cardiol 1997;29:293.
31. Maseri A, Crea F, Kaski JC, et al: Mechanisms of angina pectoris in syndrome X. J Am Coll Cardiol 1991;17:499.
32. Buffon A, Rigattieri S, Santini SA, et al: Myocardial ischemia-reperfusion damage after pacing-induced tachycardia in patients with cardiac syndrome X. Am J Physiol Heart Circ Physiol 2000;279:H2627.

33. Buchthal SD, den Hollander JA, Bairey-Merz CN, et al: Abnormal myocardial phosphorous-31 nuclear magnetic resonance spectroscopy in women with chest pain but normal coronary angiograms. N Engl J Med 2000;342:829.

34. Toivonen L, Helenius K, Viitasalo M: Electrocardiographic repolarization during stress from awakening on alarm call. J Am Coll Cardiol 1997;30:774.

35. Shapiro LM, Crake T, Poole-Wilson PA: Is altered cardiac sensation responsible for chest pain in patients with normal coronary arteries? Clinical observation during cardiac catheterization. BMJ 1988;296:170.

36. Cannon RO III, Quyyumi AA, Schenke WH, et al: Abnormal cardiac pain sensitivity in patients with chest pain and normal coronary arteries. J Am Coll Cardiol 1990;16:1359.

37. Lagerqvist B, Sylven C, Waldenstrom A: Lower threshold for adenosine-induced chest pain in patients with angina and normal coronary angiograms. Br Heart J 1992;68:282.

38. Rosen SD, Uren NG, Kaski JC, et al: Coronary vasodilator reserve, pain perception, and sex in patients with syndrome X. Circulation 1994;90:50.

39. Pasceri V, Lanza GA, Buffon A, et al: Role of abnormal pain sensitivity and behavioral factors in determining chest pain in syndrome X. J Am Coll Cardiol 1998;31:62.

40. Richter JE, Barish CF, Castell DO: Abnormal sensory perception in patients with esophageal chest pain. Gastroenterology 1986;91:845.

41. Lynn RB, Friedman LS: Irritable bowel syndrome. N Engl J Med 1993;329:1940.

42. Bass C, Wade C, Hand D, et al: Patients with angina and normal and near normal coronary arteries: Clinical and psychosocial state 12 months after angiography. BMJ 1983;287:1505.

43. Beitman BD, Mukerji V, Lamberti JW, et al: Panic disorder in patients with chest pain and angiographically normal coronary arteries. Am J Cardiol 1989;63:1399.

44. Lanza GA, Manzoli A, Bia E, et al: Acute effects of nitrates on exercise testing in patients with syndrome X: Clinical and pathophysiological implications. Circulation 1994;90:2695.

45. Lanza GA, Colonna G, Pasceri V, et al: Atenolol versus amlodipine versus isosorbide-5-mononitrate on anginal symptoms in syndrome X. Am J Cardiol 1999;84:854.

46. Bugiardini R, Borghi A, Biagetti L, et al: Comparison of verapamil versus propanolol therapy in syndrome X. Am J Cardiol 1989;63:286.

47. Kaski JC, Rosano GM, Gavrielides S, et al: Effects of angiotensin-converting enzyme inhibition on exercise-induced angina and ST segment depression in patients with microvascular angina. J Am Coll Cardiol 1994;23:652.

48. Elliott PM, Krzyzowska-Dickinson K, Calvino R, et al: Effect of oral aminophylline in patients with angina and normal coronary arteriograms (cardiac syndrome X). Heart 1997;77:523.

49. Rosano GMC, Peters NS, Lefroy D, et al: 17-Beta-estradiol therapy lessens angina in postmenopausal women with syndrome X. J Am Coll Cardiol 1996;27:1500.

50. Lerman A, Burnett JC Jr, Higano ST, et al: Long-term L-arginine supplementation improves small-vessel coronary endothelial function in humans. Circulation 1998;97:2123.

51. Cannon RO III, Quyyumi AA, Mincemoyer R, et al: Imipramine in patients with chest pain despite normal coronary angiograms. N Engl J Med 1994;330:1411.

52. Eriksson BE, Tyrni-Lenne R, Svedenhag J, et al: Physical training in syndrome X: Physical training counteracts deconditioning and pain in syndrome X. J Am Coll Cardiol 2000;36:1619.

53. Cunningham C, Brown S, Kaski JC: Effects of transcendental meditation on symptoms and electrocardiographic changes in patients with cardiac syndrome X. Am J Cardiol 2000;85:653.

54. Mayou RA, Bryant BM, Sanders C, et al: A controlled trial of cognitive behavioural therapy for non-cardiac chest pain. Psychol Med 1997;27:1021.

55. Sanderson JE, Woo KS, Chung HK, et al: The effect of transcutaneous electrical nerve stimulation on coronary and systemic hemodynamics in syndrome X. Coron Artery Dis 1996;7:547.

56. Anderson C, Hole P, Oxhoj H: Spinal cord stimulation as a pain treatment for angina pectoris. Pain Clin 1995;8:333.

57. Eliasson T, Albertsson P, Hardhammar P, et al: Spinal cord stimulation in angina pectoris with normal coronary arteriograms. Coron Artery Dis 1993;4:819.

58. Lanza GA, Sestito A, Sandric S, et al: Spinal cord stimulation in patients with refractory anginal pain and normal coronary arteries. Ital Heart J 2001;2:25.

Cocaine and Other Environmental Causes of Acute Coronary Syndromes

Audrey H. Rapp
Richard A. Lange
L. David Hillis

The term *acute coronary syndromes* (ACS) encompasses unstable angina pectoris and acute myocardial infarction (MI). Acute MI may be ST-segment elevation or non–ST-segment elevation, depending on the patient's 12-lead electrocardiogram (ECG). The pathophysiology of all three types of ACS is similar, in that a previously stable coronary arterial atherosclerotic plaque becomes ulcerated, serving as a nidus for platelet aggregation and thrombus formation. The specific ACS that subsequently evolves is determined by (1) the intensity of platelet aggregation and thrombus formation, (2) the duration of the compromise in arterial blood flow caused by platelet aggregation and thrombus formation (i.e., transient, lasting only a few minutes, or sustained, lasting several hours or more), (3) the oxygen requirements of the myocardium perfused by the involved coronary artery, and (4) the presence and magnitude of collateral blood supply to the myocardium perfused by this artery. In an occasional patient, certain exogenous factors may precipitate ACS or exacerbate previously established ACS, including cocaine, marijuana, tobacco, amphetamines, and air pollution. The identification of these exogenous factors may influence the manner in which a patient is treated.

COCAINE

Beginning in the mid-1980s, cocaine use became widespread. In a 1999 survey, an estimated 25 million Americans admitted that they had used it at least once, 3.7 million had used it within the previous year, and 1.5 million were current users.[1] These figures underestimate the true magnitude of cocaine use, since some subjects probably were reluctant to admit to previous cocaine use during a routine survey or interview. When cocaine use within the past weeks to months is assessed by hair analysis, its prevalence is estimated to be three to five times higher than that reported during standard surveys and interviews.[2,3] Cocaine is the most commonly used illicit drug among subjects seeking care in hospital emergency departments or drug treatment centers. In 1999, an estimated 30% of all drug-related emergency department visits involved cocaine. Most subjects were men in their 20s or 30s.[4]

Cardiovascular complications of cocaine use are as likely to occur in the first-time user as they are in the chronic user. Cocaine use should be considered as a possible contributing factor in nearly all patients with ACS. Apart from its illicit use, cocaine is a commonly used local anesthetic for minor rhinolaryngologic surgical procedures.[5] Occasionally, it may be responsible for cardiovascular complications perioperatively.

Cocaine (benzoylmethylecgonine) is an alkaloid that is extracted from the *Erythroxylon coca* plant.[6] It exists in two forms. The first, cocaine hydrochloride, is prepared by dissolving the alkaloid in hydrochloric acid to form a water-soluble powder or granule. It can be taken orally, intravenously, or intranasally. The second, the freebase form, is produced by processing the cocaine with ammonia or sodium bicarbonate to remove the hydrochloride. The resultant compound is heat stable and melts at 98°C, allowing it to be smoked. It is known as *crack* because of the popping sound it makes when heated.

High blood levels of cocaine may be achieved after any route of administration, with the only differences being the timing of onset, peak effect, and duration of action. Intravenously administered cocaine has an onset of action within 60 seconds, a peak effect in 3 to 5 minutes, and a duration of action of 20 to 60 minutes. When given intranasally, its onset of action occurs in 1 to 5 minutes, its peak effect occurs in 15 to 20 minutes, and its duration of action is 60 to 90 minutes. When cocaine is smoked, its onset of action is immediate, its peak effect occurs in 1 to 3 minutes, and its duration of action is 5 to 15 minutes. Cocaine is metabolized by plasma and liver cholinesterases to water-soluble metabolites, primarily benzoylecgonine and ecgonine methyl ester, which are excreted in the urine. These metabolites exert hemodynamic effects that are similar to those of cocaine (vasoconstriction), but their duration of action is substantially longer than that of the parent drug (i.e., 24 to 36 hours). The concomitant use of cocaine and ethanol results in the formation of a unique metabolite, cocaethylene, which also is a potent vasoconstrictor.

Since the first case of cocaine-associated MI was reported by Coleman and associates[7] in 1982, descriptions of more than 200 additional cases have appeared in the literature.[8] Initial small and retrospective assessments reported that ECG and enzymatic evidence of MI occurred in 0% to 31% of patients with cocaine-associated chest pain.[9-11] More recently, the COCHPA (Cocaine Associated Chest Pain) trial, a large multicenter prospective assessment, reported that 6% of subjects with cocaine-related chest pain developed enzymatic evidence of MI,[12] and Weber and colleagues[13] reported a similar percentage in a large retrospective analysis.

The typical patient with cocaine-associated MI is a young man with few risk factors for atherosclerosis other than tobacco abuse (Table 42-1).[14] He may have used any quantity of cocaine administered by any route.[15] The risk of MI is increased 24-fold within the first 60 minutes after the use of cocaine, but some subjects first may seek medical attention many hours later.[16] When cocaine users with chest pain are evaluated in the emergency department, few reliable screening tools are available to predict which of them will develop evidence of MI. The chest pain described usually is similar in character, location, and duration as that of MI unrelated to cocaine use. The ECG is abnormal in 56% to 84% of patients with cocaine-related chest pain (<10% of whom develop enzymatic evidence of MI), and 43% of cocaine users who do not develop enzymatic evidence of infarction have an initial ECG that meets criteria for the initiation of reperfusion therapy (ST-segment elevation of at least 0.1 mV in two or more contiguous leads).[17,18] These ECG findings may reflect a previous MI, or they may represent repolarization abnormalities that often occur normally in young men. Overall, the 12-lead ECG offers 36% sensitivity, 90% specificity, 18% positive predictive value, and 96% negative predictive value for detecting MI in cocaine users with chest pain.[19] Rhabdomyolysis may occur in cocaine users, causing an elevated serum creatine kinase concentration. Of patients with recent cocaine use, 14% have an elevated CK-MB fraction without other evidence of myocardial necrosis.[20] In cocaine users, serum troponin concentrations should be measured.[21]

Patients who seek medical attention with cocaine-associated chest pain often continue to use cocaine during the weeks to months after discharge.[22] Over the next 12 months, these individuals have a 75% likelihood of having recurrent chest pain and a 1% risk of MI. In contrast, individuals who abstain from subsequent cocaine use are not at increased risk of MI or death.

■ ■ ■

TABLE 42–1 CHARACTERISTICS OF THE TYPICAL PATIENT WITH COCAINE-RELATED ACUTE CORONARY SYNDROME

Young age
Male gender
Concurrent tobacco use
Unrelated to amount or route of administration
May seek medical attention 24 hours after use
Pain typical in location and character
High likelihood of abnormal electrocardiogram

Small studies attempted to examine the cardiovascular complications of cocaine-associated MI.[23] In 90% of subjects, complications occur before or within 12 hours of hospital presentation, including ventricular arrhythmias, supraventricular arrhythmias, congestive heart failure, and ongoing, sustained chest pain. In-hospital mortality is reportedly less than 2%, owing, at least in part, to the young age of the patients.

The pathophysiology of cocaine-associated myocardial ischemia and infarction is likely multifactorial and is due to a combination of (1) increased myocardial oxygen demand in the setting of limited supply, (2) intense coronary arterial vasoconstriction, and (3) enhanced platelet aggregation and thrombus formation. Cocaine increases all three determinants of myocardial oxygen demand: heart rate, systemic arterial pressure, and left ventricular contractility. It blocks the presynaptic reuptake of norepinephrine and dopamine, producing an excess of these neurotransmitters at the site of the postsynaptic receptor. In short, cocaine acts as a powerful sympathomimetic agent. In patients studied during routine diagnostic cardiac catheterization, intranasal cocaine (2 mg/kg) induced an increase in heart rate, systemic arterial pressure, and left ventricular dP/dt,[24] while it caused an 8% to 12% decrease in coronary arterial diameter and a 17% decrease in coronary sinus blood flow. This relatively small dose of cocaine is about two thirds that used for local anesthesia and substantially less than that usually used in a recreational setting.[25,26] Although vasoconstriction was noted in angiographically nondiseased and diseased coronary arterial segments, it was particularly marked in the latter. This cocaine-induced vasoconstriction was reversed with the α-adrenergic blocking agent phentolamine, suggesting that it was mediated via α-adrenergic stimulation. Subsequent studies have shown that cocaine also induces the release of endothelin-1, a potent vasoconstrictor.[27]

Some patients with cocaine-related MI have been shown to have angiographic evidence of coronary arterial thrombosis.[28] Cocaine stimulates platelet aggregation and thrombus formation by (1) increasing plasminogen activator inhibitor activity,[29] (2) increasing plasma catecholamines, and (3) stimulating β-granule release from platelets.[30]

Cigarette smoking and cocaine increase myocardial oxygen demand and diminish oxygen supply. Their combination seems to be synergistic in causing an imbalance between oxygen supply and demand.[31,32] Moliterno and colleagues[33] compared the effects of smoking alone, cocaine alone, and their combination in patients during diagnostic cardiac catheterization. Compared with either agent alone, a cocaine/tobacco combination caused a marked increase in myocardial oxygen demand (as measured by heart rate–systolic arterial pressure double product) and a substantial decline in coronary arterial dimensions.[33]

As mentioned previously, cocaethylene, the cocaine metabolite that is synthesized when cocaine is used in the presence of ethanol, is a powerful vasoconstrictor in vitro. In vivo studies showed, however, that the administration of modest amounts of cocaine and ethanol concomitantly causes coronary arterial vasodilation.[34] A cocaine/ethanol combination may exert different effects if either (or both) is given in larger amounts. In this regard, the combination of large amounts of cocaine and ethanol has been linked to increased morbidity and mortality when compared with either agent alone.[35] A cocaine/ethanol combination is the second most common combination in patients who die of substance abuse.[36]

Cocaine-related myocardial ischemia and infarction may be caused by (1) increased myocardial oxygen demand in the setting of limited supply, (2) intense coronary arterial vasoconstriction, or (3) enhanced platelet aggregation and thrombus formation. Treatment should target as many of these potential causes as possible. For the patient with cocaine-related chest pain, first-line therapy includes oxygen, aspirin, nitroglycerin, and benzodiazepines. Second-line therapy includes verapamil, phentolamine, and reperfusion therapy (thrombolytic therapy or primary angioplasty) (Table 42–2).

Lange and coworkers[37] showed that β-adrenergic blockade (in an attempt to lower systemic arterial pressure and heart rate) may potentiate cocaine-induced coronary arterial vasoconstriction, presumably by causing unopposed α-adrenergically mediated smooth muscle contraction. Labetalol, which has α-adrenergic and β-adrenergic blocking activity, alleviates cocaine-associated hypertension, but it exerts no effect (beneficial or detrimental) on coronary arterial tone.[38] The administration of a pure α-adrenergic blocking agent, such as phentolamine, is not recommended because it may cause symptomatic hypotension. Since nitroglycerin and verapamil reverse cocaine-induced hypertension and coronary arterial vasoconstriction, they are the first choice in the treatment of patients with cocaine-associated chest pain.[39,40] Hollander and associates[41] showed that sublingual nitroglycerin provided relief of chest pain in 67% of patients with cocaine-associated chest pain. Benzodiazepines, such as diazepam, are also effective in relieving cocaine-associated chest pain.[42]

All patients with cocaine-associated chest pain should receive aspirin, unless it is contraindicated. As discussed previously, some of these patients have chest pain and ECG criteria for reperfusion therapy (ST-segment elevation of at least 0.1 mV in two or more contiguous leads), but most do not develop enzymatic evidence of myocardial necrosis. The experience with thrombolytic therapy in these patients is limited, and the results are inconclusive.[43] Since these patients are often hypertensive (and may be at increased risk for intracranial hemorrhage with thrombolytic therapy), it is not recommended that such therapy be considered as first line. If the patient continues to have symptoms and ECG changes suggestive of MI, he or she should be considered for urgent coronary angiography and primary angioplasty, if appropriate.

TOBACCO

Perhaps the most common exogenous substance to which individuals are exposed is cigarette smoke. Cigarette smoking increases the risk of cardiovascular disease in general and of acute MI in particular.[44] In the Gruppo Italiano per lo Studio della sopravvivenza nell infarto miocardico (GISSI-2) study, smokers had a threefold to fourfold increased relative risk of acute MI compared with nonsmokers, and the risk was 9 to 12 times higher in smokers younger than age 50.[45] Similar to cocaine, cigarette smoking may cause (1) increased platelet aggregation, (2) increased myocardial oxygen demand in the setting of limited supply, and (3) intense coronary arterial vasoconstriction. The smoking-induced enhancement of platelet aggregation is not seen with nicotine-free cigarettes, suggesting that nicotine is the cause of enhanced platelet aggregation.[46,47] Nicotine may increase platelet aggregation directly or may do so by increasing plasma catecholamine concentrations. Cigarette smoking increases myocardial oxygen demand by increasing heart rate, systemic arterial pressure, and left ventricular contractility.[48] At the same time, it diminishes coronary arterial blood flow and myocardial oxygen supply,[49] an effect that seems to be mediated by α-adrenergic stimulation, as it is reversed with phentolamine, an α-adrenergic blocking agent.

Compared with nonsmokers, cigarette smokers are at increased risk of having a MI, but their short-term prognosis after MI is better than that of nonsmokers.[50] This so-called smokers' paradox seems to be due to the following: (1) Smokers are likely to have less severe coronary atherosclerosis[51] than are nonsmokers, (2) effective reperfusion with thrombolytic therapy occurs more often in smokers than in nonsmokers,[52] and (3) smokers with acute MI are younger (by an average of 11 years) than nonsmokers.[53] This smokers' paradox seems to be true for subjects with ST-segment elevation and non–ST-segment elevation MI.[54] In the Platelet glycoprotein IIb/IIIa in Unstable Angina: Receptor Suppression Using Integrelin Therapy (PURSUIT) study, cigarette smokers with ACS had a better short-term outcome than did nonsmokers, but this benefit seemed to be attributable to their younger age and their decreased incidence of diabetes mellitus and hypertension. Smokers and nonsmok-

■ ■ ■

TABLE 42–2 RECOMMENDED TREATMENT OF PATIENTS WITH COCAINE-ASSOCIATED CHEST PAIN OR MYOCARDIAL INFARCTION

First-Line Agents

Oxygen
Aspirin
Nitroglycerin
Benzodiazepines

Second-Line Agents

Verapamil
Phentolamine
Thrombolytic therapy or primary angioplasty

ers responded similarly to therapy with a glycoprotein IIb/IIIa inhibitor.

MARIJUANA

In 1998, more than 72 million Americans admitted that they had used marijuana at least once, making it the most widely used illicit drug in the United States.[55] Marijuana use causes an increase in heart rate and systemic arterial pressure, presumably caused by delta-9-tetrahydro-cannabinol.[56] In the setting of a limited myocardial oxygen supply, this increase in oxygen demand may cause a worsening of angina. Marijuana has been associated with acute MI in individuals considered to be at low risk.[57-59] In their study of almost 4000 patients, Mittleman and colleagues[60] found that the risk of MI was increased almost fivefold during 1 hour after marijuana use. Since these subjects subsequently were found to have no coronary arterial narrowing on angiography, coronary arterial vasospasm was hypothesized to be the cause.[61]

Published treatment guidelines for patients with acute MI and recent marijuana use do not exist. Coronary arterial vasospasm should be considered as a likely cause, and the patient should be treated with nitrates. Because β-adrenergic blockers may potentiate coronary arterial vasospasm, they should be avoided.

AMPHETAMINES

Amphetamines stimulate the release of norepinephrine and dopamine from presynaptic nerves, leading to stimulation of α-adrenergic receptors, which may induce coronary arterial vasoconstriction,[62] increase myocardial oxygen demand, and enhance platelet aggregation. The most commonly observed cardiovascular effects of amphetamines are hypertension and tachycardia, which may induce angina in a patient with underlying coronary artery disease. Amphetamines have been reported to be temporally related to the development of acute MI, particularly when they are administered intravenously.[63] At subsequent coronary angiography, some of these patients had angiographically normal coronary arteries, whereas others had evidence of intraluminal thrombosis.

OTHER MEDICATIONS

Two medications used to treat subjects with migraine headaches, ergotamine and sumatriptan, have been associated with acute MI. Although ergotamine causes vaso-constriction of intracerebral and extracranial blood vessels, it only rarely has been associated with coronary arterial vasospasm and acute MI.[64,65] Sumatriptan is a selective 5-hydroxytryptamine agonist, which also exerts its therapeutic effect through cerebral arterial vasocon-striction. Although it has been shown to cause coronary arterial vasoconstriction,[66] only a few cases of acute MI in association with its use have been reported.[67,68]

OTHER SUBSTANCES

Scattered reports have appeared in the literature of other substances believed to be responsible for acute MI, including heroin,[69] toluene,[70] intravenous penta-zocine and tripelennamine,[71] and air pollution. As worldwide levels of particulate pollution increase, its possible role in exacerbating stable cardiovascular disease and in triggering acute MI has been suggested. Peters and colleagues[72] correlated levels of air pollution in Boston with the risk of acute MI, showing an increased risk of MI at times when the levels of pollution were highest. Although the mechanism by which air pollution triggers acute MI is unknown, it may do so by increasing blood viscosity,[73] inflammation (as measured by C-reactive protein), heart rate, or shear stress.[74]

REFERENCES

1. Nicholi AM Jr: The nontherapeutic use of psychoactive drugs: A modern epidemic. N Engl J Med 1983;308:925-933.
2. Kidwell DA, Blanco MA, Smith FP: Cocaine detection in a university population by hair analysis and skin swab testing. Forensic Sci Int 1997;84:75-86.
3. Fendrich M, Johnson TP, Sudman S, et al: Validity of drug use reporting in a high-risk community sample: A comparison of cocaine and heroin survey reports with hair tests. Am J Epidemiol 1999;149: 955-962.
4. Office of Applied Studies: Year-End 1999 Emergency Department Data from the Drug Abuse Warning Network. DHHS publication no. (SMA) 00-3462. Rockville, MD, Substance Abuse and Mental Health Services Administration, 2000.
5. Fairbanks DN, Fairbanks GR: Cocaine uses and abuses. Ann Plast Surg 1983;10:452-457.
6. Catterall W, Mackie K: Local anesthetics. In Hardman JG, Gilman AG, Limbird LE (eds): Goodman and Gilman's Pharmacologic Basis of Therapeutics, 9th ed. New York, McGraw-Hill, 1996, pp 331-338.
7. Coleman DL, Ross TF, Naughton JL: Myocardial ischemia and infarction related to recreational cocaine use. West J Med 1982;136:444-446.
8. Galasko GI: Cocaine, a risk factor for myocardial infarction. J Cardiovasc Risk 1997;4:185-190.
9. Zimmerman JL, Dellinger RP, Majid PA: Cocaine-associated chest pain. Ann Emerg Med 1991;20:611-615.
10. Gitter MJ, Goldsmith SR, Dunbar DN, Sharkey SW: Cocaine and chest pain: Clinical features and outcome of patients hospitalized to rule out myocardial infarction. Ann Intern Med 1991;115: 277-282.
11. Amin M, Gabelman G, Karpel J, Butrick P: Acute myocardial infarction and chest pain syndromes after cocaine use. Am J Cardiol 1990;66:1434-1437.
12. Hollander JE, Hoffman RS, Gennis P, et al: Prospective multicenter evaluation of cocaine associated chest pain. Acad Emerg Med 1994; 1(4): 330-339.
13. Weber JE, Chudnofsky CR, Boczar M, et al: Cocaine-associated chest pain: How common is myocardial infarction? Acad Emerg Med 2000;7:873-877.
14. Hollander JE, Hoffman RS: Cocaine induced myocardial infarction: Analysis and review of the literature. J Emerg Med 1992;10: 169-177.
15. Isner JM, Estes NM, Thompson PD, et al: Acute cardiac events temporally related to cocaine abuse. N Engl J Med 1986;315: 1438-1443.
16. Mittleman MA, Mintzer D, Maclure M, et al: Triggering of myocardial infarction by cocaine. Circulation 1999;99:2737-2741.
17. Hollander JE, Hoffman RS, Gennis P, et al: Prospective multicenter evaluation by cocaine. Acad Emerg Med 1994;1:330-339.

18. Gitter MJ, Goldsmith SR, Dunbar DN, et al: Cocaine and chest pain: Clinical features and outcome of patients hospitalized to rule out myocardial infarction. Ann Intern Med 1991;115:277–282.

19. Hollander JE, Levitt MA, Young GP, et al: Effect of recent cocaine use on the specificity of cardiac markers for diagnosis of acute myocardial infarction. Am Heart J 1998;135(2 Pt 1):245–252.

20. Tokarski GF, Paganussi P, Urbanski R, et al: An evaluation of cocaine-induced chest pain. Ann Emerg Med 1990;19:1088–1092.

21. Hollander JE, Levitt MA, Young GP, et al: Effect of recent cocaine use on specificity of cardiac markers for diagnosis of acute myocardial infarction. Am Heart J 1998;135(2 Pt 1):245–252.

22. Hollander JE, Hoffman RS, Gennis P, et al: Cocaine-associated chest pain: One year follow-up. Acad Emerg Med 1995;2:179–181.

23. Hollander JE, Hoffman RS, Burstein JL, et al: Cocaine-associated myocardial infarction. Arch Intern Med 1995;155: 1081–1086.

24. Boehrer JD, Moliterno DJ, Willard JE, et al: Hemodynamic effects of intranasal cocaine in humans. J Am Coll Cardiol 1992;20:90–93.

25. Lange RA, Cigarroa RG, Yancy CW, et al: Cocaine-induced coronary-artery vasoconstriction. N Engl J Med 1989;321:1557–1562.

26. Poklis A, Mackell MA, Graham M: Disposition of cocaine in fatal poisoning in man. J Anal Toxicol 1985;9:227–229.

27. Wilbert-Lampen U, Seliger C, Zilker T, et al: Cocaine increases the endothelial release of immunoreactive endothelin and its concentrations in human plasma and urine: Reversal by coincubation with alpha-receptor antagonists. Circulation 1998;98:385–390.

28. Stenberg RG, Winniford MD, Hillis LD, et al: Simultaneous acute thrombosis of two major coronary arteries following intravenous cocaine use. Arch Pathol Lab Med 1989;113:521–524.

29. Moliterno DJ, Lange RA, Gerard RD, et al: Influence of intranasal cocaine on plasma constituents associated with endogenous thrombosis and thrombolysis. Am J Med 1994;96:492–496.

30. Rinder HM, Ault KA, Jatlow PI, et al: Platelet alpha-granule release in cocaine users. Circulation 1994;90:1162–1167.

31. Nicod P, Rehr R, Winniford MD, et al: Acute systemic and coronary hemodynamic and serologic responses to cigarette smoking in long-term smokers with atherosclerotic coronary artery disease. J Am Coll Cardiol 1984;4:964–971.

32. Lange RA, Cigarroa RG, Yancy CW, et al: Cocaine-induced coronary artery vasoconstriction. N Engl Med 1989;321:1557–1562.

33. Moliterno DJ, Willard JE, Lange RA, et al: Coronary-artery vasoconstriction induced by cocaine, cigarette smoking, or both. N Engl J Med 1994;330:454–459.

34. Pirwitz MJ, Willard JE, Landau C, et al: Influence of cocaine, ethanol or their combination on epicardial coronary arterial dimensions in humans. Arch Intern Med 1995;155:1186–1191.

35. Randall J: Cocaine, alcohol mix in body to form even longer lasting, more lethal drug. JAMA 1992;267:1043–1044.

36. Grant BF, Harford TC: Concurrent and simultaneous use of alcohol with cocaine: Results of national survey. Drug Alcohol Depend 1990;25:97–104.

37. Lange RA, Cigarroa RC, Flores ED, et al: Potentiation of cocaine-induced coronary vasoconstriction by beta-adrenergic blockade. Ann Intern Med 1990;112:897–903.

38. Boehrer JD, Moliterno DJ, Willard JE, et al: Influence of labetalol on cocaine-induced coronary vasoconstriction in humans. Am J Med 1993;94:608–610.

39. Negus BH, Willard JE, Hillis LD, et al: Alleviation of cocaine-induced coronary vasoconstriction with intravenous verapamil. Am J Cardiol 1994;73:510–513.

40. Brogan WC III, Lange RA, Kim AS, et al: Alleviation of cocaine-induced coronary vasoconstriction by nitroglycerin. J Am Coll Cardiol 1991;18:581–586.

41. Hollander JE, Hoffman RS, Gennis P, et al: Nitroglycerin in the treatment of cocaine associated chest pain: Clinical safety and efficacy. J Toxicol Clin Toxicol 1994;32:243–256.

42. Baumann BM, Perrone J, Hornig SE, et al: Randomized, double-blind, placebo-controlled trial of diazepam, nitroglycerin, or both for the treatment of patients with cocaine-associated acute coronary syndromes. Acad Emerg Med 2000;7:878–885.

43. Hollander JE, Burstein JL, Hoffman RS, et al: Cocaine-associated myocardial infarction: Clinical safety of thrombolytic therapy. Chest 1995;107:1237–1241.

44. Surgeon General: The Health Consequences of Smoking: Cardiovascular Disease. Rockville, MD, U.S. Department of Health and Human Services, 1983.

45. Negri E, Franzosi MG, La Vecchia C, et al: Tar yield of cigarettes and risk of acute myocardial infarction. BMJ 1993;306:1567–1570.

46. Davis JW, Davis RF: Acute effect of tobacco cigarette smoking on the platelet aggregate ratio. Am J Med Sci 1979;278:139–143.

47. Levine PH: An acute effect of cigarette smoking on platelet function: A possible link between smoking and arterial thrombosis. Circulation 1973;48:619–623.

48. Nicod P, Rehr R, Winniford MD, et al: Acute systemic and coronary hemodynamic and serologic responses to cigarette smoking in long-term smokers with atherosclerotic coronary artery disease. J Am Coll Cardiol 1984;4:964–971.

49. Winniford MD, Wheelan KR, Kremers MS, et al: Smoking-induced coronary vasoconstriction in patients with atherosclerotic coronary artery disease: Evidence for adrenergically mediated alterations in coronary artery tone. Circulation 1986;73:662–667.

50. Barbash GI, Reiner J, White HD, et al: Evaluation of paradoxic beneficial effects of smoking in patients receiving thrombolytic therapy for acute myocardial infarction: Mechanisms of the "smoker's paradox" from the GUSTO-1 Trial with angiographic insights. J Am Coll Cardiol 1995;26:1222–1229.

51. Ishihara M, Sato H, Tateishi H, et al: Clinical implications of cigarette smoking in acute myocardial infarction: Acute angiographic findings and long-term prognosis. Am Heart J 1997;134(5 Pt 1): 955–960.

52. Gomez MA, Karagounis LA, Allen A, Anderson JL: Effect of cigarette smoking on coronary patency after thrombolytic therapy for myocardial infarction. Am J Cardiol 1993;72:373–378.

53. Andrikopolous GK, Richter DJ, Dilaveris PE, et al: In-hospital mortality of habitual cigarette smokers after acute myocardial infarction: The "smoker's paradox" in a countrywide study. Eur Heart J 2001;22:776–784.

54. Hasdai D, Holmes DR, Criger DA, et al: Cigarette smoking status and outcome among patients with acute coronary syndromes without persistent ST-segment elevation: Effect of inhibition of platelet glycoprotein IIb/IIIa with eptifibitide. Am Heart J 2000;139:454–460.

55. Substance Abuse and Mental Health Services Administration: National Household Survey on Drug Abuse. DHHS no. (SMA) 99-3328. Rockville, MD, SAMSHA, Office of Applied Sciences, 1998.

56. Prakash R, Aronow WS, Warren M, et al: Effects of marihuana and placebo marihuana smoking on hemodynamics in coronary artery disease. Clin Pharmacol Ther 1975;18:90–95.

57. Collins JS, Higginson JD, Boyle DM, et al: Myocardial infarction during marijuana smoking in a young female. Eur Heart J 1985;6:637–638.

58. Pearl W, Choi YS: Marijuana as a cause of myocardial infarction. Int J Cardiol 1992;34:353.

59. Charles R, Holt S, Kirkhon N: Myocardial infarction and marijuana. Clin Toxicol 1979;14:433–438.

60. Mittleman MA, Lewis RA, Maclure M, et al: Triggering myocardial infarction by marijuana. Circulation 2001;103:2805–2809.

61. Heiden D, Rodvien R, Jones R, et al: Effect of oral delta-9-tetrahydrocannabinol on coagulation. Thromb Res 1980;17: 885–889.

62. Hillis LD, Braunwald E: Coronary artery spasm. N Engl J Med 1978;299:695–702.

63. Waksman J, Taylor RN, Bodor GS, et al: Acute myocardial infarction associated with amphetamine use. Mayo Clin Proc 2001;76: 323–326.

64. Klein LS, Simpson RJ, Stern R, et al: Myocardial infarction following administration of sublingual ergotamine. Chest 1982;82:372–376.

65. Benedict CR, Robertson D: Angina pectoris and sudden death in the absence of atherosclerosis following ergotamine therapy for migraine. Am J Med 1979;67:177–178.

66. MacIntyre PD, Bhargava B, Hogg KJ, et al: Effect of subcutaneous sumitriptan, a selective 5HT1 agonist on the systemic, pulmonary and coronary circulation. Circulation 1993;87:401–405.

67. Main ML, Ramaswamy K, Andrews TC: Cardiac arrest and myocardial infarction immediately after sumatriptan injection. Ann Intern Med 1998;128:874.

68. Willett F, Curzen N, Adams J, et al: Coronary vasospasm induced by subcutaneous sumatriptan. BMJ 1992;304:1415.

69. Sztajzel J, Karpuz H, Rutishauser W: Heroin abuse and myocardial infarction. Int J Cardiol 1994;47:180–182.

70. Hussain TF, Heidenreich PA, Benowitz N: Recurrent non-Q wave myocardial infarction associated with toluene abuse. Am Heart J 1996;131:615–616.

71. McGwier BW, Alpert MA, Panayiotou H, et al: Acute myocardial infarction associated with intravenous injection of pentazocine and tripelennamine. Chest 1992;101:1730–1732.

72. Peters A, Dockery DW, Muller JE, Mittleman MA: Increased particulate air pollution and the triggering of myocardial infarction. Circulation 2001;103:2810–2815.

73. Peters A, Döring A, Wichmann HE, et al: Increased plasma viscosity during the 1985 air pollution episode: A link to mortality? Lancet 1997;349:1582–1587.

74. Peters A, Perez S, Döring A, et al: Increases in heart rate during an air pollution episode. Am J Epidemiol 1999;150:1094–1098.

■ ■ ■ chapter **4 3**

Control of Risk Factors

Priscilla Hsue
David D. Waters

Coronary artery disease (CAD) is the leading cause of morbidity and mortality in the United States and the industrialized world.

PREVALENCE

Approximately 60,800,000 Americans have one or more types of cardiovascular disease, and CAD accounts for about one third of these cases, with hypertension, stroke, congestive heart failure, and congenital cardiovascular defects accounting for the remainder.[1]

MORTALITY

In 1998, coronary heart disease (CHD) caused 459,841 deaths in the United States, which is 1 out of every 5 deaths, and remains the single largest killer of American men and women.[2] Within 1 hour of the onset of symptoms, one fourth of 1 million people die each year, with approximately 50% having no symptoms. In a given year, an estimated 1 million Americans will have a new or recurrent coronary attack, and 40% of people who experience a coronary attack die of it.[3] Most people who die of CHD are 65 years old or older; in 1998, men accounted for 51% of deaths and women accounted for 49% of deaths from CHD.

ECONOMIC CONSEQUENCES

In 2001, the cost of cardiovascular diseases and stroke in the United States was estimated at $298 billion, with CHD accounting for one third of this amount.

PREVENTION

In the 1990s, the death rate from CHD declined. These reductions most likely are attributable to efforts in primary prevention and improved therapies for myocardial infarction (MI). Recognizing and treating risk factors is an effective means of preventing coronary disease in many patients.

Blood Pressure Reduction

According to NHANES (National Health and Nutrition Examination Survey), 1 in 5 Americans, which is about 50 million people, has hypertension.[1] Hypertension is defined by the Sixth Joint National Committee for Detection, Evaluation, and Treatment of Hypertension (JNC VI) as a systolic blood pressure greater than 140 mm Hg and a diastolic blood pressure greater than 90 mm Hg (with lower guidelines of 130 mm Hg and 85 mm Hg for diabetic patients) (Table 43-1).[4] An additional 13 million people may have been identified at one time or another as having hypertension. Age, sex, and race all influence the prevalence of hypertension. The prevalence of hypertension increases with age and is present in 64% of men and 66% of women older than age 75 compared with 8.6% of men and 3.4% of women between ages 20 and 34. A higher percentage of men compared with women have hypertension until the age of 55; after age 55, a higher percentage of women have hypertension. African Americans have among the highest age-adjusted prevalence of hypertension in the world. Compared with whites, African Americans develop hypertension at an earlier age and have higher average blood pressures.

Association of Blood Pressure and Risk of Cardiovascular Disease

Numerous epidemiologic studies have shown the association of elevated blood pressure with increased risk of cardiovascular disease. In a pooled analysis, 418,343 patients were followed for 10 years by MacMahon and colleagues[5] to determine the relationship between baseline blood pressure and occurrence of CHD and stroke. The diastolic blood pressure ranged from 76 to 105 mm Hg; even with this relatively small range of diastolic pressures, the risk of CHD and stroke was about fivefold and tenfold higher for patients at the higher end of the diastolic blood pressure range. Other studies showed similar increased risk with elevated systolic blood pressure in addition to diastolic blood pressure; the increased cardiovascular risk is consistent among patients of differing genders, race, and ages.[6-8] In addition, the relationship between hypertension and renal disease has been shown

■ ■ ■

TABLE 43–1 BLOOD PRESSURE
CLASSIFICATION FOR PERSONS AGED
18 YEARS AND OLDER

CATEGORY	SYSTOLIC/DIASTOLIC BLOOD PRESSURE (MM HG)
Optimal	<120/<80
Normal	<130/<85
High-normal	130–139/85–89
Hypertension	
Stage 1	140–59/90–99
Stage 2	160–179/100–109
Stage 3	≥180/≥110

in observational studies. MRFIT (Multiple Risk Factor Intervention Trial) was a prospective study of 332,544 men that examined the relationship between blood pressure and renal disease.[9] In the 16-year follow-up, hypertension was implicated in half of the 814 cases of end-stage renal disease. Among patients who did not develop end-stage renal disease, patients with a systolic blood pressure of 140 to 159 mm Hg or a diastolic blood pressure of 90 to 99 mm Hg had a 2.8 higher relative risk (RR) of eventually developing end-stage renal disease compared with patients in the study without hypertension.

Systolic Hypertension and Cardiovascular Risk

Isolated systolic hypertension becomes more prevalent after age 55. It is more common in women than men and affects 30% of persons 65 to 74 years old.[10] Data from SHEP (Systolic Hypertension in the Elderly Program)[11] show that 8% of persons who are 60 to 69 years old had isolated systolic hypertension (defined as systolic blood pressure >160 mm Hg and diastolic blood pressure <90 mm Hg) compared with 11% of persons in the 70- to 79-year age range and 22% of persons older than 80 years. For cardiovascular risk, systolic blood pressure may play a greater role than diastolic blood pressure. In the SHEP trial, treatment with antihypertensive medication resulted in net decreases of 11.1 mm Hg in systolic blood pressure and 3.4 mm Hg in diastolic blood pressure. As a result, there was a 36% reduction in the incidence of stroke ($P = .0003$) and a 27% reduction in the combined end point of nonfatal MI plus coronary death ($P = .02$). The age-adjusted 10-year mortality in MRFIT showed that systolic blood pressure was a stronger predictor of CAD events than diastolic blood pressure.[9]

Antihypertensive Trials

Collins and coworkers[12] combined the results of 17 major clinical trials that examined the effects of antihypertensive medication on clinical outcomes of 47,653 patients. The mean age of participants was 56 years with an equal representation of men and women. Patients were followed for 4 to 5 years. In 12 of the 17 trials, diuretics were used as first-line drug therapy, and the goal in most of the trials was to maintain a diastolic blood pressure of 90 mm Hg or less in the active treatment group. Patients on antihypertensive drug treatment had a 16% reduction in total CHD incidence (95% confidence interval [CI], 8% to 23%) and a 16% reduction in fatal CHD (95% CI, 5% to 26%). In addition, patients in active treatment had a 38% reduction in the odds of total stroke (95% CI, 31% to 45%; $P < .001$) and a 40% reduction in the odds of fatal stroke (95% CI, 26% to 51%; $P < .001$). In contrast to the reduction in CHD risk, which occurred only after several years of therapy, most of the reduction in stroke risk was achieved in the first year of antihypertensive treatment. There was an overall reduction of 21% (95% CI, 12% to 28%; $P < .001$) for cardiovascular disease mortality for the patients on antihypertensive medication. Patients who had a higher level of blood pressure at entry had a greater reduction in risk. Because patients with a higher level of blood pressure have a higher stroke event rate, the pooled analysis showed an impressive relationship between absolute reduction in stroke risk and blood pressure at entry for patients in the treatment arm. Taken as a whole, the estimated reduction in the risk of MI is 2% to 3% for each decline of 1 mm Hg in diastolic blood pressure.

Therapy

Nonpharmacologic Measures Clinical trials have shown that weight reduction in addition to exercise can reduce systolic and diastolic blood pressure. A salt-restricted diet may reduce the need for combination antihypertensive medication. Cessation of smoking and alcohol use also can reduce blood pressure markedly.

Medical Therapy Selection of medication includes consideration of demographic characteristics, cost, concomitant disease, and interactions with other drugs. In the HOPE (Heart Outcomes Prevention Evaluation) study, normotensive and hypertensive high-risk patients were found to have significantly reduced rates of death, stroke, and MI compared with placebo patients when treated with the angiotensin-converting enzyme (ACE) inhibitor ramipril.[13]

ALLHAT (Antihypertensive and Lipid-Lowering Treatment to Prevent Heart Attack Trial) was a randomized double-blind, active-controlled trial designed to determine whether the incidence of fatal CHD and nonfatal MI was different in patients treated with a diuretic (chlorthalidone) compared with patients treated with a calcium antagonist (amlodipine), an ACE inhibitor (lisinopril), and an α-adrenergic blocker (doxazosin).[14] After a 3.3-year follow-up, 365 patients in the doxazosin group and 608 patients in the chlorthalidone group had fatal CHD or nonfatal MI with no difference in risk between the groups (RR, 1.03; 95% CI, 0.90 to 1.17; $P = 0.71$). Patients in the chlorthalidone arm had a reduced risk of combined cardiovascular death events, especially from congestive heart failure. The JNC VI algorithm for treatment of hypertension begins with lifestyle modifications, and the selection of initial pharmacologic therapy depends on patient demographics and concomitant diseases and therapies. Hypertension in African American patients may be more responsive to treatment with diuretics and calcium antagonists. Diabetes mellitus and proteinuria are compelling indications to treat patients with ACE inhibitors. Patients with congestive heart failure should be treated with ACE inhibitors and diuretics, whereas patients with a history of MI should be placed on β-blockers and ACE inhibitors. Older patients with isolated hypertension may be candidates for therapy with diuretics or calcium antagonists.[4]

Hyperlipidemia

Aside from age, dyslipidemia is the strongest predictive factor for CAD. A continuous and graded relationship exists between total cholesterol or low-density lipoprotein (LDL) and risk for coronary events, with a 20% increase in risk of CHD for each 10% increase in serum cholesterol.[15] The relationship has been shown in men and women and across age groups.

Lipid-Lowering Trials

Primary Prevention   The strongest evidence linking the development of CAD to lipids comes from randomized clinical primary prevention trials (Table 43–2).[16,17] Researchers in WOSCOPS (West of Scotland Coronary Prevention Study)[17] randomized 6595 men with moderately elevated lipid levels to either pravastatin, 40 mg/day, or placebo. After 4.9 years of follow-up, there was a 31% reduction in CHD events and a 37% reduction in revascularization procedures and coronary related deaths. The AFCAPS/TexCAPS (Air Force/Texas Coronary Atherosclerosis Prevention Study)[16] studied patients with only modest elevations in LDL cholesterol (mean, 221 mg/dL) and low high-density lipoprotein (HDL) levels (mean, 36 mg/dL). Patients were treated with lovastatin and had a 25% reduction in LDL cholesterol. Treatment with lovastatin reduced the risk for first acute major coronary events by 36%.

Secondary Prevention Trials   The 4S (Scandinavian Simvastatin Survival Study) trial treated 4444 men and women with a history of CAD, total cholesterol levels of 212 to 309 mg/dL, and a mean LDL at baseline of 199 mg/dL (range, 130 to 255 mg/dL) (Table 43–3).[18] Treatment with simvastatin, 20 to 40 mg/day, resulted in a total mortality reduction of 30% and a 42% reduction in deaths from CAD.

In the CARE (Cholesterol and Recurrent Events) study, investigators studied 4159 patients who had had MI 3 to 20 months before randomization.[19] Patients had a plasma total cholesterol less than 240 mg/dL, LDL cholesterol between 115 and 174 mg/dL, and triglycerides less than 350 mg/dL. Patients were randomized to pravastatin, 40 mg/day, or placebo with a median follow-up of 5 years. Pravastatin therapy lowered the mean LDL cholesterol of 139 mg/dL by 32%. Primary end points of death from CAD or nonfatal MI occurred in 13.2% versus 10.2% in the placebo group. The risk of MI was 25% lower in the pravastatin group (7.5% versus 10%; 95% CI, 8% to 39%; $P = .006$). In addition, the rates of coronary artery bypass graft surgery, percutaneous transluminal coronary angioplasty, and stroke all were lower in the pravastatin-treated group. Subset analyses revealed that the benefits were similar regardless of age, sex, ejection fraction, hypertension, diabetes mellitus, and cigarette smoking. The results of this study suggested that treatment

TABLE 43–2   PRIMARY PREVENTION STATIN TRIALS

TRIAL	POPULATION AND NO. RANDOMIZED	THERAPY	END POINT	RISK REDUCTION
AFCAPS/TexCAPS[16]	6595 middle-aged men and women	Lovastatin	Fatal CAD, nonfatal MI	36%
WOSCOPS[17]	6595 middle-aged men	Pravastatin	Fatal CAD, nonfatal MI, total mortality	31% MI, 22% total mortality

CAD, coronary artery disease; MI, myocardial infarction.

TABLE 43–3   SECONDARY PREVENTION STATIN TRIALS

TRIAL	POPULATION	THERAPY	END POINT	RISK REDUCTION
4S[18]	4444 men and women aged 35–70 with a history of angina or MI	Simvastatin	Total mortality,	30%
			Fatal CAD, nonfatal MI	44%
CARE[19]	4159 men and women aged 21–75 with recent MI	Pravastatin	Fatal CAD, nonfatal MI	24%
LIPID[21]	9014 men and women aged 31–75 with history of acute MI or unstable angina	Pravastatin	CAD mortality	34%

CAD, coronary artery disease; MI, myocardial infarction.

of patients with moderately elevated total cholesterol could have important public health implications. In this study, reduction of LDL to 125 mg/dL was associated with a reduction in coronary events.

In the Heart Protection Study,[20] more than 20,000 patients with a history of MI or CAD, other occlusive arterial disease, diabetes mellitus, or hypertension were randomized to therapy with simvastatin, 40 mg/day, or placebo. Patients treated for 5 years had a reduction in major vascular events even if baseline LDL was less than 100 mg/dL, suggesting that even patients with lower levels of LDL cholesterol may benefit from additional cholesterol-lowering therapy.

The LIPID (Long-term Intervention with Pravastatin in Ischemic Disease) study enrolled 9014 patients aged 31 to 75 with a history of acute MI or unstable angina within 3 to 36 months before enrollment.[21] Patients had a baseline plasma total cholesterol of 155 to 271 mg/dL and a fasting triglyceride level of less than 445 mg/dL. The treatment regimen consisted of an 8-week single-blind placebo run in phase with a low-fat diet, and thereafter patients were randomized to either pravastatin, 40 mg/day, or placebo. Total plasma cholesterol decreased by 39 mg/dL in the pravastatin group, which was an 18% greater decrease compared with the placebo group ($P < .001$). Total mortality was 11% in the pravastatin group compared with 14.1% in the placebo group (22% risk reduction; 95% CI, 12% to 35%; $P < .001$). Cardiovascular mortality was 7.3% and 9.6% in the pravastatin and placebo groups (25% risk reduction; 95% CI, 13% to 35%; $P < .001$). Fewer patients in the pravastatin group had MI, needed coronary artery bypass graft surgery, required hospitalization for unstable angina, or had strokes.

The MIRACL (Myocardial Ischemia Reduction with Aggressive Cholesterol Lowering) study randomized 3086 patients with unstable angina or non–Q-wave MI to atorvastatin, 80 mg/day, or placebo.[22] The mean LDL cholesterol level at the end of the 16-week follow-up period was 72 mg/dL in the atorvastatin group and 135 mg/dL in the placebo group. The primary composite end point was reduced with active treatment (RR, 0.84; 95% CI, 0.7 to 1.0; $P = .048$).

Lipid Management

The National Cholesterol Education Panel (NCEP) Adult Treatment III guidelines recommend that the number of Americans treated with cholesterol-lowering drugs should increase from 13 million to 36 million.[23] The goals of each intervention are adjusted according to the level of CHD risk for an individual (Table 43–4).

The optimal LDL concentration for patients with CAD is less than 100 mg/dL, and patients should have lipids monitored annually. In addition, the new NCEP guidelines[23] include raising patients with diabetes without prior CAD to the risk of patients with CAD and identifying an LDL cholesterol less than 100 mg/dL as optimal. New features of NCEP Adult Treatment III guidelines include raising categorically low HDL cholesterol from less than 35 mg/dL to less than 40 mg/dL and recommending treatment beyond LDL lowering for patients with triglycerides greater than or equal to 200 mg/dL.

■ □ ■

TABLE 43–4   NATIONAL CHOLESTEROL EDUCATION TREATMENT GUIDELINES

	LDL GOAL	LDL LEVEL TO INITIATE LIFESTYLE CHANGES (MG/DL)	LDL LEVEL TO CONSIDER DRUG THERAPY (MG/DL)
CHD or CHD risk equivalent	<100	≥100	≥130
>2 risk factors	<130	≥130	≥160
0–1 risk factors	<160	≥160	≥190

CHD, coronary heart disease; LDL, low-density lipoprotein.

Summary

Taken as a whole, there is a causal relationship between elevated serum cholesterol and risk of CHD. A 10% increase in serum cholesterol is associated with a 20% to 30% increase in the risk of CHD, and elevations that occur earlier in life seem to be associated with even higher increases in risk. Data from randomized trials show treatment to lower cholesterol levels by 10% reduces risks of CHD death by 10% and events by 18%, whereas treatment for more than 5 years results in a 25% reduction in CHD events. Overviews of randomized trials have shown a reduction in total mortality associated with cholesterol reduction in primary and secondary prevention. Ensuring that public health measures are taken to reduce cholesterol in primary prevention with aggressive cholesterol reduction in patients with underlying atherosclerosis or patients with high risk seems warranted and will remain important in the future.

Diabetes Mellitus

Approximately 8 million people in the United States have diabetes mellitus, and 10% of Americans age 65 and older have non–insulin-dependent diabetes mellitus. Type 1 and type 2 diabetes mellitus are directly associated with dramatically increased rates of CHD. In type 1 diabetes (caused by autoimmune B-cell destruction), the risk is increased approximately 10-fold, whereas in type 2 diabetes (associated with obesity and insulin resistance), the risk is increased 2-fold to 4-fold. Multiple large angiographic trials have shown that diabetic patients undergoing cardiac catheterization or percutaneous transluminal coronary angioplasty have more severe CAD with decreased collateral circulation. Diabetes is an independent predictor for the development and progression of atherosclerotic lesions. Diabetes also increases cardiovascular risk. According to data from the Framingham study,[24] CAD accounts for 80% of all deaths and hospital admissions among persons with diabetes and is the leading cause of premature deaths in diabetic patients.

Women and Diabetes

In women, diabetes mellitus is the most powerful risk factor for CAD. Compared with women without diabetes, women with diabetes have a fivefold higher prevalence of cardiovascular disease. The incidence of CAD increases with blood glucose level and age. Women with diabetes have an equal risk for MI compared with men of similar ages without diabetes. Even after adjustment for age and other CAD risk factors, women with diabetes have a higher risk for CAD compared with men with diabetes and women without diabetes. This increased risk may be attributed partly to other risk factors that are present in female diabetics, such as lower HDL cholesterol and higher triglycerides, systolic blood pressure, and relative body weight.

Clinical Trials

Control of Hyperglycemia DCCT (Diabetes Control and Complications Trial) randomly assigned a total of 1441 patients with insulin-dependent diabetes mellitus to intensive treatment with an external insulin pump and frequent glucose monitoring or to conventional therapy with one or two daily insulin injections.[25,26] Patients were followed for an average of 6.5 years. Patients were 13 to 39 years old, and patients with known coronary disease or risk factors, such as hypertension and hyperlipidemia, were excluded. Patients with intensive treatment had beneficial effects on the occurrence of retinopathy and peripheral neuropathy. The mean total serum cholesterol, calculated LDL cholesterol, and triglycerides were significantly decreased in the intensive treatment group. After the 6.5-year follow-up, there were 50 combined major macrovascular events in the conventionally treated group compared with 23 in the intensive treatment group ($P = .08$). In insulin-dependent diabetic patients, nephropathy was found to be a strong predictor of subsequent cardiac events. Intensive treatment that also reduces the progression of proteinuria and improves the lipid profile may decrease macrovascular events. Other studies have shown that glycemic control slows diabetic renal lesions in renal grafts[27] and reduces the development of carotid intima media thickening.[28]

UKPDS (United Kingdom Prospective Diabetes Study), a randomized controlled study, compared the effects of intensive blood glucose control with either sulfonylurea or insulin over a 10-year period.[29] Investigators found that in patients with intensive glycemic control by either insulin or sulfonylureas, the risk of microvascular complications was reduced by 25% in non–insulin-requiring diabetic patients. Diabetes-related mortality was 10% lower in the intensive group (95% CI, 0.73 to 1.11; $P = .34$), whereas incidence of MI was 16% lower in the intensive group (95% CI, 0.71 to 1.00; $P = .052$). This study showed no difference in rates of MI or diabetes-related death between patients treated with sulfonylurea or insulin therapy, in contrast to UGDP (University Group Diabetes Program),[30] which previously had been the only large-scale randomized trial in type 2 diabetics and reported an increased risk of cardiovascular mortality in patients receiving tolbutamide. A similar reduction in mortality was observed among diet-treated obese non–insulin-requiring diabetic patients taking metformin.[31]

Additional Risk Factors

Hyperlipidemia In addition to the already mentioned primary and secondary prevention trials, a subgroup analysis of 4S showed in diabetic patients with hypercholesterolemia and known CAD that lowering LDL cholesterol with simvastatin was associated with a marked reduction in major CAD and associated atherosclerotic events.[32] In diabetic patients, 5-year mortality was reduced by 43% compared with 29% in nondiabetic patients. A similar outcome was found in the CARE trial,[19] which found a greater benefit of pravastatin in diabetics compared with nondiabetics with a greater RR reduction for major coronary events and revascularization procedures during a 5-year follow-up. In a subgroup of diabetics with a history of MI or unstable angina, there was a 19% reduction of the composite end point of CAD-related death and MI after a 6.1-year follow-up in diabetics treated with pravastatin in LIPID.[21] New features of the NCEP Adult Treatment Panel III recognize the significantly increased risk of diabetic patients and raises patients with diabetes to the risk level of patients who have had CAD.

Hypertension Hypertension in diabetic patients increases the risk of coronary events, congestive heart failure, stroke, and peripheral vascular disease. Lowering of blood pressure is associated with preserved renal function; also, independent of blood pressure lowering, ACE inhibitors slow the rate of progression of proteinuria.

In UKPDS, blood pressure control by β-blockers or ACE inhibitors showed an important beneficial effect on microvascular disease.[33] In particular, ACE inhibitors showed benefit in insulin-dependent and non–insulin-dependent diabetics.[34] A total of 3577 patients with diabetes, who were included in the HOPE study and had a previous cardiovascular event or one other risk factor and no low ejection fraction, were randomly assigned to ramipril, 10 mg/day, versus placebo.[35] Investigators found that ramipril lowered the risk of the combined primary outcome of MI, stroke, or cardiovascular death by 25% (95% CI, 12 to 36; $P = .0004$). Even after adjustment for changes in systolic and diastolic blood pressure, ramipril still lowered the risk of the combined primary outcome by 25% (95% CI, 12 to 16; $P = .0004$). Revised guidelines by the JNC recommend a level of 130/85 mm Hg for diabetic patients.[4]

Insulin Resistance Syndrome The insulin resistance syndrome, described by Reaven,[36] characterizes patients who do not have frank diabetes but have hyperinsulinemia and metabolic abnormalities associated with diabetes mellitus. Patients with the prediabetic condition may have an atherogenic pattern of risk factors before the onset of clinical diabetes. In the Paris Prospective Study, in which 7028 men were followed for 11 years,[37] the strongest predictor of subsequent death from CAD was plasma triglyceride concentration. Other independent predictors of CAD death were blood pressure, smoking, cholesterol level, and fasting and 2-hour post-load plasma insulin levels. The NCEP Adult Treatment Panel III Report identifies persons with the metabolic syndrome as candidates for intensified lifestyle modifications.

Summary

Patients with diabetes are at significantly increased risk for CAD. Optimal glycemic control and treatment of hypertension and dyslipidemia are essential for preventing and delaying the progression of CAD.

Cigarette Smoking

Cigarette smoking is the leading preventable cause of death in the United States.[38] In 1990, one in every five deaths was attributable to cigarette smoking.[39] Although the prevalence of smoking has declined dramatically since its peak in 1965, in 1995, about 25% of adults in the United States smoked cigarettes.[40]

Pathophysiology

Cigarette smoking has effects on a variety of physiologic and biochemical factors and has effects on the cardio-vascular system at multiple points. Cigarette smoking increases blood pressure and heart rate.[41] Nicotine is an adrenergic agonist and increases norepinephrine and epinephrine levels.[42] As a result of the nicotine-mediated increase in catecholamines and the hemodynamic changes, cigarette smoking has been shown to increase the risk of cardiac arrhythmias and is associated with an increased incidence of sudden cardiac death.[43] In addition to the effects of nicotine, other components of cigarette smoke, such as carbon monoxide, bind directly to hemoglobin, reducing oxygen carrying capacity and altering the balance between myocardial oxygen supply and demand.

Vascular Effects

Exposure to cigarette smoke has been shown to decrease distensibility in carotid and brachial arteries.[44] The smoke of a single cigarette in susceptible individuals can produce sudden marked epicardial coronary vasoconstriction and can increase acutely coronary vascular resistance and decrease flow velocity in the coronary arteries.[45] Smoking also has a direct effect on endothelial function; studies have shown that flow-mediated vascular forearm dilation, which serves as a marker for endothelial function, is impaired in cigarette smokers.[46]

Thrombotic Effects

Cigarette smoking has effects on active and chronic thrombotic activity. Enhanced platelet aggregation has been observed after experimental cigarette smoking.[47] Platelet-derived nitric oxide release is significantly impaired in long-term smokers, which further augments platelet aggregability.[48] Epidemiologic studies suggest that smoking causes an elevation in blood fibrinogen concentration, enhances platelet reactivity, and induces secondary polycythemia by increasing whole-blood viscosity.[49] Smoking also induces a small change in serum cholesterol; it increases total cholesterol by 3%, decreases HDL cholesterol by 6%, and increases triglyceride level by 9%.[50] It does not seem to alter LDL cholesterol levels directly. Smoking influences the cardiovascular system on a hemodynamic level and via thrombotic, metabolic, and vascular factors.

Epidemiologic Studies on Cigarette Smoking and Cardiovascular Disease Risk

Overwhelming epidemiologic evidence supports a causal relationship between cigarette smoking and cardiovascular disease. Numerous studies have shown a dose-responsive relationship between CAD and the duration and intensity of smoking. Current smokers have a 70% increased risk of fatal CHD and a twofold to fourfold higher risk of nonfatal CHD and sudden death.[51] In addition, cigarette smoking in combination with hypertension and hyperlipidemia has a synergistic effect to increase markedly the risk of CAD. In women, oral contraceptive use also synergistically increases the risk of MI and ischemic stroke.

Passive smoking caused by chronic environmental exposure to cigarettes also can have important consequences. In 1992, the Environmental Protection Agency identified passive smoking exposure as a carcinogen responsible for more than 3000 lung cancer deaths per year among nonsmoking Americans.[52] In nonsmokers, passive smoke exposure increases the risk of death from ischemic heart disease by 30%, and one study estimated that passive smoking was responsible for 40,000 cardiovascular deaths per year in the United States.[53] Using the Nurses' Health Study cohort, 32,046 nonsmoking women 36 to 61 years old were followed for 10 years.[54] After adjustment for risk factors, nonsmokers had a total CHD RR of 1.00, whereas women with occasional smoke exposure had an RR of 1.58, and women with regular exposure had an RR of 1.91 ($P = .002$).

Smoking Cessation and Cardiovascular Risk Numerous studies have shown the benefits of smoking cessation in reducing cardiovascular morbidity and mortality. In a large study from the American Cancer Society, more than 1 million men and women aged 30 and older were followed for 12 years.[55] The RR for CHD death was 2.66 for men and 2.23 for women who had stopped smoking for 2 to 4 years and decreased to 1.37 for men and 0.98 for women who had stopped smoking for 10 to 14 years. Numerous large observational studies have followed patients for 10 years and support the conclusion that smoking cessation reduces cardiovascular morbidity and mortality. Case-control studies in men and women have shown that within 2 to 3 years after stopping smoking, the risk of MI decreased to levels similar to those in people who had never smoked.[56,57] This decline in risk was present regardless of the amount smoked or duration of cigarette smoking. Data obtained from other cohort studies have shown reductions in risk in women and elderly patients as well.[58,59] MRFIT was a clinical trial studying the effect of smoking cessation as a component of a compound intervention program.[60] A total of 12,866 men were followed for 10.5 years. After 1 year of cessation, the RR of dying of CHD of smoking quitters compared with nonquitters was significantly lower (0.63) even after adjusting for baseline differences and changes in risk factors. Persistent quitters had a 65% 3-year risk reduction compared with persistent smokers.

Primary Prevention of Coronary Artery Disease

Data from the U.S. Department of Health and Human Services 2000 Report shows that smoking more than doubles the incidence of coronary disease and increases mortality from coronary disease by 70%.[61] There is a clear dose-response relationship between the number of cigarettes smoked and risk of heart disease in men and women.[62,63] In a cohort of more than 34,000 British physicians, the mortality rate from ischemic heart disease among men younger than 65 increased from 166 per 100,000 for nonsmokers to 278 for men smoking 1 to 14 cigarettes a day and to 427 for men who smoked 25 or more cigarettes a day.[62] In women, cigarette smoking accounts for about half of all MIs before age 55.[63] A report from the Surgeon General in 1990 summarized the major cohort and case-control studies.[64] All of the studies performed on patients in different countries and of differing ages and backgrounds show that the risks of CAD incidence and mortality are consistently lower among former smokers compared with individuals who continue to smoke. The time required for total mortality and cardiovascular mortality in former smokers to decline to the level of nonsmokers is less clear. The observational studies also support a dose-response relationship among all aspects of smoking and outcomes, with the initial benefit occurring rapidly, with half the risk reduction within 1 year of smoking cessation. The excess risk continues to decline more gradually over the following 10 to 15 years. The estimated mean reduction in risk of MI is 50% to 70% lower in former compared with current cigarette smokers within 5 years of cessation.

Secondary Prevention

A review of major studies on smoking cessation on persons with diagnosed CHD showed that survivors of MI or cardiac arrest benefit from smoking cessation, with improvements in mortality of 50%. A study following 310 survivors of out-of-hospital cardiac arrest who were smokers found that reformed smokers had a 19% incidence of recurrent arrest compared with smokers, who had a 27% incidence ($P = .038$).[65] A more recent study followed patients after acute MI over 21 months.[66] Of the patients who had quit smoking, the mortality during the next 4 years was 17% compared with 31% for patients who continued to smoke ($P < .05$). Much of this benefit was accounted for, however, by a higher baseline risk among patients who failed to quit, including history of prior MI and congestive heart failure.

In CASS (Coronary Artery Surgical Study), death rates were compared between never-smokers, current smokers, and current quitters.[67] Current quitters had a worse prognosis at baseline compared with current smokers. After adjustment for baseline characteristics, 5-year survival was better at every level of risk for quitters compared with smokers with a risk reduction of 40%. After 10 years of follow-up, survival among smokers who stopped smoking was 82% compared with 77% among continuing smokers ($P = .025$).[68] This difference in survival was more pronounced in patients randomized to coronary artery bypass graft surgery compared with medically treated patients. An observational study of about 5000 patients from the Mayo Clinic after coronary angioplasty showed a high RR of mortality (RR, 1.76) and of Q-wave MI (RR, 2.08) in persistent smokers compared with nonsmokers.[69]

Summary

Observational epidemiologic data collected for more than 40 years, including primary and secondary prevention cohort studies, multiple risk factor intervention trials, and cardiovascular treatment trials, all show that smoking cessation lowers morbidity and mortality from CAD compared with patients who continue to smoke. This effect is present regardless of how much or how long one has smoked, in men and women of all ages, and even after the diagnosis of cardiovascular disease. Data suggest that there is a rapid initial decline in cardiovascular risk within the first several years of cessation followed by a more gradual decline. After 10 to 15 years of abstinence, the risk of former smokers approaches that of never-smokers.

Estrogen Replacement Therapy

Cardiovascular disease is the leading cause of mortality in women in developed countries, causing about 500,000 deaths per year in women in the United States. Epidemiologic evidence suggests that estrogen has a cardioprotective effect in women. Premenopausal women have a low risk for CHD, young women with bilateral oophorectomy not on hormone replacement therapy have a greater CHD, and after menopause, women have a similar CHD risk compared with men.

Cholesterol Effects

In small clinical trials, oral estrogen-only replacement therapy consistently reduced LDL and raised HDL.[70,71] The observed magnitude of effect had considerable variation depending on the type, dose, and duration of therapy. Conjugated equine estrogen has been the most predominantly prescribed oral estrogen in observational studies that have shown a lower cardiovascular risk with hormone replacement therapy. Along with estrogen therapy, progestin commonly is added to protect the endometrium from unopposed estrogen. Progestin induces hepatic lipase activity and lowers HDL in direct proportion to the dose and degree of androgenicity.[72] In addition, estrogen raises triglycerides by increasing the production of very-low-density lipoprotein (VLDL), whereas progestins decrease VLDL catabolism and reduce triglycerides with short-term use.[73] The PEPI (Postmenopausal Estrogen/Progestin Interventions) trial was a 3-year randomized double-blind, placebo-controlled study in which 875 postmenopausal women aged 45 to 64 were randomized to (1) placebo; (2) 0.625 mg/day of conjugated equine estrogen (CEE); (3) 0.625 mg/day of CEE plus 10 mg medoxyprogesterone acetate (MPA) for 12 days per month; (4) 0.625 mg/day of CEE plus consecutive MPA, 2.5 mg/day; or (5) 0.625 mg/day of CEE plus micronized progesterone (MP), 200 mg/day for 12 days per month.[74] Women in the CEE-alone group had increases in HDL of 5.6 mg/dL, and women in the CEE plus cyclic MPA group had increases in HDL of 4.1 mg/dL. Cyclic MPA and continuous MPA attenuated the effect of estrogen on HDL slightly; however, all hormone-treated groups had higher HDL levels (+2.4 to 6.8 mg/dL) than the placebo groups and lower levels of LDL (−15.9 mg/dL average). In contrast to other trials in which progestins partly attenuated the rise in triglycerides with estrogen, in PEPI, all hormone-treated groups had higher triglycerides (mean +12.8 mg/dL). In observational studies, a 1 mg/dL increase in HDL is associated with a 3% lower risk of CAD and a 4.7% lower cardiovascular mortality risk.[75] HDL in women may be a stronger predictor of primary coronary disease than LDL.[76]

Hemostatic Effects

Fibrinogen may play a role in atherogenesis by serving as a substrate for thrombin and having effects on platelet aggregation, blood viscosity, and proliferation of fibroblasts. Fibrinogen may be an independent coronary risk factor in men and women.[77] In the PEPI study, fibrinogen was higher in the placebo group compared with the active treatment groups after 3 years (+0.10 g/L versus −0.02 to 0.06 g/L), which may translate to a decreased risk of CAD with hormone replacement therapy. Oral estrogen replacement therapy may have effects on factor VII, other activation peptides, fibrinolysis, and platelets; however, larger trials with longer follow-up need to be done to characterize the interactions better.

Vascular Effects

Estrogen increases cardiac output and lowers systemic vascular resistance in animal models. Estrogen may have beneficial effects on the endothelium, which would serve to regulate vascular tone. In postmenopausal women, intracoronary injections of 17β-estradiol have been shown to reverse acetylcholine-induced vasoconstriction of atherosclerotic coronary arteries.[78] A study by Roselli and colleagues[79] randomized 26 postmenopausal women to treatment with transdermal estrogen (0.05 mg/day) plus cyclic oral norethisterone acetate (1 mg/day for 12 days) or to no hormone treatment. The hormone-treated groups were found to have significantly higher nitric oxide synthetase inhibitor activity, suggesting that hormone therapy may augment nitric oxide release in postmenopausal women.

Epidemiologic Studies: Estrogen Only/Combined Hormone Replacement Therapy

Significant RRs have been seen in prospective cohort studies, hospital-based and community-based case-control studies, and cross-sectional angiographic studies in estrogen-only hormone replacement therapy. In a study by Grodstein and Stampfer[80] that combined all study types, the RR of CHD of ever-users versus never-users was 0.64 (95% CI, 0.59 to 0.68), whereas the RR of current users versus nonusers was 0.50 (95% CI, 0.45 to 0.59). A similar RR of CAD of 0.65 (95% CI, 0.59 to 0.71) was reported in a meta-analysis in ever-users versus nonusers, whereas combined hormone replacement therapy was associated with a reduced risk of MI that was similar to estrogen-only replacement therapy, with a RR of CHD of 0.65 to 0.80.[81] In the updated Nurses' Health Study, estrogen replacement therapy users had an adjusted RR of CHD of 0.60 (95% CI, 0.43 to 0.83) compared with never-users.[82] The Nurses' Health Study also compared the risk of CHD in users of combined hormone replacement therapy (adjusted RR, 0.39; 95% CI, 0.19 to 0.78) and estrogen-only replacement therapy (adjusted RR, 0.60; 95% CI, 0.43 to 0.83) compared with never-users.

Secondary Prevention

The role of hormone replacement therapy in secondary prevention of CHD was addressed in HERS (Heart and Estrogen/Progestin Replacement Study).[83] In this trial, 2763 postmenopausal women with CAD (history of MI, >50% stenosis in at least one coronary artery, coronary artery bypass graft surgery or percutaneous coronary transluminal angioplasty) were randomized to treatment with 0.625 mg of conjugated equine estrogen per day plus 2.5 mg of medroxyprogesterone daily versus placebo. The women were followed for a mean of 4.1 years. A total of 348 women reached the primary combined end point of nonfatal MI or death from CHD. There was no observed difference in the overall risk between the two groups (RR, 0.99; 95% CI, 0.80 to 1.22). Time-trend analysis showed a 52% increase in cardiovascular events during the first year of therapy in the hormone-treated group compared with placebo, with the risk decreasing in following years. Explanations for the negative effects of hormone therapy in the HERS trial include inadequate duration of follow-up, adverse effects of progesterone, possible late benefits of estrogen, older average age of women enrolled in the study (66.7 years), and the possibility that hormone replacement therapy does not prevent recurrent cardiovascular events in women with established cardiovascular disease. A longer term follow-up of the HERS cohort is in progress and may provide additional information about the role of hormone replacement therapy in secondary prevention.

The ERA (Estrogen Replacement and Atherosclerosis) trial was the first randomized trial with an angiographic end point to test the effect of hormone replacement therapy on the progression of atherosclerosis in postmenopausal women with documented coronary disease.[84] This study showed no benefit of 0.625 mg of estrogen combined with 2.5 mg/day of progesterone on angiographic progression of disease; the estrogen-only arm also showed no angiographic benefit. Prior angiographic studies, which were neither randomized nor prospective, showed an inverse relationship between hormone therapy and coronary atherosclerosis.[85] Discrepancies between these findings and the results of the ERA trial may be due to the older age of ERA patients (mean, 65.8 years) and differences in drug regimens, duration of therapy, and extent of coronary disease.

The Women's Health Initiative is a 15-year study sponsored by the National Institutes of Health examining the effects of hormone replacement therapy on the prevention of CAD. Predominantly healthy women randomized to estrogen-alone replacement therapy (0.625 mg/day) or combination therapy with estrogen (0.625 mg/day) and progesterone (2.5 mg/day) were found to have an early increased risk of cardiovascular events compared with women randomized to placebo.[86] The effect of selective estrogen-receptor modulators on cardiovascular end points is being studied currently in the RUTH (Raloxifene Use for The Heart) trial.[87]

Summary

Insufficient evidence exists to support the initiation of hormone replacement therapy for the sole purpose of primary prevention of CAD. Hormone replacement therapy should not be initiated solely for secondary prevention of cardiovascular disease, and the decision to continue or stop hormone therapy in women with established cardiovascular disease should be based on noncardiac effects and patient preference. Randomized clinical trials are ongoing to help guide decisions on the role of hormone replacement therapy for primary prevention.

Diet and Exercise

Obesity is associated with elevated cholesterol, hypertension, and glucose intolerance, all of which may increase cardiovascular mortality. In the Nurses' Health Study,[82] women with a body mass index of 25 to 29 had an age-adjusted RR for CAD of 1.8 compared with leaner women. Women with morbid obesity (body mass index >29) had an RR for CAD of 3.3. Obesity among adults is associated with increased left ventricular mass, which is a powerful independent predictor of mortality and morbidity from cardiovascular disease.

The Third Report of the NCEP[23] advocates a decrease of saturated fat and cholesterol to prevent CAD. The NCEP Step 2 diet recommends a total fat intake less than or equal to 30%, saturated fat less than 7%, carbohydrate greater than or equal to 55%, and cholesterol intake less than 200 mg/day.

Controlled dietary trials show a clear effect on cardiovascular events. All trials in which diet lowered plasma total cholesterol by at least 10% showed a decrease in coronary events. STARS (St. Thomas Atherosclerosis Regression Study)[88] compared dietary therapy with or without cholestyramine and used coronary angiography to measure luminal diameter of diseased coronary arter-

ies as the primary study end point. The study diet was designed to lower total and saturated fat and increase unsaturated oils and fruits and vegetables. LDL decreased by 16%, whereas HDL did not decrease and triglycerides decreased. Compared with the control group, dietary groups with or without cholestyramine showed significant improvement in coronary stenosis, and the diet-only group had improvement in coronary stenosis. The Lyon Diet Heart Study was a secondary prevention trial that tested the effects of a Mediterranean diet that substituted animal fats with polyunsaturated vegetable oils rich in α-linolenic acid and replaced meat, butter, and cream with fish, bread, and fruits.[89] There was no change in plasma lipid levels; however, coronary events in the treatment group were reduced by 73% ($P = .001$), suggesting that dietary aspects other than lipids may have an effect on prevention of coronary events. Several studies examined early initiation of diet after MI ranging from several days to 6 weeks after MI, and all showed reduction in coronary death ranging from 1 to 3 years. Treated groups began diverging from control groups within several months of randomization, showing a striking early benefit. The Indian Heart Study studied patients during hospitalization for acute MI.[90,91] During hospitalization, patients were taught to increase intake of fruits and vegetables and to decrease saturated fat and cholesterol. Serum cholesterol decreased by 8%, body weight decreased by 4 kg, blood pressure decreased by 8 mm Hg systolic and 6 mm Hg diastolic, and fasting glucose was reduced. At the end of 12 weeks, coronary events were reduced by 36% ($P < .01$). After 1-year follow-up, coronary death was reduced by 41%, and coronary events were reduced by 36% ($P < .01$). In one angiographic trial, diet and vigorous exercise therapy for 1 year improved coronary stenosis.[92]

Clinical trials show that diets that increase unsaturated fat and decrease saturated fat reduce coronary events. Multifactorial programs for multiple risk factors are more complicated to evaluate, but programs that improve risk factors with diet therapy and exercise are likely to be effective.

New Risk Factors

Lipoprotein(a) (Lp(a)) is structurally similar to LDL with the addition of apolipoprotein A, which is a highly glycosylated protein. Lp(a) has an amino-acid sequence similar to plasminogen and may play a role in thrombosis and atherosclerosis. Clinical studies have had mixed results, with cross-sectional and retrospective case-control studies generally supporting the role of Lp(a) in CAD, whereas several prospective studies found little association between Lp(a) and CAD risk. In young male survivors of MI, elevated Lp(a) concentrations were found, suggesting that it may be an independent risk factor for early MI, and in other studies, levels greater than 0.3 g/L were associated with a twofold greater risk for CAD.[93,94] Angiographic studies have correlated coronary lesion scores with cholesterol and Lp(a) in women of all ages and men age 55 and older.[95] Lp(a) levels are difficult to lower, and possible therapeutic options include niacin and colestipol. Therapy aimed at reducing Lp(a) with the intent to reduce CAD risk has not been well studied.

Homocysteine

Homocysteine is a metabolite derived from the breakdown of methionine. Studies have shown a positive correlation between high homocysteine levels and CAD.[96,97] Angiographic analysis of lesions show that homocysteine levels are associated with a graded increase in risk for mortality and that homocysteine may represent a risk factor in younger patients. A prospective study by Wald and associates[98] found that homocysteine levels were significantly higher in men who died of ischemic heart disease, and there was a continuous dose-response relationship, with risk increasing by 41% (95% CI, 20% to 65%) for each 5-μmol/L increase in serum homocysteine level. Although the effect of folate supplementation in reducing the risk of CAD remains unclear, some researchers recommend folate supplementation for patients.[99]

Fibrinogen

Fibrinogen is a clotting factor that aggregates platelets through the glycoprotein IIb/IIIa receptor and activates thrombin. The Framingham Study and several other prospective studies have shown a strong correlation between plasma fibrinogen levels and the occurrence of CAD and stroke.[100] Elevated fibrinogen levels are an independent risk factor for CAD and markedly increase the risk for hypercholesterolemia. In the Northwick Park Heart Study, a fibrinogen level in the upper third of the population was associated with a risk for cardiovascular disease three times higher than the level of patients in the lower third.[101] No clinical trial has identified a drug that reduces fibrinogen levels in a safe and selective manner; however, fibrates, steroids, and polyunsaturated fatty acids have been tested in various clinical settings.

C-Reactive Protein

C-Reactive protein (CRP) is an acute-phase reactant, and a high-sensitivity assay for measurement has been developed. In a study of 388 British men aged 50 to 69 years, the prevalence of CAD was found to increase 1.5-fold for each doubling of CRP level.[102] In addition, prospective studies have shown that baseline CRP is a good marker for predicting future cardiovascular events.[103] Ridker and coworkers[104] studied participants in the CARE study and found that patients who were treated with pravastatin had significantly lower median CRP concentrations compared with placebo patients after 5 years of active treatment (median change, –17.5%; P = .004).

Chlamydia pneumoniae

Chlamydia pneumoniae (formerly known as TWAR) has been implicated in CAD. A study by Gupta and associates[105] randomized 220 men after MI with positive antibody titers for C. pneumoniae to azithromycin or placebo. After 6 months of therapy, compared with patients in the placebo group, the azithromycin-treated group had a fivefold reduction in cardiovascular events, with an odds ratio of 0.2 (95% CI, 0.05 to 0.8l; P = .03).

A larger study performed by Anderson and colleagues[106] showed no decrease, however, in cardiovascular events in patients with CAD and positive C. pneumoniae titers who were treated with azithromycin for 3 months and followed for 2 years.[106]

Summary

New risk factors have been identified that may enhance risk for CAD. Further studies are needed to elucidate better the role of new risk factors in atherosclerosis and future risk.

REFERENCES

1. National Health and Nutrition Examination Survey III (NHANES III), 1988–1994.
2. American Heart Association: 2001 Heart and Stroke Statistical Update. Dallas, TX, American Heart Association, 2000.
3. Atherosclerotic Risk in Communities (ARIC) National Heart, Lung, and Blood Institute (NHLBI) publication. http://www.nhlbi.nih.gov/resources/oeca/elements.htlm
4. National Institute of Health, NHLBI: National High Blood Pressure Education Program. Sixth Report of the Joint National Committee for Detection, Evaluation, and Treatment of Hypertension. NIH publication No. 98-4080. 1997.
5. MacMahon S, Peto R, Cutler J, et al: Blood pressure, stroke, and coronary heart disease: Part 1. Prolonged differences in blood pressure: Prospective observational studies corrected for the regression dilution bias. Lancet 1990;335:765-774.
6. Sagie A, Larson MG, Levy D: The natural history of borderline isolated systolic hypertension. N Engl J Med 1993;329:1912-1917.
7. Neaton JD, Wentworth D: Serum cholesterol, blood pressure, cigarette smoking, and death from coronary artery disease: Overall findings and differences by age for 316,099 white men. Arch Intern Med 1992;152:56-64.
8. van den Hoogen PCW, Feskens EJM, Nagelkerke NJD, et al: The relation between blood pressure and mortality due to coronary heart disease among men in different parts of the world. N Engl J Med 2000; 342:1-8.
9. Klag MJ, Whelton PK, Randall BL, et al: A prospective study of blood pressure and incidence of end-stage renal disease in 332,544 men. N Engl J Med 1996;334:13-18.
10. Working Group on Hypertension in the Elderly: Statement on hypertension in the elderly. JAMA 1986;256:70-74.
11. Kostis JB, Davis BR, Cutler J, et al: Prevention of heart failure by antihypertensive drug treatment in older persons with isolated systolic hypertension. SHEP Cooperative Research Group. JAMA 1997;278:212-216.
12. Collins R, Peto R, MacMahon SW, et al: Blood pressure, stroke, and CHD: Part 2. Short-term reductions in blood pressure: Overview of randomized drug trials in their epidemiological context. Lancet 1990;335:827-838.
13. Heart Outcomes Prevention Evaluation study investigators: Effects of an angiotensin-converting-enzyme inhibitor, ramipril, on cardiovascular events in high-risk patients. N Engl J Med 2000;342: 145-153.
14. ALLHAT Officers and Coordinators for the ALLHAT Collaborative Research Group: Major cardiovascular events in hypertensive patients randomized to doxazosin vs chlorthalidone. The Antihypertensive and Lipid-Lowering Treatment to Prevent Heart Attack Trial (ALLHAT). JAMA 2000;283:1967-1975.
15. LaRosa JC, Hunninghake D, Bush TD, et al: The cholesterol facts: A summary of the evidence relating dietary fats, serum cholesterol, and coronary heart disease: A joint statement by the American Heart Association and the National Heart, Lung, and Blood Institute. AHA Medical/Scientific Statement. AHA and NHLBI publication, 1990, pp 1721-1733.
16. Downs JR, Clearfield M, Weis S, et al: Primary prevention of acute coronary events with lovastatin in men and women with average cholesterol levels. JAMA 1998;279:1615-1622.

17. Shepherd J, Cobbe SM, Ford I, et al: Prevention of coronary heart disease with pravastatin in men with hypercholesterolemia. N Engl J Med 1995;333:1301–1307.

18. Randomised trial of cholesterol lowering in 4444 patients with coronary heart disease. The Scandinavian Simvastatin Survival Study (4S). Lancet 1994;344:1383–1389.

19. Sacks FM, Pfeffer MA, Moye LA, et al: The effect of pravastatin on coronary events after myocardial infarction in patients with average cholesterol levels. N Engl J Med 1996;335:1001–1009.

20. MRC/BHF Heart Protection Study of cholesterol lowering with simostatin in 20,536 high-risk individuals: a randomized placebo-controlled trial. Lancet 2002;630:7–22.

21. Prevention of cardiovascular events and death with pravastatin in patients with coronary heart disease and a broad range of initial cholesterol levels. The Long-Term Intervention with Pravastatin in Ischaemic Disease (LIPID) Study Group. N Engl J Med 1998;339:1349–1357.

22. Schwartz GG, Olsson AG, Ezekowitz MD, et al: Effects of atorvastatin on early recurrent ischemic events in acute coronary syndromes: The MIRACL study: A randomized controlled trial. JAMA 2001;285:1711–1718.

23. Expert Panel on Detection, Evaluation, and Treatment of High Blood Cholesterol in Adults: Summary of the Third Report of the National Cholesterol Education Program (NCEP) Expert Panel on Detection, Evaluation, and Treatment of High Blood Cholesterol in Adults (Adult Treatment Panel-III). JAMA 2001;285:2486–2497.

24. Kannel WB: Lipids, diabetes, and coronary heart disease: Insights from the Framingham Study. Am Heart J 1985;110:1100–1107.

25. Diabetes Control and Complications Trial Research Group: The effect of intensive treatment of diabetes on the development and progression of long-term complications in insulin-dependent diabetes mellitus. N Engl J Med 1993;329:977–986.

26. Diabetes Control and Complications Trial Research Group: Effect of Intensive Diabetes Management on Macrovascular Events and Risk Factors in the Diabetes Control and Complications Trial. Am J Cardiol 1995;75:894–903.

27. Barbosa J, Steffes MW, Sutherland DER, et al: Effect of glycemic control on early diabetic renal lesions. JAMA 1994;272:600–606.

28. Jensen-Urstad KJ, Reichard PG, Rosfors JS, et al: Early atherosclerosis is retarded by improved long-term blood glucose control in patients with IDDM. Diabetes 1996;45:1253–1258.

29. UK Prospective Diabetes Study (UKPDS) Group: Intensive blood-glucose control with sulphonylureas or insulin compared with conventional treatment and risk of complications in patients with type 2 diabetes (UKPDS 33). Lancet 1998;352:837–853.

30. University Group Diabetes Program: A study of the effects of hypoglycemic agents on vascular complications in patients with adult-onset diabetes. Diabetes 1976;25:1129–1153.

31. UK Prospective Diabetes Study (UKPDS) Group: Effect of intensive blood-glucose control with metformin on complications in overweight patients with type 2 diabetes (UKPDS 34). Lancet 1998;352:854–865.

32. Haffner SM: The Scandinavian Simvastatin Survival Study (4S) subgroup analysis of diabetic subjects: Implications for the prevention of coronary heart disease. Diabetes Care 1997;20:469–471.

33. UK Prospective Diabetes Study (UKPDS) Group: Tight blood pressure control and risk of macrovascular and microvascular complications in type 2 diabetes (UKPDS 38). BMJ 1998;317:703–713.

34. Lewis EJ, Hunsicker LG, Bain RP, Rohde RD: The effect of angiotensin-converting enzyme inhibition on diabetic nephropathy. N Engl J Med 1993;329:1456–1462.

35. Heart Outcomes Prevention Evaluation (HOPE) Study investigators: Effects of ramipril on cardiovascular and microvascular outcomes in people with diabetes mellitus: Results of the HOPE study and MICRO-HOPE substudy. Lancet 2000;355:253–259.

36. Reaven GM: Role of insulin resistance in human disease. Diabetes 1988;37:1595–1607.

37. Charles MA, Fontbonne A, Thebult N, et al: Risk factors for NIDDM in white population. Diabetes 1991;40:796–799.

38. Bartecchi CE, MacKenzie TK, Schrier RW: The human cost of tobacco use. N Engl J Med 1994;330:907–912, 975–980.

39. Centers for Disease Control and Prevention: Cigarette-attributable mortality and years of potential life lost—United States, 1990. MMWR Morb Mortal Wkly Rep 1993;42:645–649.

40. Cigarette smoking among adults—United States, 1995. MMWR Morb Mortal Wkly Rep 1997;46:1217–1219.

41. McBride PE: The health consequences of smoking. Med Clin North Am 1992;76:333–353.

42. Cryer PE, Haymond MW, Santiago JV, et al: Norepinephrine and epinephrine release and adrenergic mediation of smoking-associated hemodynamic and metabolic events. N Engl J Med 1976;295:573–577.

43. Hallstrom AP, Cobb LA, Ray R: Smoking as a risk factor for recurrence of sudden cardiac arrest. N Engl J Med 1986;314:271–275.

44. Kool MJF, Hoeks APG, Struijker Boudier HAJ, et al: Short- and long-term effects of smoking on arterial wall properties in habitual smokers. J Am Coll Cardiol 1993;22:1881–1886.

45. Quillen JE, Rossen JD, Oskarsson HJ, et al: Acute effect of cigarette smoking on the coronary circulation: Constriction of epicardial and resistance vessels. J Am Coll Cardiol 1993;22:642–647.

46. Celermajer DS, Sorensen KE, Georgakopoulos D: Cigarette smoking is associated with dose-related and potentially reversible impairment of endothelium-dependent dilatation in healthy young adults. Circulation 1993;88:2149–2155.

47. Levine PH: An acute effect of cigarette smoking on platelet function: A possible link between smoking and arterial thrombosis. Circulation 1973;48:619–623.

48. Ichiki K, Ikeda H, Haramaki N, et al: Long-term smoking impairs platelet-derived nitric oxide release. Circulation 1996;94:3109–3114.

49. Dotevall A, Johansson S, Wilhelmsen L: Association between fibrinogen and other risk factors for cardiovascular disease in men and women: Results from the Goteborg MONICA survey 1985. Ann Epidemiol 1994;4:369–374.

50. Craig WY, Palomake GE, Haddow JE: Cigarette smoking and serum lipid and lipoprotein concentrations: An analysis of published data. BMJ 1989;298:784–788.

51. Jonas MA, Oates JA, Ockene JK, et al: Statement on smoking and cardiovascular disease for health care professionals. AHA Medical/Scientific Statement. Circulation 1992;86:1664–1669.

52. Environmental Protection Agency: Respiratory Health Effects of Passive Smoking: Lung Cancer and Other Disorders. Washington, DC, Office of Health and Environmental Assessment, 1992.

53. Glantz SA, Parmley WW: Passive smoking and heart disease: Mechanisms and risk. JAMA 1995;273:1047–1053.

54. Kawachi I, Coditz GA, Speizer FE, et al: A prospective study of passive smoking and coronary heart disease. Circulation 1997;95:2374–2379.

55. Burns DM, Shanks TG, Choi W, et al: The American Cancer Society Cancer Prevention Study: I. 12-year follow-up of 1 million men and women. In: Changes in Cigarette-Related Disease Risks and Their Implication for Prevention and Control: Smoking and Tobacco Control Monograph. NIH Publication No. 97-4213. National Cancer Institute. Washington, DC, U.S. Government Printing Office, 1997, pp 113–304.

56. Rosenberg L, Kaufman DW, Helmrich SP, Shapiro S: The risk of myocardial infarction after quitting smoking in men under 55 years of age. N Engl J Med 1985;313:1511–1514.

57. Rosenberg L, Palmer JR, Shapiro S: Decline in the risk of myocardial infarction among women who stop smoking. N Engl J Med 1990;332:213–217.

58. Kawachi I, Colditz GA, Stampfer MJ, et al: Smoking cessation in relation to total mortality rates in women: A prospective cohort study. Ann Intern Med 1993;119:992–1000.

59. LaCroix AZ, Lang J, Scherr P, et al: Smoking and mortality among older men and women in three communities. N Engl J Med 1991;324:1619–1625.

60. Ockene JK, Kuller LH, Svendsen KH, Meilahn E: The relationship of smoking cessation to coronary heart disease and lung cancer in the Multiple Risk Factor Intervention Trial (MRFIT). Am J Public Health 1990;80:954–958.

61. U.S. Department of Health and Human Services: Reducing Tobacco Use: A Report of the Surgeon General—Executive Summary. Atlanta, U.S. Department of Health and Human Services, Centers for Disease Control and Prevention, National Center for Chronic Disease Prevention and Health Promotion, Office on Smoking and Health, 2000.

62. Doll R, Peto R: Mortality in relation to smoking: 20 years' observation on male British doctors. BMJ 1976;2:1525–1536.

63. Willett WC, Green A, Stampfer MJ, et al: Relative and absolute excess risks of coronary heart disease among women who smoke cigarettes. N Engl J Med 1987;317:1303–1309.

64. Department of Health and Human Services: The Health Benefits of Smoking Cessation. A Report of the Surgeon General. DHHS Publication No. (CDC) 90-8416. Bethesda, MD, U.S. Department of Health and Human Services, Public Health Service, Centers for Disease Control, Office on Smoking and Health, 1990.

65. Hallstrom AP, Cobb LA, Ray R: Smoking as a risk factor for recurrence of sudden cardiac arrest. N Engl J Med 1986;314:271-275.

66. Herlitz J, Bengtson A, Hjalmarson A, Karlson BW: Smoking habits in consecutive patients with acute myocardial infarction: Prognosis in relation to other risk indicators and to whether or not they quit smoking. Cardiology 1995;86:496-502.

67. Vliestra RE, Kronmal RA, Oberman A, et al: Effect of cigarette smoking on survival of patients with angiographically documented coronary artery disease: Report from the CASS Registry. JAMA 1986;255:1023-1027.

68. Cavender JB, Rogers WJ, Fisher LD, et al: Effects of smoking on survival and morbidity in patients randomized to medical or surgical therapy in the coronary artery surgery study (CASS): 10-year follow-up. J Am Coll Cardiol 1992;20:287-294.

69. Hasdai D, Garatt KN, Grill DE, et al: Effect of smoking status on the long-term outcome after successful percutaneous coronary vascularization. N Engl J Med 1997;336:755-761.

70. Bush TL, Miller VT: Effects of pharmacologic agents used during menopause: Impact on lipids and lipoproteins. In Misshell DR (ed): Menopause: Physiology and Pharmacology. Chicago, Year Book Medical Publishers, 1987, pp 187-208.

71. Sacks FM, Walsh BW: The effects of reproductive hormones on serum lipoproteins: Unresolved issues in biology and clinical practice. Ann N Y Acad Sci 1990;592:272-285.

72. Tikkanen MJ, Nikkilä EA, Kuusi T, Sipinen S: Different effects of two progestins on plasma high-density lipoprotein (HDL_2) and post-heparin plasma hepatic lipase activity. Atherosclerosis 1981;40:365-369.

73. Tikkanen MJ, Kuusi T, Nikkilä EA, Sipinen S: Postmenopausal hormone replacement therapy: Effects of progestogens on serum lipids and lipoproteins—a review. Maturitas 1986;8:7-17.

74. The Writing Group for the PEPI Trial: Effects of estrogen or estrogen/progestin regimens on heart disease risk factors in postmenopausal women. The Postmenopausal Estrogen/Progestin Interventions (PEPI) Trial. JAMA 1995;273:199-208.

75. Gordon DJ, Probstfield JL, Garrison RJ, et al: High-density lipoprotein cholesterol and cardiovascular disease: Four prospective American studies. Circulation 1989;79:8-15.

76. Walsh JME, Grady D: Treatment of hyperlipidemia in women. JAMA 1995;274:1152-1158.

77. Kannel WB, D'Agostino RB, Belanger AJ: Update on fibrinogen as a cardiovascular risk factor. Ann Epidemiol 1992;2:457-466.

78. Gilligan DM, Quyyumi AA, Cannon RO: Effects of physiological levels of estrogen on coronary vasomotor function in postmenopausal women. Circulation 1994;89:2545-2551.

79. Roselli M, Imthurn B, Keller PJ, et al: Circulating nitric oxide (nitrite/nitrate) levels in postmenopausal women substituted with 17 beta-estradiol amd norethisterone acetate: A two-year follow-up study. Hypertension 1995;25(pt 2):848-853.

80. Grodstein F, Stampfer M: The epidemiology of coronary heart disease and estrogen replacement in postmenopausal women. Prog Cardiovasc Dis 1995;38:199-210.

81. Grady D, Rubin SM, Pettiti DB, et al: Hormone therapy to prevent disease and prolong life in postmenopausal women. Ann Intern Med 1992;117:1016-1037.

82. Grodstein F, Stampfer MJ, Manson JE, et al: Postmenopausal estrogen and progestin use and the risk of cardiovascular disease. N Engl J Med 1996;335:453-461.

83. Hulley S, Grady D, Bush T, et al, for the Heart and Estrogen/Progestin Replacement Study (HERS) Research Group: Randomized trial of estrogen plus progestin for secondary prevention of coronary heart disease in postmenopausal women. JAMA 1998;280:605-613.

84. Herrington DM, Reboussin DM, Brosnihan KB, et al: Effects of estrogen replacement on the progression of coronary artery atherosclerosis. N Engl J Med 2000;343:522-529.

85. Sullivan JM: Coronary arteriography in estrogen-treated postmenopausal women. Prog Cardiovasc Dis 1995;38:211-222.

86. National Institutes of Health, National Heart, Lung, and Blood Institute: Women's Health Initiative. Available at www.nhlbi.nih.gov/whi/hrt-en.htn.

87. Mosca L, Barrett-Connor E, Wenger NK, et al: Design and methods of the Raloxifene Use for the Heart (RUTH) Study. Am J Cardiol 2001;88:392-395.

88. Watts GF, Lewis B, Brunt JN, et al: Effects on coronary artery disease of lipid-lowering diet, or diet plus cholestyramine, in the St. Thomas' Atherosclerosis Regression Study (STARS). Lancet 1992;339:563-569.

89. de Lorgeril M, Renaud S, Mamelle N, et al: Mediterranean alpha-linolenic acid-rich diet in secondary prevention of coronary heart disease. Lancet 1994;343:1454-1459.

90. Singh RB, Rostogi SS, Verma R, et al: Randomised, controlled trial of cardioprotective diet in patients with recent acute myocardial infarction: Results of one-year follow-up. BMJ 1992;304:1015-1019.

91. Singh RB, Niaz MA, Ghosh S, et al: Effect on mortality and reinfarction of adding fruits and vegetables to a prudent diet in the Indian Experiment of Infarct Survival. J Am Coll Nutr 1993;12:255-261.

92. Ornish D, Brown SE, Scherwitz LW, et al: Can lifestyle changes reverse coronary heart disease? The Lifestyle Heart Trial. Lancet 1990;336:129-133.

93. Sandkamp M, Funke H, Schulte H, et al: Lipoprotein(a) is an independent risk factor for myocardial infarction at a young age. Clin Chem 1990;36:20-23.

94. Bostom AG, Cupples LA, Jenner JL, et al: Elevated plasma lipoprotein (a) and coronary heart disease in men aged 55 years and younger: A prospective study. JAMA 1996;276:544-548.

95. Dahlen GH, Guyton JR, Attar M, et al: Association of levels of lipoprotein Lp(a), plasma lipids, and other lipoproteins with coronary artery disease documented by angiography. Circulation 1986;74:758-765.

96. Stampfer MJ, Malinow R, Willett WC, et al: A prospective study of plasma homocysteine and risk of myocardial infarction in US physicians. JAMA 1992;268:877-881.

97. Genest JJ, McNamara JR, Salem DN, et al: Plasma homocyst(e)ine levels in men with premature coronary artery disease. J Am Coll Cardiol 1990;16:1114-1119.

98. Wald NJ, Watt HC, Law MR, et al: Homocysteine and ischemic heart disease: Results of a prospective study with implications regarding prevention. Arch Intern Med 1998;158:862-867.

99. Omenn GS, Beresford SAA, Motulsky AG: Preventing coronary heart disease: B vitamins and homocysteine [ed]. Circulation 1998;97:421-424.

100. Kannel WB: Lipids, diabetes, and coronary heart disease: Insights from the Framingham Study. Am Heart J 1985;110:1100-1107.

101. Meade TW, Mellow S, Brozovic M, et al: Haemostatic function and ischaemic heart disease: Principal results of the Northwick Park Heart Study. Lancet 1986;2:533-537.

102. Mendall MA, Patel P, Ballam L, et al: C-reactive protein and its relation to cardiovascular risk factor: A population based cross sectional study. BMJ 1996;312:1061-1065.

103. Ridker P, Haughie P: Prospective studies of C-reactive protein as a risk factor for cardiovascular disease. J Invest Med 1988;46:391-395.

104. Ridker P, Rifai N, Pfeffer MA, et al, for the Cholesterol and Recurrent Events (CARE) investigators: Long-term effects of pravastatin on plasma concentration of C-reactive protein. Circulation 1999;100:230-235.

105. Gupta S, Leathem EW, Carrington D, et al: Elevated *Chlamydia pneumoniae* antibodies, cardiovascular events, and azithromycin in male survivors of myocardial infarction. Circulation 1997;96:404-407.

106. Anderson JL, Mulhestein JG, Carlquist J, et al: Randomized secondary prevention trial of azithromycin in patients with coronary artery disease and serological evidence for *Chlamydia pneumoniae* infection. Circulation 1999;99:1540-1547.

chapter 44

Dietary Intervention in Coronary Care Units and in Secondary Prevention

Michel de Lorgeril
Patricia Salen

Secondary prevention of coronary heart disease (CHD) should begin immediately after the first clinical manifestation of CHD and, if it occurs, during the first stay in the coronary care unit. In more general terms, secondary prevention usually focuses on risk reduction in patients with established CHD who are at high risk of recurrent cardiac events and death from cardiac causes. The two main causes of death in these patients are sudden cardiac death (SCD) and heart failure, often resulting from myocardial ischemia and subsequent necrosis. The main mechanism underlying recurrent cardiac events is myocardial ischemia resulting from atherosclerotic plaque rupture or ulceration. Plaque rupture is usually the consequence of intraplaque inflammation associated with a high lipid content of the lesion and high concentration of leukocytes and lipid peroxidation products. In patients with established CHD, the three main aims of the preventive strategy are to prevent malignant ventricular arrhythmia and the development of severe ventricular dysfunction (and heart failure) and to minimize the risk of plaque inflammation and ulceration. The priority of secondary prevention is different from that of primary prevention. In the context of primary prevention, intervention focuses on traditional risk factors (e.g., blood cholesterol or blood pressure) and surrogate end points rather than on specific clinical complications, such as SCD. This does not mean that traditional risk factors of CHD should not be measured and, if necessary, corrected in secondary prevention because they also play a role in the occurrence of CHD complications. It simply means that because complications such as SCD and associated syndromes are often unpredictable, occur outside the hospital and far from any potential therapeutic resources in most cases, and account for about 50% of cardiac mortality in secondary prevention, they should be the priority of a secondary prevention program. This chapter focuses on recommendations and comments specifically on clinical efficacy and not on surrogate efficacy.

Whatever the specific clinical aims of the program, nutritional evaluation and counseling of each patient with CHD must be a key point of the preventive intervention. Nutrition is, however, only one component of such a program. Exercise training, behavioral interventions (particularly to help the patient abstain from smoking), and drug therapy have equally important roles. The control of risk factors has been seen traditionally in the perspective of prevention. The target is moving increasingly into the acute phase of the disease, however, considering the importance of risk factor control on one hand and a potential early benefit for acute plaque stabilization on the other.

The dietary prevention program commonly is initiated during hospitalization for a first CHD event. With shorter stays in the coronary care unit, the dietary intervention is initiated during the following days in the hospital, then continued in secondary prevention centers and included in cardiac rehabilitation programs. An individualized dietary prevention program should be developed under the guidance of a specialized dietitian and in close collaboration with the patient's cardiologist and primary care physician so that there is no discontinuity or discrepancy in dietary counseling between the hospitalization and posthospitalization phases of the rehabilitation program.

We propose a *minimum clinical priority dietary program* based on the idea that many patients (and their families) find it difficult (e.g., because they are not supported by a well-informed physician) to adopt fully and immediately an effective cardioprotective diet. The clinical priority program provides a list of simple dietary recommendations that the patient and his or her attending physician will try to follow or not, according to their own choices and possibilities. Patients and physicians should know, however, that none of these minimum changes could replace the holistic approach described in this chapter.

DIETARY PREVENTION OF SUDDEN CARDIAC DEATH

In the absence of a generally accepted definition, SCD usually is defined as death from a cardiac cause occurring within 1 hour from the onset of symptoms.[1] In many studies, however, investigators used different definitions with a time frame of 3 hours or even 24 hours in the old World Health Organization definition. SCD currently is attributed to cardiac arrhythmia, although it is well recognized that classification based on clinical circumstances only is sometimes misleading. The magnitude of the problem is considerable because SCD is a common, and often the first, manifestation of CHD, and it accounts for about 50% of cardiovascular mortality in developed countries.[1] In most cases, SCD occurs without prodromal symptoms and outside the hospital. This mode of death is a major public health issue. Because 80% of SCD patients had CHD,[2] the epidemiology and potential preventive approaches of SCD in theory should parallel those of CHD. In other words, any treatment aimed at reducing CHD should reduce the incidence of SCD.

This section examines whether diet (and, more precisely, certain dietary factors) may prevent (or help prevent) SCD in patients with established CHD. Analysis is focused on the effects of the different families of fatty acids, antioxidants, and alcohol.[2]

Fish and n-3 Fatty Acids

The hypothesis that eating fish may protect against SCD is derived from the results of a secondary prevention trial, DART (Diet And Reinfarction Trial), which showed a significant reduction in total and cardiovascular mortality (both by about 30%) in patients who had at least two servings of fatty fish per week.[3] The authors suggested that the protective effect of fish might be explained by a preventive action on ventricular fibrillation because no benefit was observed on the incidence of nonfatal acute myocardial infarction (MI). This hypothesis was consistent with experimental evidence suggesting that n-3 polyunsaturated fatty acids (PUFA), the dominant fatty acids in fish oil and fatty fish, have an important effect on the occurrence of ventricular fibrillation in the setting of myocardial ischemia and reperfusion in various in vivo and in vitro animal models.[4,5] In the same studies, it was also apparent that saturated fatty acids are proarrhythmic compared with unsaturated fatty acids. Using an elegant in vivo model of SCD in dogs, Billman and colleagues[6] showed a striking reduction of ventricular fibrillation after intravenous administration of pure n-3 PUFA, including the long-chain fatty acids present in fish oil and α-linolenic acid, their parent n-3 PUFA occurring in some vegetable oils. These authors found the mechanism of this protection to result from the electrophysiologic effects of free n-3 PUFA when these are partitioned into the phospholipids of the sarcolemma without covalently bonding to any constituents of the cell membrane. After dietary intake, these fatty acids are incorporated preferentially into membrane phospholipids.[7] Nair and colleagues[7] also showed that an important pool of free (nonesterified) fatty acids exists in the normal myocardium and that the amount of n-3 PUFA in this pool is increased by supplementing the diet in n-3 PUFA.

Table 44–1 shows the huge increases observed in n-3 PUFA concentrations, in particular for the nonesterified fraction, in the myocardium of pigs that were fed fish oil; this illustrates the potential of diet to modify the structure and biochemical composition of cardiac cells. In case of ischemia, phospholipases and lipases quickly release new fatty acids from phospholipids, including n-3 fatty acids in higher amounts than the other fatty acids,[7] further increasing the pool of free n-3 fatty acids that can exert an antiarrhythmic effect. The lipoprotein lipase is particularly active after consumption of n-3 PUFA.[8] One hypothesis is that the presence of the free form of the n-3 PUFA in the membrane of every cardiac muscle cell renders the myocardium more resistant to arrhythmias, probably by modulating the conduction of several membrane ion channels.[9] So far, it seems that the potent inhibitory effects of n-3 PUFA on the fast sodium current, I_{Na},[10,11] and the L-type calcium current, I_{CaL},[12] are the major contributors to the antiarrhythmic actions of these fatty acids in ischemia. Briefly, n-3 PUFA act by shifting the steady-state inactivation potential to more negative values, as also was observed in other excitable tissues such as neurons.

Another important aspect of the implication of n-3 PUFA in SCD is their role in the metabolization of eicosanoids. In competition with n-6 PUFA, they are the precursors to a broad array of structurally diverse and potent bioactive lipids (including eicosanoids, prostaglandins, and thromboxanes), which are thought to play a role in the occurrence of ventricular fibrillation during myocardial ischemia and reperfusion.[13,14]

Other clinical data show suppression (by >70%) of ventricular premature complexes in middle-aged patients

■ ■ ■

TABLE 44–1 FATTY ACID CONCENTRATION OF THE PHOSPHOLIPID FRACTION AND NONESTERIFIED FATTY ACID FRACTION IN THE MYOCARDIUM OF PIGS FED FISH OIL FOR 6 WEEKS

	PHOSPHOLIPIDS (μMOL/G HEART)		NEFA (NMOL/G HEART)	
	Control	Fish Oil	Control	Fish Oil
18:0	3.2 ± 0.4	3.5 ± 0.1	478 ± 44	648 ± 68
18:1 (n-9)	2.6 ± 0.2	2.5 ± 0.2	963 ± 89	774 ± 119
18:2(n-6)	6.1 ± 0.6	3.4 ± 0.2*	729 ± 77	679 ± 129
20:4(n-6)	3.1 ± 0.2	1.5 ± 0.1*	387 ± 38	227 ± 21*
20:5(n-3)	0.2 ± 0.03	2.4 ± 0.1*	35 ± 6	415 ± 34*
22:6(n-3)	0.3 ± 0.02	1.1 ± 0.1*	45 ± 4	246 ± 33*

* $P < .05$.
NEFA, nonesterified fatty acid.
Modified from Nair SD, Leitch J, Falconer J, et al: Cardiac (n-3) nonesterified fatty acids are selectively increased in fish oil–fed pigs following myocardial ischemia. J Nutr 1999; 129:1518–1523.

with frequent ventricular extrasystoles randomly assigned to take either fish oil or placebo.[15] Also, survivors of acute MI[16] and healthy men[17] receiving fish oil were shown to have improved measurements of heart rate variability, suggesting other mechanisms by which n-3 PUFA may be antiarrhythmic.

Support for the hypothesis of a clinically significant antiarrhythmic effect of n-3 PUFA in the secondary prevention of CHD, as put forward in DART,[3] came from two randomized trials testing the effect of ethnic dietary patterns (instead of a single food or nutrient)—a Mediterranean type of diet and an Asian vegetarian diet—in the secondary prevention of CHD.[18,19] The two experimental diets included a high intake of essential α-linolenic acid, the main vegetable n-3 PUFA. Although the incidence of SCD was reduced markedly in both trials, the number of cases was small, and the antiarrhythmic effect cannot be entirely attributed to α-linolenic acid because these experimental diets also were high in other nutrients with potential antiarrhythmic properties, including various antioxidants. These findings were extended by the population-based, case-control study conducted by Siscovick and colleagues[20] on the intake of n-3 PUFA among patients with primary cardiac arrest compared with that of age-matched and sex-matched controls. Their data indicated that the intake of about 5 to 6 g of n-3 PUFA per month (an amount provided by consuming fatty fish once or twice a week) was associated with a 50% reduction in the risk of cardiac arrest. In that study, the use of a biomarker, the red blood cell membrane level of n-3 PUFA, considerably enhanced the validity of the findings, which also were consistent with the results of many (but not all) cohort studies suggesting that consumption of one to two servings of fish per week is associated with a marked reduction in CHD mortality compared with no fish intake.[21,22] In most studies, however, the SCD end point is not reported.

In a large prospective study (>20,000 participants with a follow-up of 11 years), Albert and colleagues[23] examined the specific point that fish has antiarrhythmic properties and may prevent SCD. They found that the risk of SCD was 50% lower for men who consumed fish at least once a week than for men who consumed fish less than once a month. The consumption of fish was not related to nonsudden cardiac death, suggesting that the main protective effect of fish (or n-3 PUFA) is related to an effect on arrhythmia. These results are consistent with those of DART[3] but differ from those of the Chicago Western Electric Study, in which there was a significant inverse association between fish consumption and nonsudden cardiac death but not SCD.[24] Several methodologic factors may explain the discrepancy between the two studies, especially the way of classifying deaths in the Western Electric Study[24]; this illustrates the limitations of observational studies and the obvious fact that only randomized trials definitely can provide a clear demonstration of causal relationships.

The GISSI-Prevenzione trial was aimed at helping to address the question of the health benefits of foods rich in n-3 PUFA (and in vitamin E) and their pharmacologic substitutes.[25] Patients (n = 11,324) surviving a recent acute MI (<3 months) and having received the prior

advice to consume a Mediterranean type of diet were randomly assigned supplements of n-3 PUFA (0.8 g daily), vitamin E (300 mg daily), both, or none (control) for 3.5 years. The primary efficacy end point was the combination of death and nonfatal acute MI and stroke. Secondary analyses included overall mortality, cardiovascular mortality, and SCD. The exact definition of SCD was not given in the article. The clinical events were validated, however, by an ad-hoc committee of expert cardiologists,[25] who presumably used the current definition of SCD. Treatment with n-3 PUFA significantly lowered the risk of the primary end point (the relative risk decreased by 15%). Secondary analyses provided a clearer profile of the clinical effects of n-3 PUFA (Table 44-2). Overall mortality was reduced by 20% and cardiovascular mortality by 30%. The effect on SCD (45% lower) accounted for most of the benefits seen in the primary combined end point and overall and cardiovascular mortality. There was no difference across the treatment groups for nonfatal cardiovascular events, a result comparable to that of DART.[3] The results obtained in this randomized trial are consistent with previous controlled trials,[3,18,19] large-scale observational studies,[21-24] and experimental studies,[4-7] which together strongly support an effect of n-3 PUFA in relation to SCD. The protective effect of n-3 PUFA on SCD was greater in the groups of patients who complied more strictly with the Mediterranean diet. This finding suggests a positive interaction between n-3 PUFA and some components of the Mediterranean diet, which is, by definition, not high in n-6 PUFA and low in saturated fats but rich in oleic acid, various antioxidants, and fiber and associated with a moderate consumption of alcohol (see later for further comments).

Existing evidence suggests that an intake of n-3 PUFA (about 1 g daily), either in the form of supplements or by eating at least two large (about 200 g) servings of fatty fish per week, would help to prevent SCD. At present, there is no reason to encourage (or prescribe) intakes exceeding 1 to 2 g of n-3 PUFA per day. The dosage to be recommended in high-risk patients and in secondary prevention of SCD warrants further investigation.

■ ■ ■

TABLE 44–2 CLINICAL EFFICACY OF (N-3) POLYUNSATURATED FATTY ACIDS IN THE GISSI-PREVENZIONE TRIAL

	RELATIVE RISK (95% CI)
Death, nonfatal acute myocardial infarction, and stroke	0.85 (0.70–0.99)
Overall mortality	0.80 (0.67–0.94)
Cardiovascular mortality	0.70 (0.56–0.87)
Sudden cardiac death	0.55 (0.40–0.76)
Nonfatal cardiovascular events	0.96 (0.76–1.21)
Fatal and nonfatal stroke	1.30 (0.87–1.96)

CI, confidence interval.
Modified from GISSI-Prevenzione investigators: Dietary Supplementation with n-3 polyunsaturated fatty acids and vitamin E after myocardial infarction: Results of the GISSI-Prevenzione trial. Lancet 1999;354:447–455.

Saturated Fatty Acids, Oleic Acid, Trans Fatty Acids, and n-6 Fatty Acids

Regarding the other dietary fatty acids, animal experiments have indicated that a diet rich in saturated fatty acids is associated with a high incidence of ischemia-induced and reperfusion-induced ventricular arrhythmia, whereas PUFA of either the n-6 or n-3 family reduce that risk.[4-6] Some large epidemiologic studies have shown consistent associations between the intake of saturated fatty acids and CHD mortality.[26] The SCD end point is usually not analyzed in these studies, however. In addition, a clear demonstration of a causal relationship between dietary saturated fatty acids and SCD would require the organization of a randomized trial, which is not ethically acceptable. Besides the effect of saturated fatty acids on blood cholesterol levels, the exact mechanisms by which saturated fats increase CHD mortality are unclear. If animal data, showing a proarrhythmic effect of saturated fatty acids, are confirmed in humans, the first thing to do to prevent SCD in humans would be to reduce drastically the intake of saturated fats. This reduction has been done in randomized dietary trials, and, as expected, the rate of SCD decreased in the experimental groups.[18,19] The beneficial effect cannot be attributed entirely to the reduction of saturated fats, however, because other potentially antiarrhythmic dietary factors, including n-3 PUFA, also were modified in these trials.[22,23]

In contrast with n-3 PUFA, few data have been published so far in humans regarding the effect of n-6 PUFA on the risk of SCD. Roberts and associates[27] reported that the percentage content of linoleic acid (the dominant n-6 PUFA in the diet) in adipose tissue (an indicator of long-term dietary intake) was inversely related to the risk of SCD, which was defined in that study as instantaneous death or death within 24 hours of the onset of symptoms.[27] This study is in line with most animal data and may suggest that patients at risk of SCD would benefit from increasing their dietary intake of n-6 PUFA, in particular linoleic acid, in the same way as for n-3 PUFA. n-3 PUFA were more effective on SCD than n-6 PUFA, however, in most animal experiments.[4-6] In addition, diets high in n-6 PUFA increase the linoleic acid content of lipoproteins and render them more susceptible to oxidation,[28] which would be an argument against such diets. Lipoprotein oxidation is a major step in the inflammatory process that renders atherosclerotic lesions unstable and prone to rupture.[29-31] Erosion and rupture of atherosclerotic lesions were shown to trigger CHD complications (see the section on plaque inflammation and rupture) and myocardial ischemia and to enhance considerably the risk of SCD.[32-35] In the secondary prevention of CHD, diets high in n-6 PUFA failed to improve the overall prognosis of the patients.[36] Also, in the Dayton study, a mixed primary and secondary prevention trial, in which the chief characteristic of the experimental diet was the substitution of n-6 PUFA for saturated fat, the number of SCDs was apparently lower in the experimental group than in the control group (18 versus 27), but the number of deaths from other causes, in particular cancers, was higher in the experimental group (85 versus 71), offsetting the potential protective effect of n-6 PUFA on SCD and resulting in no effect at all on mortality.[37] Such negative effects were not reported with n-3 PUFA. Despite the beneficial effect of n-6 PUFA on lipoprotein levels, which in theory could reduce SCD in the long-term by reducing the development of atherosclerosis, it seems preferable not to increase the consumption of n-6 PUFA beyond the amounts required to prevent deficiencies in the essential n-6 fatty acid, linoleic acid (approximately 4% to 6% of the total energy intake), which are found in the current average Western diet. As a substitute for saturated fat, the best choice is to increase the intake of vegetable monounsaturated fat (oleic acid) in accordance with the Mediterranean diet pattern. If oleic acid has no apparent effect on the risk of SCD (at least by comparison with n-3 and n-6 PUFA), its effects on blood lipoprotein levels are similar to those of n-6 PUFA, and it has the advantage of protecting lipoproteins against oxidation.[38] The best fatty acid combination to prevent SCD (and the other complications of CHD) and to accumulate antiarrhythmic, antioxidant, and hypolipidemic effects would result from the adoption of a diet close to the Mediterranean diet pattern as described[38,39] (Table 44-3).

Roberts and colleagues[40] reported no significant relationship between trans isomers of oleic and linoleic acids in adipose tissue and the risk of SCD, whereas Lemaitre and coworkers[41] found that cell membrane trans isomers of linoleic acid (but not of oleic acid) are associated with a large increase in the risk of primary cardiac arrest.[41] As for the role of trans fatty acids on ventricular arrhythmias, it has not been investigated in experimental models.

Although specific human data on the effect of saturated fatty acids on SCD are lacking, results of several trials suggest that it is important to reduce their intake in the secondary prevention of CHD. Despite a possible beneficial effect on the risk of SCD, increasing consumption of n-6 PUFA should not be recommended in clinical practice for patients with established CHD. Diets including low intakes in saturated fatty acid (and trans isomers of linoleic acid) and n-6 PUFA (but enough to provide the essential linoleic acid) and high intakes in n-3 PUFA

■ ■ ■

TABLE 44–3   THE MAIN CHARACTERISTICS OF THE MODERN MEDITERRANEAN DIET PATTERN

NUTRIENTS	AMOUNTS (% TOTAL ENERGY)
Total lipids	27–35
Saturated fats	7–10
Polyunsaturated fats	4–6
Oleic acid	12–16
(n-3) Fatty acids	0.8–1.2
Alcohol	4–10
Vitamin C (mg/day)	80–200
Selenium (µg/day)	80–200
Fibers (g/day)	18–25
Folates (µg/day)	300–800

Data from references 39 and 40.

and oleic acid (Mediterranean diet pattern) seem to be the best option to prevent SCD and nonfatal acute MI recurrence.[19,38]

Alcohol

The question of the effect of alcohol on heart and vessel diseases has been the subject of intense controversy. The consensus is now that moderate alcohol drinking is associated with reduced cardiovascular mortality, although the exact mechanisms by which alcohol is protective are still unclear. In contrast, chronic heavy drinking has been incriminated in the occurrence of atrial and ventricular arrhythmias in humans, an effect called "the holiday heart" because it often is associated with binge drinking by healthy people, specifically during the weekend. Studies in animals have shown varying and apparently contradictory effects of alcohol on cardiac rhythm and conduction, depending on the animal species, the experimental model, and the dose of alcohol. If given acutely to nonalcoholic animals, ethanol may have antiarrhythmic properties.

In humans, few studies specifically have investigated the effect of alcohol on SCD. The hyperadrenergic state resulting from binge drinking and from withdrawal in alcoholics seems to be the main mechanism by which alcohol induces arrhythmias in humans. In the British Regional Heart Study, the relative risk of SCD in heavy drinkers (>6 drinks per day) was twice as high as in occasional or light drinkers.[42] The effect of binge drinking on SCD was more evident, however, in men with no preexisting CHD than in men with established CHD. In contrast, in the Honolulu Heart Program,[43] the risk of SCD among healthy middle-aged men was positively related to blood pressure, serum cholesterol, smoking, and left ventricular hypertrophy (LVH) but inversely related to alcohol intake. The effect of moderate social drinking on the risk of SCD in nonalcoholic subjects has been addressed so far in only one study. Investigators of the Physicians' Health Study assessed whether light-to-moderate alcohol drinkers apparently free of CHD at baseline have a decreased risk of SCD.[44] After controlling for multiple confounders, men who consumed 2 to 4 drinks per week or 5 to 6 drinks per week at baseline had a significantly reduced risk of SCD (by 60% to 80%) compared with men who rarely or never consumed alcohol. Analyses were repeated after excluding deaths occurring during the first 4 years of follow-up (to exclude the possibility that some men who refrained from drinking at baseline did so because of early symptoms of heart disease) and using the updated measure of alcohol intake ascertained at year 7 to address potential misclassification in the baseline evaluation of alcohol drinking.[44] These secondary analyses basically provided the same results and confirmed the potential protective effect of moderate drinking on the risk of SCD. Despite limitations (the selected nature of the cohort, an exclusively male study group, no information on beverage type and drinking pattern), this study suggests that a significant part of the cardioprotective effect of moderate drinking is related to the prevention of SCD. Further research should be directed at understanding the mechanisms by which moderate alcohol drinking may prevent ventricular arrhythmias and SCD.

In practice, current knowledge suggests that in CHD patients at risk of SCD, there is no reason not to allow moderate alcohol drinking. From a practical point of view, we advise drinking 1 or 2 drinks per day, preferably wine, preferably during the evening meal, and never before driving a car or partaking in dangerous work.

Antioxidants

The issue about the effect of dietary antioxidants on the risk of CHD in general and on SCD in particular is more controversial. Regarding vitamin E, the most widely studied dietary antioxidant, discrepant findings between the expected benefits based on epidemiologic observations[45,46] and the results of clinical trials[47,48] were published. In a controlled trial, a significant decrease in nonfatal acute MI and a nonsignificant increase in cardiovascular mortality (in particular in the rate of SCD) were reported with a daily regimen of 400 to 800 mg of vitamin E in patients with established CHD.[49] Because of certain methodologic shortcomings (not discussed here), this trial was said to confuse rather than clarify the question of the usefulness of vitamin E supplementation in CHD and provided no indication about possible links between vitamin E and the prevention of SCD.

The GISSI-Prevenzione trial brings new information in this regard. In contrast to studies of (n-3) PUFA, the results of vitamin E supplementation do not support a significant effect on the primary end point—a combination of death and nonfatal acute MI and stroke.[25] The secondary analysis provides a clearer view, however, of the clinical effect of vitamin E in CHD patients, which cannot be dismissed easily (Table 44-4). Among the 193 and 155 cardiac deaths that occurred in the control and vitamin E group during the trial (a difference of 38, $P < .05$), there were 99 and 65 SCDs (a difference of 34, $P < .05$), which indicated that the significant decrease in cardiovascular mortality (by 20%) in the vitamin E group was almost entirely due to a decrease in the incidence of SCD (by 35%). In contrast, nonfatal cardiac events and nonsudden cardiac deaths were not influenced.[25] These data suggest that vitamin E may be useful for the primary prevention of SCD in patients with established CHD.

The vitamin E data of the GISSI trial do not stand in isolation. In an in vivo dog model of myocardial ischemia,[50] we reported a protective effect of vitamin E on the incidence of ventricular fibrillation (the main mechanism of SCD) with a 16% rate in the vitamin E group and 44% in the placebo group ($P < .05$). Also in line with the GISSI results, infarct size, which is the main determinant of acute heart failure and nonsudden cardiac death, was larger in the supplemented group (58.5% of the ischemic area) than in the placebo group (41.9%, $P < .05$). Such ambivalent effects of vitamin E may explain at least partly why its effects were neutral or nonsignificant in many studies, with the negative effects hiding the beneficial ones. Nevertheless, the GISSI trial showed that cardiovascular mortality and SCD were reduced significantly by vitamin E, and the effect on overall mortality showed a favorable trend ($P = .07$). Finally, the HOPE (Heart

■ ■ ■

TABLE 44–4   CLINICAL EFFICACY OF VITAMIN E IN THE GISSI-PREVENZIONE TRIAL

	RELATIVE RISK (95% CI)
Death, nonfatal acute myocardial infarction, and stroke	0.89 (0.77–1.03)
Overall mortality	0.86 (0.72–1.02)
Cardiovascular mortality	0.80 (0.65–0.99)
Sudden cardiac death	0.65 (0.48–0.89)
Nonfatal cardiovascular events	1.02 (0.81–1.28)
Fatal and nonfatal stroke	0.95 (0.61–1.47)

CI, confidence interval.
Modified from GISSI-Prevenzione investigators: Dietary supplementation with n-3 polyunsaturated fatty acids and vitamin E after myocardial infarction: Results of the GISSI-Prevenzione trial. Lancet 1999;354:447–455.

Outcome Prevention Evaluation) trial, testing the effect of 400 IU of vitamin E daily in patients at high risk of CHD (in primary prevention) and reporting an apparent lack of effect of vitamin E, does not help us to solve the issue of whether or not vitamin E is protective against SCD.[51] In that trial, it is not clear whether the patients took the capsules during meals (a prerequisite for intestinal absorption of vitamin E), whether the patients were more or less deficient in vitamin E (no blood measurement), and whether some of them were taking vitamin supplements (a current practice nowadays among certain populations), and SCD apparently was not among the predefined end points. Patients with left ventricular dysfunction, a major determinant of the risk of SCD, were not eligible.

Further clinical and experimental studies, specifically designed to test the antiarrhythmic effect of vitamin E during myocardial ischemia, are warranted. In particular, the issue of the interactions between vitamin E (either α-tocopherol or γ-tocopherol), the different fatty acids, and the various antioxidants have to be addressed. At present, however, vitamin E supplementation has no obvious harmful effect on the risk of SCD, but no general recommendations can be given yet.

DIET AND THE RISK OF HEART FAILURE AFTER ACUTE MYOCARDIAL INFARCTION

The incidence of chronic heart failure, the common end result of most cardiac diseases, is increasing steadily in many countries despite (and probably because of) considerable improvements in the acute and long-term treatment of CHD, which today is the main cause of chronic heart failure in most countries.[52] In recent years, most research efforts in chronic heart failure have been focused on drug treatment, and there has been little attention paid to nonpharmacologic management. Some unidentified factors may contribute to the rise in the prevalence of chronic heart failure and should be recognized and corrected if possible. Chronic heart failure now is considered a metabolic problem with endocrine and immunologic disturbances potentially contributing

to the progression of the disease.[53,54] In particular, the role of tumor necrosis factor (TNF) is discussed subsequently. It also has been recognized that increased oxidative stress may contribute to the pathogenesis of chronic heart failure.[55] The intimate link between diet and oxidative stress is obvious, knowing that the major antioxidant defenses of the body are derived from essential nutrients.[56] Antioxidant nutrients are discussed later.

Although it generally is considered that a high-sodium diet is detrimental (and may result in acute decompensation of heart failure through a volume overload mechanism), little is known about other aspects of diet in chronic heart failure in terms of general nutrition and micronutrients, such as vitamins and minerals. In these patients, it is important not only to diagnose and treat the chronic heart failure syndrome itself and identify and aggressively manage traditional risk factors of CHD, such as high blood pressure and cholesterol (because they can aggravate the syndrome), but also to recognize and correct malnutrition and deficiencies in specific micronutrients.

The importance of micronutrients for health and the fact that several micronutrients have antioxidant properties are fully recognized. These antioxidant properties may be as direct antioxidants, such as vitamins C and E, or as components of antioxidant enzymes, such as superoxide dismutase or glutathione peroxidase.[56] It is widely believed (but still not causally shown) that diet-derived antioxidants may play a role in the development (and in the prevention) of chronic heart failure. Clinical and experimental studies have suggested that chronic heart failure may be associated with increased free radical formation[57] and reduced antioxidant defenses[58] and that vitamin C may improve endothelial function in patients with chronic heart failure.[59] In the secondary prevention of CHD, in dietary trials in which the tested diet included high intakes of natural antioxidants, the incidence of new episodes of chronic heart failure was reduced in the experimental groups.[18,60] Taken together, these data suggest (but do not show) that antioxidant nutrients may help prevent chronic heart failure in post-MI patients.

Other nutrients also may be involved in certain cases of chronic heart failure. Although deficiency in certain micronutrients, whatever the reason, can cause chronic heart failure and should be corrected (see later), patients suffering from chronic heart failure also have symptoms that can affect their food intake and result in deficiencies. These symptoms include tiredness when strained; breathing difficulties; and gastrointestinal symptoms, such as nausea, loss of appetite, and early feeling of satiety. Drug therapy can lead to loss of appetite and excess urinary losses in case of diuretic use. All of these are mainly consequences, not causative factors, of chronic heart failure. The basic treatment of chronic heart failure in theory should improve these nutritional anomalies. Because they can contribute to the development and severity of chronic heart failure, however, they should be recognized and corrected as early as possible.

Finally, it has been shown that 50% of patients with chronic heart failure are malnourished to some degree,[61] and chronic heart failure often is associated with weight loss. There may be multiple causes to the weight loss,[62] in particular, lack of activity resulting in loss of muscle bulk and increased resting metabolic rate. There is also a shift toward catabolism with insulin resistance and increased catabolic relative to anabolic steroids.[63] TNF, sometimes called *cachectin*, is more abundant in many patients with chronic heart failure,[53,63] which may explain weight loss in these patients. There is a positive correlation between TNF and markers of oxidative stress in the failing heart,[64] suggesting a link between TNF and antioxidant defenses in chronic heart failure (the potential importance of TNF in chronic heart failure is discussed later in the section on dietary fatty acids and chronic heart failure). Finally, cardiac cachexia is a well-recognized complication of chronic heart failure, its prevalence increases as symptoms worsen,[65] and it is an independent predictor of mortality in chronic heart failure patients. The pathophysiologic alteration leading to cachexia is unclear, however, and at present, there is no specific treatment apart from the treatment of the basic illness and correction of the associated biologic abnormalities.

Deficiency in Specific Micronutrients

As mentioned earlier, an important practical point is that deficiencies in specific micronutrients can cause chronic heart failure, or at least aggravate it. The prevalence of these deficiencies among patients with chronic heart failure (and post-MI patients) is unknown. Whether we should search systematically for them also is unclear. In particular, we do not know whether the association of several borderline deficiencies that do not result individually in chronic heart failure may result in chronic heart failure, especially in the elderly. For certain investigators, there is sufficient evidence to support a large-scale trial of dietary micronutrient supplementation in chronic heart failure.[66]

Detailed discussion of the present knowledge regarding micronutrient deficiencies is beyond the scope of this chapter. Nonetheless, if we restrict our comments only to human data, things can be summarized as follows.

Cases of hypocalcemia-induced cardiomyopathy (usually in children with a congenital cause for hypocalcemia) that can respond dramatically to calcium supplementation have been reported.[67] Hypomagnesemia often is associated with a poor prognosis in chronic heart failure,[68] and correction of the magnesium levels (e.g., in anorexia nervosa) leads to an improvement in cardiac function. Low serum and high urinary zinc levels are found in chronic heart failure,[69] possibly as a result of diuretic use, but there are no data regarding the clinical effect of zinc supplementation in that context. In one study, plasma copper was slightly higher and zinc slightly lower in chronic heart failure subjects than in healthy controls.[58] As expected, dietary intakes were in the normal range, and no significant relationship was found between dietary intakes and blood levels in the two groups. It is not possible to say whether these copper and zinc abnormalities may contribute to the development of chronic heart failure or are simple markers for the chronic inflammation known to be associated with chronic heart failure.[53,63] Further studies are needed to address the point because the implications for prevention are substantial.

Selenium deficiency has been identified as a major factor in the cause of certain nonischemic chronic heart failure syndromes, especially in low-selenium soil areas such as Eastern China and Western Africa.[70] In Western countries, cases of congestive cardiomyopathy associated with low antioxidant nutrients (vitamins and trace elements) have been reported in malnourished, human immunodeficiency virus (HIV)–infected patients and in patients on long-term parenteral nutrition.[71] Selenium deficiency is also a risk factor for peripartum cardiomyopathy.

In China, an endemic cardiomyopathy called *Keshan disease* seems to be a direct consequence of selenium deficiency. Although the question of the mechanism by which selenium deficiency results in chronic heart failure is open, data suggest that selenium may be involved in skeletal (and cardiac) muscle deconditioning (and in chronic heart failure symptoms, such as fatigue and low exercise tolerance) rather than in left ventricular dysfunction.[58] In the Keshan area, the selenium status coincides with the clinical severity rather than with the degree of left ventricular dysfunction as assessed by echocardiographic studies. When the selenium levels of residents were raised to the typical levels in the nonendemic areas, the mortality rate declined significantly, but clinically latent cases still were found, and the echocardiographic prevalence of the disease remained high.[70] What can be learned from Keshan disease and other studies conducted elsewhere[58] is that in patients with a known cause of chronic heart failure, even a mild deficiency in selenium may influence the clinical severity of the disease (e.g., tolerance to exercise).

These data should serve as a strong incentive for the initiation of studies testing the effects of natural antioxidants on the clinical severity of chronic heart failure. In the meantime, physicians would be well advised to measure selenium in patients with an exercise inability disproportionate to their cardiac dysfunction. Finally, low whole-blood thiamine (vitamin B_1) levels have been documented in patients with chronic heart failure on loop diuretics and hospitalized elderly patients, and thiamine supplementation induced a significant improvement in cardiac function and symptoms.[72]

Dietary Fatty Acids, Sodium Intake, Cytokines, Left Ventricular Hypertrophy, and Chronic Heart Failure

Beyond the well-known effect of high sodium intake in the clinical course of chronic heart failure (and the occurrence of acute episodes of decompensation), another important issue is the role of diet in the development of LVH, a major risk factor for chronic heart failure (and SCD) as well as for cardiovascular and all-cause mortality and morbidity.[73,74]

The cause of LVH is largely unknown. Although male gender, obesity, heredity, and insulin resistance may explain some of the variance in LVH, hypertension generally is regarded as the primary culprit.[75] The risks associated with LVH and hypertension are intimately linked. Data also suggest that low dietary intake of PUFA and high intake of saturated fatty acids, hypertension, and obesity at age 50 predicted the prevalence of LVH 20 years later.[76] Although the source of saturated fatty acids is usually animal fat, the source of unsaturated fatty acids in that specific Scandinavian population and at that time was less clear, and there was no adjustment for other potential dietary confounders, such as magnesium, potassium, calcium, and sodium. This study did not provide data to conclude definitely the dietary lipid determinants of LVH.[76] It does suggest, however, that dietary fatty acids may be involved in the development of LVH and that this "diet-heart connection" may explain partially the harmful effect of animal saturated fatty acids on the heart.

Another diet-heart connection in the context of advanced chronic heart failure relates to the theory that chronic heart failure also is a low-grade chronic inflammatory disease with elevated circulating levels of cytokines and cytokine receptors that are otherwise independent predictors of mortality.[53,63] High-dose angiotensin-converting enzyme inhibition with enalapril, a treatment that reduces mechanical overload and shear stress (two stimuli for cytokine production in patients with chronic heart failure), was shown to decrease cytokine bioactivity and left ventricular wall thickness.[77] Finally, various anticytokine and immunomodulating agents were shown to have a beneficial effect on heart function and clinical functional class in patients with advanced chronic heart failure,[78] suggesting a causal relationship between high cytokine production and chronic heart failure. This study also suggests there is a potential for therapies altering cytokine production in chronic heart failure. In that regard, it has been shown that dietary supplementation with n-3 fatty acids (either fish oil or vegetable oil rich in n-3 fatty acid) reduces cytokine production at least in healthy volunteers.[79,80] An inverse exponential relationship between leukocyte n-3 fatty acid content and cytokine production by these cells was found, with most of the reduction in cytokine production being seen with eicosapentanoic acid in cell membrane less than 1%, a level obtained with moderate n-3 fatty acid supplementation.[80] Further studies are warranted, however, to test whether (and at which dosage) dietary n-3 fatty acids may influence the clinical course of chronic heart failure through an anticytokine effect.

Sodium intake is the environmental factor that currently is most suspected of influencing blood pressure and the prevalence of hypertension. The full damaging potential of high sodium intake for the heart (and the kidney) seems to be largely independent of the pressor effect of sodium, however. Animal experiments and clinical studies consistently have shown that high sodium intake is a powerful and independent determinant of LVH and that such an arterial pressure–independent effect of salt is not confined to the heart.[81,82] The multiple pathophysiologic effects of high sodium intake are summarized in Figure 44–1.

Although the long-term effect of a reduced sodium intake after a recent acute MI is unknown, in particular

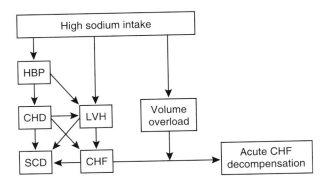

FIGURE 44–1. Schematic representation of the complex relationships between coronary heart disease (CHD), left ventricular hypertrophy (LVH), chronic heart failure (CHF), and sudden cardiac death (SCD). The potential impact of high sodium intake through its effects on blood pressure and high blood pressure (HBP), LVH, and plasma volume also is illustrated.

on LVH, experts claim that even a 50-mmol reduction in the daily sodium intake would reduce the average systolic blood pressure by at least 5 mm Hg (in patients aged >50 years) and CHD mortality by about 16%. Regarding the damaging effect of high sodium intake on the heart, and despite the lack of strong data showing the beneficial effect of reducing sodium intake in that specific group of patients, we believe that cardiologists should extend their dietary counseling about sodium not only to the patients with hypertension or chronic heart failure, but also to all post-MI patients.

DIET AND THE PREVENTION OF PLAQUE INFLAMMATION AND RUPTURE

For several decades, the prevention of CHD (including the prevention of ischemic recurrence after a prior acute MI) has focused on the reduction of the traditional risk factors: smoking, hypertension, and hypercholesterolemia. Priority was given to the prevention (or reversion) of vascular atherosclerotic stenosis. As discussed earlier, it has become clear in secondary prevention that clinical efficiency needs to prevent primarily the fatal complications of CHD, such as SCD. This does not mean, however, that we should not try slowing down the atherosclerotic process, in particular plaque inflammation and rupture. It is crucial to prevent the occurrence of new episodes of myocardial ischemia, whose repetition in a recently injured heart can precipitate SCD or chronic heart failure. Myocardial ischemia is usually the consequence of coronary occlusion caused by plaque rupture and subsequent thrombotic obstruction of the artery. Progress in the understanding of the cellular and biochemical pathogenesis of atherosclerosis suggests that, in addition to the traditional risk factors of CHD, there are other important targets of therapy to prevent plaque inflammation and rupture. In this regard, the most important question is how and why does plaque rupture occur?

Coronary Heart Disease—an Inflammatory Disease

Most investigators agree that atherosclerosis is a chronic inflammatory disease.[29] Proinflammatory factors (free radicals produced by cigarette smoking, hyperhomocysteinemia, diabetes, peroxidized lipids, hypertension, elevated and modified blood lipids) contribute to injure the vascular endothelium, which results in alterations of its antiatherosclerotic and antithrombotic properties. This is thought to be a major step in the initiation and formation of arterial fibrostenotic lesions.[29] From a clinical point of view, however, an essential distinction should be made between unstable, lipid-rich, and leukocyte-rich lesions and stable, acellular fibrotic lesions poor in lipids because the propensity of these two types of lesion to rupture into the lumen of the artery, whatever the degree of stenosis and lumen obstruction, is different.

In 1987, we proposed that inflammation and leukocytes play a role in the onset of acute CHD events.[83] This proposal has been confirmed.[32-35] It now is accepted that one of the main mechanisms underlying the sudden onset of acute CHD syndromes, including unstable angina, MI, and SCD, is the erosion or rupture of an atherosclerotic lesion,[32,33] which triggers thrombotic complications and considerably enhances the risk of malignant ventricular arrhythmias.[34,35] Leukocytes also have been implicated in the occurrence of ventricular arrhythmias in clinical and experimental settings,[84,85] and they contribute to myocardial damage during ischemia and reperfusion.[103] Clinical and pathologic studies showed the importance of inflammatory cells and immune mediators in the occurrence of acute CHD events,[29,86] and prospective epidemiologic studies showed a strong, consistent association between acute CHD and systemic inflammation markers.[87,88] A major question is why there are macrophages and activated lymphocytes[29] in atherosclerotic lesions and how they get there. Discussion of issues such as local inflammation, plaque rupture, and attendant acute CHD complications follows.

Lipid Oxidation Theory of Coronary Heart Disease

In 1989, Steinberg and associates[89] proposed that oxidation of lipoproteins causes accelerated atherogenesis. Elevated plasma levels of low-density lipoproteins (LDLs) are a major factor of CHD, and reduction of blood LDL levels (e.g., by drugs) results in less CHD. The mechanisms behind the effect of high LDL levels are not fully understood, however. The concept that LDL oxidation is a key characteristic of unstable lesions is supported by many reports.[29] Two processes have been proposed. First, when LDL particles become trapped in the artery wall, they undergo progressive oxidation and are internalized by macrophages, leading to the formation of typical atherosclerotic foam cells. Oxidized LDL is chemotactic for other immune and inflammatory cells and up-regulates the expression of monocyte and endothelial cell genes involved in the inflammatory reaction.[29,89] The inflammatory response itself can have a profound effect on LDL,[29] creating a vicious circle of LDL oxidation, inflammation, and further LDL oxidation. Second, oxidized LDL circulates in the plasma for a period sufficiently long to enter and accumulate in the arterial intima, suggesting that the entry of oxidized lipoproteins within the intima may be another mechanism of lesion inflammation, in particular, in patients without hyperlipidemia.[30,31,90] Elevated plasma levels of oxidized LDL are associated with CHD, and the plasma level of malondialdehyde-modified LDL is higher in patients with unstable CHD syndromes (usually associated with plaque rupture) than in patients with clinically stable CHD.[30] In the accelerated form of CHD typical of post-transplantation patients, higher levels of lipid peroxidation[91-93] and of oxidized LDL[94] were found compared with the stable form of CHD in nontransplanted patients. Reactive oxygen metabolites and oxidants influence thrombus formation,[95] and platelet reactivity is significantly higher in transplanted patients than in nontransplanted CHD patients.[96]

The oxidized LDL theory is consistent with the well-established, lipid-lowering treatment of CHD because there is a positive correlation between plasma levels of LDL and markers of lipid peroxidation,[92,97] and low absolute LDL level results in reduced amounts of LDL available for oxidative modification. LDL levels can be lowered by drugs or by reducing saturated fats in the diet. Reduction of the oxidative susceptibility of LDL was reported when replacing dietary fat with carbohydrates. Pharmacologic/quantitative (lowering of cholesterol) and nutritional/qualitative (high antioxidant intake) approaches toward the prevention of CHD are not mutually exclusive but additive and complementary. An alternative way to reduce LDL concentrations is to replace saturated fats with polyunsaturated fats in the diet. Diets high in PUFA increase the PUFA content of LDL particles, however, and render them more susceptible to oxidation[28] (which would argue against use of such diets; see earlier section on SCD and n-6 PUFA). In the secondary prevention of CHD, such diets failed to improve the prognosis of the patients.[36] In that context, the traditional Mediterranean diet, with low saturated fat and polyunsaturated fat intakes, seems to be the best option. Diets rich in oleic acid increase the resistance of LDL to oxidation independent of the content in antioxidants[98,99] and results in leukocyte inhibition.[100] Oleic acid–rich diets decrease the proinflammatory properties of oxidized LDL. Constituents of olive oil other than oleic acid also may inhibit LDL oxidation.[101] Various components of the Mediterranean diet also may affect LDL oxidation. α-Tocopherol or vitamin C or a diet combining reduced fat, low-fat dairy products, and a high intake of fruits and vegetables was shown to affect favorably either LDL oxidation itself or the cellular consequences of LDL oxidation.[102,103]

Finally, significant correlation was found between certain dietary fatty acids and the fatty acid composition of human atherosclerotic plaques,[104,105] which suggests that dietary fatty acids are incorporated rapidly into the plaques. This incorporation implies a direct influence of dietary fatty acids on plaque formation and the process of plaque rupture. It is conceivable that fatty acids that stimulate oxidation of LDL (n-6 fatty acids) induce plaque rupture, whereas fatty acids that inhibit LDL oxidation (oleic acid) inhibit leukocyte function (n-3 fatty acids)[106] or prevent "endothelial activation," and the expression of proinflammatory proteins (oleic acid and n-3 fatty acids)[107,108] contributes to pacifying and stabilizing the dangerous lesions. In that regard, moderate alcohol consumption, a well-known cardioprotective factor, was shown to be associated with low blood levels of systemic markers of inflammation,[109] suggesting a new protective mechanism to explain the inverse relationship between alcohol and CHD rate. The potential of dietary n-3 fatty acids to reduce the production of inflammatory cytokines[79,80] by leukocytes (as discussed in the section on dietary fatty acids and chronic heart failure) should be emphasized. Because dietary n-3 fatty acids and moderate alcohol consumption are major characteristics of the Mediterranean diet, it is not surprising to observe that this diet was associated with a lower rate of new episodes of chronic heart failure in the Lyon Diet Heart Study.[60]

Any dietary pattern combining a high intake of natural antioxidants, a low intake of saturated fatty acids, a high intake of oleic acid, a low intake of omega-6 fatty acids, and a high intake of omega-3 fatty acids logically would produce a highly cardioprotective effect. This idea is consistent with what we know about the Mediterranean diet pattern[38,39] and with the results of the Lyon Diet Heart Study[19,60,110] and was confirmed by the GISSI investigators.[111]

DIETARY PREVENTION OF POSTANGIOPLASTY RESTENOSIS

Patients treated with percutaneous transluminal coronary angioplasty (PTCA) have a high (15% to 50%, depending on studies) risk of developing restenosis within the first 6 months after the procedure. At present, with the exception of stents coated with antifibrotic substances[112] and probucol (the latter with many unacceptable side effects), there is no drug treatment to prevent that complication. A dietary approach with either n-3 fatty acid or folate supplementation has been proposed.

Several small studies suggested that supplementation with n-3 fatty acids may inhibit restenosis. More recent larger trials set up to prove that effect failed to do so, however.[113-115] In the Coronary Angioplasty Restenosis Trial, in particular, 500 patients were randomly allocated to 5 g/day of a fish oil concentrate or placebo (corn oil) from at least 2 weeks before until 2 months after PTCA.[115] Compliance was documented by measuring the content of n-3 fatty acids in the blood, and patients receiving n-3 fatty acids had a significant reduction in serum triglyceride levels. No effect could be shown, however, on the restenosis rate or coronary atherosclerosis assessed by quantitative coronary angiography after 6 months of treatment.

In these negative trials, patients were treated with high doses of n-3 fatty acids, up to 8 g/day,[114] and no previous data supported the use of such doses in the prevention of CHD. These studies all were performed in patients having had conventional balloon PTCA, and there are no data on patients receiving any type of stent. Finally, one major limitation of the dietary approach of the prevention of restenosis is the theoretical requirement to start supplementation at least a few days before PTCA, whereas many PTCAs are performed in emergency settings or during the subacute phase of acute MI, with no time for a presenting supplementation.

Finally, data suggest that high homocysteine levels could be associated with restenosis and accelerated atherosclerosis,[116,117] and a combination of folic acid, vitamin B_{12}, and pyridoxine (known to decrease homocysteine levels) was shown to reduce the rate of restenosis in a double-blind randomized trial.[117] In that trial, the need for revascularization also was significantly lower in patients receiving the treatment (10.8% versus 22.3%). This finding underlines the potential clinical benefit of the dietary approach to the prevention of restenosis and should be compared with the data of the Lyon Diet Heart Study, in which the patients randomized in the experimental group and following a Mediterranean diet, which is typically a folate-rich diet, also had a lower rate of restenosis after PTCA.[60] Further studies are needed to clarify which component of the vitamin cocktail of the Swiss trial[117] was preventive and which dosage should be the most appropriate. The potential impact of dietary folates in the various clinical manifestations of CHD also is discussed in the section on endothelial dysfunction.

DIETARY APPROACH TO REDUCE CONVENTIONAL RISK FACTORS

Diet and Blood Cholesterol

Cholesterol is a determinant of CHD mortality, and its blood level is regulated at least partly by diet. Few epidemiologic studies have included prospectively analyses of the dietary habits of the studied populations in the evaluation of their risk, however.[118] In the Seven Countries Study, marked differences in CHD mortality, dietary habits, and cholesterol distribution were observed in the different cohorts.[118] Cholesterol levels were high in Northern Europe and in the United States (an average level of 7 mmol/L) and low in rural Japan (an average of 4 mmol/L), and population cholesterol levels were positively associated with CHD mortality (Fig. 44-2). Secondary prevention trials with statins in Northern Europe[119] and Australia[120] confirmed the importance of cholesterol by showing a reduction by 25% to 30% of the relative risk of CHD death in patients taking these drugs. Whether the effect of statins was related entirely to their effect on cholesterol is unknown.

A major (and often underestimated) finding of the Seven Countries Study was the large difference in absolute risk of CHD death at the same level of serum cholesterol in the different cohorts. At a cholesterol level of about 6 mmol/L (see Fig. 44-2), CHD mortality was three times as high in Northern Europe as in Mediterranean Europe (18% versus 6%). This finding sug-

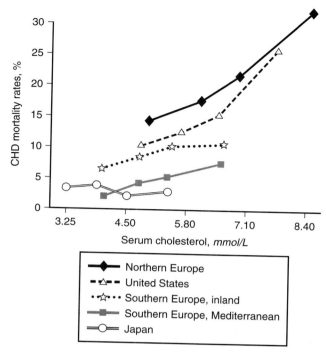

FIGURE 44–2. Coronary heart disease (CHD) mortality in the different cohorts of the Seven Countries Study. Rates of 25-year mortality owing to CHD (adjusted for age, smoking, blood pressure) per quartile of serum cholesterol are shown. The cohorts have been pooled into five populations according to similarities in mortality rates, dietary patterns, and geographic features. (From Kromhout D: On the waves of the Seven Countries Study: A public health perspective on cholesterol. Eur Heart J 1999;20:796–802.)

gested that factors other than cholesterol were playing an important role. Because of the similarity of the other traditional risk factors and the large differences in the dietary habits of the cohorts,[121] it was proposed that the difference in CHD mortality between populations was related mainly to their dietary habits, through biologic effects independent of cholesterol.[122] This was the basis of a new "diet-heart hypothesis," in which cholesterol was not the central issue.[36,122] In fact, the first dietary trials designed for the secondary prevention of CHD were based on the hypothesis that a cardioprotective diet primarily should reduce cholesterol.[36] Although the investigators succeeded in reducing cholesterol, they failed to reduce CHD mortality.[41] This failure was attributed mainly to an insufficient effect of the tested diets on cholesterol, and the conclusion was that cholesterol-lowering drugs should be preferred. None of the diets tested in these old trials was patterned, however, on the traditional diets of populations protected from CHD (e.g., vegetarian, Asian, or Mediterranean), although these diets are associated with low cholesterol.[118,121] Also, no trial was aimed at testing the cholesterol-lowering effect of a typical Mediterranean diet, probably because this diet was (and often still is) regarded mistakenly as a high-fat diet, allegedly not appropriate to reduce cholesterol. Studies investigated, however, the effect of the main lipid-related features of Mediterranean diets, for instance, diets low in saturated and polyunsaturated fat but relatively high in monounsaturated fat.[122-124] Certain

aspects of the Mediterranean diet not related to lipids (e.g., the amount of fiber) were not investigated, although they influence lipid metabolism. The consensus now is, however, that a diet low in saturated and polyunsaturated fat but rich in oleic acid results in a significant reduction of total and LDL cholesterol and has an effect on triglycerides and a small positive or no effect on high-density lipoprotein cholesterol.[122-124] It is not certain whether these results can be reproduced completely in patients with established CHD because none of these studies were conducted in such patients. Finally, as discussed elsewhere in this chapter, the Mediterranean diet was shown to reduce the risk of CHD complications (Fig. 44–3) in secondary prevention[19,60] and should be one of the preferred dietary patterns adopted by post-MI patients. In the Lyon trial, the lipid-lowering effect of the Mediterranean diet was not different from that of the prudent Western diet followed by the control group because lipid-lowering drugs were used widely in the two randomized groups. This finding nonetheless suggested that the Mediterranean diet was cardioprotective through biologic effects independent of its effect on cholesterol. In particular, data from the Lyon trial suggested that the Mediterranean diet might prevent SCD (see earlier section about dietary prevention of SCD).

Diet and Blood Pressure

Blood pressure is related to CHD mortality, and hypertension is a common problem in many Western countries. The relationship between blood pressure and CHD

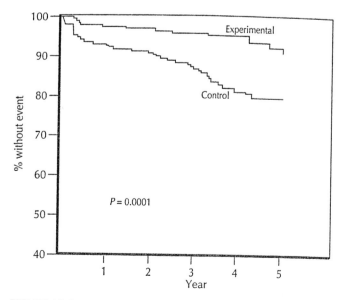

FIGURE 44–3. Results of the Lyon Diet Heart Study. Data are cumulative survivals without recurrent nonfatal acute myocardial infarction in the experimental (Mediterranean group) patients and the control subjects. Patients were randomized an average of 2 months after acute myocardial infarction. Note the early separation of the survival curves. (From de Lorgeril M, Salen P, Martin JL, et al: Mediterranean diet, traditional risk factors and the rate of cardiovascular complications after myocardial infarction: Final report of the Lyon Diet Heart Study. Circulation 1999;99:779–785.)

is continuous, and there is no abrupt increase in risk at levels of blood pressure regarded as criteria for hypertension.[125] This finding suggests that efforts toward the prevention of the blood pressure–related diseases should be focused on hypertensive and on nonhypertensive persons. In secondary prevention, most patients are taking some blood pressure–lowering drugs (often β-blockers) as systematic post-MI treatment. Traditional approaches to control the epidemic of blood pressure–related CHD have concentrated largely on drug therapy in persons with hypertension. Because of the many side effects, however, the rate of discontinuation is high with these classes of drugs.[126] A nondrug therapy, including lifestyle modifications, may have an important and expanding role as a complement of drug therapy, especially in the long-term. Another point is the importance of small differences in blood pressure in terms of outcome. A 5-mm Hg reduction in diastolic blood pressure has been shown to result in a 35% to 40% lower risk of stroke.[127] A significant clinical benefit can be expected even from a small decrease in blood pressure resulting from a dietary change.

Regarding the influence of diet on blood pressure–related CHD complications, data from the Seven Countries Study provide major information.[128] As shown in Figure 44–4, CHD mortality varies greatly among populations at each level of systolic or diastolic blood pressure. At a diastolic blood pressure level of 90 mm Hg, CHD mortality was three times as low among Mediterraneans as among the populations from the United States and Northern Europe. On the same reasoning as for cholesterol, it is presumed that the protective factor is the diet of Mediterraneans. The same reasoning probably applies for the Asian (Japanese) diet. Another question is whether dietary factors influence blood pressure. High sodium intake and binge alcohol drinking certainly increase blood pressure.[129] Whether the Mediterranean diet pattern specifically may influence (decrease?) blood pressure is unknown, although this dietary pattern has been reported to protect the arterial endothelium that is responsible for the production and release of several major vasodilators, including nitric oxide (NO).[130] In the (Mediterranean diet) Lyon trial, the extensive use of blood pressure–lowering drugs in both groups prevented any effect on blood pressure from becoming apparent.

Research has emphasized the powerful role of total diet in hypertension.[129] An adequate intake of minerals (sodium, potassium, magnesium, and calcium), rather than the sole restriction of sodium, was proposed as the focus of dietary recommendations.[131] In this approach, the direct role of high sodium intake on the myocardium is not taken fully into account, however (see section on chronic heart failure and LVH). Other studies suggested that dietary n-3 fatty acids may lower blood pressure in subjects with hypertension.[132] The responses were proportional to the changes in phospholipid n-3 fatty acids, whereas n-6 fatty acids had no effect, which suggests that the effect did result specifically from the n-3 family. These data implied that in addition to their benefits through mechanisms such as the prevention of ventricular arrhythmias (see section on SCD), n-3 fatty acids may be

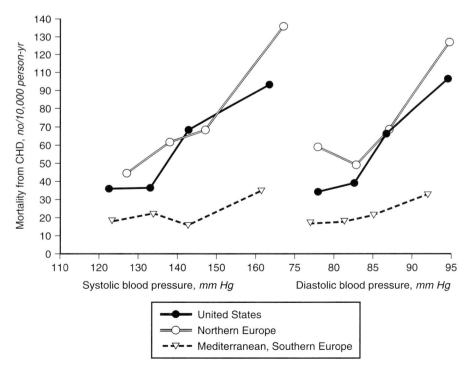

FIGURE 44–4. Mortality resulting from coronary heart disease per quartile of systolic and diastolic blood pressure in three populations with large differences in the prevalence of the disease. Values shown are 25-year rates, adjusted for age, serum cholesterol level, and smoking status. (Modified from Van den Hoogen PCW, Feskens EJM, Nagelkerke NJD, et al: The relation between blood pressure and mortality due to coronary heart disease among men in different parts of the world. N Engl J Med 2000;342:1–8.)

helpful in modulating (endothelial) factors regulating blood pressure.

The DASH (Dietary Approaches to Stop Hypertension) trial tested the effect on blood pressure of either a diet rich in fruits and vegetables or a combination diet rich in fruits, vegetables, and low-fat dairy products, and with reduced saturated and total fat.[133] Although this combination diet was not a typical Mediterranean diet, its main characteristics can be included among those recommended in a Mediterranean diet trial. In the first DASH trial, sodium intake was kept constant, and the combination diet decreased systolic blood pressure by 5 to 6 mm Hg in subjects with normal blood pressure; in subjects with mild hypertension, the blood pressure reduction was twice as great—about 12 mm Hg. Reductions of this magnitude (Fig. 44–5) are similar to those observed with antihypertensive medications, but they are obtained at a much lower cost, particularly in terms of side effects. The first DASH trial confirmed the meta-analyses and earlier indications from observational studies suggesting that dietary factors other than sodium markedly affect blood pressure.[131] In a second trial, the DASH investigators studied the effects of different levels of dietary sodium in conjunction with the DASH diet.[134] As before, the DASH diet substantially lowered systolic and diastolic blood pressure. In addition, at any level of sodium intake, blood pressure was lower among patients following the DASH diet than among those following the control diet.[134] Combining a reduction of sodium intake to levels less than 100 mmol/day and the DASH diet lowers blood pressure to a greater extent than either of the two separately. Whether these dietary changes may reduce the risk of CHD remains to be shown.

Diet and Endothelial Dysfunction

One mechanism that may contribute to the association between high blood pressure and CHD is called *endothelial dysfunction*. The endothelium, the innermost layer of all blood vessels, is crucial in determining the contractile state of the underlying smooth muscle.[135] Through the release of many substances, the endothelium modulates several other functions, including platelet aggregation, leukocyte adhesion and migration, smooth muscle cell proliferation, and lipid oxidation, all of which participate in the atherosclerotic process. The term *endothelial dysfunction* has been used to describe a constellation of abnormalities in these regulatory actions of the endothelium, and endothelial dysfunction has been reported in conditions such as hypercholesterolemia, hypertension, diabetes, and hyperhomocysteinemia. In patients with hypertension, there is an imbalance in the bioactivity of endothelial factors with proatherosclerotic (endothelin-1) and antiatherosclerotic (NO) actions[136] that may explain why hypertension is a risk factor for CHD, regardless of whether endothelial dysfunction is a cause or a consequence of hypertension. Coronary endothelial dysfunction by itself was shown to be of prognostic significance in patients with CHD.[137] Endothelium-derived NO plays an important role in the regulation of tissue perfusion, and evidence is accumulating that NO-dependent vasodilation and NO availability are impaired in the coronary arteries of patients with CHD or with CHD risk factors such as high blood cholesterol or homocysteine levels. Folic acid therapy, either as long-term oral supplementation or as acute intra-arterial administration of the active form of folic acid (5-methyltetrahydrofolate), restores the impaired endothelial function even in patients with CHD risk factors but normal serum folic acid and homocysteine levels.[138,139] Also, a deficient NO-synthase cofactor, tetrahydrobiopterin (BH4), may be involved in blunted endothelium-dependent vasodilation in humans.[140] In the case of BH4 deficiency, uncoupling of the L-arginine-NO pathway is observed, resulting in increased formation of oxygen radicals. Intra-arterial or intracoronary infusion of BH4 was shown to improve endothelial dysfunction in patients with various clinical manifestations.[140,141] The key point here is that the active

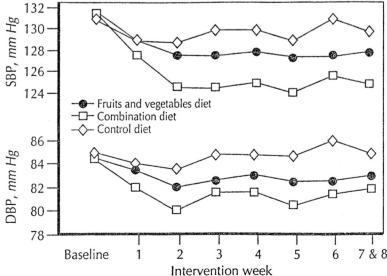

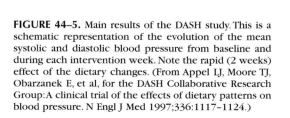

FIGURE 44–5. Main results of the DASH study. This is a schematic representation of the evolution of the mean systolic and diastolic blood pressure from baseline and during each intervention week. Note the rapid (2 weeks) effect of the dietary changes. (From Appel LJ, Moore TJ, Obarzanek E, et al, for the DASH Collaborative Research Group: A clinical trial of the effects of dietary patterns on blood pressure. N Engl J Med 1997;336:1117–1124.)

form of folic acid is involved in the endogenous regeneration of BH4, suggesting a major interaction between the arginine-NO-synthase pathway and folic acid. An adequate amount of folates in the diet seems to be crucial to protect the endothelium (and for the prevention of endothelial dysfunction) and, in general, for the prevention and treatment of CHD far beyond a simple effect on homocysteine (see earlier).

Another cause of endothelial dysfunction in the context of traditional risk factors of CHD (including hypertension, dyslipidemias, and insulin resistance) is an elevated level of asymmetric dimethyl arginine (ADMA), which also inhibits the production of NO.[142] Although blood ADMA levels seem under the influence of dietary fats, further studies are required to clarify the relationship between the dietary factors (folates, antioxidants) involved in the regulation of NO-synthase and ADMA metabolism.

A diet rich in vegetables and fruits and the traditional Mediterranean diet provide large amounts of folates. Consumption of legumes (dry beans and peas, peanuts, peanut butter, lentils), which is another typical Mediterranean habit, is a major source of folates and has been shown to be associated with a reduced risk of CHD.[143] Also, tree nuts, such as walnut and hazelnut (also a usual ingredient of vegetarian and Mediterranean diets), can help supply patients with folates. Most nuts also are rich in arginine, an amino acid serving as substrate for the synthesis of NO. Because of the importance of NO in cardiovascular diseases, there has been growing interest in using arginine to prevent and treat cardiovascular diseases.[144] Compelling evidence shows that enteral or parenteral administration of arginine reverses endothelial dysfunction associated with major CHD risk factors in a way similar to that observed with folic acid and BH4. Endothelial arginine is derived from the plasma, via intracellular synthesis with citrulline as a precursor, and from the net degradation of intracellular proteins. Food is the ultimate source of arginine for the body, however. Dietary arginine intake (the main source being animal products for the Western population) by an adult has been estimated to be around 5 g/day.[144] Because of arginase activity in the intestine and of the limited digestibility of protein-bound arginine, it is assumed that only 50% of dietary arginine enters the systemic circulation. The adequate daily arginine requirement is difficult to assess and probably varies in accordance with the presence or absence of CHD risk factors, which often are associated with the presence of endogenous NO-synthase inhibitors. It probably also varies with the amount of folates in the diet because the active form of folic acid is indispensable for the regeneration of BH4. The amount of arginine found in the typical Western diet seems at best barely sufficient to cover the daily requirements of a healthy individual.

In the presence of CHD risk factors or established CHD, the intake of arginine would tend to decrease as patients turn away from animal foods, which, though protein-rich, are considered "unhealthy for the heart" in other respects. The exact requirements of these patients are yet to be determined, but previous studies suggested that to reverse endothelial dysfunction, an amount on the order of 6 to 9 g

above dietary supplies might be necessary. Other factors, such as impaired intestinal absorption, competition with other amino acids (in particular, lysine) for cell transport, and the amount of folates in the diet, were not taken into account in these calculations. Whatever the clinical condition, nuts are a convenient natural source of arginine, not only because of the high concentration of arginine in most nuts, but also because nuts have high levels of folates and vitamin B_6, the major cofactors involved in the catabolism or recycling of homocysteine.

Diet and Type 2 Diabetes

Patients with type 1 diabetes are rare among patients considered for secondary prevention of CHD. Apart from the dietary prevention recommended for nondiabetic patients, patients with type 1 diabetes do not raise specific dietary issues beyond the usual diabetic diet to control blood glucose when insulin treatment is correctly administered. In contrast, the number of patients with type 2 diabetes or insulin resistance is increasing rapidly, and cardiologists have to manage that specific problem in more post-MI patients.

Type 2 diabetes mellitus is associated with a threefold to fourfold increase in the incidence of CHD,[145] and the risk of CHD death is as high in diabetics without CHD as in nondiabetic patients with established CHD.[146] The decline in CHD mortality in most Western populations has been attributed mainly to reduction of risk factors, owing to dietary changes in particular. The smaller decline in CHD mortality among diabetics, particularly women, may be due to less effective changes in risk factors for those patients. Apart from calorie restriction, the composition of the diet of patients with type 2 diabetes is controversial. The emphasis currently is on a diet low in saturated fatty acids. A reduction of the total fat intake also is suggested when weight loss is a primary issue. Because most type 2 diabetics should lose weight, a low-fat diet commonly is prescribed. Many physicians are still reluctant to recommend such a diet, however, because they think that a diet high in monounsaturated fats improves metabolic control in these patients better than a low-fat, high-carbohydrate diet and should be preferred.[147] On the basis of a meta-analysis, diets high in monounsaturated fat improve the lipoprotein and blood glucose profiles and lower blood pressure.[147] This type of diet also may reduce the susceptibility of LDL particles to oxidation and reduce their atherogenic potential; in addition, it does not induce weight gain, provided that energy intake is controlled. In theory, diets low in saturated fatty acids but rich in monounsaturated fats (two of the main characteristics of the Mediterranean diet) are advantageous for the prevention of CHD in diabetics. No diabetic diet has been tested in this way for the prevention of CHD.

An important message from UKPDS and other trials is that in the prevention of CHD in type 2 diabetics, it is unwise to focus on single risk factors.[148] All known risk factors should be addressed simultaneously, including hyperlipemia and hypertension. Also, because of a high risk of SCD in diabetics, specific recommendations aimed at preventing SCD should be given (see earlier).

Classic risk factors fail to explain the excess CHD rate in Indians compared with Europeans, although the high prevalence of diabetes in India may play a part.[149] When exploring the contribution of dietary fatty acids in Indian diabetics, large differences in phospholipid fatty acids were noted, with lower concentrations of n-3 fatty acids among Indians,[150] suggesting an explanation for their high CHD mortality.

Considering all of these observations, it seems that the optimal diabetic diet may be a low-calorie Mediterranean diet. Not only does this diet protect the heart, improve lipid profiles, and reduce blood pressure, but also certain components of the Mediterranean diet (n-3 fatty acids in association with vegetables and legumes) have been shown to improve glucose tolerance and prevent the apparition of overt diabetes.[151] These human data confirm animal research that showed the importance of n-3 fatty acids in the action of insulin in various experimental models.[152] Although further studies are required, in particular, about the physical structure of foods to modulate glucose metabolism and insulin resistance,[153] it is clear that diabetics should be instructed in the basic principles of the Mediterranean diet.

Diet, Overweight, and Obesity

Another question is why the incidence of type 2 diabetes has increased so rapidly. Considerable epidemiologic evidence points to excess caloric intake and physical inactivity as the major reasons. The problem of obesity and overweight in patients with established CHD and specifically after a recent acute MI is beyond the scope of this chapter. Obesity and overweight are associated with a clustering of CHD risk factors, and weight reduction results in favorable changes in the risk factor profile of most individuals. Weight reduction efforts have met with limited success in the general population, however, and the treatment of obesity is complex and difficult. There is no reason (and no published data) to believe that the situation is different among patients with CHD. There are controversies regarding the efficacy, benefits, and consequences of high-carbohydrate, low-fat, very-low-fat, or high-protein diets, all of which have been proposed as the best way to reduce weight. Despite the fact that having (or maintaining or reaching) a healthy body weight has been claimed a major goal of the dietary prevention of CHD in primary prevention,[154] we do not believe that this is true in secondary prevention as well. As discussed in the previous sections (and summarized in the last section), there are other dietary priorities for which we have scientific evidence showing that the patients with CHD get immediate and major clinical benefits by adhering to them. In CHD patients with extreme obesity or asking spontaneously for a slimming diet, that issue should be addressed appropriately. Keeping in line with the principle of "clinical rather than surrogate efficacy," we admit that we have only a few scientific data on the topic "slimming diet in CHD patients." No dietary (or pharmacologic) trial has been conducted so far to test whether weight loss is associated with improved prognosis in patients with CHD. Finally, whether a high-protein or high-carbohydrate diet or any other diet, in addition to a low-energy diet, is preferable is an open question.

MINIMUM CLINICAL PRIORITY DIETARY PROGRAM

Despite the increased evidence that dietary prevention is crucial in the post–acute MI patient, many physicians (and patients) remain poorly informed about the potential of diet to reduce cardiac mortality, the risk of new CHD complications, and the need for recurrent hospitalization and investigation. There are many reasons for that, the main one probably being an insufficient knowledge of nutrition.[155] For that reason (and knowing the resistance of many physicians to accept the idea that diet is important in CHD), we propose a minimum dietary program that every CHD patient, whatever his or her medical and familial environment, should know and follow. Based on the clinical priorities of secondary prevention discussed in this chapter, the minimum Mediterranean dietary program should include the following:

1. Reduced consumption of animal saturated fat (e.g., by totally excluding butter and cream from the daily diet and drastic reduction of fatty meat) and increased consumption of n-3 fatty acids through increased intakes of fatty fish (about 200 g, twice a week). For patients who cannot eat fish (for any reason), taking capsules of n-3 fatty acids (e.g., a mix of α-linolenic acid and long-chain n-3 fatty acids) is the best alternative option. With this comprehensive approach, some ways of presenting or cooking fish (salted, deeply fried with saturated or polyunsaturated fat) should be avoided. Importantly, the patients (and their physicians) should be aware that n-3 fatty acid supplementation will be more cardioprotective if associated with adequate dietary modifications discussed earlier.[156]

2. Increased intake of anti-inflammatory fatty acids (oleic acid and n-3 fatty acids) and decreased intake of proinflammatory fatty acids (n-6 fatty acids). The best way is to use exclusively olive oil and canola oil for cooking and salad dressing and canola oil–based margarine instead of butter and polyunsaturated oils and margarines.[157-159] Patients also should systematically reject convenience food prepared with fats rich in saturated, polyunsaturated, and trans fatty acids.

3. Increased intake of natural antioxidants (vitamins and trace elements) and folates through increased consumption of fresh fruits and vegetables and tree nuts.[160]

4. Moderate intake of alcoholic beverages (1 or 2 drinks per day), preferably wine, preferably during the evening meal, and never before driving or engaging in a dangerous technical manipulation.

5. Reduction of sodium intake (<100 mmol/day if possible). This is a difficult task at present because of the high sodium content of many natural (including typical Mediterranean foods such as olives and cheeses) and convenience foods.

Patients (and physicians) should keep in mind that an optimal (and individual) dietary prevention program should be managed under the guidance of a professional dietician aware of the most recent scientific advances in the field.

REFERENCES

1. Zipes DP, Wellens HJ: Sudden cardiac death. Circulation 1998;98: 2234-2251.
2. de Lorgeril M, Salen P, Defaye P, et al: Dietary prevention of sudden cardiac death. Eur Heart J 2002;23:277-285.
3. Burr ML, Fehily AM, Gilbert JF, et al: Effects of changes in fat, fish, and fibre intakes on death and myocardial reinfarction. Diet And Reinfarction Trial (DART). Lancet 1989;2:757-761.
4. McLennan PL, Abeywardena MY, Charnock JS: Reversal of arrhythmogenic effects of long term saturated fatty acid intake by dietary n-3 and n-6 polyunsaturated fatty acids. Am J Clin Nutr 1990;51:53-58.
5. McLennan PL, Abeywardena MY, Charnock JS: Dietary fish oil prevents ventricular fibrillation following coronary occlusion and reperfusion. Am Heart J 1988;16:709-716.
6. Billman GE, Kang JX, Leaf A: Prevention of sudden cardiac death by dietary pure omega-3 polyunsaturated fatty acids in dogs. Circulation 1999;99:2452-2457.
7. Nair SD, Leitch J, Falconer J, et al: Cardiac (n-3) non-esterified fatty acids are selectively increased in fish oil-fed pigs following myocardial ischemia. J Nutr 1999;129:1518-1523.
8. Harris SW, Lu G, Rambjor GS, et al: Influence of (n-3) fatty acid supplementation on the endogenous activities of plasma lipases. Am J Clin Nutr 1997;66:254-260.
9. Kang JX, Xiao Y-F, Leaf A: Free, long-chain, polyunsaturated fatty acids reduce membrane electrical excitability in neonatal rat cardiomyocyte. Proc Natl Acad Sci U S A 1995;92:3997-4001.
10. Xiao Y-F, Kang JX, Morgan JP, et al: Blocking effects of polyunsaturated fatty acids on Na channels of neonatal rat ventricular myocytes. Proc Natl Acad Sci U S A 1995;92:1100-1104.
11. Xiao Y-F, Wright SN, Wang GK, et al: n-3 fatty acids suppress voltage-gated Na currents in HEK293t cells transfected with the alpha-subunit of the human cardiac Na channel. Proc Natl Acad Sci U S A 1998;95:2680-2685.
12. Xiao Y-F, Gomez AM, Morgan JP, et al: Suppression of voltage-gated L-type Ca currents by polyunsaturated fatty acids in neonatal and adult cardiac myocytes. Proc Natl Acad Sci U S A 1997;94: 4182-4187.
13. Corr PB, Saffitz JE, Sobel BE: What is the contribution of altered lipid metabolism to arrhythmogenesis in the ischemic heart? In Hearse DJ, Manning AS, Janse MJ (eds): Life Threatening Arrhythmias During Ischemia and Infarction. New York, Raven Press, 1987, pp 91-114.
14. Parratt JR, Coker SJ, Wainwright CL: Eicosanoids and susceptibility to ventricular arrhythmias during myocardial ischemia and reperfusion. J Mol Cell Cardiol 1987;19(Suppl 5):55-66.
15. Sellmayer A, Witzgall H, Lorenz RL, et al: Effects of dietary fish oil on ventricular premature complexes. Am J Cardiol 1995;76:974-977.
16. Christensen JH, Gustenhoff P, Korup E, et al: Effect of fish oil on heart rate variability in survivors of myocardial infarction: A double blind randomised controlled trial. BMJ 1996;312:677-678.
17. Christensen JH, Christensen MS, Dyerberg J, et al: Heart rate variability and fatty acid content of blood cell membranes: A dose-response study with n-3 fatty acids. Am J Clin Nutr 1999;70: 331-337.
18. Singh RB, Rastogi SS, Verma R, et al: Randomised controlled trial of cardioprotective diet in patients with recent acute myocardial infarction: Results of one year follow-up. BMJ 1992;304:1015-1019.
19. de Lorgeril M, Renaud S, Mamelle N, et al: Mediterranean alpha-linolenic acid-rich diet in secondary prevention of coronary heart disease. Lancet 1994;343:1454-1459.
20. Siscovick DS, Raghunathan TE, King I, et al: Dietary intake and cell membrane levels of long-chain n-3 polyunsaturated fatty acids and the risk of primary cardiac arrest. JAMA 1995;274:1363-1367.
21. Kromhout D, Bosschieter EB, de Lezenne Coulander C: The inverse relation between fish consumption and 20-year mortality from coronary heart disease. N Engl J Med 1985;312:1205-1209.
22. Shekelle RB, Missel L, Paul O, et al: Fish consumption and mortality from coronary heart disease. N Engl J Med 1985;313:820.
23. Albert CM, Hennekens CH, O'Donnel CJ, et al: Fish consumption and the risk of sudden cardiac death. JAMA 1998;279:23-28.
24. Daviglus ML, Stamler J, Orencia AJ, et al: Fish consumption and the 30-year risk of fatal myocardial infarction. N Engl J Med 1997;336:1046-1053.
25. GISSI-Prevenzione investigators: Dietary supplementation with n-3 polyunsaturated fatty acids and vitamin E after myocardial infarction: Results of the GISSI-Prevenzione trial. Lancet 1999;354: 447-455.
26. Keys A: Seven Countries: A Multivariate Analysis of Death and Coronary Heart Disease. A Commonwealth Fund Book. Cambridge, Harvard University Press, 1980.
27. Roberts TL, Wood DA, Riemersma RA, et al: Linoleic acid and risk of sudden cardiac death. Br Heart J 1993;70:524-529.
28. Louheranta AM, Porkkala-Sarataho EK, Nyyssönen MK, et al: Linoleic acid intake and susceptibility of very-low-density and low-density lipoproteins to oxidation in men. Am J Clin Nutr 1996;63:698-703.
29. Ross R: Atherosclerosis: An inflammatory disease. N Engl J Med 1999;340:115-126.
30. Holvoet P, Vanhaecke J, Janssens S, et al: Oxidized LDL and malondialdehyde-modified LDL in patients with acute coronary syndromes and stable coronary artery disease. Circulation 1998;98:1487-1494.
31. Juul K, Nielsen LB, Munkholm K, et al: Oxidation of plasma low-density lipoprotein accelerates its accumulation in the arterial wall in vivo. Circulation 1996;94:1698-1704.
32. Moreno PR, Falk E, Palacios JF, et al: Macrophage infiltration in acute coronary syndromes: Implications for plaque rupture. Circulation 1994;90:775-778.
33. Van der Wal AC, Becker EC, Van der los DS, et al: Site of intimal rupture or erosion of thrombosed coronary atherosclerotic plaques is characterized by an inflammatory process irrespective of the dominant plaque morphology. Circulation 1994;89:36-44.
34. Farb A, Burk AP, Tang AL, et al: Coronary plaque erosion without rupture into a lipid core: A frequent cause of coronary thrombosis in sudden coronary death. Circulation 1996;93:1354-1363.
35. Davies MJ, Thomas A: Thrombosis and acute coronary-artery lesions in sudden cardiac ischemic death. N Engl J Med 1984;310: 1137-1140.
36. de Lorgeril M, Salen P, Monjaud I, et al: The diet heart hypothesis in secondary prevention of coronary heart disease. Eur Heart J 1997;18:14-18.
37. Dayton S, Pearce ML, Hashimoto S, et al: A controlled trial of a diet high in unsaturated fat in preventing complications of atherosclerosis. Circulation 1969;34(Suppl II):1-63.
38. de Lorgeril M, Salen P: Modified Mediterranean diet in the prevention of coronary heart disease and cancer. World Rev Nutr Diet 2000;87:1-23.
39. Simopoulos AP, Sidossis LS: What is so special about the traditional diet of Greece: The scientific evidence. World Rev Nutr Diet 2000;87:24-42.
40. Roberts TL, Wood DA, Riemersma RA, et al: Trans isomers of oleic and linoleic acids in adipose tissue and sudden cardiac death. Lancet 1995;345:278-282.
41. Lemaitre RN, King IB, Raghunathan TE, et al: Cell membrane trans-fatty acids and the risk of primary cardiac arrest. Circulation 2002;105:697-701.
42. Wannamethee G, Shaper AG: Alcohol and sudden cardiac death. Br Heart J 1992;68:443-448.
43. Kagan A, Yano K, Reed DM, et al: Predictors of sudden cardiac death among Hawaiian-Japanese men. Am J Epidemiol 1989;130: 268-277.
44. Albert CM, Manson JE, Cook NR, et al: Moderate alcohol consumption and the risk of sudden cardiac death among US male physicians. Circulation 1999;100:944-950.
45. Rimm EB, Stampfer MJ, Ascherio A, et al: Vitamin E consumption and the risk of coronary heart disease in men. N Engl J Med 1993;328:1450-1456.
46. Stampfer MJ, Hennekens CH, Manson JE, et al: Vitamin E consumption and the risk of coronary heart disease in women. N Engl J Med 1993;328:1444-1449.

47. Alpha-Tocopherol, Beta-Carotene Cancer Prevention Study Group: The effect of vitamin E and beta-carotene on the incidence of lung cancer and other cancers in male smokers. N Engl J Med 1994;330:1029-1035.

48. Rapola JM, Virtamo J, Ripatti S, et al: Randomised trial of alpha-tocopherol and beta-carotene supplements on incidence of major coronary events in men with previous myocardial infarction. Lancet 1997;349:1715-1720.

49. Stephens NG, Parsons A, Schofield PM, et al: Randomised controlled trial of vitamin E in patients with coronary heart disease. The Cambridge Heart Antioxidant Study (CHAOS). Lancet 1996;347:781-786.

50. Sebbag L, Forrat R, Canet E, et al: Effect of dietary supplementation with alpha-tocopherol on myocardial infarct size and ventricular arrhythmias in a dog model of ischemia and reperfusion. J Am Coll Cardiol 1994;24:1580-1585.

51. Heart Outcome Prevention Evaluation (HOPE) study investigators: Vitamin E supplementation and cardiovascular events in high-risk patients. N Engl J Med 2000;342:154-160.

52. Cowie MR, Mostred A, Wood DA, et al: The epidemiology of heart failure. Eur Heart J 1997;18:208-225.

53. Levine B, Kalman J, Mayer L, et al: Elevated circulating levels of tumor necrosis factor in severe chronic heart failure. N Engl J Med 1990;323:236-241.

54. Swan JW, Anker SD, Walton C, et al: Insulin resistance in chronic heart failure: Relation to severity and etiology of heart failure. J Am Coll Cardiol 1997;30:527-532.

55. Keith M, Geranmayegan A, Sole MJ, et al: Increased oxidative stress in patients with congestive heart failure. J Am Coll Cardiol 1998;31:1352-1356.

56. Evans P, Halliwell B: Micronutrients: Oxidant/antioxidant status. Br J Nutr 2001;85:S67-S74.

57. Dhalla AK, Hill M, Singal PK: Role of oxidative stress in transition of hypertrophy to heart failure. J Am Coll Cardiol 1996;28:506-514.

58. de Lorgeril M, Salen P, Accominotti M, et al: Dietary blood antioxidants in patients with chronic heart failure: Insights into the potential importance of selenium in heart failure. Eur J Heart Fail 2001;3:661-669.

59. Hornig B, Arakawa N, Kohler C, Drexler H: Vitamin C improves endothelial function of conduit arteries in patients with chronic heart failure. Circulation 1998;97:363-368.

60. de Lorgeril M, Salen P, Martin JL, et al: Mediterranean diet, traditional risk factors and the rate of cardiovascular complications after myocardial infarction: Final report of the Lyon Diet Heart Study. Circulation 1999;99:779-785.

61. Jacobson A, Pihl-Lindgren E, Fridlund B: Malnutrition in patients suffering from chronic heart failure: The nurse's care. Eur J Heart Failure 2001;3:449-456.

62. Pittman JG, Cohen P: The pathogenesis of cardiac cachexia. N Engl J Med 1964;271:453-460.

63. Anker SD, Clark AL, Kemp M, et al: Tumor necrosis factor and steroid metabolism in chronic heart failure: Possible relation to muscle wasting. J Am Coll Cardiol 1997;30:997-1001.

64. Tsutamoto T, Atsuyuki W, Matsumoto T, et al: Relationship between tumor necrosis factor-alpha and oxidative stress in the failing hearts of patients with dilated cardiomyopathy. J Am Coll Cardiol 2001;37:2086-2092.

65. Anker SD, Ponikowski P, Varney S, et al: Wasting as independent risk factor for mortality in chronic heart failure. Lancet 1997;349:1050-1053.

66. Witte KK, Clark AL, Cleland JG: Chronic heart failure and micronutrients. J Am Coll Cardiol 2001;37:1765-1774.

67. Rimailho A, Bouchard P, Schaison G, et al: Improvement of hypocalcemic cardiomyopathy by correction of serum calcium level. Am Heart J 1985;109:611-613.

68. Gottlieb SS, Baruch L, Kukin ML, et al: Prognostic importance of the serum magnesium concentration in patients with congestive heart failure. J Am Coll Cardiol 1990;16:827-831.

69. Golik A, Cohen N, Ramot Y, et al: Type II diabetes mellitus, congestive cardiac failure and zinc metabolism. Biol Trace Elem Res 1993;39:171-175.

70. Ge K, Yang G: The epidemiology of selenium deficiency in the etiological study of endemic diseases in China. Am J Clin Nutr 1993;57(Suppl):259S-263S.

71. Chariot P, Perchet H, Monnet I: Dilated cardiomyopathy in HIV-infected patients. N Engl J Med 1999;340:732.

72. Shimon I, Shlomo A, Vered Z, et al: Improved left ventricular function after thiamine supplementation in patients with congestive heart failure receiving long-term furosemide therapy. Am J Med 1995;98:485-490.

73. Levy D, Garrison RJ, Savage DD, et al: Prognostic implications of echocardiographically determined left ventricular mass in the Framingham Heart Study. N Engl J Med 1990;322:1561-1566.

74. Koren MJ, Devereux RB, Casale NB, et al: Relation of left ventricular mass and geometry to morbidity and mortality in uncomplicated essential hypertension. Ann Intern Med 1991;114:345-352.

75. Dahlof B, Pennert K, Hansson L: Reversal of left ventricular hypertrophy in hypertensive patients: A meta-analysis of 109 treatment studies. Am J Hypertens 1992;5:95-110.

76. Sundström J, Lind L, Vessby B, et al: Dyslipidemia and an unfavorable fatty acid profile predict left ventricular hypertrophy 20 years later. Circulation 2001;103:836-841.

77. Gullestad L, Aukrust P, Ueland T, et al: Effect of high versus low-dose angiotensin converting enzyme inhibition on cytokine levels in chronic heart failure. J Am Coll Cardiol 1999;34:2061-2067.

78. Bozkurt B, Torre-Amione G, Warren MS, et al: Results of targeted anti-tumor necrosis factor therapy with etanercept (ENBREL) in patients with advanced heart failure. Circulation 2001;103:1044-1046.

79. Endres S, Ghorbani R, Kelley VE, et al: The effect of dietary supplementation with n-3 polyunsaturated fatty acids on the synthesis of interleukine-1 and tumor necrosis factor by mononuclear cells. N Engl J Med 1989;320:265-271.

80. Caughey GE, Mantzioris E, Gibson RA, et al: The effect on human tumor necrosis factor and interleukine-1 production of diets enriched in n-3 fatty acids from vegetable oil or fish oil. Am J Clin Nutr 1996;63:116-122.

81. Frohlich ED, Chien EY, Sesoko S, Pegram BL: Relationship between dietary sodium intake, hemodynamics, and cardiac mass in SHR and WKY rats. Am J Physiol 1993;264:30-34.

82. Schmieder RE, Messerli FH, Caravaglia GE, Nunez BD: Dietary salt intake: A determinant of cardiac involvement in essential hypertension. Circulation 1988;78:951-956.

83. de Lorgeril M, Latour JG: Leukocytes, thrombosis and unstable angina. N Engl J Med 1987;316:1161.

84. de Lorgeril M, Basmadjian A, Lavallée M, et al: Influence of leukopenia on collateral flow, reperfusion flow, reflow ventricular fibrillation, and infarct size in dogs. Am Heart J 1989;117:523-532.

85. Kuzuya T, Hoshida S, Suzuki K, et al: Polymorphonuclear leukocyte activity and ventricular arrhythmia in acute myocardial infarction. Am J Cardiol 1988;62:868-872.

86. Liuzzo G, Biasucci LM, Gallimore JR, et al: The prognostic value of C-reactive protein and serum amyloid A protein in severe unstable angina. N Engl J Med 1994;331:417-424.

87. Ernst E, Hammerschmidt DE, Bagge U, et al: Leukocytes and the risk of ischemic heart diseases. JAMA 1987;257:2318-2324.

88. Kruskal JB, Commerford PJ, Franks JJ, Kirsch RE: Fibrin and fibrinogen-related antigens in patients with stable and unstable coronary artery disease. N Engl J Med 1987;317:1361-1365.

89. Steinberg D, Parthasarathy S, Carew TE, et al: Beyond cholesterol: Modifications of low-density lipoproteins that increase its atherogenicity. N Engl J Med 1989;320:915-924.

90. Hodis HN, Kramsch DM, Avogaro P, et al: Biochemical and cytotoxic characteristics of an in vivo circulating oxidized low density lipoprotein. J Lipid Res 1994;35:669-677.

91. Holvoet P, Stassen JM, Van Cleemput J, et al: Correlation between oxidized low density lipoproteins and coronary artery disease in heart transplant patients. Arterioscler Thromb Vasc Biol 1998;18:100-107.

92. Chancerelle Y, de Lorgeril M, Viret R, et al: Increased lipid peroxidation in cyclosporin-treated heart transplant recipients. Am J Cardiol 1991;68:813-817.

93. de Lorgeril M, Richard MJ, Arnaud J, et al: Lipid peroxides and antioxidant defenses in accelerated transplantation-associated arteriosclerosis. Am Heart J 1992;125:974-980.

94. Holvoet P, Perez G, Zhao Z, et al: Malondialdehyde-modified low density lipoproteins in patients with atherosclerotic disease. J Clin Invest 1995;95:2611-2619.

95. Ambrosio G, Tritto I, Golino P: Reactive oxygen metabolites and arterial thrombosis. Cardiovasc Res 1997;34:445-452.

96. de Lorgeril M, Dureau G, Boissonnat P, et al: Platelet function and composition in heart transplant recipients compared with

nontransplanted coronary patients. Arterioscler Thromb 1992;12: 222–230.

97. Zock PL, Katan MB: Diet, LDL oxidation and coronary artery disease. Am J Clin Nutr 1998;68:759–760.

98. Bonamone A, Pagnan A, Biffanti S, et al: Effect of dietary monounsaturated and polyunsaturated fatty acids on the susceptibility of plasma low density lipoproteins to oxidative modification. Arterioscler Thromb 1992;12:529–533.

99. Tsimikas S, Reaven PD: The role of dietary fatty acids in lipoprotein oxidation and atherosclerosis. Curr Opin Lipidol 1998;9: 301–307.

100. Mata P, Alonso R, Lopez-Farre A, et al: Effect of dietary fat saturation on LDL and monocyte adhesion to human endothelial cells in vitro. Arterioscler Thromb Vasc Biol 1996;16:1347–1355.

101. Visioli F, Bellomo G, Montedoro G, et al: Low density lipoprotein oxidation is inhibited in vitro by olive oil constituents. Atherosclerosis 1995;117:25–32.

102. Jialal I, Grundy SM: Effect of combined supplementation with alpha-tocopherol, ascorbate and beta-carotene on low density lipoprotein oxidation. Circulation 1993;88:2780–2786.

103. Miller ER III, Appel LJ, Risby TH: Effect of dietary patterns on measures of lipid peroxidation: Results of a randomized clinical trial. Circulation 1998;98:2390–2395.

104. Felton CV, Crook D, Davies MJ, Oliver MF: Dietary polyunsaturated fatty acids and composition of human aortic plaques. Lancet 1994;344:1195–1196.

105. Rapp JH, Connor WE, Lin DS, Porter JM: Dietary eicosapentanoic acid and docosahexaenoic acid from fish oil: Their incorporation into advanced human atherosclerotic plaques. Arterioscler Thromb 1991;11:903–911.

106. Lee TH, Hoover RL, Williams JD, et al: Effect of dietary enrichment with eisosapentanoic and docosahexaenoic acids on in-vitro neutrophil and monocyte leukotriene generation and neutrophile function. N Engl J Med 1985;312:1217–1224.

107. De Caterina R, Cybulsky MI, Clinton SK, et al: The omega-3 fatty acid docosahexaenoate reduces cytokine-induced expression of proatherogenic and proinflammatory proteins in human endothelial cells. Arterioscler Thromb Vasc Biol 1994;14: 1829–1836.

108. Carluccio MA, Massaro M, Bonfrate C, et al: Oleic acid inhibits endothelial cell activation. Arterioscler Thromb Vasc Biol 1999;19:220–228.

109. Imhof A, Froehlich M, Brenner H, et al: Effect of alcohol consumption on systemic markers of inflammation. Lancet 2001;357:763–767.

110. Kris-Etherton P, Eckel R, Howard B, et al: Lyon Diet Heart Study: Benefits of a Mediterranean-style, National Cholesterol Education Program/American Heart Association Step I Dietary Pattern on cardiovascular disease. Circulation 2001;103:1823–1825.

111. Marchioli R, Valagussa F, Del Pinto M, et al: Mediterranean dietary habits and risk of death after myocardial infarction. Circulation 2000;102(Suppl II):379.

112. Morice MC, Serruyis PW, Sousa JE, et al: A randomized comparison of a sirolimus-eluting stent with a standard stent for coronary revascularization. N Engl J Med 2002;346:1773–1780.

113. Cairns JA, Gill J, Morton B, et al: Fish oils and low-molecular-weight heparin for the reduction of restenosis after percutaneous transluminal coronary angioplasty. Circulation 1994;94:1553–1560.

114. Leaf A, Jorgensen MB, Jacobs AK, et al: Do fish oils prevent restenosis after coronary angioplasty? Circulation 1994;90:2248–2257.

115. Johansen O, Brekke M, Seljeflot I, et al: n-3 fatty acids do not prevent restenosis after coronary angioplasty: Results from the CART study. J Am Coll Cardiol 1999;33:1619–1626.

116. Homocysteine Lowering Trialists' Collaboration: Lowering blood homocysteine with folic acid based supplements: Meta-analysis of randomised trials. BMJ 1998;316:894–898.

117. Schnyder G, Roffi M, Pin R, et al: Decreased rate of coronary restenosis after lowering of plasma homocysteine levels. N Engl J Med 2001;345:1593–1600.

118. Kromhout D: On the waves of the Seven Countries Study: A public health perspective on cholesterol. Eur Heart J 1999;20: 796–802.

119. Scandinavian Simvastatin Survival Study Group: Randomized trial of cholesterol lowering in 4444 patients with coronary heart disease. The Scandinavian Simvastatin Survival Study (4S). Lancet 1994;344:1383–1389.

120. Long-term Intervention with Pravastatin in Ischaemic Disease (LIPID) study group: Prevention of cardiovascular events and death with pravastatin in patients with coronary heart disease and a broad range of initial cholesterol levels. N Engl J Med 1998;339:1349–1357.

121. Kromhout D, Keys A, Aravanis C, et al: Food consumption patterns in the 1960s in seven countries. Am J Clin Nutr 1989;49: 889–894.

122. Renaud S, de Lorgeril M: Dietary lipids and their relation to ischaemic heart disease: From epidemiology to prevention. J Intern Med 1989;225(Suppl 1):39–46.

123. Grundy SM, Denke MA: Dietary influences on serum lipids and lipoproteins. J Lipid Res 1990;31:1149–1172.

124. Clarke R, Frost C, Collins R, et al: Dietary lipids and blood cholesterol: Quantitative meta-analysis of metabolic ward studies. BMJ 1997;314:112–117.

125. Macmahon S: Blood pressure and the risk of cardiovascular disease. N Engl J Med 2000;342:50–52.

126. EUROASPIRE: A European Society of cardiovascular survey of secondary prevention of coronary heart disease: Principal results. Eur Heart J 1997;18:1569–1582.

127. Guidelines Subcommittee: 1999 World Health Organisation–International Society of Hypertension guidelines for the management of hypertension. J Hypertens 1999;17:151–183.

128. Van den Hoogen PCW, Feskens EJM, Nagelkerke NJD, et al: The relation between blood pressure and mortality due to coronary heart disease among men in different parts of the world. N Engl J Med 2000;342:1–8.

129. INTERSALT Cooperative Research Group: Intersalt: An international study of electrolyte excretion and blood pressure: Results for 24-hour urinary sodium and potassium excretion. BMJ 1988;297:319–328.

130. Fuentes F, Lopez-Miranda J, Sanchez E, et al: Mediterranean and low-fat diets improve endothelial function in hypercholesterolemic men. Ann Intern Med 2001;134:1115–1119.

131. McCarron DA: Diet and blood pressure: The paradigm shift. Science 1998;281:933–934.

132. Bonaa KH, Bjerve KS, Straume B, et al: Effect of eicosapentanoic and docosahexanoic acids on blood pressure in hypertension. N Engl J Med 1990;322:795–801.

133. Appel LJ, Moore TJ, Obarzanek E, et al, for the DASH Collaborative Research Group: A clinical trial of the effects of dietary patterns on blood pressure. N Engl J Med 1997;336:1117–1124.

134. Sacks FM, Svetkey LP, Vollmer WM, et al: Effects on blood pressure of reduced dietary sodium and the Dietary Approaches to Stop Hypertension (DASH) diet. N Engl J Med 2001;344:3–10.

135. Furchgott RF, Zawadski JV: The obligatory role of endothelial cells in the relaxation of arterial smooth muscle by acetylcholine. Nature 1980;288:373–376.

136. Panza JA, Quyyumi AA, Brush JE, Epstein SE: Abnormal endothelium-dependent vascular relaxation in patients with essential hypertension. N Engl J Med 1990;323:22–27.

137. Schachinger V, Britten MB, Zeiher AM: Prognostic impact of coronary vasodilator dysfunction on adverse long-term outcome of coronary heart disease. Circulation 2000;101:1899–1906.

138. Verhaar MC, Wever RMF, Kastelein JJP, et al: 5-Methyltetrahydrofolate, the active form of folic acid, restores endothelial function in familial hypercholesterolemia. Circulation 1998;97:237–241.

139. Verhaar MC, Wever RMF, Kastelein JJP, et al: Effects of oral folic acid supplementation on endothelial function in familial hypercholesterolemia: A randomised placebo-controlled trial. Circulation 1999;100:335–338.

140. Stroes E, Kastelein J, Cosentino F, et al: Tetrahydrobiopterin restores endothelial function in hypercholesterolemia. J Clin Invest 1997;99:41–46.

141. Setoguchi S, Mohri M, Shimokawa H, Takeshita A: Tetrahydrobiopterin improves endothelial dysfunction in coronary microcirculation in patients without epicardial coronary heart disease. J Am Coll Cardiol 2001;38:493–498.

142. Nash DT: Insulin resistance, ADMA levels, and cardiovascular disease. JAMA 2002;287:1451–1452.

143. Bazzano L, He J, Ogden LG, et al: Legume consumption and risk of coronary heart disease in US men and women. Arch Intern Med 2001;161:2573–2578.

144. de Lorgeril M: Dietary arginine and the prevention of cardiovascular diseases. Cardiovasc Res 1998;37:560–563.

145. Kannel WB, McGee DL: Diabetes and glucose tolerance as risk factors for cardiovascular diseases: The Framingham Study. Diabetes Care 1979;2:120–126.

146. Haffner SM, Lehto S, Rönnemaa T, et al: Mortality from coronary heart disease in subjects with type 2 diabetes and in nondiabetic subjects with and without prior myocardial infarction. N Engl J Med 1998;339:229–234.

147. Garg A: High-monounsaturated-fat diets for patients with diabetes mellitus: A meta-analysis. Am J Clin Nutr 1998;67(Suppl): 577S–582S.

148. Laakso M: Benefits of strict glucose and blood pressure control in type 2 diabetes: Lessons from the UK Prospective Diabetes Study. Circulation 1999;99:461–462.

149. McKeigue PM, Shah B, Marmot MG: Relation of central obesity and insulin resistance with high diabetes prevalence and cardiovascular risk in South Asians. Lancet 1991;1:382–386.

150. Peterson DB, Fisher K, Carter RD, Mann J: Fatty acid composition of erythrocytes and plasma triglyceride and cardiovascular risk in Asian diabetic patients. Lancet 1994;343:1528–1530.

151. Toft I, Bonaa KH, Ingebretsen OC, et al: Effects of n-3 fatty acids on glucose homeostasis and blood pressure in essential hypertension. Ann Intern Med 1995;123:911–918.

152. Storlien LH, Kraegen EW, Chisholm DJ, et al: Fish oil prevents insulin resistance induced by high-fat feeding in rats. Science 1987;237:885–888.

153. Riccardi G, Rivellese AA: Diabetes: Nutrition in prevention and management. Nutr Metab Cardiovasc Dis 1999;9(Suppl):33–36.

154. Krauss RM, Eckel RH, Howard B, et al: AHA Dietary Guidelines: Revision 2000: A statement for healthcare professionals from the Nutrition Committee of the American Heart Association. Circulation 2000;102:2296–2311.

155. Guagnano MT, Merlitti D, Pace-Palitti V, et al: Clinical nutrition: Inadequate teaching in medical schools. Nutr Metab Cardiovasc Dis 2001;11:104–107.

156. de Lorgeril M, Salen P: Fish and n-3 fatty acids in the prevention and treatment of coronary heart disease: Nutrition is not pharmacology. Am J Med 2002;112:316–319.

157. Kris-Etherton P: Monounsaturated fatty acids and the risk of cardiovascular disease. Circulation 1999;100:1253–1258.

158. de Lorgeril M, Salen P, Laporte F, de Leiris J: Alpha-linoleic acid in the prevention and treatment of coronary heart disease. Eur Heart J 2001;3(Suppl D):26–32.

159. de Lorgeril M, Salen P, Laporte F, et al: Rapeseed oil and rapeseed oil-based margarine in the prevention and treatment of coronary heart disease. Eur J Lipid Sci Technol 2001;103:490–495.

160. de Lorgeril M, Salen P, Laporte F, de Leiris J: Potential use of nuts for the prevention and treatment of coronary heart disease: From natural to functional foods. Nutr Metab Cardiovasc Dis 2001;11:362–371.

■ ■ ■ chapter 45

Perspectives for Gene and Cell-Based Therapy

Lúis G. Melo
Abeel A. Mangi
Alok S. Pachori
Victor J. Dzau

Despite the identification of multiple risk factors for coronary artery disease (CAD), the preponderance of current therapeutic approaches for management of the disease aim at treating overt symptoms of ischemia, such as angina or infarction, with the goal of restoring blood flow to the ischemic myocardium. However, the efficacy of these "rescue" therapies is hampered by the narrow time window for successful intervention following an acute ischemic event, often resulting in poor long-term prognosis and survival after myocardial infarction.[1] Furthermore, thrombolytic and anticoagulant therapies, although successful in restoring flow to the ischemic region, do not prevent the postreperfusion pathologic sequelae, such as the activation of pro-inflammatory and pro-oxidant processes that may lead to subsequent ventricular failure.[2] Likewise, the long-term success of acute surgical revascularization procedures such as percutaneous coronary angioplasty and coronary artery bypass grafting may be limited by restenosis and graft atherosclerosis, and the potential need for multiple revascularizations may lead to the depletion of native conduits in the absence of a suitable prosthetic alternative.[3]

The current availability of cardiotropic vectors for gene transfer[4,5] and the recent identification of several gene targets involved in the pathologic mechanism leading to CAD[6] offers an opportunity for the design of gene-based therapeutic strategies for protection of the myocardium from ischemic injury and failure. The ability of vector systems such as adeno-associated virus (AAV) to confer stable and long-term protein expression with a single administration of the therapeutic gene[7,8] renders them ideally suited to the treatment of patients afflicted with or at risk for CAD, whereas vectors such as alphaviruses capable of very rapid transgene expression[9,10] may allow therapeutic genetic manipulation in acute myocardial infarction. The ability to isolate, expand, and genetically modify cardiomyocyte and endothelial progenitor cells from adult bone marrow and peripheral blood[11-13] may allow the repair and vascularization of injured myocardium using autologous cell transplantation. Strategies have also been devised for

inhibition of genes whose overactivity may lead to myocardial injury. Antisense and decoy deoxyoligonucleotides and ribozymes are effective tools for acute blockade of gene function.[14-16] In many instances, the acute inhibition of a pathogenic gene is sufficient to prevent disease. We anticipate that advances in the field will be propelled by genomic research. The emergence of genomic profiling and screening technology will lead to the discovery of new therapeutic targets and facilitate the detection of disease-causing polymorphisms and the design of individualized gene and cell-based therapies.

In this chapter, we review the current state of gene and cell-based therapies for heart disease, with emphasis on strategies for the protection and rescue of the heart from acute injury, their clinical feasibility, and a perspective on future developments. We highlight the major breakthroughs, the opportunities lying ahead in this exciting field, and the potential difficulties in making the successful transition from the preclinical phase to clinical trials and therapeutic application.

TARGETS FOR GENE AND CELL-BASED THERAPIES FOR ACUTE CORONARY SYNDROMES AND CORONARY ARTERY DISEASE

Despite major advances in understanding the molecular mechanisms underlying the pathologic processes leading to CAD and subsequent heart failure, the difficulty in identifying specific predisposing genetic markers for heart disease has hampered the development of therapeutic strategies for preventing the disease. Consequently, the focus has been on the design of rescue therapies for treatment. However, as the genetic and molecular mechanisms of CAD unravel, the impetus will be on the development of novel "protective" gene and cell-based therapeutic strategies aimed at preventing acute ischemic episodes. Ideally, such strategies should confer a sustained therapeutic benefit with one single administration of the therapeutic gene. These requirements are met, at least in part, by the availability of AAV vectors. These vectors are highly cardiotropic and are capable of long-term transgene expression with minimal immunologic consequences to the host.[11-13,17,18]

In the setting of acute myocardial ischemia, the over-expression of cytoprotective and survival genes (e.g., antioxidant enzymes,[19-23] anti-apoptotic proteins,[24-26] and protein kinase B/Akt[27-29]) and the inhibition of pro-inflammatory cytokines[30-32] and pro-apoptotic[33-35] and pro-oxidant[36,37] genes have emerged as potential therapeutic targets for cardioprotection from studies of various animal and cellular models of myocardial ischemic injury (Table 45-1). Gene manipulations yielding overexpression of vasodilator substances[38-40] and thrombolytic proteins[41-43] or inhibition of vasoconstrictor pathways[44-48] have also shown beneficial protective effects. Gene therapy strategies for plaque stabilization and inhibition of platelet adhesion should also prove to be of benefit in reducing thrombotic events and myocardial infarction. Potential strategies include the inhibition of pro-inflammatory mediator CD40/CD40L[49,50] signaling and the glycoprotein IIb/IIIa receptor.[51,52] Other potential strategies in the postinfarction period include manipulation of genes involved in regulation of cardiac remodeling. Among these, the inhibition of matrix metalloproteinases involved in extracellular matrix degradation is emerging as a useful target for prevention of pathologic ventricular remodeling after myocardial infarction.[53-55] Another relevant gene therapy strategy is therapeutic angiogenesis by the delivery of proangiogenic genes such as vascular endothelial growth factor (VEGF),[56-58] fibroblast growth factor (FGF),[59,60] and hepatocyte growth factor.[61,62] An exciting new field is emerging with the recent identification and isolation of endothelial and cardiomyocyte precursor stem cells from adult bone marrow.[11-13] The ability to expand and genetically modify these cells ex vivo[63] offers the opportunity to use them as an autologous cellular substrate for the generation of new blood vessels (therapeutic vasculogenesis) and the regeneration of infarcted myocardium.

VECTORS AND STRATEGIES FOR GENETIC MANIPULATION OF THE CARDIOVASCULAR SYSTEM

A major hindrance to the development of effective gene therapies for heart disease has been the unavailability of efficient tools for genetic manipulation of the myocardium and blood vessels. A variety of vectors and delivery strategies has evolved for the introduction of

■ ■ ■

TABLE 45–1 TARGETS OF GENE-BASED THERAPY FOR CORONARY ARTERY DISEASE

STRATEGY	THERAPEUTIC TARGET	GENETIC MANIPULATION	VECTOR	APPLICATION
Protection/Prevention				
Antioxidant enzymes	HO-1, SOD, catalase, GPx	Overexpression	AAV, LV	CAD, MI
Heat shock proteins	HSP70, HSP90, HSP27	Overexpression	AAV, LV	CAD, MI
Anti-inflammatory agents	I-CAM, V-CAM, NF-κB, TNF-α	Inhibition	AS-ODN	Graft atherosclerosis
			Decoy ODN	Transplantation
			AAV-AS-ODN	
			RV-AS-ODN	
Survival genes	Bcl-2, Akt	Overexpression	AAV, LV	CAD, MI, HF
Pro-apoptotic genes	Bad, p53, Fas ligand	Inhibition	AS-ODN	MI, HF
			Decoy ODN	
			AAV-AS-ODN	
Coronary vessel tone	eNOS, adenosine (P1, P3) receptors	Overexpression	RV, AAV(?)	CAD, HF
Rescue				
Pro-angiogenic genes	VEGF, FGF, HGF	Overexpression	AAV	CAD, MI, HF
Plaque stabilization	CD40	Overexpression	RV, AAV(?)	CAD
Thromboprotection	PAI-1, plasminogen activator Tissue factor	Inhibition	AS-ODN	CAD, MI
	TPA, hirudin, urokinase Thrombomodulin, COX-1, PGI₂ synthase	Overexpression	AAV	CAD, MI
Blood pressure	Kallikrein, eNOS, ANP	Overexpression	AAV, RV	Hypertension, CAD
	ACE, AGT, AT₁	Inhibition	AAV-AS-ODN	
Inhibition of neointimal hyperplasia	NOS, Ras dominant negative	Overexpression	AD, RV, AAV(?)	Graft atherosclerosis
	E2F, c-myb, c-myc, PCNA	Inhibition	AS-ODN, decoy-ODN	Restenosis

AAV, adeno-associated virus; AS-ODN, antisense oligodeoxynucleotide; CAD, coronary artery disease; HF, heart failure; LV, lentivirus; MI, myocardial infarction; α-MHC, alpha myosin heavy chain; RV, retrovirus, HO-1, heme oxygenase-1; SOD, superoxide dismutase; GPx, glutathione peroxidase; HSP70, 70 KD heat shock protein; HSP90, 90 kD heat shock protein; I-CAM, intracellular adhesion molecule; V-CAM, vascular adhesion molecule; NF-κB, nuclear factor κB; TNF-α, tumor necrosis factor α; eNOS, endothelial nitric oxide synthase; VEGF, vascular endothelial growth factor; FGF, fibroblast growth factor; HGF, hematopoietic growth factor; V1, vasopressin-1 receptor; βARK, β-adrenergic receptor kinase; PAI-1, plasminogen activator inhibitor-1; TPA, tissue plasminogen activator; COX-1, cyclooxygenase-1; PGI₂ synthase, prostacyclin synthase; ANP, atrial natriuretic peptide; ACE, angiotensin-converting enzyme; AGT, angiotensinogen; AT₁, angiotensin II type 1 receptor; NOS, nitric oxide synthase; PCNA, proliferating cell nuclear antigen.

genetic material into cardiovascular tissues, with widely varying efficiencies (Table 45–2; Fig. 45–1).[14,64,65] As a general rule, the efficiency of gene transfer is determined by the type of vector used for delivery of the therapeutic gene, the route of delivery, the permissiveness of the target cells to the vector,[64,65] and, to a lesser extent, the dosage and volume of delivery of the genetic material.[66] The choice of vector and delivery method is determined in part by the pathologic features of the disease being treated, the cycling status of the target cells, and the biologic properties of the vector. For terminally differentiated cells such as adult cardiomyocytes, the exclusive use of vectors capable of transferring genetic material to quiescent cells is essential.

Strategies for Delivery of Genetic Material to Myocardium

With regard to the route of administration, intracoronary delivery of the therapeutic material is favored for global myocardial diseases such as heart failure and cardiomyopathy. For regional myocardial disease such as coronary ischemia or myocardial infarction, the localized delivery of the therapeutic material by intramyocardial injection may be preferred. This approach has been used for delivery of angiogenic and cytoprotective genes to ischemic myocardium.[67,68] Other methods, such as pericardial injection and catheter-mediated delivery, have shown limited efficacy and consequently are not widely employed in myocardial gene transfer.[69,70] The overall safety and specificity of gene transfer protocols may be enhanced by incorporating regulatory elements that can direct tissue-specific expression of the transgene in response to underlying pathophysiologic cues such as hypoxia, oxidative stress, or inflammation.[71,72] This degree of physiologic control of transgene expression could avert potential cytotoxic effects associated with constitutive expression of the therapeutic protein.[73]

Nonviral Vectors

Gene transfer vectors may be classified under three broad categories as *nonviral, viral,* and *cell-based* (see Table 45–2). Nonviral vectors include naked plasmids and a variety of cationic liposome and hybrid formulations and several physical methods.[74-78] Myocardial gene transfer using a nonviral vector, however, is generally characterized by low transfection efficiency, rapid degradation of the vector, and transient transgene expression.[79,80] Nevertheless, there have been reports in which

■ ■ ■

TABLE 45–2 VECTORS USED FOR TRANSFER AND MANIPULATION OF GENETIC MATERIAL IN CARDIOVASCULAR TISSUES

VECTOR POTENTIAL	CHROMOSOMAL INTEGRATION	TRANSFER EFFICIENCY IN VIVO	ONSET OF TRANSGENE EXPRESSION	SUSTAINABILITY OF THERAPEUTIC EFFECT	LEVEL OF EXPRESSION	TARGET CELLS	HOST IMMUNE RESPONSE	RISKS
Nonviral								
Cationic liposomes cytotoxicity	No	+	Rapid	Short	+	Quiescent and dividing	+	
HVJ-liposomes cytotoxicity	No	+++	Rapid	Short	++	Quiescent and dividing	+	
Naked plasmid cytotoxicity	No	+	Moderate	Short	+	Quiescent and dividing	+	
Viral								
Retrovirus cytotoxicity oncogenesis	Yes	++	Rapid	Life-long	++	Dividing	+	
Lentivirus cytoxicity mutation	Yes	+++	Rapid	Life-long	+++	Quiescent and dividing	+	Viral
Adenovirus cytotoxicity mutation	No	+++++	Rapid	Moderate	+++++	Quiescent and dividing	++++	Viral
Adenosine–associated virus oncogenesis mutation	Yes	+++	Slow	Life-long	+++	Quiescent and dividing	+	Viral
Herpes simplex virus cytotoxicity mutation	No	+++	Moderate	Long	+++	Quiescent and dividing	+++	Viral
Alphavirus cytotoxicity mutation	No	++	Very rapid	Short	+++	Quiescent and dividing	+++	Viral

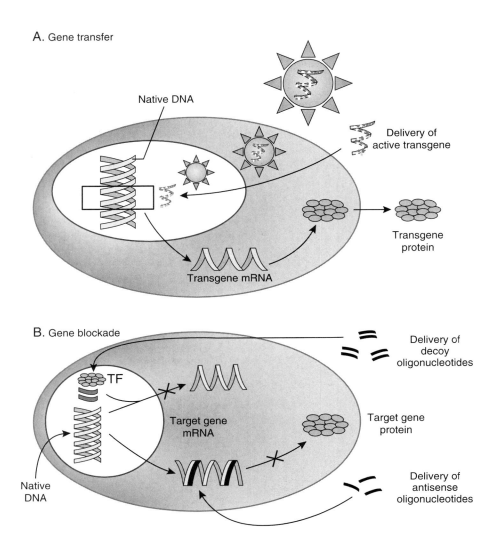

A. Gene transfer

Native DNA

Delivery of active transgene

Transgene protein

Transgene mRNA

B. Gene blockade

Delivery of decoy oligonucleotides

TF

Target gene mRNA

Target gene protein

Native DNA

Delivery of antisense oligonucleotides

FIGURE 45–1. Strategies for genetic manipulation in the cardiovascular system. *A,* Gene transfer involves the delivery of one or several exogenous genes (transgenes) by a vector capable of expressing the therapeutic protein in the host cells. The overall goal is to increase the activity of a gene or genes (gain of function) whose endogenous function may be deficient and cause disease. *B,* Gene blockade involves inhibition of genes whose overactivity may lead to disease. Two strategies are commonly used to inhibit gene activity at the transcriptional or translational level. Short single-stranded deoxyoligonucleotides complementary to the target gene mRNA (antisense oligonucleotides) are delivered to the target cells or tissue by transfection or with the aid of a vector. The antisense deoxyoligonucleotide binds to the target mRNA transcript and prevents it from being translated. The second strategy employs double-stranded deoxyoligonucleotides containing the consensus binding sequences (decoy oligonucleotides) for transcriptional factors involved in the activation of pathogenic genes. Transfection of a molar excess of the decoy oligonucleotide prevents the binding and transactivation of the genes regulated by the target transcriptional factor. Less commonly, short segments of RNA with enzymatic activity (ribozymes) are used to degrade target mRNA transcripts.

plasmid gene transfer into the myocardium translated into a sustained therapeutic effect.[81,82] The efficiency of plasmid gene transfer can be increased by encapsulating the plasmid in neutral liposomes fused to the viral coat of the Sendai virus (hemagglutinating virus of Japan),[83] but transgene expression with this vector system is transient, rendering it unsuitable for use in chronic heart disease. Electroporation has been used for transfer of naked DNA into embryonic chick hearts ex vivo with moderate efficiency,[84] but this protocol appears to be impractical for myocardial gene transfer in humans. Application of nondistending pressure in an enclosed environment has been used to deliver oligonucleotides ex vivo to the heart[85] and vein grafts,[86] highlighting a potential application of this technique for genetic engineering of blood vessels and other organs in preparation for transplantation.

Viral Vectors

Recombinant viruses have become the favored vectors for myocardial gene transfer because they are more efficient than nonviral vectors at delivering genetic material into cells[63,87–89] and are capable, in general, of sustaining expression of the therapeutic gene for greater periods of time.[87] However, in some instances, a robust immunogenic response may be mounted by the host in response to the viral proteins synthesized by the vector, which could significantly reduce the efficiency of gene transfer and the sustainability of transgene expression. Furthermore, the possibility, although remote, that the vector may revert to replication proficiency raises safety concerns about biologic hazards such as oncogenesis and insertional mutagenesis.

Of the currently available viral vectors, adenovirus are the most widely used and efficient vectors.[89] These viruses can transduce a wide variety of myocardial cell types and can accommodate large DNA inserts. The vector infects both dividing and terminally differentiated cells. However, the cytotoxicity associated with induction of the immune response and the episomal localization of the viral genomes results in rapid loss of transgene expression even in the absence of cell division.[89] More recently, a new generation of "gutted" adenoviral vectors has been developed in which the host inflammatory response is attenuated by removing all of the adenoviral coding sequences.[90] These adenoviral vectors can accommodate very large DNA fragments and may be useful for delivering multiple genes. AAV has emerged as the vector of choice for myocardial gene transfer because of its high myocardial tropism and ability to stably transduce terminally differentiated myocytes with high efficiency.[11-13,17,18,91] The major limitation of the vector is its inability to accommodate large DNA inserts (transgene size is restricted to 4 kb or less); however, trans-splicing between two separate AAV vectors has recently been used as a strategy for delivery of genes greater than 4 kb.[92]

RNA-based retroviral and lentiviral vectors have not found widespread application in cardiovascular gene transfer protocols for several biologic and technical reasons.[93-94] These vectors integrate into the host genome, leading to the possibility of long-term transgene expression.[93] However, retroviral integration requires cell division, rendering these vectors inefficient in the transduction of adult cardiomyocytes. Furthermore, retrovirally delivered transgenes are prone to transcription silencing, which may significantly shorten the duration of transgene expression. Production of high-titer retrovirus preparations is difficult, although recent improvements in packaging systems, such as the use of pseudotyped viral coats incorporating the vesicular stomatitis virus G protein, has greatly improved the stability of the viral particles and has allowed transduction of a wider spectrum of cell types with relatively high efficiency.[94] Lentiviruses are relative newcomers in cardiovascular gene therapy.[95] In contrast with the oncoretroviruses, these HIV-1–related retroviruses can infect both dividing and quiescent cells.[95,96] Moderate transgene expression was noted in the heart following transduction with a pseudotyped lentivirus.[97]

Other viral vector systems currently used for gene transfer, such as herpes simplex viruses and alphaviruses, have had limited application in myocardial gene transfer. The ability of herpes simplex virus–based vectors to accommodate very large DNA fragments would provide an advantage for the transfer of very large genes such as dystrophin or sarcoglycans for treatment of inherited cardiomyopathies.[98] Recombinant alphaviruses have been used for very rapid and efficient transduction of several cells and tissues in vitro.[99] These viruses can express transgenes within 24 hours of transduction in the heart with minimal cytoxicity, suggesting a potential application of these vectors for gene manipulation in acute myocardial disease such as myocardial infarction.

A number of cell types have also been used as vectors for delivery of genetic material to tissues. The recent identification and isolation of endothelial and cardiomyocyte precursor stem cells from adult bone marrow and peripheral blood[11-13] provides a nondepleting, self-renewing autologous cell source that can simultaneously be used as substrate for regeneration and reconstruction of injured myocardium and blood vessels and as vehicles for delivery of therapeutic genes.[14-16,100] For example, the cells could be engineered ex vivo to express cytoprotective or proangiogenic genes (or both) that would promote survival of the grafted cells and neovascularization of the infarcted myocardium. Macrophages, erythro-cytes, and vascular endothelial cells have also been successfully transduced ex vivo with retroviral vectors and used as "shuttles" for efficient delivery of therapeutic genes into tissues.[101-103] Macrophages genetically engineered to express protective genes under endogenous regulation by hypoxia may have potential application for targeted delivery of genes in myocardial ischemia.

GENE THERAPY FOR MYOCARDIAL PROTECTION

The continuum of myocardial injury, commonly called *ischemia/reperfusion (I/R) injury,* that is initiated by a coronary ischemic event and propagated by reperfusion,[19,104] may be clinically manifested in patients undergoing thrombolytic therapy after an acute coronary episode.[105] Reoxygenation of the ischemic myocardium leads to a robust increase in free radical species that may eventually deplete the buffering capabilities of endogenous antioxidant systems, thereby exacerbating the deleterious effects of these reactive species (Fig. 45-2).[106] The development of thrombolytic gene therapies for acute myocardial infarction has been difficult because the time required for transcription and translation of therapeutic genes with the vectors currently used in gene transfer exceeds the time window for successful intervention. In view of these limitations, an alternative gene therapy approach for acute coronary syndromes is to "prevent" I/R by the transfer of cytoprotective genes into the myocardium of high-risk patients prior to ischemia, using a gene delivery method that could confer long-term therapeutic gene expression. This novel concept of preventive gene therapy would protect the heart from future I/R injury, thereby minimizing the need for acute intervention. Given the prominent role of oxidative stress in I/R injury, a therapeutic approach aimed at increasing endogenous antioxidant reserves should, in principle, prove useful as a strategy for prevention and protection in patients at risk for acute myocardial infarction. In principle, this strategy should potentiate the native protective response of the myocardium,[107] rendering it more resistant to future ischemic insults.

Gene Therapy for Protection from Ischemia/Reperfusion-Induced Injury

As a means of evaluating the feasibility of antioxidant enzyme gene transfer as a long-term first line of defense against I/R-induced oxidative injury, we used an rAAV vector for intramyocardial delivery of the heme oxygenase 1 (HO-1) gene in a rat coronary artery ligation/release model of I/R injury.[108] Our findings showed that intramyocardial delivery of the HO-1 gene to the left-ventricular risk area several weeks in advance of myocardial infarction resulted in approximately 80% reduction in infarct size in the treated animals. The reduction in myocardial injury in the treated animals was accompanied by decreases in oxidative stress, inflammation, and interstitial fibrosis. Consistent with the histopathologic picture, echocardiographic assessment showed

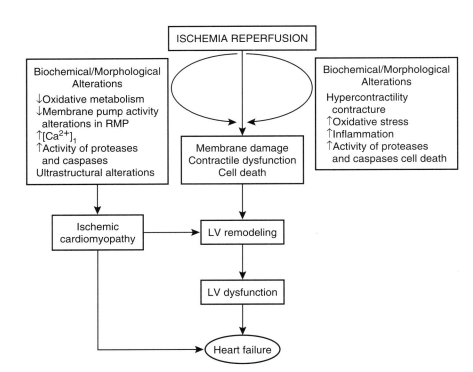

FIGURE 45–2. Pathophysiology of coronary artery disease. Myocardial ischemia subsequent to coronary artery occlusion, if sufficiently prolonged, results in irreversible cellular damage highlighted by alterations in membrane fluidity and pump activity, mitochondrial damage, and depressed metabolic and contractile activity. Reperfusion introduces a separate set of cellular stresses that may exacerbate the damage initiated during ischemia. Reoxygenation of the ischemic myocardium results in the formation of reactive free radical oxygen species, leading to activation of the inflammatory cascade, myocyte injury, and endothelial dysfunction. The end result of ischemia/reperfusion is a continuum of myocardial injury that culminates with myocardial infarction caused by membrane damage, contractile dysfunction, and eventual cell death. In time, these changes lead to ventricular remodeling, a process characterized by myocyte hypertrophy, interstitial fibrosis, chamber dilatation, and increased propensity for contractile dysfunction and failure. Acute coronary syndromes are a clinical manifestation of coronary artery disease. Chronic coronary artery disease leads to ischemic cardiomyopathy heart failure and premature death. RMP, rest membrane potential.

postinfarction recovery of left-ventricular function in the HO-1–treated animals, whereas the untreated control animals presented evidence of ventricular enlargement and significantly depressed fractional shortening and ejection fraction. Comparable findings were noted with extracellular superoxide dismutase (ecSOD) gene transfer.[23,109-111] This secreted metalloenzyme plays an essential role in maintenance of redox homeostasis by dismutating the oxygen free radical superoxide. Our findings showed that long-term survival after acute myocardial infarction is improved in the ecSOD-treated animals relative to the animals treated with the control vector, in parallel with smaller infarcts and decreased myocardial inflammation. Efficient protection from I/R injury has also been achieved by overexpression of other major antioxidant enzyme systems, such as Cu/Zn SOD,[20,112] catalase,[20,113] and glutathione peroxidase;[114] of stress-induced heat shock proteins such as HSP 70[21,115] and HSP 27;[116] of survival genes such as Bcl-2 and Akt;[24-29,117,118] and of immunosuppressive cytokines,[30-32,119] adenosine A_1 and A_3 receptors,[120,121] kallikrein,[122] caspase inhibitor,[35] and hepatocyte growth factor.[123]

The inhibition of pro-inflammatory genes involved in the pathogenesis of I/R injury offers another option for cardioprotection. Morishita et al[124] showed that pretreatment with a decoy oligonucleotide capable of inhibiting the trans-activating activity of the pro-inflammatory transcription factor NF-κB reduces myocardial infarct after coronary artery ligation in rats. Similarly, intravenous administration of antisense oligonucleotide against angiotensin-converting enzyme mRNA[125] or angiotensin AT_1 receptor[126] significantly reduces myocardial dysfunction and injury following ischemia and reperfusion. Although the rapid in vivo degradation of oligonucleotides precludes their use in long-term myocardial protection, they may be useful in the treatment of acute myocardial ischemia and cardiac transplantation[127] by providing a tool for inhibiting pro-oxidant, pro-inflammatory, and immunomodulatory genes activated by ischemia and reperfusion. For example, treatment with antisense oligonucleotide directed against intercellular adhesion molecule 1 was shown to prolong cardiac allograft tolerance and long-term survival when administered ex vivo prior to transplantation into the host.[128] Such an approach could be beneficial in the preparation of donor hearts for transplantation. For example, oligonucleotide-mediated inhibition of anti-inflammatory genes and adhesion molecules in donor organs in advance of transplantation could be used to suppress the acute inflammatory response that ensues upon reperfusion of the transplanted organ in the recipient.

The suitability of these experimental therapies for myocardial protection in humans remains to be established. Further work is required in order to elucidate the mechanism by which exogenous gene delivery of antioxidant enzymes confers myocardial protection from ischemic injury. It is conceivable that the increase in basal pro-oxidant scavenging activity imparted by constitutive overexpression of antioxidant enzymes confers cytoprotection by preconditioning the myocardium to future I/R episodes. Nevertheless, these preclinical studies provide compelling evidence that antioxidant gene therapy may be a viable strategy for protection from ischemic myocardial injury.

Gene Therapy for Atherosclerosis, Thromboresistance, and Plaque Stabilization

Plaque rupture and subsequent coronary thrombosis and occlusion are the major causes of acute coronary episodes that result in myocardial infarction and sudden cardiac death.[1] Hyperlipidemias, in both acquired and inherited forms, are the predominant risk factor for CAD, leading to the appearance of lipid- and macrophage-rich plaque. These "vulnerable" plaques have reduced collagen content and smooth muscle number, resulting in poor tensile strength. This renders these highly susceptible plaques to rupture and thrombosis in response to extrinsic factors such as hypertension or vasospasm.[129] Lipid-lowering and antithrombotic pharmacologic therapies, such as statins and aspirin/heparin, favor plaque stabilization and reduce the incidence of acute coronary events by decreasing serum cholesterol levels and conferring thromboresistance.[130] Gene therapy strategies aimed at decreasing cholesterol levels or increasing thromboresistance and tensile strength within the plaque may offer a novel and potentially effective alternative option to achieve long-term plaque stabilization and to prevent acute coronary events.[131]

The effect of lipid-lowering gene therapy has been evaluated mainly in inherited disorders of lipid metabolism, such as familial hypercholesterolemia and apoE deficiency. Initial attempts at correcting familial hypercholesterolemia involved transplantation of autologous hepatocytes stably transduced ex vivo with a retroviral vector constitutively expressing the low-density lipoprotein receptor in Watanabe heritable hyperlipidemic rabbits.[132] This initial study showed a 30% to 50% decrease in plasma cholesterol levels for up to 6 months. The success of this animal study led to a small clinical trial, but the outcome was less impressive, showing a reduction of 6% to 23% in plasma low-density lipoprotein levels in three of five treated patients,[133] with a relatively short duration. Other potential targets for correction of genetic hyperlipidemia include replacement of lipoprotein lipase and hepatic lipase genes,[134,135] apoE,[136] very-low-density lipoprotein receptor,[137] and scavenger receptor B-1.[138] In most cases, the improvement in serum lipid profiles was transient, probably due to the immune response to the vector used. The low immunogenicity of AAV provides and advantage in this regard, and Chen et al[139] showed that AAV-mediated delivery of very-low-density lipoprotein receptor into low-density lipoprotein receptor–deficient mice leads to sustained reduction of serum lipid levels and inhibition of aortic atherosclerosis. Other potential lipid-lowering strategies for gene therapy are emerging. Overexpression of apoprotein apoA-1 in mice by intravenous adenoviral gene delivery increases serum high-density lipoprotein levels.[140] The increase in serum high-density lipoprotein may lead to plaque stabilization by reducing the amount of cholesterol and macrophage accumulation in the plaque.

Various strategies have been developed for transfer of therapeutic genes into atherosclerotic vessels. Local expression of genes in the arterial wall has been achieved using catheters for delivery of plasmid and viral vectors in vivo and ex vivo,[141-143] and the vascular endothelium may be selectively targeted for delivery of anticoagulant, antifibrinolytic, and antiplatelet genes such as thrombomodulin,[144] tissue-specific plasminogen activator,[43,145] tissue factor pathway inhibitor,[146] prostacyclin synthase,[147] and cyclo-oxygenase I.[148] Overexpression of antithrombotic genes at sites in the vessel wall at risk for thrombosis may be a feasible protective strategy for vulnerable plaque and prevention of acute coronary events. Gene transfer to coronary arteries, however, is technically challenging, and refinements to the delivery catheters currently in use are necessary in order to improve the efficiency of gene transfer. Nevertheless, genes have successfully been delivered into the coronary arteries of dogs and pigs using perfusion balloon catheters.[141] As a primary thrombolytic therapy for acute myocardial infarction, gene transfer of anticoagulant genes is not feasible, at least with the current generation of vectors, because the time required for production of the therapeutic protein is too long for successful intervention after coronary thrombosis. However, antithrombotic gene therapy may have a role as an adjuvant to primary thrombolytic therapy to prevent the reoccurrence of thrombosis and reocclusion of the affected vessel.

Gene Therapy for Restenosis and Vascular Proliferative Disease

Because acute revascularization using primary percutaneous coronary angioplasty or bypass grafting are treatment options for CAD, we discuss the recent developments in gene therapy for these procedures. The ability to deliver antiproliferative genes locally or to inhibit pro-proliferative genes in the vessel wall allows genetic engineering of native vessels or grafts to render them resistant to atherosclerosis and neointimal hyperplasia. Genetic strategies to inhibit neointimal smooth muscle proliferation have major implications for the treatment of vascular proliferative diseases, given the high incidence of restenosis associated with revascularization procedures such as percutaneous transluminal coronary angioplasty and coronary artery bypass grafting. Using an ex vivo approach, Kim et al[149] employed adenovirus to deliver thrombomodulin to jugular vein segments prior to interpositional grafting in rabbits. The authors reported that genetic engineering of the graft led to thromboresistance and graft survival. Zoldhelyi et al showed that delivery of tissue factor pathway inhibitor to balloon-injured atherosclerotic carotid arteries of Watanabe rabbits reduced neointima proliferation and inhibited thrombus formation.[150] Similarly, adenoviral delivery of the suicide gene thymidine kinase into carotid arteries of Watanabe rabbits inhibits neointimal proliferation after balloon angioplasty,[151] thus demonstrating the potential of cytotoxic gene therapy for inhibition of restenosis.

Cytostatic gene therapy has also yielded promising results in the treatment of vasculoproliferative disease. In vivo treatment of jugular veins with hemagglutinating virus of Japan/liposome complexes containing antisense oligonucleotide against cell cycle regulators proliferating cell nuclear antigen and cdc2 kinase inhibited atherosclerosis and neointimal hyperplasia after carotid artery interpositional grafting in rabbits maintained on a high-cholesterol diet.[152] We have shown that ex vivo genetic engineering of vein grafts with a decoy deoxyoligonucleotide consisting of the consensus binding sequence of E2F-1, a transcriptional factor involved in cell-cycle progression, resulted in prolonged resistance to neointimal hyperplasia and improved graft patency.[153] These findings led to a large-scale, phase I, prospective, randomized, double-blind trial of human saphenous vein graft treatment with E2F decoy (PREVENT-1).[154] Using nondistending pressure to deliver the E2F decoy oligonucleotide ex vivo prior to arterial interpositional grafting in this safety and feasibility trial, the authors reported that E2F decoy treatment prevented neointimal hyperplasia concomitant with inhibition of cell-cycle progression, resulting in improved long-term survival of the graft. These results have been confirmed in a phase II trial designed to evaluate the effect of E2F decoy treatment on failed coronary artery bypass grafting.[155]

Other cytostatic strategies have yielded variable degrees of success in experimental models of restenosis. Treatment with antisense against cell-cycle regulatory genes cdk2 kinase and proliferating cell nuclear antigen,[156] p21 cyclin–dependent kinase inibitor,[157] non-phosphorylatable retinoblastoma gene product[158] p53,[159] and the proto-oncogenes c-myb[160] and c-myc[161] have all been reported to inhibit neointimal hyperplasia in animal models of arterial injury, as was the case with inhibition of intracellular signaling mediators of mitogen dependent kinases, NF-κB, Bcl-xL protein, or overexpression of Fas ligand and gax and GATA-6 transcription factors.[162] Local delivery of angiotensin-converting enzyme antisense oligonucleotide was also reported to reduce neointima formation in a rat carotid injury model,[163] suggesting that locally derived angiotensin may play a role in vascular injury. In vivo delivery of endothelial and inducible nitric oxide synthase genes is quite efficacious in reducing neointimal thickening in balloon injured vessels.[164-166] This has led to at least one phase I clinical trial currently underway (REstenosis GENe Therapy trial [REGENT]) to evaluate the efficacy of catheter-based iNOS gene delivery to prevent restenosis of coronary arteries treated by percutaneous transluminal coronary angioplasty.[164]

Despite the promising preclinical data and early phase trials, the use of gene therapy as a therapeutic modality for vasculoproliferative disease still has to overcome various feasibility, safety, and efficacy issues. Improvements in vector and delivery technologies are warranted. The development of physiologically responsive vectors capable of cell-specific transgene targeting will play a fundamental role in overcoming some of the safety and efficacy issues associated with vascular gene transfer. Vascular cell types such as endothelial cells may be genetically modified ex vivo to express cytoprotective or antiproliferative genes and used for repair of damaged vessels and bioengineering of vascular prostheses and stents, rendering them thromboresistant and less susceptible to restenosis. Preclinical studies have already demonstrated proof of concept for some of these strategies, and future clinical trials should determine their feasibility and safety for use in humans.

GENE THERAPY FOR MYOCARDIAL RESCUE

Although preventive/protective therapy would be the ideal approach to the management of CAD, the preponderance of gene therapy protocols have been designed for the purpose of rescue from myocardial ischemia and heart failure. This preference has been conditioned on one hand by the lack of definitive genetic markers that could be used to reliably identify patients at risk for CAD and on the other hand by the availability of knowledge on the molecular mechanisms underlying many of the functional and morphologic alterations associated with CAD, which has provided a repertoire of targets for therapeutic intervention. Genetherapy protocols for neovascularization of the ischemic myocardium are being intensively pursued as an alternative for patients deemed unsuited for surgical revascularization, such as those with advanced CAD; in some cases, the preclinical studies have made the transition to early-phase clinical trials with variable success. Strategies for manipulation of the activity of genes involved in regulation of myocardial contractility have shown promise for improvement of the inotropic state in the failing heart. Grafting of myocyte lineage cells is emerging as an option for regeneration of infarcted myocardium, and the recent isolation of cardiomyocyte progenitor mesenchymal stem cells from adult bone marrow provides a source of autologous cells that can be expanded and genetically modified ex vivo and used for both organ repair and tissue engineering.

Gene Therapy for Myocardial Ischemia

With the exception of the female reproductive tract and neoplastic disease, postnatal neovascularization is rare.[167] The vascular endothelium, which usually remains in a quiescent, nonproliferative state, is activated in pathologic conditions characterized by wounding, inflammation, and oxidative stress, resulting in endothelial cell proliferation, migration, and formation of new vascular networks by angiogenesis.[167] Gradual occlusion of the coronary artery in animals and patients with ischemic heart disease leads to a chronic imbalance of myocardial oxygen supply and demand, which results in the adaptive development of collateral vessels aimed at maintaining tissue perfusion and oxygenation. This native protective response of the myocardium, however, does not provide adequate compensation in the face of severe ischemia, and depression of cardiac function ensues. In time, chronic myocardial ischemia leads to heart failure.

Several animal and human studies have provided evidence of enhanced neovascularization and functional recovery of ischemic myocardium after exogenous supplementation of proangiogenic cytokines by gene transfer.[57-61,168-171] This novel strategy, commonly known as *therapeutic angiogenesis,* offers a potentially efficacious therapeutic modality for treatment of CAD in clinical cases wherein percutaneous angioplasty or surgical revascularization alternatives have been excluded. Proof of principle for therapeutic angiogenesis has been demonstrated in several animal models of hindlimb and myocardial ischemia by gene transfer of VEGF,[169,170,172] FGF,[59,60,173] and hepatocyte growth factor.[61,62,174] In all cases, improvement in tissue perfusion was accompanied by morphologic and angiographic evidence of new vessel formation, thus establishing a relationship between improved tissue viability and neovascularization. For example, Mack et al[58] showed that intramyocardial delivery of $VEGF_{121}$ by adenovirus led to an improvement in regional myocardial perfusion and left-ventricular function in response to stress in an amaroid constrictor model of chronic myocardial ischemia in pigs. Using intracoronary injection of an adenovirus vector encoding human FGF-5, Giordano et al[59] showed a significant improvement in blood flow and a reduction in stress-induced functional abnormalities as early as 2 weeks after amaroid placement around the proximal left circumflex coronary artery in pigs, in association with an increase in capillary to fiber ratios.

A combinatorial approach using pro-angiogenic gene transfer with transmyocardial laser therapy has also been tested as a potentially synergistic approach to stimulate angiogenesis. Transmyocardial laser revascularization has been reported to provide relief of angina in patients with ischemic heart disease by forming channels that may improve collateral blood flow.[175] Sayeed-Shah and colleagues[176] demonstrated that intramyocardial delivery of plasmid encoding VEGF in the region treated by transmyocardial laser revascularization yielded superior recovery of ventricular function than either therapy alone. To our knowledge, this strategy has not been tested in human patients.

The success of these preclinical studies has led to several phase I and II clinical trials of angiogenic gene therapy in human patients suffering from myocardial and limb ischemia.[169,170,177–179,180] These safety trials, although consisting of small nonrandomized patient samples, demonstrate the potential of angiogenic gene therapy for treatment of ischemic heart disease. Losordo et al[81] carried out a phase I study in five male patients 53 to 71 years old with angiographic evidence of CAD in whom conventional anti-anginal therapy failed. The authors reported that direct intramyocardial delivery of naked plasmid encoding $VEGF_{165}$ into the ischemic myocardium resulted in significant reduction of anginal symptoms and modest improvement in left-ventricular function concomitant with reduced ischemia and improved Rentrop score.

Using adenovirus for intramyocardial delivery of $VEGF_{121}$ into an area of reversible ischemia in the left ventricle as sole or adjunct therapy in patients undergoing conventional coronary artery bypass grafting, Rosengart et al[169] showed improvements in regional ventricular function and wall motion in the region of vector administration in both groups of patients. Vale and colleagues[177] carried out a randomized, single-blinded, placebo-controlled phase I trial in patients with chronic myocardial ischemia using catheter-based delivery of naked $VEGF_{165}$ assisted by electromechanical NOGA

mapping of the left ventricle. The results of this study indicated significant reductions in weekly anginal attacks for as long as 1 year after gene delivery in the treated patients, in contrast with the patients receiving placebo. The reduction in anginal episodes was accompanied by improved myocardial perfusion as evidenced by SPECT-sestamibi perfusion scanning and electromechanical mapping. More recently, Grines and colleagues[178] undertook the Angiogenic GENe Therapy (AGENT) double-blinded, randomized, placebo-controlled trial using dose-escalating adenovirus-mediated intracoronary delivery of FGF-4 in patients with angina in order to evaluate the safety and efficacy of this protocol in reducing ischemic symptoms. The authors reported increased exercise tolerance and improved stress echocardiograms at 4 and 12 weeks after gene transfer in the patients who received FGF-4 gene therapy compared with the patients receiving placebo.

Clearly, the success of these small-scale phase I and phase II trials warrants larger and more adequately controlled later-phase trials. Several issues relating to feasibility, safety, and sustainability require further investigation before therapeutic angiogenesis can gain acceptance as a viable therapeutic alternative for treatment of ischemic heart disease. The broad issue of feasibility and safety of the approach requires systematic evaluation. This is particularly relevant in light of recent evidence that transplantation of myoblasts constitutively expressing VEGF under a retroviral promoter into mouse hearts led to intramural angiomas followed by heart failure and death,[73] thus underscoring the necessity for regulated expression of pro-angiogenic cytokines. Such a strategy may require the incorporation of promoter sequences such as hypoxia-sensitive responsive elements capable of rendering expression of the therapeutic transgene subservient to the pathophysiologic changes in myocardial oxygen tension.[71,72] This may allow endogenous regulation of angiogenesis so that the magnitude of neovascularization is graded to the severity of the ischemic insult. It will also be necessary to determine the safest route and method of gene delivery in order to avert potentially hazardous side effects, such as neovascularization of occult neoplasms or peripheral vascular effects, that may result in edema and hypotension. In this context, the desired approach may encompass targeted tissue delivery by incorporation of cell-specific promoters for expression of the transgene at the sites of interest. Regarding long-term therapeutic sustainability, it will be necessary to determine whether a single administration of the therapeutic gene is sufficient to achieve the desired long-term therapeutic effect or whether multiple treatments may be required. This potential problem may be circumvented by the use of regulated AAV vectors.[181,182]

Cell-Based Therapy for Myocardial Ischemia

An alternative strategy for therapeutic angiogenesis involves the use of endothelial precursor cells as angiogenic substrate. Several reports have documented the existence of blood-borne endothelial progenitor cells (EPCs) originating from a common hemangioblast precursor in adult bone marrow.[13,183–186] These endothelial lineage cells have the properties of an endothelial progenitor (CD34[+], Flk-1[+]) and are recruited to foci of neo-vascularization such as ischemic muscle[187] and the myocardium,[188] where they differentiate into functional endothelial cells, indicating that they may play a role in postembryonic vasculogenesis in ischemic tissues. The therapeutic potential of these cells as vehicles for tissue salvage or regeneration from ischemia has been demonstrated. Local implantation of autologous bone marrow–derived cells in rat[189] and mouse[190,191] ischemic hindlimb induces angiogenesis and partially restores blood flow and exercise capacity in the ischemic limb. Similarly, transplantation of ex vivo–expanded human EPCs into nude rats[188,192] and pigs[193] with myocardial ischemia leads to increased capillary density and improved ventricular function. More recently, it was reported that the number of circulating EPCs increases in patients with acute myocardial infarction[194] and is lower in patients with CAD,[195] indicating that these cells may be essential to neovascularization of the myocardium in response to ischemia.

The ability to culture and genetically engineer EPCs ex vivo with vectors expressing therapeutic genes suggests that these cells may be ideally suited as a substrate for cell-based gene therapy for neovascularization of ischemic tissues. In this scheme, EPCs genetically modified to express angiogenic growth factors could serve as a cell substrate for new vessel growth by vasculogenesis, driven by local proliferation and differentiation of the transplanted cells, and as a source of pro-angiogenic growth factors for growth of preexisting vessels by sprouting. This concept was validated by Iwaguro et al.[100] Using athymic mice with hindlimb ischemia, this group showed that transplantation of murine EPCs transduced ex vivo with an adenoviral vector expressing VEGF resulted in more efficient neovascularization and blood flow recovery that treatment with untransduced EPCs. The improved neovascularization in the animals treated with VEGF-transduced EPCs appears to be, at least in part, due to enhanced EPC proliferation and adhesion. Thus, VEGF gene transfer exerts phenotypic modulation of the EPCs, thereby potentiating biologic properties that favor the angiogenic response.

A potential noninvasive approach to angiogenesis of ischemic myocardium in CAD may involve the mobilization of EPCs to the ischemic region using conventional pharmacologic therapeutic agents used in the treatment of CAD, such as statins. Several groups showed that statin therapy increases the number of EPCs in patients with stable CAD,[196,197] suggesting that the beneficial therapeutic effect of these drugs may be mediated, at least in part, via mobilization of EPCs and subsequent neovascularization of ischemic myocardium. Walter et al[198] showed that statin therapy accelerates re-endothelialization of balloon-injured arterial segments in rats, leading to a reduction in neointimal thickening.

Cell-Based Therapy for Myocardial Regeneration

Despite evidence of myocyte replication in the heart,[199,200] the vast majority of adult cardiomyocytes are terminally differentiated and thus are unable to divide.[201] Consequently, the regenerative capacity of the infarcted myocardium is limited.[202] Hypertrophy and, possibly, hyperplasia of the surviving myocytes may provide initial structural and functional compensation, but in time these processes lead to maladaptive remodeling of the ventricle and heart failure.[203] Cell transplantation (cellular cardiomyoplasty) offers a potential alternative to reconstitution of infarcted myocardium and recuperation of cardiac function.[204] The basic premise of this approach is that repopulation of the necrotic myocardium with replication-competent cells capable of generating force should rescue contractile function and the structural integrity that is disrupted by myocardial infarction. Several cell-based regenerative strategies have evolved using a variety of substrates, such as skeletal muscle myoblasts,[205] fetal[206] and embryonic[207] cardiomyocytes, and autologous marrow-derived mesenchymal cardiomyocyte progenitors.[208] However, the therapeutic efficacy of cellular cardiomyoplasty has been inconsistent, and several technical and safety issues remain to be resolved. The optimal time for grafting after injury, the source and availability of cellular substrate, the delivery method, and the immunotolerance of the host to the grafted cells are important technical and safety considerations.

The use of an adult self-regenerating autologous source of progenitor cells with the potential for differentiation into cardiomyocytes that would graft and electrically couple to the native myocardium appears ideal. Mesenchymal cells from the bone marrow stroma of long bones may provide the best option for cellular cardiomyoplasty using autologous cells.[209] These cells are multipotent and have been shown to differentiate into functional cardiomyocytes under specific culture conditions.[210-212] Mononuclear cell preparations can be induced to differentiate into cardiomyocytes in vitro after treatment with the cytosine analog 5-azacytidine.[11,211] Synchronously beating myotube structures were observed in primary cultures of mouse bone marrow grown in the presence of 5-azacytidine. The differentiated cells present ultrastructural, genetic, and biophysical characteristics of fetal ventricular myocytes, namely, the presence of sarcomeres and atrial granules around a central nucleus, the expression of a fetal cardiac gene profile and prolonged action potentials,[11] and expression of functional adrenergic and muscarinic receptors.[210] Administration of mononuclear cell preparations harvested from bone marrow has been reported to improve cardiac function in various models of myocardial injury.[211-213]

Bone marrow mobilization with cytokines is being investigated as a potential strategy for treatment of acute myocardial infarction. Treatment with stem cell factor and granulocyte colony–stimulating factor before and immediately after infarction led to significant regeneration of infarcted myocardium and improvement in ventricular function, chamber dimensions, and long-term survival in mice.[214] These findings suggest that mobilization and "homing" of bone marrow–derived cardiogenic precursors to sites of injury in the heart may constitute a natural repair mechanism that complements native reparative processes.[215,216] The mobilization of cardiogenic precursors would then constitute a therapeutic approach to potentiating this indigenous repair mechanism. However, the regenerative capability of this cardiac "self-repair" mechanism has been questioned by two groups[217,218] who have argued that the number of extracardiac progenitors that are capable of migrating to the heart is too small to induce effective long-term regeneration of the myocardium.

From a clinical perspective, the effectiveness and simplicity of bone marrow mobilization protocols is attractive and may hold therapeutic potential as a noninvasive strategy for the treatment of acute myocardial infarction. However, further work is required to establish the lineage of these precursors, the nature of the migratory and homing signals, the mechanism of transdifferentiation, and the optimal timing for therapeutic intervention. Despite these outstanding issues, one group has treated a patient who had suffered an acute myocardial infarct with unfractionated bone marrow.[219] The authors reported that intracoronary delivery of autologous mononuclear bone marrow cells 6 days after infarction led to a reduction in infarct size and improvement in ventricular function and chamber geometry assessed at 10 weeks after transplantation. Although this study illustrates the therapeutic potential of bone marrow stem cell transplantation for treatment of myocardial infarction in humans, the general consensus of those working in the field is that the biology of these cells must be better characterized before larger clinical trials are undertaken.

PERSPECTIVES AND FUTURE DIRECTIONS

Recent years have witnessed the elucidation of many molecular mechanisms of cardiovascular diseases that has led to the development of an array of gene and cell-based strategies with potential therapeutic value for treatment of cardiovascular diseases. Some of these strategies have already made the transition from the preclinical phase to clinical trials and are now being considered for use in human patients; several others are currently undergoing safety and feasibility evaluation in early-phase trials. Notwithstanding these significant advances, we recognize the need for further developments in several aspects of cardiovascular gene therapy. Progress in vector and delivery technologies has not kept up with the identification of novel therapeutic targets, which continues to occur swiftly. All vectors currently in use for transfer of genetic material lack some of the desired features of the ideal vector. We need to emphasize the development of vectors that are amenable to endogenous regulation and that can confer tissue specificity of transgene expression. Such a degree of spatial and temporal control over transgene expression will enhance the safety of human gene therapy protocols and potentially overcome many of the potential ethical issues that arise from nonspecific transgene expression, such as germ cell line transmission. Much of this development can be carried out using current vector platforms. Rigorous systematic evaluation of the

safety and efficacy of delivery strategies and improvement of delivery devices are also prerequisites for human gene therapy protocols. The optimal genetic therapy for a complex disease such as myocardial infarction may require a combination of cell transplantation and pro-angiogenic gene therapy for long-term sustenance of the regenerated myocardium. Such potentially synergistic combinatorial approaches have seldom been considered in the design of cardiovascular gene therapy strategies, which have traditionally been developed around a single therapeutic target.

ACKNOWLEDGMENTS

Dr. Melo is a New Investigator of the Heart and Stroke Foundation of Canada and is supported by grants from the Canadian Institutes of Health Research, Canadian Foundation of Innovation, and the Health and Services Utilization and Research Commission of Saskatchewan. Dr. Dzau is supported by grants from the National Institutes of Health and is the recipient of their MERIT award. Dr. Pachori is the recipient of a postdoctoral fellowship from the American Heart Association. Dr. Mangi is the recipient of the Linton Research Fellowship from the Department of Surgery, Massachusetts General Hospital, Boston.

REFERENCES

1. Rentrop KP: Thrombi in acute coronary syndromes. Revisited and revised. Circulation 2000;101:1619.
2. Stein EA: Identification and treatment of individuals at high risk of coronary artery disease. Am J Med 2002;112:3S–9S.
3. Pitt M, Lewis ME, Bonser RS: Coronary artery surgery for ischemic heart failure: Risks, benefits, and the importance of assessment of myocardial viability. Prog Cardiovasc Dis 2001;43:373.
4. Svensson E, Marshall DJ, Woodard K, et al: Efficient and stable transduction of cardiomyocytes after intramyocardial injection or intracoronary perfusion with recombinant adeno-associated virus vectors. Circulation 1999;99:201.
5. Kaplitt MG, Xiao X, Samulski J, et al: Long-term gene transfer in porcine myocardium after coronary infusion of an adeno-associated virus vector. Ann Thorac Surg 2000;62:1669.
6. Colucci WS: Molecular and cellular mechanisms of myocardial failure. Am J Cardiol 1997;80:15L.
7. Monahan PE, Samulski RJ: Adeno-associated virus vectors for gene therapy: More pros than cons? Mol Med Today 2000;6:433.
8. Fisher KJ, Joos K, Alston J, et al: Recombinant adeno-associated virus for muscle directed gene therapy. Nat Med 1997;3:306.
9. Lundstrom K, Schweitzer C, Rotmann D, et al: Semliki Forest virus vectors: Efficient vehicles for in vitro and in vivo gene delivery. FEBS Lett 2001;504:99.
10. Schlesinger S: Alphavirus vectors: Development and potential therapeutic applications. Expert Opin Biol Ther 2001;1:177.
11. Makino S, Fukuda K, Miyoshi S, et al: Cardiomyocytes can be generated from marrow stromal cells in vitro. J Clin Invest 1999;103:697.
12. Wang JS, Shum-Tim D, Galipeau J, et al: Marrow stromal cells for cellular cardiomyoplasty: Feasibility and potential clinical advantages. J Thorac Cardiovasc Surg 2000;120:999.
13. Asahara T, Murohara T, Sullivan A, et al: Isolation of putative progenitor endothelial cells for angiogenesis. Science 1997;275:964.
14. Li S, Huang L: Nonviral gene therapy: Promises and challenges. Gene Ther 2000;7:31.
15. Akhtar S, Hughes MD, Khan A, et al: The delivery of antisense therapeutics. Adv Drug Del Rev 2000;44:3.

16. Morishita R, Higaki J, Tomita N, et al: Application of transcription factor "decoy" strategy as means of gene therapy and study of gene expression in cardiovascular disease. Circ Res 1998;82:1023.

17. Chirmule N, Propert K, Magosin S, et al: Immune responses to adenovirus and adeno-associated virus in humans. Gene Ther 1999;6:1574.

18. Hernandez YJ, Wang J, Kearns WG, et al: Latent adeno-associated virus infection elicits humoral but not cell-mediated immune responses in a nonhuman primate model. J Virol 1999;73:8549.

19. Carden DL, Granger DN: Pathophysiology of ischemia-reperfusion injury. Am J Pathol 2000;190:255.

20. Woo YJ, Zhang JC, Vijayasarathy C, et al: Recombinant adenovirus-mediated cardiac gene transfer of superoxide dismutase and catalase attenuates postischemic contractile dysfunction. Circulation 1998;98(Suppl II):255.

21. Okudo SO, Wildner MR, Shah JC, et al: Gene transfer of heat shock-protein 70 reduces infarct size in vivo after ischemia/reperfusion in the rabbit heart. Circulation 2001;103:877.

22. Hangaishi M, Ishizaka N, Aizawa T, et al: Induction of heme oxygenase-1 can act protectively against cardiac ischemia/reperfusion in vivo. Biochem Biophys Res Commun 2000;279:582.

23. Li Q, Bolli R, Qiu Y, et al: Gene therapy with extracellular superoxide dismutase protects conscious rabbits against myocardial infarction. Circulation 2001;103:1893.

24. Chen Z, Chua CC, Ho Y-S, et al: Overexpression of Bcl-2 attenuates apoptosis and protects against myocardial I/R injury in transgenic mice. Am J Physiol 2001;280:H2313.

25. Brocheriou V, Hagege AA, Oubenaissa A, et al: Cardiac functional improvement by a human Bcl-2 transgene in a mouse model of ischemia/reperfusion injury. J Gene Med 2000;2:326.

26. Hattori R, Hernanderz TE, Zhu L, et al: An essential role of the antioxidant gene Bcl-2 in myocardial adaptation to ischemia: An insight with antisense Bcl-2 therapy. Antioxid Redox Signal 2001;3:403.

27. Miao, W, Luo Z, Kitsis RN, et al: Intracoronary adenovirus-mediated Akt gene transfer in heart limits infarct size following ischemia-reperfusion injury in vivo. J Mol Cell Cardiol 2000;32:2397.

28. Brar BK, Stephanou A, Knight R: Activation of protein kinase B/Akt by urocortin is essential for its ability to protect cardiac cells against hypoxia/reoxygenation-induced cell death. J Mol Cell Cardiol 2002;34:483.

29. Matsui T, Tao J, del Monte F, et al: Akt activation preserves cardiac function and prevents injury after transient cardiac ischemia in vivo. Circulation 2001;104:330.

30. Brauner R, Nonoyama M, Laks H, et al: Intracoronary adenovirus-mediated transfer of immunosuppressive cytokine genes prolongs allograft survival. J Thorac Cardiovasc Surg 1997;114:923.

31. Qin L, Ding Y, Bromberg JS: Gene transfer of transforming growth factor-beta 1 prolongs murine cardiac allograft survival by inhibiting cell-mediated immunity. Hum Gene Ther 1996;7:1981.

32. Qin L, Chavin D, Ding Y, et al: Retrovirus-mediated transfer of viral IL-10 gene prolongs murine cardiac allograft survival. J Immunol 1996;156:2316.

33. Maulik N, Sasaki H, Addya S: Regulation of cardiomyocyte apoptosis by redox-sensitive transcription factors. FEBS Lett 2000;485:7.

34. Leri A, Fiordaliso F, Setoguchi M, et al: Inhibition of p53 function prevents renin-angiotensin system activation and stretch-mediated myocyte apoptosis. Am J Pathol 2000;157:843.

35. Holly TA, Drincic A, Byun Y, et al: Caspase inhibition reduces myocyte cell death induced by myocardial ischemia and reperfusion in vivo. J Mol Cell Cardiol 1999;31:1709.

36. Wang QD, Pernow J, Sjoquist PO, et al: Pharmacological possibilities for protection against myocardial reperfusion injury. Cardiovasc Res 2002;55:25.

37. Fukui T, Yoshiyama M, Hanatani A, et al: Expression of p22-phox and gp91-phox, essential components of NADPH oxidase, increases after myocardial infarction. Biochem Biophys Res Commun 2001;281:1200.

38. Lin KF, Chao J, Chao L: Human atrial natriuretic peptide gene delivery reduces blood pressure in hypertensive rats. Hypertension 1995;26:847.

39. Lin KF, Chao L, Chao J: Prolonged reduction of high blood pressure with human nitric oxide synthase delivery. Hypertension 1997;30:307.

40. Yoshida H, Zhang JJ, Chao L, et al: Kallikrein gene delivery attenuates myocardial infarction and apoptosis after myocardial ischemia and reperfusion. Hypertension 2000;35:25.

41. Nishida T, Ueno H, Atsuchi N, et al: Adenovirus-mediated local expression of human tissue factor pathway inhibitor eliminates shear stress–induced recurrent thrombosis in the injured carotid artery of the rabbit. Circ Res 1999;84:1446.

42. Zoldhelyi P, Chen ZQ, Shelat HS, et al: Local gene transfer of tissue factor pathway inhibitor regulates intimal hyperplasia in atherosclerotic arteries. Proc Natl Acad Sci U S A 2001;98:4078.

43. Waugh JM, Kattash M, Li J, et al: Gene therapy to promote thromboresistance: Local overexpression of tissue plasminogen activator to prevent arterial thrombosis in an in vivo rabbit model. Proc Natl Acad Sci U S A 1999;96:1065.

44. Gelband CH, Katovich MJ, Raizada MK: Current perspectives on the use of gene therapy for hypertension. Circ Res 2000;87:1118.

45. Makino N, Sugano M, Ohtsuka S, et al: Chronic antisense therapy for angiotensinogen on cardiac hypertrophy in spontaneously hypertensive rats. Cardiovasc Res 1999;44:543.

46. Wang H, Katovich MJ, Gelband CH, et al: Sustained inhibition of angiotensin I–converting enzyme (ACE) expression and long-term antihypertensive action by virally mediated delivery of ACE antisense cDNA. Circ Res 1999;85:614.

47. Reaves PY, Gelband GH, Wang H, et al: Permanent cardiovascular protection from hypertension by the AT1 receptor antisense gene therapy in hypertensive rat offspring. Circ Res 1999;85:e44.

48. Zhang YC, Bui JD, Shen L, et al: Antisense inhibition of β1-adrenergic receptor mRNA in a single dose produces a profound and prolonged reduction in high blood pressure in spontaneously hypertensive rats. Circulation 2000;101:682.

49. Lee Y, Lee WH, Lee SC, et al: CD40L activation in circulating platelets in patients with acute coronary syndrome. Cardiology 1999;92:11.

50. Schonbeck U, Mach F, Sukhova GK, et al: Regulation of matrix metalloproteinase expression in human vascular smooth muscle cells by T lymphocytes: A role for CD40 signaling in plaque rupture? Circ Res 1997;81:448.

51. Kereiakes DJ: Preferential benefit of platelet glycoprotein IIb/IIIa receptor blockade: Specific considerations by device and disease state. Am J Cardiol 1998;81:49E.

52. Kingma JG Jr, Plante S, Bogaty P: Platelet GPIIb/IIIa receptor blockade reduces infarct size in a canine model of ischemia-reperfusion. J Am Coll Cardiol 2000;36:2317.

53. Spinale FG: Matrix metalloproteinases. Regulation and dysregulation in the failing heart. Circ Res 2002;90:520.

54. Lee RT: Matrix metalloproteinase inhibition and the prevention of heart failure. Trends Cardiovasc Med 2001;11:202.

55. Lindsey ML, Gannon J, Aikawa M, et al: Selective matrix metalloproteinase inhibition reduces left ventricular remodeling but does not inhibit angiogenesis after myocardial infarction. Circulation 2002;105:753.

56. Koransky ML, Robbins RC, Blau HM: VEGF gene delivery for treatment of ischemic cardiovascular disease. Trends Cardiovasc Med 2002;12:108.

57. Tio RA, Tkebuchava T, Scheuermann, TH, et al: Intramyocardial gene therapy with naked DNA encoding vascular endothelial growth factor improves collateral flow to ischemic myocardium. Hum Gene Ther 1999;10:2953.

58. Mack CA, Patel SR, Schwarz EA, et al: Biological bypass with the use of adenovirus-mediated gene transfer of the complementary deoxyribonucleic acid for vascular endothelial growth factor 121 improves myocardial perfusion and function in the ischemic porcine heart. J Thorac Cardiovasc Surg 1998;115:168.

59. Giordano FJ, Ping P, McKirnan MD, Nozaki S, et al: Intracoronary gene transfer of fibroblast growth factor-5 increases blood flow and contractile function in an ischemic region of the heart. Nat Med 1996;2:534.

60. Ueno H, Li JJ, Masuda S, et al: Adenovirus-mediated expression of the secreted form of basic fibroblast growth factor (FGF-2) induces cellular proliferation and angiogenesis in vivo. Arterioscler Thromb Vasc Biol 1997;17:2453.

61. Ueda H, Sawa Y, Matsumoto K, et al: Gene transfection of hepatocyte growth factor attenuates reperfusion injury in the heart. Ann Thorac Surg 1999;67:1726.

62. Taniyama Y, Morishita R, Aoki M, et al: Angiogenesis and antifibrotic action by hepatocyte growth factor in cardiomyopathy. Hypertension 2002;40:47.

63. Luttun A, Carmeliet G, Carmeliet P: Vascular progenitors: From biology to treatment. Trends Cardiovasc Med 2002;12:88.

64. Robbins PD, Ghivizzani SC: Viral vectors for gene therapy. Pharmacol Ther 1998;80:35.

65. Lam PYP, Breakefield XO: Hybrid vector designs to control the delivery, fate and expression of transgenes. J Gene Med 2000;2:395.

66. Sinnaeve P, Varenne O, Collen D, et al: Gene therapy in the cardiovascular system; An update. Cardiovasc Res 1999;44:498.

67. Isner JM: Myocardial gene therapy. Nature 2002;415:234.

68. Alexander MY, Webster KA, McDonald PH, et al: Gene transfer and models of gene therapy for the myocardium. Clin Exp Pharmacol Physiol 1999;26:661.

69. Sylven C, Sarkar N, Insulander P, et al: Catheter-based transendocardial myocardial gene transfer. J Interv Cardiol 2002;15:7.

70. Lamping KG, Rios CD, Chun JA, et al: Intrapericardial administration of adenovirus for gene transfer. Am J Physiol 1997;272:H310.

71. Shibata T, Giaccia AJ, Brown JM: Development of a hypoxia-responsive vector for tumour-specific gene therapy. Gene Ther 2000;7:493.

72. Prentice H, Bishopric N, Hicks MN, et al: Regulated expression of a foreign gene targeted to the ischemic myocardium. Cardiovasc Res 1997;35:567.

73. Lee RJ, Springer ML, Blanco-Bose WE, et al: VEGF gene delivery to myocardium. Deleterious effects of upregulated expression. Circulation 2000;102:898.

74. Herttuala SY, Martin JF: Cardiovascular gene therapy. Lancet 2000;355:213.

75. Wright MJ, Wightman LML, Lilley C, et al: In vivo myocardial gene transfer: Optimization, evaluation and direct comparison of gene transfer vectors. Basic Res Cardiol 2001;96:227.

76. Wright MJ, Rosenthal E, Stewart L, et al: beta-Galactosidase staining following intracoronary infusion of cationic liposomes in the in vivo rabbit heart is produced by microinfarction rather than effective gene transfer: A cautionary tale. Gene Ther 1998;5:301.

77. Song YK, Liu F, Chu S, et al: Characterization of cationic liposome-mediated gene transfer in vivo by intravenous administration. Hum Gene Ther 1997;8:1585.

78. Labhasetwar V, Bonadio J, Goldstein S, et al: A DNA controlled-release coating for gene transfer: Transfection in skeletal and cardiac muscle. J Pharm Sci 1998;87:1347.

79. Buttrick PM, Kass A, Kitsis RN, et al: Behavior of genes directly injected into the rat heart in vivo. Circ Res 1992;70:193.

80. Sarkar N, Blomberg P, Wardell E, et al: Nonsurgical direct delivery of plasmid DNA into rat heart: Time course, dose response, and the influence of different promoters on gene expression. J Cardiovasc Pharmacol 2002;39:215.

81. Losordo DW, Vale PR, Symes JF, et al: Gene therapy for myocardial angiogenesis: Initial clinical results with direct myocardial injection of phVEGF165 as sole therapy for myocardial ischemia. Circulation 1998;98:2800.

82. Shyu KG, Wang MT, Wang BW, et al: Intramyocardial injection of naked DNA encoding HIF-1alpha/VP16 hybrid to enhance angiogenesis in an acute myocardial infarction model in the rat. Cardiovasc Res 2002;54:576.

83. Sawa Y, Kadoba K, Suzuki K, et al: Efficient gene transfer method into the whole heart through the coronary artery with hemagglutinating virus of Japan liposome. J Thorac Cardiovasc Surg 1997;113:512.

84. Harrison RL, Byrne BJ, Tung L: Electroporation-mediated gene transfer in cardiac tissue. FEBS Lett 1998;435:1.

85. Mann MJ, Gibbons GH, Hutchinson H, et al: Pressure-mediated oligonucleotide transfection of rat and human cardiovascular tissues. Proc Natl Acad Sci U S A 1999;96:6411.

86. Poston RS, Tran KP, Mann MJ, et al: Prevention of ischemically induced neointimal hyperplasia using ex vivo antisense oligodeoxynucleotides. J Heart Lung Transplant 1998;17:349.

87. Mah C, Byrne BJ, Flotte TR: Virus-based gene delivery systems. Clin Pharmacokin 2002;41:901.

88. Krasnykh VN, Douglas JT, van Beusechem VW: Genetic targeting of adenoviral vectors. Mol Ther 2000;1:391.

89. Bowles NE, Wang Q, Towbin JA: Prospects for adenovirus-mediated gene therapy of inherited diseases of the myocardium. Cardiovasc Res 1997;35:422.

90. Hartigan-O'Connor D, Barjot C, Salvatori G, et al: Generation and growth of gutted adenoviral vectors. Methods Enzymol 2002;346:224.

91. Maeda Y, Ikeda U, Shimpo M, et al: Adeno-associated virus-mediated vascular endothelial growth factor gene transfer into cardiac myocytes. J Cardiovasc Pharmacol 2000;36:438.

92. Yan Z, Zhang Y, Duan D, et al: Trans-splicing vectors expand the utility of adeno-associated virus for gene therapy. Proc Natl Acad Sci U S A 2000;97:6716.

93. Hu W-S, Pathak VK: Design of retroviral vectors and helper cells for gene therapy. Pharmacol Rev 2000;52:493.

94. Daly G, Chernajovski Y: Recent developments in retroviral-mediated gene transduction. Mol Ther 2000;2:423.

95. Trono D: Lentiviral vectors: Turning a deadly foe into a therapeutic agent. Gene Ther 2000;7:20.

96. Zhao J, Pettigrew GJ, Thomas J, et al: Lentiviral vectors for delivery of genes into neonatal and adult ventricular cardiac myocytes in vitro and in vivo. Basic Res Cardiol 2002;97:348.

97. Sakoda T, Kasahara N, Hamamori Y, et al: A high titer lentiviral production system mediates transduction of differentiated cells including beating cardiac myocytes. J Mol Cell Cardiol 1999;31:2037.

98. Coffin RS, Howard MK, Cummings DV, et al: Gene delivery to the heart in vivo and to cardiac myocytes and vascular smooth muscle cells in vitro using herpes virus vectors. Gene Ther 1996;3:560.

99. Datwyler DA, Eppenberger HM, Koller D, et al: Efficient gene delivery into adult cardiomyocytes by recombinant Sindbis virus. J Mol Med 1999;77:859.

100. Iwaguro H, Yamaguchi J, Kalka C, et al: Endothelial progenitor cell vascular endothelial growth factor gene transfer for vascular regeneration. Circulation 2002;105:732.

101. Griffiths I, Binley K, Iqball S, et al: The macrophage—a novel system to deliver gene therapy to pathological hypoxia. Gene Ther 2001;7:255.

102. Pastorino S, Massazza S, Cilli M, et al: Generation of high titer retroviral vector-producing macrophages as vehicles for in vivo gene transfer. Gene Ther 2001;8:431.

103. Howrey RP, El-Alfondi M, Phillips KL, et al: An in vitro system for efficiently evaluating gene therapy approaches to hemoglobinopathies. Gene Ther 2000;7:215.

104. Vanden Hoek TL, Shao Z, Li C, et al: Reperfusion injury on cardiac myocytes after simulated ischemia. Am J Physiol 1996;270:H1334.

105. Yeghiazarians Y, Braunstein JB, Askari A, et al: Unstable angina pectoris. N Engl J Med 2000;342:101.

106. Park JL, Lucchesi BR: Mechanisms of myocardial reperfusion injury. Ann Thorac Surg 1999;68:1905.

107. Dhalla NS, Elmoselhi AB, Hata T: Status of myocardial antioxidants in ischemia-reperfusion injury. Cardiovasc Res 2000;47:446.

108. Melo LG, Agrawal R, Zhang L, et al: Gene therapy strategy for long-term myocardial protection using adeno-associated virus-mediated delivery of heme oxygenase gene. Circulation 2002;105:602.

109. Li Q, Bolli R, Qiu Y, et al: Gene therapy with extracellular superoxide dismutase attenuates myocardial stunning in conscious rabbits. Circulation 1998;98:1438.

110. Chen EP, Bittner HB, Davis RD, et al: Physiologic effects of extracellular superoxide dismutase transgene overexpression on myocardial function after ischemia and reperfusion injury. J Thorac Cardiovasc Surg 1998;115:450.

111. Chen EP, Bittner HB, Davis RD, et al: Extracellular superoxide dismutase transgene overexpression preserves postischemic myocardial function in isolated murine hearts. Circulation 1996;94(Suppl II):412.

112. Yoshida T, Maulik N, Engelman RM: Targeted disruption of the mouse SOD I gene makes the hearts vulnerable to ischemic reperfusion injury. Circ Res 2000;86:264.

113. Zhu HL, Stewart AS, Taylor MD: Blocking free radical production via adenoviral gene transfer decreases cardiac ischemia-reperfusion injury. Mol Ther 2000;2:470.

114. Yoshida T, Watanabe M, Engelman DT, et al: Transgenic mice overexpressing glutathione peroxidase are resistant to myocardial ischemia reperfusion injury. J Mol Cell Cardiol 1996;28:1759.

115. Suzuki K, Sawa Y, Kaneda Y: In vivo gene transfer with heat shock protein 70 enhances myocardial tolerance to ischemia-reperfusion injury in rat. J Clin Invest 1997;99:1645.

116. Vander Heide RS: Increased expression of HSP27 protects canine myocytes from simulated ischemia-reperfusion injury. Am J Physiol 2002;282:H935.

117. Chatterjee S, Stewart AS, Bish LT, et al: Viral gene transfer of the antiapoptotic factor Bcl-2 protects against chronic postischemic heart failure. Circulation 2002;106(Suppl 1):I212.

118. Jonassen AK, Sack MN, Mjos OD, et al: Myocardial protection by insulin at reperfusion requires early administration and is mediated via Akt and p70s6 kinase cell-survival signaling. Circ Res 2001;89:1191.

119. David A, Chetritt J, Guillot C, et al: Interleukin-10 produced by recombinant adenovirus prolongs survival of cardiac allografts in rats. Gene Ther 2000;7:505.

120. Yang Z, Cerniway RJ, Byford AM: Cardiac overexpression of A1-adenosine receptor protects intact mice against myocardial infarction. Am J Physiol 2002;282:H949.

121. Liang BT, Jacobson KA: A physiological role of the adenosine A3 receptor: Sustained cardioprotection. Proc Natl Acad Sci U S A 1998;95:6995.

122. Agata J, Chao L, Chao J: Kallikrein gene delivery improves cardiac reserve and attenuates remodeling after myocardial infarction. Hypertension 2002;40:653.

123. Ueda, H, Sawa Y, Matsumoto K, et al: Gene transfection of hepatocyte growth factor attenuates reperfusion injury in the heart. Ann Thorac Surg 1999;67:1726.

124. Morishita R, Sugimoto T, Aoki M, et al: In vivo transfection of cis element "decoy" against nuclear factor-κB binding site prevents myocardial infarction. Nat Med 1997;3:894.

125. Chen H, Mohuczy D, Li D: Protection against ischemia/reperfusion injury and myocardial dysfunction by antisense-oligodeoxynucleotide directed at angiotensin-converting enzyme mRNA. Gene Ther 2001;8:804.

126. Yang Z, Bove CM, French BA, et al: Angiotensin II type 2 receptor overexpression preserves left ventricular function after myocardial infarction. Circulation 2002;106:106.

127. Stepkowski SM: Development of antisense oligodeoxynucleotides for transplantation. Curr Opin Mol Ther 2000;2:304.

128. Poston RS, Mann MJ, Hoyt EG, et al: Antisense oligodeoxynucleotides prevent acute cardiac allograft rejection via a novel, nontoxic, highly efficient transfection method. Transplantation 1999;68:825.

129. Yasue H, Kugiyama K: Coronary spasm: Clinical features and pathogenesis. Intern Med 1997;36:760.

130. Sposito AC, Chapman MJ: Statin therapy in acute coronary syndromes: Mechanistic insight into clinical benefit. Arterioscler Thromb Vasc Biol 2002;22:1524.

131. Feldman LJ, Isner JM: Gene therapy for vulnerable plaque. J Am Coll Cardiol 1995;26:826.

132. Chowdhury JR, Grossman M, Gupta S, et al: Long-term improvement of hypercholesterolemia after ex vivo gene therapy in LDLR-deficient rabbits. Science 1991;254:1802.

133. Grossman M, Rader DJ, Muller DW, et al: A pilot study of ex vivo gene therapy for homozygous familial hypercholesterolaemia. Nat Med 1995;1:1148.

134. Zsigmond E, Kobayashi K, Tzung KW, et al: Adenovirus-mediated gene transfer of human lipoprotein lipase ameliorates the hyperlipidemias associated with apolipoprotein E and and LDL receptor deficiencies in mice. Hum Gene Ther 1997;8:1921.

135. Applebaum-Bowden D, Kobayashi J, Kashyap VS, et al: Hepatic lipase gene therapy in hepatic lipase-deficient mice: Adenovirus-mediated replacement of a lipolytic enzyme to the vascular endothelium. J Clin Invest 1996;97:799.

136. Rinaldi M, Catapano AL, Parrella P, et al: Treatment of severe hypercholesterolemia in apolipoprotein E–deficient mice by intramuscular injection of plasmid DNA. Gene Ther 2000;7:1795.

137. Oka K, Pastore L, Kim IH, et al: Long-term stable correction of low density lipoprotein receptor-deficient mice with a helper dependent adenoviral vector expressing the very low density lipoprotein receptor. Circulation 2001;103:1274.

138. Laukkanen J, Lehtolainen P, Gough PJ, et al: Adenovirus-mediated gene transfer of a secreted form of human macrophage scavenger receptor inhibits modified low-density lipoprotein degradation and foam cell formation in macrophages. Circulation 2000;101:1091.

139. Chen SJ, Rader DJ, Tazelaar J, et al: Prolonged correction of hyperlipidemia with familial hypercholesterolemia using an adeno-associated viral vector expressing very low-density lipoprotein receptor. Mol Ther 2000;2:256.

140. Tangirala RK, Tsukamoto K, Chun SH, et al: Regression of atherosclerosis induced by liver-directed gene transfer of apolipoprotein A-1 in mice. Circulation 1999;100:1816.

141. Kullo IJ, Simari RD, Schwartz RS: Vascular gene transfer. From bench to bedside. Arterioscler Thromb Vasc Biol 1999;19:196.

142. Vassalli G, Dichek DA: Gene therapy for arterial thrombosis. Cardiovasc Res 1997;35:459.

143. Rekhter MD, Simari RD, Work CW, et al: Gene transfer into normal and atherosclerotic human blood vessels. Circ Res 1998;82:1243.

144. Kupfer J, Lei W, Pan T: Adenovirus-mediated gene transfer of thrombomodulin to human endothelial cells: Effects on thromboresistance and in vitro clotting. Circulation 1996;96(Suppl I):741.

145. Dichek DA, Anderson J, Kelly AB: Enhanced anithrombotic effects of endothelial cells expressing recombinant plasminogen activators transduced with retroviral vectors. Circulation 1996;93:301.

146. Golino P, Cirillo P, Calabro P, et al: Expression of exogegnous tissue factor pathway inhibitor in vivo suppresses thrombus formation in injured rabbit carotid arteries. J Am Coll Cardiol 2001;38:569.

147. Numaguchi Y, Naruse K, Harada M: Prostacyclin synthase gene transfer accelerates reendothelialization and inhibits neointimal formation in rat carotid arteries after balloon injury. Arterioscler Thromb Vasc Biol 1999;19:727.

148. Zoldhelyi P, McNatt J, Xu X-M: Prevention of arterial thrombosis by adenovirus-mediated transfer of cyclooxygenase gene. Circulation 1996;93:10.

149. Kim AY, Walinsky PL, Kolodgie FD: Early loss of thrombomodulin expression impairs vein graft thromboresistance: Implications for vein graft resistance. Circ Res 2002;90:205.

150. Zoldhelyi P, McNatt J, Shelat HS: Thromboresistance of balloon-injured porcine carotid arteries after local gene transfer of human tissue factor pathway. Circulation 2000;101:289.

151. Steg PG, Tahlil O, Aubailly N, et al: Reduction of restenosis after angioplasty in an atheromatous rabbit model by suicide gene therapy. Circulation 1997;96:408.

152. Morishita R, Gibbons, GH, Ellison KE, et al: Single intraluminal delivery of antisense cdc2 kinase and proliferating-cell nuclear antigen oligonucleotides results in chronic inhibition of neointimal hyperplasia. Proc Natl Acad Sci U S A 1993;90:8474.

153. Morishita R, Gibbons GH, Horiuchi M, et al: A gene therapy strategy using a transcription factor decoy of the E2F binding site inhibits smooth muscle proliferation in vivo. Proc Natl Acad Sci U S A 1995;92:5855.

154. Mann MJ, Whittemore AD, Donaldson MC, et al: Ex-vivo gene therapy of human vascular bypass grafts with E2F decoy: The PREVENT single-centre, randomized, controlled trial. Lancet 1999;354:1493.

155. Grube E, Gerckens U, Yeung AC, et al: prevention of distal embolization during coronary angioplasty in saphenous vein grafts and native vessels using porous filter protection. Circulation 2001; 104:2436–2441.

156. Morishita R, Gibbons, GH, Ellison KE, et al: Intimal hyperplasia after vascular injury is inhibited by antisense cdk2 kinase oligonucleotides. J Clin Invest 1994;93:1458.

157. Chang MW, Barr E, Lu MM, et al: Adenovirus-mediated overexpression of the cyclin/cyclin dependent kinase inhibitor, p21 inhibits vascular smooth muscle proliferation and neointima formation in the rat carotid artery model of balloon angioplasty. J Clin Invest 1995;96:2260.

158. Chang MW, Barr E, Seltzer J, et al: Cytostatic gene therapy for vascular proliferative disorders with a constitutively active form of the retinoblastoma gene product. Science 1995;267:518.

159. Yonemitsu Y, Kaneda Y, Tanaka S, et al: Transfer of wild-type p53 gene effectively inhibits vascular smooth muscle proliferation in vitro and in vivo. Circ Res 1998;82:147.

160. Gunn J, Holt CM, Francis SE, et al: The effect of oligonucleotides to c-myb on vascular smooth muscle proliferation and neointima formation after porcine coronary angioplasty. Circ Res 1997;80:520–531.

161. Shi Y, Fard A, Galeo A, et al: Transcatheter delivery of c-myc antisense oligomers reduces neointimal formation in a porcine model of coronary artery balloon injury. Circulation 1994;90:944.

162. Morishita R, Yamada S, Yamamoto K, et al: Novel therapeutic strategy for atherosclerosis. Circulation 1998;98:1898.

163. Morishita R, Gibbons GH, Tomita N, et al: Antisense oligodeoxynucleotide inhibition of vascular angiotensin-converting enzyme expression attenuates neointimal formation. Arterioscler Thromb Vasc Biol 2000;20:915.

164. Tzeng E, Shears LL, Robbins PD, et al: Vascular gene transfer of the human inducible nitric oxide synthase: Characterization of activity and effects of myointimal hyperplasia. Mol Med 1996;2:211.

165. von der Leyen HE, Gibbons GH, Morishita R, et al: Gene therapy inhibiting neointimal vascular lesion: In vivo transfer of endothelial cell nitric oxide synthase gene. Proc Natl Acad Sci U S A 1995;92:1137.

166. von der Leyen HE, Dzau VJ: Therapeutic potential of nitric oxide synthase gene manipulation. Circulation 2001;103:2760.

167. Carmeliet P: Mechanisms of angiogenesis and arteriogenesis. Nat Med 2000;6:389.

168. Baumgartner I, Isner JM: Somatic gene therapy in the cardiovascular system. Annu Rev Physiol 2001;63:427.

169. Rosengart TK, Lee LY, Patel SR, et al: Angiogenesis gene therapy. Phase I assessment of direct intramyocardial administration of an adenovirus vector expressing VEGF121 cDNA to individuals with clinically significant severe coronary artery disease. Circulation 1999;100:468.

170. Symes JF, Losordo DW, Vale PR, et al: Gene therapy with vascular endothelial growth factor for inoperable coronary artery disease. Ann Thorac Surg 1999;68:830.

171. Hammond HK, McKirnan MD: Angiogenic gened therapy for heart disease: A review of animal studies and clinical trials. Cardiovasc Res 2001;49:561, 2001.

172. Lee LY, Patel SR, Hackett NR, et al: Focal angiogenesis therapy using intramyocardial delivery of an adenovirus vector coding for vascular endothelial growth factor 121. Ann Thorac Surg 2000;69:14.

173. Tabata H, Silver M, Isner JM: Arterial gene transfer of acidic fibroblast growth factor for therapeutic angiogenesis in vivo: Critical role of secretion signal in use of naked DNA. Cardiovasc Res 1997;35:470.

174. Aoki M, Morishita R, Taniyama Y: Therapeutic angiogenesis induced by hepatocyte growth factor: Potential gene therapy for ischemic diseases. J Atheroscler Thromb 2000;7:71.

175. Yamamoto N, Kohmoto T, Roethy W: Histological evidence that fibroblast growth factor enhances the angiogenic effects of transmyocardial laser revascularization. Basic Res Cardiol 2000;95:55.

176. Sayeed-Shah U, Mann MJ, Martin J: Complete reversal of ischemic wall motion abnormalities by combined use of gene therapy with transmyocardial laser revascularization. J Thorac Cardiovasc Surg 1998;116:763.

177. Vale PR, Losordo DW, Milliken CE, et al: Randomized, single-blind, placebo-controlled pilot study of catheter-based myocardial gene transfer for therapeutic angiogenesis using left ventricular electromechanical mapping in patients with chronic myocardial ischemia. Circulation 2001;103:2138.

178. Grines CL, Watkins MW, Helmer G, et al: Angiogenic gene therapy (AGENT) trial in patients with stable angina pectoris. Circulation 2002;105:1291.

179. Losordo DW, Vale PR, Isner JM: Gene therapy for myocardial angiogenesis. Am Heart J 1999;138:S132.

180. Bashir R, Vale PR, Isner JM, et al: Angiogenic gene therapy: Preclinical studies and phase I clinical data. Kidney Int 2002; 61(Suppl 1):110.

181. Su H, Lu R, Kan YW: Adeno-associated viral vector-mediated vascular endothelial growth factor gene transfer induces neovascular formation in ischemic heart. Proc Natl Acad Sci U S A 2000;97: 13801.

182. Su H, Arakawa-Hoyt J, Kan YW: Adeno-associated viral vector-mediated hypoxia response element-regulated gene expression in mouse ischemic heart model. Proc Natl Acad Sci U S A 2002; 99:9480.

183. Boyer M, Townsend LE, Vogel LM, et al: Isolation of endothelial cells and their progenitor cells from human peripheral blood. J Vasc Surg 2000;31:181.

184. Lin Y, Weisdorf DJ, Solovey A, et al: Origins of circulating endothelial cells and endothelial outgrowth from blood. J Clin Invest 2000;105:71.

185. Shi Q, Raffi S, Wu MH, et al: Evidence for circulating bone-marrow derived endothelial cells. Blood 1998;92:362.

186. Asahara T, Masuda H, Takahashi T, et al: Bone marrow origin of endothelial progenitor cells responsible for postnatal vasculogenesis in physiological and pathological neovascularization. Circ Res 1999;85:221.

187. Shintani S, Murohara T, Ikeda I, et al: Augmentation of postnatal neovascularization with autologous bone marrow transplantation. Circulation 2001;103:897.

188. Kawamoto A, Gwon H-C, Iwaguro H, et al: Therapeutic potential of ex vivo expanded endothelial progenitor cells for myocardial ischemia. Circulation 2001;103:634.

189. Ikenaga S, Hamano K, Nishida M, et al: Autologous bone marrow implantation induced angiogenesis and improved deteriorated exercise capacity in a rat ischemic hindlimb model. J Surg Res 2001;96:277.

190. Murohara T, Ikeda H, Duan J, et al: Transplanted chord blood-derived endothelial percursor cells augment postnatal neovascularization. J Clin Invest 2000;105:1527.

191. Kalka C, Matsuda H, Takahashi T, et al: Transplantation of ex vivo expanded endothelial progenitor cells for therapeutic neovascularization. Proc Natl Acad Sci U S A 2000;97:3422.

192. Kocher AA, Schuster MD, Szabolcs MJ, et al: Neovascularization of ischemic myocardium by human bone-marrow derived angioblasts prevents cardiomyocyte apoptosis, reduces remodelling and improves cardiac function. Nat Med 2001;4:430.

193. Fuchs S, Baffour R, Zhou YF, et al: Transendocardial delivery of autologous bone marrow enhances collateral perfusion and regional function in pigs with chronic experimental myocardial ischemia. J Am Coll Cardiol 2001;37:1726.

194. Shintani S, Murohara T, Ikeda H, et al: Mobilization of endothelial progenitor cells in patients with acute myocardial infarction. Circulation 2001;103:2776.

195. Vasa M, Fichtlscherer S, Aiccher A, et al: Number and migratory activity of circulating endothelial progenitor cells inversely correlate with risk factors for coronary artery disease. Circ Res 2001;89:e1.

196. Vasa M, Fichtlscherer S, Adler K, et al: Increase in circulating endothelial progenitor cells by statin therapy in patients with stable coronary artery disease. Circulation 2001;103:2885.

197. Dimmeler S, Aicher A, Vasa M, et al: HMG-CoA reductase inhibitors (statins) increase endothelial progenitor cells via the PI 3-kinase/Akt pathway. J Clin Invest 2001;108:391.

198. Walter DH, Rittig K, Bahlmann FH, et al: Statin therapy accelerates reendothelialization. A novel effect involving mobilization and incorporation of bone marrow–derived endothelial progenitor cells. Circulation 2002;105:3017.

199. Anversa P, Kajstura J: Ventricular myocytes are not terminally differentiated in the adult mammalian heart. Circ Res 1998;83:1.

200. Beltrami AP, Urbanek K, Kajstura J, et al: Evidence that human cardiac myocytes divide after myocardial infarction. N Engl J Med 2001;344:1750.

201. Soonpaa MH, Field LJ: Survey of studies examining mammalian cardiomyocyte DNA synthesis. Circ Res 1998;83:15.

202. Li F, Wang X, Capasso JM, et al: Rapid transition of cardiac myocytes from hyperplasia to hypertrophy during postnatal development. J Mol Cell Cardiol 1996;28:1737.

203. Sutton MG, Sharpe N: Left ventricular remodelling after myocardial infarction. Pathophysiology and therapy. Circulation 2000;101:2981.

204. Reinlib L, Field L: Cell transplantation as future therapy for cardiovascular disease? Circulation 2000;101:e192.

205. Taylor DA, Atkins BZ, Hungspreugs P, et al: Regenerating functional myocardium: Improved performance after skeletal myoblast transplantation. Nat Med 1998;4:929.

206. Li RK, Mickle DA, Weisel RD, et al: Natural history of fetal rat cardiomyocytes transplanted into adult rat myocardial scar tissue. Circulation 1997;96(Suppl II):179.

207. Min JY, Yang Y, Converso KL, et al: Transplantation of embryonic stem cells improves cardiac function in postinfarcted rats. J Appl Physiol 2002;92:288.

208. Toma C, Pittenger MF, Cahill KS, et al: Human mesenchymal stem cells differentiate to a cardiomyocyte phenotype in the adult murine heart. Circulation 2002;105:93.

209. Jiang Y, Jahagirdar BN, Reinhardt RL, et al: Pluripotency of mesenchymal stem cells derived from adult marrow. Nature 2002;418:41.

210. Hakuno D, Fukuda K, Makino S, et al: Bone-marrow-derived regenerated cardiomyocytes (CMG cells) express functional adrenergic and muscarinic receptors. Circulation 2002;105:380.

211. Tomita S, Li RK, Weisel RD, et al: Autologous transplantation of bone marrow cells improves damaged heart function. Circulation 1999;100(Suppl II):247.

212. Jackson K, Majka SM, Wang H, et al: Regeneration of ischemic cardiac muscle and vascular endothelium by adult stem cells. J Clin Invest 2001;107:1395.

213. Orlic D, Kajstura J, Chimenti S, et al: Bone marrow cells regenerate infarcted myocardium. Nature 2001;410:701–705.

214. Orlic D, Kajstura J, Chimenti S, et al: Mobilized bone marrow cells repair the infarcted heart, improving function and survival. Proc Natl Acad Sci U S A 2001;98:10344.

215. Quaini F, Urbanek K, Beltrami AP, et al: Chimerism of the transplanted heart. N Engl J Med 2002;346:5.

216. Muller P, Pfeiffer P, Koglin J, et al: Cardiomyocytes of noncardiac origin in myocardial biopsies of human transplanted hearts. Circulation 2002;106:31.

217. Taylor DA, Hruban R, Rodriguez ER, et al: Cardiac chimerism as a mechanism for self-repair: Does it happen and if so to what degree? Circulation 2002;106:2.

218. Laflamme MA, Myerson D, Saffitz JE, et al: Evidence for cardiomyocyte progenitors in transplanted human hearts. Circ Res 2002;90:634.

219. Strauer BE, Brehm M, Zeus T, et al: Myocardial regeneration after intracoronary transplantation of human autologous stem cells following acute myocardial infarction. Dtsch Med Wochenschr 2001;126:932.

Cardiovascular Regeneration and Stem Cell Differentiation

Susan M. Majka
Kathyjo A. Jackson
Margaret A. Goodell
Karen K. Hirschi

Myocardial infarction (MI) is a leading cause of heart failure and death in developed countries. Heart failure affects approximately 4 to 5 million Americans, has a 4-year mortality rate of about 50%, and results in health care costs of approximately $12 billion per year.[1] Research efforts have focused on preventing chronic heart disease and improving recovery from acute myocardial infarction.

The failing heart is characterized by ischemic damage, the transition into a dilated state, ventricular remodeling, collagen deposition, and reduced contractility. Acute onset of myocardial ischemia, such as occurs in response to occlusion of a coronary vessel, results in myocardial cell death, necrosis, and scar formation. The heart is thought to lack a resident stem cell population capable of contributing to regeneration of the injured tissue; the damage is largely irreversible, yielding a permanent impairment of cardiac function. Contemporary clinical interventions, such as angiotensin-converting enzyme inhibitors or β-blockers, do not adequately prevent left ventricular remodeling and ultimately heart failure. Advances in cell plasticity and the stem cell field may offer adjunct or alternative therapies.

Circulating and bone marrow–derived stem cells have been found to contribute to the regeneration of differentiated cardiomyocytes and vascular endothelial and smooth muscle cells and, in model systems, have been associated with the restoration of cardiac function after ischemic injury. This newly identified potential of adult stem cells may prove useful as adjunct therapy for current treatment modalities. The continued evolution of strategies to manipulate adult stem cells for cardiovascular cell and gene therapy may lead to autologous preventive and restorative therapies. This chapter discusses cardiovascular regeneration in response to ischemic damage and the contribution of adult stem cells to this process.

REGENERATIVE POTENTIAL OF THE CARDIOVASCULAR SYSTEM

The repair of cardiac and vascular tissue after ischemia-reperfusion injury is a complex process. Repair involves local and systemic immune responses; invasion of the damaged tissue by circulating cells; and alterations in proliferation, migration, and phenotype of resident cell types, including cardiac myocytes, cardiac fibroblasts, and vascular endothelial and smooth muscle cells. The contribution of each of these responses is discussed in this section.

Immune Response

In the cardiovascular system, the host response to ischemia-reperfusion injury can be divided into stages that take place within a 6- to 8-week postinfarct repair period.[2] Initially the infarcted region of the heart undergoes local necrosis and myocyte apoptosis, resulting in secretion of cytokines and an accumulation of cellular debris, which stimulates an inflammatory response. The cellular debris is scavenged by infiltrating immune cells, such as macrophages and neutrophils, that also produce cytokines, such as tumor necrosis factor (TNF), transforming growth factor (TGF)-β, and interleukin (IL)-6. These factors promote the proliferation and migration of endothelial cells from existing vascular structures to form new blood vessels,[3,4] in a process referred to as *angiogenesis*, and aid in the repair of the ventricular wall.

During the postinflammatory response, there is migration and localization of differentiated myofibroblasts and deposition of fibrillar collagen types I and III,[2] which replace the immune cells and granulation tissue in the infarcted region.[5-7] The presence of myofibroblasts producing abnormal levels of collagen leads to scar formation and fibrosis, which results in abnormal ventricular function.[8,9] The fibrotic tissue accumulation in the injured heart is a continual one, and after infarction, depending on the extent of insult, fibrous tissue also may be identifiable in the noninfarcted muscle, leading to stiffness in remote parts of the heart.[2] This repair process allows the ventricle to function but is associated with irreversible deficits in cardiac output secondary to reduced cardiac contractility.[10-13]

The type of myocardial fibrosis characteristic of an infarct and associated with cardiomyocyte necrosis[7] is termed *replacement fibrosis*. In contrast, *reactive fibrosis*, which occurs in the absence of necrosis, involves collagen deposition in the perivascular space that adversely affects the functioning of arteries and arterioles in the damaged regions after injury.[7] Perivascular and interstitial myocardial fibrosis are associated with cardiac hypertrophy and a high risk of mortality.[14]

The extent of host inflammatory response; absorbance of necrotic foci; and extent of neovascularization and ensuing fibroblast proliferation, collagen production, and fibrosis determine the degree of ventricular remodeling that occurs in response to ischemic injury. One study[15] focused on the contribution of the inflammatory response, comparing the ability of two inbred mouse strains, with differing immune responses (C57Bl/6 versus MRL/MpJ), to regenerate functional ventricular tissue in response to injury. The C57Bl/6 mouse strain characteristically mounts a type 2 immune response, which is associated with TNF release and tissue destruction.[16] The inflammatory response exhibited by the MRL/MpJ mice results in relatively less tissue destruction and earlier transition to tissue repair.[17] The MRL/MpJ mouse strain has been described as having an extraordinary capacity to heal surgical wounds with little to no scarring; genes that mediate this response have been mapped to seven different genetic loci.[15] The differences in the immune response and ensuing tissue remodeling may play a pivotal role in the restoration of the injured region of the heart.

Relative to the MRL mice, the C57Bl/6 mice exhibit fewer new cardiomyocytes but enhanced neovascularization in the injury site, which may facilitate the early movement of existing cardiomyocytes into the wound followed by their DNA synthesis and proliferation.[15] The mitotic index of cardiomyocytes in the marginal zone, at 60 days postinjury, is 1% to 3% in the C57Bl/6 mice compared with 10% to 20% in the MRL mice. MRL mice also exhibit a decrease in hydroxyproline synthesis at 60 days postinjury, relative to the levels in C57Bl/6 mice. When functional analyses were performed on the MRL mice at 1 to 3 months postinjury, the left ventricle showed early dilation followed by right ventricular end-diastolic dimension shrinkage.[15] These data suggest that the capacity to regenerate after dramatic cardiac injury depends on the degree and nature of the immune response and subsequent remodeling of the wound site.

The immune response also elicits the release of cytokines and growth factors that may stimulate the mobilization and homing of circulating cells. Stem cell factor is secreted by a small subset of macrophages and promotes mast cell and myeloid precursor accumulation in the remodeling myocardium. Mast cells, in turn, affect differentiation and proliferation of fibroblasts and endothelial cells.[18] Other factors, such as vascular endothelial growth factor (VEGF), have been shown to promote the mobilization and accumulation of circulating endothelial progenitor cells. The potential of such recruited cells to give rise to cardiovascular tissue and their role in the repair of ischemic damaged tissue are discussed later.

Regeneration of Heart Tissue

Cardiac Myocytes

Cardiac myocytes are the contractile cells of the heart, and there is a large decrease in myocyte number after ischemia-reperfusion injury.[19-21] Loss of functional cardiomyocytes is devastating to the structural integrity and the contractile function of the heart. Fibrotic tissue that replaces the functional myocardium is noncontractile and does not propagate electrical conduction through the heart muscle.

Cell-cell transmission of action potentials is mediated via intercellular gap junction communication, and disruption of gap junction–mediated communication in the heart leads to arrhythmia. Gap junction channels are composed of connexin (Cx) proteins; Cx43 is the most abundant in cardiac myocytes, whereas Cx40 and Cx45 are expressed in the Purkinje fibers of the heart and allow impulse distribution through the working ventricular myocardium.[22-26] Factors contributing to a proarrhythmic condition, in response to ischemia-reperfusion injury, include localized disordering of gap junction distribution at the border zone of the infarct[25,26] and decreased Cx43 mRNA and protein levels.[25,26] To diminish such devastating effects of cardiac myocyte loss or malfunction, ongoing research efforts have focused on the preservation of myocyte viability after injury and promotion of their reentry into the cell cycle, although their replicative capacity is controversial.[27-32]

Myocyte death, in response to ischemia-reperfusion injury, results from necrosis and apoptosis in the infarcted region and apoptosis in the noninfarcted myocardium.[19,33] Apoptosis of cardiac myocytes is mediated via the up-regulation of p53, Bax, and caspase 3, in response to oxidative stress.[34-37] Antioxidant therapy has been found to attenuate oxidative stress and right ventricular hypertrophy, decreasing myocyte programmed death.[33]

Preventing death of cardiac myocytes has been an important focus because they are thought to have limited replicative capacity resulting from irreversible cell cycle exit.[28] Little evidence of DNA synthesis (0.015% in humans; 0.05% to 1% is believed to be clinically significant[27]) is observed in cardiac myocytes after injury.[29-32] Efforts have been made to enhance their capacity for replication and survival, however. Oh and colleagues[28] analyzed the effect of telomerase activity on replicative senescence in cardiac myocytes. Telomerase reverse transcriptase was expressed in the myocardium by way of a viral vector. The expression of telomerase reverse transcriptase in myocytes results in delayed exit from the cell cycle, protection from apoptosis, and progression to hypertrophy without fibrosis or impaired function.[28]

Myocardial hypertrophy is a compensatory response of the heart to deal with an increased mechanical load (pressure and volume) in an attempt to maintain cardiac contractile function.[38] Initially, cardiac function is augmented in response to hypertrophy; however, there is a gradual transition to heart failure. Cardiac hypertrophy is characterized by an increase in cardiomyocyte size in the absence of cell division, an accumulation of ribosomal RNA and messenger RNA, and increased protein synthesis and degradation, with the balance favoring synthesis. Contractile changes are due to myocyte loss of myofilaments and sarcomeric skeleton, causing contractile and diastolic dysfunction.[38,39] Chronic heart failure in humans is characterized by cardiomyocytes that have doubled in size; when that limit is reached, no further enlargement of the heart occurs.[27] The mouse displays a 46% increase in heart weight and 19.3% increase in cardiomyocyte area.[29] Familial hypertrophic cardiomyopathy is caused by mutations in components of the sarcomere, which functions as the contractile apparatus.[39,40]

Cardiac Myofibroblasts

Myofibroblasts participate in healing and remodeling of the heart and the vasculature in response to hemodynamic stress and locally released cytokines after ischemia-reperfusion injury. In the heart, cardiac fibroblasts constitute 60% of the total cells, and in the vasculature these cells are localized in the vessel wall.[41] Myofibroblasts contribute to normal collagen turnover[7] and are thought to differentiate from fibroblasts,[42] or represent "dedifferentiated" smooth muscle cells that are capable of modulating their phenotype in response to environmental cues.[43] The differentiation involves the accumulation of stress fibers or microfilaments and the expression of cytoskeletal proteins, such as smooth muscle α-actin, followed by the development of extensive interactions with extracellular matrix.[42,44,45]

The interaction of myofibroblasts with extracellular matrix and adjacent cells allows these cells to develop a contractile assembly and facilitates remodeling of the tissue microenvironment.[5-7] Their contractile activity then prevents dilation in the affected area.[46] The myofibroblast cells also orient themselves strictly parallel to the epicardium and endocardium.[47,48] This parallel alignment is thought to be modulated via the up-regulation of a tissue polarity gene, *frizzled*.[46] In this circumstance, the matrix-producing and contractile functions of the myofibroblasts are beneficial; however, they also can contribute to the progression of pathologic conditions.

Myofibroblasts play a central role in fibrogenesis during myocardial scar formation, stenosis of vascular grafts, and atherosclerosis.[48,49] In these circumstances, the myofibroblasts do not undergo apoptosis as occurs during normal wound healing, but instead they persist, express and deposit collagen,[8,9,42,44,48,50] and produce a condition referred to as *constrictive remodeling*. Such deposition of collagen is seen in the left ventricle scar after infarct and in the scarring of the hypertensive adventitia of coronary arteries.[8,9] The abnormal activity of myofibroblasts impairs functioning of the heart and surrounding vasculature and leads to apoptosis of surrounding parenchymal cells.[7]

Neovascularization of the Heart

The vasculature is a dynamic organ system, with the ability to remodel and regenerate through autocrine and paracrine means. In response to coronary occlusion and the resulting decreased distribution of oxygen and nutrients, epicardial collateral arterioles expand to maintain blood flow to the ischemic tissue.[51] When the onset of insult is gradual, the formation of new blood vessels, from the preexisting vasculature, contributes to the neovascularization of ischemic tissue.[51] Such neovascularization involves the migration, proliferation, and differentiation of endothelial and mural (pericytes and smooth muscle) cells and is crucial for repair of injured heart tissue.

Typically, uninjured adult blood vessels comprise mitotically inactive vascular endothelial and smooth muscle cells.[51,52] In response to pathologic stresses, such as hypoxia and inflammation, that cause the up-regulation of growth factors including VEGF, vascular cells are stimulated to divide and migrate. Initially, endothelial cells dissolve cell-cell contacts, detach from their basement membranes, and migrate to form neovascular sprouts. The newly formed endothelial tubes then recruit mural cells to form the surrounding vessel wall. Mural cells are thought to be recruited from either existing vessel structures, along with the endothelial cells,[53] or the surrounding mesenchyme in response to endothelial-secreted chemoattractant and mitogen, platelet-derived growth factor-B.[54,55] Direct interactions of recruited mesenchymal cells with endothelial cells leads to the activation of TGF-β,[56] which promotes the differentiation of mesenchymal cells toward a mural cell phenotype,[54,57] in a process mediated via the up-regulation of serum response factor.[58] Continued interaction between these cell types promotes quiescence[55] and ensures vessel stability. Factors involved in this multifaceted angiogenic response are summarized in Table 46–1.

Communication Between Endothelial Cells and Cardiomyocytes

Endothelial cells of different vascular beds are specialized for their particular tissue or organ system to carry out diversified functions.[59] Heterogeneity also occurs within a given vascular bed. The microenvironment of the endothelial cells may be responsible for variations in mitotic rates and responses to growth factors and hypoxia.[60,61] Endothelial cell gene expression in the heart is known to be regulated by adjacent cardiomyocytes. Myocytes stimulate expression of von Willebrand factor in a fraction of the cardiac microvascular endothelial cells.[62] Von Willebrand factor expression characteristically is elevated at microvascular sites of angiogenesis[63,64] and functions to enhance platelet adhesion to collagen fibers, preventing bleeding.[65] In turn, endothelial cells promote the differentiation of fibroblasts into myofibroblasts and promote their contractile properties.[66] This intimate interaction between cardiac myocytes and endothelial cells is crucial to maintaining muscle integrity.

CONTRIBUTION OF STEM CELLS AND MUSCLE PRECURSORS TO CARDIOVASCULAR REGENERATION

Although cardiac tissue may have a limited capacity to regenerate itself, studies show that stem cells and muscle progenitors resident in other tissues may aid in the regeneration of cardiac myocytes and blood vessels after

■ ■ ■

TABLE 46–1   CYTOKINES/GROWTH FACTORS INVOLVED IN NEOVASCULARIZATION

SOLUBLE EFFECTOR	FUNCTION
Ang-1	Binds Tie-2 and induces phosphorylation; essential for vessel wall assembly and stabilization; secreted by perivascular mesenchyme and mural cells[66]
Ang-2	Antagonist of Ang-1; destabilizes vessels to allow remodeling; secreted by perivascular mesenchyme and mural cells[66]
a-FGF	Promotes fibroblast and endothelial and mural cell migration and proliferation; secreted by fibroblasts and endothelial and mural cells[66]
b-FGF	Increased expression in response to ischemia; stored in cytoplasm of endothelial and mural cells; promotes fibroblast and endothelial and mural cell migration and proliferation[51,66]
GM-CSF	Mobilizes circulating endothelial precursor cells; secreted by macrophages[4]
HGF/SF	Stimulates endothelial cell migration, proliferation, and tube formation; secreted by fibroblasts[66]
IGF-1 and 2	Up-regulated in response to vascular injury and potentiate angiogenic response; mural cell production stimulated by PDGF-B and b-FGF; secreted by fibroblasts and endothelial and mural cells[66]
IL-6	Modulates VEGF expression; secreted by macrophages[3,4]
PDGF-B	Stimulates mural cell migration and proliferation; necessary for vessel wall assembly; stimulates mural cell and fibroblast production of VEGF and bFGF; secreted by fibroblasts and endothelial cells[66,115]
PlGF	Amplifies the activity of VEGF in ischemic heart tissue; plays a crucial role in postnatal wound healing[116]
Statin drugs	Increase the number of circulating endothelial precursor cells[89,114]
TGF-β1	Regulates migration and proliferation of fibroblasts and endothelial and mural cells; modulates VEGF expression; induces mural cell differentiation[51,66]
TNF	Procoagulant and proinflammatory; induces leukocyte adhesion and IL-1 production; inhibits endothelial cell proliferation; secreted by macrophages, mast cells, and smooth muscle cells[3,4,66]
VEGF-A	Increased expression in response to ischemia; increases vascular permeability; induces endothelial cell migration and proliferation and myocardial angiogenesis; required for cardiovascular development; secreted by macrophages, fibroblasts, and endothelial and mural cells[66,111,112,115,116]

Ang, angiopoietin; FGF, fibroblast growth factor; GM-CSF, granulocyte-macrophage colony-stimulating factor; HGF/SF, hepatocyte growth factor and scatter factor; IGF, insulin-like growth factor; IL-6, interleukin-6; PDGF, platelet-derived growth factor; PlGF, placental growth factor; TGF-β, transforming growth factor-β; TNF, tumor necrosis factor; VEGF, vascular endothelial growth factor.

ischemic injury and contribute to functional restoration of injured heart tissue. Circulating progenitors, bone marrow–derived hematopoietic stem cells (HSC), and bone marrow–derived mesenchymal cells (MSC) have been shown to engraft into cardiac muscle, neovessels, or both (Fig. 46-1). These studies show that such adult stem cells may be useful for autologous treatment of cardiovascular disease and injury. These and related studies of cardiac engraftment of other cell types, including myocytes derived from neonatal heart and skeletal muscle, embryonic stem cells, and fibroblasts, are summarized in Table 46-2 and discussed subsequently. Also discussed is the potential of differentiated cells within heart tissue to transdifferentiate into other cell types after injury.

Transdifferentiation

Transdifferentiation involves the conversion of a "fate-specified" cell into another cell type with a distinctly different phenotype.[67] Instances of transdifferentiation have been reported; however, in most cases, stringent controls have not been done to rule out the possibility that the population under investigation did not contain multiple cell types or "uncommitted" cells that then differentiate and not "transdifferentiate."

Most reports of transdifferentiation involve cell types within mammalian muscle (Fig. 46-2). Muscle cells have been reported to convert from smooth to striated phenotypes and to an adipocytic lineage.[68,69] Some evidence suggests that vascular smooth muscle cells may be derived from endothelial cells.[70] More recently, reports

of embryonic vascular endothelial cells transdifferentiating into cardiac myocytes suggest that such a process

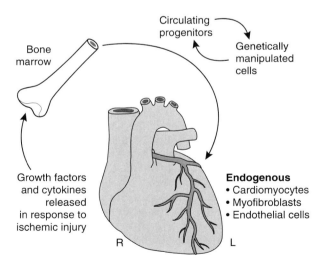

FIGURE 46–1. Mechanisms of cardiovascular regeneration. In response to ischemia-reperfusion injury, growth factors and cytokines are released into circulation from the injured site, presumably inducing mobilization of undifferentiated stem cells that home to the site of injury and contribute to the regeneration of damaged cardiovascular tissue. When the true progenitors are identified, it is hoped that they can be isolated, expanded, and genetically manipulated efficiently to express therapeutic agents, which accelerate and extend the healing process. Endogenous cells within heart tissue also may contribute to regeneration in response to injury; however, their abilities are limited, as evidenced by the large number of fatalities resulting from ischemia-reperfusion injury.

TABLE 46–2   CARDIOVASCULAR CELL THERAPY

PRECURSOR CELL	ADMINISTRATION	ENGRAFTMENT	IMPROVED FUNCTION (Y/N/NT)*	REFERENCE
Myoblasts and Fibroblasts				
Skeletal myoblasts	Direct injection	Myocytes	Y	75
Dermal fibroblasts	Direct injection	Myocytes	N	75
Skeletal myoblasts	Direct injection	Cardiac myocytes	NT	74
Skeletal myoblasts	Transventricular injection	Cardiac myocytes	NT	73
Skeletal myoblasts	Direct injection	Myocytes	Y	113
Skeletal myoblasts	Direct injection	Myocytes	Y	106
Fetal and Embryonic Cells				
Cardiomyocytes†	Direct injection	Cardiac myocytes	NT	108,109
Cardiomyocytes	IV injection	Cardiac myocytes	Y	107
Cardiomyocytes	Direct injection	Cardiac myocytes	NT	29,118,119
Cardiomyocytes	Patch	Cardiac myocytes	NT	117
Cardiomyocytes	IV injection	Cardiac myocytes	Y	110
ESC-derived cardiomyocytes	Direct injection	Cardiac myocytes	NT	81
ESC-derived cardiomyocytes	Direct injection	Cardiac myocytes	Y	80
Endothelial Cells and Precursors				
Endothelial cells or precursors	Direct injection	Cardiac myocytes	NT	71
Circulating EPC	IV injection	Endothelial cells	Y	94
BM-derived	BM transplant	Endothelial cells	NT	83,84
EPC (Flk-1+,Tie-2+)				
Bone Marrow–Derived Cells				
BM-SP cells (lin−/CD34−/low/c-kit+/Sca+)	BM transplant	Cardiac myocytes Vascular endothelium	NT	72
BM-angioblasts (CD34+)	IV injection	Endothelial cells Smooth muscle cells	Y	85
BM subpopulation (lin−/c-kit−)	Direct injection	Myocardium Vascular endothelium Vascular smooth muscle	Y	96
BM-stromal cells	IV injection	Cardiac myocytes Myofibroblasts Endothelium Endocardium	NT	103
huMSC	Direct injection	Cardiac myocytes	NT	104

* Y, yes; N, no; NT, not tested.
† Fetal, neonatal—viable, adult—nonviable.
BM, bone marrow; EPC, endothelial precursor cells; SP, side population; ESC, embryonic stem cells; huMSC, human mesenchymal stem cells; IV, intravenous.

may contribute to myocyte regeneration in response to injury.

Condorelli and associates[71] isolated endothelial cells from embryonic (E9) mouse dorsal aortas and showed that cells within this population expressed markers of

Original cell type → Resulting cell type		Reference
Smooth muscle	Striated muscle	69
Skeletal myocyte	Cardiac myocyte	67, 106, 113
Endothelium	Cardiac myocyte	71
Embryonic dorsal aorta endothelium	Smooth muscle and mesenchymal cells	70

FIGURE 46–2. Reported transdifferentiation of differentiated cell types to cardiovascular cells. Transdifferentiation involves the conversion of a "fate-specified" cell into another cell type with a distinctly different phenotype.

cardiomyocytes in vivo and in vitro. These studies suggest that nonconventional pathways of cell differentiation, completely independent of the accepted developmental paradigms, may contribute to cellular regeneration in response to injury. These findings are confounded, however, by the fact that the starting population of endothelial cells was characterized by expression of markers, such as PE-CAM-1, that also are expressed on endothelial progenitors and multipotent stem cells.[72] True transdifferentiation of a committed cell type was not shown and would require a thorough characterization of the molecular phenotype of the cell population in question and evaluation of differentiation on a single-cell, or clonal, level.

Myoblasts and Fibroblasts

In efforts to identify autologous sources of cells for cardiac repair, muscle precursor cells, or myoblasts, derived from noncardiac sources have been tested for their ability to engraft into cardiac muscle and become functionally integrated into the myocardium. Robinson and coworkers[73] showed that myoblasts derived from skeletal muscle and administered intravenously stably engraft into host myocardium.[73] Desmosomes and Cx43-containing gap junctions are present between transplanted cells and adjacent cardiac myocytes,[73] suggesting the potential for cell-cell communication and electrical coupling. In subsequent studies, Reinecke and coworkers[74] and others[67] determined that although skeletal myoblasts engraft into myocardium and are capable of contracting, they are not electrically coupled to cardiac myocytes. In contrast, in vitro coculture of neonatal or adult cardiomyocytes with skeletal myoblasts results in the synchronous contraction of 10% of the skeletal myoblasts; expression of Cx43 between these cell types is detectable using electron microscopy.[74]

Despite the fact that in vivo studies indicate that transplanted skeletal myoblasts do not form functional junctions with cardiomyocytes, other in vivo studies report an increase in cardiac function after myoblast transplantation (see Table 46-2). The mechanism by which transplanted myoblasts promoted improved function was not clear. To investigate whether it was the contractile properties of the myoblasts that enhanced cardiac function, Hutcheson and coworkers[75] directly compared the abilities of transplanted skeletal myoblasts versus noncontractile dermal fibroblasts to restore cardiac muscle function in injured rabbit hearts. Diastolic and systolic performances were evaluated in both groups at 3 weeks after transplant. Diastolic performance was improved after transplantation of both cell types, whereas the systolic function was improved only by the myoblast engraftment; fibroblast engraftment decreased performance.[76] These results suggest that the contractile properties of the myoblasts may promote cardiac function. Differences in functional outcome resulting from differences in extracellular matrix synthesis and deposition by the distinct cell types were not evaluated, however. Fibroblasts are known to make abnormally high levels of collagen I, which can adversely affect myocardial function, as previously discussed; the true limitation of these cells in contributing to functional myocytes is still not entirely clear.

Stem Cell Origins

Stem cells can be isolated from several sources, including embryonic, fetal, and adult tissues. Although embryonic stem cells are known to be pluripotent, adult stem cells previously were thought to replenish only the tissue in which they reside. More recent studies show, however, that progenitors from other organ systems can regenerate cardiac tissue in the absence of endogenous cells with ample regenerative capacity. Circulating and bone marrow–derived stem cells have been shown to engraft into cardiac muscle and blood vessels in the regenerating myocardium. These studies suggest that the transplanta-

tion of such precursor cells may be of therapeutic value. The potential use of adult stem cells and embryonic and fetal cells for cardiovascular therapy is discussed subsequently.

Fetal Cells

In contrast to the previously discussed adult skeletal myoblasts, cardiac myocytes derived from fetal tissue proliferate and form stable cell-cell communication channels with cardiac myocytes on transplantation into injured murine myocardium.[77] Sakai and associates[78] found that fetal cardiomyocyte transplantation into the scar region of an ischemia-reperfusion injury improved cardiac function; however, the engraftment was not stable, and the cells eventually were rejected.[78]

The influence of the developmental stage of the transplanted cardiomyocytes on graft survival and functional integration was investigated.[74] These studies revealed that fetal and neonatal cardiac myocytes engraft into normal and acutely injured myocardium and granulation tissue, whereas adult cardiomyocytes do not engraft stably into these tissues.[74] The engrafted fetal and neonatal cardiomyocytes expressed Cx43 and N-cadherin and were coupled electrically to the host myocytes. Although fetal myocytes have an apparent functional advantage over adult myocytes in the repair of damaged heart tissue, they would not be available for autologous cardiovascular therapies. In the clinical setting, their use may be limited.

Embryonic Stem Cells

In contrast to fetal cells, which are isolated from specific organ systems prenatally embryonic stem cells are isolated much earlier in development from the inner cell mass of blastocysts. Embryonic stem cells are known to give rise to all cell types of the body and represent an attractive cell source for many clinical therapies. Additionally, embryonic stem cells can be propagated and maintained as undifferentiated cells in culture indefinitely, and it was shown that human embryonic stem cells can be differentiated into cardiomyocytes in vitro.[79] Embryonic stem cell–derived cardiomyocytes were identified in culture by their spontaneous contraction (8.1% of the population) and were characterized further by their ability to propagate calcium currents and express cardiac-specific proteins, including cardiac myosin heavy chain, α-actinin, desmin, cardiac troponin I, and atrial natriuretic peptide.[79] The structural and functional properties of the embryonic stem cell–derived cardiomyocytes were similar to previously characterized embryonic and fetal cardiomyocytes.[79]

Transplantation of mouse embryonic stem cell–derived cardiomyocytes in vivo, after injury, has been shown to improve functional restoration of cardiac tissue. Green fluorescent protein (GFP)-labeled embryonic stem cell–derived cardiomyocytes were injected directly into mouse myocardium after coronary ligation.[80] The transplanted cells were found to engraft into the myocardium and express sarcomeric α-actin, cardiac α-myosin heavy chain, and troponin I.[80] Six weeks after injury and transplantation, the embryonic stem cell–derived cells comprised 7.3% of the left ventricular myocardium, and the engrafted heart tissue exhibited improved ventricular contractility, although electrical coupling to the preexisting cardiomyocytes was not documented. A similar study using genetically selected embryonic stem cell–derived cardiac myocytes injected into the ventricles of mdx mice (dystrophin–/–) found dystrophin-positive cardiac myocytes engrafted into the myocardium and expressing sarcomeric myosin, desmin, and α-actinin.[81]

Embryonic stem cells also are known to give rise to vascular endothelium and smooth muscle and may promote nascent blood vessel formation in injured tissues and stimulate the release of cardioprotective vascular-specific growth factors, such as VEGF.[80,82] VEGF has been shown to enhance the mobilization of circulating endothelial cell precursors and vascularization of ischemia-injured tissues,[83,84] as discussed subsequently.

Circulating Endothelial Precursor Cells

In addition to progenitors that reside in fetal and embryonic tissues, precursor populations are retained within tissues postnatally and may contribute to cardiovascular regeneration throughout life. Bone marrow and peripheral blood are two well-studied sources of such cells that may prove beneficial for autologous cardiovascular cell therapies.

Peripheral blood is known to contain a population of cells that can regenerate vascular endothelium in response to injury. These so-called circulating endothelial precursor cells are thought to be bone marrow derived and are likened to the angioblast, with which they share common antigenic markers, such as CD34, VEGF receptor-2 (Flk-1), PE-CAM-1, and Tie-2.[83,85,86] Circulating endothelial precursor cells are capable of incorporating into foci of postnatal neovascularization,[86,87] via a process more similar to embryonic vasculogenesis than the previously described angiogenic sprouting and remodeling of the existing vasculature. The contribution of nonresident circulating endothelial precursor cells to de novo vessel formation illuminated the potential for the existence of an easily accessible, autologous source of vascular precursors that may be used to modulate blood vessel formation in adults.

The contribution of circulating endothelial precursor cells to repair after ischemic injury has been well documented. The mobilization of circulating endothelial precursor cells can be promoted in response to ischemic insult or via exogenous administration of cytokines.[83,85,86] In an animal model, hindlimb ischemia increases the number of circulating endothelial precursor cells greater than 400-fold.[86] The growth factors granulocyte-macrophage colony-stimulating factor (GM-CSF) and VEGF, present in ischemic myocardium and statin drugs, augment circulating levels of these cells that maintain their ability to integrate into new blood vessels.[86,88–92] VEGF alone in mice and humans elicits a 245-fold and 154-fold increase in circulating endothelial precursor cells 1 to 28 days post-treatment.[83,90] Increased neovascularization evoked by these cells, in response to myocardial ischemia, has been shown to improve postinjury cardiac function.[85,94]

Studies by Vasa and coworkers[93] examined the effects of coronary artery disease and statin therapy on the number and migratory capacity of human circulating endothelial precursor cells because atherosclerotic risk factors have been shown to decrease neovascularization in response to tissue ischemia. Hypertension was found to reduce endothelial precursor cell migration, whereas smoking decreased the number of circulating cells, possibly as a result of apoptosis in response to oxidative stress.[89,92] The cells' migratory response to VEGF also was impaired; however, there was no decrease in VEGF receptor-2 expression (Flk-1).[92] Statin treatment of patients increased the numbers of circulating endothelial precursor cells by 1.5-fold to 3-fold over the course of the 4-week study without altering serum levels of VEGF, TNF, and GM-CSF.[93] These cells have been isolated from the peripheral circulation, cultured ex vivo, reintroduced, and found to contribute to therapeutic angiogenesis in an infarcted heart, helping to restore function.[90,94] Statin drug therapies may be beneficial on multiple levels.

Bone Marrow–Derived Stem Cells

Bone marrow is a well-documented source of multipotent cells containing HSC and MSC. Studies have shown the potential for HSC and MSC to incorporate into injured myocardium and blood vessels and restore some degree of cardiac function (see Table 46–2).

Hematopoietic Cells. HSC are capable of self-renewal and the production and replenishment of all hematopoietic lineages over the course of an organism's lifetime. They may be distinguished from other stem cells by bone marrow transplantation analysis. In murine models, recipients are lethally irradiated and transplanted with putative HSC, which repopulates the bone marrow and reconstitutes all blood cell lineages. Bone marrow transplantation of non-HSC does not rescue the mouse from lethal irradiation.

Bone marrow–derived HSC may be isolated based on their expression of specific cell surface antigens, which differ between mouse-derived and human-derived cells, and lack of expression of differentiated hematopoietic lineage markers (lin-).[95] Studies by Jackson and colleagues[72] and Orlic and associates[96,97] showed the ability of two different marrow-derived populations, enriched for HSC, to contribute to the regenerating myocardium.

Jackson and colleagues[72] transplanted murine LacZ-marked, enriched HSC, the so-called side population (SP) of cells, into lethally irradiated mice. SP cells represent a purified (CD34-/low, c-kit+, Sca-1+, lin-) HSC population that is selected by Hoechst dye efflux and the resultant fluorescence activated cell sorter (FACS) profile.[98] After the lethally irradiated recipients were stably engrafted with bone marrow–derived SP cells, they underwent surgery to induce myocardial ischemia by occlusion of the left anterior descending branch of the coronary artery for 1 hour followed by reperfusion. The engrafted SP cells, or their progeny, migrated into the ischemic left

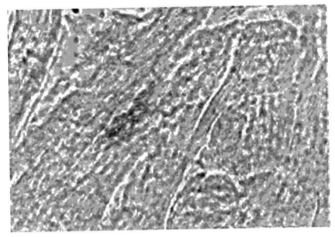

A

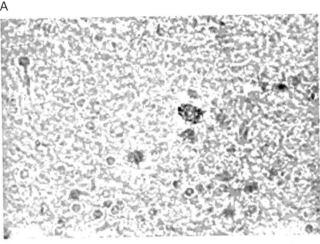

B

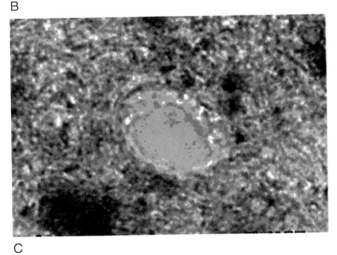

C

FIGURE 46–3. Bone marrow–derived SP cell engraftment into infarcted myocardium. Stably engrafted bone marrow–derived SP cells were mobilized from the bone marrow, homed to the site of cardio-vascular injury, and engrafted into cardiac myofibers (A), vascular endothelium (B), and fibrotic tissue (C) in the infarcted and border zones after ischemia-reperfusion injury. (Magnification ×65.)

ventricle, as evidenced by the presence of LacZ-marked cells in this region. The donor SP cells participated in the regeneration of cardiomyocytes and myofibers and vas-

cular endothelium and fibrotic tissue (Fig. 46–3). The LacZ-positive cells expressed markers of lineage commitment, α-actinin, or Flt-1 and ICAM-1, indicative of cardiac myocyte and endothelial cell differentiation. Donor-derived cardiomyocytes were found predominantly in the peri-infarct region with an incorporation rate of 0.02% throughout the entire heart. Endothelial engraftment occurred at a rate of 3.3%, primarily in small vessels adjacent to the infarct. Bone marrow–derived SP cells did not stably engraft into uninjured sham-operated hearts. The incorporation of marrow-derived SP cells into endothelial and cardiomyocyte lineages in response to injury suggests that stem cells within bone marrow naturally contribute to the repair of heart tissue.

Orlic and coworkers[96] used a lin-, c-kit+ population of murine bone marrow cells, enriched for HSC but containing other progenitors as well. After coronary ligation, these cells were injected directly into the wall bordering the infarct in the heart and were found to replace 68% of the infarcted myocardium. These investigators[97] went on to study the impact of stem cell mobilization on tissue recovery. GM-CSF and stem cell factor (SCF) were injected intravenously immediately after cardiac injury and presumed to enhance the mobilization of stem cells from bone marrow. The cytokine treatment after infarction was associated with a 68% decrease in mortality, 40% decrease in infarct diameter, 26% decrease in cavity dilation, 70% decrease in diastolic stress, and a progressive increase in ejection fraction. In this study, cells within the bone marrow were not labeled, so it is impossible to determine if marrow-derived "stem" cells engrafted into the site of injury and contributed to functional restoration of the cardiac tissue. The possibility that postinfarction cytokine treatment improves postinjury cardiac recovery via other mechanisms cannot be ruled out.

The different methods of stem cell delivery used in these studies, bone marrow transplantation versus direct injection, may have contributed to variations in observed stem cell engraftment levels. The differences in the stem cell populations under investigation also must be considered. The bone marrow–derived SP cells are highly purified and homogeneous, relative to the lin-/c-kit+ fraction of whole bone marrow. Whether simultaneous delivery of multiple stem cell types, as occurs with the injection of heterogeneous populations, is required for clinically significant levels of engraftment and functional integration into injured tissues remains to be determined. Nonetheless, these studies suggest that bone marrow transplantation of HSC and mobilization strategies may be useful for autologous repair of injured heart tissue.

Mesenchymal Cells. Bone marrow also contains precursor cells for nonhematopoietic cell types, which are referred to as stromal cells or MSC. MSC are multipotential in nature with the ability to differentiate into osteoblasts, chondrocytes, adipocytes, and myotubes[99,100] and are isolated from whole bone marrow based on their ability to adhere to tissue culture plastic.[1]

A cardiomyogenic cell line was isolated and characterized from murine bone marrow stroma.[102] The cultures were evaluated for their ability to propagate action potentials and express cardiac isoforms of the contractile proteins actin and myosin and cardiomyocyte-specific genes MEF2A and MEF2D.[102] The cultured cells were likened to fetal ventricular cardiomyocytes.

MSC isolated from murine and human bone marrow have been found to contribute to myocyte regeneration in vivo. MSC were isolated from murine tissue, based solely on their adherence properties in culture, labeled with lacZ, and introduced intravenously 4 weeks after coronary ligation–induced injury.[103] LacZ-positive cells were observed to engraft into fibroblasts in the scar region and into cardiomyocytes, vascular endothelium, and endocardium in the peri-infarct region. MSC derived from human bone marrow and transplanted into mice exhibited similar behavior.[104] LacZ-labeled huMSC were injected into the ventricle of immunodeficient mice, and over time, the surviving cells expressed α-actinin, β-myosin heavy chain, and cardiac troponin T with sarcomeric organization of the contractile proteins.[104]

Although engraftment of MSC into myocardial tissue is evident from these studies, the true cardiovascular progenitor cells within the heterogeneous MSC populations are unknown. To develop MSC populations further for clinical use, molecular characterization and subcloning of specific stem cell types would be necessary.

Progenitors of Unspecified Origin

Most of the previously discussed studies examined the potential of a specific population of putative stem cells to engraft cardiovascular tissue in vivo, using such techniques as bone marrow transplantation or direct injection of genetically labeled progenitors. In contrast, another study[105] evaluated the engraftment of donor hearts with recipient cells, which may have been derived from multiple sources. In these human studies, donor hearts derived from female patients were transplanted into male patients with from congestive heart failure.[105] Engraftment of the donor hearts with recipient cells was determined via Y-chromosome localization within cardiac and vascular cells post mortem.

The hypothesis of these studies was that undifferentiated (stem) cells would translocate from the recipient to the grafted tissue and contribute to ventricular remodeling and neovascularization and sustain cardiac performance. Y chromosome–positive cells were reported to constitute 4% to 15% of the cardiac myocytes, 7% to 12% of the arterioles, and 5% to 9% of the capillaries in the transplanted female hearts, although engraftment levels were inversely correlated with length of transplantation, suggesting instability of engrafted cardiac and vascular cells, which normally have long half-lives. Nonetheless the average levels of engraftment into cardiovascular tissue by nonresident cells in this study are higher than those reported in studies of specific, marked populations. It is likely that the cells that engrafted into the transplanted hearts were derived from multiple tissue sources within the recipient (muscle, bone marrow, and blood circulation), as discussed previously, and this may contribute to the apparent discrepancy. The lack of evaluation of functional restoration of the transplanted hearts precludes determination of whether high levels of engraftment of nonresident cells would prove clinically beneficial. Further studies of the functional integration and stability of known, marked populations of progenitor cells are needed.

SUMMARY

In response to ischemia-reperfusion injury, heart tissue has limited ability to regenerate healthy, functional myocardium. Through compensatory mechanisms, the injured tissue is replaced by fibrotic scar and hypertrophied cardiomyocytes, which initially maintain some degree of structural integrity; however, the ultimate result of these processes is heart failure.

The aforementioned studies provide evidence that nonresident cell populations (differentiated, immature, and multipotent cells) from multiple tissue sources (embryonic and fetal tissue, skeletal muscle, bone marrow, and blood circulation) can contribute to the remodeling myocardium. The best source of these cells for the production of stable, functional heart tissue remains to be determined.

Areas of ongoing and future study focus on enhancing mobilization of autologous progenitors, improving homing to sites of injury, and assessing the long-term stability and functional integration of such cells into cardiovascular tissues. Optimization of these parameters is necessary to achieve clinically significant levels of engraftment and functional restoration of injured tissues. Standardization of functional tests would enable the comparison of many trials, including trials that assess levels of incorporation of endogenously mobilized cells and transplanted cells engineered to deliver therapeutic agents.

REFERENCES

1. Delling U, Sussman M, Molkentin J: Re-evaluating sarcoplasmic reticulm function in heart failure. Nat Med 2000;6:942-943.
2. Sun Y, Weber K: Infarct scar: A dynamic tissue. Cardiovas Res 2000;46:250-256.
3. Sack M, Smith R, Opie L: TNF in myocardial hypertrophy and ischaemia—an anti apoptotic perspective. Cardiovasc Res 2000;45:688-695.
4. Entman M, Smith C: Postreperfusion inflammation: A model for reaction to injury in cardiovascular disease. Cardiovasc Res 1994;28:1301-1311.
5. Gabbiani G, Hirschel B, Ryan G, et al: Granulation tissue as contractile organ: Structure and function. J Exp Med 1972;135:719-734.
6. Gabbiani G, Ryan G, Majno G: Presence of modified fibroblasts in granulation tissue and their possible role in wound contraction. Experientia 1971;27:549-550.
7. Weber K, Sun Y, Katwa L: Myofibroblasts and local angiotensin II in rat cardiac tissue repair. Int J Biochem Cell Biol 1997;29:31-42.
8. Cleutjens J, Verluyten M, Smits J, et al: Collagen remodeling after myocardial infarction in rat heart. Am J Pathol 1995;147:325-338.
9. Silver M, Pick R, Brilla C, et al: Reactive and reparative fibrillar collagen remodeling in the hypertrophied rat left ventricle: Two experimental modes of myocardial fibrosis. Cardiovasc Res 1990;24:741-747.
10. Irwin M, Mak S, Mann D: Tissue expression and immunolocalization of tumor necrosis factor alpha in postinfarction dysfunctional myocardium. Circulation 1999;99:1492-1498.

11. Meldrum D, Meng X, Dinarello C: Human myocardial tissue TNF expression following acute global ischemia in vivo. J Mol Cell Cardiol 1998;30:1683–1689.

12. Szabolcs M, Michler R, Yang X: Apoptosis of cardiac myocytes during cardiac allograft rejection: Relation to induction of nitric oxide synthase. Circulation 1996;94:1665–1673.

13. Tracey K, Beutler B, Lowry S: Shock and tissue injury induced by recombinant human cachectin. Science 1986;234:470–474.

14. Staufenberger S, Jacobs M, Brandstatter K, et al: Angiotensin II type I receptor regulation and differential trophic effects on rat cardiac myofibroblasts after acute myocardial infarction. J Cell Physiol 2001;187:326–335.

15. Leferovich J, Bedelbaeva K, Samulewicz S, et al: Heart regeneration in adult MRL mice. Proc Natl Acad Sci U S A 2001;98:9830–9835.

16. Majka S, Kasimos J, Izzo A: MMP expression in pulmonary inflammation varies with the immune response: Granuloma formation is associated with MMP-2 expression. J Med Mycol 2002;40:323–328.

17. Li X, Mohan S, Gu W, et al: Analysis of gene expression in the wound repair/regeneration process. Mamm Genome 2001;12:52–59.

18. Frangogiannis N, Perrard J, Mendoza L, et al: Stem cell factor induction is associated with mast cell accumulation after canine myocardial ischemia and reperfusion. Circulation 1998;98:687–698.

19. Cheng W, Kajstura J, Nitahara J, et al: Programmed cell death contributes to ventricular remodeling after myocardial infarction in rats. Exp Cell Res 1996;226:316–327.

20. Beltrami A, Urbanek K, Kajstura J, et al: Evidence that human cardiac myocytes divide after myocardial infarction. N Engl J Med 2001;344:1750–1757.

21. Beltrami C, Finato N, Rocco M, et al: Structural basis of end stage failure in ischemic cardiomyopathy in humans. Circulation 1994;89:151–163.

22. Beyer E, Kistler J, Paul D, et al: Antisera directed against connexin 43 peptides react with a 43 kD protein localized to gap junctions in myocardium and other tissues. J Cell Biol 1989;108:595–605.

23. Coppen S, Dupont E, Rothery S, Severs N: Connexin 45 expression is preferentially associated with the ventricular conduction system in mouse and rat heart. Circ Res 1998;8:232–243.

24. Gros D, Jongsma H: Connexins in mammalian heart function. BioEssays 1996;18:719–730.

25. Severs N: The cardiac muscle cell. Bioessays 2000;22:188–199.

26. Severs N: Gap junctions and coronary heart disease. In DeMello WC, Janse MJ (eds): Heart Cell Communication in Health and Disease. Boston, Kluwer, 1998, pp 175–194.

27. Anversa P, Kajstura J: Ventricular myocytes are not terminally differentiated in the adult mammalian heart. Circ Res 1998;83:1–14.

28. Oh H, Taffet G, Youker K, et al: Telomerase reverse transcriptase promotes cardiac muscle cell proliferation, hypertrophy and survival. Proc Natl Acad Sci U S A 2001;98:10308–10313.

29. Soonpaa M, Field L: Assessment of cardiomyocyte DNA synthesis during hypertrophy in adult mice. Am J Physiol 1994;266:1439–1445.

30. Soonpaa M, Kim K, Pajak L, et al: Cardiomyocyte DNA synthesis in binucleation during murine development. Am J Physiol 1996;271:2183–2189.

31. Soonpaa M, Field L: Assessment of cardiomyocyte DNA synthesis in normal and injured adult mouse hearts. Am J Physiol 1997;272:220–226.

32. Soonpaa M, Field L: Survey of studies examining mammalian cardiomyocyte DNA synthesis. Circ Res 1998;83:15–26.

33. Oskarsson H, Coppey L, Weiss R, Li W: Antioxidants attenuate myocyte apoptosis in the remote noninfarcted myocardium following large myocardial infarction. Cardiovasc Res 2000;45:679–687.

34. Didenko V, Wang X, Yang L, et al: Expression of p21 and p53 in apoptotic cells in adrenal cortex and induction by ischemia/reperfusion injury. J Clin Invest 1996;97:1723–1731.

35. von Harsdorf R, Li P, Dietz R: Signaling pathways in reactive oxygen species induced cardiomyocyte apoptosis. Circulation 1999;99:2934–2941.

36. Matsura T, Kai M, Fujii Y, et al: Hydrogen peroxide induced apoptosis in HL-60 cells requires caspase 3 activation. Free Rad Res 1999;30:73–83.

37. Sandau K, Pfeilschifter J, Brune B: Nitric oxide and super oxide induced p53 ans Bax accumulation during mesangial cell apoptosis. Kidney Int 1997;52:378–386.

38. Puri P, Natoli G, Avantaggiati M, et al: The molecular basis of myocardial hypertrophy. Ann Ital Med Int 1994;9:160–165.

39. Nicol RL, Frey N, Olson EN: From the sarcomere to the nucleus: Role of genetics and signaling in structural heart disease. Ann Rev Genomics Hum Genet 2000;1:179–223.

40. Schaub M, Hefti M, Harder B, Eppenberger H: Various hypertrophic stimuli induce distinct phenotypes in cardiomyocytes. J Mol Med 1997;75:901–920.

41. Dubey R, Gillespie D, Zacharia L, et al: A2B receptors mediate the antimitogenic effects of adenosine in cardiac fibroblasts. Hypertension 2001;37:716–721.

42. Zalewski A, Shi Y: Vascular myofibroblasts: Lessons from coronary repair and remodeling. Arterioscler Thromb Vasc Biol 1997;17:417–422.

43. Nobuyoshi M, Kimura T, Ohishi H, et al: Restenosis after percutaneous transluminal coronary angioplasty. J Am Coll Cardiol 1991;17:433–439.

44. Darby I, Skalli O, Gabianni G: Smooth muscle alpha actin is transiently expressed by myofibroblasts during experimental wound healing. Lab Invest 1990;63:21–29.

45. Welch M, Odland G, Clark R: Temporal relationships of F-actin bundles formation, collagen and fibronectin matrix assembly, and fibronectin receptor expression to wound contraction. J Cell Biol 1990;110:133–145.

46. Blankesteijin W, Essers-Janssen Y, Verluyten M, et al: A homologue of Drosophila tissue polarity gene frizzled is expressed in migrating myofibroblasts in the infarcted rat heart. Nat Med 1997;3:541–544.

47. Vracko R, Thorning D: Contractile cells in myocardial scar tissue. Lab Invest 1991;65:214–227.

48. Willems I, et al: The alpha smooth muscle actin positive cells in healing human myocardial scars. Am J Pathol 1994;145:868–875.

49. Schwartz S, deBlois D, O'Brien E: The intima: Soil for atherosclerosis and restenosis. Circ Res 1995;77:445–465.

50. Johnson R, Iida H, Alpers C, et al: Expression of smooth muscle phenotype by rat mesangial cells in immune complex nephritis: SmaA is a marker of mesangial cell proliferation. J Clin Invest 1991;87:847–858.

51. Hariawala M, Sellke F: Angiogenesis and the heart: Therapeutic implications. J R Soc Med 1997;90:307–311.

52. Schwartz SM, Benditt EP: Clustering of replicating cells in aortic endothelium. Proc Natl Acad Sci U S A 1976;73:651–653.

53. Lindahl P, Hellstrom M, Kalen M, Betsholtz C: Endothelial-perivascular cell signaling in vascular development: Lessons from knockout mice. Curr Opin Lipidol 1998;9:407–411.

54. Hirschi KK, Rohovsky SA, D'Amore P: PDGF, TGF beta and heterotypic cell-cell interactions mediate the recruitment and differentiation of 10T1/2 cells to a smooth muscle cell fate. J Cell Biol 1998;141:805–814.

55. Hirschi K, Rohovsky S, Beck L, et al: Endothelial cells modulate the proliferation of mural cell precursors via PDGF-BB and heterotypic cell contact. Circ Res 1999;84:298–305.

56. Antonelli-Orlidge A, Saunders KB, Smith SR, D'Amore PA: An activated form of transforming growth factor beta is produced by cocultures of endothelial cells and pericytes. Proc Natl Acad Sci U S A 1989;86:4544–4548.

57. Hungerford JE, Owens GK, Argraves WS, Little CD: Development of the aortic vessel wall as defined by vascular smooth muscle and extracellular matrix markers. Dev Biol 1996;178:375–392.

58. Hirschi KK, Lai L, Belaguli NS, et al: TGF-β induction of a smooth muscle cell phenotype requires transcriptional and translational control of serum response factor. J Biol Chem 2002;277:6287–6295.

59. Aird W, Edelberg J, Weiler-Guettler H, et al: Vascular bed-specific expression of endothelial cell gene is programmed by the tissue microenvironment. J Cell Biol 1997;138:1117–1124.

60. Beekhuizen H, van Furth R: Growth characteristics of cultured human macrovascular venous and arterial endothelial cells. J Vasc Res 1994;31:230–239.

61. Rupnick M, Carey A, Williams S: Phenotypic diversity in cultured cerebral microvascular endothelial cells. In Vitro Cell Dev Biol 1988;4:435–444.

62. Edelberg J, Aird W, Wu W, et al: PDGF mediates cardiac microvascular communication. J Clin Invest 1998;102:837–843.

63. Horak E, Leek R, Klenk N, et al: Angiogenesis, assessed by platelet/endothelial cell adhesion molecule antibodies. Lancet 1992;340:1120-1124.

64. Weidner N, Semple J, Welch W, Folkman J: Tumor angiogenesis and metastasis-correlation in invasive breast carcinoma. N Engl J Med 1991;324:1-8.

65. Brass L: VWF meets the ADAMTS family. Nat Med 2001;7: 1177-1178.

66. Nicosia R, Vilaschi S: Autoregulation of angiogenesis by cells of the vessel wall. Int Rev Cytol 1999;185:1-43.

67. Kessler P, Byrne B: Myoblast cell grafting into heart muscle: Cellular biology and potential applications. Annu Rev Physiol 1999;61:219-242.

68. Hu E, Tontonoz P, Spiegelman B: Transdifferentiation of myoblasts by the adipogenic transcription factors PPAR gamma and C/EBP alpha. Proc Natl Acad Sci U S A 1995;92:9856-9860.

69. Patapoutian A, Wold B, Wagner R: Evidence for developmentally programmed transdifferentiation in mouse esophageal muscle. Science 1995;270:1818-1821.

70. DeRuiter M, Poelmann R, VanMunsteren J, et al: Embryonic endothelial cells transdifferentiate into mesenchymal cells expressing smooth muscle actins in vivo and in vitro. Circ Res 1997;80:444-451.

71. Condorelli G, Borello U, DeAngelis L, et al: Cardiomyocytes induce endothelial cells to transdifferentiate into cardiac muscle: Implications for myocardium regeneration. Proc Natl Acad Sci U S A 2001;98:10733-10738.

72. Jackson K, Majka S, Wang H, et al: Regeneration of ischemic cardiac muscle and vascular endothelium by adult stem cells. J Clin Invest 2001;107:1395-1402.

73. Robinson S, Cho P, Levitsky H, et al: Arterial delivery of genetically labeled skeletal myoblasts to the murine heart: Long term survival and phenotypic modification of implanted myoblasts. Cell Transplant 1996;5:77-91.

74. Reinecke H, MacDonald G, Hauschka S, Murry C: Electromechanical coupling between skeletal and cardiac muscle: Implications for infarct repair. J Cell Biol 2000;149:731-740.

75. Hutcheson K, Atkins B, Hueman M, et al: Comparison of benefits on myocardial performance of cellular cardiomyoplasty with skeletal myoblasts and fibroblasts. Cell Transplant 2000;9:359-368.

76. Goodell M, Jackson K, Majka S, et al: Stem cell plasticity in muscle and bone marrow. Ann N Y Acad Sci 2001;938:208-220.

77. Soonpa M, Koh G, Klug M, Field L: Formation of nascent intercalated disks between grafted fetal cardiomyocytes. Science 1994;264:98-101.

78. Sakai T, Li R, Weisel R, et al: Autologous heart cell transplantation improves cardiac function after myocardial injury. Ann Thorac Surg 1999;68:2074-2080.

79. Kehat I, Kenyagin-Karesenti D, Snir M, et al: Human embryonic stem cells can differentiate into myocytes with structural and functional properties of cardiomyocytes. J Clin Invest 2001;108:407-414.

80. Min J, Yang Y, Converso K, et al: Transplantation of embryonic stem cells improves cardiac function in post infarcted hearts. J Appl Physiol 2002;92:288-296.

81. Klug M, Soonpa M, Koh G, Field L: Genetically selected cardiomyocytes from differentiating ES cells form stable intracardiac grafts. J Clin Invest 1996;98:216-224.

82. VanMeter C, Claycomb W, Delcarpio J, et al: Myoblast transplantation in the porcine model: A potential technique for myocardial repair. J Thorac Cardiovasc Surg 1995;110:1442-1448.

83. Asahara T, Takahashi T, Masuda H, et al: VEGF contributes to postnatal neovascularization by mobilizing bone marrow derived endothelial progenitor cells. EMBO J 1999;18:3964-3972.

84. Asahara T, Masuda H, Takahashi T, et al: Bone marrow origin of endothelial progenitor cells responsible for postnatal vasculogenesis in physiological and pathological neovascularization. Circ Res 1999;85:221-228.

85. Kocher A, Schuster M, Szabolcs S, et al: Neovascularization of ischemic myocardium by human bone marrow derived angioblasts prevents cardiomyocyte apoptosis, reduces remodeling and improves cardiac function. Nat Med 2001;7:430-436.

86. Takahashi T, Kalka C, Masuda H, et al: Ischemia- and cytokine induced mobilization of bone marrow-derived endothelial progenitor cells for neovascularization. Nat Med 1999;5:434-438.

87. Asahara T, et al: Isolation of putative progenitor endothelial cells for angiogenesis. Science 1997;275:965-967.

88. Altieri D: Statins' benefits begin to sprout. J Clin Invest 2001;108: 365-366.

89. Dimmeler S, Aicher A, Vasa M, et al: HMG-CoA reductase inhibitors (statins) increase endothelial progenitor cells via the PI3 kinase/Akt pathway. J Clin Invest 2001;108:391-397.

90. Kalka C, et al: VEGF 165 gene transfer augments cEPC in human subjects. Circ Res 2000;86:1198-2002.

91. Llevadot J, Murasawa S, Kureishi Y, et al: HMG-CoA reductase inhibitor mobilizes bone marrow derived endothelial progenitor cells. J Clin Invest 2001;108:399-405.

92. Vasa M, Fichtlscherer S, Adler K, et al: Increase in circulating endothelial progenitor cells by statin therapy in patients with stable coronary artery disease. Circulation 2001;103:2885-2890.

93. Vasa M, Fichtlscherer S, Aicher A, et al: Number and migratory activity of circulating endothelial progenitor cells inversely correlates with risk factors for coronary artery disease. Circ Res 2001;89:e1-e7.

94. Kawamoto A, Gwon H, Iwaguro H, et al: Therapeutic potential of ex vivo expanded endothelial progenitor cells for myocardial ischemia. Circulation 2001;103:634-636.

95. Spangrude GJ, Heimfeld S, Weissman IL: Purification and characterization of mouse hematopoietic stem cells. Science 1988;241: 58-62.

96. Orlic D, Kajstura J, Chimenti S, et al: Bone marrow cells regenerate infarcted myocardium. Nature 2001;410:701-705.

97. Orlic D, Kajstura J, Chimenti S, et al: Mobilized bone marrow cells repair the infarcted heart, improving function and survival. Proc Natl Acad Sci U S A 2001;98:10344-10349.

98. Goodell M, Rosenzweig M, Kim H, et al: Dye efflux studies suggest that HSCs expressing low or undetectable levels of CD34 antigen exist in multiple species. Nat Med 1997;3:1337-1345.

99. Colter D, Class R, DiGirolamo CM, Prockop D: Rapid expansion of recycling stem cells in cultures of plastic-adherent cells from human bone marrow. Proc Natl Acad Sci U S A 2000;97:3213-3218.

100. Prockop D: Marrow stromal cells as stem cells for non-hematopoietic tissues. Science 1997;276:7174-7185.

101. Deans R, Moseley A: Mesenchymal stem cells: Biology and potential clinical uses. Exp Hematol 2000;28:875-884.

102. Fukuda K: Development of regenerative cardiomyocytes from mesenchymal stem cells for cardiovascular tissue engineering. Artif Organs 2001;25:187-193.

103. Wang J, Tim D, Chedrawy E, Chiu R: The coronary delivery of marrow stromal cells for myocardil regeneration: Pathophysiologic and therapeutic implications. J Thorac Cardiovasc Surg 2001;122:699-670.

104. Toma C, Pittenger M, Cahill K, et al: Human mesenchymal stem cells differentiate into a cardiomyocyte phenotype in adult murine heart. Circulation 2002;105:93-98.

105. Quiani F, Urbanek K, Beltrami A, et al: Chimerism of the transplanted heart. N Engl J Med 2002;346:5-15.

106. Taylor D, et al: Regenerating functional myocardium: Improved performance after skeletal myoblast transplantation. Nat Med 1998;4:929-933.

107. Sakai T, Li R, Weisel R, et al: Fetal cell transplantation: A comparasion of 3 cell types. J Thorac Cardiovasc Surg 1999;118:715-725.

108. Reinecke H, Zhang M, Bartosek T, Murry C: Survival, integration, and differentiation of cardiomyocyte grafts: A study in normal and injured rat hearts. Circulation 1999;100:193-202.

109. Zhang M, Methot D, Poppa V, et al: Cardiomyocyte grafting for cardiac repair: Graft cell death and anti death strategies. J Mol Cell Cardiol 2001;33:907-921.

110. Li R, Jia Z, Weisel R, et al: Cardiomyocyte transplantation improves heart function. Ann Thorac Surg 1996;62:654-661.

111. Lee R, Springer M, Blanco-Bose W, et al: VEGF gene delievery to myocardium: Deleterious effects of unregulated expression. Circulation 2000;102:898-901.

112. Lee S, Wolf P, Escudero R, et al: Early expression of angiogenesis factors in acute myocardial ischemia and infarction. N Engl J Med 2000;342:626-633.

113. Jain M, DerSimonian H, Brenner D, et al: Myoblast cell therapy attenuates deleterious ventricular remodling and improves cardiac performance post-myocardial infarction. J Card Fail 2000;6:10.

114. Dimmeler S, Zeiher A: Reactive oxygen species and vascular cell apoptosis in response to angiotensin II and pro atherosclerotic factors. Regul Pept 2000;90:19-25.
115. Carmeliet P: Clotting factors build blood vessels. Science 2001;293:1602-1604.
116. Carmeliet P: Creating unique blood vessels. Nature 2001;412: 868-869.
117. Leor J, Etzion S, Dar A, et al: Bioengineered cardiac grafts. Circulation 2001;102:56-60.
118. Leor J, Patterson M, Quinones MJ, et al: Transplantation of fetal myocardial tissue into the infarcted myocardium of rat: A potential method for repair of infarcted myocardium? Circulation 1996;94:II32-II36.
119. Connold AL, Frischknecht R, Dimitrakos M, Vrbova G: The survival of embryonic cardiomyocytes transplanted into damaged host rat myocardium. J Muscle Res Cell Motil 1997;18:63-70.

■ ■ ■ chapter **47**

Identifying the Vulnerable Plaque and the Vulnerable Patient

Herbert D. Aronow
Eric J. Topol

IDENTIFYING THE VULNERABLE ARTERY AND THE VULNERABLE PATIENT

Atherogenesis begins early in life.[1] By the age of 15 to 19 years, half of individuals already have detectable coronary artery intimal lesions.[2] By mid to late adulthood, atherosclerotic cardiovascular disease is ubiquitous and accounts for more death and disability than any other disease entity in the Western world.[3] Tremendous advances have been made in the treatment of individuals who develop clinically manifest atherosclerotic cardiovascular disease. Coronary care units, antiplatelet and antithrombotic agents, and the advent and widespread use of mechanical and pharmacologic reperfusion therapies in eligible individuals have reduced significantly the morbidity and mortality associated with acute coronary syndromes (ACS). Although novel pharmacologic agents and combination therapies promise to improve further on these outcomes, many individuals who develop coronary disease die suddenly without exhibiting prior disease manifestations, and individuals who do survive remain at elevated risk of recurrent adverse events. The ability to identify atherosclerotic plaque at risk of disruption, superimposed thrombosis, or distal embolization (i.e., the vulnerable plaque) and the ability to identify individuals who are at increased risk for developing these processes (i.e., the vulnerable patient)

would have a much greater impact than watchful waiting. With an eye to the future, this chapter highlights advances in identifying the vulnerable artery and the vulnerable patient.

THE VULNERABLE ARTERY

Many invasive and noninvasive imaging modalities that are capable of detecting vulnerable atherosclerotic plaque have emerged. Each modality attempts to identify one or more characteristic structural, cellular, or molecular features underlying plaque vulnerability (Table 47-1).

Invasive Imaging Modalities

Angiography

Angiography has been used to identify vulnerable coronary atherosclerotic plaque through assessments of lesion severity and morphology. Plaque disruption resulting in ACS occurs more commonly at sites that have only mild or moderate angiographic narrowing.[4-8] Because these less severe stenoses are more prevalent, it is difficult to predict accurately which of these will disrupt or result in ACS.[9] In contrast, the risk of future plaque progression and instability has been tied to

■ ■ ■

TABLE 47-1 CHARACTERIZATION OF VULNERABLE ATHEROSCLEROTIC PLAQUE

	% LUMINAL STENOSIS	VESSEL WALL	LIPID	FIBROUS	CALCIUM	THROMBUS	INFLAMMATION	PREDICT EVENTS
Angiography	+	−	−	−	+/−	+/−	−	+/−
IVUS	+	+	+/−	+	+	+/−	−	+/−
Angioscopy	−	−	+	+	+	+	−	+/−
OCT	+	+	+	+	−	+	−	+/−
Thermography	−	−	?	?	?	?	−	?
Raman/NIR spectroscopy	−	−	+	+	+	−	+	+/−
Nuclear/Scintigraphy	−	−	+	−	−	+	−	?
EBCT	+	−	−	−	+	−	−	+/−
MSCT	+	+	+	+	+	−	−	?
MRI	+	+	+	+	+	−	−	?

EBCT, electron-beam (ultrafast) computed tomography; IVUS, intravascular ultrasound; MRI, magnetic resonance imaging; MSCT, multislice spiral (helical) computed tomography; NIR, near-infrared spectroscopy; OCT, optical coherence tomography. Modified from[236] Fayad ZA, Fuster V: Clinical imaging of the high-risk or vulnerable atherosclerotic plaque. Circ Res 2001; 89:305–316.

many prospectively identified lesion morphologic characteristics. These include lesions that are irregular in contour, are longer, have steeper inflow and outflow angles, are bifurcated, are ulcerated, or have superimposed thromboses.[10-14] These associations have not been observed consistently[15]; there is significant overlap in lesion behavior; and angiographically complex lesions, although more likely to progress than other lesions, typically remain stable over long periods.[16] As a result of these and other limitations, the ability of angiography to predict future coronary events is limited.[17-20]

High-Frequency Intravascular Ultrasound

Intravascular ultrasound (IVUS) has been employed for the identification of vulnerable atherosclerotic plaque (Fig. 47-1), and many cross-sectional studies have characterized lesion appearance by IVUS in temporal proximity to ACS. Patients with ACS have culprit lesions that are more frequently echolucent and less frequently mixed or calcified than in patients with stable angina.[21-23] Additionally, eccentric lesions are more prevalent in the setting of ACS.[24] Culprit lesions also have larger plaque and vessel areas in patients with unstable compared with stable angina.[25-28] Nevertheless, others have found that some of these IVUS characteristics poorly discriminate between stable and unstable culprit lesions.[29]

Prospective studies using IVUS to identify markers of plaque vulnerability are scarce. Preliminary IVUS data suggest that vessel regions with greater peak circumferential tensile stress are most susceptible to plaque rupture during balloon angioplasty (Fig. 47-2).[30] In the setting of spontaneous plaque rupture, only one study has shown that eccentric, large, or echolucent plaques on IVUS are more prone to instability.[31] The ability of IVUS to predict plaque instability accurately is limited at present.

Angioscopy

Similar to IVUS studies, most angioscopic studies of vulnerable plaque are of cross-sectional design, evaluating patients in proximity to ACS. Yellow plaques with disruption and associated thrombi are more prevalent in patients with ACS than stable angina,[26,29,32-36] and these characteristics may persist for at least 1 month after an acute myocardial infarction (MI).[37-39]

There are few prospective angioscopic studies predicting clinical outcome. One small study of patients with stable angina found that patients with yellow plaques identified on angioscopy were more likely to develop ACS over the following 12 months than patients with white plaques, a relationship that was even stronger for glistening than nonglistening yellow plaques.[18] In a second study of patients with ACS, angioscopy was compared with angiography and IVUS to predict clinical outcome after percutaneous coronary intervention. Plaque rupture on preprocedure angioscopy and postintervention lesion thrombus were significant multivariate predictors of recurrent ischemia during the 12-month follow-up. In contrast, angiography and IVUS findings were not predictive of recurrent ischemic events in this study.[19]

Despite these encouraging findings, the ability of angioscopy to detect and characterize vulnerable coronary atherosclerotic plaque is hampered by its inability to image vessels of small or moderate caliper, to traverse severe stenoses, and to image beyond the vessel lumen.[40]

Optical Coherence Tomography

Optical coherence tomography (OCT) is an emerging technology that holds promise for characterizing vulnerable plaque at the microstructural level (see Chapter 21). Micron-level tomographic images are acquired in a manner similar to IVUS, but back-reflected infrared light rather than acoustical waves are measured.[41] OCT also

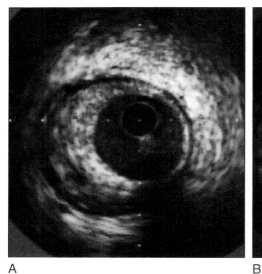
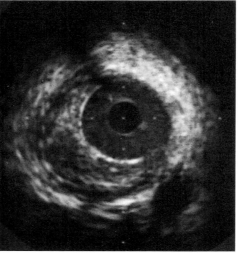

A   B

FIGURE 47–1. Intravenous ultrasound images of stable and vulnerable coronary atherosclerotic plaque. Stable plaque is characterized by a small lipid core and thick fibrous cap *(left)*, whereas vulnerable plaque is notable for its large lipid core and thin fibrous cap. (From[237] Nissen SE, Yock P: Intravascular ultrasound: Novel pathophysiological insights and current clinical applications. Circulation 2001;103:604–616.)

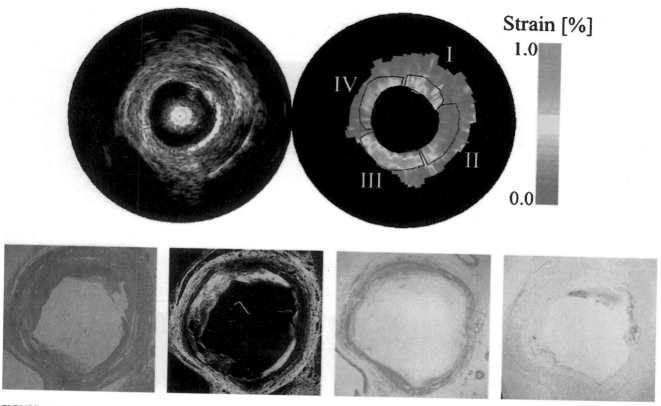

FIGURE 47–2. (See color section.) Intravenous ultrasound (IVUS) *(top left)*, IVUS elastogram *(top right)*, and corresponding histologic images *(bottom)* of an atherosclerotic human femoral artery. IVUS elastography was performed by acquiring IVUS images at two intraluminal pressures (80 and 100 mm Hg) and performing cross-correlational analysis on local strain levels determined from radiofrequency data. Red represents low; yellow, intermediate; and green, high local strain. Standard IVUS image reveals concentric plaque with varying echogenicity. IVUS elastogram shows two hard (II, IV) and two soft (I, III) regions. Histologic sections *(left to right)* are stained with picro-Sirius red for collagen, picro-Sirius red with polarized light microscopy for fatty tissue, anti-α-actin antibody for smooth muscle cells, and anti-CD68 antibody for macrophages. By histology, soft regions on IVUS elastography contain fatty material with increased macrophage density, whereas harder regions are composed of fibrous material. (From[238] de Korte CL, Pasterkamp G, van der Steen AF, et al: Characterization of plaque components with intravascular ultrasound elastography in human femoral and coronary arteries in vitro. Circulation 2000;102:617–623.)

may be used to perform tissue biochemical analyses.[42] This intravascular imaging modality can penetrate plaque to the same degree as IVUS, but its image resolution is nearly an order of magnitude greater (approximately 10 μm).[43] Systems in development have the capacity to image at less than 4 μm.[44] In humans, OCT has identified accurately plaque characterized as fibrous, lipid-rich with a well-defined fibrous cap, or calcified-fibrous by IVUS.[45,46]

At present, the in vivo clinical application of intravascular OCT is limited by its requirement for intravascular saline flushing for adequate image acquisition. Prospective studies have not yet assessed the ability of OCT to image vulnerable plaque or to predict adverse clinical outcome.

Thermography

Intravascular catheter-based thermography has established that thermal heterogeneity is present within the arteries and atherosclerotic plaques of patients with coronary disease but not in controls free of coronary disease (Fig. 47–3).[47] Among patients with coronary disease, temperature differences are greatest in patients with MI, intermediate in patients with unstable angina, and least in patients with stable angina. C-reactive protein (CRP) and serum amyloid A (SAA), acute phase reactants that are markers of inflammation and patient vulnerability, are highly correlated with the degree of thermal heterogeneity.[48] That histologic studies have positively associated the density of inflammatory cells, presence of endothelial denudation, and superimposition of fibrin-platelet thrombosis with plaque thermal heterogeneity also suggests that increased plaque surface temperature reflects inflammation and plaque vulnerability.[49] Thermal heterogeneity is greater in vessels with positive remodeling or greater plaque area,[50,51] IVUS characteristics that have been prospectively associated with an increased likelihood of plaque disruption and ischemic events.[31]

Preliminary data suggest that thermal heterogeneity can predict clinical outcome. In a group of patients undergoing percutaneous coronary intervention for stable angina, unstable angina, or acute MI, the difference in temperature between the culprit lesion and proximal reference segment accurately discriminated between

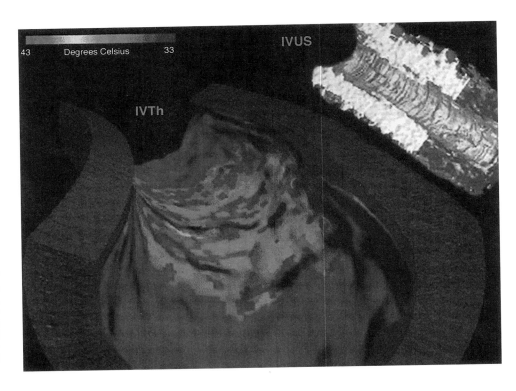

FIGURE 47–3. (See color section.) Three-dimensional reconstruction of catheter-based thermography *(left)* and intravenous ultrasound *(right)* in rabbit aorta. The color scale *(upper left)* is bounded by red (43°C) and dark blue (33°C). Three-dimensional intravenous ultrasound yields important structural detail, whereas thermography localizes inflammation by detecting thermal heterogeneity, highlighting the complementary nature of these two imaging modalities. (From[239] Diamantopoulos LD, Van Langenhove G, de Feyter P, et al: 3-D thermal reconstruction of the atherosclerotic plaque: A new insight into plaque vulnerability by means of thermography and advanced computer algorithms. J Am Coll Cardiol 2001;37:382A.)

patients who suffered in-hospital MI, recurrent angina, or death and patients who remained free of events over 18 months.[52]

Raman and Near-Infrared Spectroscopy

Raman spectroscopy employs laser energy to characterize the structure and chemical composition of biologic tissue. After illuminating the tissue of interest, photons contained in the emitted light are characteristically scattered (i.e., in molecule-specific Raman spectra) as the result of their interaction with vibrational energy of individual molecules (see Chapter 21).[53]

In ex vivo studies, Raman spectroscopy has differentiated between lipids, cholesterol, elastin, collagen, and calcium apatite[54]; has quantified free cholesterol, cholesterol esters, triglycerides, phospholipids, and calcium salts[55,56]; and has accurately classified coronary arteries as atherosclerotic or nonatherosclerotic.[57] More recently, in vivo human studies of Raman spectroscopy have been performed. Raman spectra, obtained from the aortic wall during abdominal aortic aneurysm repair surgery, permitted the accurate quantification of vessel wall proteins, cholesterol, and calcium.[58] Finally, IVUS and Raman spectroscopy may yield complementary information about the structural and chemical composition of atherosclerotic plaque[59]; the development of a catheter capable of simultaneously performing IVUS and Raman spectroscopy is currently under way.[59]

Near-infrared spectroscopy (NIRS) employs near-infrared light to illuminate a biologic tissue and relates the recovered light to the amount of tissue chromophores.[60,61] By doing so, NIRS can characterize quali-tatively and quantitatively the components of atherosclerotic plaque.

In ex vivo studies, NIRS accurately determined levels of tissue cholesterol[62]; correctly identified thin fibrous caps, lipid pools, macrophages, and calcium[63]; and accurately classified lipid-rich plaques.[64] NIRS detected features of plaque vulnerability with high sensitivity and specificity, including lipid pools, thin fibrous caps, and inflammatory cells.[65] In human atherosclerotic plaques imaged before carotid endarterectomy, NIRS successfully differentiated between American Heart Association lesion types I/II, III/IV, and V/VI.[66] Catheter-based NIRS is also in development. In an animal model, an intravascular NIRS catheter correctly identified simulated vulnerable plaque,[67] and in human cadavers, a NIRS fiberoptic probe successfully classified coronary plaques according to their lipid content.[64] Whether catheter-based Raman spectroscopy or NIRS, by themselves or in conjunction with other imaging modalities, will facilitate the detection of vulnerable plaque or provide important prognostic information remains to be seen.

Noninvasive Imaging Modalities

Nuclear Scintigraphy

Nuclear scintigraphic imaging also has been used to characterize noninvasively vulnerable atherosclerotic plaque. This approach has been employed for the detection of native and oxidized lipoproteins and apolipoproteins,[68-73] identification of proliferating smooth muscle cells,[74-78] estimation of macrophage density,[79-81] and assessment of apoptosis.[82] Arterial thrombi also have been identified using nuclear scintigraphic techniques that radiolabel platelets,[83-85] activated platelet glycoprotein IIb/IIIa receptors,[86] platelet glycoprotein P-selectin,[80] platelet ADP receptor-mediated aggregation,[87] platelet receptor binding peptides,[88,89] fibrin,[90] fibrinogen,[91] fibronectin,[92] and fibrin degradation products.[93]

Despite their great potential, few of these agents have been tested in humans, and most have not been sensitive enough for routine clinical use because of poor target-to-background and target-to-blood ratios.[80,81] Whether any of the aforementioned nuclear scintigraphic techniques or those as yet to emerge will identify and characterize coronary atherosclerotic plaque or facilitate prognostication is unknown.

Computed Tomography

The electron-beam computed tomography (EBCT) coronary artery calcium score is related to the overall burden of coronary atherosclerosis[94,95] and can predict coronary events to a modest degree.[96,97] Nevertheless, it is likely that noncalcified, less advanced vulnerable plaques elsewhere in the coronary arterial tree pose the greatest risk.[98] This idea is supported by in vitro data that have shown that plaque calcium content provides little information about vulnerability[99] or biomechanical stability.[100] As a result, EBCT, although it does convey prognostic information, does not seem to have a role in detecting or characterizing vulnerable coronary atherosclerotic plaque at present.

Contrast-enhanced EBCT is being developed for noninvasive coronary angiography, and its accuracy continues to improve.[101-107] Nevertheless, using contemporary scanning protocols, 20% to 25% of arterial segments cannot be imaged adequately.[108] Even if this technology could approximate the accuracy and resolution of invasive coronary angiography, it would provide information only about the coronary artery lumen and likewise would have only limited ability to detect and characterize vulnerable plaque or to convey important prognostic information.

Similar to contrast-enhanced CT, multislice spiral CT (MSCT) is being evaluated for noninvasive coronary angiography[109-111] and can detect severe coronary arterial stenoses.[112] MSCT also may be useful for the characterization of atherosclerotic plaque composition. Single-slice spiral CT (an earlier MSCT cousin) can differentiate between fibrous tissue, lipid, and calcium in atheroma from carotid arteries,[113] and MSCT density measurements differ significantly between coronary plaques classified as soft, intermediate, or calcified by IVUS (Fig. 47–4).[114] The utility of MSCT for identifying vulnerable coronary artery plaque or predicting clinical events on that basis awaits further study.

Magnetic Resonance Imaging

Coronary magnetic resonance imaging (MRI) is emerging as a potentially useful tool for evaluating coronary artery disease.[115] Advances in imaging techniques have allowed MRI to visualize the coronary artery lumen and wall. Although promising, MRI coronary angiography is limited by its inability to image distal epicardial coronary vessels and its failure to visualize nearly 15% of proximal or mid coronary artery segments.[116] Nevertheless, given its ability to characterize plaque at the submillimeter level and the use of newer protocols that employ multicontrast imaging,[117] MRI may be useful for vulnerable plaque imaging.

In vivo MRI studies have identified lipid, fibrocellular, calcific, and thrombotic components in atheroma from human thoracic aorta[118] and lipid core, fibrous cap, calcium, and normal vessel structures in carotid artery atheroma.[119] Accurate measurements of carotid plaque size[120] and fibrous cap thickness and visualization of

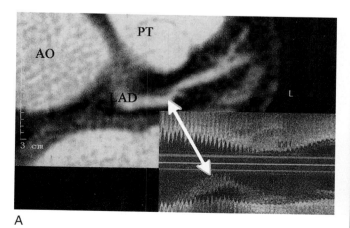

A

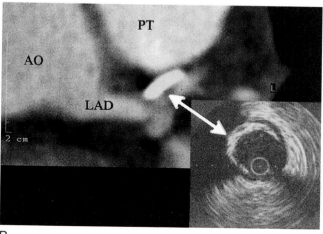

B

FIGURE 47–4. Soft *(A)* and calcified *(B)* plaque as assessed by multislice computed tomography *(upper left)* and longitudinal or sagittal intravenous ultrasound slices *(lower right)*. Plaques characterized as soft and calcified by intravenous ultrasound had significantly different densities (measured in Hounsfield units) on multislice computed tomography. AO, aorta; LAD, left anterior descending coronary artery; PT, pulmonary arterial trunk. (From Schroeder S, Kopp AF, Baumbach A, et al: Noninvasive detection and evaluation of atherosclerotic coronary plaques with multislice computed tomography. J Am Coll Cardiol 2001;37:1430–1435.)

ruptured carotid atherosclerotic plaque are also possible with MRI.[121] Although the use of MRI to characterize plaque in the coronary arteries is feasible, this modality has been employed to date primarily for measurements of wall thickness and area.[122,123] Although these measurements are important and have been related to plaque vulnerability in prior studies, further advances are needed if vulnerable coronary atherosclerotic plaque is to be identified and characterized with MRI. Technologic advances, such as improved receiver coils,[124] may enable this possibility.

THE VULNERABLE PATIENT

Evidence is accumulating that coronary atherosclerotic plaque disruption with superimposed thrombosis is a multifocal process.[125-127] If so, it may be as important to identify vulnerable patients as it is to localize and characterize vulnerable plaque. Although characterizing vulnerable plaque may permit the application of local (i.e., lesion-directed) therapies, characterizing vulnerable patients may facilitate the targeting of systemic (i.e., patient-directed) therapies. Because the processes of plaque disruption, thrombosis, and distal embolization seem to be pan-vascular, the identification of systemic perturbations that predispose persons to develop clinically manifest disease is paramount.

From a public health standpoint, it is at least as important to detect markers of vulnerability in apparently healthy individuals as it is in individuals who have clinically manifest disease who are at increased risk of recurrent events (e.g., after MI or unstable angina). Numerous studies have examined the ability of various serum markers to predict adverse cardiac events in these cohorts and are discussed subsequently. Some of these markers are innocent bystanders, whereas others play an active role in the pathophysiology of atherosclerosis. Their division into lipid, thrombotic/fibrinolytic, inflammatory, endothelial, and other markers is an oversimplification intended for illustrative purposes only; many of these markers are involved directly in or reflect indirectly multiple simultaneous pathophysiologic processes that underlie atherosclerosis initiation, progression, and vulnerability (e.g., the roles of monocytes and platelet CD154 in inflammation and thrombosis[128,129]).

Lipid Markers

Measurement of lipid fractions and calculation of lipid ratios was one of the earliest means used to predict incident coronary disease among healthy individuals.[130] Despite the emphasis placed on measurement and targeting of low-density lipoprotein (LDL) cholesterol in current National Cholesterol Education Program Adult Treatment Panel III guidelines,[131] the total cholesterol–to-high-density lipoprotein (HDL) cholesterol ratio has consistently borne out as the most powerful lipid marker of future coronary events. In the Framingham study, the likelihood ratios for developing coronary disease over 14 years were significantly higher for the total cholesterol–to-HDL cholesterol ratio than LDL cholesterol.[130]

This was also the case in the Chinese Chin-Shan Community Cardiovascular Cohort study, the Copenhagen Male Study,[132] and the Quebec Cardiovascular Study.[133] When added to models including traditional coronary risk factors and contemporary plasma inflammatory markers, the total cholesterol–to-HDL ratio remains independently predictive of future cardiovascular events.[134,135]

Thrombotic/Fibrinolytic Markers

A host of thrombotic/fibrinolytic markers have been evaluated as predictors of future coronary events in individuals with and without overt coronary disease. During fibrinolysis, tissue plasminogen activator cleaves plasminogen into plasmin, which subsequently degrades cross-linked fibrin, yielding fibrin degradation products, including D-dimer. Many studies have explored these and other elements of the thrombotic/fibrinolytic cascade as they relate to incident or prevalent coronary disease and are worthy of mention.

One of the most promising thrombotic/fibrinolytic markers of vulnerability is fibrin D-dimer. Increased fibrin D-dimer levels have been associated with prevalent coronary disease[136,137] and incident coronary death or nonfatal MI.[138] In a meta-analysis of this study and six earlier prospective studies of patients with and without vascular disease,[139-144] D-dimer levels were independently predictive of incident coronary disease.

Other thrombotic/fibrinolytic markers, such as plasminogen, have been associated with incident coronary disease as well.[145,146] Increased plasminogen levels were associated with incident coronary events in the 4-year ARIC (Atherosclerosis Risk in Communities)[136] and 7-year FINRISK 1992[146] cohort studies. Thrombotic/fibrinolytic markers, such as tissue plasminogen activator, plasminogen activator inhibitor-1, the activation peptides of factors IX and X, activity and antigen of factor VII, activated factor XII, and prothrombin fragment 1+2, have been associated with incident coronary disease, but these associations are most often negated or minimized on inclusion of traditional risk factors into multivariate models.[145-147]

Inflammatory Markers

Atherosclerosis is in large part a chronic inflammatory condition,[148] and inflammation has become one of the most intensively studied areas in this field. A large contingent of cytokines and other proinflammatory mediators, cell adhesion molecules (CAMs), and acute phase reactants have been examined as harbingers of future cardiovascular events.

Cytokines

Most prominent among the cytokines studied are interleukin (IL)-6 and tumor necrosis factor (TNF)-α. IL-6 is a proinflammatory cytokine that is the primary initiator of the acute phase response, culminating in hepatocyte production of acute phase reactants, including CRP.[149] Several studies have observed that IL-6 conveys important prognostic information among individuals with and without prevalent atherosclerotic cardiovascular disease. Elevated IL-6 levels are associated independently with increased long-term all-cause mortality among elderly men and women[150] and MI among men without prevalent vascular disease.[151] Likewise, higher IL-6 levels are associated with a greater incidence of long-term mortality among elderly women with prevalent cardiovascular disease[152] and more frequent in-hospital adverse coronary events among patients with unstable angina.[153]

Increased levels of TNF-α, another pleiotropic cytokine similar to IL-6 that amplifies the inflammatory cascade, have been associated independently with an increased incidence of recurrent events after MI,[154] and TNF receptor (but not TNF-α) levels have been associated with greater maximal carotid plaque thickness among individuals younger than age 70.[155]

Cell Adhesion Molecules

Among their manifold functions, CAMs mediate leukocyte adhesion and transmigration across the vascular endothelium, processes integral in the initiation and progression of atherosclerosis.[156] After cytokine activation, CAMs are shed from endothelial cell, platelet, and leukocyte surfaces. Although it is difficult to quantify cell surface expression of CAMs in vivo,[157] soluble forms in serum or plasma may serve as markers of vascular inflammation and endothelial or platelet activation.[158] Many soluble CAMs have been studied to predict vulnerability to coronary events, including the selectins and CAMs belonging to the immunoglobulin superfamily.

Adhesion molecules from the selectin family mediate rolling and tethering, the first step in leukocyte adhesion to the vascular endothelium.[156] P-selectin is stored in platelet α granules and endothelial Weibel-Palade bodies; increased P-selectin levels predicted incident cardiovascular events (cardiovascular death, MI, stroke, or coronary revascularization) during 3.5 years of follow-up in a study of women without apparent vascular disease at baseline.[159] In contrast, elevated soluble P-selectin levels were not predictive of incident coronary events (coronary death or nonfatal MI) in another study of apparently healthy men during 16 years of follow-up.[157] Although P-selectin levels are higher in patients with unstable angina[160,161] and acute MI[162-164] than in patients who have stable angina, P-selectin has not predicted cardiovascular outcome among patients with manifest atherosclerotic vascular disease.[165,166]

E-selectin is synthesized de novo by endothelial cells in response to IL-1 and TNF-α.[156] Few studies have evaluated E-selectin as a predictor of cardiovascular outcome. In persons without coronary disease at baseline, elevated E-selectin levels have not independently predicted coronary events.[157,167] The relationship between E-selectin and cardiovascular events has been less consistent. Among patients with stable or unstable angina, elevated E-selectin levels independently predicted cardiovascular death in one study[168] but did not predict major adverse cardiovascular events in a smaller study of patients with unstable angina or non–Q-wave MI.[165]

Intercellular adhesion molecule-1 (ICAM-1) and vascular adhesion molecule-1 (VCAM-1) are CAMs from the immunoglobulin superfamily that act as ligands for leukocyte and platelet integrins, mediate signal transduction, and facilitate endothelial transmigration of leukocytes.[156] ICAM and VCAM expression is stimulated by cytokines such as IL-1 and TNF-α. Among patients without evident atherosclerotic vascular disease, higher baseline levels of soluble ICAM-1 have independently predicted greater risk of subsequent fatal and nonfatal cardiac events in some studies[167,169] but not in others.[135,157,170] Similarly, in one study of patients with stable or unstable angina, elevated soluble ICAM-1 was independently associated with greater risk of death, but this association was no longer significant when levels of other adhesion molecules were entered into multivariate models.[168] Another small study of patients with unstable angina failed to show an independent relationship between soluble ICAM-1 and incident major adverse cardiovascular events.[165]

Studies on the relationship between VCAM-1 and coronary disease also have been mixed. Elevated baseline levels of soluble VCAM-1 have not independently predicted incident fatal or nonfatal coronary events in studies of patients with coronary disease.[157,167,171] In contrast, among patients with a history of stable or unstable angina, elevated soluble VCAM-1 levels have independently predicted cardiovascular death,[168] and in another study of patients with unstable angina or non–Q-wave MI, soluble VCAM-1 levels were independently correlated with the ischemic events during follow-up.[165]

Acute Phase Reactants

Concentrations of acute phase reactants vary widely in reaction to tissue damage.[106] Numerous studies have assessed the predictive capacity of acute phase reactants, including CRP, SAA, fibrinogen, white blood cell count, and albumin, to predict coronary events. Collectively, these studies suggest that increasing CRP, fibrinogen (Fig. 47-5),[172] white blood cell count (Fig. 47-6),[172] and SAA predict incident coronary disease in individuals with and without vascular disease at baseline, whereas increasing albumin is associated with an increased incidence of coronary disease among individuals with preexisting vascular disease.[172,173] Fibrinogen levels may be more valuable for predicting risk when viewed with glycoprotein IIIa (i.e., fibrinogen receptor) gene polymorphisms. Although platelet aggregability is impaired among patients harboring the PlA2 polymorphism regardless of fibrinogen level, increasing fibrinogen levels are associated with greater platelet aggregability among individuals who are homozygous for the PlA1 genotype.[174]

As a marker of patient vulnerability, CRP warrants special attention for several reasons. First, CRP has been studied more extensively than any other inflammatory marker. To this end, multiple prospective studies have shown its ability to predict independently all-cause and vascular mortality, MI, stroke, and peripheral vascular disease (Fig. 47-7).[135,150,158,173,175-182] It also is associated with major adverse cardiovascular events among

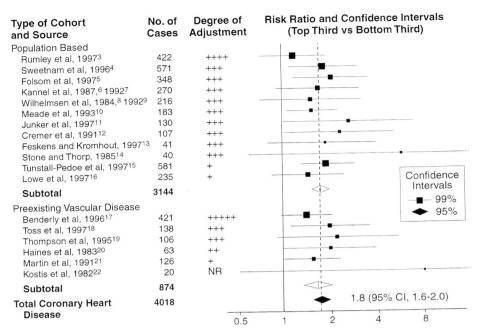

FIGURE 47–5. Risk ratio plot relating baseline fibrinogen level to incident coronary disease in population-based studies and in studies of patients with preexisting vascular disease. Risk ratios compare the top and bottom fibrinogen tertiles. Black squares (size proportional to number of cases) represent risk ratios with horizontal lines indicating 99% confidence intervals (CIs). Combined risk ratios with 95% CIs are indicated by open (subtotals) and shaded (overall) diamonds. NR, not reported; +, adjusted for age and gender; ++, adjusted for these factors and smoking; +++, adjusted for these factors and some standard vascular risk factors; ++++, adjusted for these factors and markers of social class; +++++, adjusted for these factors and baseline prevalent chronic disease. (From Danesh J, Collins R, Appleby P, Peto R: Association of fibrinogen, C-reactive protein, albumin, or leukocyte count with coronary heart disease: Meta-analyses of prospective studies. JAMA 1998;279:1477–1482.)

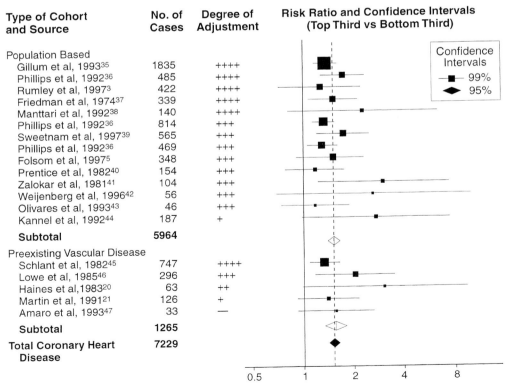

FIGURE 47–6. Risk ratio plot relating baseline white blood cell count to incident coronary disease in population-based studies and in studies of patients with preexisting vascular disease. Risk ratios compare the top and bottom white blood cell count tertiles. Black squares (size proportional to number of cases) represent risk ratios with horizontal lines indicating 99% confidence intervals (CIs). Combined risk ratios with 95% CIs are indicated by open (subtotals) and shaded (overall) diamonds. NR, not reported; +, adjusted for age and gender; ++, adjusted for these factors and smoking; +++, adjusted for these factors and some standard vascular risk factors; ++++, adjusted for these factors and markers of social class; +++++, adjusted for these factors and baseline prevalent chronic disease. (From Danesh J, Collins R, Appleby P, Peto R: Association of fibrinogen, C-reactive protein, albumin, or leukocyte count with coronary heart disease: Meta-analyses of prospective studies. JAMA 1998;279:1477–1482.)

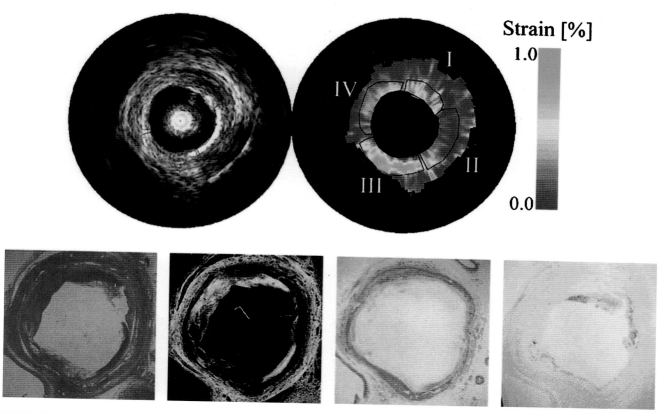

FIGURE 47–2. Intravenous ultrasound (IVUS) *(top left)*, IVUS elastogram *(top right)*, and corresponding histologic images *(bottom)* of an atherosclerotic human femoral artery. IVUS elastography was performed by acquiring IVUS images at two intraluminal pressures (80 and 100 mm Hg) and performing cross-correlational analysis on local strain levels determined from radiofrequency data. Red represents low; yellow, intermediate; and green, high local strain. Standard IVUS image reveals concentric plaque with varying echogenicity. IVUS elastogram shows two hard (II, IV) and two soft (I, III) regions. Histologic sections *(left to right)* are stained with picro-Sirius red for collagen, picro-Sirius red with polarized light microscopy for fatty tissue, anti-α-actin antibody for smooth muscle cells, and anti-CD68 antibody for macrophages. By histology, soft regions on IVUS elastography contain fatty material with increased macrophage density, whereas harder regions are composed of fibrous material. (From de Korte CL, Pasterkamp G, van der Steen AF, et al: Characterization of plaque components with intravascular ultrasound elastography in human femoral and coronary arteries in vitro. Circulation 2000;102:617–623.)

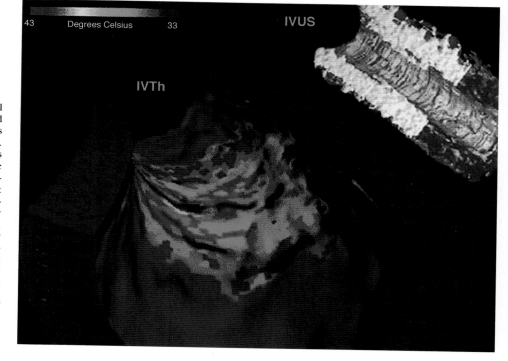

FIGURE 47–3. Three-dimensional reconstruction of catheter-based thermography *(left)* and intravenous ultrasound *(right)* in rabbit aorta. The color scale *(upper left)* is bounded by red (43°C) and dark blue (33°C). Three-dimensional intravenous ultrasound yields important structural detail, whereas thermography localizes inflammation by detecting thermal heterogeneity, highlighting the complementary nature of these two imaging modalities. (From Diamantopoulos LD, Van Langenhove G, de Feyter P, et al: 3-D thermal reconstruction of the atherosclerotic plaque: A new insight into plaque vulnerability by means of thermography and advanced computer algorithms. J Am Coll Cardiol 2001;37:382A.)

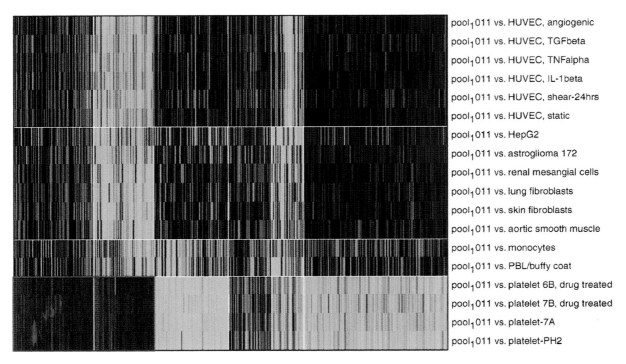

pool₁011 vs. HUVEC, angiogenic
pool₁011 vs. HUVEC, TGFbeta
pool₁011 vs. HUVEC, TNFalpha
pool₁011 vs. HUVEC, IL-1beta
pool₁011 vs. HUVEC, shear-24hrs
pool₁011 vs. HUVEC, static
pool₁011 vs. HepG2
pool₁011 vs. astroglioma 172
pool₁011 vs. renal mesangial cells
pool₁011 vs. lung fibroblasts
pool₁011 vs. skin fibroblasts
pool₁011 vs. aortic smooth muscle
pool₁011 vs. monocytes
pool₁011 vs. PBL/buffy coat
pool₁011 vs. platelet 6B, drug treated
pool₁011 vs. platelet 7B, drug treated
pool₁011 vs. platelet-7A
pool₁011 vs. platelet-PH2

FIGURE 47–9. Gene chip showing the platelet transcriptome of 1700 platelet-selective mRNAs. HUVEC, human umbilical vein endothelial cell. (Courtesy of Dr. James Topper.)

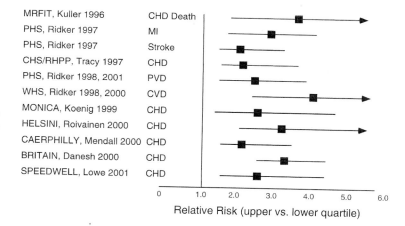

FIGURE 47–7. Risk ratio plot relating baseline C-reactive protein to future cardiovascular risk in persons without established coronary disease. Squares and horizontal bars represent risk ratio and 95% confidence intervals comparing the fourth with the first quartile of baseline C-reactive protein. CHD, coronary heart disease; CVD, cardiovascular disease; MI, myocardial infarction; PVD, peripheral vascular disease. (From Blake GJ, Ridker PM: Novel clinical markers of vascular wall inflammation. Circ Res 2001;89:763–771.)

patients with stable and unstable angina,[183-191] recent or remote MI,[192-194] and in the setting of percutaneous[195-199] or surgical[200] coronary revascularization. Second, CRP is unique in that it adds incremental prognostic information beyond that provided by traditional risk factors, lipids, and other markers of thrombosis/fibrinolysis and inflammation.[134,182] Finally, although it seems to be the most predictive inflammatory marker, when considered with the total cholesterol-to-HDL cholesterol ratio, it is even more valuable (Fig. 47–8).[201] Third, and perhaps most importantly, CRP is more than a marker of risk, it is a pivotal player in the development and progression of atherosclerotic disease. To this end, it has been shown to activate complement,[202] induce CAM expression,[203] mediate macrophage LDL cholesterol uptake,[204] recruit monocytes into the arterial wall,[205] increase production of monocyte-chemoattractant protein-1,[206] induce the expression of tissue factor in monocytes,[207] and sensitize T cells to kill endothelial cells.[208]

Other Immune Mediators

CD40, a member of the TNF receptor superfamily, and its ligand CD40L (CD154) are found on endothelial cells, platelets, smooth muscle cells, and macrophages and are believed to play a prominent role in the initiation, progression, and acute complications of atherosclerosis.[209,210] The CD40L occurs in a cell-associated and soluble form. In the only prospective study relating soluble CD40L to coronary disease, increased levels of soluble CD40L were independently associated with the development of MI, stroke, or cardiovascular death among apparently healthy middle-aged women over 4 years of follow-up.[210] Further assessment of this biomarker in a broader patient population, with and without prevalent vascular disease at baseline and in the presence of other lipid, thrombotic/fibrinolytic, and inflammatory markers, seems warranted.

Markers of Endothelial Dysfunction

Endothelial dysfunction seems to be an integral step in the development and progression of atherosclerosis.[148] Elevated levels of von Willebrand factor are believed to reflect generalized endothelial dysfunction[211] and have been independently associated with incident MI and death among patients with angina pectoris or a history of prior MI.[212,213] In addition, although they failed to predict cardiovascular mortality in two population-based studies,[140,214] increased von Willebrand factor levels were independently associated with increased cardiovascular and all-cause mortality at 5 years in a third general population study.[215]

Other Markers

In one study of patients with ACS, brain (B-type) natriuretic peptide, a neurohormone synthesized by the ventricular myocardium during ventricular dilation and pressure overload, was independently predictive of death, MI, and heart failure at 10 months.[216] Pregnancy-

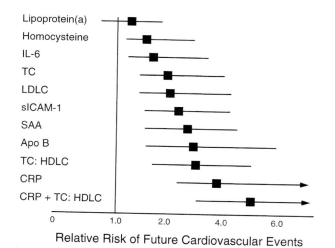

FIGURE 47–8. Comparison of risk ratios for future cardiovascular events according to lipid and inflammatory markers measured in the Women's Health Study. Simultaneously considering the total cholesterol-to-high-density lipoprotein cholesterol ratio (TC:HDLC) and C-reactive protein (CRP) level enabled the most powerful prediction of future cardiovascular risk. Risk ratios and 95% confidence intervals are indicated by squares and horizontal bars. Apo B, apolipoprotein B-100; IL-6, interleukin 6; LDLC, low-density lipoprotein cholesterol; SAA, serum amyloid A; sICAM, soluble intercellular adhesion molecule. (From Ridker PM: High-sensitivity C-reactive protein: Potential adjunct for global risk assessment in the primary prevention of cardiovascular disease. Circulation 2001;103:1813–1818.)

associated plasma protein A (PAPP-A), a metalloproteinase and an activator of insulin-like growth factor,[217] has been identified histologically in vulnerable (i.e., ruptured or eroded) plaque but only to a limited extent in stable coronary atheroma.[218] PAPP-A levels are higher in patients with ACS than in patients with stable coronary disease or in healthy controls.[218] It remains to be seen whether PAPP-A levels will predict recurrent events after ACS or first-time events among otherwise healthy adults. Leptin, a protein that is hypothesized to regulate body weight and that may reflect underlying insulin resistance, was an independent predictor of incident death, nonfatal MI, and coronary revascularization among hyperlipidemic men in one large study.[219] In the same study, lipoprotein-associated phospholipase A$_2$, an enzyme that is regulated by inflammatory mediators and circulates bound to LDL, also independently predicted incident coronary events.[220] Additional risk markers are currently under investigation.

Whether a single biomarker will capture sufficient prognostic information when used in conjunction with traditional lipid and nonlipid risk factors remains to be seen. It is more probable that a multiple biomarker approach will provide incremental predictive value (see Fig. 22–8).[221]

Genetics

Many genes potentially involved in plaque and patient vulnerability have been identified. Genetic loci associated with coronary disease and MI have been eluci-dated,[222-224] as have genetic variations (single nucleotide polymorphisms) that are associated with thrombosis,[225-227] inflammation,[228] and lipid metabolism.[229-231] Finally, genes involved in plaque rupture are under investigation, and preliminary data have been published to this effect.[232, 233] The profiling of multiple single nucleotide polymorphisms simultaneously (i.e., haplotypes) or of overall genetic expression using microarray technology[234] may facilitate the identification of persons with poorer prognoses or lower likelihood of responding to treatment. Topper[235] identified the full platelet *transcriptome* of 1700 platelet-selective mRNAs (Fig. 47–9). This transcriptome lays the groundwork to determine specific genes conferring aspirin resistance or genes with a predisposition to platelet thrombosis. Each of the aforementioned strategies are complementary and may enable better assessment of risk and selection of appropriate therapies.

CONCLUSION

A multitude of imaging technologies, established and emerging, are being evaluated for the detection of vulnerable plaque in individuals with established coronary disease. Simultaneously, a vast array of biomarkers and many genetic variants are being measured in individuals with and without clinically manifest atherosclerotic cardiovascular disease in an effort to identify the vulnerable patient. Ultimately, some combination of biomarker,

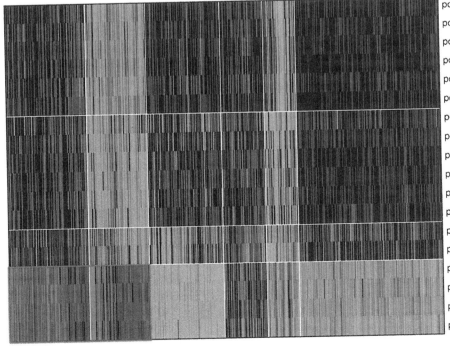

FIGURE 47–9. (See color section.) Gene chip showing the platelet transcriptome of 1700 platelet-selective mRNAs. HUVEC, human umbilical vein endothelial cell. (Courtesy of Dr. James Topper.)

genetic, imaging, and traditional coronary risk factor data will be used to estimate an individual's global risk. Endeavors in this arena are already bearing fruit and likely will usher in the next frontier in cardiovascular medicine.

REFERENCES

1. Strong JP, Malcom GT, McMahan CA, et al: Prevalence and extent of atherosclerosis in adolescents and young adults: Implications for prevention from the Pathobiological Determinants of Atherosclerosis in Youth Study. JAMA 1999;281:727–735.
2. Tuzcu EM, Kapadia SR, Tutar E, et al: High prevalence of coronary atherosclerosis in asymptomatic teenagers and young adults: Evidence from intravascular ultrasound. Circulation 2001;103:2705–2710.
3. Murray CJ, Lopez AD: Alternative projections of mortality and disability by cause 1990–2020: Global Burden of Disease Study. Lancet 1997;349:1498–1504.
4. Moise A, Theroux P, Taeymans Y, et al: Unstable angina and progression of coronary atherosclerosis. N Engl J Med 1983;309:685–689.
5. Ambrose JA, Winters SL, Arora RR, et al: Angiographic evolution of coronary artery morphology in unstable angina. J Am Coll Cardiol 1986;7:472–478.
6. Ambrose JA, Tannenbaum MA, Alexopoulos D, et al: Angiographic progression of coronary artery disease and the development of myocardial infarction. J Am Coll Cardiol 1988;12:56–62.
7. Hackett D, Davies G, Maseri A: Pre-existing coronary stenoses in patients with first myocardial infarction are not necessarily severe. Eur Heart J 1988;9:1317–1323.
8. Little WC, Constantinescu M, Applegate RJ, et al: Can coronary angiography predict the site of a subsequent myocardial infarction in patients with mild-to-moderate coronary artery disease? Circulation 1988;78(5 Pt 1):1157–1166.
9. Giroud D, Li JM, Urban P, et al: Relation of the site of acute myocardial infarction to the most severe coronary arterial stenosis at prior angiography. Am J Cardiol 1992;69:729–732.
10. Ellis S, Alderman EL, Cain K, et al: Morphology of left anterior descending coronary territory lesions as a predictor of anterior myocardial infarction: A CASS Registry Study. J Am Coll Cardiol 1989;13:1481–1491.
11. Taeymans Y, Theroux P, Lesperance J, Waters D: Quantitative angiographic morphology of the coronary artery lesions at risk of thrombotic occlusion. Circulation 1992;85:78–85.
12. Kaski JC, Chester MR, Chen L, Katritsis D: Rapid angiographic progression of coronary artery disease in patients with angina pectoris: The role of complex stenosis morphology. Circulation 1995;92:2058–2065.
13. Chen L, Chester MR, Crook R, Kaski JC: Differential progression of complex culprit stenoses in patients with stable and unstable angina pectoris. J Am Coll Cardiol 1996;28:597–603.
14. Ledru F, Theroux P, Lesperance J, et al: Geometric features of coronary artery lesions favoring acute occlusion and myocardial infarction: A quantitative angiographic study. J Am Coll Cardiol 1999;33:1353–1561.
15. Tousoulis D, Davies G, Stefanadis C, Toutouzas P: Can angiography predict the vulnerable lesion that progresses to myocardial infarction? J Am Coll Cardiol 2000;35:261–262.
16. Haft JI, al-Zarka AM: The origin and fate of complex coronary lesions. Am Heart J 1991;121(4 Pt 1):1050–1061.
17. Topol EJ, Nissen SE: Our preoccupation with coronary luminology: The dissociation between clinical and angiographic findings in ischemic heart disease. Circulation 1995;92:2333–2342.
18. Uchida Y, Nakamura F, Tomaru T, et al: Prediction of acute coronary syndromes by percutaneous coronary angioscopy in patients with stable angina. Am Heart J 1995;130:195–203.
19. Feld S, Ganim M, Carell ES, et al: Comparison of angioscopy, intravascular ultrasound imaging and quantitative coronary angiography in predicting clinical outcome after coronary intervention in high risk patients. J Am Coll Cardiol 1996;28:97–105.

20. Little WC, Applegate RJ: Coronary angiography before myocardial infarction: Can the culprit site be prospectively recognized? Am Heart J 1998;136:368–370.
21. Hodgson JM, Reddy KG, Suneja R, et al: Intracoronary ultrasound imaging: Correlation of plaque morphology with angiography, clinical syndrome and procedural results in patients undergoing coronary angioplasty. J Am Coll Cardiol 1993;21:35–44.
22. Rasheed Q, Nair RN, Sheehan HM, Hodgson JM: Coronary artery plaque morphology in stable angina and subsets of unstable angina: An in vivo intracoronary ultrasound study. Int J Card Imaging 1995;11:89–95.
23. Kearney P, Erbel R, Rupprecht HJ, et al: Differences in the morphology of unstable and stable coronary lesions and their impact on the mechanisms of angioplasty: An in vivo study with intravascular ultrasound. Eur Heart J 1996;17:721–730.
24. Bocksch W, Schartl M, Beckmann S, et al: Intravascular ultrasound imaging in patients with acute myocardial infarction. Eur Heart J 1995;16(Suppl J):46–52.
25. Smits PC, Pasterkamp G, Quarles van Ufford MA, et al: Coronary artery disease: Arterial remodelling and clinical presentation. Heart 1999;82:461–464.
26. Smits PC, Pasterkamp G, de Jaegere PP, et al: Angioscopic complex lesions are predominantly compensatory enlarged: An angioscopy and intracoronary ultrasound study. Cardiovasc Res 1999;41:458–464.
27. Schoenhagen P, Ziada KM, Kapadia SR, et al: Extent and direction of arterial remodeling in stable versus unstable coronary syndromes: An intravascular ultrasound study. Circulation 2000;101:598–603.
28. Schoenhagen P, Vince DG, Ziada KM, et al: Association of arterial expansion (expansive remodeling) of bifurcation lesions determined by intravascular ultrasonography with unstable clinical presentation. Am J Cardiol 2001;88:785–787.
29. de Feyter PJ, Ozaki Y, Baptista J, et al: Ischemia-related lesion characteristics in patients with stable or unstable angina: A study with intracoronary angioscopy and ultrasound. Circulation 1995;92:1408–1413.
30. Ohayon J, Teppaz P, Finet G, Rioufol G: In-vivo prediction of human coronary plaque rupture location using intravascular ultrasound and the finite element method. Coron Artery Dis 2001;12:655–663.
31. Yamagishi M, Terashima M, Awano K, et al: Morphology of vulnerable coronary plaque: Insights from follow-up of patients examined by intravascular ultrasound before an acute coronary syndrome. J Am Coll Cardiol 2000;35:106–111.
32. Sherman CT, Litvack F, Grundfest W, et al: Coronary angioscopy in patients with unstable angina pectoris. N Engl J Med 1986;315:913–919.
33. Mizuno K, Miyamoto A, Satomura K, et al: Angioscopic coronary macromorphology in patients with acute coronary disorders. Lancet 1991;337:809–812.
34. White CJ, Ramee SR, Collins TJ, et al: Percutaneous coronary angioscopy: Applications in interventional cardiology. J Intervent Cardiol 1993;6:61–67.
35. Waxman S, Mittleman MA, Zarich SW, et al: Angioscopic assessment of coronary lesions underlying thrombus. Am J Cardiol 1997;79:1106–1109.
36. Nesto RW, Waxman S, Mittleman MA, et al: Angioscopy of culprit coronary lesions in unstable angina pectoris and correlation of clinical presentation with plaque morphology. Am J Cardiol 1998;81:225–228.
37. Tabata H, Mizuno K, Arakawa K, et al: Angioscopic identification of coronary thrombus in patients with postinfarction angina. J Am Coll Cardiol 1995;25:1282–1285.
38. Ueda Y, Asakura M, Hirayama A, et al: Intracoronary morphology of culprit lesions after reperfusion in acute myocardial infarction: Serial angioscopic observations. J Am Coll Cardiol 1996;27:606–610.
39. Van Belle E, Lablanche JM, Bauters C, et al: Coronary angioscopic findings in the infarct-related vessel within 1 month of acute myocardial infarction: Natural history and the effect of thrombolysis. Circulation 1998;97:26–33.
40. Waxman S: Characterization of the unstable lesion by angiography, angioscopy, and intravascular ultrasound. Cardiol Clin 1999;17:295–305.

41. Huang D, Swanson EA, Lin CP, et al: Optical coherence tomography. Science 1991;254:1178–1181.
42. Tearney GJ, Brezinski ME, Boppart SA, et al: Images in cardiovascular medicine: Catheter-based optical imaging of a human coronary artery. Circulation 1996;94:3013.
43. Brezinski M, Saunders K, Jesser C, et al: Index matching to improve optical coherence tomography imaging through blood. Circulation 2001;103:1999–2003.
44. Boppart SA, Bouma BE, Pitris C, et al: In vivo cellular optical coherence tomography imaging. Nat Med 1998;4:861–865.
45. Jang IK, Bouma BE, Kang DH, et al: Identification of different coronary plaque types in living patients using optical coherence tomography. Circulation 2000;102:II-410.
46. Jang IK, Tearney GJ, Kang DH, et al: Comparison of optical coherence tomography and intravascular ultrasound for detection of coronary plaques with large lipid-core in living patients. Circulation 2000;102:II-509.
47. Stefanadis C, Diamantopoulos L, Vlachopoulos C, et al: Thermal heterogeneity within human atherosclerotic coronary arteries detected in vivo: A new method of detection by application of a special thermography catheter. Circulation 1999;99:1965–1971.
48. Stefanadis C, Diamantopoulos L, Dernellis J, et al: Heat production of atherosclerotic plaques and inflammation assessed by the acute phase proteins in acute coronary syndromes. J Mol Cell Cardiol 2000;32:43–52.
49. Casscells W, Hathorn B, David M, et al: Thermal detection of cellular infiltrates in living atherosclerotic plaques: Possible implications for plaque rupture and thrombosis. Lancet 1996;347:1447–1451.
50. Toutouzas K, Stefanadis C, Vavuranakis M, et al: Arterial remodeling in acute coronary syndromes: Correlation of IVUS characteristics with temperature of the culprit lesion. Circulation 2000;102:II-707.
51. Verheye S, Van Langenhove G, Knaapen MW, et al: Thermal heterogeneity correlates with distribution and severity of atherosclerotic plaques. Circulation 2001;104:II-459.
52. Stefanadis C, Toutouzas K, Tsiamis E, et al: Increased local temperature in human coronary atherosclerotic plaques: An independent predictor of clinical outcome in patients undergoing a percutaneous coronary intervention. J Am Coll Cardiol 2001;37:1277–1283.
53. Carey PR: Raman spectroscopy, the sleeping giant in structural biology, awakes. J Biol Chem 1999;274:26625–26628.
54. Baraga JJ, Feld MS, Rava RP: In situ optical histochemistry of human artery using near infrared Fourier transform Raman spectroscopy. Proc Natl Acad Sci U S A 1992;89:3473–3477.
55. Brennan JF 3rd, Romer TJ, Lees RS, et al: Determination of human coronary artery composition by Raman spectroscopy. Circulation 1997;96:99–105.
56. Romer TJ, Brennan JF 3rd, Schut TC, et al: Raman spectroscopy for quantifying cholesterol in intact coronary artery wall. Atherosclerosis 1998;141:117–124.
57. Romer TJ, Brennan JF 3rd, Fitzmaurice M, et al: Histopathology of human coronary atherosclerosis by quantifying its chemical composition with Raman spectroscopy. Circulation 1998;97:878–885.
58. van de Poll SWE, Buschman HPJ, Visser MJ, et al: Raman spectroscopy provides characterization of human atherosclerotic plaque composition in vivo. J Am Coll Cardiol 2000;35:52A.
59. Romer TJ, Brennan JF 3rd, Puppels GJ, et al: Intravascular ultrasound combined with Raman spectroscopy to localize and quantify cholesterol and calcium salts in atherosclerotic coronary arteries. Arterioscler Thromb Vasc Biol 2000;20:478–483.
60. Owen-Reece H, Smith M, Elwell CE, Goldstone JC: Near infrared spectroscopy. Br J Anaesth 1999;82:418–426.
61. Simonson SG, Piantadosi CA: Near-infrared spectroscopy: Clinical applications. Crit Care Clin 1996;12:1019–1029.
62. Jaross W, Neumeister V, Lattke P, Schuh D: Determination of cholesterol in atherosclerotic plaques using near infrared diffuse reflection spectroscopy. Atherosclerosis 1999;147:327–337.
63. Moreno PR, Lodder RA, O'Connor WN, et al: Characterization of vulnerable plaques by near-infrared spectroscopy in an atherosclerotic rabbit model. J Am Coll Cardiol 1999;33:66A.
64. Moreno PR, Ryan SE, Hopkins D, et al: Identification of lipid-rich plaques in human coronary artery autopsy specimens by near-infrared spectroscopy. J Am Coll Cardiol 2001;37:648A.
65. Moreno PR, Lodder RA, Purushothaman KR, et al: Detection of lipid pool, thin fibrous cap, and inflammatory cells in human aortic atherosclerotic plaques by near-infrared spectroscopy. Circulation 2002;105:923–927.
66. Wang J, Geng YJ, Guo B, et al: Near-infrared spectroscopic characterization of human advanced atherosclerotic plaques. J Am Coll Cardiol 2002;39:1305–1313.
67. Charash WE, Lodder RA, Moreno PR, et al: Detection of simulated vulnerable plaque using a novel near infrared spectroscopy catheter. J Am Coll Cardiol 2000;35:38A.
68. Lees RS, Lees AM, Strauss HW: External imaging of human atherosclerosis. J Nucl Med 1983;24:154–156.
69. Lees AM, Lees RS, Schoen FJ, et al: Imaging human atherosclerosis with 99mTc-labeled low density lipoproteins. Arteriosclerosis 1988;8:461–470.
70. Virgolini I, Rauscha F, Lupattelli G, et al: Autologous low-density lipoprotein labelling allows characterization of human atherosclerotic lesions in vivo as to presence of foam cells and endothelial coverage. Eur J Nucl Med 1991;18:948–951.
71. Hardoff R, Braegelmann F, Zanzonico P, et al: External imaging of atherosclerosis in rabbits using an 123I-labeled synthetic peptide fragment. J Clin Pharmacol 1993;33:1039–1047.
72. Iuliano L, Signore A, Vallabhajosula S, et al: Preparation and biodistribution of 99m technetium labelled oxidized LDL in man. Atherosclerosis 1996;126:131–141.
73. Tsimikas S, Palinski W, Halpern SE, et al: Radiolabeled MDA2, an oxidation-specific, monoclonal antibody, identifies native atherosclerotic lesions in vivo. J Nucl Cardiol 1999;6(1 Pt 1):41–53.
74. Prat L, Torres G, Carrio I, et al: Polyclonal 111In-IgG, 125I-LDL and 125I-endothelin-1 accumulation in experimental arterial wall injury. Eur J Nucl Med 1993;20:1141–1145.
75. Narula J, Petrov A, Bianchi C, et al: Noninvasive localization of experimental atherosclerotic lesions with mouse/human chimeric Z2D3 F(ab)2 specific for the proliferating smooth muscle cells of human atheroma: Imaging with conventional and negative charge-modified antibody fragments. Circulation 1995;92:474–484.
76. Carrio I, Pieri PL, Narula J, et al: Noninvasive localization of human atherosclerotic lesions with indium 111-labeled monoclonal Z2D3 antibody specific for proliferating smooth muscle cells. J Nucl Cardiol 1998;5:551–557.
77. Dinkelborg LM, Duda SH, Hanke H, et al: Molecular imaging of atherosclerosis using a technetium-99m-labeled endothelin derivative. J Nucl Med 1998;39:1819–1822.
78. Tepe G, Duda SH, Meding J, et al: Tc-99m-labeled endothelin derivative for imaging of experimentally induced atherosclerosis. Atherosclerosis 2001;157:383–392.
79. Fischman AJ, Rubin RH, Khaw BA, et al: Radionuclide imaging of experimental atherosclerosis with nonspecific polyclonal immunoglobulin G. J Nucl Med 1989;30:1095–1100.
80. Vallabhajosula S, Fuster V: Atherosclerosis: Imaging techniques and the evolving role of nuclear medicine. J Nucl Med 1997;38:1788–1796.
81. Ohtsuki K, Hayase M, Akashi K, et al: Detection of monocyte chemoattractant protein-1 receptor expression in experimental atherosclerotic lesions: An autoradiographic study. Circulation 2001;104:203–208.
82. Blankenberg FG, Katsikis PD, Tait JF, et al: In vivo detection and imaging of phosphatidylserine expression during programmed cell death. Proc Natl Acad Sci U S A 1998;95:6349–6354.
83. Davis HH 2nd, Siegel BA, Sherman LA, et al: Scintigraphic detection of carotid atherosclerosis with indium-111-labeled autologous platelets. Circulation 1980;61:982–988.
84. Minar E, Ehringer H, Dudczak R, et al: Indium-111-labeled platelet scintigraphy in carotid atherosclerosis. Stroke 1989;20:27–33.
85. Moriwaki H, Matsumoto M, Handa N, et al: Functional and anatomic evaluation of carotid atherothrombosis: A combined study of indium 111 platelet scintigraphy and B-mode ultrasonography. Arterioscler Thromb Vasc Biol 1995;15:2234–2240.
86. Mitchel J, Waters D, Lai T, et al: Identification of coronary thrombus with a IIb/IIIa platelet inhibitor radiopharmaceutical, technetium-99m DMP-444: A canine model. Circulation 2000;101:1643–1646.
87. Elmaleh DR, Narula J, Babich JW, et al: Rapid noninvasive detection of experimental atherosclerotic lesions with novel 99mTc-labeled diadenosine tetraphosphates. Proc Natl Acad Sci U S A 1998;95:691–695.

88. Lister-James J, Vallabhajosula S, Moyer BR, et al: Pre-clinical evaluation of technetium-99m platelet receptor-binding peptide. J Nucl Med 1997;38:105–111.

89. Lister-James J, Knight LC, Maurer AH, et al: Thrombus imaging with a technetium-99m-labeled activated platelet receptor-binding peptide. J Nucl Med 1996;37:775–781.

90. Stratton JR, Cerqueira MD, Dewhurst TA, Kohler TR: Imaging arterial thrombosis: Comparison of technetium-99m-labeled monoclonal antifibrin antibodies and indium-111-platelets. J Nucl Med 1994;35:1731–1737.

91. Mettinger KL, Larsson S, Ericson K, Casseborn S: Detection of atherosclerotic plaques in carotid arteries by the use of 123I-fibrinogen. Lancet 1978;1:242–244.

92. Uehara A, Isaka Y, Hashikawa K, et al: Iodine-131-labeled fibronectin: Potential agent for imaging atherosclerotic lesion and thrombus. J Nucl Med 1988;29:1264–1267.

93. Knight LC: Scintigraphic methods for detecting vascular thrombus. J Nucl Med 1993;34(3 Suppl):554–561.

94. Sangiorgi G, Rumberger JA, Severson A, et al: Arterial calcification and not lumen stenosis is highly correlated with atherosclerotic plaque burden in humans: A histologic study of 723 coronary artery segments using nondecalcifying methodology. J Am Coll Cardiol 1998;31:126–133.

95. Schmermund A, Baumgart D, Gorge G, et al: Coronary artery calcium in acute coronary syndromes: A comparative study of electron-beam computed tomography, coronary angiography, and intracoronary ultrasound in survivors of acute myocardial infarction and unstable angina. Circulation 1997;96:1461–1469.

96. Raggi P, Callister TQ, Cooil B, et al: Identification of patients at increased risk of first unheralded acute myocardial infarction by electron-beam computed tomography. Circulation 2000;101:850–855.

97. Keelan PC, Bielak LF, Ashai K, et al: Long-term prognostic value of coronary calcification detected by electron-beam computed tomography in patients undergoing coronary angiography. Circulation 2001;104:412–417.

98. Fiorino AS: Electron-beam computed tomography, coronary artery calcium, and evaluation of patients with coronary artery disease. Ann Intern Med 1998;128:839–847.

99. Moreno PR, Purushothaman K, O'Connor WN, et al: Lack of association between calcification and vulnerability in human atherosclerotic plaques. J Am Coll Cardiol 2000;35:303A.

100. Huang H, Virmani R, Younis H, et al: The impact of calcification on the biomechanical stability of atherosclerotic plaques. Circulation 2001;103:1051–1056.

101. Moshage WE, Achenbach S, Seese B, et al: Coronary artery stenoses: Three-dimensional imaging with electrocardiographically triggered, contrast agent-enhanced, electron-beam CT. Radiology 1995;196:707–714.

102. Schmermund A, Rensing BJ, Sheedy PF, et al: Intravenous electron-beam computed tomographic coronary angiography for segmental analysis of coronary artery stenoses. J Am Coll Cardiol 1998;31:1547–1554.

103. Reddy GP, Chernoff DM, Adams JR, Higgins CB: Coronary artery stenoses: Assessment with contrast-enhanced electron-beam CT and axial reconstructions. Radiology 1998;208:167–172.

104. Rensing BJ, Bongaerts A, van Geuns RJ, et al: Intravenous coronary angiography by electron beam computed tomography: A clinical evaluation. Circulation 1998;98:2509–2512.

105. Achenbach S, Moshage W, Ropers D, et al: Value of electron-beam computed tomography for the noninvasive detection of high-grade coronary-artery stenoses and occlusions. N Engl J Med 1998;339:1964–1971.

106. Budoff MJ, Oudiz RJ, Zalace CP, et al: Intravenous three-dimensional coronary angiography using contrast enhanced electron beam computed tomography. Am J Cardiol 1999;83:840–845.

107. Achenbach S, Ropers D, Regenfus M, et al: Contrast enhanced electron beam computed tomography to analyse the coronary arteries in patients after acute myocardial infarction. Heart 2000;84:489–493.

108. Achenbach S, Ropers D, Regenfus M, et al: Noninvasive coronary angiography by magnetic resonance imaging, electron-beam computed tomography, and multislice computed tomography. Am J Cardiol 2001;88:70E–73E.

109. Achenbach S, Ulzheimer S, Baum U, et al: Noninvasive coronary angiography by retrospectively ECG-gated multislice spiral CT. Circulation 2000;102:2823–2828.

110. Knez A, Becker C, Ohnesorge B, et al: Noninvasive detection of coronary artery stenosis by multislice helical computed tomography. Circulation 2000;101:E221–E222.

111. Nieman K, van Ooijen P, Rensing B, et al: Four-dimensional cardiac imaging with multislice computed tomography. Circulation 2001;103:E62.

112. Achenbach S, Giesler T, Ropers D, et al: Detection of coronary artery stenoses by contrast-enhanced, retrospectively electrocardiographically-gated, multislice spiral computed tomography. Circulation 2001;103:2535–2538.

113. Estes JM, Quist WC, Lo Gerfo FW, Costello P: Noninvasive characterization of plaque morphology using helical computed tomography. J Cardiovasc Surg (Torino) 1998;39:527–534.

114. Schroeder S, Kopp AF, Baumbach A, et al: Noninvasive detection and evaluation of atherosclerotic coronary plaques with multislice computed tomography. J Am Coll Cardiol 2001;37:1430–1435.

115. Task Force of the European Society of Cardiology, in collaboration with the Association of European Paediatric Cardiologists: The clinical role of magnetic resonance in cardiovascular disease. Eur Heart J 1998;19:19–39.

116. Kim WY, Danias PG, Stuber M, et al: Coronary magnetic resonance angiography for the detection of coronary stenoses. N Engl J Med 2001;345:1863–1869.

117. Yuan C, Mitsumori LM, Beach KW, Maravilla KR: Carotid atherosclerotic plaque: Noninvasive MR characterization and identification of vulnerable lesions. Radiology 2001;221:285–299.

118. Fayad ZA, Nahar T, Fallon JT, et al: In vivo magnetic resonance evaluation of atherosclerotic plaques in the human thoracic aorta: A comparison with transesophageal echocardiography. Circulation 2000;101:2503–2509.

119. Toussaint JF, LaMuraglia GM, Southern JF, et al: Magnetic resonance images lipid, fibrous, calcified, hemorrhagic, and thrombotic components of human atherosclerosis in vivo. Circulation 1996;94:932–938.

120. Yuan C, Beach KW, Smith LH Jr, Hatsukami TS: Measurement of atherosclerotic carotid plaque size in vivo using high resolution magnetic resonance imaging. Circulation 1998;98:2666–2671.

121. Hatsukami TS, Ross R, Polissar NL, Yuan C: Visualization of fibrous cap thickness and rupture in human atherosclerotic carotid plaque in vivo with high-resolution magnetic resonance imaging. Circulation 2000;102:959–964.

122. Fayad ZA, Fuster V, Fallon JT, et al: Noninvasive in vivo human coronary artery lumen and wall imaging using black-blood magnetic resonance imaging. Circulation 2000;102:506–510.

123. Botnar RM, Stuber M, Kissinger KV, et al: Noninvasive coronary vessel wall and plaque imaging with magnetic resonance imaging. Circulation 2000;102:2582–2587.

124. Fayad ZA, Hardy CJ, Giaquinto R, et al: Improved high resolution MRI of human coronary lumen and plaque with a new cardiac coil. Circulation 2000;102:II-399.

125. Goldstein JA, Demetriou D, Grines CL, et al: Multiple complex coronary plaques in patients with acute myocardial infarction. N Engl J Med 2000;343:915–922.

126. Asakura M, Ueda Y, Yamaguchi O, et al: Extensive development of vulnerable plaques as a pan-coronary process in patients with myocardial infarction: An angioscopic study. J Am Coll Cardiol 2001;37:1284–1288.

127. Finet G, Rioufol G, Ajani AE, et al: Does more than one plaque rupture in acute coronary syndromes? An intravascular ultrasound analysis. Eur Heart J 2001;22:273.

128. Libby P, Simon DI: Inflammation and thrombosis: The clot thickens. Circulation 2001;103:1718–1720.

129. Lindemann S, Tolley ND, Dixon DA, et al: Activated platelets mediate inflammatory signaling by regulated interleukin 1beta synthesis. J Cell Biol 2001;154:485–490.

130. Castelli WP: Epidemiology of coronary heart disease: The Framingham study. Am J Med 1984;76:4–12.

131. Executive Summary of the Third Report of the National Cholesterol Education Program (NCEP) Expert Panel on Detection, Evaluation, and Treatment of High Blood Cholesterol in Adults (Adult Treatment Panel III). JAMA 2001;285:2486–2497.

132. Jeppesen J, Hein HO, Suadicani P, Gyntelberg F: Relation of high TG-low HDL cholesterol and LDL cholesterol to the incidence of ischemic heart disease: An 8-year follow-up in the Copenhagen Male Study. Arterioscler Thromb Vasc Biol 1997;17:1114–1120.

133. Lemieux I, Lamarche B, Couillard C, et al: Total cholesterol/HDL cholesterol ratio vs LDL cholesterol/HDL cholesterol ratio as indices of ischemic heart disease risk in men: The Quebec Cardiovascular Study. Arch Intern Med 2001;161:2685–2692.

134. Ridker PM, Glynn RJ, Hennekens CH: C-reactive protein adds to the predictive value of total and HDL cholesterol in determining risk of first myocardial infarction. Circulation 1998;97:2007–2011.

135. Ridker PM, Hennekens CH, Buring JE, Rifai N: C-reactive protein and other markers of inflammation in the prediction of cardiovascular disease in women. N Engl J Med 2000;342:836–843.

136. Salomaa V, Stinson V, Kark JD, et al: Association of fibrinolytic parameters with early atherosclerosis: The ARIC Study. Atherosclerosis Risk in Communities Study. Circulation 1995;91:284–290.

137. Koenig W, Rothenbacher D, Hoffmeister A, et al: Plasma fibrin D-dimer levels and risk of stable coronary artery disease: Results of a large case-control study. Arterioscler Thromb Vasc Biol 2001;21:1701–1705.

138. Danesh J, Whincup P, Walker M, et al: Fibrin D-dimer and coronary heart disease: Prospective study and meta-analysis. Circulation 2001;103:2323–2327.

139. Lowe GD, Yarnell JW, Sweetnam PM, et al: Fibrin D-dimer, tissue plasminogen activator, plasminogen activator inhibitor, and the risk of major ischaemic heart disease in the Caerphilly Study. Thromb Haemost 1998;79:129–133.

140. Smith FB, Lee AJ, Fowkes FG, et al: Hemostatic factors as predictors of ischemic heart disease and stroke in the Edinburgh Artery Study. Arterioscler Thromb Vasc Biol 1997;17:3321–3325.

141. Ridker PM, Hennekens CH, Cerskus A, Stampfer MJ: Plasma concentration of cross-linked fibrin degradation product (D-dimer) and the risk of future myocardial infarction among apparently healthy men. Circulation 1994;90:2236–2240.

142. Cushman M, Lemaitre RN, Kuller LH, et al: Fibrinolytic activation markers predict myocardial infarction in the elderly. The Cardiovascular Health Study. Arterioscler Thromb Vasc Biol 1999;19:493–498.

143. Smith FB, Rumley A, Lee AJ, et al: Haemostatic factors and prediction of ischaemic heart disease and stroke in claudicants. Br J Haematol 1998;100:758–763.

144. Moss AJ, Goldstein RE, Marder VJ, et al: Thrombogenic factors and recurrent coronary events. Circulation 1999;99:2517–2522.

145. Folsom AR, Aleksic N, Park E, et al: Prospective study of fibrinolytic factors and incident coronary heart disease: The Atherosclerosis Risk in Communities (ARIC) Study. Arterioscler Thromb Vasc Biol 2001;21:611–617.

146. Salomaa V, Rasi V, Kulathinal S, et al: Hemostatic factors as predictors of coronary events and total mortality: The FINRISK '92 Hemostasis Study. Arterioscler Thromb Vasc Biol 2002;22:353–358.

147. Cooper JA, Miller GJ, Bauer KA, et al: Comparison of novel hemostatic factors and conventional risk factors for prediction of coronary heart disease. Circulation 2000;102:2816–2822.

148. Ross R: Atherosclerosis—an inflammatory disease. N Engl J Med 1999;340:115–126.

149. Heinrich PC, Castell JV, Andus T: Interleukin-6 and the acute phase response. Biochem J 1990;265:621–636.

150. Harris TB, Ferrucci L, Tracy RP, et al: Associations of elevated interleukin-6 and C-reactive protein levels with mortality in the elderly. Am J Med 1999;106:506–512.

151. Ridker PM, Rifai N, Stampfer MJ, Hennekens CH: Plasma concentration of interleukin-6 and the risk of future myocardial infarction among apparently healthy men. Circulation 2000;101:1767–1772.

152. Volpato S, Guralnik JM, Ferrucci L, et al: Cardiovascular disease, interleukin-6, and risk of mortality in older women: The women's health and aging study. Circulation 2001;103:947–953.

153. Biasucci LM, Liuzzo G, Fantuzzi G, et al: Increasing levels of interleukin (IL)-1Ra and IL-6 during the first 2 days of hospitalization in unstable angina are associated with increased risk of in-hospital coronary events. Circulation 1999;99:2079–2084.

154. Ridker PM, Rifai N, Pfeffer M, et al: Elevation of tumor necrosis factor-alpha and increased risk of recurrent coronary events after myocardial infarction. Circulation 2000;101:2149–2153.

155. Elkind MS, Cheng J, Boden-Albala B, et al: Tumor necrosis factor receptor levels are associated with carotid atherosclerosis. Stroke 2002;33:31–37.

156. Price DT, Loscalzo J: Cellular adhesion molecules and atherogenesis. Am J Med 1999;107:85–97.

157. Malik I, Danesh J, Whincup P, et al: Soluble adhesion molecules and prediction of coronary heart disease: A prospective study and meta-analysis. Lancet 2001;358:971–976.

158. Blake GJ, Ridker PM: Novel clinical markers of vascular wall inflammation. Circ Res 2001;89:763–771.

159. Ridker PM, Buring JE, Rifai N: Soluble P-selectin and the risk of future cardiovascular events. Circulation 2001;103:491–495.

160. Ikeda H, Takajo Y, Ichiki K, et al: Increased soluble form of P-selectin in patients with unstable angina. Circulation 1995;92:1693–1696.

161. Xu DY, Zhao SP, Peng WP: Elevated plasma levels of soluble P-selectin in patients with acute myocardial infarction and unstable angina: An inverse link to lipoprotein(a). Int J Cardiol 1998;64:253–258.

162. Ikeda H, Nakayama H, Oda T, et al: Soluble form of P-selectin in patients with acute myocardial infarction. Coron Artery Dis 1994;5:515–518.

163. Sakurai S, Inoue A, Koh CS, et al: Soluble form of selectins in blood of patients with acute myocardial infarction and coronary intervention. Vasc Med 1997;2:163–168.

164. Shimomura H, Ogawa H, Arai H, et al: Serial changes in plasma levels of soluble P-selectin in patients with acute myocardial infarction. Am J Cardiol 1998;81:397–400.

165. Mulvihill NT, Foley JB, Murphy RT, et al: Risk stratification in unstable angina and non-Q wave myocardial infarction using soluble cell adhesion molecules. Heart 2001;85:623–627.

166. Barbaux SC, Blankenberg S, Rupprecht HJ, et al: Association between P-selectin gene polymorphisms and soluble P-selectin levels and their relation to coronary artery disease. Arterioscler Thromb Vasc Biol 2001;21:1668–1673.

167. Hwang SJ, Ballantyne CM, Sharrett AR, et al: Circulating adhesion molecules VCAM-1, ICAM-1, and E-selectin in carotid atherosclerosis and incident coronary heart disease cases: The Atherosclerosis Risk In Communities (ARIC) study. Circulation 1997;96:4219–4225.

168. Blankenberg S, Rupprecht HJ, Bickel C, et al: Circulating cell adhesion molecules and death in patients with coronary artery disease. Circulation 2001;104:1336–1342.

169. Ridker PM, Hennekens CH, Roitman-Johnson B, et al: Plasma concentration of soluble intercellular adhesion molecule 1 and risks of future myocardial infarction in apparently healthy men. Lancet 1998;351:88–92.

170. Wallen NH, Held C, Rehnqvist N, Hjemdahl P: Elevated serum intercellular adhesion molecule-1 and vascular adhesion molecule-1 among patients with stable angina pectoris who suffer cardiovascular death or non-fatal myocardial infarction. Eur Heart J 1999;20:1039–1043.

171. de Lemos JA, Hennekens CH, Ridker PM: Plasma concentration of soluble vascular cell adhesion molecule-1 and subsequent cardiovascular risk. J Am Coll Cardiol 2000;36:423–426.

172. Danesh J, Collins R, Appleby P, Peto R: Association of fibrinogen, C-reactive protein, albumin, or leukocyte count with coronary heart disease: Meta-analyses of prospective studies. JAMA 1998;279:1477–1482.

173. Danesh J, Whincup P, Walker M, et al: Low grade inflammation and coronary heart disease: Prospective study and updated meta-analyses. BMJ 2000;321:199–204.

174. Feng D, Lindpaintner K, Larson MG, et al: Platelet glycoprotein IIIa Pl(a) polymorphism, fibrinogen, and platelet aggregability: The Framingham Heart Study. Circulation 2001;104:140–144.

175. Kuller LH, Tracy RP, Shaten J, Meilahn EN: Relation of C-reactive protein and coronary heart disease in the MRFIT nested case-control study. Multiple Risk Factor Intervention Trial. Am J Epidemiol 1996;144:537–547.

176. Koenig W, Sund M, Frohlich M, et al: C-Reactive protein, a sensitive marker of inflammation, predicts future risk of coronary heart disease in initially healthy middle-aged men: Results from the MONICA (Monitoring Trends and Determinants in Cardiovascular Disease) Augsburg Cohort Study, 1984 to 1992. Circulation 1999;99:237–242.

177. Ridker PM, Cushman M, Stampfer MJ, et al: Inflammation, aspirin, and the risk of cardiovascular disease in apparently healthy men. N Engl J Med 1997;336:973–979.

178. Tracy RP, Lemaitre RN, Psaty BM, et al: Relationship of C-reactive protein to risk of cardiovascular disease in the elderly: Results from the Cardiovascular Health Study and the Rural Health Promotion Project. Arterioscler Thromb Vasc Biol 1997;17: 1121-1127.

179. Ridker PM, Buring JE, Shih J, et al: Prospective study of C-reactive protein and the risk of future cardiovascular events among apparently healthy women. Circulation 1998;98:731-733.

180. Ridker PM, Cushman M, Stampfer MJ, et al: Plasma concentration of C-reactive protein and risk of developing peripheral vascular disease. Circulation 1998;97:425-428.

181. Lowe GD, Yarnell JW, Rumley A, et al: C-reactive protein, fibrin D-dimer, and incident ischemic heart disease in the Speedwell study: Are inflammation and fibrin turnover linked in pathogenesis? Arterioscler Thromb Vasc Biol 2001;21:603-610.

182. Ridker PM, Stampfer MJ, Rifai N: Novel risk factors for systemic atherosclerosis: A comparison of C-reactive protein, fibrinogen, homocysteine, lipoprotein(a), and standard cholesterol screening as predictors of peripheral arterial disease. JAMA 2001;285: 2481-2485.

183. Liuzzo G, Biasucci LM, Gallimore JR, et al: The prognostic value of C-reactive protein and serum amyloid a protein in severe unstable angina. N Engl J Med 1994;331:417-424.

184. Toss H, Lindahl B, Siegbahn A, Wallentin L: Prognostic influence of increased fibrinogen and C-reactive protein levels in unstable coronary artery disease: FRISC study group. Fragmin during Instability in Coronary Artery Disease. Circulation 1997;96: 4204-4210.

185. Morrow DA, Rifai N, Antman EM, et al: C-reactive protein is a potent predictor of mortality independently of and in combination with troponin T in acute coronary syndromes: A TIMI 11A substudy. Thrombolysis in Myocardial Infarction. J Am Coll Cardiol 1998;31:1460-1465.

186. Biasucci LM, Liuzzo G, Grillo RL, et al: Elevated levels of C-reactive protein at discharge in patients with unstable angina predict recurrent instability. Circulation 1999;99:855-860.

187. Ferreiros ER, Boissonnet CP, Pizarro R, et al: Independent prognostic value of elevated C-reactive protein in unstable angina. Circulation 1999;100:1958-1963.

188. Lindahl B, Toss H, Siegbahn A, et al: Markers of myocardial damage and inflammation in relation to long-term mortality in unstable coronary artery disease: FRISC study group. Fragmin during Instability in Coronary Artery Disease. N Engl J Med 2000;343: 1139-1147.

189. Haverkate F, Thompson SG, Pyke SD, et al: Production of C-reactive protein and risk of coronary events in stable and unstable angina. European Concerted Action on Thrombosis and Disabilities Angina Pectoris Study Group. Lancet 1997;349: 462-466.

190. Heeschen C, Hamm CW, Bruemmer J, Simoons ML: Predictive value of C-reactive protein and troponin T in patients with unstable angina: A comparative analysis. CAPTURE Investigators. Chimeric c7E3 AntiPlatelet Therapy in Unstable angina REfractory to standard treatment trial. J Am Coll Cardiol 2000;35:1535-1542.

191. Zebrack JS, Muhlestein JB, Horne BD, Anderson JL: C-reactive protein and angiographic coronary artery disease: Independent and additive predictors of risk in subjects with angina. J Am Coll Cardiol 2002;39:632-637.

192. Ridker PM, Rifai N, Pfeffer MA, et al: Inflammation, pravastatin, and the risk of coronary events after myocardial infarction in patients with average cholesterol levels. Cholesterol and Recurrent Events (CARE) investigators. Circulation 1998;98: 839-844.

193. Tommasi S, Carluccio E, Bentivoglio M, et al: C-reactive protein as a marker for cardiac ischemic events in the year after a first, uncomplicated myocardial infarction. Am J Cardiol 1999;83: 1595-1599.

194. Mueller C, Buettner HJ, Hodgson JM, et al: Inflammation and long-term mortality after non-ST elevation acute coronary syndrome treated with a very early invasive strategy in 1042 consecutive patients. Circulation 2002;105:1412-1415.

195. Gaspardone A, Crea F, Versaci F, et al: Predictive value of C-reactive protein after successful coronary-artery stenting in patients with stable angina. Am J Cardiol 1998;82:515-518.

196. Buffon A, Liuzzo G, Biasucci LM, et al: Preprocedural serum levels of C-reactive protein predict early complications and late restenosis after coronary angioplasty. J Am Coll Cardiol 1999;34: 1512-1521.

197. Versaci F, Gaspardone A, Tomai F, et al: Predictive value of C-reactive protein in patients with unstable angina pectoris undergoing coronary artery stent implantation. Am J Cardiol 2000;85:92-95, A8.

198. Chew DP, Bhatt DL, Robbins MA, et al: Incremental prognostic value of elevated baseline C-reactive protein among established markers of risk in percutaneous coronary intervention. Circulation 2001;104:992-997.

199. Walter DH, Fichtlscherer S, Sellwig M, et al: Preprocedural C-reactive protein levels and cardiovascular events after coronary stent implantation. J Am Coll Cardiol 2001;37:839-846.

200. Milazzo D, Biasucci LM, Luciani N, et al: Elevated levels of C-reactive protein before coronary artery bypass grafting predict recurrence of ischemic events. Am J Cardiol 1999;84:459-461, A9.

201. Ridker PM: High-sensitivity C-reactive protein: Potential adjunct for global risk assessment in the primary prevention of cardiovascular disease. Circulation 2001;103:1813-1818.

202. Wolbink GJ, Brouwer MC, Buysmann S, et al: CRP-mediated activation of complement in vivo: Assessment by measuring circulating complement-C-reactive protein complexes. J Immunol 1996; 157: 473-479.

203. Pasceri V, Willerson JT, Yeh ET: Direct proinflammatory effect of C-reactive protein on human endothelial cells. Circulation 2000;102:2165-2168.

204. Zwaka TP, Hombach V, Torzewski J: C-reactive protein-mediated low density lipoprotein uptake by macrophages: Implications for atherosclerosis. Circulation 2001;103:1194-1197.

205. Torzewski M, Rist C, Mortensen RF, et al: C-reactive protein in the arterial intima: Role of C-reactive protein receptor-dependent monocyte recruitment in atherogenesis. Arterioscler Thromb Vasc Biol 2000;20:2094-2099.

206. Pasceri V, Cheng JS, Willerson JT, et al: Modulation of C-reactive protein-mediated monocyte chemoattractant protein-1 induction in human endothelial cells by anti-atherosclerosis drugs. Circulation 2001;103:2531-2534.

207. Nakagomi A, Freedman SB, Geczy CL: Interferon-gamma and lipopolysaccharide potentiate monocyte tissue factor induction by C-reactive protein: Relationship with age, sex, and hormone replacement treatment. Circulation 2000;101:1785-1791.

208. Nakajima T, Schulte S, Warrington KJ, et al: T-cell-mediated lysis of endothelial cells in acute coronary syndromes. Circulation 2002;105:570-575.

209. Schonbeck U, Libby P: CD40 signaling and plaque instability. Circ Res 2001;89:1092-1103.

210. Schonbeck U, Varo N, Libby P, et al: Soluble CD40L and cardiovascular risk in women. Circulation 2001;104:2266-2268.

211. Mannucci PM: von Willebrand factor: A marker of endothelial damage? Arterioscler Thromb Vasc Biol 1998;18:1359-1362.

212. Jansson JH, Nilsson TK, Johnson O: von Willebrand factor in plasma: A novel risk factor for recurrent myocardial infarction and death. Br Heart J 1991;66:351-355.

213. Thompson SG, Kienast J, Pyke SD, et al: Hemostatic factors and the risk of myocardial infarction or sudden death in patients with angina pectoris. European Concerted Action on Thrombosis and Disabilities Angina Pectoris Study Group. N Engl J Med 1995;332:635-641.

214. Folsom AR, Wu KK, Rosamond WD, et al: Prospective study of hemostatic factors and incidence of coronary heart disease: The Atherosclerosis Risk in Communities (ARIC) study. Circulation 1997;96:1102-1108.

215. Jager A, van Hinsbergh VW, Kostense PJ, et al: von Willebrand factor, C-reactive protein, and 5-year mortality in diabetic and nondiabetic subjects: The Hoorn Study. Arterioscler Thromb Vasc Biol 1999;19:3071-3078.

216. de Lemos JA, Morrow DA, Bentley JH, et al: The prognostic value of B-type natriuretic peptide in patients with acute coronary syndromes. N Engl J Med 2001;345:1014-1021.

217. Lawrence JB, Oxvig C, Overgaard MT, et al: The insulin-like growth factor (IGF)-dependent IGF binding protein-4 protease secreted by human fibroblasts is pregnancy-associated plasma protein-A. Proc Natl Acad Sci U S A 1999;96:3149-3153.

218. Bayes-Genis A, Conover CA, Overgaard MT, et al: Pregnancy-associated plasma protein A as a marker of acute coronary syndromes. N Engl J Med 2001;345:1022-1029.

219. Wallace AM, McMahon AD, Packard CJ, et al: Plasma leptin and the risk of cardiovascular disease in the West of Scotland Coronary Prevention Study (WOSCOPS). Circulation 2001;104:3052-3056.

220. Packard CJ, O'Reilly DS, Caslake MJ, et al: Lipoprotein-associated phospholipase A2 as an independent predictor of coronary heart disease. West of Scotland Coronary Prevention Study group. N Engl J Med 2000;343:1148-1155.

221. Sabatine MS, Morrow DA, de Lemos JA, et al: Multimarker approach to risk stratification in non-ST elevation acute coronary syndromes: Simultaneous assessment of troponin I, C-reactive protein, and B-type natriuretic peptide. Circulation 2002;105:1760-1763.

222. Pajukanta P, Cargill M, Viitanen L, et al: Two loci on chromosomes 2 and X for premature coronary heart disease identified in early-and late-settlement populations of Finland. Am J Hum Genet 2000;67:1481-1493.

223. Francke S, Manraj M, Lacquemant C, et al: A genome-wide scan for coronary heart disease suggests in Indo-Mauritians a susceptibility locus on chromosome 16p13 and replicates linkage with the metabolic syndrome on 3q27. Hum Mol Genet 2001;10:2751-2765.

224. Broeckel U, Hengstenberg C, Mayer B, et al: A comprehensive linkage analysis for myocardial infarction and its related risk factors. Nat Genet 2002;30:210-214.

225. Ardissino D, Mannucci PM, Merlini PA, et al: Prothrombotic genetic risk factors in young survivors of myocardial infarction. Blood 1999;94:46-51.

226. Girelli D, Russo C, Ferraresi P, et al: Polymorphisms in the factor VII gene and the risk of myocardial infarction in patients with coronary artery disease. N Engl J Med 2000;343:774-780.

227. Topol EJ, McCarthy J, Gabriel S, et al: Single nucleotide polymorphisms in multiple novel thrombospondin genes may be associated with familial premature myocardial infarction. Circulation 2001;104:2641-2644.

228. Andreotti F, Porto I, Crea F, Maseri A: Inflammatory gene polymorphisms and ischaemic heart disease: Review of population association studies. Heart 2002;87:107-112.

229. Kuivenhoven JA, Jukema JW, Zwinderman AH, et al: The role of a common variant of the cholesteryl ester transfer protein gene in the progression of coronary atherosclerosis. The Regression Growth Evaluation Statin Study Group. N Engl J Med 1998;338:86-93.

230. Imai Y, Morita H, Kurihara H, et al: Evidence for association between paraoxonase gene polymorphisms and atherosclerotic diseases. Atherosclerosis 2000;149:435-442.

231. Lambert JC, Brousseau T, Defosse V, et al: Independent association of an APOE gene promoter polymorphism with increased risk of myocardial infarction and decreased APOE plasma concentrations—the ECTIM study. Hum Mol Genet 2000;9:57-61.

232. Schwartz SM, Hatsukami TS, Yuan C: Molecular markers, fibrous cap rupture, and the vulnerable plaque: New experimental opportunities. Circ Res 2001;89:471-473.

233. Faber BC, Cleutjens KB, Niessen RL, et al: Identification of genes potentially involved in rupture of human atherosclerotic plaques. Circ Res 2001;89:547-554.

234. Schena M, Heller RA, Theriault TP, et al: Microarrays: Biotechnology's discovery platform for functional genomics. Trends Biotechnol 1998;16:301-306.

235. Topper JN: Genes, matrix, and restenosis. Arterioscler Thromb Vasc Biol 2000;20:2173-2174.

236. Fayad ZA, Fuster V: Clinical imaging of the high-risk or vulnerable atherosclerotic plaque. Circ Res 2001;89:305-316.

237. Nissen SE, Yock P: Intravascular ultrasound: Novel pathophysiological insights and current clinical applications. Circulation 2001;103:604-616.

238. de Korte CL, Pasterkamp G, van der Steen AF, et al: Characterization of plaque components with intravascular ultrasound elastography in human femoral and coronary arteries in vitro. Circulation 2000;102:617-623.

239. Diamantopoulos LD, Van Langenhove G, de Feyter P, et al: 3-D Thermal reconstruction of the atherosclerotic plaque: A new insight into plaque vulnerability by means of thermography and advanced computer algorithms. J Am Coll Cardiol 2001;37:382A.

The Modern Coronary Care Unit

Robert M. Califf
Galen S. Wagner
Christopher B. Granger
L. Kristin Newby
Wanda Bride

Despite the many advances in recent years in the care of acute coronary syndromes (ACSs), acute cardiac ischemia and its complications remain major public health problems. The cardiac care unit (CCU) is the center for the receipt, organization, and treatment of patients with acute cardiovascular problems in most hospitals. However, CCUs must continue to expand in two directions: management of acute cardiac situations of all types, especially the broad spectrum of ACSs and heart failure, and extension into the community. At the same time, because of various economic forces, CCUs must focus on efficiency.

In many ways, the CCUs will be a center of convergence for the population and economic trends relating to health care in our society. Our longevity continues to improve steadily and dramatically,[1] but this effect is modest compared with the increase in our functionality.[2] Thus, we have a population that is healthier until the time of acute vascular events, which constitute the leading cause of death and disability by a growing margin. At the same time, societal investment has resulted in an ever-increasing arsenal of expensive biotechnology. The drug-coated stent,[3] the implantable defibrillator,[4,5] and the left-ventricular assist device[6] are just now hitting the clinical arena, and the advent of cell-replacement therapy[7] will greatly affect the cost of care and expectations of the population. With more and more previously functional elderly patients making up the bulk of CCU patients and rapidly advancing technologic capacity, the issue of effectiveness relative to cost and, perhaps more than in younger populations, patient preferences will become dominant in coming years. Clearly, we will not be able to afford to do everything that could prolong life in every patient, nor may that always be an appropriate or even desired goal. Therefore, it will become paramount to develop more systematic approaches to delivering the most effective therapy to patients who will benefit most from it.

The massive increase in heart failure[8] is straining the capacity of CCUs and bringing up issues of specialized heart-failure units in addition to the prevalent chest-pain centers. Particularly with the impending widespread availability of the left-ventricular assist device, the CCU is likely to become the focus of decision-making for an increasing number of people who are ineligible for cardiac transplantation but who still need decisions made about treatment that will require enormous expenditures but may significantly lengthen life.

The trends in out-of-hospital outcomes are more difficult to gauge than the inpatient trends. We do know that out-of-hospital cardiac arrest remains the leading cause of death by far, and we know that extension of technology formerly available only in the hospital can significantly reduce mortality and morbidity in communities. Automated external defibrillators, community cardiopulmonary resuscitation (CPR), and performance of electrocardiograms (ECGs) at the scene to identify ST-segment elevation myocardial infarction (MI) or high-risk non–ST-segment elevation (NSTE) ACSs are initial examples of the extension of the CCU into the community. Inadequate effort has been expended to organize these technologies into a comprehensive, evidence-based approach. Such an effort is needed in the next few years!

PREHOSPITAL CARE

The extension of the CCU into the prehospital phase involves a shift in thinking from the CCU as a fortress, inside of which excellent clinical care can be divorced from the chaos of the external world. Instead, we now know that applying the same principles of evidence, using outcomes studies and clinical trials, can improve the fate of patients in the highest-risk situation—before reaching the hospital—and that we can have a major effect in the period of highest risk in the hospital, the emergency department (ED).

The system begins with the basic principle of encouraging those with symptoms to enter the care system as quickly and efficiently as possible. Most people with symptoms of myocardial ischemia do not seek help quickly, and when they do, the majority do not call 911 or other emergency medical services (EMS); rather, they arrange nonmedical transport to an emergency facility. Though these statements simply present the facts, they belie the underlying complexity of this principle. First, it is based on the assumption that the public really understands or can recognize the symptoms of ischemia and the implications of delay. Without those two concepts, people at risk will not enter the system quickly or efficiently. Although the implications of delay may be relatively simple to teach, we know that accurate symptom recognition is difficult even for medically trained personnel, which has largely fueled the widespread use of chest pain units. Further, our understanding of what influences even knowledgeable people in the decisions they make when confronted with potential ischemic symptoms is limited. Coupled with wide variability in EMS and patient perceptions of them, fulfilling this basic principle is a great challenge to successful prehospital cardiac care.

The National Heart, Lung, and Blood Institute–sponsored Rapid Early Action for Coronary Treatment (REACT) trial[9] randomized communities to a massive public-relations effort or conventional approaches to attempting to improve reactions to symptoms of possible ischemia. Disappointingly, the trial showed no effect on time to treatment, appropriate diagnoses, or improved outcomes, but it did show an improvement in the use of EMS as the mode of transport. These results and those of previous studies suggest a need for more-targeted education and refocus of these efforts. Patient delay (prehospital delay) is the major factor of treatment delay, and this component has not changed substantially in the reperfusion era.[10,11] Efforts to understand the factors predisposing to delay and to define and target educational efforts to high-risk, high-yield people or populations may ultimately be a better approach than massive public-education efforts.

In a substudy, the REACT investigators[12] showed that the decision to use EMS depended on the person's thinking about the symptoms: those who lived alone, those who thought that their symptoms were serious enough to take nitroglycerin, and those who were prompted to "go quickly" by others used EMS. Of interest, those who called their doctors were less likely to use EMS. Further, communities that had an EMS prepayment plan tended to experience greater EMS use than communities in which individuals paid out of pocket (as fee for service) for EMS.

Despite these difficulties, given that the risk of death declines with time from onset of the acute event, earlier access to life-saving technology is a crucial part of any community cardiac-care program. This technology includes four main elements, extensions of interventions available in the hospital: the defibrillator, the 12-lead ECG, acute reperfusion therapy, and other drugs.

Time to defibrillation is a critical variable in determining the likelihood of surviving a cardiac arrest. Of course, the ultimate approach to this problem is implantation of an automated internal cardioverter/defibrillator. Even with the expanded Multicenter Automatic Defibrillator Implantation Trial (MADIT-2) criteria,[4,13] this approach is unlikely to meet the full extent of the need for primary prophylaxis against sudden death because a patient must have already experienced major dysrhythmia or MI to meet these criteria. Another approach is wider distribution of automated external cardioverter defibrillators (AECDs). A recent pilot study from Germany reported a threefold improvement in meaningful recovery from cardiac arrest in the community when AECDs were introduced,[14] and the positive results of the deployment of AECDs in the casinos in Las Vegas have been much discussed.[15]

The standard 12-lead ECG for decision support of the on-call cardiologist completes the loop for modern acute care of people with thrombosis-induced MI, given that both pathophysiology and definitive therapies have been established for this condition. The standard 12-lead ECG that provides key diagnostic information in patients with ACS symptoms now is commonly performed before hospital arrival by EMS personnel. More-modern technology can even provide wireless ECG transmission from the scene to a handheld liquid crystal display (LCD) to provide support for the on-call cardiologist to make the required triage decisions directly.[16] A recent study has shown that 50% of patients with ECG interpretation of "acute MI" by trained emergency medical technologists and 85% with cardiologist concurrence of "acute MI" will have an acute thrombotic occlusion confirmed during attempted primary percutaneous coronary intervention (PCI).[17] Further, the ability of practicing cardiologists to make both the same ECG diagnosis and the same reperfusion triage decision on paper and on the LCD of a handheld device has been reported.[18,19]

The ST segment has been the portion of the ECG typically used to provide both diagnostic and prognostic information. Ischemia-induced terminal distortion of the QRS complex, however, has been shown to be superior to ST-segment measurements in predicting final acute MI size and assessing the possible effects of fibrinolytic therapy.[20] Also, comparative quantitative changes in T waves and infarction-induced initial distortion of the QRS complex have been shown to add to historical timing in the prediction of limiting MI size through reperfusion therapy.[21]

When the prehospital ECG is perceived to indicate acute coronary thrombosis and the clinical situation is appropriate, early reperfusion therapy can be started intravenously by the emergency medical technologists, by rapid administration in the ED, or by PCI by the cardiologist in the catheterization laboratory. Electronic transmission of 12-lead ECGs to the hospital ED has been shown to reduce the time to reperfusion via primary PCI by 30 minutes.[22] The administration of fibrinolytic therapy in the field, also predicated on the availability of 12-lead ECGs at the scene, now has been tested in multiple clinical trials. A systematic overview showed reduced mortality with prehospital versus hospital administration of fibrinolytic therapy,[23] and a pilot trial of field fibrinolysis has suggested outcomes comparable with direct PCI.[24] For the most part, field administration of fibrinolytic therapy in the United States has been limited by concerns about liability and the absence of physicians on ambulances. In countries such as France, the system supports the effort, but it is unclear in the United States whether appropriately trained nonphysician personnel can safely give prehospital fibrinolytic or other medical therapy unless there is direct exchange of clinical and ECG information with an on-call physician. The results of the ASsessment of the Safety and Efficacy of a New Thrombolytic Agent (ASSENT) III Plus study, in which patients from around the world were treated with fibrinolytic therapy in the field by personnel with various clinical backgrounds, should help to address these concerns.

In the United States, then, until reforms in medical liability can be addressed and the safety of prehospital therapy given by nonphysicians is clearly shown and accepted, the first consideration should be to ensure that all EMS units can capture and transmit in-field 12-lead ECGs. Prehospital services then can focus on timely transfer of patients with acute MI to regional centers capable of rapid administration of fibrinolytic therapy or performance of PCI. For rural areas with long transit times to the nearest hospital, however, improved technology, including electronic transmission of ECGs from the field to on-call physicians, should drive consideration of in-field treatment if qualified nonphysician personnel are available. Development of hybrid, but perhaps safer, alternative approaches to full-dose fibrinolysis also could be an answer. Regardless, in addition to understanding patient-related factors in responding to symptoms and using EMS, broad standardization of EMS services and their improved coordination with regional acute cardiac care facilities will be necessary as a first step in enhancing prehospital care.

In patients with ACS who are not candidates for acute reperfusion therapy, the amount of depression in the ST segment of the initial ECG has been shown to have value in early risk stratification.[25] Unlike ST-segment elevation MI, it has been difficult to show a dramatic time-dependency of outcome after giving effective therapies in NSTE ACSs. Thus, it is difficult to know whether the expense of supplies and training needed for prehospital administration of pharmacologic therapy, other than aspirin and acute therapies such as oxygen, nitrates, and morphine, is warranted. However, having the ECG information available from the field should aid in patient triage on arrival and inform decisions for early invasive management strategies. Such information also could improve the likelihood of evidenced-based therapies being started early on arrival as well as aid in the identification of patients eligible for clinical trials, particularly if integrated with input from on-call cardiology services at the receiving hospital.

Future prehospital cardiac care of patients with ACSs may be enhanced by the availability of both practice guidelines and access to the medical literature via handheld devices. Even a simple innovation—such as a new way to provide quantitative information from the 12-lead ECG to the handheld device of the on-call cardiologist—might be useful. A new display of the ECG with all available 24 views around "clock faces" surrounding schematic images of the heart, in both the frontal and transverse planes, has been introduced.[26] This might provide added decision support for the cardiologist's interpretation of the initial ECG by indicating the spatial location of the acute ST-segment deviation for more precise localization of the culprit lesion within the coronary artery. A substudy of the Global Use of Strategies To Open occluded coronary arteries

(GUSTO) I and II trials has suggested the value of this method.[27]

THE EMERGENCY DEPARTMENT

Although geographically distinct, the ED, and even EDs at separate referral hospitals, must be effectively integrated with the CCU for patients progressing from the outpatient to the critical-care setting. An example of success in a joint ED-cardiology initiative was the Heart Attack Alert Program, which resulted in a 50% reduction in time from ED arrival until fibrinolysis during the 1990s.[28] Because the immediate needs of EDs and CCUs are different and at times even contradictory, regular communication among the two sets of physician and nurse leaders is essential to provide optimal acute cardiac care. Common standards and algorithms should be established (e.g., for reperfusion therapy for acute ST-segment elevation MI). Regular meetings of staff representatives, in which cases are reviewed to highlight problems and successes in integration of emergency and intensive care, constitute one mechanism for continuous improvement.

Hospital-wide ACS protocols should begin in the ED. These protocols should include clear direction on the preferred initial evaluation, the immediate therapeutic approach, and the clinical trials in which the institution is participating. Examples of the Duke ACS protocols are shown in Figure 48-1. Another important issue for facilities without full cardiac services should be development of a standard approach to determining who should be transferred to a higher-intensity facility and when transfer should occur. In an ideal world, this would be done regionally so that the criteria are standard and the roles and responsibilities of participating facilities (and of the transport links between them and the EMS linking them with the public) are clear. The system would allow such decisions to be made as early as possible after patient arrival in the ED, and with central coordination and input from the EMS and 12-lead ECG in the field, these protocols might be applied even earlier, eliminating the need for transfer to another facility after arrival at the first ED.

Quality measures, as described later, should be viewed jointly by the ED and the CCU. For example, time to reperfusion therapy could be delayed at multiple points, ranging from obtaining the initial ECG to the availability of consultation for difficult cases. Ultimately, because time from symptom onset to reperfusion is critical to preservation of myocardium and, ultimately, to patient outcome in ST-segment elevation MI, understanding and eliminating delays at all levels in the system is essential. This can be done only with collaborative review and discussion of the results of quality measures.

CHEST PAIN UNITS

After a patient is evaluated in the ED, one of several triage routes must be considered: discharge to home, admission

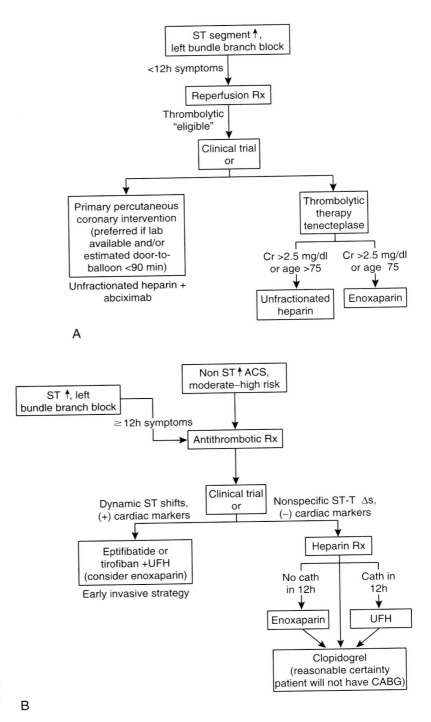

FIGURE 48–1. Algorithms for management of patients with ST-segment elevation MI (*A*) and NSTE ACS (*B*) at Duke.

to a standard hospital bed, admission to the CCU, or, the newest option, admission to a chest pain unit.

One of the greatest challenges facing the ED physician is the management of chest pain or other symptoms of possible acute coronary ischemia. Each year, an estimated 5 million people arrive at EDs in the United States with such symptoms, only a minority of whom actually have an ACS.[29] Among 10,689 patients presenting to EDs with acute chest pain in the multicenter Acute Coronary Ischemia–Time-Insensitive Predictive

Instrument (ACI-TIPI) study, only 8% had acute MI and only 9% had unstable angina.[30] The challenge, then, is to rapidly identify those who would benefit from immediate intervention and hospitalization while limiting unnecessary resource use for the majority who do not have ACSs.

Using the basic tools of the history, physical examination, and 12-lead ECG, physicians are remarkably sensitive in their admission of patients with acute coronary ischemia, admitting 90% to 98% of patients with the diagnosis.[30-37] This sensitivity comes at the expense of specificity, however—only 30% to 40% of patients admitted with a suspected ACS ultimately are found to have one.[38,39] Admission of these patients, often to intensive care units, competes for limited inpatient resources and generates an estimated $600 million per year in unnecessary costs in the United States.[40]

Equally important are the clinical and medicolegal consequences arising among the small minority of patients with true ACS who are mistakenly released from the ED. In the ACI-TIPI study, 2.1% of patients with MI and 2.3% of patients with unstable angina were released from the ED.[30] Among these patients, the adjusted odds ratios for 30-day mortality were 1.7 and 1.9, respectively. Although this represents only a minority of all patients with chest pain, the consequences of missed MI account for 21% of all malpractice claims in the United States against ED physicians.[41]

Over the past 20 years, a systematic approach has gradually evolved to address the conflicting pressures and needs of managing patients with chest pain in the ED. Conceived in 1981 as specialized chest pain ERs to encourage earlier arrival after chest-pain onset, to prevent cardiac arrest, and later to aid in the rapid recognition and time-sensitive treatment of ST-segment elevation MI,[42] these programs now have been developed at many hospitals into tiered chest-pain–center approaches to managing the spectrum of chest pain, from acute ST-segment elevation MI to low-risk chest pain with normal or nondiagnostic initial evaluation results.[43-46] In such systems, rather than being admitted to inpatient beds or released directly, patients with low clinical risk based on the standard history, physical examination, 12-lead ECG, and cardiac-marker results, but for whom diagnostic uncertainty remains, are evaluated further in chest pain units. There are now more than 520 chest-pain units in hospitals throughout the United States.[47]

The structure of a chest pain unit and its size and physical location vary among hospitals, but the central theme is one of systematic, protocol-driven observation and evaluation, usually over 6 to 12 hours. In general, nurse/patient ratios of 3:1 or 4:1 during chest pain unit observation are acceptable. During this time, either serial 12-lead ECG or ST-segment trend monitoring is performed along with serial cardiac-marker testing. The National Academy of Clinical Biochemistry recommends a two-marker approach, using a marker such as myoglobin, which is likely to be positive within 6 hours of symptom onset, in combination with a highly specific marker, such as troponin T or I, which remains elevated in the serum for several days.[48] The diagnostic and prognostic utility of such an approach was shown in the CHest pain Evaluation by Creatine Kinase-MB, Myoglobin And Troponin I Evaluation (CHECKMATE).[49] Algorithms for treatment of patients in the Duke chest pain unit are shown in Figure 48–2. Functional assessment (stress testing with or without imaging) should be performed before patients with negative cardiac markers and ECG evaluation results are discharged. Patients who experience positive cardiac markers or ECG changes consistent with ischemia should be admitted to intensive care units and treated according to American College of Cardiology/ American Heart Association (ACC/AHA) guidelines, and those with positive stress test results should be triaged for further evaluation. The specifics of the protocol used are dictated by local expertise and existing infrastructure, but all emphasize this basic, systematic approach to evaluation.

Acute imaging as an adjunct to cardiac marker testing and ST-segment trend monitoring or serial ECG has been evaluated. Although acute echocardiography may reveal wall-motion abnormalities that aid in diagnosis of acute ischemia, up to 27% of patients with acute ischemia have nondiagnostic echocardiogram results,[50] and no benefit of routine echocardiography has been shown in protocols that incorporate serial cardiac marker testing.[51] In facilities with services available 24 hours a day, 7 days a week, technetium-99 sestamibi imaging often is used in

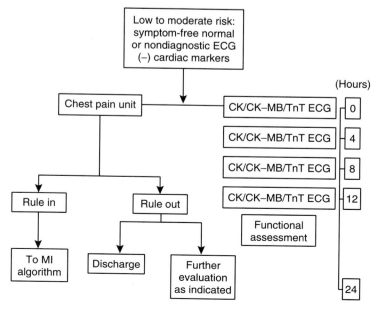

FIGURE 48–2. Algorithms for patient management in the Duke Chest Pain Unit.

combination with standard chest-pain evaluation protocols. This approach has been shown to be within the acceptable range of incremental cost-effectiveness.[52-54] The sensitivity of technetium-99 sestamibi imaging ranges from 94% to 100%; specificity, from 78% to 93%; and negative predictive value, from 94% to 100%.[55] Diagnostic sensitivity depends greatly on injection during pain, however.[56]

Just as protocols may differ from hospital to hospital, so, too, may the physical location of the chest pain unit. Although the unit ideally would be in or adjacent to the ED, either as a dedicated space or as a virtual unit within the ED, in some centers, space constraints dictate other arrangements. A systematic, protocol-driven approach administered by trained personnel (physicians, physician-extenders, and nurses) still should function effectively regardless of physical location and existing infrastructure.

THE CARDIAC CARE UNIT

The contemporary CCU is faced with the challenge of providing efficient care for patients with complex cardiac conditions using an increasingly extensive and complicated set of medical and device options. To succeed, key elements include effective teamwork and communication, systematic approaches, and the use of computer technology to improve performance.

Although major cardiology society guidelines provide a detailed framework for applying evidence-based treatment in a spectrum of patients and situations, their complexity and length—91 pages for the 2002 AHA/ACC MI guidelines[57]—essentially preclude their use by physicians in a busy patient-care environment. The guidelines can direct systematic approaches to patient care that can be customized to a hospital or unit, especially when information systems can help track how care is being provided. For example, a poster outlining a systematic approach to early antithrombotic and interventional care of the spectrum of patients with ACS can be placed in both the ED and the CCU to establish standard approaches that incorporate guidelines and evidence-based approaches. This could include strategies for reperfusion therapy in patients with ST-elevation MI and how to use platelet glycoprotein IIb/IIIa inhibitors and low-molecular-weight heparins for patients with NSTE ACSs. For institutions participating in clinical trials, such a poster also can highlight which patients are eligible for which ongoing trials. In the near future, the goal should be to have such algorithms available to the care team by means of handheld computers with direct links to the supporting guidelines or literature and to specific dosing guidelines and caveats. Registries such as the National Registry of Myocardial Infarction (NRMI),[28] the Global Registry of Acute Coronary Events (GRACE),[58] and the Can Rapid risk stratification of Unstable angina patients Suppress ADverse outcomes with Early implementation of the ACC/AHA guidelines? (CRUSADE),[59] as well as internal quality-assurance data collection, are essential tools in establishing whether treatments are being effectively applied in cardiac emergency and critical care.

After decades of generating negative feelings in the medical community, standardized orders have gained acclaim as part of an effective strategy to reduce medical errors. Standard admission orders can help ensure that common evidence-based treatments, such as aspirin for all patients with ACSs, are not forgotten. Standard dosing guidelines for unfractionated heparin, which customize the dose of heparin according to patient weight and sex and call for adjustments according to an algorithm, can improve therapeutic heparin use.[60] Algorithm-driven replacement of potassium and magnesium likewise can allow more accurate and efficient normalization of electrolytes. The ACC-sponsored Guidelines Applied in Practice (GAP) project showed that patients whose doctors were exposed to standard order forms were more likely to be sent home with therapies in alignment with the ACC/AHA guidelines.[61]

The Team Approach

Strong physician leadership of a CCU is required so that medical decisions, reflecting consensus, can be applied systematically to ensure the highest-quality care. In many practice situations, because physicians who admit patients to the CCU may belong to competing practice groups, systematic application of standards of care is possible only if a mechanism (preferably a unit medical director) exists to adjudicate differences. For day-to-day care, some units may have one attending physician responsible for the care of all patients admitted to the unit, a situation better suited to central decision-making, whereas others may have separate physicians responsible for each patient with no formal alignment of the providers. Given the growing complexity of acute cardiac care, the ever-increasing arsenal of expensive biotechnology and pharmacologic treatment options, and the increasing demands on the CCU and its physicians to make decisions regarding their use, this situation is no longer tenable in most modern CCUs.

In addition to focusing delivery of such care in highly specialized centers, only cardiologists experienced with substantial volumes and spectra of critically ill patients should care directly for cardiology patients in intensive care units. At centers that do not provide these services, protocols defining the appropriate transfer of patients should be developed in conjunction with their referral centers. In addition, modern CCU physicians should be expected to meet high standards for clinical competency and compliance with practice guidelines. Obviously, widespread implementation of this change in the model will require the skills of a strong physician-leader able to traverse the political minefield inherent in such an approach, which ultimately has the best interests of patient care as its focus. Outside interests may drive such organization as well. The Leapfrog group, which represents a coalition of organizations that pay for health care in the United States, has made the presence of full-time intensivists and computerized physician order entry criteria of quality for referral of patients by the employers who constitute this group.[62]

When attending physicians are not immediately available in person, they should have fax machine or Internet access to ECGs (and, ideally, coronary angiography and echocardiogram data) for immediate interpretation at home or office, or this responsibility should be delegated to someone physically present. In addition to competence in standard invasive intensive-care-unit procedures, physicians staffing CCUs should be capable in performance and interpretation of echocardiograms. Training in advanced cardiac life support is advisable.

Nursing

Competent and compassionate nurses are the most important team members of the successful CCU. After accounting for the fixed costs of facilities, more than 80% of the direct CCU budget can be attributed to nursing personnel. The complexity of the CCU calls for a team of specially trained, relatively independent practitioners. In our environment, the CCU nurse is the defender of the standard of care. Given that physicians spend limited time in the CCU, it is the nurse who identifies when variations in prescribing or procedure use are reasonable and when they deviate from the standard of care. The nurse is the gatekeeper for the patient, ensuring that the right thing is being done at the right time. Timely and effective communication between nurses and physician leaders in real time is critical to avoiding conflict between nurses and doctors when differences of opinion arise.

Because the demand for CCU beds varies uncontrollably, it is critical to develop and maintain standards for flexibility in staffing. This can be done by maintaining a core of "budgeted" nurses based on analysis of occupancy and severity-of-illness trends. Shifts in the patient census then can be handled by cross-training with other cardiology units so that nurses can move to and from those areas when needed, maintaining a flexible workforce that can be tapped when overflow occurs and allowing judicious filling of empty beds with selected non-CCU patients. Each unit must develop a specific solution, but common to all approaches is the need for intensive, standards-based education of nurses.

In a large CCU, in addition to the usual nurse management and educator system, a nurse-clinician focused on family and physician communication has been and remains a critical feature. The nurse-clinician plays critical roles in maintaining quality data regarding performance improvement and in being the liaison between the families and the health care team. In many cases, miscommunications among the patient, family, nurses, and doctors can be avoided or resolved with external oversight from an experienced nurse-clinician. The compelling results from the Study to Understand Prognoses and Preferences for Outcomes and Risks of Treatments (SUPPORT) study[63] caused us to conclude that significant resources must be put toward the end of life as well as improving longevity. The nurse-clinician is critical in developing and maintaining a multidisciplinary protocol for the withdrawal of life support and end-of-life care.

Pharmacist Role

The clinical pharmacist is an essential partner in the CCU. The publicity about patient harm from medication errors has emphasized the importance of expert review and advice regarding use of drugs. Using the definition of medical errors put forward by the Institute of Medicine—having the wrong plan or making an error in the execution of the correct plan[64]—few patients make it through a CCU experience without at least one medical error. Given the age of this population and the high prevalence of comorbidity, including variable renal and hepatic function, they are particularly at risk for bleeding, arrhythmias, and other adverse effects.

Pharmacy support should address three areas: education of physicians and nurses as to safe use of common medications and their combinations, establishment of systems to guide effective and safe use of drugs, and personal review of medication use in patients in the CCU. As electronic pharmacy, laboratory, and medical-order systems become more sophisticated, algorithms programmed into the system can flag potential problems. Recent studies have shown that dosing errors in administration of fibrinolytic therapy can result in catastrophic patient outcomes,[65] which might be avoided with built-in electronic checks and feedback to the physician about dosing before drug administration. One area of extreme importance is dose adjustment for renally excreted drugs. In recent research done by the Centers for Education and Research on Therapeutics, the dose of dofetilide was correctly given in less than 40% of patients.[66] Integrated electronic systems in both the CCU and the cardiology ward could substantially reduce these types of prescribing errors. Until such systems are widely available, however, pharmacist oversight of prescribing for the individual patient's clinical situation and changes in condition remains essential.

Effective sedation of the agitated patient is a special challenge in the intensive-care setting. This can be addressed by including pharmacist input on developing a systematic approach for this population. Further, as the use of invasive procedures, mechanical prostheses, and ventilators in the CCU continues to escalate, antibiotics are becoming ubiquitous, but cardiologists have difficulty staying abreast of the latest information about antibiotic prescribing and overuse, leading to significant risk of resistant organisms in the local environment. We think that a clinically knowledgeable pharmacist should review drug orders on all CCU patients at least daily and that special attention should be paid to renally excreted drugs, sedation, and antibiotics.

Other Team Members

Ideally, members of the entire care team participate in the discussion and design of the care plan. Respiratory technicians play an important role in optimizing ventilator management, and physical and occupational therapists can ensure early and consistent rehabilitation. Maintaining adequate nutritional support, balancing increased metabolic demands against possible renal or hepatic impairment, is essential to the recovery of the critically ill patient, and recovering patients with ACSs and their families are most available for and attuned to education about dietary modification and its role in long-term management of coronary disease and heart failure in the CCU.

The importance of "hotel functions" in a system of cardiac care cannot be underestimated. Maintenance of facilities and supplies and efficient cleaning and turnover of rooms is critical. Additionally, the unscheduled nature of CCU admissions calls for extensive communication efforts within and between hospitals. In the United States, the criteria for transfer and admission seem to vary as a function of whether the unit is full.[67] Given the growing epidemic of vascular disease in the aging, it seems unlikely that facilities will be built at the same pace as the demand on those facilities. This inevitable fact demands a regional system to ensure that patients are not caught between hospitals or transferred inappropriately when beds may be empty at different hospitals.

Communication with the Family

Similar to the need for a pediatrician to communicate with the parents of a young sick child, the CCU physicians and staff must effectively communicate with and support the families of critically ill patients. More liberal, flexible visiting hours tend to provide better support for families. A particularly important time for intensive support and counseling of families is at the end of life, including situations in which life support is withdrawn from a patient with a terminal and irreversible illness. A nurse with interest and expertise in critical care and in family communication and support can be an invaluable part of the care team when extensive family interactions are needed. A related need, for less acutely ill patients, is patient and family teaching. A patient in the early days of recovery after an acute MI, for example, is a captive and generally receptive audience for teaching about smoking cessation,

diet, lifestyle changes, and what to expect from upcoming procedures. A patient-education booklet customized to the institution is an important adjunct for patient education.

Assessment of Quality

Understanding the quality of medical care has been potentiated by focus from various organizations, most notably, the Institute of Medicine. Its two seminal reports—*To Err Is Human*[64] and *Crossing the Quality Chasm*[68]—lay out an approach to providing quality health care that is forming the basis for research in and measurement of quality.

A broad approach in cardiovascular medicine,[69] into which the CCU readily fits, has been to attempt to develop a cycle of quality (Fig. 48–3). Given an excellent idea based on a plausible biologic construct, multiple studies are needed before a definitive phase III or phase IV trial can be performed. If this trial or series of trials is of adequate quality, the results can be used to create a clinical practice guideline. Particular trials of adequate power, done in a relevant environment with modern background therapy and producing a robust result, can result in a class I (proven to be effective), level of evidence A (based on multiple trials or a megatrial) or B (based on less definitive trials) recommendation. Definitive clinical practice guideline recommendations can be translated into performance indicators that measure whether a practitioner, practice, hospital, or system is adhering to guideline standards, and aggregates of performance indicators can be used to characterize clinical performance.

The CCU is an ideal environment in which to test approaches to the cycle of quality and an important

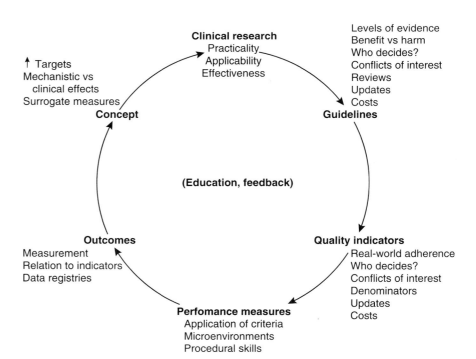

FIGURE 48–3. Model for the integration of quality into the therapeutic development cycle. (From Califf RM, Peterson ED, Gibbons RM, et al: Integration of quality into the cycle of therapeutic development. J Am Coll Cardiol 2003 [in press].)

place to develop constructs that work because of the massive public health implications. In fact, many of the standards of care that currently exist are based on clinical trials in acute cardiac care.

Members of the care provider team should meet regularly to address optimizing care of the CCU patient. For example, systems should be established to ensure success in the six Oryx performance measures established by the U.S. Joint Commission for the Accreditation of Healthcare Organizations (JCAHO) that apply to the first days of treatment of acute MI—rapid reperfusion with either fibrinolysis or primary angioplasty; the use of aspirin, β-blockers, and angiotensin-converting enzyme inhibitors; and smoking cessation counseling.[70]

Rapid use of cardioversion/defibrillation for pulseless ventricular arrhythmias also should be ensured. One of the most important functions of a CCU is highly effective intervention for treatable life-threatening cardiac arrhythmias. In fact, the concept of the CCU was originally established in large part for that capability.[71] For each minute of delay in defibrillation, there is an approximately 10% decrease in survival[72,73]; thus, every CCU should establish that ventricular fibrillation is treated with defibrillation within 1 minute of its occurrence. To do so, the unit must establish a system to respond to ventricular fibrillation and must measure the time from onset of ventricular fibrillation until first defibrillator shock to ensure that the goal is accomplished.

Table 48–1 lists a set of performance indicators for MI adopted by the JCAHO.[70] Our goal is to exceed the criteria for adherence to guidelines by a wide margin.

For NSTE ACS, Peterson and colleagues have shown a broad variance in adherence to the ACC/AHA guidelines.[74] However, the hospitals that most closely adhered to guideline recommendations had the lowest mortality rates.[74] Figure 48–4 illustrates this finding for the use of glycoprotein IIb/IIIa inhibitors. Whether these better outcomes result directly from the therapies studied or represent a marker of the ability to organize complex therapeutic schemes among multiple practitioners remains to be discovered.

■ ■ ■

TABLE 48–1   JCAHO CORE PERFORMANCE MEASURES FOR MYOCARDIAL INFARCTION[70]

1. Aspirin given at arrival
2. Aspirin prescribed at discharge
3. Patients with left-ventricular ejection fraction < 40% prescribed an ACE inhibitor at discharge
4. Adult smoking cessation advice/counseling
5. β-Blocker prescribed at discharge
6. β-Blocker given at arrival
7. Time from arrival to start of fibrinolysis
8. Time from arrival to start of primary percutaneous coronary intervention
9. Inpatient mortality

ACE, angiotensin-converting enzyme.

Our approach to quality measurement in the CCU has been to use existing registries to produce measures of adherence to performance indicators. In the ST-elevation setting, we have registered our data with the NRMI, a commercially based effort.[28] This registry has collected data on hundreds of thousands of patients and now includes more than 500 hospitals in North America. Thus, it provides a robust source for peer comparisons. In the NSTE ACS setting, we participate in the CRUSADE registry, now involving 300 hospitals in North America, with the goal of increasing to more than 500 hospitals this year.[59]

In addition, the CCU Morbidity and Mortality Conference is used to review issues of coordination of care and communication. When a major incident occurs with a patient, consideration is given to a sentinel event analysis in conjunction with the hospital's quality system. An ultimate measure of quality for the CCU of the future would be the morbidity and mortality rates for the community. Such a measure obviously would require collaboration between the CCU and EMS.

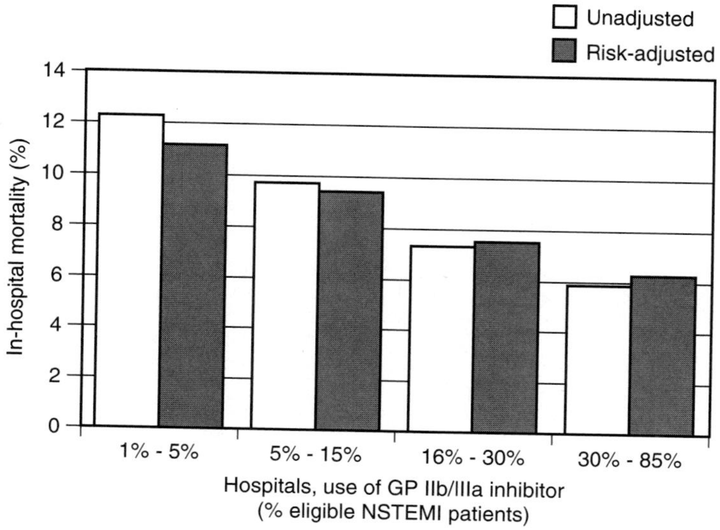

FIGURE 48–4. In-hospital mortality versus adherence to ACC/AHA guidelines for use of GP IIb/IIIa inhibitors in management of NSTE ACS.[74]

Finances

The CCU is a major cost center for hospitals, but it also serves as a source of patient throughput that generates substantial revenue. Major percutaneous intervention and cardiac surgical programs are not sustainable without adequate CCU support. Thus, the efficient management of CCU services, personnel, and supplies plays a major role in the financial stability of hospitals. Because the CCU is integrated with other cardiovascular services, it is critical to view financial reports for cardiac services as a whole, rather than simply evaluating the CCU as a "tub on its own bottom."

Most costs in the CCU are attributable to facilities, equipment, and personnel. Management of facilities and equipment requires a sophisticated understanding of fixed and variable costs and an ability to estimate the effect of having or not having these components on clinical outcomes and other costs. For example, given a fixed investment in CCU beds, the rapid availability of cardiac-intervention facilities becomes a major determinant of whether the beds will be filled to spread the fixed costs adequately. Management of nursing personnel has been discussed, but the quality of care may depend more on this factor than any other. A recent study showed that 30-day mortality increases by 7% with each additional patient per nurse, at the same time increasing the risk of nurse "burnout" by 23% and the odds of job dissatisfaction by 15%.[75] Thus, the nurse-manager and CCU director must work incessantly to ensure that adequate nurses are staffed for first-rate patient care while maintaining fiscal responsibility.

Ultimately, given the likelihood of progressive dissociation between what is possible and the costs of effective therapy, the fate of the CCU will depend on how well its leaders can make the case for incremental spending for more benefit. This advocacy will be more effective if the CCU can set the standard within the hospital for efficient resource use. We think that participation in the research enterprise is a critical component of identifying which approaches provide enough benefit to justify the cost and which should be eschewed.[76]

CONCLUSIONS

The CCU is an increasingly complex entity, and it must be integrated into a broad community and hospital approach to prevention and treatment of cardiovascular disease. A focus on standards of care, with derivative rational allocation of costs to provide the greatest benefit, will enable the CCU of the future to do more good for more people. To meet this demand, the CCU must be led by physicians and nurses with a broad view of clinical medicine, finance, and management.

REFERENCES

1. Murray CJ, Lopez AD: Global mortality, disability, and the contribution of risk factors: Global Burden of Disease Study. Lancet 1997;349:1436–1442.

2. Manton KG, Stallard E, Corder LS: The dynamics of dimensions of age-related disability 1982 to 1994 in the U.S. elderly population. J Gerontol Ser A–Biol Sci Med Sci 1998;53:B59–B70.

3. Morice MC, Serruys PW, Sousa JE, et al, for the RAVEL Study Group: A randomized comparison of a sirolimus-eluting stent with a standard stent for coronary revascularization. N Engl J Med 2002;346:1773–1780.

4. Moss AJ, Zareba W, Hall J, et al: Prophylactic implantation of a defibrillator in patients with myocardial infarction and reduced ejection fraction. N Engl J Med 2002;346:877–883.

5. Buxton AE, Lee KL, Fisher JD, et al: A randomized study of the prevention of sudden death in patients with coronary artery disease. N Engl J Med 1999;341:1882–1890.

6. Rose EA, Gelijns AC, Moskowitz AJ, et al: Long-term use of a left ventricular assist device for end-stage heart failure. N Engl J Med 2001;345:1435–1443.

7. Taylor DA, Hruban R, Rodriguez ER, et al: Cardiac chimerism as a mechanism for self-repair: Does it happen and if so to what degree? Circulation 2002;106:2–4.

8. Massie BM, Shah NB: Evolving trends in the epidemiologic factors of heart failure: Rationale for preventive strategies and comprehensive disease management. Am Heart J 1997;133:703–712.

9. Luepker RV, Raczynski JM, Osganian S, et al: Effect of a community intervention on patient delay and emergency medical service use in acute coronary heart disease: The Rapid Early Action for Coronary Treatment (REACT) Trial. JAMA 2000;284:60–67.

10. Alexander JH, Poku MB, Card TL, et al: Randomization in a clinical trial only modestly delays time to treatment in acute myocardial infarction patients undergoing thrombolysis: Results from the ASSENT-2 emergency department registry [Abstract]. Circulation 2002;102:II-796.

11. Gibler WB, Armstrong PW, Ohman EM, et al: Persistence of delays in presentation and treatment for patients with acute myocardial infarction: The GUSTO-I and -III experience. Ann Emerg Med 2002;39:123–130.

12. Brown AL, Mann NC, Daya M, et al: Demographic, belief, and situational factors influencing the decision to utilize emergency medical services among chest pain patients. Circulation 2000;102:173–178.

13. Lee KL, Hafley G, Fisher JD, et al: Effect of implantable defibrillators on arrhythmic events and mortality in the Multicenter UnSustained Tachycardia Trial. Circulation 2002;106:233–238.

14. Cummins RO, Eisenberg MS, Bergner L, et al: Automatic external defibrillation: Evaluations of its role in the home and in emergency medical services. Ann Emerg Med 1984;13(9 Pt 2):789–801.

15. Valenzuela TD, Roe DJ, Nichol G, et al: Outcomes of rapid defibrillation by security officers after cardiac arrest in casinos. N Engl J Med 2000;343:1206–1209.

16. Pettis KS, Kwong M, Wagner GS: Prehospital diagnosis and management of patients with acute myocardial infarction using remote transmission of electrocardiograms to palmtop computers. In Clements IP (ed): ECG in Acute Myocardial Infarction. Armonk, N.Y., Futura, 1998, pp 223–234.

17. Sejersten M, Young D, Clemmensen P, et al: Comparison of the ability of paramedics with that of cardiologists in diagnosing ST-segment elevation acute myocardial infarction in patients with acute chest pain. Am J Cardiol 2002;90:995–998.

18. Pettis KR, Savona MR, Leibrandt PN, et al: Evaluation of the efficacy of hand-held computer screens for cardiologists' interpretations of 12 lead electrocardiograms. Am Heart J 1999;138:765–770.

19. Leibrandt PN, Bell SJ, Savona MR, et al: Validation of cardiologist's decisions to initiate reperfusion therapy for acute myocardial infarction using ECGs on liquid crystal displays hand held computer as decision support regarding reperfusion therapy for acute myocardial infarction. Am Heart J 2000;140:747–752.

20. Birnbaum Y, Maynard C, Wolfe S, et al: Terminal QRS distortion on admission is better than ST segment measurements in predicting final infarct size and assessing the potential effect of thrombolytic therapy in anterior wall acute myocardial infarction. Am J Cardiol 1999;84:530–534.

21. Corey KE, Maynard C, Pahlm O, et al: Combined historical and electrocardiographic timing of anterior and inferior wall acute myocardial infarcts for prediction of reperfusion achievable size limitation. Am J Cardiol 1999;83:826–831.

22. Wall TC, Albright J, Jacobowitz S, et al: The TIME (Timely Intervention in Myocardial Emergency) Trial: Reducing time to pri-

mary PTCA with the use of prehospital ECGs for patients with acute MI. N C Med J 2000;61:104–108.

23. Morrison LJ, Verbeek PR, McDonald AC, et al: Mortality and prehospital thrombolysis for acute myocardial infarction: A meta-analysis. JAMA 2000;283:2686–2692.

24. Bonnefoy E, Lapostolle F, Leizorovicz A, et al: Primary angioplasty versus prehospital fibrinolysis in acute myocardial infarction: A randomised study. Lancet 2002;360:825–829.

25. Holmvang L, Clemmensen P, Wagner GS, et al: Admission standard ECG for early risk stratification in patients with unstable coronary artery disease not eligible for acute revascularization therapy: A TRIM substudy. Am Heart J 1999;137:24–33.

26. Pahlm-Webb U, Pahlm O, Sadanandan S, et al: A new method for using the direction of ST segment deviation to localize the site of acute coronary occlusion: The 24-view standard ECG. Am J Med 2002:113:75–78.

27. Sadanandan S, Hochman JS, Kolodziej A, et al: Clinical and angiographic characteristics of patients with combined anterior and inferior ST segment deviation on the initial ECG during acute MI. Am Heart J 2003 (in press).

28. Rogers WJ, Canto JG, Lambrew CT, et al: Temporal trends in the treatment of over 1.5 million patients with myocardial infarction in the US from 1990 through 1999: The National Registry of Myocardial Infarction 1, 2 and 3. J Am Coll Cardiol 2000;36: 2056–2063.

29. Burt CW: Summary statistics for acute cardiac ischemia and chest pain visits to United States EDs, 1995–1996. Am J Emerg Med 1999;17:552–559.

30. Pope JH, Aufderheide TP, Ruthazer R, et al: Missed diagnoses of acute cardiac ischemia in the emergency department. N Engl J Med 2000;342:1163–1170.

31. Howell JM, Hedges JR: Differential diagnosis of chest discomfort and general approach to myocardial ischemia decision making. Am J Emerg Med 1991;9:571–579.

32. Tierney WM, Fitzgerald J, McHenry R, et al: Physicians' estimates of the probability of myocardial infarction in emergency room patients with chest pain. Med Decis Making 1986;6:12–17.

33. Eagle KA: Medical decision making in patients with chest pain. N Engl J Med 1991;324:1282–1283.

34. Lee TH, Rouan GW, Weisberg MC, et al: Sensitivity of routine clinical criteria for diagnosing myocardial infarction within 24 hours of hospitalization. Ann Intern Med 1987;106:181–186.

35. Lee TH: Chest pain in the emergency department: uncertainty and the test of time. Mayo Clin Proc 1991;66:963–965.

36. McCarthy BD, Wong JB, Selker HP: Detecting acute cardiac ischemia in the emergency department: A review of the literature. J Gen Intern Med 1990;5:365–373.

37. Villanueva FS, Sabia PJ, Afrooktch A, et al: Value and limitations of current methods of evaluating patients presenting to the emergency room with cardiac-related symptoms for determining long-term prognosis. Am J Cardiol 1992;69:746–750.

38. Gibler WB, Lewis LM, Erb RE, et al: Early detection of acute myocardial infarction in patients presenting with chest pain and non-diagnostic ECGs: Serial CK-MB sampling in the emergency department. Ann Emerg Med 1990;19:1359–1366.

39. Gibler WB, Young GP, Hedges JR, et al: Acute myocardial infarction in chest pain patients with nondiagnostic ECGs: Serial CK-MB sampling in the emergency department. Ann Emerg Med 1992;21: 504–512.

40. Jesse RL, Kontos MC: Evaluation of chest pain in the emergency department. Curr Prob Cardiol 1997;22:149–236.

41. Rusnak RA, Stair TO, Hansen K, et al: Litigation against the emergency department physician: Common features in cases of missed myocardial infarction. Ann Emerg Med 1989;18:1029–1034.

42. Bahr RD: Growth of chest pain emergency departments throughout the United States: A cardiologist's spin on solving the heart attack problem. Coron Artery Dis 1995;6:827–838.

43. Nichol G, Walls R, Goldman L, et al: A critical pathway for management of patients with acute chest pain who are at low risk for myocardial ischemia: Recommendations and potential impact. Ann Intern Med 1997;127:996–1005.

44. Ornato JP: Critical pathways for triage and treatment of chest pain patients in the emergency department. Clinician 1996;14:53–55.

45. Storrow AB, Gibler WB, Walsh RA, et al: An emergency department chest pain rapid diagnosis and treatment unit: Results from a 6-year experience [Abstract]. Circulation 1998;98:I-425.

46. Farkouh ME, Smars PA, Reeder GS, et al: A clinical trial of a chest-pain observation unit for patients with unstable angina. N Engl J Med 1998;339:1882–1888.

47. Zalenski RJ, Selker HP, Cannon CP, et al: National Heart Attack Alert Program position paper: Chest pain centers and programs for the evaluation of acute cardiac ischemia. Ann Emerg Med 2000;35: 462–471.

48. Wu AHB, Apple FS, Gibler WB, et al: National Academy of Clinical Biochemistry Standards of Laboratory Practice: Recommendations for use of cardiac markers in coronary artery disease. Clin Chem 1999;45:1104–1121.

49. Newby LK, Storrow AB, Gibler WB, et al: Bedside multimarker testing for risk stratification in chest pain units: The Chest Pain Evaluation by Creatine Kinase-MB, Myoglobin, and Troponin I (CHECKMATE) study. Circulation 2001;103:1832–1837.

50. Ewy GA, Ornato JP, chairs: 31st Bethesda Conference: Emergency cardiac care. J Am Coll Cardiol 2000;35:825–880.

51. Levitt MA, Promes SB, Bullock S, et al: Combined cardiac marker approach with adjunct two-dimensional echocardiography to diagnose acute myocardial infarction in the emergency department. Ann Emerg Med 1996;27:1–7.

52. Radensky PW, Stowers SA, Hilton TC, et al: Cost-effectiveness of acute myocardial perfusion imaging with Tc-99m sestamibi for risk stratification of emergency strategies in unstable angina and non-Q-wave myocardial infarction [Abstract]. Circulation 1994;90: I-528.

53. Weismann IA, Dickinson CZ, Dworkin HJ, et al: Cost-effectiveness of myocardial perfusion imaging with SPECT in the emergency department evaluation of patients with unexplained chest pain. Radiology 1996;199:353–357.

54. Kontos MC, Jesse RL, Ornato JP, et al: Cost effectiveness of a comprehensive strategy for the evaluation and triage of the chest pain patient [Abstract]. Circulation 1999;100:I-290.

55. Kim SC, Adams SL, Hendel RC: Role of nuclear cardiology in the evaluation of acute coronary syndromes. Ann Emerg Med 1997;30:210–218.

56. Bilodeau L, Theroux P, Gregoire J, et al: Technetium-99m sestamibi tomography in patients with spontaneous chest pain. J Am Coll Cardiol 1991;18:1684–1691.

57. Ryan TJ, Antman EM, Brooks NH, et al: ACC/AHA guidelines for the management of patients with acute myocardial infarction: 1999 update. Available at http://www.acc.org/clinical/guidelines/nov96/1999/index.htm. Accessed 22 October 2002.

58. The GRACE Investigators: Rationale and design of the GRACE (Global Registry of Acute Coronary Events) Project: A multinational registry of patients hospitalized with acute coronary syndromes. Am Heart J 2001;141:190–199.

59. Roe MT, Staman KL, Pollack C, et al: A practical guide to understanding the 2002 ACC/AHA guidelines for the management of patients with non-ST-segment elevation acute coronary syndromes. Crit Pathways Cardiol 2002;1:129–149.

60. Cruickshank MK, Levine MN, Hirsh J, et al: A standard heparin nomogram for the management of heparin therapy. Arch Intern Med 1991;151:333–337.

61. Mehta RH, Montoye CK, Gallogly M, et al: Improving quality of care for acute myocardial infarction: The Guidelines Applied in Practice (GAP) initiative. JAMA 2002;287:1269–1276.

62. The Leapfrog Group. Available at http://www.leapfroggroup.org. Accessed 28 October 2002.

63. The SUPPORT Principal Investigators: A controlled trial to improve care for seriously ill hospitalized patients: The Study to Understand Prognoses and Preferences for Outcomes and Risks of Treatments (SUPPORT) [erratum published JAMA 1996;275:1232]. JAMA 1995; 274:1591–1598.

64. Kohn LT, Corrigan JM, Donaldson MS (eds): To Err Is Human: Building a Safer Health System. Washington, D.C., Institute of Medicine/National Academy Press, 2000.

65. Murphy SA, Gibson CM, Van de Werf F, et al: Comparison of errors in estimating weight and in dosing of single-bolus tenecteplase with tissue plasminogen activator (TIMI 10B and ASSENT I). Am J Cardiol 2002;90:51–54.

66. Allen LaPointe NM, Kramer JM, Weinfurt K, et al: Practitioner acceptance of dofetilide risk-management program. Pharmacotherapy 2002;22:1041–1046.

67. Singer DE, Carr PL, Mulley AG, Thibault GE: Rationing intensive care—physician responses to a resource shortage. N Engl J Med 1983;309:1155–1160.

68. Committee on Quality of Health Care in America: Crossing the Quality Chasm: A New Health System for the 21st Century. Washington, D.C., Institute of Medicine/National Academy Press, 2001.

69. Califf RM, Peterson ED, Gibbons RM, et al: Integration of quality into the cycle of therapeutic development. J Am Coll Cardiol 2003 (in press).

70. Joint Commission on Accreditation of Health Care Organization: Core Measures. Available at http://www.jcaho.org/pms/core+measures. Accessed 28 October 2002.

71. Day HW: History of coronary care units. Am J Cardiol 1972;30: 405–440.

72. Cummins RO, Hazinski MF, eds: Guidelines 2000 for cardiopulmonary resuscitation and emergency cardiovascular care: An international consensus on science. Circulation 2000;102 (Suppl I):1.

73. Capucci A, Aschieri D, Piepoli MF, et al: Tripling survival from sudden cardiac arrest via early defibrillation without traditional education in cardiopulmonary resuscitation. Circulation 2002;106: 1065–1070.

74. Peterson ED, Canto JG, Pollack CV, et al, for the NRMI-4 Investigators: Early use of glycoprotein IIb/IIIa inhibitors and outcomes in non-ST–elevation acute myocardial infarction: Observations from the National Registry of Myocardial Infarction 4 [Abstract]. J Am Coll Cardiol 2002;39:279A.

75. Aiken LH, Clarke SP, Sloane DM, et al: Hospital nurse staffing and patient mortality, nurse burnout, and job dissatisfaction. JAMA 2002;288:1987–1993.

76. Califf RM, DeMets DL: Principles from clinical trials relevant to clinical practice. Parts 1 and 2. Circulation 2002;106:1015–1021 and 1172–1175.

■ ■ ■ chapter **4 9**

Guidelines of the European Society of Cardiology

Michel E. Bertrand

Acute coronary syndromes (ACSs) have become a major health care problem in recent years, with millions of patients hospitalized annually in the world. A European survey conducted in 103 centers of 25 European countries recorded 10,484 patients within an 8-month period.[1]

ACSs—namely unstable angina and evolving myocardial infarction (MI)—share a common anatomic substrate: pathologic, angioscopic, and biologic observations have demonstrated that unstable angina and MI are different clinical presentations that result from a common underlying pathophysiological mechanism, namely, atherosclerotic plaque rupture or erosion, with differing degrees of superimposed thrombosis and distal embolization.[2-4]

Clinical criteria have been developed to allow the clinician to make timely decisions and to choose the best treatment based on risk stratification and a targeted approach to intervention.

In practice, two categories of patients may be encountered:

- Patients with a presumed ACS with ongoing chest discomfort and persistent ST-segment elevation (or new-onset left bundle branch block). Persistent ST-segment elevation generally reflects acute total coronary occlusion. The therapeutic objective is rapid, complete, and sustained recanalization by primary angioplasty (if technically feasible) or fibrinolytic treatment (if not contraindicated).
- Patients who present with chest pain with ECG abnormalities suggesting acute ischemic heart disease. They do not have persistent ST-segment elevation but rather persistent or transient ST-segment depression or T-wave inversion, flat T waves, pseudonormalization of T waves, or nonspecific ECG changes; the ECG may also be normal at presentation. Patients with ischemic ECG abnormalities but without symptoms (silent ischemia) may be included in this category.

The treatment of patients without persistent ST-segment elevation was addressed in the ESC Guidelines for management of acute MI published in 2000 in the European Heart Journal (volume 21, pages 1406 to 1432). In this rapidly evolving field, an update was considered: The revision started in October 2001, was completed and

reviewed by the members of the committee for practice guidelines at the end of July 2002 and published in the December issue of the European Heart Journal.

DIAGNOSIS

Clinical Presentation

The clinical presentation of ACSs encompasses a wide variety of symptoms. Traditionally, several clinical presentations have been distinguished:

- Prolonged (>20 minutes) anginal pain at rest
- New onset (de novo)
- Severe (class III of the Canadian Cardiovascular Society [CCS] classification) angina
- Recent destabilization of previously stable angina with at least CCS III angina characteristics (crescendo angina)

Prolonged pain occurs in 80% of patients; de novo or accelerated angina occurs in only 20%.[5] The classic features of typical ischemic cardiac pain are well known and are not further described here. However, atypical presentations of ACSs are not uncommon. They are often observed in younger (25 to 40 years old) and older (>75 years old) patients, diabetic patients, and women.

Physical Examination

Physical examination results are most often normal, including chest examination, auscultation, and measurement of heart rate and blood pressure. The purpose of the examination is to exclude noncardiac causes of chest pain, nonischemic cardiac disorders (pericarditis, valvular disease), potential precipitating extracardiac causes, and pneumothorax, and to search for signs of potential hemodynamic instability and left-ventricular (LV) dysfunction.

Electrocardiogram

The resting electrocardiogram is fundamental in the assessment of patients with suspected ACSs. Ideally, a tracing should be obtained when the patient is symptomatic and compared with a tracing obtained when symptoms have resolved. Comparison with a previous ECG, if available, is valuable, particularly in patients with coexisting cardiac disease such as LV hypertrophy or a previous MI.[6,7] Significant Q waves, consistent with previous MI, are highly suggestive of the presence of significant coronary atherosclerosis but do not necessarily imply current instability.

ST-segment shift and T-wave changes are the most reliable electrocardiographic indicators of unstable coronary disease.[8,9] In the appropriate clinical context, ST-segment depression greater than 1 mm (0.1 mV) in two or more contiguous leads is highly suggestive of an ACS, as are inverted T waves (>1 mm) in leads with predominant R waves, although the latter finding is less specific. Deep symmetrical inversion of the T waves in the anterior chest leads is often related to significant stenosis of the proximal left anterior descending coronary artery. Nonspecific ST-segment shift and T-wave changes (<0.1 mV) are less specific. Indeed, in the Multicenter Chest Pain Study, such nonspecific changes were often noted in patients in whom ACSs were ultimately ruled out. It should be appreciated that a completely normal-appearing electrocardiogram does not exclude the possibility of an ACS. In several studies, approximately 5% of patients with normal-appearing electrocardiograms who were discharged from the emergency department were ultimately found to have either an acute MI or unstable angina.[10-12] However, a completely normal-appearing ECG recorded during an episode of significant chest pain should direct attention to other possible causes for the patient's complaints.

Biochemical Markers of Myocardial Damage

Cardiac troponin T and troponin I are the preferred markers of myocardial necrosis because they are more specific and more reliable than traditional cardiac enzymes such as creatine kinase (CK) or its isoenzyme MB (CK-MB) in this setting. Any elevation of cardiac troponin T or I is thought to reflect irreversible myocardial cellular necrosis. In the setting of myocardial ischemia (chest pain, ST-segment changes), such elevation should be labeled as MI according to the recent consensus document of the European Society of Cardiology (ESC) and the American College of Cardiology (ACC).[13,14]

The troponin complex is formed by three distinct structural proteins (troponin I, C, and T) and is located on the thin filament of the contractile apparatus in both skeletal and cardiac muscle, regulating the calcium-dependent interaction of myosin and actin. Cardiac isoforms for all three troponins are encoded by different genes and thus can be distinguished by monoclonal antibodies that recognize the distinct amino acid sequence. The cardiac isoforms of troponin T and I are exclusively expressed in cardiac myocytes. Accordingly, the detection of cardiac troponin T and troponin I is specific for myocardial damage, attributing these markers the role of a new gold standard.[15] In conditions of "false positive" elevated CK-MB such as skeletal muscle trauma, tro-

ponins clarify any cardiac involvement. In patients with MI, an initial rise in troponins in peripheral blood occurs after 3 to 4 hours and is due to release from the cytosolic pool; persistent elevation for up to 2 weeks is caused by proteolysis of the contractile apparatus. The high proportional rise of troponins, reflecting the low plasma troponin concentrations in healthy persons, allows the detection of myocardial damage in about one third of patients presenting with an ACS without elevated CK-MB. It is important to stress that other life-threatening conditions presenting with chest pain, such as dissecting aortic aneurysm or pulmonary embolism, may also result in elevated troponin and should always be considered in the differential diagnosis.

A single test for troponins on arrival of the patient in hospital is not sufficient: In 10% to 15% of patients, troponin deviations can be detected in subsequent hours. To demonstrate or to exclude myocardial damage, repeated blood sampling and measurements are required 6 to 12 hours after admission and after any further episodes of severe chest pain. If the patient's last episode of chest pain was more than 12 hours before the initial determination of troponin, a second sample may be omitted in the absence of any other index of suspicion.

Elevation of cardiac troponins also occurs in the setting of nonischemic myocardial injury, e.g., myocarditis, severe congestive heart failure, pulmonary embolism, or cardiotoxic chemotherapeutic agents.[16-18] This should not be labeled as false-positive test results but rather reflects the sensitivity of the marker. True false-positive results have been documented for troponin T in the setting of skeletal myopathies or chronic renal failure and for troponin I related to interaction of the immunoassays with fibrin strands or heterophilic antibodies. Current assays have largely overcome these deficiencies, although infrequent false-positive results may still occur.

There is no fundamental difference between troponin T and troponin I testing. Differences between study results are predominantly explained by varying inclusion criteria, differences in sampling pattern, and use of assays with different diagnostic cutoffs. Only one manufacturer produces the troponin T assays whereas several manufacturers provide assays for troponin T. The consensus committee's recommendations specify a diagnostic cutoff for MI using cardiac troponins based on the 99th percentile of levels among healthy controls rather than in comparison with CK-MB. Acceptable imprecision (coefficient of variation) at the 99th percentile for each assay should be below 10%. Each laboratory should regularly assess the range of reference values in the specific setting. For troponin T, cutoff levels between 0.01 and 0.03 μg/L have been shown to be associated with adverse cardiac outcomes in ACSs.[19,20] For troponin I, the decision limits must be based on carefully conducted clinical studies for individual troponin I assays and should not be generalized from different troponin I assays. Slight or moderate elevations of troponins appear to carry the highest early risk in patients with ACSs.[21]

Therapy is started in patients with ACS without ST elevation before the diagnosis is confirmed. This may not be as critical as in ST-elevation MI. Nevertheless, point-of-care testing for biochemical markers may aid rapid, correct diagnosis for prompt triage. Point-of-care tests are assays that can be performed either directly at the bedside or at "near patient" locations such as the emergency department, chest pain evaluation center, or intensive care unit. The rationale for point-of-care testing is the potential for such tests to speed up diagnosis and treatment. Point-of-care testing should be implemented when a central laboratory can not consistently provide test results within 45 to 60 minutes.[22] No special skill or prolonged training is required to read the result of these assays. Accordingly, these tests can be performed by a variety of members of the health care team after adequate training. However, most of these tests are qualitative and read visually and, therefore, are observer-dependent. A potential limitation is that visual assessment only allows a binary classification of test results without definitive information regarding the concentration of the marker in the blood. Careful reading, exactly at the assay-specific indicated time and under good illumination, is essential to reduce observer misinterpretation, especially in case of marginal antibody binding. Even the faintest coloring should be read as a positive test result.

Myoglobin is a relatively early marker; elevations in CK-MB or troponin appear later. Troponin may remain elevated for 1 or 2 weeks in patients with a large infarct, which may complicate the detection of recurrent necrosis (re-infarction) in patients with recent infarction. In such a case, repeated CK-MB or myoglobin measurements are the preferred markers to detect re-infarction.

Clinical Practice Recommendations

In patients with suspected acute ischemic heart disease:

- An ECG should be obtained with the patient at rest, and multilead continuous ST-segment monitoring should be initiated (or frequent ECGs recordings where monitoring is unavailable)
- Troponin T or I should be measured on admission and, if the level is normal, repeated 6 to 12 hours later
- Myoglobin or CK-MB mass, or both, may be measured in patients with recent (<6 hours) symptoms as an early marker of MI and in patients with recurrent ischemia after recent (<2 weeks) infarction to detect further infarction
- Level of evidence: A

TREATMENT OPTIONS

The treatment options described in this discussion are based on the evidence from numerous clinical trials and meta-analyses. Five categories of treatment are discussed: anti-ischemic agents, antithrombotic therapy, antiplatelet agents, fibrinolytics, and coronary revascularization.

Anti-Ischemic Agents

Anti-ischemic drugs decrease myocardial oxygen utilization (lowering heart rate and blood pressure, reducing LV contractility) or induce vasodilatation.

β-Blockers

Evidence for the beneficial effects of β-blockers in unstable angina is based on limited randomized trial data, along with pathophysiologic considerations and extrapolation from experience in stable angina and acute MI. β-Blocking agents competitively inhibit the effects of circulating catecholamines. In ACSs without ST elevation, the primary benefits of β-blocker therapy are related to its effects on β_1 receptors that result in a decrease in myocardial oxygen consumption.

Initial studies of β-blocker benefits in acute ischemic heart disease were small and uncontrolled. Three double-blind randomized trials have compared β-blockers to placebo in unstable angina.[23,24] A meta-analysis suggested that β-blocker treatment was associated with a 13% relative reduction in risk of progression to acute MI.[25] Although no significant effect on mortality in unstable angina has been demonstrated in these relatively small trials, larger randomized trials of β-blockers in patients with acute or recent MI have shown a significant reduction in mortality.[26]

β-Blockers are recommended in ACSs in the absence of contraindications; the intravenous route should be preferred in patients at high risk (evidence level B). There is no evidence that any specific β-blocking agent is more effective in producing beneficial effects in unstable angina. If there are concerns regarding patient tolerance—for example, in patients with preexisting pulmonary disease or LV dysfunction—a short-acting agent is preferred for initial therapy. Initiation of parenteral β-blocker therapy requires frequent monitoring of vital signs and preferably continuous ECG monitoring. Oral therapy should subsequently be instituted to achieve a target heart rate between 50 and 60 beats per minute. Patients with significantly impaired atrioventricular conduction, a history of asthma, or a history of acute LV dysfunction should not receive β-blockers.[27]

Nitrates

The use of nitrates in unstable angina is largely based on pathophysiologic considerations and clinical experience. The therapeutic benefits of nitrates and similar drug classes such as sydnonimins are related to their effects on the peripheral and coronary circulation. The major therapeutic benefit is probably related to the venodilator effects that lead to a decrease in myocardial preload and LV end-diastolic volume, resulting in a decrease in myocardial oxygen consumption. In addition, nitrates dilate normal and atherosclerotic coronary arteries, increase coronary collateral flow, and inhibit platelet aggregation.

Trials of nitrates in unstable angina have been small and observational.[27-29] No randomized placebo-controlled trials have confirmed the benefits of this class of drugs either in relieving symptoms or in reducing major adverse cardiac events. A randomized trial that included only 40 patients compared intravenous, oral, and buccal preparations of nitrates and found no significant difference with regard to symptom relief.[30] Another small randomized trial compared intravenous nitroglycerin with buccally administered nitroglycerin and found no difference.[31] There are no data from controlled trials to indicate the optimal intensity or duration of therapy.

In patients with an ACS who require hospital admission, intravenous nitrates may be considered in the absence of contraindications (evidence level C). The dose should be titrated upwards until symptoms are relieved or side effects (notably headache or hypotension) occur. A limitation of continuous nitrate therapy is the phenomenon of tolerance, which is related both to the dose administered and to the duration of treatment.[32-34]

When symptoms are controlled, intravenous nitrates should be replaced by nonparenteral alternatives with appropriate nitrate-free intervals. An alternative is to use nitrate-like drugs, such as sydnonimins or potassium channel activators.

Potassium Channel Activators

A randomized, double-blind, placebo-controlled trial, the Impact Of Nicorandil in Angina (IONA) study, involved 5126 patients with stable angina and showed that nicorandil (10 mg three times a day for 2 weeks increased to 20 mg three times a day for 1.6 years) reduced cardiovascular death, nonfatal MI, and unplanned hospitalization for angina from 15.5% under placebo to 13.1% under nicorandil (hazard ratio, 0.83; 95% CI, 0.72 to 0.97; $P = .014$).[35] However, coronary heart disease mortality and nonfatal MI were not significantly reduced, changing from 5.2% to 4.2% (hazard ratio, 0.79; 95% CI, 0.61 to 1.02; $P = .068$). No specific data are available for ACSs.

Calcium Channel Blockers

Calcium channel blockers are vasodilating drugs. In addition, some have significant direct effects on atrioventricular conduction and heart rate.

Several small randomized trials have tested calcium channel blockers in unstable angina. Generally, they show efficacy in relieving symptoms that appears equivalent to β-blockers.[36,37] The largest randomized trial, the Holland Interuniversity Nifedipine/metoprolol Trial (HINT) study, tested nifedipine and metoprolol in a 2×2 factorial design.[24] Although no statistically significant differences were observed, there was a trend toward an increased risk of MI or recurrent angina with nifedipine (compared with placebo), whereas treatment with metoprolol or with a combination of both drugs was associated with a reduction in these events. In one study, patients with unstable angina were discharged on a regimen of β-blocker or diltiazem and were followed for 51 months.[38] Diltiazem was associated with a nonsignificant increase in the adjusted death rate (33% vs. 20%) and in the risk of rehospitalization or death (hazard

ratio, 1.4), but in two other trials the drug seems to be slightly beneficial.[39,40]

A meta-analysis of the effects of calcium channel blockers on death or nonfatal infarction in unstable angina suggests that this class of drugs does not prevent acute MI or reduce mortality.[41] In particular, several analyses of pooled data from observational studies suggest that short-acting nifedipine might be associated with a dose-dependent detrimental effect on mortality in patients with coronary artery disease.[42,43] On the other hand, there is evidence for a protective role of diltiazem in non–ST-segment elevation MI (evidence level C).[44]

Calcium channel blockers provide symptom relief in patients already receiving nitrates and β-blockers; these drugs are useful in some patients with contraindications to β-blockade and in the subgroup of patients with variant angina. Nifedipine, or other dihydropyridines, should not be used without concomitant β-blocker therapy. Calcium channel blockers should be avoided in patients with significantly impaired LV function or atrioventricular conduction.

Antithrombotic Therapy

Intracoronary thrombosis plays a major role in ACSs. Thrombus consists of fibrin and platelets. Thrombus formation may be reduced and thrombus resolution facilitated by one of the following measures:

- Drugs that inhibit thrombin directly (hirudin) or indirectly (unfractionated heparin or low-molecular-weight heparin [LMWH])
- Antiplatelet agents (aspirin, ticlopidine, glycoprotein [GP] IIb/IIIa receptor blockers)
- Fibrinolytic agents

Heparin and Low-Molecular-Weight Heparin

Unfractionated heparin has been adopted as antithrombin therapy in previous guidelines for the treatment of unstable angina and non–ST-elevation MI. Even so, the evidence for the use of unfractionated heparin is less robust than for other treatment strategies.[45] In clinical practice, maintenance of therapeutic antithrombin control is hampered by unpredictable levels of heparin binding to plasma proteins (the latter is amplified by the acute phase response). In addition, heparin has limited effectiveness against platelet-rich and clot-bound thrombin.

A study showed that in the absence of aspirin, heparin treatment is associated with a lower frequency of refractory angina/MI and death (as a combined end point) compared with placebo (relative risk reduction, 0.29); the relative risk reduction for aspirin compared with placebo in the same study was 0.56. The combination of aspirin and heparin did not have a significantly greater protective effect than aspirin alone.[46] The initial event reduction by heparin was lost after discontinuation of the latter (rebound effect). Accordingly, there was no evidence of a sustained protective effect by heparin.

In a meta-analysis of the effect of heparin added to aspirin among patients with unstable angina (six randomized trials), there was 7.9% rate of death or MI in the aspirin plus heparin group and 10.3% in the aspirin-alone group (absolute risk reduction, 2.4%; odds ratio, 0.74; 95% CI, 0.5 to 1.09; P = .10) (evidence level B).[45] Thus, these results do not provide conclusive evidence of benefit from adding heparin to aspirin, but it must be stressed that appropriately powered, larger-scale trials have not been conducted. Nevertheless, clinical guidelines recommend a strategy including administration of unfractionated heparin with aspirin as a pragmatic extrapolation of the available evidence. LMWH possesses enhanced anti-Xa activity in relation to anti-IIa (antithrombin) activity compared with unfractionated heparin. In addition, LMWH exhibits decreased sensitivity to platelet factor 4 and a more predictable anticoagulant effect, with lower rates of thrombocytopenia. These agents can be administered subcutaneously based on a weight-adjusted dose and do not require laboratory monitoring. Different LMWHs appear to have similar activity in the prevention and treatment of venous thrombosis in spite of some differences in pharmacology and half-life. Several clinical trials of patients with ACSs treated with aspirin have compared LMWHs and placebo or unfractionated heparins.

The benefit of LMWH over placebo in the presence of aspirin and the feasibility of administering such treatment over a prolonged time was demonstrated in the FRagmin and Fast Revascularization during InStability in Coronary artery disease (FRISC) trial, which tested dalteparin against placebo in aspirin-treated patients with unstable angina/non–ST-elevation MI.[47]

Four randomized trials compared different LMWHs to unfractionated heparin. A meta-analysis of the four trials showed no convincing evidence of difference in efficacy and safety between LMWH and unfractionated heparin. The meta-analysis showed that long-term LMWH was associated with a significantly increased risk of major bleeding (odds ratio, 2.26; 95% CI, 1.63 to 3.41; P < .0001).[48]

In summary, there is convincing evidence that in aspirin-treated patients, LMWH is better than placebo (evidence level A).[47] Two trials have provided data in favor of LMWH (enoxaparin) over unfractionated heparin when administered as an acute regimen (Fig. 49–1).[49-52] These results have been confirmed at 1-year follow-up.[51] Thus, for LMWHs, it can be concluded that acute treatment is at least as effective as unfractionated heparin (evidence level A). However, enoxaparin was superior to unfractionated heparin in the two head-to-head comparisons (for the combined end point of death/MI/recurrent angina).

LMWHs offer significant practical advantages, with simplicity of administration, more consistent antithrombin effects, lack of the need for monitoring, and a safety profile similar to that of unfractionated heparin. Observational studies have also suggested similar safety profiles to unfractionated heparin when used with GP IIb/IIIa inhibitors (National Investigators Collaborating on Enoxaparin [NICE] studies).[53] A moderate-sized, randomized trial (N = 750 patients) of enoxaparin versus unfractionated heparin suggests superior safety and efficacy in eptifibatide treated patients (INTACT[536]). However, the evidence to support longer-term outpatient treatment with LMWH is less convincing.

Direct Thrombin Inhibitors

The Global Use of Strategies to Open Occluded Coronary Arteries (GUSTO) IIb study tested the direct thrombin inhibitor hirudin against heparin in patients with ACSs but not receiving a thrombolytic agent. Early benefits (24 hours and 7 days) were observed, which were no longer significant at 30 days.[54]

The second Organization to Assess Strategies for Ischemic Syndromes (OASIS-2) trial tested a higher dose of hirudin for 72 hours against unfractionated heparin; the rate of cardiovascular death or new MI at 7 days was

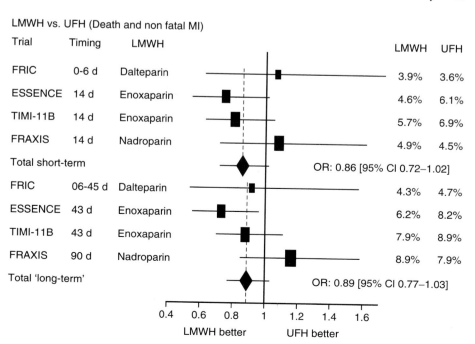

FIGURE 49–1. Comparison of low-molecular-weight heparins with unfractionated heparins in patients with acute coronary syndromes. Odds ratio and 95% confidence interval.

4.2% for unfractionated heparin group and 3.6% for hirudin ($P = .077$). There was an excess of major bleeding (1.2% vs. 0.7%) but no excess of life-threatening bleeds or strokes.

A combined analysis of the OASIS-1 pilot studies, OASIS-2, and GUSTO IIb indicates a 22% relative risk reduction in cardiovascular death or MI at 72 hours, 17% at 7 days, and 10% at 35 days (evidence level B).[54,55] This combined analysis is statistically significant at 72 hours and 7 days and of borderline significance at 35 days ($P = .057$). Hirudin has been approved for patients with heparin-induced thrombocytopenia, but none of the hirudines is licensed for ACSs.

Management of Bleeding Complications Related to Antithrombin Treatment

Minor bleeding is usually treated by simply stopping the treatment. Major bleedings such as hematemesis, melena, or intracranial hemorrhage may require the use of heparin antagonists. The risk of inducing a rebound thrombotic phenomenon should be assessed for such patients individually.

The anticoagulant and hemorrhagic effects of unfractionated heparin are reversed by an equimolar concentration of protamine sulfate, which neutralizes the anti–factor IIa activity but results in only partial neutralization of the anti–factor Xa of LMWH.

Antiplatelet Agents

Aspirin

Acetylsalicylic acid inhibits cyclooxygenase-1 and blocks the formation of thromboxane A_2. Thus, platelet aggregation induced via this pathway is blocked. Three trials have consistently shown that aspirin decreases death or MI in patients with unstable angina.[46,56,57] A meta-analysis showed that 75 to 150 mg of aspirin was as effective as higher doses. For acute MI, antiplatelet therapy (almost exclusively aspirin) results in fewer vascular events per 1000 treated patients.[58] In addition to the early benefit established in those studies, a long-term benefit is achieved by continuation of aspirin. Gastrointestinal side effects are relatively infrequent with these low doses. There a few contraindications, including active peptic ulcer, local bleeding, or hemorrhagic diatheses. Allergy is rare. Accordingly, acute treatment with aspirin is recommended in all patients with suspected ACSs in the absence of contraindications and for long-term treatment thereafter (evidence level A).

ADP Receptor Antagonists: Thienopyridines

Ticlopidine and clopidogrel are inhibitors of ADP, resulting in inhibition of platelet aggregation. Ticlopidine has been investigated in a single study,[59] but intolerance to this drug is relatively frequent because of gastrointestinal disorders or allergic reactions. In addition, neutropenia or thrombocytopenia may occur. Ticlopidine has been superseded by clopidogrel.

Clopidogrel has been investigated in aspirin-treated (75 to 325 mg) patients with ACSs in a large clinical trial (CURE) of 12,562 patients.[60] Patients hospitalized within 24 hours after the onset of symptoms with ECG changes or cardiac enzyme rise were randomized to a loading dose of 300 mg of clopidogrel followed by 75 mg once daily versus placebo for a median of 9 months. The first primary outcome (cardiovascular death, nonfatal MI, or stroke) was significantly reduced from 11.4% to 9.3% (adjusted risk, 2.1%; relative risk, 0.80; 95% CI, 0.72 to 0.90; $P < .001$). The rate of each component also tended to be lower in the clopidogrel group, but the most important difference was observed in the rates of MI (adjusted relative risk, 1.5%; relative risk, 0.77; 95% CI, 0.67 to 0.89). The rate of refractory ischemia during initial hospitalization significantly ($P = .007$) decreased from 2.0% to 1.4% (adjusted relative risk, 0.6%; relative risk, 0.68; 95% CI, 0.52 to 0.90) but did not significantly differ after discharge (7.6% in both groups). Major bleeding was significantly more common in the clopidogrel group (3.7% vs. 2.7% relative risk, 1.38; 95% CI, 1.13 to 1.67; $P = .001$); the number of patients who required transfusion of 2 or more units was higher in the clopidogrel group than in the placebo group (2.8% vs. 2.2%; $P = .02$). Major bleedings were approximately as frequent (2.0% during early treatment [<30 days after randomization]) as it was later (1.7% [>30 days after randomization]). Minor bleedings were significantly higher in the clopidogrel group than in the placebo group (5.1% vs. 2.4%; $P < .001$).

It is interesting to consider the 1822 patients of the clopidogrel group who underwent bypass surgery. Overall, there was no significant excess of major bleeding episodes (1.3% vs. 1.1%) after coronary artery bypass graft (CABG). In the 912 patients who did not stop study medication until 5 days before surgery, however, the rate of major bleeding was higher in the clopidogrel group (9.6% vs. 6.3%; $P = .06$).

Bleeding risk clearly increased as the dose of aspirin increased from less than 100 mg, to 100 to 300 mg, to greater than 300 mg in both placebo-treated (2.0%, 2.2%, 4.0% major bleeds, respectively) and clopidogrel-treated patients (2.5%, 3.5%, 4.9%, respectively). There was no clear evidence in CURE or in the Anti Platelet Trialists' Collaboration of improved outcome with higher doses of aspirin. Thus, it is recommended that clopidogrel be used in conjunction with maintenance doses of less than 100 mg aspirin.

For patients with an ACS, clopidogrel is recommended for acute treatment and for longer-term treatment for at least 9 to 12 months (evidence level B). Beyond this period, treatment depends on the risk status of the patient and individual clinical judgment. Clopidogrel should be given to patients with ACSs who are scheduled for angiography unless the patient will likely proceed to urgent surgery (within 5 days).

Clopidogrel may also be recommended for immediate and long-term therapy in patients who do not tolerate aspirin (according to the Clopidogrel versus Aspirin in Patients at Risk of Ischemic Events study, or CAPRIE)[61] and is recommended in patients receiving a stent.[62]

Glycoprotein IIb/IIIa Receptor Inhibitors

Activated GP IIb/IIIa receptors connect with fibrinogen to form bridges between activated platelets, leading to formation of platelet thrombi. Direct inhibitors of the GP IIb/IIIa receptors have been developed and have been tested in various conditions in which platelet activation plays a major role, particularly in patients undergoing percutaneous coronary intervention (PCI), patients admitted with ACSs, and patients receiving thrombolytic therapy for acute MI.

Four intravenous GP IIb/IIIa receptor blockers have been studied extensively in ACSs. Abciximab is a monoclonal antibody. It is a nonspecific blocker, with a tight receptor binding and slow reversibility of platelet inhibition after cessation of treatment. Eptifibatide is a cyclic peptide inhibiting selectively the GP IIb/IIIa receptors: It has short half-life, and platelet function recovers 2 to 4 hours after cessation of the treatment. Tirofiban is a small nonpeptide antagonist that mimics the tripeptide sequence of fibrinogen. Blockade of the receptors is rapid (5 minutes), selective, and rapidly reversible (4 to 6 hours). Lamifiban is a synthetic nonpeptide selective receptor blocker with a half-life of approximately 4 hours.

Several oral GP IIb/IIIa receptor blockers have been recently studied, including orbobifan, sibrafiban, and lefradafiban.[63]

Intravenous GP IIb/IIIa Receptor Inhibitors in Acute Coronary Syndromes   In patients admitted with ACSs, systematic use of GP IIb/IIIa receptor blockers in addition to aspirin and "standard" unfractionated heparin was studied in seven large randomized trials: C7E3 AntiPlatelet Therapy in Unstable REfractory angina (CAPTURE), Platelet Receptor Inhibition in Ischemic Syndrome Management (PRISM), PRISM in Patients Limited by Unstable Signs and symptoms (PRISM-PLUS), Platelet Glycoprotein IIb/IIIa in Unstable Angina: Receptor Suppression Using Integrilin Therapy (PURSUIT), Platelet IIb/IIIa Antagonism for the Reduction of Acute coronary syndrome events in a Global Organization Network A (PARAGON-A), PARAGON-B, and GUSTO IV ACS.[64-70] Different meta-analyses were conducted, and one can summarize the results as follows.[71]

A. Overall, the use of GP IIb/IIIa inhibitors is associated with a modest but significant reduction in death or MI at 30 days in patients with ACSs without persistent ST-segment elevation, as demonstrated by the meta-analysis from Boersma et al conducted in 27,051 patients (Fig. 49–2).[71] Medical therapy with a GP IIb/IIIa receptor blocker during the first days after admission, followed by PCI or bypass surgery, yields a significant reduction (4.3% to 2.9%) in death and nonfatal MI at 72 hours.

Subsequently, in patients undergoing PCI in CAPTURE as well as the subgroup of patients undergoing a similar procedure in PURSUIT and PRISM-PLUS, procedure-related events were reduced from 8.0% to 4.9% (P = .001). Few events occurred more than 2 days after PCI in these patients, and no additional treatment effect was apparent up to 30 days' follow-up (Fig. 49–3).

B. In the larger placebo-controlled trials of GP IIb/IIIa receptor blockers in patients with ACSs, the treatment benefit was particularly apparent in patients who underwent early coronary revascularization.[64,72,73] A meta-analysis from Boersma et al showed a strong treatment effect (death and MI in patients undergoing PCI) but no effect in those not undergoing intervention[71] (Fig. 49–4): Intervention (PCI or CABG) performed within 5 days in combination with GP IIb/IIIa receptor inhibitors induced a 3% absolute reduction of death and MI (relative risk reduction, 0.79; 95% CI, 0.68 to 0.91). When performed within 30 days, absolute risk reduction was 1.7% (relative risk reduction, 0.89; 95% CI, 0.80 to 0.98).

C. In three trials (CAPTURE, PRISM, PARAGON-B),[64,69,72] the benefits of a treatment with a GP IIb/IIIa receptor blocker were particularly apparent among patients admitted with elevated levels of cardiac troponin T or cardiac troponin I. This observation agrees with the notion that such elevated cardiac troponin levels reflect minimal myocardial damage resulting from platelet emboli. These patients seem to have active ongoing intracoronary thrombosis, which can be

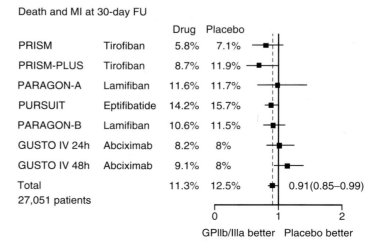

Multicenter Randomized Trials
Comparing GPIIb/IIIa vs Placebo in ACS

Death and MI at 30-day FU

		Drug	Placebo	
PRISM	Tirofiban	5.8%	7.1%	
PRISM-PLUS	Tirofiban	8.7%	11.9%	
PARAGON-A	Lamifiban	11.6%	11.7%	
PURSUIT	Eptifibatide	14.2%	15.7%	
PARAGON-B	Lamifiban	10.6%	11.5%	
GUSTO IV 24h	Abciximab	8.2%	8%	
GUSTO IV 48h	Abciximab	9.1%	8%	
Total 27,051 patients		11.3%	12.5%	0.91(0.85–0.99)

GPIIb/IIIa better   Placebo better

FIGURE 49–2. Glycoprotein IIb/IIIa inhibitors versus conventional treatment in six trials. Odds ratio and 95% confidence interval.

CAPTURE,PRISM+,PURSUIT combined

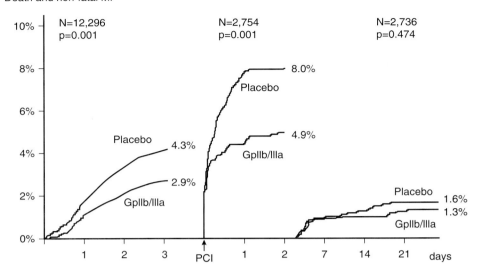

Death and non-fatal MI

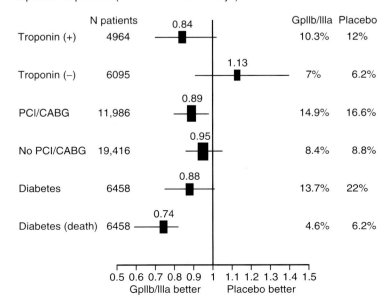

FIGURE 49–3. Glycoprotein IIb/IIIa inhibitors versus placebo in patients with acute coronary syndromes who are undergoing percutaneous coronary interventions.

effectively reduced by powerful antiplatelet therapy. In contrast, no benefit was observed in GUSTO IV patients with elevated troponin. Treatment with a GP IIb/IIIa receptor blocker in addition to aspirin and weight-adjusted low-dose heparin should be considered in all patients with ACSs and an elevated troponin T or troponin I level who are scheduled for early revascularization (evidence level A). There was no benefit for patients with negative troponins.

D. From a meta-analysis of the six randomized trials, it was demonstrated that diabetic patients with an ACS derive particular benefit from GP IIb/IIIa receptor inhibitors. Among 6458 diabetics, this antiplatelet treatment was associated with a significant mortality reduc-

tion at 30 days, from 6.2% to 4.6% (relative risk, 0.74; 95% CI, 0.59 to 0.92; P = .007) (see Fig. 49–4). Among 1279 diabetic patients undergoing PCI during index hospitalization, the use of GP IIb/IIIa receptor blockers was associated with a mortality reduction at 30 days from 4.0% to 1.2% (adjusted relative risk, 2.8; relative risk, 0.30; 95% CI, 0.14 to 0.69; P = .002).[74] Thus, GP IIb/IIIa blockers are particularly recommended in patients with diabetes and an ACS.

Oral GP IIb/IIIa Receptor Inhibitors

Four trials addressed prolonged treatment with oral GP IIb/IIIa receptor blockers in patients with ACSs or after coronary

FIGURE 49–4. Glycoprotein IIb/IIIa inhibitors in patients with acute coronary syndromes: Death or myocardial infarction in patients with positive or negative troponin levels, patients undergoing (or not) percutaneous coronary interventon or coronary artery bypass graft, diabetics; mortality rate in diabetic patients.

intervention. Such prolonged treatment did not show evidence of benefit in the Orbofiban in Patients with Unstable coronary Syndromes (OPUS–TIMI-16), Evaluation of oral Xemilofiban in Controlling Thrombotic Events (EXCITE), and first and second Sibrafiban versus Aspirin to Yield Maximum Protection from Ischemic Heart Events Post acute Coronary syndromes (SYMPHONY 1 and 2) trials. In fact, a modest but significant increase in mortality was apparent in a meta-analysis of patients receiving oral GP IIb/IIIa receptor blockers.[63]

Management of Complications Related to Administration of GP IIb/IIIa Inhibitors

With antiplatelet drugs and particularly with GP IIb/IIIa receptor inhibitors, the bleeding risk is clearly related to the dose of adjunctive heparin, and specific reduced heparin dosing schedules are recommended. In the setting of PCI, it is recommended that the doses of heparin be significantly restricted to 70 IU/kg, with a target activated clotting time of 200 seconds. When local complications such as important hematoma or continuous bleeding at the puncture site occur, surgical intervention may be required.

Thrombocytopenia may occur in a small percentage of patients during administration of parenteral GP IIb/IIIa receptor inhibitors: Platelet counts decreased to less than 50,000/mm^3 in less than 1% of patients in PRISM-PLUS and GUSTO IV ACS (over 24 hours). Stopping treatment usually results in a return to normal platelet levels.[70,73] Finally, readministration might be an issue for abciximab because of its inherent immunogenicity. In practice, the readministration registry shows similar safety and efficacy for repeat administration as compared with first-time administration.[75,76]

Most of the trials with GP IIB/IIIA receptor inhibitors have been performed in combination with unfractionated heparin, however, the bleeding risk of combined LMWH and GP IIB/IIIA receptor inhibitors must be assessed. In the Antithrombotic Combination using Trophiban and Enoxaparin (ACUTE-2) trial, conducted with tirofiban combined with enoxaparin, no difference was found in the rates of major and minor bleedings.[77] An observational study (NICE 3) showed that treatment with enoxaparin and GP IIB/IIIA receptor inhibitors (abciximab, eptifibatide, or tirofiban) does not result in an excess of non-CABG major bleeding and that patients receiving this combination can safely undergo PCI. However, in GUSTO IV ACS, major bleeds tended to be more frequent for patients receiving abciximab than placebo in both the dalteparin and the unfractionated heparin cohort (3.8%)[70]; furthermore, minor bleeds were considerably more frequent for patients on abciximab in the dalteparin cohort (46.4% vs. 27.4%; $P < .001$). Minor bleeds were considerably more common for elderly persons and females, who are at the greatest risk.[78]

Fibrinolytic Treatment

Fibrinolytic treatment has been shown to decrease the amount of intracoronary thrombus and to significantly improve survival in patients with ACSs and ST-segment elevation.[79] In contrast, a deleterious effect has consistently been observed in patients with unstable angina in several studies conducted with streptokinase, anisoylated plasminogen streptokinase activator, tissue plasminogen activator, or urokinase.[80-82] The risk of death and MI in a pooled series of 2859 patients was 9.8% in the fibrinolytic group and 6.9% in the control group. The Fibrinolytic Therapy Trialists' overview showed that in 3563 patients with suspected MI and ST-segment depression, the mortality rate was 15.2% versus 13.8% for control patients.[83] Therefore, thrombolytic therapy is not recommended for patients with ACSs without persistent ST-segment elevation.

Coronary Revascularization

Revascularization (either PCI or CABG) for unstable coronary artery disease is performed to treat recurrent or ongoing myocardial ischemia and to avoid progression to MI or death. The indications for myocardial revascularization and the preferred approach depend on the extent and angiographic characteristics of the lesions identified by coronary angiography.

Coronary Angiography

Coronary angiography is the sole examination able to address the presence and extent of significant coronary disease. Countries vary widely in the use of coronary angiography. The Euro Heart Survey demonstrated that among 5367 patients admitted with suspicion of ACSs without ST-segment elevation, 52% underwent coronary angiography with significant regional variation.[1]

Decisions to perform interventions are based on coronary angiography. The indications and timing of coronary angiography are discussed in Chapters 34 and 35. No special precautions are needed when performing coronary angiography except in hemodynamically very unstable patients (pulmonary edema, hypotension, severe life-threatening arrhythmias), in whom it may be advisable to perform the examination with placement of an intra-aortic balloon pump, to limit the number of coronary injections, and not to perform LV cineangiography, which might destabilize a fragile hemodynamic state. In such cases, LV function may be estimated by echocardiography.

Data from TIMI IIIB and FRISC II show that 30% to 38% of patients with unstable coronary syndromes have single-vessel disease and that 44% to 59% have multivessel disease. The rate of nonsignificant coronary disease varies from 14% to 19%. The incidence of left main narrowing varies from 4% to 8%. FRISC II investigators,[20] and the TIMI IIIB investigators.[83b] The pattern of ECG changes, when present, may help to identify the culprit lesion. The presence of thrombus at the lesion is an important risk marker. Eccentricity, irregular borders, ulceration, haziness, and filling defects characteristic of intracoronary thrombus are markers of high risk (see Chapter 17). However, compared with angioscopy, coronary angiography has good specificity but poor sensitivity for detection of thrombi.[84]

Description of the culprit lesion is of paramount importance in choosing the appropriate interventions.

Extreme tortuosity, calcification, or location in a bend are important findings because they can preclude PCI with stent implantation. These aspects are frequent in elderly people.

Percutaneous Coronary Interventions

The safety and success of PCI in ACSs have been markedly improved with the use of stenting and administration of GP IIb/IIIa receptor inhibitors.

In the Euro Heart Survey, 25% of the total population underwent PCI, with stent implantation in 74% of cases and administration of GP IIb/IIIa receptor inhibitors in 27% of cases.[1]

Stent implantation in the setting of unstable coronary artery helps to mechanically stabilize the disrupted plaque at the site of the lesion. This benefit is particularly obvious in high-risk lesions. In a prespecified subanalysis of the Benestent II trial involving patients with unstable angina, it was shown that stent implantation was safe and associated with a lower 6-month restenosis rate than balloon dilatation.[85] Stents coated with different drugs are still more promising: In the RAndomized double-blind study with the sirolimus eluting BX VElocity stent in the treatment of de novo coronary artery Lesions (RAVEL) trial, which included 220 patients with unstable angina, no restenosis (>50% stenosis) occurred in the group treated with a rapamycin-coated stent.

All patients undergoing PCI receive aspirin and heparin. A subanalysis of patients with unstable angina from the EPIC and Evaluation in PTCA to Improve Long-term Outcome with abciximab GPIIb/IIIa blockade (EPI-LOG) trials and the CAPTURE trial convincingly demonstrated that intravenous abciximab significantly reduced the major complication rate during balloon angioplasty. This initial benefit was sustained at 6-month follow-up and beyond.[64,86-90] Similar but smaller reductions in acute complications were achieved with eptifibatide or tirofiban, but these initial effects were not sustained at 30 days.[91,92]

From subanalyses of CAPTURE and PURSUIT, it appears that the beneficial effect of GP IIb/IIIa inhibitors was already evident 6 to 12 hours before and during planned PCI.[64,67] It is therefore recommended that adjunctive treatment with GP IIb/IIIa antagonists be started before PCI and to continue abciximab for 12 hours and other GP IIb/IIIa inhibitors for 24 hours after the procedure.[64,67]

The EPISTENT trial demonstrated that the combination of stent implantation and abciximab was associated with a significantly lower rate of major complications than the combination of stent and placebo, as well as that the combination of stent and abciximab was superior to balloon and abciximab. These findings were also observed in the subset of patients with unstable coronary disease.[88]

The novel dosing regimen of eptifibatide in the planned coronary stent implantation (ESPRIT) trial confirmed the benefit of stent implantation and eptifibatide: The composite of death, MI, and urgent target-vessel revascularization was reduced from 15% with placebo to 7.9% with eptifibatide ($P = .0015$) within 48 hours after randomization in patients with ACSs.[93]

The recently published PCI-CURE study (a subgroup prespecified analysis of CURE) studied the benefit of a pretreatment with clopidogrel.[94] At 30 days, there was a significant ($P = .04$) reduction of cardiovascular death and MI (4.4% to 2.9%); between 30 days and the end of follow-up, long-term administration of clopidogrel also reduced the rate of cardiovascular death, MI, or rehospitalization (25.3% vs. 28.9%).

In all trials of ACS with PCI, the mortality rate associated with PCI is very low.

After stent implantation, patients are usually discharged quickly on combination of clopidogrel and aspirin for 1 month.[62] PCI-CURE suggests that long-term (8 months on average in PCI-CURE) administration of clopidogrel after PCI is associated with a lower rate of cardiovascular death, MI, or any revascularization.[94]

In a limited number of cases, special tools such as thrombectomy devices and distal protection devices may be beneficial, but properly randomized trials are needed to validate the use of such devices and to define the appropriate indications.

Coronary Artery Bypass Surgery

The Euro Heart Survey showed that the current rate of CABG is overall very low (5.4%),[95] although countries vary widely. In contrast, in the FRISC II and TACTICS trials, CABG was used in 35.2% and 20% of patients in the invasive arm, respectively.[19,20] Modern surgical techniques result in low operative mortality.[96] In FRISC II, the mortality rate of surgically treated patients was 2% at 1 month of follow-up and 1.7% in TACTICS.[19,20] Surgery for postinfarction (<30 days) unstable angina carries higher (6.8%) operative mortality rates (range, 0% to 16%) and perioperative MI (5.9%) rates (range, 0% to 15%). Risk profiles vary among patients with unstable coronary artery disease undergoing bypass grafting. Perioperative mortality and morbidity are higher in patients with severe unstable angina and in patients with unstable angina after a recent (<7 days) MI. Even so, in the most recent trials of invasive treatment (FRISC II, TACTICS), CABG was associated with a low risk of mortality (2.1%),[19,20] although the majority of these surgical procedures were performed in patients with left main or multivessel disease and early after infarction (<7 days).

It is important to consider the risk of bleeding complications in patients who underwent surgery and who were initially treated with aggressive antiplatelet treatment: In the PURSUIT trial, a total of 78 patients underwent immediate CABG within 2 hours of cessation of the study drug. Major bleeding was not different between groups, occurring in 64% of patients receiving placebo and 63% of patients receiving eptifibatide.[97] The rate of blood transfusion was also similar (57% vs. 59%). Bizzarri et al made similar observations with tirofiban.[98]

In the CURE study, 1822 patients of the clopidogrel group underwent bypass surgery. Overall, there was no significant excess of major bleeding episodes after CABG (1.3% vs. 1.1%), but in the 912 patients who stopped clopidogrel within 5 days before surgery, the rate of major bleedings was higher in the clopidogrel group (9.6% vs. 6.3%; $P = .06$).[60]

Overall, pretreatment with aggressive antiplatelet regimens should be considered as only a relative contraindication to early CABG but may require specific surgical measures to minimize bleeding and sometimes may require platelet transfusions. Nevertheless, if an emergency operation is not required, it is better to stop the drug and to perform intervention 5 days later.

Comparing patients with unstable angina undergoing CABG within or after 12 hours after stopping Fragmin, Clark et al demonstrated that patients receiving dalteparin within 12 hours of operation had significantly greater blood loss than the others and recommended that dalteparin be stopped more than 12 hours before the operation.[99]

Respective Indications for Percutaneous Coronary Intervention or Surgery

Patients with single-vessel disease and an indication for revascularization are usually treated by PCI with stent implantation and adjunctive treatment with GP IIb/IIIa inhibitors. In these patients, surgical revascularization is only considered if unsuitable anatomy (e.g., extreme tortuosity of the vessel, marked angulation) precludes safe PCI.

Patients with left main or three-vessel disease, especially those with associated LV dysfunction, are usually treated with CABG. In this situation, CABG is well documented to prolong survival, improve quality of life, and reduce readmissions.[100,101] Furthermore it is a more cost-effective alternative than PCI because of better symptom relief and a decreased need for repeat intervention.[102,103]

In patients with two-vessel disease (or three-vessel disease with lesions suitable for stenting), the relative merits of surgery compared with PCI need to be evaluated individually. A subgroup analysis of the Bypass Angioplasty Revascularization Investigation (BARI) and Coronary Angioplasty versus Bypass Revascularization Investigation (CABRI) trials of patients in unstable condition did not show a significant difference in the combined end point of in-hospital mortality and MI between the angioplasty and surgical groups.[103-107] However, the rate of repeat revascularization procedures differed significantly in both trials, which was higher for the PTCA strategy (40% to 60%) than for the CABG strategy (5% to 10%). The BARI investigators followed their patients for 7 years; during that period there was no difference in the mortality rate, except for patients with diabetes mellitus, who had a better outcome with surgery than with PTCA.[102]

Interventional cardiology and surgical techniques continue to improve. Current state-of-the-art PCI is best presented in the Arterial Revascularization Therapy Study (ARTS) trial.[108] This study was a randomized trial comparing the efficacy and cost-effectiveness of stenting versus CABG in patients with multivessel CAD. A total of 1200 patients were randomized. The proportion of patients in unstable condition was approximately 36% in each group, but there was no difference between patients in stable and unstable condition. Treatment was successful in 97% of the stent group and 96% of the surgical group. The composite adverse event rate (death, MI,

stroke, and need for revascularization) at 30 days was 8.7% in the stent group and 6.8% in the surgery group (P = NS). At 2-year follow-up, there was a difference (20.5% vs. 15.2%) due to the need for subsequent revascularization in the stented group. Other trials have produced conflicting results. The Stent or Surgery (SOS) trial showed higher cardiac mortality in the PCI group than in the surgery group at 1-year follow-up (1.6% vs. 0.6%),[108b] whereas the Argentine randomized trial of percutaneous transluminal coronary angioplasty versus coronary artery bypass surgery in multivessel disease (ERACI II) trial came to the opposite conclusion (5.7% in the surgical group vs. 0.9% in the PCI group).[107]

It is difficult to extrapolate from these results in highly selected patients, but overall there seems to be no firm evidence that one strategy is superior to the other. However, in many patients with multivessel disease, some of the lesions cannot be appropriately managed with angioplasty and stenting, and therefore surgery is the obvious first-line choice.

In a few patients with multivessel disease who require total revascularization that is not achievable with PCI but in whom early surgery poses an extremely high risk, one might prefer a strategy of initial percutaneous treatment of the culprit lesion only. Also patients with severe comorbidity that precludes surgery may undergo "staged percutaneous treatment." In patients with left main narrowing who have severe associated comorbidity, angioplasty with stent implantation is acceptable in selected cases.

In patients undergoing interventions (PCI or CABG), it is important to note that it is difficult to compare rates of peri-interventional MI. In previous trials (FRISC II and TACTICS), different thresholds for enzyme rise were used after an intervention than with conservative management.[19,20] In several trials, standardized but different definitions have been adopted for specific situations: an enzyme rise greater than 3 times the upper limit of normal for PCI, a rise greater than 2 times after medical treatment, and a rise greater than 5 times the upper limit of normal after CABG. However, these different thresholds have no physiopathologic basis. Accordingly, the consensus document for the redefinition of MI suggests the use of similar thresholds for all conditions.[5]

Invasive Treatment Strategy Versus Conservative Strategy

Three large randomized trials compared modern surgery and modern angioplasty with current medical therapy. The FRISC II trial enrolled 2457 high-risk patients in unstable condition with chest pain within 48 hours of admission; the patients had ST-segment depression or T-wave inversion or biochemical markers above the normal range.[20] Patients allocated to the early invasive strategy underwent a procedure at an average of 4 days (PTCA) or 8 days (CABG), and the noninvasive arm received intervention only for severe angina. Revascularization procedures were carried out within the first 10 days in 71% of the invasive and 9% of the conservative arms and within 12 months in 78% of the invasive and 43% of the conservative arms. At 1 year, PCI was performed in 44% of patients in the invasive arm and in

21% of those in the conservative arm. Two thirds underwent stent implantation; only 10% received abciximab. CABG was performed in 38% of patients in the invasive arm and in 23% of those in the conservative arm. After 1-year follow-up, total mortality was significantly reduced in the invasive arm (2.2% vs. 3.9%; relative reduction, 0.57; 95% CI, 0.36 to 0.90), as was MI (8.6% vs. 11.6%; relative reduction, 0.74; 95% CI, 0.59 to 0.9). Accordingly, the composite end point of death or MI was significantly reduced in the invasive compared with the noninvasive group: 10.4% versus 14.1% (relative risk, 0.74; 95% CI, 0.60 to 0.92). This favorable effect on mortality was observed in men but not in women. Furthermore, the symptoms of angina and the need for readmissions were halved by the invasive strategy.

The TACTICS trial enrolled 2220 patients with ACSs without persistent ST-segment elevation who were randomly assigned to an early (2 to 48 hours) invasive strategy, including routine coronary angiography followed by revascularization as appropriate, or to a more conservative strategy in which catheterization was used only if the patient had objective evidence of recurrent ischemia or an abnormal stress test result.[19] In the trial, 60% of patients allocated to invasive therapy did undergo a procedure in the hospital; 36% of patients allocated to medical therapy underwent a revascularization procedure. Nevertheless, the rate of the primary end point (a composite of death, nonfatal MI, and rehospitalization for ACS) was significantly reduced at 6-month follow-up from 19.4% to 15.4% (adjusted relative risk, 4%; relative risk reduction, 0.78; 95% CI, 0.62 to 0.97; $P = .025$). The rate of death or nonfatal MI at 6 months was similarly reduced (7.3% vs. 9.5%; adjusted relative risk, 2.2%; relative risk reduction, 0.74; 95% CI, 0.54 to 1.00; $P < .05$). Patients with a troponin T level greater than 0.01 ng/mL significantly benefited from this invasive strategy, a benefit not observed with troponin T–negative patients.

The third Randomized Intervention Treatment of Angina (RITA-3) trial enrolled 1810 patients: 915 underwent conservative management, whereas 895 were randomized to intervention.[109] In this group, coronary angiography was performed at a median of 2 days, PCI at a median of 3 days after randomization. The predefined primary end point at 4 months was the combined incidence of death, nonfatal MI, or refractory ischemia. The rate of the primary end point was significantly lower in the invasive group compared with the conservative group: 9.6% versus 14.5% (relative risk reduction, 0.66; 95% CI, 0.51 to 0.85; $P = .001$). The coprimary end point of death or nonfatal MI within 1 year of randomization occurred in the same proportion in both groups. It should be noted that the definition of MI differed from the definition used in the TACTICS and FRISC II trials. RITA-3 data that were analyzed according to the ESC/ACC definition of MI showed the significant reduction of death and MI at 4 months (from 14.9% to 10.6%; relative reduction, 0.71; 95% CI, 0.56 to 0.91) and at 1 year (from 17.1% to 12.5%; relative reduction, 0.71; 95% CI, 0.59 to 0.92).[109]

From FRISC II, TACTICS, and RITA-3, it appears that a modern invasive strategy, preceded by modern anti-ischemic and antithrombotic medication (tirofiban in TACTICS, dalteparin in FRISC II, and enoxaparin in RITA-3), in high-risk patients with unstable coronary artery disease reduces death, MI, symptoms, and readmissions compared with a conservative strategy (evidence level A).[19,20,109]

The level of evidence of the different treatments is summarized in Table 49–1.

STRATEGY

In patients with an established diagnosis of ACS, the selection of a management strategy in a particular patient depends on the perceived risk of progression to MI or death.

ACSs encompass a heterogeneous group of patients with different clinical presentations, patients who have differences in terms of the extent and severity of underlying coronary atherosclerosis and who are at differing degrees of acute "thrombotic" risk (i.e., risk of progression to infarction).[49] To select the appropriate treatment for an individual patient, the risk of subsequent events should be assessed repeatedly. Such evaluation needs to be done early, at the time of initial diagnosis or

---

TABLE 49–1 EVIDENCE LEVELS OF VARIOUS TREATMENTS

TREATMENT	EARLY BENEFIT REDUCTION OF ISCHEMIA	EARLY BENEFIT PREVENTION OF DEATH/MI	SUSTAINED EFFECTS OF EARLY BENEFIT	ADDITIONAL LONG-TERM REDUCTION OF DEATH/MI	CLASS
β-Blockers	A	B	B	A	I
Nitrates	C	—	—	—	I
Calcium antagonists	B	B	—	—	II
Aspirin	—	A	A	A	I
Thienopyridine	B	B	B	B	I
GpIIb/IIIa receptor inhibitors	A	A	A	A	I
Unfractionated heparin	C	B	—	—	I
LMWH	A	A	A	C*	I
Specific antithrombins	—	A	A	—	I
Revascularization	A	A	A	A	I

*In a selected group of patients
LMWH, low-molecular-weight heparin; MI, myocardial infarction.

admission to the hospital, and based on immediately available clinical information and easily obtained laboratory data. This primary assessment should later be modified in the light of continuing symptoms, additional information based on ECG evidence of ischemia, the results of laboratory tests, and assessment of LV function. Apart from age and a previous history of coronary artery disease, clinical examination, ECG, and biologic measurements provide the key elements for risk assessment.

It is important to separate the acute risk, which is the thrombotic risk (i.e., the risk to die or to suffer a large MI) from the long-term risk. Risk assessment should be precise, reliable, and, preferably, easily and rapidly available at low cost. The following methods are recommended:

Markers of thrombotic risk, i.e., acute risk:

- Recurrence of chest pain
- ST-segment depression
- Dynamic ST-segment changes
- Elevated level of cardiac troponins
- Diabetes
- Thrombus on angiography

Markers of underlying disease, i.e., long-term risk:

Clinical markers

- Age
- History of previous MI, prior CABG, congestive heart failure, hypertension

Biologic markers

- Renal dysfunction (elevated creatinine or reduced creatinine clearance)
- Inflammatory markers, C-reactive protein elevation, fibrinogen elevation, interleukin-6 elevation

Angiographic markers

- LV dysfunction
- Extent of coronary artery disease

Management Strategy in Acute Coronary Syndromes

The following section outlines a strategy that is applicable to most patients admitted with a suspected ACS. Deviations from the standard strategies are, however, expected in many patients. The physician should make an individual decision for every patient, specific to the history, presentation, findings during observation or investigation in the hospital, and available treatment facilities. The guidelines are produced to orient and help the decision-making process.

Initial Assessment at Presentation

In most patients, only chest discomfort (chest pain) might be present and suspicion of ACS is only a working diagnosis. The initial assessment includes the four following steps (Fig. 49–5):

1. It is important to obtain a careful history and a precise description of the symptoms. A physical examination with particular attention to the possible presence of valvular heart disease (aortic stenosis), hypertrophic cardiomyopathy, heart failure, and pulmonary disease is required.
2. An ECG is recorded. Comparison with a previous ECG, if available, is highly valuable, particularly in patients with preexisting cardiac disease such as LV hypertrophy or known coronary disease. The ECG allows differentiation of patients with a suspicion of ACS in two categories requiring different therapeutic approaches:

- ST-segment elevation signifies complete occlusion of a major coronary artery, and immediate reperfusion therapy is usually indicated. This condition accounted for 42% of the cases in the European Heart Survey on ACSs.[1] Treatment of these patients falls outside the scope of these guidelines.

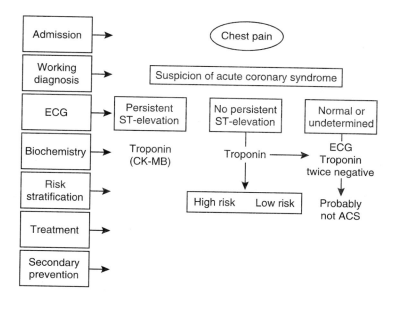

FIGURE 49–5. Acute coronary syndromes: initial assessment.

- In 51% of cases, there were ST-segment changes but without persistent ST-segment elevation or a normal-appearing ECG.
- A few cases (7%) allow no definite characterization and involve undetermined ECG changes such as bundle branch block or pacemaker rhythm.

3. In the latter two cases, biochemical markers are required for further characterization: Laboratory assessments should include hemoglobin (to detect anemia) and markers of myocardial damage, preferably troponin T or troponin I. If concentrations of troponins or cardiac enzymes rise, irreversible cell damage has occurred and these patients must be regarded as having suffered MI according to the definition of the consensus conference.[13]

4. Then starts an observational period, which includes multilead ECG ischemia monitoring. If the patient experiences a new episode of chest pain, a 12-lead ECG should be obtained and compared with a tracing obtained when symptoms have resolved spontaneously or with nitrate administration. In addition, an echocardiogram may be recorded to assess LV function and to eliminate other cardiovascular causes of chest pain. Finally, a second troponin measurement should be obtained after 6 to 12 hours.

Patients can then be classified as having ACS, distinguishing MI (with elevated markers of necrosis), or unstable angina (ECG changes but no signs of necrosis), with another cause for symptoms.

Once diagnosed, ACSs without persistent ST-segment elevation (ST-segment depression, negative T waves, pseudonormalization of T waves, or normal-appearing ECG) require an initial medical treatment including aspirin (75 to 150 mg daily), clopidogrel 300 mg loading dose followed by 75 mg daily, LMWH or unfractionated heparin, β-blockers, and oral or intravenous nitrates in case of persistent or recurrent chest pain. Clopidogrel should replace aspirin in patients with hypersensitivity or major gastrointestinal intolerance to aspirin. Calcium antagonists may be preferred over β-blockers in patients who have contraindications to, or who are known intolerant to β-blockers. In the subsequent observation period (8 to 12 hours), specific attention is paid to recurrence of chest pain, during which an ECG is recorded. Signs of hemodynamic instability (hypotension, pulmonary rales) are carefully noted and treated.

Within this initial period, risk can be assessed according to the clinical, electrocardiographic, and biochemical data and classified as high or low.

Strategies According to Risk Stratification

Figure 49–6 depicts strategies according to risk stratification.

Patients Judged to Be at High Risk for Progression to Myocardial Infarction or Death

High-risk patients include those:

- With recurrent ischemia (either recurrent chest pain or dynamic ST-segment changes (in particular ST-segment depression, or transient ST-segment elevation)
- With early postinfarction unstable angina
- With elevated troponin levels

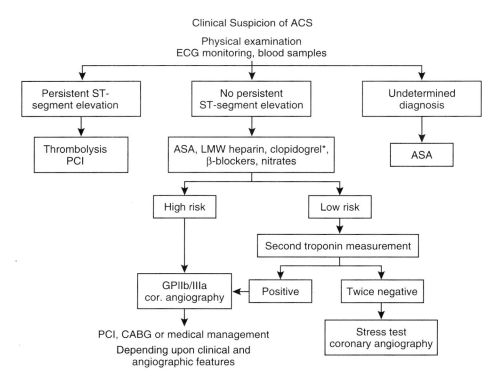

*omit clopidogrel if the patient is likely to go to CABG within 5 days

FIGURE 49–6. Recommended strategy in acute coronary syndromes.

- Who develop hemodynamic instability within the observation period
- With major arrhythmias (repetitive ventricular tachycardia, ventricular fibrillation)
- With diabetes mellitus
- With an ECG pattern that precludes assessment of ST-segment changes

In these patients, the following strategy is recommended:

- During the wait and preparation for angiography, treatment with LMWH should be continued. Administration of a GP IIb/IIIa receptor inhibitor is started and continued for 12 (abciximab) or 24 (tirofiban, eptifibatide) hours after PCI, if performed.
- Coronary angiography should be planned as soon as possible, but without undue urgency. A relatively small group of patients require a coronary angiogram within the first hour. This includes patients with severe ongoing ischemia, major arrhythmias, or hemodynamic instability. In most cases, coronary angiography is performed within the 24 hours or at least during the hospitalization. In patients with lesions suitable for myocardial revascularization, the decision regarding the most suitable procedure is made after careful evaluation of the extent and characteristics of the lesions, when appropriate, in consultation with surgical colleagues. In general, recommendations for the choice of a revascularization procedure in unstable angina are similar to those for elective revascularization procedures. In patients with single-vessel disease, PCI of the culprit lesion is the first choice. In patients with left main or triple-vessel disease, CABG is the recommended procedure, particularly in patients with LV dysfunction, except in case of serious comorbidity, which contraindicates surgery. In double-vessel and in some cases of triple-vessel coronary disease, either PCI or coronary bypass surgery may be appropriate. In some patients, a staged procedure may be considered, with immediate balloon angioplasty and stenting of the culprit lesion and subsequent reassessment of the need for treatment of other lesions, either by PCI or by CABG. If PCI is selected, it may be performed immediately after angiography in the same session.

Patients with suitable lesions for PCI receive clopidogrel. In patients for whom CABG is planned, clopidogrel is stopped, except if the operation is deferred. In that case, clopidogrel should be stopped about 5 days before the operation.

If angiography shows no options for revascularization owing to the extent of the lesions or to poor distal runoff or if it reveals no major coronary stenosis, patients are referred for medical therapy. Diagnosis of an ACS may need to be reconsidered, and particular attention should be given to possible other reasons for the presenting symptoms. However, the absence of significant stenosis does not preclude the diagnosis of an ACS. In selected patients, an ergonovine test may detect or rule out excessive coronary vasoconstriction.

Patients Considered to Be at Low Risk for Rapid Progression to Myocardial Infarction or Death

Low-risk patients include those:

- Who have no recurrence of chest pain within the observational period
- Without ST-segment depression or elevation but rather negative T waves, flat T waves, or a normal-appearing ECG
- Without elevation of troponin or other biochemical markers of myocardial necrosis on the initial and repeat measurement (performed between 6 and 12 hours)

In these patients, oral treatment should be recommended, including aspirin, clopidogrel (loading dose of 300 mg followed by 75 mg daily), β-blockers, and possibly nitrates or calcium antagonists. Secondary preventive measures should be instituted as discussed later. LMWH may be discontinued when, after the observational period, no ECG changes are apparent and a second troponin measurement is negative.

A stress test is recommended. Such a test (1) confirms or establishes a diagnosis of coronary artery disease and, when this is yet uncertain, (2) assesses the risk of future events in patients with coronary artery disease.

In patients with significant ischemia during the stress test, coronary angiography and subsequent revascularization should be considered, particularly when this occurs at a low workload on the bicycle or treadmill. A standard exercise test may be inconclusive (no abnormalities at a relatively low workload). In such patients, an additional stress echocardiogram or stress myocardial perfusion scintigram may be appropriate.

In some patients, the diagnosis may remain uncertain, particularly in patients with a normal-appearing electrocardiogram throughout the observation period, without elevated markers of myocardial necrosis, and with a normal stress test result and good exercise tolerance. The symptoms resulting in presentation to the hospital were probably not caused by myocardial ischemia, and additional investigations of other organ systems may be appropriate. In any case, the risk of cardiac events in such patients is very low. Therefore, additional tests can usually be performed later at the outpatient clinic.

LONG-TERM MANAGEMENT

Observational studies show that most recurrent cardiac events take place within a few months following the initial presentation of ACSs.[5,110] Early stabilization of a patient's clinical condition does not imply that the underlying pathologic process has stabilized. Data concerning the duration of the healing process of ruptured plaques are sparse. Some studies have shown a potential for rapid progression of culprit lesions in ACSs despite initial clinical stability on medical therapy.[111] Increased thrombin generation has been observed for as long as 6 months following unstable angina or MI.[112]

In addition, trials that examined the efficacy of heparin in addition to aspirin reported an increase in clinical events after heparin withdrawal.[46,113] In FRISC II, continuation of LMWH was beneficial only in patients waiting for an invasive procedure. Aggressive risk-factor modification is warranted in all patients following a diagnosis of ACS.

Patients must quit smoking. Patients should be clearly informed that smoking is a major risk factor. Referral to smoking cessation clinics is recommended, and the use of nicotine replacement therapy should be considered. Blood pressure control should be optimized. Aspirin should be prescribed (75 to 150 mg). According to the antiplatelet trialists meta-analysis, higher doses of aspirin confer no advantage.[58] For patients with a history of MI, a mean of 27 months of treatment results in 36 fewer vascular events per 1000 patients, including 18 fewer nonfatal MIs per 1000 patients and 14 fewer deaths per 1000 patients with aspirin treatment.[58] The results of the CURE trial show that clopidogrel (75 mg) should be prescribed for at least 9 and possibly 12 months and that the dose of aspirin should be reduced to 75 to 100 mg.[60]

β-Blockers improve prognosis in patients after MI and should be continued after ACSs. Lipid-lowering therapy should be initiated without delay. HMG-CoA reductase inhibitors substantially decrease mortality and coronary events in patients with high, intermediate, or even low (<3.0 mmol/L) levels of LDL cholesterol[113b]. Small subgroups of patients from PURSUIT, PRISM, PRISM-PLUS, and TACTICS suggest that statins may provide an immediate benefit in ACSs, but these data are nonrandomized. The MIRACL trial compared atorvastatin (80 mg daily given on average 63 hours after admission and for 16 weeks) to placebo in 3086 randomized patients.[114] The primary end point (a composite end point of death, nonfatal MI, rehospitalization for worsening angina at 16 weeks) was marginally (P = .0459) positive—14.8% versus 17.4%—but robust end points like death/MI were similar in both groups (10.1% vs. 10.9%). The difference in the primary end point was driven by rehospitalization for recurrent angina (6.2% vs. 8.4%). In the Register of Information and Knowledge about Swedish Intensive Care Admissions, the 1-year mortality rate was lower in patients with non–ST-elevation MI discharged with statin therapy than in the group not given that treatment.[115,116] Other specific trials are ongoing to assess whether statins indeed provide immediate benefit in ACSs (A to Z) and whether high doses are more effective than intermediate doses (Treating to New Targets [TNT], and Incremental Disease in Endpoints through Aggressive Lipid Lowering [IDEAL]). Several lipid intervention angiographic trials suggest that improved clinical outcome was not necessarily related to atherosclerosis regression but might relate to passivation of inflamed plaque, reversal of endothelial dysfunction, or a decrease in prothrombotic factors.

A role for angiotensin-converting enzyme (ACE) inhibitors in secondary prevention of coronary syndromes has been suggested. The Survival And Ventricular Enlargement (SAVE) and Studies On Left Ventricular Dysfunction (SOLVD) randomized trials, performed in subjects with LV impairment, reported a reduction in cardiac events in patients with known CAD treated with ACE inhibitors.[117-119] The decrease in MI

rate became apparent after 6 months of active treatment. These data strongly suggest that the beneficial effect of ACE inhibition goes beyond blood pressure control.[120,121] This concept is supported by experimental data indicating that the advantage may also be related to plaque stabilization and by the Heart Outcomes Prevention Evaluation (HOPE) trial, which showed a reduction of cardiovascular death from 8.1% to 6.1% (adjusted relative risk, 2%; relative risk, 0.74; 95% CI, 0.64 to 0.87; P < .001) and MI (relative risk, 0.80; 95% CI, 0.70 to 0.90; P < .001) over 4 to 6 years.[122] However, in the HOPE trial, no benefit was demonstrated in the subcategory of unstable angina as defined by ST and T-wave changes, but this may be due to chance.[123] Other trials are ongoing to confirm these findings: the EUropean trial of Reduction Of cardiac events with Perindopril in stable coronary Artery disease (EUROPA) and the Prevention of Events with ACE inhibitors (PEACE) study, which may establish new strategies to prevent ACSs.

Because coronary atherosclerosis and its complications are multifactorial, much attention should be paid to treating all modifiable risk factors to reduce the recurrence of cardiac events.

COMPARISON OF EUROPEAN GUIDELINES WITH ACC/AHA GUIDELINES

The updated version of the ACC/AHA guidelines has been published recently and is summarized in the next chapter of this book.[124,125] On average, the two guidelines are similar. They differ in risk assessment with three levels of risk in the ACC/AHA guidelines: low, intermediate, and high, and two in the European guidelines: low and high, the latter being associated with major cardiac events, death, or large MI. The European guidelines also include diabetic patients in the high risk category, because of a high thrombogenic state in these patients and an impaired prognosis.

Treatment strategies are also similar in the two sets of guidelines. The ACC/AHA gives priority to enoxaparin over unfractionated heparins, whereas the European guidelines recognize the advantages of low-molecular-weight heparin without a specific recommendation. The European guidelines recommend prompt initiation of a GPIIb/IIIa antagonist in the high-risk patient while planning coronary angioplasty; a GPIIb/IIIa antagonist is also recommended in the ACC/AHA guidelines, initiated either before cardiac catheterization or in the catheterization laboratory when PCI is performed.

Clopidogrel is recommended at hospital admission in all patients in whom an early noninterventional approach is planned in the ACC/AHA guidelines; clopidogrel is also recommended in patients in whom a PCI is planned and continued for at least one month and up to 9 months in patients who are not at high risk for bleeding. If CABG is planned, clopidogrel should be witheld, if possible, for at least 5 days, preferably for 7 days. The ESC guidelines recommend clopidogrel in patients with lesions suitable for PCI and in patients with coronary artery lesions not suitable for any form of revascularization. Patients scheduled for CABG will not receive clopidogrel except if the operation is postponed, but in that case clopidogrel should be stopped at least 5 days before the operation.

In spite of these minor differences, both guidelines are based on risk stratification and recognize that an aggressive antiplatelet treatment associated with antithrombins are necessary in high-risk patients who benefit from an invasive strategy if they have lesions suitable for myocardial revascularization.

ACSs are an important part of cardiovascular medicine and a very rapidly evolving field: There is no doubt that both guidelines will need to be updated frequently.

REFERENCES

1. Hasdai D, Behar S, Wallentin L, et al: A prospective survey of the characteristics, treatments and outcomes of patients with acute coronary syndromes in Europe and the Mediterranean basin; the Euro Heart Survey of Acute Coronary Syndromes (Euro Heart Survey ACS). Eur Heart J 2002;23:1190-1201.
2. Bertrand ME, Simoons ML, Fox KA, et al: Management of acute coronary syndromes in patients presenting without persistent ST-segment elevation. The Task Force for the Management of Acute Coronary Syndromes of the European Society of Cardiology. Europ Heart J 2002;23:1809-1840.
3. Davies M: Acute coronary thrombosis: The role of plaque disruption and its initiation and prevention. Eur Heart J 1995;16(Suppl L):3-7.
4. Davies M: The composition of coronary artery plaque. N Engl J Med 1997;336:1312-1313.
5. van Domburg RT, van Miltenburg-van Zijl AJ, Veerhoek RJ, Simoons ML: Unstable angina: Good long-term outcome after a complicated early course. J Am Coll Cardiol 1998;31:1534-1539.
6. Lee TH, Cook EF, Weisberg M, et al: Acute chest pain in the emergency room. Identification and examination of low-risk patients. Arch Intern Med 1985;145:65-69.
7. Fesmire FM, Percy RF, Bardoner JB, et al: Usefulness of automated serial 12-lead ECG monitoring during the initial emergency department evaluation of patients with chest pain. Ann Emerg Med 1998;31:3-11.
8. Fisch C: The Clinical ECG: Sensitivity and Specificity. Philadelphia, Elsevier Science, 1997.
9. Savonitto S, Ardissino D, Granger CB, et al: Prognostic value of the admission electrocardiogram in acute coronary syndromes. JAMA 1999;281:707-713.
10. McCarthy BD, Wong JB, Selker HP: Detecting acute cardiac ischemia in the emergency department: A review of the literature. J Gen Intern Med 1990;5:365-373.
11. Pozen MW, D'Agostino RB, Selker HP, et al: A predictive instrument to improve coronary-care-unit admission practices in acute ischemic heart disease. A prospective multicenter clinical trial. N Engl J Med 1984;310:1273-1278.
12. Rouan GW, Lee TH, Cook EF, et al: Clinical characteristics and outcome of acute myocardial infarction in patients with initially normal or nonspecific electrocardiograms (a report from the Multicenter Chest Pain Study). Am J Cardiol 1989;64:1087-1092.
13. Myocardial infarction redefined—a consensus document of The Joint European Society of Cardiology/American College of Cardiology Committee for the redefinition of myocardial infarction. J Am Coll Cardiol 2000;36:959-969.
14. Davies E, Gawad Y, Takahashi M, et al: Analytical performance and clinical utility of a sensitive immunoassay for determination of human cardiac troponin I. Clin Biochem 1997;30:479-490.
15. Jaffe AS, Ravkilde J, Roberts R, et al: It's time for a change to a troponin standard. Circulation 2000;102:1216-1220.
16. Giannitsis E, Muller-Bardorff M, Kurowski V, et al: Independent prognostic value of cardiac troponin T in patients with confirmed pulmonary embolism. Circulation 2000;102:211-217.
17. Missov E, Calzolari C, Pau B: Circulating cardiac troponin I in severe congestive heart failure. Circulation 1997;96:2953-2958.
18. Lauer B, Niederau C, Kuhl U, et al: Cardiac troponin T in patients with clinically suspected myocarditis. J Am Coll Cardiol 1997;30:1354-1359.
19. Cannon CP, Weintraub WS, Demopoulos LA, et al: Comparison of early invasive and conservative strategies in patients with unstable coronary syndromes treated with the glycoprotein IIb/IIIa inhibitor tirofiban. N Engl J Med 2001;344:1879-1887.
20. FRISC II investigators: Invasive compared with non-invasive treatment in unstable coronary-artery disease: FRISC II prospective randomised multicentre study. FRagmin and Fast Revascularisation during InStability in Coronary artery disease Investigators. Lancet 1999;354:708-715.
21. Lindahl B, Diderholm E, Lagerqvist B, et al: Mechanisms behind the prognostic value of troponin T in unstable coronary artery disease: a FRISC II substudy. J Am Coll Cardiol 2001;38:979-986.
22. Wu AH, Apple FS, Gibler WB, et al: National Academy of Clinical Biochemistry Standards of Laboratory Practice: Recommendations for the use of cardiac markers in coronary artery diseases. Clin Chem 1999;45:1104-1121.
23. Telford AM, Wilson WC: Trial of heparin versus atenolol in prevention of myocardial infarction in intermediate coronary syndrome. Lancet 1981;1:1225-1228.
24. Lubsen JTJ: Efficacy of nifedipine and metoprolol in the early treatment of unstable angina in the coronary care unit: Findings from the Holland Interuniversity Nifedipine/metoprolol Trial (HINT). Am J Cardiol 1987;60:18A-25A.
25. Yusuf S, Wittes J, Friedman L: Overview of results of randomized clinical trials in heart disease. II: Unstable angina, heart failure, primary prevention with aspirin, and risk factor modification. JAMA 1988;260:2259-2263.
26. Miami Trial research group: Metoprolol in myocardial infarction. Eur Heart J 1985;6:199-226.
27. Kaplan KDR, Parker M, Przybylek J, et al: Intravenous nitroglycerin for the treatment of angina at rest unresponsive to standard nitrate therapy. Am J Cardiol 1983;51:694-698.
28. DePace N, Herling IM, Kotler MN, et al: Intravenous nitroglycerin for rest angina. Potential pathophysiologic mechanisms of action. Arch Intern Med 1982;142:1806-1809.
29. Roubin GSHP, Eckhardt I, et al: Intravenous nitroglycerine in refractory unstable angina pectoris. Aust N Z J Med 1982;12:598-602.
30. Curfman G, Heinsimr JA, Lozner EC, Fung HL: Intravenous nitroglycerin in the treatment of spontaneous angina pectoris: A prospective randomized trial. Circulation 1983;67:276-282.
31. Dellborg M, Gustafsson G, Swedberg K: Buccal versus intravenous nitroglycerin in unstable angina pectoris. Eur J Clin Pharmacol 1991;41:5-9.
32. May DCPJ, Black WH, et al: In vivo induction and reversal of nitroglycerin tolerance in human coronary arteries. N Engl J Med 1987;317:805-809.
33. Reichek N, Priest C, Zimrin D, et al: Antianginal effects of nitroglycerin patches. Am J Cardiol 1984;54:1-7.
34. Thadani U, Hamilton SF, Olsen E, et al: Transdermal nitroglycerin patches in angina pectoris. Dose titration, duration of effect, and rapid tolerance. Ann Intern Med 1986;105:485-492.
35. Iona study group: Effect of Nicorandil on coronary events in patients with stable angina: The Impact Of Nicorandil in Angina (IONA) randomised trial. Lancet 2002;359:1269-1275.
36. Theroux P, Taeymans Y, Morissette D, et al: A randomized study comparing propranolol and diltiazem in the treatment of unstable angina. J Am Coll Cardiol 1985;5:717-722.
37. Parodi O, Simonetti I, Michelassi C: Comparison of verapamil and propanolol therapy for angina pectoris at rest. A randomized, multiple crossover, controlled trial in the coronary care unit. Am J Cardiol 1986;57:899-906.
38. Smith NL Reiber GE, Psaty BM, et al: Health outcomes associated with beta-blocker and diltiazem treatment of unstable angina. J Am Coll Cardiol 1998;32:1305-1311.
39. Gibson RS, Young PM, Boden WE, et al: Prognostic significance and beneficial effect of diltiazem on the incidence of early recurrent ischemia after non-Q-wave myocardial infarction: Results from the Multicenter Diltiazem Reinfarction Study. Am J Cardiol 1987;60:203-209.
40. Gibson RS, Hansen JF, Messerli F, et al: Long-term effects of diltiazem and verapamil on mortality and cardiac events in non-Q-wave acute myocardial infarction without pulmonary congestion: Post hoc subset analysis of the multicenter diltiazem postinfarction trial and the second Danish Verapamil Infarction Trial studies. Am J Cardiol 2000;86:275-279.

41. Held PYS, Furberg CD: Calcium channel blockers in acute myocardial infarction and unstable angina: An overview. Br Med J 1989;299:1187–1192.

42. Psaty BM, Heckbert SR, Koepsell TD, et al: The risk of myocardial infarction associated with antihypertensive drug therapies. JAMA 1995;274:620–625.

43. Yusuf S, Held P, Furberg C: Update of effects of calcium antagonists in myocardial infarction or angina in light of the second Danish Verapamil Infarction Trial (DAVIT-II) and other recent studies [editorial]. Am J Cardiol 1991;67:1295–1297.

44. Boden WE, van Gilst WH, Scheldewaert RG, et al: Diltiazem in acute myocardial infarction treated with thrombolytic agents: A randomised placebo-controlled trial. Incomplete Infarction Trial of European Research Collaborators Evaluating Prognosis post-Thrombolysis (INTERCEPT). Lancet 2000;355:1751–1756.

45. Oler A, Whooley MA, Oler J, Grady D: Adding heparin to aspirin reduces the incidence of myocardial infarction and death in patients with unstable angina. A meta-analysis. JAMA 1996;276: 811–815.

46. Theroux P, Ouimet H, McCans J, et al: Aspirin, heparin, or both to treat acute unstable angina. N Engl J Med 1988;319:1105–1111.

47. FRISC study group: Low-molecular-weight heparin during instability in coronary artery disease, Fragmin during Instability in Coronary Artery Disease (FRISC) study group. Lancet 1996;347:561–568.

48. Eikelboom JW, Anand SS, Malmberg K, et al: Unfractionated heparin and low-molecular-weight heparin in acute coronary syndrome without ST elevation: A meta-analysis. Lancet 2000;355: 1936–1942.

49. Cohen M, Demers C, Gurfinkel E, et al: A comparison of low-molecular weight heparin with unfractionated heparin for unstable coronary artery disease. N Engl J Med 1997;337:447–452.

50. Antman EM, Cohen M, Radley D, et al: Assessment of the treatment effect of enoxaparin for unstable angina/non-Q-wave myocardial infarction: TIMI 11B-ESSENCE meta-analysis. Circulation 1999;100: 1602–1608.

51. Antman EM, Cohen M, McCabe C, et al: Enoxaparin is superior to unfractionated heparin for preventing clinical events at 1-year follow-up of TIMI 11B and ESSENCE. Eur Heart J 2002;23:308–314.

52. Antman EM, McCabe CH, Gurfinkel EP, et al: Enoxaparin prevents death and cardiac ischemic events in unstable angina/non-Q-wave myocardial infarction. Results of the thrombolysis in myocardial infarction (TIMI) IIB trial. Circulation 1999;100:1593–1601.

53. Ferguson JJ: Combining low-molecular-weight heparin and glycoprotein IIb/IIIa antagonists for the treatment of acute coronary syndromes: The NICE 3 story. National Investigators Collaborating on Enoxaparin. J Invasive Cardiol 2000;12(Suppl E):E10–E13; discussion, E25–E28.

53b. Goodman SG, Fitchett D, Armstrong PW, et al: Randomized evaluation of the safety and efficiency of enoxaparin versus unfractionated heparin in high-risk patients with non–ST-segment elevation acute coronary syndromes receiving the glycoprotein IIb/IIIa inhibitor ephfibatide. Circ 2003;107:238–244.

54. GUSTO-IIB investigators: A comparison of recombinant hirudin with heparin for the treatment of acute coronary syndromes. The Global Use of Strategies to Open Occluded Coronary Arteries (GUSTO) IIb investigators. N Engl J Med 1996;335:775–782.

55. Fox KA: Implications of the Organization to Assess Strategies for Ischemic Syndromes-2 (OASIS-2) study and the results in the context of other trials. Am J Cardiol 1999;84:26M–31M.

56. Theroux P, Waters D, Qiu S, et al: Aspirin versus heparin to prevent myocardial infarction during the acute phase of unstable angina. Circulation 1993;88:2045–2048.

57. Cairns JA, Singer J, Gent M, et al: One year mortality outcomes of all coronary and intensive care unit patients with acute myocardial infarction, unstable angina or other chest pain in Hamilton, Ontario, a city of 375,000 people. Can J Cardiol 1989;5:239–246.

58. Antithrombotic Trialist Collaboration: Collaborative meta-analysis of randomised trials of antiplatelet therapy for prevention of death, myocardial infarction, and stroke in high risk patients. BMJ 2002;324:71–86.

59. Balsano F, Rizzon P, Violi F, et al: Antiplatelet treatment with ticlopidine in unstable angina. A controlled multicenter clinical trial. The Studio della Ticlopidina nell'Angina Instabile Group. Circulation 1990;82:17–26.

60. Yusuf S, Zhao F, Mehta SR, et al: Effects of clopidogrel in addition to aspirin in patients with acute coronary syndromes without ST-segment elevation. N Engl J Med 2001;345:494–502.

61. CAPRIE: A randomised, blinded, trial of clopidogrel versus aspirin in patients at risk of ischaemic events (CAPRIE). CAPRIE Steering Committee. Lancet 1996;348:1329–1339.

62. Bertrand ME, Rupprecht HJ, Urban P, et al: Double-blind study of the safety of clopidogrel with and without a loading dose in combination with aspirin compared with ticlopidine in combination with aspirin after coronary stenting: The Clopidogrel Aspirin Stent International Cooperative Study (CLASSICS). Circulation 2000;102: 624–629.

63. Leebeek FW, Boersma E, Cannon CP, et al: Oral glycoprotein IIb/IIIa receptor inhibitors in patients with cardiovascular disease: Why were the results so unfavourable? Eur Heart J 2002;23: 444–457.

64. The CAPTURE Investigators: Randomised placebo-controlled trial of abciximab before and during coronary intervention in refractory unstable angina: The CAPTURE Study. Lancet 1997;349:1429–1435.

65. PRISM study investigators: A comparison of aspirin plus tirofiban with aspirin plus heparin for unstable angina. Platelet Receptor Inhibition in Ischemic Syndrome Management (PRISM) Study Investigators. N Engl J Med 1998;338:1498–1505.

66. PRISM-PLUS study investigators: Inhibition of the platelet glycoprotein IIb/IIIa receptor with tirofiban in unstable angina and non-Q-wave myocardial infarction. Platelet Receptor Inhibition in Ischemic Syndrome Management in Patients Limited by Unstable Signs and Symptoms (PRISM-PLUS) Study Investigators. N Engl J Med 1998;338:1488–1497.

67. PURSUIT study investigators: Inhibition of platelet glycoprotein IIb/IIIa with eptifibatide in patients with acute coronary syndromes. The PURSUIT Trial Investigators. Platelet Glycoprotein IIb/IIIa in Unstable Angina: Receptor Suppression Using Integrilin Therapy. N Engl J Med 1998;339:436–443.

68. PARAGON Investigators: International, randomized, controlled trial of lamifiban (a platelet glycoprotein IIb/IIIa inhibitor), heparin, or both in unstable angina. The PARAGON Investigators. Platelet IIb/IIIa Antagonism for the Reduction of Acute coronary syndrome events in a Global Organization Network. Circulation 1998;97: 2386–2395.

69. The PARAGON-B Investigators: Randomized, placebo-controlled trial of titrated intravenous lamifiban for acute coronary syndrome. Circulation 2002; 105: 316–321.

70. The GUSTO-IV ACS Investigators: Effect of glycoprotein IIb/IIIA receptor blocker abciximab on outcome of patients with acute coronary syndromes without early revascularization: The GUSTO-IV ACS randomised trial. Lancet 2001;357:1915–1924.

71. Boersma E, Harrington R, Moliterno D, et al: Platelet glycoprotein IIb/IIIa inhibitors in acute coronary syndromes: A meta-analysis of all major randomised clinical trials. Lancet 2002;359:189–198.

72. The PRISM Investigators: A comparison of aspirin plus tirofiban with aspirin plus heparin for unstable angina. Platelet Receptor Inhibition in Ischemic Syndrome Management (PRISM) Study Investigators. N Engl J Med 1998;338:1498–1505.

73. The PRISM-PLUS study investigators: Inhibition of the platelet glycoprotein IIb/IIIa receptor with tirofiban in unstable angina and non-Q-wave myocardial infarction. Platelet Receptor Inhibition in Ischemic Syndrome Management in Patients Limited by Unstable Signs and Symptoms (PRISM-PLUS) Study Investigators [published erratum appears in N Engl J Med 1998;339:415]. N Engl J Med 1998;338:1488–1497.

74. Roffi M, Chew DP, Mukherjee D, et al: Platelet glycoprotein IIb/IIIa inhibitors reduce mortality in diabetic patients with non-ST-segment-elevation acute coronary syndromes. Circulation 2001;104: 2767–2771.

75. Madan M, Tcheng JE: Update on abciximab readministration during percutaneous coronary interventions. Curr Interv Cardiol Rep 2000;2:244–249.

76. Madan M, Kereiakes DJ, Hermiller JB, et al: Efficacy of abciximab readministration in coronary intervention. Am J Cardiol 2000;85: 435–440.

77. Cohen M, Théroux P, Borzak S et al: Randomized double blind safety study of enoxaparin versus unfractionated heparin in patients with non–ST-segment elevation acute coronary syndromes treated with tirofiban and aspirin: The ACUTE II study. Am Heart J 2002;144:470–477.

78. James S, Armstrong P, Califf R, et al: Safety of abciximab combined with dalteparin in treatment of acute coronary syndromes. Eur Heart J 2002; 23:1538–1545.

79. TIMI IIIA investigators: Early effects of tissue-type plasminogen activator added to conventional therapy on the culprit coronary lesion in patients presenting with ischemic cardiac pain at rest. Results of the Thrombolysis in Myocardial Ischemia (TIMI IIIA) Trial. Circulation 1993;87:38–52.

80. Karlsson JE, Berglund U, Bjorkholm A, et al: Thrombolysis with recombinant human tissue-type plasminogen activator during instability in coronary artery disease: Effect on myocardial ischemia and need for coronary revascularization. TRIC Study Group. Am Heart J 1992;124:1419–1426.

81. Schreiber TL, Macina G, McNulty A, et al: Urokinase plus heparin versus aspirin in unstable angina and non-Q-wave myocardial infarction. Am J Cardiol 1989;64:840–844.

82. Schreiber TL, Macina G, Bunnell P, et al: Unstable angina or non-Q-wave infarction despite long-term aspirin: Response to thrombolytic therapy with implications on mechanisms. Am Heart J 1990;120:248–255.

83. Indications for fibrinolytic therapy in suspected acute myocardial infarction: Collaborative overview of early mortality and major morbidity results from all randomised trials of more than 1000 patients. The Fibrinolytic Therapy Trialists' (FTT) Collaboration Group. Lancet 1994;343:311–322.

83b. The TIMI-3B Investigators. Effects of tissue plasminogen activator and a comparison of early invasive and conservative strategies in unstable angina and non-Q-wave myocardial infarction. Results of the TIMI-3B trial. Circ 1994;89:1545–1556.

84. Van Belle E, Lablanche JM, Bauters C, et al: Coronary angioscopic findings in the infarct-related vessel within 1 month of acute myocardial infarction: Natural history and the effect of thrombolysis. Circulation 1998;97:26–33.

85. Serruys PW, van Hout B, Bonnier H, et al: Randomised comparison of implantation of heparin-coated stents with balloon angioplasty in selected patients with coronary artery disease (Benestent II). Lancet 1998;352:673–681.

86. The EPIC investigators: Use of a monoclonal antibody directed against the platelet glycoprotein IIb/IIIa receptor in high-risk angioplasty. N Engl J Med 1994;330:956–961.

87. The EPILOG investigators: Platelet glycoprotein IIb/IIIa receptor blockade and low-dose heparin during percutaneous coronary revascularization. The EPILOG Investigators. N Engl J Med 1997;336:1689–1696.

88. The EPISTENT Investigators: Randomised placebo-controlled and balloon-angioplasty-controlled trial to assess safety of coronary stenting with use of platelet glycoprotein-IIb/IIIa blockade. The EPISTENT Investigators. Evaluation of Platelet IIb/IIIa Inhibitor for Stenting. Lancet 1998;352:87–92.

89. Lincoff AM, Califf RM, Anderson KM, et al: Evidence for prevention of death and myocardial infarction with platelet membrane glycoprotein IIb/IIIa receptor blockade by abciximab (c7E3 Fab) among patients with unstable angina undergoing percutaneous coronary revascularization. EPIC Investigators. Evaluation of 7E3 in Preventing Ischemic Complications. J Am Coll Cardiol 1997;30:149–156.

90. Lincoff AM: Trials of platelet glycoprotein IIb/IIIa receptor antagonists during percutaneous coronary revascularization. Am J Cardiol 1998;82:36P–42P.

91. The IMPACT-II Investigators: Randomised placebo-controlled trial of effect of eptifibatide on complications of percutaneous coronary intervention: IMPACT-II. Integrilin to Minimise Platelet Aggregation and Coronary Thrombosis-II. Lancet 1997;349:1422–1428.

92. The RESTORE Investigators: Effects of platelet glycoprotein IIb/IIIa blockade with tirofiban on adverse cardiac events in patients with unstable angina or acute myocardial infarction undergoing coronary angioplasty. The RESTORE Investigators. Randomized Efficacy Study of Tirofiban for Outcomes and REstenosis. Circulation 1997;96:1445–1453.

93. The ESPRIT Investigators: Novel dosing regimen of eptifibatide in planned coronary stent implantation (ESPRIT): A randomised, placebo-controlled trial. Lancet 2000;356:2037–4204.

94. Mehta SR, Yusuf S, Peters RJ, et al: Effects of pretreatment with clopidogrel and aspirin followed by long-term therapy in patients undergoing percutaneous coronary intervention: The PCI-CURE study. Lancet 2001;358:527–533.

95. Battler A: European Heart Survey of Acute Coronary syndromes. Eur Heart J 2002;23:1190–1201.

96. Bjessmo S, Ivert T, Flink H, Hammar N: Early and late mortality after surgery for unstable angina in relation to Braunwald class. Am Heart J 2001;141:9–14.

97. Dyke CM, Bhatia D, Lorenz TJ, et al: Immediate coronary artery bypass surgery after platelet inhibition with eptifibatide: Results from PURSUIT. Platelet Glycoprotein IIb/IIIa in Unstable Angina: Receptor Suppression Using Integrelin Therapy. Ann Thorac Surg 2000;70:866–871, discussion 871–872.

98. Bizzarri F, Scolletta S, Tucci E, et al: Perioperative use of tirofiban hydrochloride (Aggrastat) does not increase surgical bleeding after emergency or urgent coronary artery bypass grafting. J Thorac Cardiovasc Surg 2001;122:1181–1185.

99. Clark SC, Vitale N, Zacharias J, Forty J: Effect of low molecular weight heparin (fragmin) on bleeding after cardiac surgery. Ann Thorac Surg 2000;69:762–764;764–765.

100. Yusuf S, Zucker D, Chalmers TC: Ten-year results of the randomized control trials of coronary artery bypass graft surgery: Tabular data compiled by the collaborative effort of the original trial investigators. Part 2 of 2. Online J Curr Clin Trials 1994; Doc No. 144.

101. Yusuf S, Zucker D, Chalmers TC: Ten-year results of the randomized control trials of coronary artery bypass graft surgery: Tabular data compiled by the collaborative effort of the original trial investigators. Part 1 of 2. Online J Curr Clin Trials 1994; Doc No. 145.

102. BARI investigators. Five-year clinical and functional outcome comparing bypass surgery and angioplasty in patients with multivessel coronary disease. A multicenter randomized trial. Writing Group for the Bypass Angioplasty Revascularization Investigation (BARI) Investigators. JAMA 1997;277:715–721.

103. King SB III, Lembo NJ, Weintraub WS, et al: A randomized trial comparing coronary angioplasty with coronary bypass surgery. Emory Angioplasty versus Surgery Trial (EAST). N Engl J Med 1994;331:1044–1050.

104. The CABRI Investigators: First-year results of CABRI (Coronary Angioplasty versus Bypass Revascularization Investigation) [news]. Circulation 1996;93:847.

105. The RITA investigators: Coronary angioplasty versus coronary artery bypass surgery: The Randomized Intervention Treatment of Angina (RITA) trial. Lancet 1993;341:573–580.

106. Hamm CW, Reimers J, Ischinger T, et al: A randomized study of coronary angioplasty compared with bypass surgery in patients with symptomatic multivessel coronary disease. German Angioplasty Bypass Surgery Investigation (GABI). N Engl J Med 1994;331:1037–1043.

107. Rodriguez A, Boullon F, Perez-Balino N, et al: Argentine randomized trial of percutaneous transluminal coronary angioplasty versus coronary artery bypass surgery in multivessel disease (ERACI): In-hospital results and 1-year follow-up. ERACI Group. J Am Coll Cardiol 1993;22:1060–1067.

108. Serruys PW, Unger F, Sousa JE, et al: Comparison of coronary-artery bypass surgery and stenting for the treatment of multivessel disease. N Engl J Med 2001;344:1117–1124.

108b. Stables RH: Results of the Stent or Surgery study presented at the 50th Annual Scientific Sessions of the American College of Cardiology. Orlando, FL, March 2001.

109. Fox KA, Poole-Wilson PA, Henderson RA, et al: Interventional versus conservative treatment for patients with unstable angina or non-ST-elevation myocardial infarction: The British Heart Foundation RITA 3 randomised trial. Randomized Intervention Trial of unstable Angina. Lancet 2002;360:743–751.

110. Theroux P, Fuster V: Acute coronary syndromes: Unstable angina and non-Q-wave myocardial infarction. Circulation 1998;97:1195–1206.

111. Kontny F: Reactivation of the coagulation system: rationale for long-term antithrombotic treatment. Am J Cardiol 1997;80:55E–60E.

112. Falk E, Shah P, Fuster V: Coronary plaque disruption. Circulation 1995;92:657–671.

113. RISC G: Risk of myocardial infarction and death during treatment with low dose aspirin and intravenous heparin in men with unstable coronary artery disease. The RISC Group. Lancet 1990;336:827–830.

113b. The Heart Protection Study Collaboration Group. MRC/BHF Heart Protection Study of Cholesterol lowering with Simvostatin in 20,536 high-risk individuals: A randomized placebo-controlled trial. Lancet 2002;360:7–22.

114. Schwartz GG, Olsson AG, Ezekowitz MD, et al: Effects of atorvastatin on early recurrent ischemic events in acute coronary syndromes. The MIRACL study: A randomized controlled trial. JAMA 2001;285:1711–1718.

115. Stenestrand U, Wallentin L: Early statin treatment following acute myocardial infarction and 1-year survival. JAMA 2001;285:430–436.

116. Stenestrand U, Wallentin L: Early revascularization and 1-year survival in 14-days survivors of acute myocardial infarction: A prospective cohort study. Lancet 2002;359:1805–1811.

117. SOLVD investigators: Effect of enalapril on survival in patients with reduced left ventricular ejection fractions and congestive heart failure. The SOLVD Investigators. N Engl J Med 1991;325:293–302.

118. SOLVD investigators: Effect of enalapril on mortality and the development of heart failure in asymptomatic patients with reduced left ventricular ejection fractions. The SOLVD Investigators. N Engl J Med 1992;327:685–691.

119. Collins R, Peto R, MacMahon S, et al: Blood pressure, stroke, and coronary heart disease. Part 2: Short-term reductions in blood pressure: Overview of randomised drug trials in their epidemiological context. Lancet 1990;335:827–838.

120. Rabbani R, Topol EJ: Strategies to achieve coronary arterial plaque stabilization. Cardiovasc Res 1999;41:402–417.

121. Yusuf S, Kostis JB, Pitt B: ACE inhibitors for myocardial infarction and unstable angina. Lancet 1993;341:829.

122. Yusuf S, Sleight P, Pogue J, et al: Effects of an angiotensin-converting-enzyme inhibitor, ramipril, on cardiovascular events in high-risk patients. The Heart Outcomes Prevention Evaluation Study Investigators. N Engl J Med 2000;342:145–153.

123. Dagenais GR, Yusuf S, Bourassa MG, et al: Effects of ramipril on coronary events in high-risk persons: Results of the Heart Outcomes Prevention Evaluation Study. Circulation 2001;104:522–526.

124. Braunwald E, Antman E, Beasley J, et al: ACC/AHA 2002 guideline update for the management of patients with unstable angina and non-ST-segment elevation myocardial infarction-summary article. A report of the American College of Cardiology/American Heart Association task force on practice guidelines (Committee on the Management of Patients With Unstable Angina). J Am Coll Cardiol 2002;40:1366.

125. Braunwald E, Antman EM, Beasley JW, et al: ACC/AHA Guideline Update for the Management of Patients With Unstable Angina and Non-ST-Segment Elevation Myocardial Infarction—2002. Summary Article: A Report of the American College of Cardiology/American Heart Association Task Force on Practice Guidelines (Committee on the Management of Patients With Unstable Angina). Circulation 2002;106:1893–1900.

■■■ chapter**50**

ACC/AHA 2002 Guideline Update for the Management of Patients with Unstable Angina and Non–ST-Segment Elevation Myocardial Infarction—Summary Article

A REPORT OF THE AMERICAN COLLEGE OF CARDIOLOGY/AMERICAN HEART ASSOCIATION TASK FORCE ON PRACTICE GUIDELINES
(Committee on the Management of Patients With Unstable Angina)

Committee Members
EUGENE BRAUNWALD, MD, FACC, FAHA, Chair

Elliott M. Antman, MD, FACC, FAHA
John W. Beasley, MD, FAAFP
Robert M. Califf, MD, FACC
Melvin D. Cheitlin, MD, FACC
Judith S. Hochman, MD, FACC, FAHA
Robert H. Jones, MD, FACC
Dean Kereiakes, MD, FACC

Joel Kupersmith, MD, FACC, FAHA
Thomas N. Levin, MD, FACC
Carl J. Pepine, MD, MACC, FAHA
John W. Schaeffer, MD, FACC, FAHA
Earl E. Smith III, MD, FACEP
David E. Steward, MD, FACP
Pierre Theroux, MD, FACC, FAHA

Task Force Members
RAYMOND J. GIBBONS, MD, FACC, FAHA, Chair
ELLIOTT M. ANTMAN, MD, FACC, FAHA, Vice Chair

Joseph S. Alpert, MD, FACC, FAHA
David P. Faxon, MD, FACC, FAHA
Valentin Fuster, MD, PhD, FACC, FAHA
Gabriel Gregoratos, MD, FACC, FAHA

Loren F. Hiratzka, MD, FACC, FAHA
Alice K. Jacobs, MD, FACC, FAHA
Sidney C. Smith, Jr., MD, FACC, FAHA

INTRODUCTION

The American College of Cardiology (ACC)/American Heart Association (AHA) guidelines for the management of unstable angina and non–ST-segment elevation myocardial infarction (UA/NSTEMI) were published in September 2000.[1] Since then, a number of clinical trials and observational studies have been published or presented that, when taken together, alter significantly the recommendations made in that document. Therefore,

The ACC/AHA Task Force on Practice Guidelines makes every effort to avoid any actual or potential conflicts of interest that might arise as a result of an outside relationship or personal interest of a member of the writing panel. Specifically, all members of the writing panel are asked to provide disclosure statements of all such relationships that might be perceived as real or potential conflicts of interest. These statements are reviewed by the parent task force, reported orally to all members of the writing panel at the first meeting, and updated as changes occur.

This document was approved by the American College of Cardiology Foundation Board of Trustees in September 2002 and by the American Heart Association Science Advisory and Coordinating Committee in August 2002.

When citing this document, the American College of Cardiology Foundation and the American Heart Association would appreciate the following citation format: Braunwald E, Antman EM, Beasley JW, Califf RM, Cheitlin MD, Hochman JS, Jones RH, Kereiakes D, Kupersmith J, Levin TN, Pepine CJ, Schaeffer JW, Smith EE III, Steward DE, Theroux P.

ACC/AHA 2002 guideline update for the management of patients with unstable angina and non–ST-segment elevation myocardial infarction: summary article: a report of the American College of Cardiology/American Heart Association Task Force on Practice Guidelines (Committee on the Management of Patients With Unstable Angina). J Am Coll Cardiol 2002;40:1366–1374.

This document is available on the World Wide Web sites of the ACC (www.acc.org) and the AHA (www.americanheart.org). Single copies of this document are available for $5 each by calling 800-253-4636 (US only) or writing the American College of Cardiology Foundation, Resource Center, 9111 Old Georgetown Road, Bethesda, MD 20814-1699 (product code 71-0227). This document and the companion full-text guidelines (product code 71-0240), are available on the ACC web site at www.acc.org and the AHA web site at www.americanheart.org. To purchase additional reprints (specify version): up to 999 copies, call 800-611-6083 (US only) or fax 413-665-2671; 1000 or more copies, call 214-706-1466, fax 214-691-6342; or e-mail pubauth@heart.org.

the ACC/AHA Committee on the Management of Patients with Unstable Angina, with the concurrence of the ACC/AHA Task Force on Practice Guidelines, revised these guidelines. These revisions were prepared in December 2001, reviewed and approved, and then published on the ACC World Wide Web site (www.acc.org) and AHA World Wide Web site (www.americanheart.org) on March 15, 2002. The present article describes these revisions and provides further updates in this rapidly moving field. Minor clarifications in the wording of three recommendations that now appear differently from those that were previously published on the ACC and AHA web sites are noted in footnotes.

The ACC/AHA classifications I, II, and III are used to summarize indications as follows:

Class I: Conditions for which there is evidence and/or general agreement that a given procedure or treatment is useful and effective

Class II: Conditions for which there is conflicting evidence and/or a divergence of opinion about the usefulness/efficacy of a procedure or treatment

> *IIa:* Weight of evidence/opinion is in favor of usefulness/efficacy
>
> *IIb:* Usefulness/efficacy is less well established by evidence/opinion

Class III: Conditions for which there is evidence and/or general agreement that the procedure/treatment is not useful/effective and in some cases may be harmful

The weight of the evidence was ranked highest (A) if the data were derived from multiple randomized clinical trials that involved large numbers of patients and intermediate (B) if the data were derived from a limited number of randomized trials that involved small numbers of patients or from careful analyses of nonrandomized studies or observational registries. A lower rank (C) was given when expert consensus was the primary basis for the recommendation.

RISK ASSESSMENT

Clinical Features

UA and NSTEMI are heterogeneous disorders in which patients have widely varying risks. Risk is an important "driver" of management decisions, and accurate yet simple methods of risk assessment are important for patient care.

Risk was assessed by multivariable regression techniques in patients presenting with UA/NSTEMI in several large clinical trials. Boersma et al analyzed the relation between baseline characteristics and the incidence of death and the composite of death or myocardial (re)infarction at 30 days in patients who entered the PURSUIT (Platelet IIb/IIIa in Unstable angina: Receptor Suppression Using Integrilin Therapy) trial.[2] The most important baseline features associated with death were age, heart rate, systolic blood pressure, ST-segment depression, signs of heart failure, and elevation of cardiac biomarkers. From

this analysis, a simple risk estimation score was developed.

Antman et al developed a seven-point risk score, the "TIMI Risk Score" (age $\geq$ 65 years, more than three coronary risk factors, prior angiographic coronary obstruction, ST-segment deviation, more than two angina events within 24 h, use of aspirin [ASA] within 7 days, and elevated cardiac markers).[3] The score was defined as the simple sum of these individual prognostic variables. The risk of developing an adverse outcome—death, (re)infarction, or recurrent severe ischemia that required revascularization—ranged from 5% with a score of 0 or 1 to 41% with a score of 6 or 7. The score was derived from data in the TIMI 11B (Thrombolysis In Myocardial Infarction 11B) trial[4] and then validated in three additional trials—ESSENCE (Efficacy and Safety of Subcutaneous Enoxaparin in Non–Q-wave Coronary Events study)[5] and PRISM-PLUS (Platelet Receptor inhibition for Ischemic Syndrome Management in Patients Limited by Unstable Signs and symptoms)[6] and prospectively in one TACTICS-TIMI 18 (Treat angina with Aggrastat and determine Cost of Therapy with an Invasive or Conservative Strategy—Thrombolysis In Myocardial Infarction) 18.[7] A progressively greater benefit from newer therapies such as low-molecular-weight heparin (LMWH),[4, 5] platelet glycoprotein (GP) IIb/IIIa receptor antagonists,[6] and an invasive strategy[7] with increasing risk score have been reported.

Biomarkers

The Joint European Society of Cardiology/American College of Cardiology Committee for the Redefinition of Myocardial Infarction[8] emphasized the use of troponins as critical markers of the presence of myocardial necrosis. Although troponins are accurate in identifying myocardial necrosis, the latter is not always secondary to atherosclerotic coronary artery disease. Therefore, in establishing the diagnosis of NSTEMI, cardiac troponins should be used in conjunction with appropriate clinical features and electrocardiographic changes. Myocardial injury of diverse origins (e.g., myocarditis, trauma, or cardioversion) may cause necrosis and release of troponins. Although these may be considered instances of NSTEMI, they should be distinguished on clinical grounds from the more common form of NSTEMI secondary to coronary atherosclerosis.

Antiplatelet Therapy

Antiplatelet therapy is a cornerstone in the management of UA/NSTEMI. Three classes of antiplatelet drugs (ASA, thienopyridines, and GP IIb/IIIa antagonists) have been found useful in the management of these patients and are the subject of continued intensive investigation and analysis.

Clopidogrel. Given its more rapid onset of action[9,10] and better safety profile compared with ticlopidine, clopidogrel is now the preferred thienopyridine. The CURE (Clopidogrel in Unstable angina to prevent Recurrent ischemic Events) trial[11] randomized 12,562 patients with UA/STEMI who presented within 24 h to placebo or clopidogrel (loading dose of 300 mg followed by 75 mg daily) and followed them for 3 to 12 months; all patients were given aspirin. Cardiovascular death, myocardial infarction (MI), or stroke occurred in 11.5% of patients assigned to placebo and 9.3% of those assigned to clopidogrel (relative risk [RR] 0.80; $P < .001$). Looking at the individual components of the primary composite and end point, there was a trend in favor of clopidogrel for cardiovascular death and stroke (5.5% and 1.4%, respectively, for placebo vs. 5.1% and 1.2% for clopidogrel), and there was a significant reduction in MI (6.7% vs. 5.2% RR = 0.77; $P < .001$). However, there was no significant difference in the incidence of non–Q-wave MI (3.8% vs. 3.5%). A reduction in recurrent ischemia was noted within the first few hours after randomization. These salutary results were observed across all subgroups of patients. There was, however, a significant excess of major bleeding (2.7% in the placebo group vs. 3.7% in the clopidogrel group; $P = .003$) and of minor bleeding, as well as a (nonsignificant) trend for an increase in life-threatening bleeding. The risk of bleeding was increased in patients who underwent coronary artery bypass grafting (CABG) within the first 5 days after clopidogrel was discontinued.

The CURE trial was performed in hospitals in which there was *no* routine policy of early invasive procedures, and therefore, revascularization was performed during the initial admission in only 23% of the patients, a substantially lower percentage than currently receive this therapy at most U S hospitals. Although the addition of a GP IIb/IIIa antagonist appeared to be well tolerated in patients who were given ASA, clopidogrel, and heparin in CURE, fewer than 10% of patients received this combination. Therefore, additional information on the safety of "quadruple therapy" (heparin [unfractionated or low-molecular-weight], ASA, clopidogrel, and a GP IIb/IIIa antagonist) should be obtained.

The CURE trial provides strong support for the addition of clopidogrel to ASA on admission in the management of patients with UA and NSTEMI. Clopidogrel appears to be especially useful in hospitals that do not have a routine policy of early invasive procedures and in patients who are not candidates or who do not wish to be considered for revascularization. The optimal duration of therapy with clopidogrel has not been determined. The major benefits in CURE were observed at 30 days, with small additional benefits observed over the subsequent treatment period, which averaged 8 months.

In PCI-CURE, a substudy of CURE, 2658 patients who underwent percutaneous coronary intervention (PCI) had been randomly assigned to double-blind treatment with clopidogrel (n = 1313) or placebo (n = 1345);[12] all patients also received ASA. Patients were pretreated with placebo or study drug for a median of 10 days before PCI. After the procedure, most patients received open-label thienopyridine (clopidogrel or ticlopidine) for approximately 4 weeks, after which the study drug (placebo or clopidogrel) was again administered for an average of 8 months. The primary end point, a composite of cardiovascular death, MI, or urgent target-vessel revas-

cularization within 30 days of PCI, occurred in 86 patients (6.4%) in the placebo group compared with 59 (4.5%) in the clopidogrel group (RR 0.70; $P = .03$). When events that occurred before and after PCI were considered, there was a 31% reduction in cardiovascular death or MI with assignment to clopidogrel ($P = .002$). Thus, in patients with UA and NSTEMI who are given ASA and are undergoing PCI, a strategy of clopidogrel pretreatment followed by at least 1 month and probably longer-term therapy is beneficial in reducing major cardiovascular events.[12]

There now appears to be an important role for clopidogrel in patients with UA/NSTEMI, both those who are managed conservatively and those who undergo PCI, especially stenting. However, it is not entirely clear how long therapy should be maintained. Because clopidogrel, when added to ASA, increases the risk of bleeding during major surgery in patients who are scheduled for CABG, if possible, clopidogrel should be withheld for at least 5 days[11] and preferably for 7 days before surgery.[13] In many hospitals in which patients with UA/NSTEMI undergo diagnostic catheterization within 24 to 36 h of admission, clopidogrel is not started until it is clear that CABG will *not* be scheduled within the next several days. A loading dose of clopidogrel can be given to a patient on the catheterization table if a PCI is to be performed immediately. If PCI is not performed, clopidogrel can be begun after the catheterization.

Glycoprotein IIb/IIIa Antagonists in PCI. The introduction of platelet GP IIb/IIIa antagonists represents an important advance in the treatment of patients with UA/NSTEMI who are undergoing PCI. These drugs take advantage of the fact that platelets play an important role in the development of ischemic complications that may occur in patients with UA/NSTEMI during coronary revascularization procedures. The September 2000 guidelines emphasized the value of GP IIb/IIIa antagonists in patients with UA/NSTEMI who were undergoing PCI.[1]

Two trials of GP IIb/IIIa inhibitors have been published since September 2000. The ESPRIT trial (Enhanced Suppression of the Platelet IIb/IIIa Receptor with Integrilin Therapy) was a placebo-controlled trial designed to assess whether eptifibatide improved outcome in patients undergoing stenting.[14] Fourteen percent of the 2064 patients enrolled in ESPRIT had UA/NSTEMI. The primary end point (the composite of death, MI, target-vessel revascularization, and "bailout" GP IIb/IIIa antagonist therapy) was reduced from 10.5% to 6.6% with treatment ($P = .0015$). There was consistency in the reduction of events in all components of the end point and in all major subgroups, including patients with UA/NSTEMI. Major bleeding occurred more frequently in patients who received eptifibatide (1.3%) than in those who received placebo (0.4%; $P = .027$); however, no significant difference in the transfusion rate occurred. At 1 year of follow-up, death or MI occurred in 12.4% of patients assigned to placebo and 8.0% of eptifibatide-treated patients (hazard ratio, 0.63; 95% confidence interval [CI], 0.48 to 0.83; $P = .001$).[15]

In the only head-to-head comparison of GP IIb/IIIa antagonists, the TARGET trial (Do Tirofiban And ReoPro Give similar Efficacy? Trial) randomized 5308 patients to tirofiban or abciximab before PCI with the intent to perform stenting.[16] The primary end point, a composite of death, nonfatal MI, and urgent target-vessel revascularization at 30 days, occurred less frequently in those given abciximab than in those given tirofiban (6.0% vs. 7.6%; P = .038). There was a similar direction and magnitude for each component of the end point. The difference in outcome between the two treatment groups may be related to a suboptimal dose of tirofiban resulting in inadequate platelet inhibition. However, by 6 months, the primary end point occurred in a similar percentage of patients in each group (14.9% tirofiban vs. 14.3 % abciximab, NS). Mortality was also similar (1.9% vs. 1.7%, NS).[17]

Glycoprotein IIb/IIIa Antagonists Without Scheduled PCI. The Global Utilization of Strategies to Open Occluded Coronary Arteries IV-Acute Coronary Syndromes (GUSTO IV-ACS) trial[18] enrolled 7800 patients with UA/NSTEMI who were admitted to the hospital with more than 5 min of chest pain and ST-segment depression and/or elevated troponin T or I concentration and in whom early (<48 h) revascularization was not intended to be conducted. All received ASA and either unfractionated heparin (UFH) or LMWH. They were randomized to placebo, an abciximab bolus and 24-h infusion, or an abciximab bolus and 48-h infusion. The primary end point, death or MI at 30 days, occurred in 8.0% of patients given placebo, 8.2% given 24-h abciximab, and 9.1% given 48-h abciximab, differences that were not statistically significant. At 48 h, death occurred in 0.3%, 0.7%, and 0.9% in these groups, respectively (placebo vs. abciximab 48 h, P = .008). The lack of benefit of abciximab was observed in most subgroups, including patients with elevated concentrations of troponin who were at higher risk. Although the explanation for these results is not clear, they indicate that abciximab, at least at the dosing regimen used in GUSTO IV-ACS, is *not* indicated in the management of patients with UA or NSTEMI in whom an early invasive management strategy is not planned.

In the PRISM-PLUS trial, 1069 patients did not undergo early PCI. Although tirofiban treatment was associated with a lower incidence of death, MI or death, and MI or refractory ischemia at 30 days, these reductions were not statistically significant.[19] In a high-risk subgroup of these patients not undergoing PCI (TIMI risk score ≥ 4),[3] tirofiban appeared to be beneficial whether they underwent PCI (odds ratio [OR] 0.60; 95% CI, 0.35 to 1.01) or not (OR, 0.69; 95% CI, 0.49 to 0.99). However, no benefit was observed in the patients at lower risk.[6] In the PURSUIT trial, eptifibatide reduced the incidence of death or MI from 15.7% to 14.2% (RR, 0.91; 95% CI, 0.79 to 1.00; P = .032).[20]

Boersma et al performed a meta-analysis of GP IIb/IIIa antagonists in all six large, randomized, placebo-controlled trials, including GUSTO IV-ACS,[18] which involved 31,402 patients with UA/NSTEMI who were not

routinely scheduled to undergo coronary revascularization.[21] A small reduction in the odds of death of MI in the active treatment arm (11.8% vs. 10.8%; OR, 0.91; 95% CI, 0.84 to 0.98; P = .015) was observed. Unexpectedly, no benefit was observed in women (test for interaction between treatment assignment and gender; P < .0001). However, women with positive troponins derived a treatment benefit that was similar to men. In the meta-analysis, reductions in the end points of death or nonfatal MI considered individually did *not* achieve statistical significance.

Although not scheduled for coronary revascularization procedures, 11,965 of the 31,402 patients (38%) actually underwent PCI or CABG within 30 days, and in this subgroup, the OR for death or MI in patients assigned to GP IIb/IIIa antagonists was 0.89 (95% CI, 0.80 to 0.98). In the other 19,416 patients who did not undergo coronary revascularization, the OR for death or MI in the GP IIb/IIIa group was 0.95 (95% CI, 0.86 to 1.05; P = NS). Major bleeding complications were increased in the GP IIb/IIIa antagonist–treated group compared with those who received placebo (1.4% vs. 2.4%; P < .0001). The authors concluded that in patients with UA/NSTEMI who were not routinely scheduled for early revascularization and who were at high risk of thrombotic complications, "treatment with a GP IIb/IIIa inhibitor might therefore be considered."[21] Thus, GP IIb/IIIa inhibitors are of benefit in high-risk patients with UA/NSTEMI, and their administration, in addition to ASA and heparin, to patients in whom catheterization and PCI are planned, received a class I recommendation. These agents are of questionable benefit in patients who do not undergo PCI. However, the revised guidelines recommend broader indications for a routine invasive strategy (see following text).

Thus, clopidogrel (in addition to aspirin and heparin or LMWH) is recommended for patients with UA/NSTEMI in whom a noninterventional approach is planned (class I recommendation). In patients in whom an interventional approach is planned, a GP IIb/IIIa inhibitor (in addition to aspirin and heparin or LMWH) is recommended (class I recommendation). No head-to-head comparison of clopidogrel, a GP IIb/IIIa inhibitor, and their combination has been reported. The addition of a GP IIb/IIIa inhibitor to a subset of patients in the CURE trial who were receiving aspirin, clopidogrel, and heparin appeared to be well tolerated, and current practice frequently involves the use of this combination of drugs. However, until further information on the safety and efficacy of such quadruple therapy becomes available, a class IIa recommendation is made for the addition of a GP IIb/IIIa inhibitor for patients with UA/NSTEMI who are receiving aspirin, clopidogrel, and UFH or LMWH and who are referred for an invasive strategy. A class I recommendation is made for a GP IIb/IIIa inhibitor at the time of PCI in patients receiving heparin and aspirin. Specific updated recommendations for the use of antiplatelet regimens in the revised guidelines are as follows:

Class I

1. Antiplatelet therapy should be initiated promptly. ASA should be administered as soon as possible

after presentation and continued indefinitely. *(Level of Evidence: A)*

2. Clopidogrel should be administered to hospitalized patients who are unable to take ASA because of hypersensitivity or major gastrointestinal intolerance. *(Level of Evidence: A)*

*3. In hospitalized patients in whom an early noninterventional approach is planned, clopidogrel should be added to ASA as soon as possible on admission and administered for at least 1 month *(Level of Evidence: A)*, and for up to 9 months. *(Level of Evidence: B)*

*4. A platelet GP IIb/IIIa antagonist should be administered, in addition to ASA and heparin, to patients in whom catheterization and PCI are planned. The GP IIb/IIIa antagonist may also be administered just prior to PCI. *(Level of Evidence: A)*

*†5. In patients for whom a PCI is planned and who are not at high risk for bleeding, clopidogrel should be started and continued for at least 1 month *(Level of Evidence: A)* and for up to 9 months. *(Level of Evidence: B)*

*6. In patients taking clopidogrel in whom elective CABG is planned, the drug should be withheld for 5 to 7 days. *(Level of Evidence: B)*

Class IIa

*1. Epitifibatide or tirofiban should be administered, in addition to ASA and LMWH or UFH, to patients *with* continuing ischemia, an elevated troponin, or with other high-risk features in whom an invasive management strategy is *not* planned. *(Level of Evidence: A)*

*2. A platelet GP IIb/IIIa antagonist should be administered to patients already receiving heparin, ASA, *and clopidogrel* in whom catheterization and PCI are planned. The GP IIb/IIIa antagonist may also be administered just prior to PCI. *(Level of Evidence: B)*

Class IIb

*1. Eptifibatide or tirofiban, in addition to ASA and LMWH or UFH, to patients *without* continuing ischemia who have no other high-risk features and in whom PCI is *not* planned. *(Level of Evidence: A)*

Class III

1. Intravenous fibrinolytic therapy in patients without acute ST-segment elevation, a true posterior MI, or a presumed new left bundle-branch block. *(Level of Evidence: A)*

*2. Abciximab administration in patients in whom PCI is not planned. *(Level of Evidence: A)*

Anticoagulant Therapy

The September 2000 guidelines[1] reviewed the evidence regarding the use of intravenous UFH or subcutaneous

LMWH. It provided the following class I recommendation:

Parenteral anticoagulation with intravenous UFH or subcutaneous LMWH should be added to antiplatelet therapy with ASA or a thienopyridine. *(Level of Evidence: B)*

In the interim, a number of studies have appeared that support the use of enoxaparin. In the EVET trial (Enoxaparin VErsus Tinzaparin in the management of unstable coronary artery disease), two LMWHs, enoxaparin and tinzaparin, administered for 7 days, were compared in 438 patients with UA/NSTEMI. A preliminary report stated that both the recurrence of unstable angina and the need for revascularization were significantly lower in the enoxaparin group.[22] Because the level of anticoagulant activity cannot be easily measured in patients given LMWH (e.g., activated partial thromboplastin time or activated clotting time), interventional cardiologists have expressed concern about the substitution of LMWH for UFH in patients scheduled for catheterization with possible PCI. However, Collet et al[23] have shown in a small nonrandomized observation study in 293 patients that PCI can be performed safely with UA/NSTEMI patients who received the usual dose of enoxaparin. In NICE-1 (National Investigators Collaborating on Enoxaparin), an observational study, intravenous enoxaparin (1.0 mg/kg) was used in 828 patients undergoing elective PCI without an intravenous GP IIb/IIIa antagonist.[24] The rates of bleeding (1.1% major bleeding and 6.2% minor bleeding in 30 days) were comparable to those observed in historical controls with UFH.

An alternative approach is to use LMWH during the period of initial stabilization and to withhold the dose on the morning of the procedure. If an intervention is required and more than 8 h has elapsed since the last dose of LMWH, UFH can be used for PCI according to usual practice patterns. Because the anticoagulant effect of UFH can be more readily reversed than that of LMWH, UFH is preferred in patients likely to undergo CABG within 24 h.

The September 2000 guidelines reflected concern regarding the combined use of LMWH and GP IIb/IIIa antagonists. Although the data are not definitive, it now appears that GP IIb/IIIa antagonists can be used with LMWH. In the ACUTE II (Anti-thrombotic Combination Using Tirofiban and Enoxaparin II) study,[25] UFH and enoxaparin were compared in patients with UA/NSTEMI who were given tirofiban. The frequencies of both major and minor bleeding were similar, and there was a trend to fewer adverse events in the patients given enoxaparin. A number of other open-label studies have examined the safety of combining enoxaparin with abciximab, eptifibatide, or tirofiban in patients with UA/NSTEMI who are treated with PCI or conservatively; of combining enoxaparin with abciximab in patients undergoing elective PCI[26]; and of combining dalteparin with abciximab in patients with UA/NSTEMI who are treated conservatively and during PCI.[27] Although the majority of these studies relied on historical controls, none suggested that the combination of enoxaparin and a GP IIb/IIIa antagonist was associated with excess bleeding, whether or not the patient also underwent PCI.

---

*New indication, not included in the September 2000 guidelines.
†Minor clarification different from full-text version on web site.

Specific recommendations for the use of heparins in the revised guidelines are as follows:

Class I

*1. Anticoagulation with subcutaneous LMWH or intravenous UFH should be added to antiplatelet therapy with ASA and/or clopidogrel. *(Level of Evidence: A)*

Class IIa

*†1. Enoxaparin is preferable to UFH as an anticoagulant in patients with UA/NSTEMI, in the absence of renal failure and unless CABG is planned within 24 h. *(Level of Evidence: A)*

EARLY CONSERVATIVE VERSUS EARLY INVASIVE STRATEGIES

The September 2000 guidelines indicated that two different treatment strategies, termed *early conservative* and *early invasive*, may be used in patients with UA/NSTEMI.[1] In the *early conservative strategy*, coronary angiography is reserved for patients with evidence of recurrent ischemia (angina at rest or with minimal activity or dynamic ST-segment changes) or a strongly positive stress test despite vigorous medical therapy. In the *early invasive strategy*, patients without clinically obvious contraindications to coronary revascularization are routinely recommended for coronary angiography and angiographically directed revascularization, if possible.

Several trials comparing these two strategies were reviewed, but greatest attention was paid to the then-most-recent trial, FRISC II (Fragmin and Fast Revascularization during InStability in Coronary artery disease II).[28] At 1 year, the mortality rate in the invasive strategy group was 2.2% compared with 3.9% in the noninvasive strategy group (P = .016).[29] However, in FRISC II, the invasive strategy involved treatment for an average of 6 days in the hospital with LMWH, ASA, nitrates, and β-blockers before coronary angiography, an approach that would be difficult to adopt in U.S. hospitals.

In the interim, the TACTICS-TIMI 18 trial was reported.[7] In this trial, 2220 patients with UA or NSTEMI were treated with ASA, heparin, and the GP IIb/IIIa antagonist tirofiban. They were then randomized to an early invasive strategy with routine coronary angiography within 48 h followed by revascularization if the coronary anatomy was deemed suitable or to a more conservative strategy. In the latter, catheterization was performed only if the patient had recurrent ischemia or a strongly positive stress test. Death, myocardial (re)infarction, or rehospitalization for an acute coronary syndrome at 6 months occurred in 19.4% of patients assigned to the conservative strategy vs. 15.9% assigned to the invasive strategy (OR, 0.78; 95% CI, 0.62 to 0.97; P = .025). Occurrence of death or MI was also reduced at 6 months (9.5% vs. 7.3%;

P < .05). The beneficial effects on outcome were particularly evident in medium- and high-risk patients, as defined by an elevation of troponin T greater than 0.01 ng/mL or of troponin I greater than 0.1 ng/mL, the presence of ST-segment deviation, or a TIMI risk score greater than or equal to 3.[7,30] In the absence of these high-risk features, outcomes in patients assigned to the two strategies were similar. Rates of major bleeding were similar, and lengths of hospital stay were reduced in patients assigned to the invasive strategy. The benefits of the invasive strategy were achieved at no significant increase in the cost of care over the 6-month follow-up period.

Thus, both the FRISC II[28,29] and TACTICS-TIMI 18[7,30] trials, the two most recent trials comparing invasive versus conservative strategies in patients with UA/NSTEMI, showed a benefit in patients assigned to the invasive strategy. In contrast to earlier trials, a large majority of patients undergoing PCI in these two trials received coronary stents as opposed to balloon angioplasty alone. In TACTICS-TIMI 18, treatment included the GP IIb/IIIa antagonist tirofiban, which was administered for an average of 22 h before coronary angiography. The routine use of the GP IIb/IIIa antagonist in this trial may have eliminated the excess risk of early (within 7 days) acute MI in the invasive arm, an excess risk that was observed in FRISC II and other trials in which there was no routine "upstream" use of a GP IIb/IIIa antagonist. Therefore, an invasive strategy is associated with a better outcome in UA/NSTEMI patients at high risk who receive a GP IIb/IIIa antagonist.[7] Although the benefit of GP IIb/IIIa antagonists is well established for patients with UA/NSTEMI who undergo PCI, the optimum time of commencing these drugs—as early as possible after presentation, i.e. "upstream," as in TACTICS-TIMI 18, or just before the PCI—has not been established.

Specific recommendations for the use of an invasive strategy in the revised guidelines are as follows:

Class I

†1. An early invasive strategy in patients with UA/NSTEMI without serious comorbidity and who have any of the following high-risk indicators: *(Level of Evidence: A)*
   *a) Recurrent angina/ischemia at rest or with low-level activities despite intensive anti-ischemic therapy
   *b) Elevated troponin T or I
   *c) New or presumably new ST-segment depression
   d) Recurrent angina/ischemia with CHF symptoms, an S_3 gallop, pulmonary edema, worsening rales, or new or worsening MR
   e) High-risk findings on noninvasive stress testing
   f) Depressed LV systolic function (e.g., EF <0.40 on noninvasive study)
   g) Hemodynamic instability

---

*New indication, not included in the September 2000 guidelines.
†Minor clarification different from full-text version on web site.

*New indication, not included in the September 2000 guidelines.
†Minor clarification different from full-text version on web site.

h) Sustained ventricular tachycardia
i) PCI within 6 months
j) Prior CABG

2. In the absence of any of these findings, either an early conservative or an early invasive strategy may be offered in hospitalized patients without contraindications for revascularization. *(Level of Evidence: B)*

RISK-FACTOR MODIFICATION

The September 2000 guidelines pointed out that despite the overwhelming evidence for the benefits of β-hydroxy–β-methylglutaryl–coenzyme A (HMG-CoA) reductase (statin) therapy in patients with elevated low-density lipoprotein (LDL) cholesterol levels, almost no data existed about the timing of initiation of therapy in patients with acute coronary syndromes.[1] Indeed, the secondary prevention trials of statins specifically excluded patients with UA/NSTEMI in the acute phase. Fewer than 300 patients had been entered into the trials within 4 months of an acute coronary syndrome.

The Lipid-Coronary Artery Disease (L-CAD) study was a small trial that randomized 126 patients with an acute coronary syndrome to early treatment with pravastatin, alone or in combination with cholestyramine or niacin, or to usual care. At 24 months, the patients who received early aggressive treatment had a lower incidence of clinical events (23%) than the usual-care group (52%; P = .005).[31] In the MIRACL (Myocardial Ischemia Reduction with Aggressive Cholesterol Lowering) trial, 3086 patients were randomized to treatment with an aggressive lipid-lowering regimen of atorvastatin 80 mg per day or placebo 24 to 96 h after an acute coronary syndrome.[32] At 16 weeks of follow-up, the primary end point of death, nonfatal MI, resuscitated cardiac arrest, or recurrent severe myocardial ischemia was reduced from 17.4% in the placebo group to 14.8% in the atorvastatin group (P = .048). There were *no* significant differences between the two groups in the risk of the following individual end points: death, nonfatal MI, cardiac arrest, or worsening heart failure, however, there were fewer strokes and a lower risk of severe recurrent ischemia in patients assigned to atorvastatin.

Although the evidence from these two trials of a beneficial effect of predischarge initiation of lipid-lowering therapy is not yet robust or definitive, observational studies support this policy. In the Swedish Registry of Cardiac Intensive Care of almost 20,000 patients, the adjusted relative risk of mortality was 25% lower in patients in whom statin therapy was initiated before hospital discharge.[33] In addition, patients in whom lipid-lowering therapy is begun in the hospital are much more likely to be undergoing such therapy at a later time. In one demonstration project, the Cardiovascular Hospitalization Atherosclerosis Management Program (CHAMP), the in-hospital initiation of lipid-lowering therapy was associated with an increased percentage of patients treated with statins 1 year later (from 10% to 1%) and with a higher frequency of patients whose

LDL cholesterol was less than 100 mg/dL (from 6% to 58%).[34] Although additional trials are ongoing, there appear to be no adverse effects and substantial advantages to the initiation of lipid-lowering therapy before hospital discharge.[35-37] Such early initiation of therapy has also been recommended in the third report of the National Cholesterol Education Program (NCEP III), which also raised the threshold of high-density lipoprotein cholesterol concentration that required therapy.[38] Similar considerations apply to the early initiation of statin therapy following PCI. In the Lescol Intervention Prevention Study (LIPS), 1669 patients were randomized to receive 80 mg fluvastatin or placebo, beginning 2 days after PCI. After a follow-up of 3.9 years, the statin-treated group had a lower incidence of clinical events (21.4%) than the placebo group (26.7%), P = .01.[39]

In addition to maintaining the original class I recommendations for LDL cholesterol reduction, specific additional recommendations for the use of lipid-lowering therapy in UA/NSTEMI in the revised guidelines are as follows:

Class I

*1. A fibrate or niacin if high-density lipoprotein cholesterol is less than 40 mg/dL, occurring as an isolated finding or in combination with other lipid abnormalities. *(Level of Evidence: B)*

Class IIa

*1. HMG-CoA reductase inhibitors and diet for LDL cholesterol greater than 100 mg/dL begun 24 to 96 h after admission and continued at hospital discharge. *(Level of Evidence: B)*

CONCLUSIONS

These guidelines address the diagnosis and management of patients with UA and the closely related condition NSTEMI. These life-threatening disorders are a major cause of emergency medical care and are responsible for more than 1.4 million hospitalizations annually in the United States.[40] Nearly 60% of these admissions are among persons greater than 65 years old, and almost half occur in women. In 1997, there were 5,315,000 visits to U.S. emergency departments for the evaluation of chest pain and related symptoms.[41]

Because of the high incidence of UA/NSTEMI and the seriousness of this condition (approximately 15% rate of death or [re]infarction at 30 days),[1,20] continued research in this field is of the greatest importance. It is encouraging that in the 21 months since the publication of the September 2000 guidelines, a considerable body of additional useful information about these conditions has emerged. Indeed, the progress between September 2000 and June 2002 equals that between 1994, when the first guidelines were published,[42] and Setpermber 2000.

---

*New indication, not included in the September 2000 guidelines.

REFERENCES

1. Braunwald E, Antman EM, Beasley JW, et al: ACC/AHA guidelines for the management of patients with unstable angina and non–ST-segment elevation myocardial infarction: A report of the American College of Cardiology/American Heart Association Task Force on Practice Guidelines (Committee on the Management of Patients With Unstable Angina). J Am Coll Cardiol 2000;36:970-1062.

2. Boersma E, Pieper KS, Steyerberg EW, et al: Predictors of outcome in patients with acute coronary syndromes without persistent ST-segment elevation: Results from an international trial of 9461 patients. The PURSUIT Investigators. Circulation 2000;101: 2557-2567.

3. Antman EM, Cohen M, Bernink PJ, et al: The TIMI risk score for unstable angina/non-ST elevation MI: A method for prognostication and therapeutic decision making. JAMA 2000;284:835-842.

4. Antman EM, McCabe CH, Gurfinkel EP, et al: Enoxaparin prevents death and cardiac ischemic events in unstable angina/non–Q-wave myocardial infarction: Results of the Thrombolysis In Myocardial Infarction (TIMI) 11B trial. Circulation 1999;100:1593-1601.

5. Cohen M, Demers C, Gurfinkel EP, et al: A comparison of low-molecular-weight heparin with unfractionated heparin for unstable coronary artery disease. Efficacy and Safety of Subcutaneous Enoxaparin in Non–Q-Wave Coronary Events Study Group. N Engl J Med 1997;337:447-452.

6. Morrow DA, Antman EM, Snapinn SM, et al: An integrated clinical approach to predicting the benefit of tirofiban in non-ST elevation acute coronary syndromes: Application of the TIMI Risk Score for UA/NSTEMI in PRISM-PLUS. Eur Heart J 2002;23:223-229.

7. Cannon CP, Weintraub WS, Demopoulos LA, et al: Comparison of early invasive and conservative strategies in patients with unstable coronary syndromes treated with the glycoprotein IIb/IIIa inhibitor tirofiban. N Engl J Med 2001;344:1879-1887.

8. Alpert JS, Thygesen K, Antman E, Bassand JP: Myocardial infarction redefined—a consensus document of the Joint European Society of Cardiology/American College of Cardiology Committee for the redefinition of myocardial infarction. J Am Coll Cardiol 2000;36: 959-969.

9. Cadroy Y, Bossavy JP, Thalamas C, et al: Early potent antithrombotic effect with combined aspirin and a loading dose of clopidogrel on experimental arterial thrombogenesis in humans. Circulation 2000;101:2823-2828.

10. Helft G, Osende JI, Worthley SG, et al: Acute antithrombotic effect of a front-loaded regimen of clopidogrel in patients with atherosclerosis on aspirin. Arterioscler Thromb Vasc Biol 2000;20: 2316-2321.

11. Yusuf S, Zhao F, Mehta SR, Chrolavicius S, et al: Effects of clopidogrel in addition to aspirin in patients with acute coronary syndromes without ST-segment elevation. N Engl J Med 2001;345: 494-502.

12. Mehta SR, Yusuf S, Peters RJ, et al: Effects of pretreatment with clopidogrel and aspirin followed by long-term therapy in patients undergoing percutaneous coronary intervention: The PCI-CURE study. Lancet 2001;358:527-533.

13. Physicians' Desk Reference. 56th ed. Montvale, NJ, Medical Economics, 2002, p 3085.

14. The ESPRIT Investigators: Novel dosing regimen of eptifibatide in planned coronary stent implantation (ESPRIT): A randomised, placebo-controlled trial. Lancet 2000;356:2037-2044.

15. O'Shea JC, Hafley GE, Greenberg S, et al: Platelet glycoprotein IIb/IIIa integrin blockade with eptifibatide in coronary stent intervention: The ESPRIT trial: A randomized controlled trial. JAMA 2001;285:2468-2473.

16. Topol EJ, Moliterno DJ, Herrmann HC, et al: Comparison of two platelet glycoprotein IIb/IIIa inhibitors, tirofiban and abciximab, for the prevention of ischemic events with percutaneous coronary revascularization. N Engl J Med 2001;344:1888-1894.

17. Roffi M, Moliterno DJ, Meier B, et al: Impact of different platelet glycoprotein IIb/IIIa receptor inhibitors among diabetic patients undergoing percutaneous coronary intervention: Do Tirofiban and ReoPro Give Similar Efficacy Outcomes Trial (TARGET) 1-year follow-up. Circulation 2002;105:2730-2736.

18. Simoons ML: Effect of glycoprotein IIb/IIIa receptor blocker abciximab on outcome in patients with acute coronary syndromes without early coronary revascularisation: The GUSTO IV-ACS randomised trial. Lancet 2001;357:1915-1924.

19. Inhibition of the platelet glycoprotein IIb/IIIa receptor with tirofiban in unstable angina and non-Q-wave myocardial infarction. Platelet Receptor Inhibition in Ischemic Syndrome Management in Patients Limited by Unstable Signs and Symptoms (PRISM-PLUS) Study investigators. N Engl J Med 1998;338: 1488-1497.

20. Inhibition of platelet glycoprotein IIb/IIIa with eptifibatide in patients with acute coronary syndromes. The PURSUIT Trial Investigators. Platelet Glycoprotein IIb/IIIa in Unstable Angina: Receptor Suppression Using Integrilin Therapy. N Engl J Med 1998;339:436-443.

21. Boersma E, Harrington RA, Moliterno DJ, et al: Platelet glycoprotein IIb/IIIa inhibitors in acute coronary syndromes: A meta-analysis of all major randomised clinical trials. Lancet 2002;359:189-198.

22. Michalis LK, Papamichail N, Katsouras C: Enoxaparin Versus Tinzaparin in the Management of Unstable Coronary Artery Disease (EVET Study) [Abstract]. J Am Coll Cardiol 2001;37 (Suppl):365a.

23. Collet JP, Montalescot G, Lison L, et al: Percutaneous coronary intervention after subcutaneous enoxaparin pretreatment in patients with unstable angina pectoris. Circulation 2001;103:658-663.

24. Kereiakes DJ, Grines C, Fry E, et al: Enoxaparin and abciximab adjunctive pharmacotherapy during percutaneous coronary intervention. J Invasive Cardiol 2001;13:272-278.

25. Cohen M, Theroux P, White HD: Anti-Thrombotic Combination Using Tirofiban and Enoxaparin: The ACUTE II Study [Abstract]. Circulation 2000;102:II826.

26. Young JJ, Kereiakes DJ, Grines CL: Low-molecular-weight heparin therapy in percutaneous coronary intervention: The NICE 1 and NICE 4 trials. National Investigators Collaborating on Enoxaparin Investigators. J Invasive Cardiol 2000;12(Suppl F): E14-E18.

27. Kereiakes DJ, Kleiman NS, Fry E, et al: Dalteparin in combination with abciximab during percutaneous coronary intervention. Am Heart J 2001;141:348-352.

28. The FRagmin and Fast Revascularisation during InStability in Coronary artery disease Investigators. Invasive compared with non-invasive treatment in unstable coronary-artery disease: FRISC II prospective randomised multicentre study. Lancet 1999;354: 708-715.

29. Wallentin L, Lagerqvist B, Husted S, et al: Outcome at 1 year after an invasive compared with a non-invasive strategy in unstable coronary artery disease: The FRISC II invasive randomised trial. FRISC II Investigators. Fast Revascularisation during Instability in Coronary artery disease. Lancet 2000;356:9-16.

30. Morrow DA, Cannon CP, Rifai N, et al: Ability of minor elevations of troponins I and T to predict benefit from an early invasive strategy in patients with unstable angina and non-ST elevation myocardial infarction: Results from a randomized trial. JAMA 2001;286: 2405-2412.

31. Arntz HR, Agrawal R, Wunderlich W, et al: Beneficial effects of pravastatin (+/-colestyramine/niacin) initiated immediately after a coronary event (the randomized Lipid-Coronary Artery Disease [L-CAD] Study). Am J Cardiol 2000;86:1293-1298.

32. Schwartz GG, Olsson AG, Ezekowitz MD, et al: Effects of atorvastatin on early recurrent ischemic events in acute coronary syndromes: The MIRACL study. A randomized controlled trial. JAMA 2001:285: 1711-1718.

33. Stenestrand U, Wallentin L: Early statin treatment following acute myocardial infarction and 1-year survival. JAMA 2001;285: 430-436.

34. Fonarow GC, Gawlinski A, Moughrabi S, Tillisch JH: Improved treatment of coronary heart disease by implementation of a Cardiac Hospitalization Atherosclerosis Management Program (CHAMP). Am J Cardiol 2001;87:819-822.

35. Muhlestein JB, Horne BD, Bair TL, et al: Usefulness of in-hospital prescription of statin agents after angiographic diagnosis of coronary artery disease in improving continued compliance and reduced mortality. Am J Cardiol 2001;87:257-261.

36. Fonarow GC, Ballantyne CM: In-hospital initiation of lipid-lowering therapy for patients with coronary heart disease: The time is now. Circulation 2001;103:2768-2770.

37. Michels KB, Braunwald E: Estimating treatment effects from observational data: Dissonant and resonant notes from the SYMPHONY trials. JAMA 2002;287:3130-3132.

38. Executive Summary of the Third Report of the National Cholesterol Education Program (NCEP) Expert Panel on Detection Evaluation, and Treatment of High Blood Cholesterol in Adults (Adult Treatment Panel III). JAMA 2001;285:2486-2497.

39. Serruys PW, de Feyter P, Macaya C, et al: Fluvastatin for prevention of cardiac events following successful first percutaneous coronary intervention: A randomized controlled trial. JAMA 2002;287: 3215-3222.

40. National Center for Health Statistics. Detailed diagnoses and procedures: National Hospital Discharge Survey, 1996. Hyattsville, MD, National Center for Health Statistics, 1998, p 13. Data from Vital and Health Statistics.

41. Nourjah P: National Hospital Ambulatory Medical Care Survey: 1997 Emergency department summary. Hyattsville, MD, National Center for Health Statistics; 1999, p 304. Advance Data from Vital and Health Statistics.

42. Braunwald E, Mark, DB, Jones, RH, et al: Unstable Angina: Diagnosis and Management. AHCPR Publication No 94-0602, 1-154. 3-1-1994. Rockville, Md, Agency for Health Care Policy and Research and the National Heart, Lung, and Blood Institute, Public Health Service, U.S. Department of Health and Human Services.